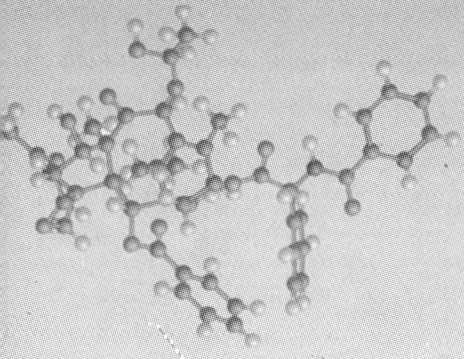

Textbook of
Medicinal
Chemistry

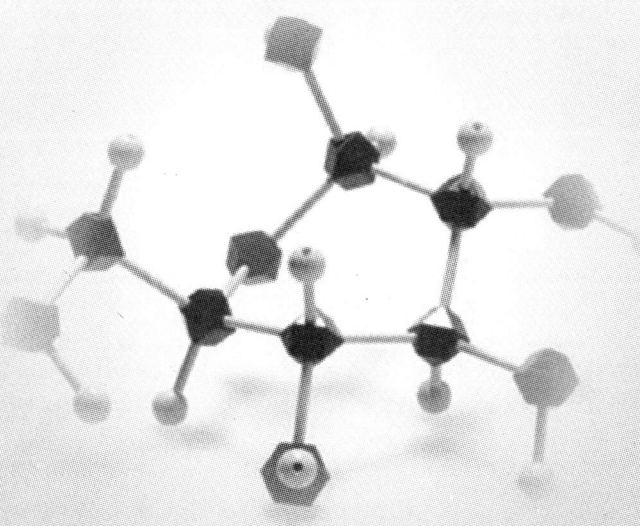

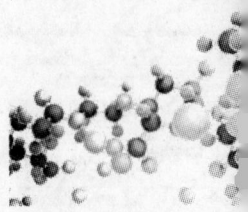

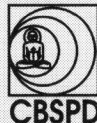

Textbook of
Medicinal
Chemistry

Malleshappa N. Noolvi PhD

Professor, Department of Pharmaceutical Chemistry
Shree Dhanvantary Pharmacy College, Surat, Gujarat

Anurekha Jain PhD

BR Nahata College of Pharmacy
Mandsaur, Madhya Pradesh

Harun M Patel PhD

Medicinal Chemist
Division of Computer Aided Drug Design and Discovery
Department of Pharmaceutical Chemistry
RC Patel Institute of Pharmaceutical Education and Research
Shirpur (Dhule), Maharashtra

CBSPD

CBS Publishers & Distributors Pvt Ltd

New Delhi • Bengaluru • Chennai • Kochi • Kolkata • Lucknow • Mumbai
Gujarat • Hyderabad • Jharkhand • Nagpur • Patna • Pune • Uttarakhand

Textbook of
Medicinal Chemistry

ISBN: 978-81-239-2359-8

Copyright © Authors and Publishers

First Edition: 2014

Reprint: 2019, **2025**

Published by **Satish Kumar Jain** and produced by **Varun Jain** for

CBS Publishers & Distributors Pvt Ltd

4819/XI Prahlad Street, 24 Ansari Road, Daryaganj, New Delhi 110 002, India
Ph: 011-23289259, 23266838   Website: www.cbspd.com
                                    e-mail: delhi@cbspd.com
Corporate Office: 204 FIE, Industrial Area, Patparganj, Delhi 110 092
Ph: 011-4934 4934   Fax: 011-4934 4935   e-mail: publishing@cbspd.com; publicity@cbspd.com

Branches

- **Bengaluru:** Seema House 2975, 17th Cross, K.R. Road, Banasankari 2nd Stage, Bengaluru 560 070, Karnataka, India
  Ph: +91-80-26771678/79   Fax: +91-80-26771680   e-mail: bangalore@cbspd.com

- **Chennai:** 18/8B, Subbarayan Street, Shenoy Nagar, Chennai 600 030, Tamil Nadu, India
  Ph: +91-44-42032115, 26681266   e-mail: chennai@cbspd.com

- **Kochi:** 42/1325, 1326, Power House Road, Opp KSEB, Power House, Ernakulam 682 018, Kerala, India
  Ph: +91-484-4059061-65   Fax: +91-484-4059065   e-mail: kochi@cbspd.com

- **Kolkata:** 147, Hind Ceramics Compound, 1st Floor, Nilgunj Road, Belghoria, Kolkata-700056, West Bengal, India
  Ph: 033-25633055, 033-25633056   e-mail: kolkata@cbspd.com

- **Lucknow:** Basement, Khushnuma Complex, 7-Meerabai Marg (Behind Jawahar Bhawan), Lucknow 226001, India
  Ph: 0522-4000032   e-mail: tiwari.lucknow@cbspd.com

- **Mumbai:** PWD Shed. Gala no. 25/26, Ramchandra Bhatt Marg, Next to JJ Hospital Gate no. 2 Opp. Union Bank of India Noorbaug Mumbai-400009, Maharashtra, India
  Ph: 022-66661880/89   e-mail: mumbai@cbspd.com

Representatives

- **Gujarat**   0-9879558667   • **Hyderabad** 0-9885175004   • **Jharkhand**   0-9811541605   • **Nagpur**   0-8692091830
- **Patna**   0-9334159340   • **Pune**   0-9664372571   • **Uttarakhand** 0-9716462459

Printed at Rashtriya Printers, Dilshad Garden, Delhi, India

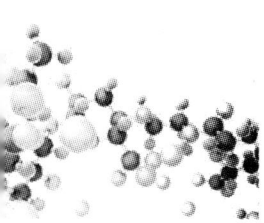

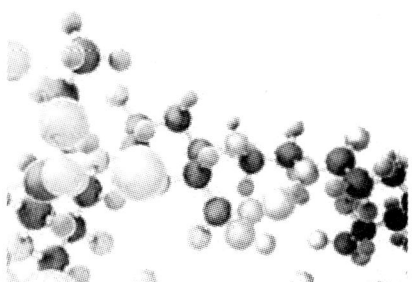

*Dr Harun M. Patel
dedicates this textbook to
his late mother
Ms. Ajija Patel
for her unconditional love
and inspiration*

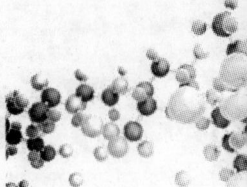

Acknowledgements

The authors are particularly grateful to Ms. Pallavi K. J. for necessary corrections in textbook and Mr. Channabasappa Noolvi, for design and text alignment. Authors are also thankful to the CBS Publishers & Distributors, for bringing out this book.

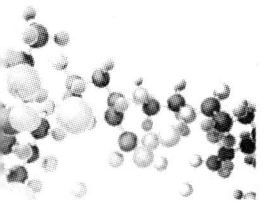

Preface

The prime focus of **Textbook of Medicinal Chemistry** is an educational introduction into the current knowledge of methodological aspects and basic principles in the rapidly developing field of medicinal chemistry. Potentials and limitations of the techniques are critically and comparatively discussed and comprehensively exemplified. It is intended to provide the reader with diagrammatic as well as schematic explanation of the concepts of medicinal chemistry. It is going to motivate the students to read the book.

The **Textbook** has two objectives in view. The first objective is to attract the interest of the undergraduate students in developing countries so that they feel a spontaneous urge to explore and understand the basic theories of medicinal chemistry. These students often encounter enormous difficulties in grasping the fundamentals of synthesis of simple as well as complex compounds including those belonging to the therapeutic group, and they often get confused when they are supplied with inadequate information of vitally important medicinal compounds, their chemical formulae and chemical names. This book aims at removing this inadequacy by furnishing copious information about medicinal compounds and pointing out the interrelations wherever they exist. This method, it is believed, will add new incentive to the study of the subject, and will boost the spirit of research and provide a new dimension to the study of medicinal chemistry. Thus, in this book an attempt has been made to include and correlate detailed accounts of most of the important categories of drugs usually taught in various Universities of developing countries offering diploma, degree and honors courses in pharmacy.

The second objective that has been kept in view is to make this a handy reference for the professional class. With a view to fulfilling this objective, the author has adopted a specific style.

The entire text of the book is divided into 12 units, each unit has multiple chapters and each chapter has been subdivided into four sections* in the following manner.

- The first section has a brief introduction.
- The second section follows classification based on either chemical or pharmacological basis in both diagrammatic and schematic way.
- The third section is pharmacology and mechanism of actions of drugs in both diagrammatic and explanatory way.
- The fourth section, the most significant, contains the synthesis of various important members treated individually, brief description of the synthesis, therapeutic applications of each compound, together with name of the reactants.

The mode of action of various classes of medicinal compounds, in addition to the structure–activity relationship (SAR), has also been elaborated wherever relevant. Greater emphasis has been laid on the chemistry of various compounds treated in this book so that an undergraduate student may acquire a comprehensive knowledge on the basic concepts of the medicinal chemistry.

For the reasons mentioned above, it is believed that this book will enjoy equal favour and confidence with pharmacy students, practising pharmacists, and also medical service representatives. Manufacturing pharmacists engaged in basic drug manufacture may also find it as a useful reference book and will appreciate its originality of approach and its significant departure from similar books available on the subject.

Malleshappa N. Noolvi
Anurekha Jain
Harun M. Patel

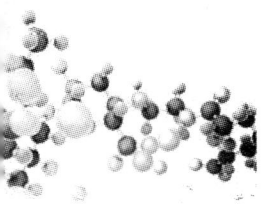

Contents

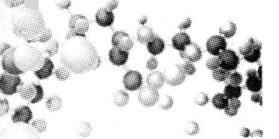

Unit **X ANTI-INFLAMMATORY DRUGS AND AUTACOIDS**

Unit **XI CHEMOTHERAPEUTIC AGENTS**

Unit **XII MISCELLANEOUS**

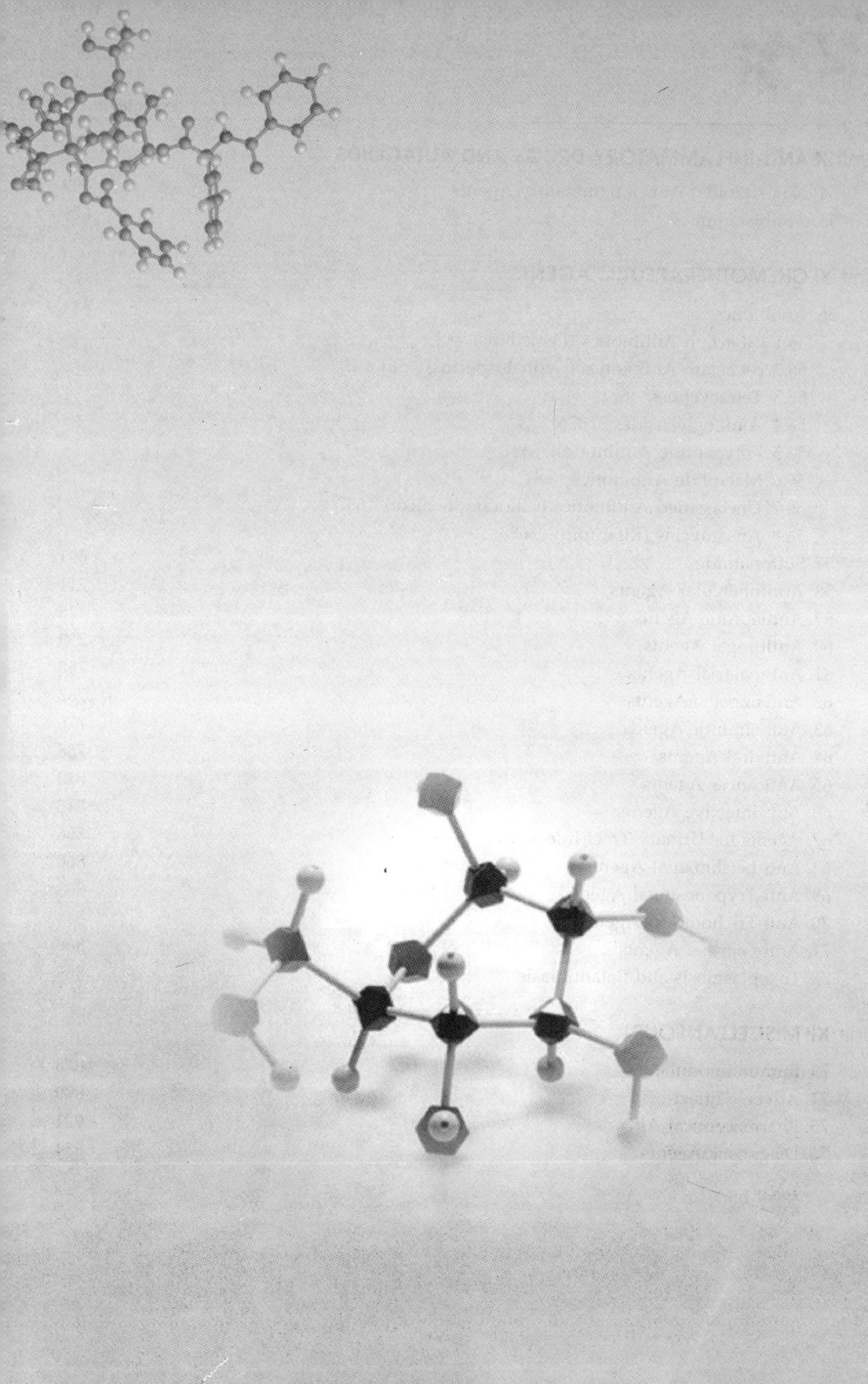

Unit I

Introduction to Medicinal Chemistry

History of
Medicinal Chemistry

It is so-called prescientific era, natural products having a history as folk remedies were in use. Some of the natural products that are used today, either as extracts or derivatives, were often used for various purposes, e.g. arrow poison and other cosmetics. Examples of such products are opium, belladonna, cinchona bark, ergot, nutmeg, foxglove and squill.

▦ EARLY INVESTIGATION OF NATURAL PRODUCTS

- Before the development of chemistry as a science, drugs that have been used were either natural organic products or inorganic materials. Herbal pharmacopoeia was published thousands of years ago. Bartholomeus Anglicus published one of the first herbal in Basel in 1470. The first London Pharmacopoeia was published in 1618.

- Among the earliest recorded use of plant medicines were those of the herb called '*ma huang*' a species of Ephedra. The use of Squill as a cardiac tonic was recorded in the Ebers papyrus (Egypt, 1500 BC). With the gradual decline of the magic and superstition that had accompanied the use of substance believed to have medicinal properties, English physicians had also experimented with the use of Priestley's 'fixed air' or carbon dioxide for dissolving kidney stones.

- Opium was among the first plant drugs investigated by the method of plant analysis introduced by Fourcroy. Later, Serturner, an Austrian apothecary followed Derosne work and showed that the narcotic principle of opium had an alkali-like character and forms salt with the acids. Antoine Fourcroy instituted the use of specific reagent to determine the presence of minerals, and analysis of various barks. Thomas Anderson determined the composition of codeine, a mild analgesic opium alkaloid.

- Thomas Fraser, found that the quaternary salts of strychnine, brucine, thebaine, codeine, morphine, atropine all have curare-like paralyzing activity.

- In 1887, Ralph Stockman established that the ethyl ether of morphine was almost identical to the methyl ether in pharmacological tests. In 1898, Heinrich Dreser of Fridrich Bayer introduced diacetylmorphine as a safer pain reliever than morphine. It was known as Heroin.

- In 1820, quinine from Cinchona bark had been introduced in Europe. Since it was first described by an Augustinian monk, who had lived in Peru, it become known as 'Jesuit's bark'. Following isolation of quinine, Pelltier and Caventon urged medical practitioners to study the pure plant principle Francois Magendi utilized animal tests and then treated patients with quinine, thus setting the present course of drug development.

- Pelletier and Caventon then started the manufacture of quinine on a large scale and by 1826, they were producing 3600 kg of quinine sulfate yearly.

▨ DRUG DISCOVERY AND DEVELOPMENT

Drugs are chemicals that prevent disease or assist in restoring health of diseased individuals. They have an indispensable role in modern medicine. Medicinal chemistry is the branch of science that provides these drugs through discovery or through design. Medicinal chemist should have the knowledge of biochemistry, cell biology, biophysics, anatomy, computers and genetics. The central objectives of each branch of chemistry are to possess the relationship between chemical structure and molecular properties of a drug molecule.

Historical Prospective

In the prehistoric times, wide variety of organic drugs originated from natural materials (crude drugs), e.g. the use of opium, liquorices, digitalis, cocoa and others.

1. About 100 years ago, an idea by Langley and Ehrlich that only certain cells contained receptor molecule that served as host for the drugs. The resulting combination created a super molecule that has new therapeutic values.
2. Later lock and key mechanism came into picture. Drug acts as a key that fits into lock that is receptor. Most common receptors are transdermal glycoprotein, contain certain specific amino acids arranged in 3D space. This indicates that receptor is a rigid structure.
3. Modern picture is that both receptor and drug do not have any rigid structure. Thus, the docking interaction takes place between the receptor and drug. The non-rigid structures are known as *zipper model*.

Thus in many cases, it is important to determine 3D aspects of receptor-ligand complex. Enzymes can also act as receptor. DNA and RNA can also act as receptor, so it is important to design the ligands for them. The earliest applications of DNA liganding lie in inhibiting its formation (DNA) and cause the cell death. Newer targets like; neurotransmitter, receptors on cell surface (Table 1.1).

Table 1.1: Total molecular targets for various drugs

Cellular receptors	45%
Enzymes	28%
Hormones and factors	11%
Ion channels	5%
DNA	2%
Nuclear receptors	2%
Unknown	7%

Various methods are available in screening the 3D structure of many enzymes and receptors such as molecular spectroscopy, NMR and computer graphics.

Thus the medicinal chemist's motto is **"Good enough–soon enough"**.

What Kind of Compounds become Drugs?

The majority of effective oral drugs follow the Lipinski rule of five.

There are four criteria:

1. The substance should have a molecular weight of 500 or less.
2. It should have fewer than five H-bond donating function.
3. It should have fewer than ten H-bond accepting functions.
4. The substance should have a calculated Log P between 1 and 5.

Thus, in short compounds should have a low molecular weight, be non-polar and partition between an aqueous and lipid phase, but should also have proper water solubility.

▓ PREPARATION AND ORGANIZATION OF DRUG DISCOVERY PROCESS

Various steps in drug seeking are as follows:

1. Year 0–1   →   Identify the suitable disease, start pharmacology and chemistry then obtain a satisfactory budget.
2. Year 1–2   →   Confirm potential utility of hits in animals.
3. Year 3–5   →   Detailed pharmacology such as mode of action, teratogenicity, adjust absorption, distribution, metabolism and excretion characteristics.
4. Year 4–9   →   Phase 1 clinical studies safety of new drug and its dosage.
5. Phase 2   →   Clinical studies (side effects, effectiveness).
6. Phase 3   →   Clinical studies (interaction studies).
7. Year 8–11   →   Regulatory review.
8. Year 10–15 →   Marketing and phase 4 clinical studies.
9. Year 17–20 →   Renewal of patent or making new patent, generic competition.

Various orphan drugs are also come into picture; these drugs are for rare disease treatment. Now, a novel gene product is also selected that appears to be involved in pathology of disease. Lead molecules are modified synthetically to identify the pharmacophore and to increase potency and selectivity.

▓ DEVELOPMENT LEADING TO VARIOUS CLASSES OF DRUGS

— Anesthetic agents
— Hypnotic and analgesics
— Antipyretics
— Local anesthetics
— Antiseptics
— Cardiac stimulants
— Antianginal drugs
— Antiarrhythmic drugs
— Chemotherapeutic agents

Anesthetic agents: Nitrous oxide, ether, chloroform were introduced as anesthetic agents during 1840s. Later on, various anesthetic agents are also discovered, e.g. N_2O, $C_2H_5OC_2H_5$, $CHCl_3$.

Hypnotics and analgesic: Opium was first drug used to relive pain and induce natural sleep. Later on morphine was isolated from opium in pure form. Later on, chloral hydrate, paraldehyde, acetaldehyde, sulphone were used for their hypnotic and analgesic actions. Research suggested that 5,5-diethylbarbituric acids used as hypnotic agent.

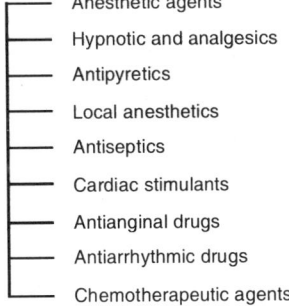
Morphine

Antipyretics: Salicylic acid was first introduced by Carl Buss in Switzerland for possible cure of thyroid fever. It was found to be very effective antipyretic. Later on, aspirin derived, here "a" means acetyl and spirin from the name of plant from which salicylic acid was first obtained, *Spirea Ulmaria*. Aspirin has disadvantage of causing ulcers. Nowadays, dispersible and effervescent formulation are developed and widely used.

Another antipyretics like, antipyrin, phenazone were synthesized by Ludwig Knorrin 1884 with the mistaken assumption that he was preparing a portion of quinine molecule. The methoxy derivative of acetanilide was synthesized and was marketed as phenacetin. Later on salicin, the active principle from Millow Bark was used to treat a patient with rheumatic fever. Phenylbutazone, oxphenbutazone were used as safer drugs but causing aganulocytosis, aplastic anemias. Safer derivatives like azapropazone, feprazone were developed latter.

Local anesthetics: Local anesthetics were also developmented during fruitful period of drug discovery. Cocaine was first discovered as local anesthetic but it had systemic toxic effects and addictive property, thus Eucaine was discovered. Later on more safer analogues were prepared that are orthocaine, benzocaine, nupercaine, procaine were safer spinal anesthetics, bupivacaine latter on widely used as epidural anesthesia.

Antiseptic: The antiseptic property of coal tar was recognized in 1815. The chemical constitution known as 'acid phenique'. Phenol was used to control the growth of bacteria. Mercuric chloride was used as sporicidal. Methyl violet was used as internal antiseptic. Mercuric benzoate, carbolated and salicylate were introduced in late 1880s. Thiomersal, phenyl mercuric nitrate and acetate were used as effective antiseptic.

Cardiac stimulants: Foxglove was used first for treatment of dropsy. Later on, digitalis purpurea was used as powdered leaf. Various attempts were made to isolate the active, crystalline material that is digitoxin. This isolated product was known as glycosides of digitalis and cardiac stimulants.

Later on, active principal from Strophanthus gratus was extracted and used as cardiac glycosides.

Antianginal drugs: Amyl nitrate was firstly used as antianginal drug. It caused dilation of blood vessels leading to a drop in blood pressure. Various derivatives of local anesthetics like lidocaine (lignocaine) were used as antianginal drug.

Antiarrhythmic drugs: This agent is quinidine from cinchona used for depressant action on the heart. Various other antiarrhythmic agents are procaine, procainamide which are effectively used.

EARLY DEVELOPMENT IN CHEMOTHERAPEUTIC AGENTS

A. Antiprotozoal agents.
B. Antimonials.
C. Antimalarials.
D. Schistosomicidal agents.

Aspirin

Phenacetin

Procaine

Phenol

Mercuric chloride

Digitoxigenin

Lignocaine

Quinidine

Antiprotozoal agents: An agent like naphthalene urea was tested and effectively used as antiprotozoal agents and latter on given the name Suramin. It was principal drug for prevention and treatment of some forms of trypanosomiasis.

Diamidines were used as principal drug for trypanosomiasis. Later on, arsenicals were used as antiprotozoal agents, but they have deleterious effects on skin because they can get absorbed through skin and hydrolyze to form arsenite.

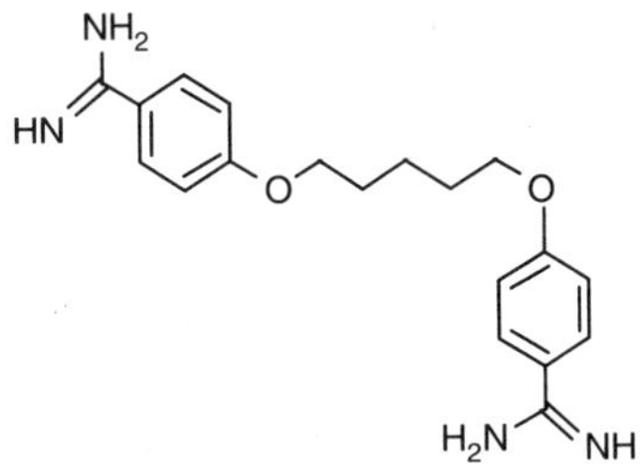

Antimonials: Leishmaniasis is a group of disease, common form of kala-azar. In this case, sodium antimony gluconate was used as antimonials.

Antimalarials: Quinoline and its derivative used effectively as antimalarial. Various 4-aminoquinolines, aminoacridines derivatives were used as effective antimalarials, but are superior to quinidine derivative. Later on, pyrimethamine (daraprine) was used as antimalarial agent.

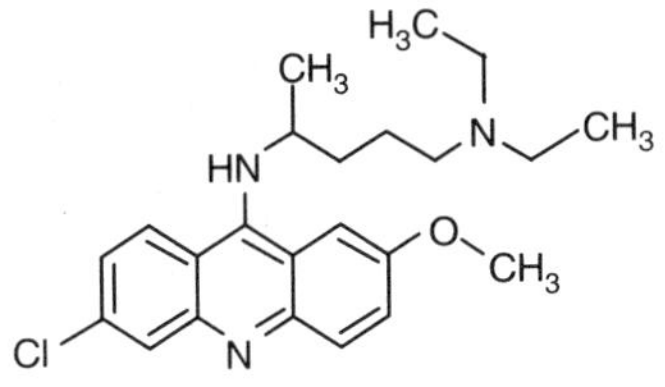

Schistosomicidal agents: These drugs are used against the schistosomiasis. It was believed that Lucanthone was used as schistosomiasics drug. Its hydroxy derivative is most widely used and is very effective.

Pentadiamidine

9-aminoacridine (quinacrine)

▨ CONCLUSION

These discoveries described in short, forms the basis for many successes in the drug development. These early researchers deserve our gratitude; admiration and the role of human imagination in the drug research should not be forgotten.

Principles of Drug Discovery

In the earlier days, purely randomized search procedures were involved in the discovery of new drugs. In such methods, the experience and intuition of medicinal chemist were the important factors to reduce the stochastic nature of search techniques. In view of the ever increasing number of chemical compounds and in particular the heavier demands to be met by new chemicals, randomized search is no longer effective; it is too time consuming; guarantees too little success and is too expensive.

- The chance of discovering a new agent has diminished to 1 in 10,000 and will decrease even further, whereas development costs have risen to more than 40 millions dollars per new drug. Those necessitated the development of a new logical and scientific approach in discovery of new drug which is known as drug design.

- Drug design is an integrated developing discipline which pretends an era of 'tailored drug'. It involves the study of effects of biologically active compounds on the basis of molecular interaction in terms of molecular structure or its physico-chemical properties involved. It studies the process by which the drugs produce their effects, how they react with protoplasm to elicit a particular pharmacological effect or response, how they are modified or detoxified, metabolized or eliminated by the organism?

- Disposition of drugs in individual regions of biosystems is one of the main factors determining the place, mode and intensity of their action. The biological activity may be positive as in drug design or negative as in toxicology. Thus drug designs involve either total innovation of lead or an optimization of already available lead. This built up the concept of drug design.

APPROACHES FOR DRUG DISCOVERY

There are two approaches by which we can discover the new drugs (Fig. 2.1):

1. Analogue aproach
2. Rational approach

1. ANALOGUE APPROACH

An analogue is normally accepted as being that modification which brings about a carbon skeletal transformation or substituent synthesis. In simple language, we can say that here we are preparing different analogues of lead compound to develop clinically effective agent through structural modification. These include the following:

a. Discovery of lead: It involves the search for the lead compound from various resources.

b. Exploration of lead: It involves improvement and extension of lead.

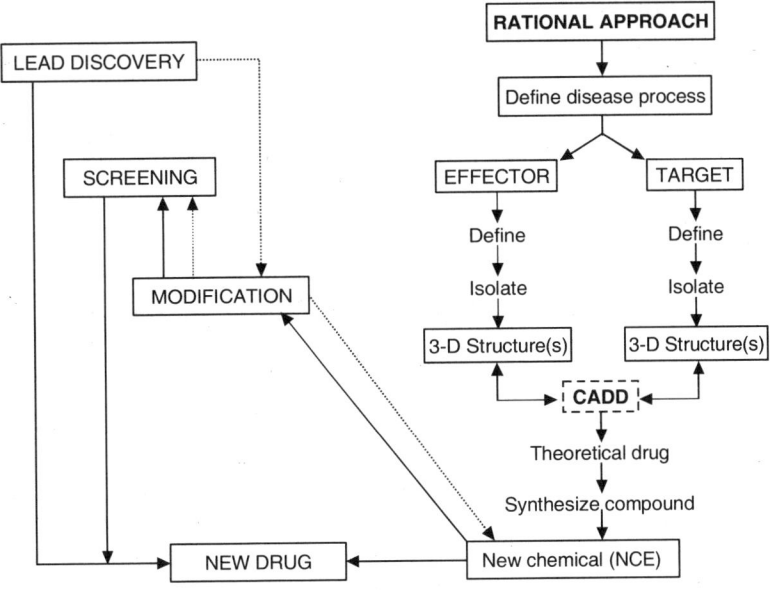

Fig. 2.1: Analogue and rational approach of drug discovery

LEAD

- The lead is prototype compound that has the desired biological or pharmacological activity but may have many undesirable characteristics like;
    1. A high toxicity.
    2. Insolubility problem.
    3. Metabolism problem.
- By exploring lead compound, we can minimize such unwanted effect and make a drug a good candidate for therapeutic use.

Examples of lead

Antipyretic analgesic: Bio-oxidation (metabolism) of acetanilide into p-aminophenol, which subsequently on chemical manipulation yield antipyretic-analgesic like 'paracetamol and phenacetin'.

Sources of Lead Compound

Sources of lead compound are shown in Fig. 2.2.

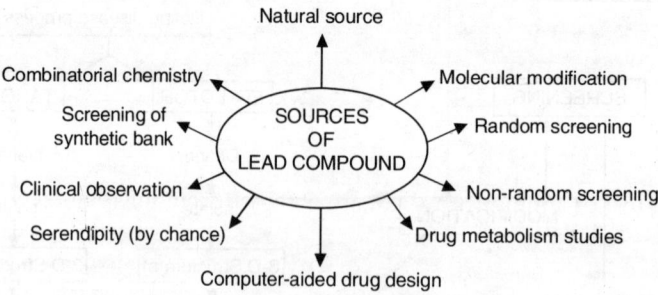

Fig. 2.2: Sources of lead compound

Random screening

- In this method, all compounds (including synthetic chemical, natural product of plant, marine and microbial origin) from a given series are tested. Besides the age old example of morphine, cocaine, digitalis, nicotine, muscarine, tubocurarine, quinine and anti-malarial agent artimisnin have been discovered from plant source.

- Inspite of budgetary and manpower overuse, this method may be used to discover drugs or leads that have unexpected activities.

- Antibiotics like, streptomycin, tetracyclines, fungal metabolites like lovastatin and cyclosporine were found out by this method. Similarly potent anti-cancer agent, euracin A was obtained from a marine cyanobacterium.

Non-random screening

It is a modified form of the random screening, which was developed because of budgetary and manpower restriction. In this method, only such compounds having similar structural skeletons with that of the lead are tested.

Natural sources

Here we can obtain the lead compound from the following sources.

1. Plant
2. Microbes
3. Animals
4. Marine

The plant kingdom: Following lead compounds have been obtained from the plant source.

Morphine

Cocaine

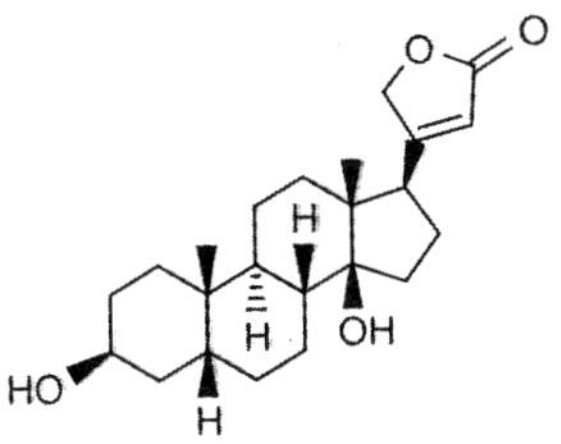

Digitoxigenine

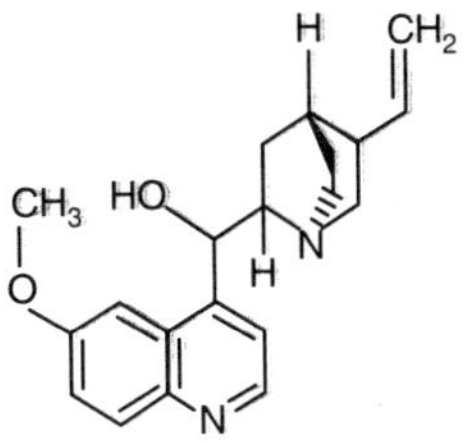

Quinine

From microbes: Most of antibiotics as lead are obtained from microbes as follows.

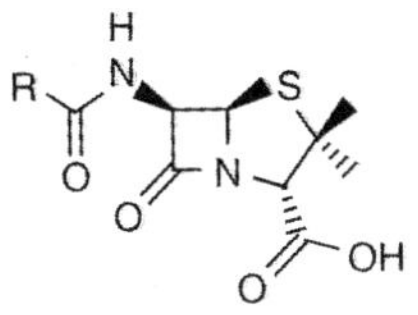

Penicillin

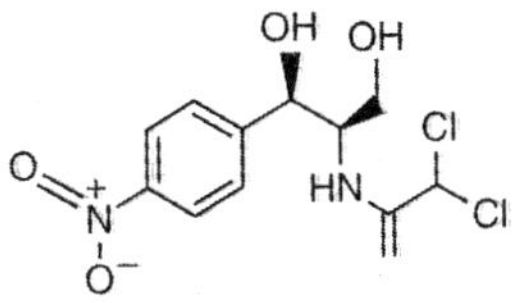

Chloramphenicol

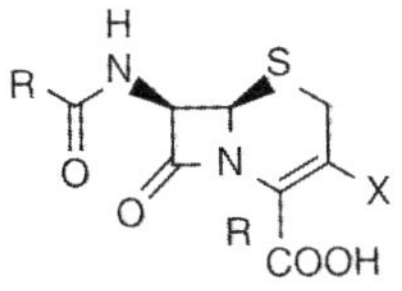

Cephalosporines

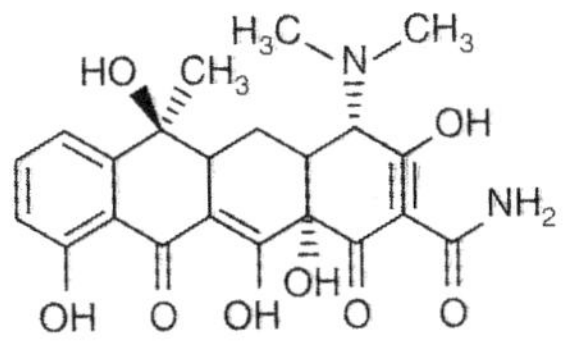

Tetracycline

Animal source: Epibatidine is obtained from frog skin.

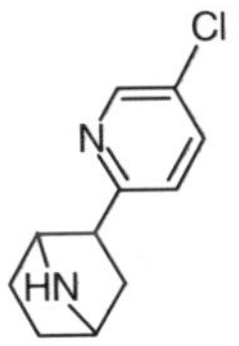

Epibatidine

Marine source:
- Laminine is obtained from *Laminaria angustata*, it is having hypotensive activity.
- Ara – C is obtained from Caribben sponge, which is having anticancer activity.

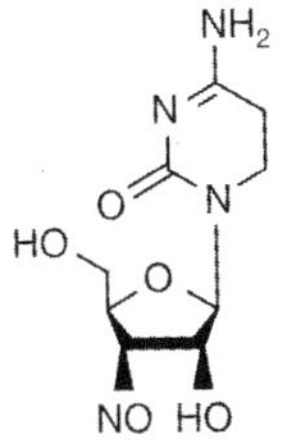

Ara-C

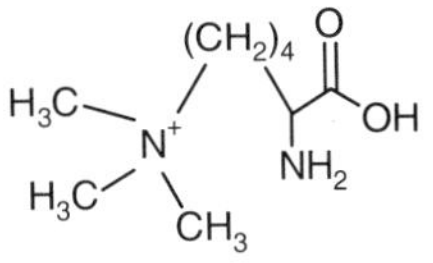

Laminine

- 2 – cyano, 4, 5 dibromopyrole is obtained from *Agela oroids*, it's having antimicrobial activity.

2-cyano, 4,5 dibromopyrole

- Aeroplysinine is obtained from *Asparogopsis toxiformis*, having antimicrobial activity.

Aeroplysinine

Drug metabolism studies

Metabolism of drug occurs as an attempt by metabolizing enzymes to cut short the period of stay of the drug in the body. Structural modification (i.e. metabolic transformation) is done in drug molecule by the enzymes to increase its polarity.

It is brought about regardless of whether the resulting drug metabolite possesses more activity or toxicity. The discovery of sulfanilamide is reported through the metabolic studies of protonsil.

Acetanilide → Metabolism → Paracetamol

The antipyretic action of acetanilide was discovered by chance when a nurse by mistake dispensed acetanilide to a patient. Due to its toxicities, acetanilide could not stand in the market. Metabolic studies showed that the toxicities are due to its in vivo metabolite, p-aminophenol. This observation leads to development of phenacetin and paracetamol.

Clinical observation

- Many times the drug possesses more than one pharmacological activity. The main activity is called as therapeutic effect while rests of the actions are known as side effects of the drug. Such drug may be used as lead compound for structural modification to improve the potency of secondary effects.

Tolbutamide

- Sulphonamides oral hypoglycemic arose directly from the clinical observation in 1942, that a sulphathiazole derivative, which was being used specifically for treating typhoid, lowered the blood sugar drastically.

- The pronounced hypoglycemia exerted by 5-isopropyl-2 sulphaniamido-1, 3, 4-thiadiazole indicate that an aryl sulfonyl thioureas moiety present in thiadiazoles is responsible for their blood glucose lowering effect. This observation led to the development of carbutamide by Frank and Fuchs through opening of thiazole ring to give a thioureas moiety in which =S was then replaced by =O.

Tolazamide

- In order to nullify the toxicity and antibacterial activity of the 4-amino group, it was replaced by other substituents resulting into tolbutamide, chlorpropramide and tolazamide.

Serendipty (by chance)

Frequently lead compounds are found as a result of accidental discovery or serendipity.

1. Penicillin

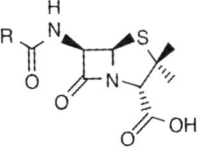

Penicillin

- The examples of drug discovery without a lead are quite few in number. The most prominent examples include Penicilium and Librium. In 1928, Alexander Fleming noticed a green mould growing in a culture of *Staphylococcus aureus* and where the two had converged, the bacteria were lysed.

- This led to the accidental discovery of penicillin, which was produced by the mold. Dr. Ronald Hare, colleague of Dr. Fleming found that very special conditions were required to produce the phenomenon initially observed by Fleming. Another extraordinary circumstance was that the particular strain of the mould on Fleming culture was a relatively good penicillin producer, although most strains of that mould (Penicilium) produce no penicillin at all.

- The mold presumably came from the laboratory just below Fleming's laboratory where research on molds was going on. Thus, the discovery of penicillin could be possible because a combination of all unlikely events took place simultaneously.

- The full extent of the value of penicillin was not revealed until late 1940s because of emergence of the sulfonamide antibacterial in 1935 and outbreak of World War II. Thereafter, the original mould (*Penicilium notatum*) was replaced by *Penicillium chrysogenum* because of relatively low yield of penicillin from the former. The correct structure of penicillin was reported in 1943 by Sir Robert and Karl Folkeres. Once the structure was known, penicillin became lead nucleus for future analogue.

2. Benzodiazepine

- Yet another example of drug discovered without lead is Librium, the first benzodiazepines tranquilizer. A series of quinazoline-3-oxides was synthesized by Dr. Leo Steinbach at Roche in a programme to develop a new class of tranquilizer drug.

(2) Librium

- Since none of these compounds was found to be active, the scheme was terminated in 1955. However, a vial from the above scheme which remains untested was found in 1957 during general laboratory cleanup.

- The compound (2) present in it, was submitted for pharmacological testing to complete official formalities. Surprisingly, it gave very promising results during preliminary screening for tranquilizing activity. It was found to be benzodiazepine-4-oxide, presumably produced in an unexpected reaction of the corresponding chloromethyl quinazoline-3-oxide with methylamine.

- If that vial had not been found in the laboratory clean-up, the benzodiazepines may not have been discovered for many years to come. Thus, Librium once identified as a lead, was then exploited to develop future analogs like diazepam. The latter is about 10 times more potent than the lead.

3. Mustard gas

The alkylating agent stood as the first systemically approach to cancer chemotherapy especially in leukemia where leucocytes multiply in an uncontrolled fashion.

They were developed to lower down high toxicity of mustard gas whose anti-leucocytic action was evidenced when a ship loaded with mustard gas was bombed in an Italian harbor. The military personnel who came in contact with this gas showed an unusually low blood cell count.

Molecular modification

This is one of the approaches by which lead compound can be mined. In this method, modification of already existing compound is done. This is useful for minimizing the side effect.

Example: From phentolamine, tolazoline was obtained.

Phentolamine   Tolazoline

Natural Ligand for the Receptor

Here we are elucidating the structure of natural agonist. After that we are preparing the synthetic analogue of them which can bind to the same receptor as that of natural ligand.

Example: Adrenaline, noradrenaline were the starting point for development of adrenergic β-agonist such as salbutamol.

Noradrenaline

Adrenaline

Salbutamol

Enzyme product as lead compound

Enzyme catalyze the reaction in both direction, so product of enzymatic reaction may be used as lead compound, as excess of product cause feedback inhibition.

$$A + B \underset{\text{Enzyme}}{\rightleftarrows} C + D$$

Example: L-benzyl succinic acid is used as inhibitor of carboxypeptidase

$$\text{Peptide} \xrightarrow{\text{Carboxypeptidase}} \text{L - Benzyl succinic acid}$$

Combinatorial synthesis

By this method, a large number of compounds in a short time period using defined reaction route and large variety of starting material and reagent can be generated.

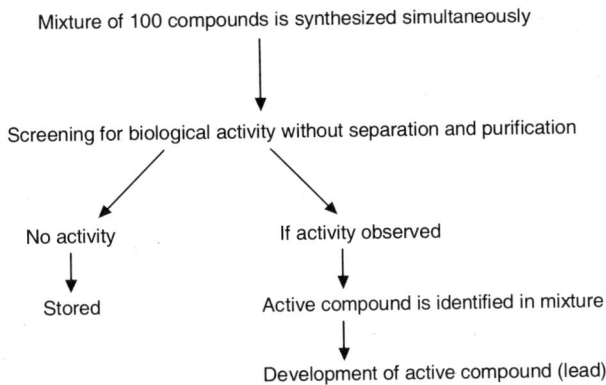

Mixture of 100 compounds is synthesized simultaneously

Screening for biological activity without separation and purification

No activity → Stored

If activity observed → Active compound is identified in mixture → Development of active compound (lead)

Optimization of Lead

Once the lead nucleus is identified, it is easy to exploit. This process is rather straight forward. Various approaches are employed in order to improve the desired pharmacological properties of the lead nucleus. Important amongst them are as follows;

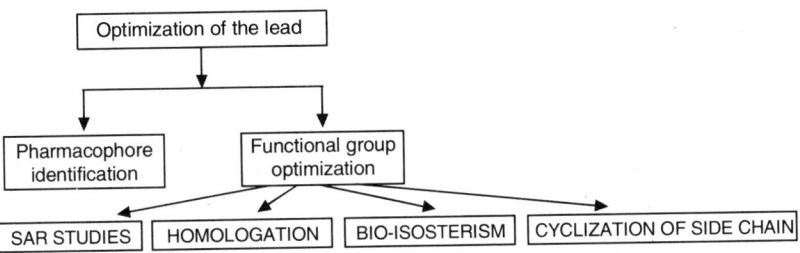

Optimization of the lead

Pharmacophore identification

Functional group optimization

SAR STUDIES | HOMOLOGATION | BIO-ISOSTERISM | CYCLIZATION OF SIDE CHAIN

Pharmacophore identification

Any drug molecule consists of both, essential and non-essential parts. Essential part is important in governing pharmacodynamic (drug-receptor interaction) property while non-essential part influences pharmacokinetic features. The relevant groups on a molecule that interact with a receptor are known as bioactive functional groups. They are responsible for the activity. The schematic representation of nature of such bioactive functional group along with their interatomic distance is known as pharmacophore.

Pharmacophore for narcotic ring

Example:

- One such pharmacophore is identified; structure modification can be done to improve pharmacokinetic properties of the drug, e.g. the presence of a phenyl ring, asymmetric carbon, ethylene bridge and tertiary nitrogen are found to be minimum structural requirement for a narcotic analgesic to become active.

- Morphine the prototype narcotic agent has a pentacyclic structure. The complexity of structure leads to appearance of several adverse effects. Hence the pharmacophore of morphine has been recognized through

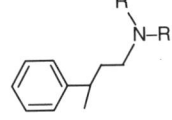

Methadone

molecular dissection and was used to develop still simpler and even acyclic analogues, e.g. methadone is as potent as analgesic as morphine.

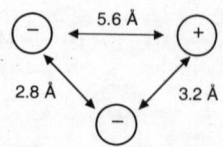

Pharmacophore for cholinergic drug

- Similarly, the presence of two anionic sites and one cationic site must be present in cholinergic agent.

- Similarly in estrogenic compounds, two bio-active sites, having ability to undergo H-bonding, should be separated by a minimum distance of 8.5 Å. In 17- estradiol, the distance is 10.9 Å while in diethyl stilbesterol, it is 12.1 Å.

Functional group optimization

- The activity of a drug can be correlated to its structure in terms of the contribution of its functional groups to the lipophillicity, electronic and steric features of the drug skeleton. Hence, by selecting proper functional group, one can govern the drug distribution pattern and can avoid the occurrence of side effect.

Carbutamide   Tolbutamide

- For example, the amino group of carbutamide (antibacterial agent) was replaced by a methyl group to give tolbutamide (antidiabetic agent). Similarly removal of sulfonamide side chain of chlorthiazide (an antihypertensive drug with diuretic activity) helped to design diazoxide (an antihypertensive drug without diuretic activity).

Chlorthiazide   Diazoxide

- Since a neuroleptic activity runs parallel with the α-adrenoreceptor blocking activity, piperoxan an alpha adrenoreceptor blocking agent was chosen as a lead to get pentamoxane which showed high neuroleptic activity in animal studies.

Piperoxan   Pentamoxane

- The replacement of Cl by CF_3 in ring position 2 and the modification of the basic side chain to include a piperazine moiety is thought to enhance neuroleptic potency by increasing lipophillicity so that CNS-entry of the drug is facilitated.

Structure activity relationship (SAR) studies

- The physiological action of a molecule is a function of its chemical constituent. This observation is the basis of SAR studies. SAR studies usually involve the interpretation of activity in terms of the structural features of a drug molecule.

- Generalized conclusion then can be made after examining a sufficient number of drug analogues. For example, sulphonamides are found to be associated with diuretic and antidiabetic activities in addition to their antibacterial activity. The generalized structures need for individual activity is represented below.

Antibacterial sulphonamide   Diuretic sulphonamide

- Because of hepatotoxic side effects of hydrazine and hydrazides, structurally diversified compounds were synthesized resulting into the introduction of paragyline and tranylcypromine.
- Tranylcypromine was developed as a structural analog of amphetamine and is used as an antidepressant agent. Further structural modification of paragyline skeleton resulted into cyclogyline.

Paragyline   Cyclogyline

Homoligation

- The variation in the substituent can be used to increase or decrease the polarity, alter the pKa and change the electronic properties of a molecule. Exploration of homologous series is one of the most often used methods to induce these changes in a very gradual manner. A homologous series is a group of compounds that differ by a constant unit, generally a CH_2 group. For example, the alkyl substituents of ethers, amines, esters and amides are easily varied. Such variation helps to judge the depth and width of hydrophobic cavity present in the target receptor. Usually increasing the length of a saturated carbon side chain from one (CH_3) to 5–9 atoms (pentyl to nonyl) produces an increase in pharmacological effects. Further increase in side chain decrease the activity.
- This is probably either due to increase in lipophillicity beyond optimum value (hence decreased absorption and distribution) or decrease in concentration of free drug (i.e. micelle formation). For example, maximum hypnotic activity is seen from 1-hexanol to 1-octanol. Thereafter activity decreases for higher homologs.
- Similarly in a series of 4-alkyl substituted resorcinol derivatives, 4-n-hexyl-resorcinol (clinically used topical anesthetic in throat lozenges) was found to possess maximum antibacterial activity. While in a series of mandelate esters, n-nonyl ester has maximum antispasmodic activity. In the same series, branching leads to decrease in the activity, probably due to interference with receptor binding. For example, primaquine (an antimalarial agent) is much more potent than its secondary or tertiary homologs.

Cyclization of side chain

- Over simplification of the structure may sometimes be responsible for increased side effect and reduced activity or selectivity. Two straight forward strategies for enhancing binding affinity involve reducing conformational flexibility and incorporating substituents that bring additional binding interaction. Change in the potency or change in the activity spectra can be brought about by transformation of alkyl side chain into cyclic analogs.

- For example, chlorpromazine (a) has more neuroleptic activity than its cyclic analog; (b) similarly the compound (c) has anti-depressant (imipramine activity) like activity than neuroleptic activity. Similarly, partial rigidity may be incorporated by introducing a double bond, alkyne, amide or aromatic ring in the flexible side chain.

- Locking a rotatable bond into a ring is not the only way to rigidify the structure. Sometimes bridging of two carbons (secondary cyclization) also leads to an increase in potency or change in activity spectrum.

- Examples include thebaine derivatives, atropine, and bridged piperazine derivatives of phenothiazine.

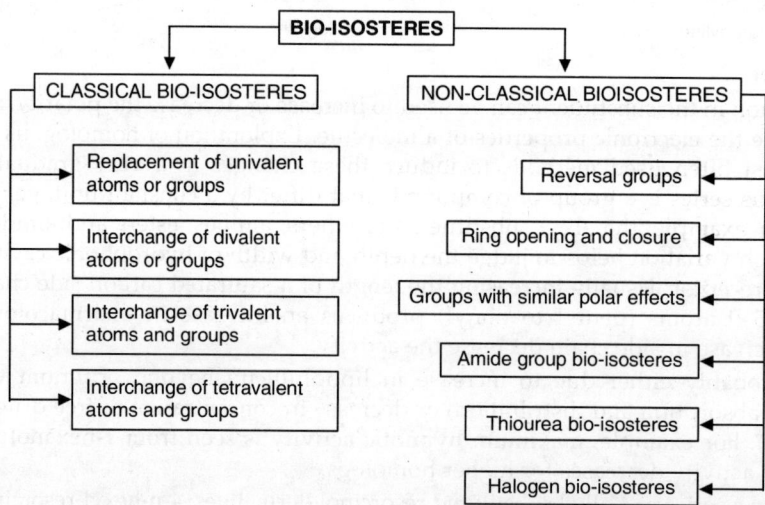

| A | B | C |

Bio-isosteres

```
                        ┌─────────────────┐
                        │  BIO-ISOSTERES  │
                        └─────────────────┘
              ┌──────────────────┴──────────────────┐
   ┌──────────────────────────┐        ┌────────────────────────────┐
   │ CLASSICAL BIO-ISOSTERES  │        │ NON-CLASSICAL BIOISOSTERES │
   └──────────────────────────┘        └────────────────────────────┘
```

CLASSICAL BIO-ISOSTERES:
- Replacement of univalent atoms or groups
- Interchange of divalent atoms or groups
- Interchange of trivalent atoms and groups
- Interchange of tetravalent atoms and groups

NON-CLASSICAL BIOISOSTERES:
- Reversal groups
- Ring opening and closure
- Groups with similar polar effects
- Amide group bio-isosteres
- Thiourea bio-isosteres
- Halogen bio-isosteres

- Bio-isosteres are groups or molecules that impart similar physical, chemical and biological properties to a molecule due to similarities in size, electronegativity or stereochemical aspect.

- The purpose of molecular modification is usually to improve potency, selectivity, duration of action and reduce toxicity. Bio-isosteres are substituents or groups that have similar physical or chemical properties and hence similar biological activity pattern. Isosteric groups according to Erlenmeyer's are isoelectronic in their outmost electron shell. Bioisosteric replacement may help to decrease toxicity or to change activity spectra. It may also alter the metabolic pattern of the drug.

- The parameters being changed are molecular size, steric shape (bond angles, hybridization), electron distribution, lipid solubility, water solubility, the pKa of the chemical reactivity to cell components and capacity to undergo H-bonding (receptor interaction). Even if the bio-isosteric replacements relatively minor (Cl for CH_3). Cl may block metabolic hydroxylation, whereas CH_3 may be oxidized and the compound may have shorter half-life. For example, tolbutamide (R=CH_3) has shorter half-life than chlorpropramide (R=Cl).

- These are known as classical bio-isosteres, where same valency and biological activity are important. However, it is the retention of same biological activity which determines whether a group is bio-isosteres and not the valency. Hence non-isosteric groups can also be used as bio-isosteres.

- They are known as non-classical bio-isosteres. Non-classical bio-isosteres do not have the same number of atoms and do not fit the steric and electronic rules of classical isosteres, but they do produce a similarity in biological activity. Fluorine has the same size as hydrogen but is more electronegative.

- Hence, fluorine is used as an isoster of hydrogen to vary the electronic properties of the drug without changing steric parameters. Moreover C-F bonds are not easily broken during metabolism.

- Hence the anti-tumour drug 5-fluorouracil is a powerful blocker of the target enzyme than its natural substrate, uracil. Pyrrole ring may be sometimes used as non-classical isosteres for an amide to increase the activity and selectivity of the drug.

1. Classical bio-isosteres

Replacement of univalent atoms or groups: The analogous groups consider here –F(Cl), –OH, –NH_2 and CH_3. Programme modification of the oral hypoglycemic has involved the successive replacement of the amino (–NH_2) group by methyl or chlorine –Cl, to give tolbutamide and chlorpropramide respectively, which possess extended biological half-lives and reduced toxicity.

Carbutamide   Tolbutamide   Chlorpheniramine

Fluorine vs hydrogen replacement

- The substitution of hydrogen by fluorine is one of the more commonly employed monovalent isosteric replacement. Steric parameters for hydrogen and fluorine are similar.

- The anti-neoplastic agent 5-fluorouracil represents a classical example of how fluorine substitution of normal enzyme substrate can result in a derivative which can alter select enzymatic processes.

- The metabolite of 5-fluorouracil, 5-fluoro -2-deoxyuridylic acid is more reactive relative to 2′-deoxyuridylic acid (normal metabolite) to thymidylate synthase, enzyme involved in the conversion of uridylic acid to thymidylic acid and critical for DNA synthesis.

2-deoxyuridylic acid

5-fluoro 2-deoxyuridylic acid

- Fluorine exerts inductive effect which is responsible for its more covalent binding to thymidylate synthase and inhibition of the enzyme.

Interchange of hydroxyl and thiols groups: The replacement of OH with SH is based on the ability of both these functional groups to be hydrogen bond acceptors or donors. A classical illustration of this replacement being guanine and 6-thioguanine.

Guanine

6-thioguanine

6-thioguanine acts as a fraudulent nucleic acid and inhibits hypoxanthine – guanine phosphoribosyl transferase and thus blocking the synthesis of DNA.

Interchange of divalent atoms or groups

- Bio-isosterism occurs more frequently between divalent atoms and groups. Steric similarities here are aided by similarities in bond angles, so that attached groups are specially oriented in a like manner. This is born out in the isomeric relationship of esters and amides. In esters, the rotation of C–O–C bonds is restricted by resonance and aliphatic esters exist, predominantly in the *cis*-configuration rather than the *trans*.

Procaine

Procainamide

- Structure on amides has also revealed similar planner structure and a predominant *cis* configuration, analogous to the *cis* ester. This explains the ability by structurally related esters, e.g. procaine and amide, procainamide to function as local an asthetics. The local anesthetic activity of procaine is, however, greater than that of procainamide.

- Since, in the former, the dipolar character of the carbonyl group, required for activity, is more pronounced. In procainamide, the amino group resonance is offset by the amide resonance. So that the magnitude of the C=O dipole is decreased. Procaine is believed to owe its local anesthetic activity to an optimum conformation of lipid solubility for transport across the phospholipids, nerve membrane and polarity for charge transfer complex formation involving dipolar C=O and a thiazolinium ion of thiamine pyrophosphate, which has a specific role in nerve conduction.

Interchange of trivalent atoms and groups

- The substitution of –CH= by –N= in aromatic ring has one of the most successful application of classical isosterism. One of the most potent antihistamines, mepyramine, has evolved from the replacement of a phenyl group in antegran by pyridyl.

- The π-electron deficiency of the pyridine nucleus enables the nitrogen electron pair to hydrogen bond with a water molecule, affecting an increase in hydrophillicity which is significant in determining the high level of biological activity.
- Substitution of the pyridinyl amino –N= by –CH= in mepyramine and 4-methoxy-benzyl by 4-chlorophenyl produces chlorpheniramine, valued for its short, powerful action and relative freedom from sedation, which is an undesirable side effect of antihistaminic drugs.
- The electron withdrawing effect of the pyridyl and p-Cl phenyl substitution on the –CH= group promotes formation of an electron deficient centre, which may determine the mechanism by which bioreceptor interaction occurs.

Antegran   Mepyramine   Chlorpheniramine

Interchange of tetravalent atoms and groups: In this, interchange of a quaternary charged atom with a tertiary carbon atom has been attempted. In case of cholinergic agonist, replacement of quaternary ammonium group with the phosphonium and arsonium analogues has resulted in greater toxicity.

2. Non-classical isosteres

Non-classical isosteres do not obey the steric and electronic definition of classical isosteres. They do not have the same number of atoms as a replacement.

Reversal of groups: Trimaperidine is the propanoate ester of a piperidyl alcohol, while pethidine, meperidine, is an ethyl ester of a piperidyl carboxylic acid. Thus the first compound is related to the second by reversal of an ester group.

Trimaperidine

Pethidine

Ring opening and closure: Sulphathiazole derivative lowered the blood sugar almost to a fatal level. Sulfonamide oral hypoglycemic agents arose based on this observation. Modification involves opening of the thiazole ring to give thioureas unit in which =S was ultimately replaced by =O yielded carbutamide which was later replaced by the less toxic tolbutamide.

Carbutamide

Tolbutamide

A vast number of profitable modifications have evolved from the closure of rings. Thus, the lying back of the aromatic rings of a diphenyl methyl ester to produce a fluorine analogue markedly increases anti-cholinergic spamolytic activity.

Group with similar polar-effects: The correlation of metabolite – anti-metabolite relationship in the antagonism of PABA by sulfonamides has focused attention on groups with similar polar effects, e.g. –COOH and –SO$_2$NHR. Thus, the interchange of such groups was pursued in a search for antagonistic or analogous biological effects. The antagonism of nikethemide by pyridine-3-sulphonic acid and the simulation of its respiratory stimulant effects by the nitrophenyl analogue are example.

| Nikethamide | Pyridine -3 - sulphonic acid | Nitrophenyl analouge |

Carbenicillin: A broad spectrum semisynthetic antibiotic is not administered orally. Since the β-carboxyl acid readily decarboxylates in the acidic environment of the stomach. The α-(5-tetrazolyl) derivative represents an attempt to overcome this stability.

| Carbenicillin | Tetrazolyl derivatives of carbenicillin |

Amide group bio-isosteres: Amide bond is important for the peptide chemistry. It is possible to convert amide bond into chemically stable and orally available molecules. Table 2.1 shows the possible bioisosteric replacement for the amide bond.

Table 2.1: Possible bio-isoster for the amide

Bio-isoster	Formula
Amide	-NHCO-
Reversed amide	-CONH-
Thioamide	-NH-CS-
Amide homologue	-CH$_2$NHCO-
Ketomethylene	-COCH$_2$-
Urea	-NHCONH-
Methylene amine	-CH$_2$-NH-

The ability of these groups to be suitable bioisosteres depends on the role of amide group plays in eliciting the biological activity and the ability of the bio-isosteres to mimic this role as closely as possible. Amide bond is required as hydrogen donor and receptor functionalities for maintaining biological activity.

In the design of anticonvulsant semicarbazones, alkyl and amide are postulated to act as hydrogen donor/acceptor and the compound is found active. Replacement of the amide with $-OCH_2-$ completely abolishes the activity, emphasizing the importance of hydrogen bonding.

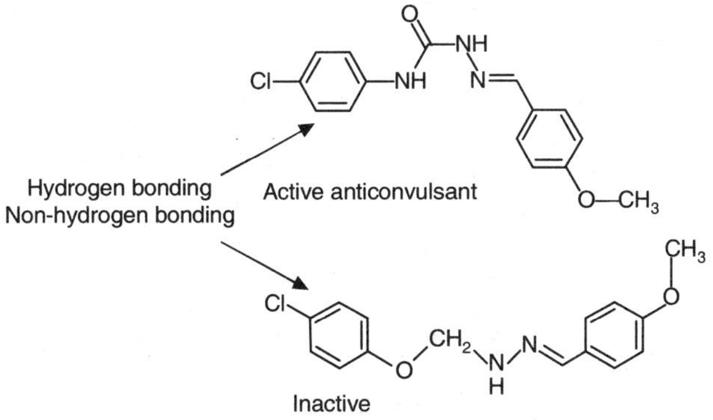

Hydrogen bonding
Non-hydrogen bonding
Active anticonvulsant

Inactive

In another example, where amide bond in benzoic acid appears to be in the positioning or spacing of the m-dialkyl phenyl and the p-carboxy phenyl groups. It was observed that amide (-NHCO-) group replacements such as –CONH-, SO_2NH-, N=N-, retained activity, regardless of their electronic properties or activity to act as hydrogen bond donors.

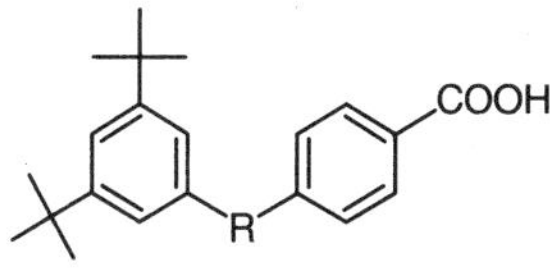

Thiourea bio-isosteres: Thiourea bio-isosteres have been successfully employed in the development of H_2-receptor antagonist (for the treatment of peptic ulcer disease). The early drug metiamide with thioureas moiety in the side chain produced agranulocytosis.

Replacement with a guanidine group gave a compound with improved H_2-antagonist activity but resulted in absorption problems. Further bioisosteric substitution with a cyanoguanidino derivative provided first clinically useful drug cimetidine. Isosteric modification of the imidazole nucleus in cimetidine gave ranitidine without side effects associated with cimetidine.

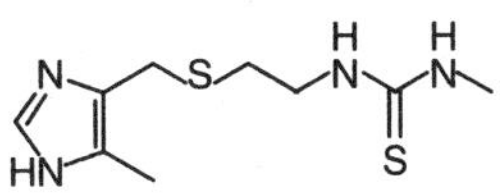

Metiamide 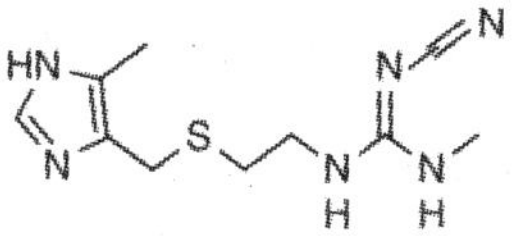   Cimetidine 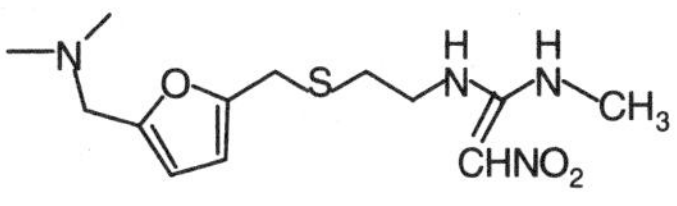   Ranitidine

Halogen bio-isosteres: Halogen has replaced by electron withdrawing groups such as a cyano or trifluoromethyl group. In a series of 5-benzyluracil developed as uridinephosphorylase inhibitors the activity is decreased by strong electron withdrawing groups like CF_3.

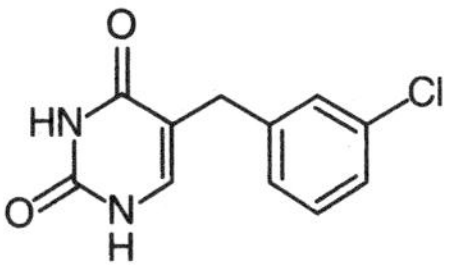

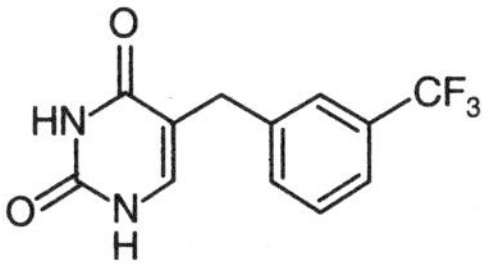

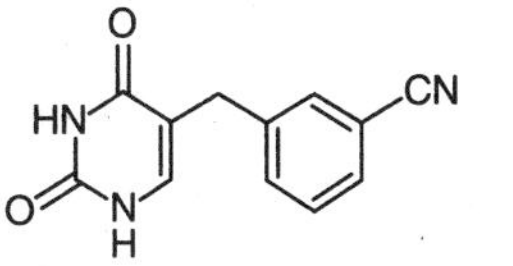

2. RATIONAL APPROACH OF DRUG DISCOVERY (Fig. 2.3)

- The knowledge about the receptors and their mode of interaction with drug molecules plays an important role in drug design. This knowledge may be used to develop conformationally bioactive skeletons having exact three-dimensional complementary to a receptor.

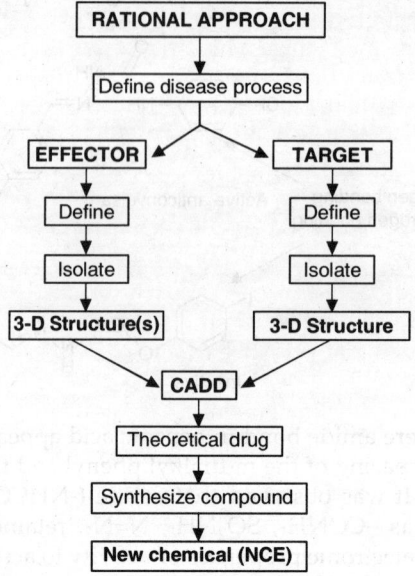

Fig. 2.3: Rational approach for drug discovery

- Greater potency, higher selectivity and less adverse effects are expected by reducing the flexibility of the drug structure. For example, replacement of a terminal N, N-dimethylamino group by piperidino exploits the decreasing valency angle at the tertiary nitrogen of the latter so that access of the basic group to anionic sites might be improved.
- This modification leads to the development of major tranquilizers, local anesthetic, anti-histaminics and spasmolytics. Incorporating a rigid ring leads to altered pharmacokinetic and pharmacodynamic features due to altered pKa of the amine and lipophillicity of the molecule.
- This approach is of greater importance in identification of lead nucleus. It involves the use of signs and symptoms of the disease. Most diseases, at least in part, arise from an imbalance of particular endogenous bioactive substance in the body.
- This imbalance may be corrected by agonism or antagonism of receptor or by inhibition of a particular enzyme. Once the real site of such imbalance is identified, the natural enzyme substrate or endogenous substance may be used as a lead nucleus. For example, endogenous hormones, progesterone and 17–β-estradiol were used for developing oral contraceptive. The development of an anti-inflammatory drug, indomethacin from the led nucleus, serotonin is a possible mediator of inflammation.

  A rational approach to drug design may be viewed from different angles, viz.

Quantum Mechanical Approach

Quantum mechanics (or wave mechanics) is composed of certain vital principles derived from fundamental assumptions describing the natural phenomenon effectively. The properties of protons, neutrons and electrons are adequately explained under quantum mechanics. The electronic features of the molecule responsible for chemical alteration from the basis of drug molecule phenomenon.

Molecular Orbital Approach

Based on the assumption that electrons present in molecules seem to be directly linked with orbitals engulfing the entire molecules which set forth the molecular orbital theory. The molecular orbital approach shows dependence on electronic charge as evidenced by the study of three volatile inhalation anesthetics and also on molecular conformation studied with respect to acetylcholine by such parameters as bond lengths and angles including tensional angles.

Molecular orbital calculations are achievable by sophisticated computers and after meticulous interpretation of result the molecular structure in respect of structure –activity analysis is established.

Molecular Connectivity Approach

This approach establishes the presence of structural features like cyclization, unsaturation, skeletal branching, the position and presence of heteroatom in molecules with the aid of series of numerical indices. For example, an index determined to possess a correlative factor in the SAR study of amphetamine type hallucinogenic drugs.

Molecular connectivity has some definite limitation such as electronegativity variance between atoms, non-distinguishable entity of *cis-trans* isomerism.

Linear Free Energy Approach

This method establishes the vital link between the proper selections of physicochemical parameters with a specific biological phenomenon. However, such a correlation may not guarantee and allow a direct interpretation with regard to molecular structure, but may positively offer a possible clue towards the selection of candidate molecules for synthesis. Examples are hypoglycemic and anorectic agents.

Hypoglycemic Agents

Insulin analouge: Attempt was made to synthesize various insulin analogues by specific amino acid substitution of the β-chain of insulin molecule using recombinant DNA techniques. These analogues have different pharmacokinetic properties than the clinically used insulin. The monomeric insulin analogues appeared to be less immunogenic and allergic than insulin.

Somatostatin analogues: Somatostatin a tetradecapeptide is an inhibitor of growth hormone release. It may also improve glycemic control by slowing down nutrient absorption from gut. Several somatostatin analogues have been synthesized. However, the high cost of production of these peptides may limit their clinical utility.

Fatty acid oxidation inhibitors: In diabetic person, always an increased utilization of fatty acids occurs. The fatty acid oxidation inhibitors exert hypoglycemic activity by promoting increased carbohydrate utilization and inducing a reduction in fatty acid oxidation. These agents selectively block carnitine palmitoyl transferase (CPT), a key enzyme in the oxidation of long-chain fatty acyl groups.

sodium 2-[5-(4-chlorophenyl)pentyl]oxiran-2-yl carbonate   2-tetradecylglycidate

Anorectic Agents

Weight loss is an effective means to achieve improved glycemic control in the treatment of obese non-insulin dependent diabetes mellitus. A variety of anorectic agents which may be used for short-term therapy includes mazindal and ciclazindal.

Inhibitors of carbohydrate metabolism: The intestinal carbohydrate digestion can be delayed by inhibiting the enzymes which cleave the terminal glucose. Acarbose is clinically used example.

Mazindal   Ciclazindal

Aldose reductase inhibitors: Glucose is mainly metabolized in body by two pathways.

1. Glycolic pathway involving an initial phosphorylation by the enzyme, hexokinase.

2. Polyol pathway by the enzyme, aldose reductase which reduces glucose to fructose via sorbitol. Glucose is preferentially metabolized by glycolytic pathway in normal person. In diabetic patient, the high glucose concentration leads to saturation of glycolytic pathway.

Excess glucose is then metabolized by Polyol pathway resulting into production of sorbitol and fructose. Since the rate of formation of sorbitol is higher than its rate of conversion to fructose, sorbitol selectively accumulates and causes complication of chronic diabetes like cataract, neuropathy and retinopathy. Tolrestat is an example of clinically used agent useful in the prophylaxis of diabetic neuropathy, retinopathy and cataract.

Tolrestat

Drug–Receptor Interaction

The vast majority of drugs show a remarkably high correlation of structure and specificity to produce pharmacological effects. Experimental evidence indicates that drugs interact with receptor sites localized in macromolecules which have protein-like properties and specific three-dimensional shapes.

- A minimum three-point attachment of a drug to a receptor site is required. In most cases, a rather specific chemical structure is required for the receptor site. Slight changes in the molecular structure of the drug may drastically change specificity.

- Several chemical forces may result in a temporary binding of the drug to the receptor. Essentially any bond could be involved with the drug–receptor interaction. Covalent bonds would be very tight and practically irreversible. Since by definition the drug–receptor interaction is reversible, covalent bond formation is rather rare except in a toxic situation. Since many drugs contain acid or amine functional groups, which are ionized at physiological pH, ionic bonds are formed by the attraction of opposite charges in the receptor site.

- Polar–polar interactions as in hydrogen bonding are a further extension of the attraction of opposite charges. The drug–receptor reaction is essentially an exchange of the hydrogen bond between a drug molecule, surrounding water and the receptor site.

- Finally hydrophobic bonds are formed between non-polar hydrocarbon groups on the drug and those in the receptor site. These bonds are not very specific but the interactions do occur to exclude water molecules. Repulsive forces which decrease the stability of the drug–receptor interaction include repulsion of like charges and steric hindrance. Steric hindrance refers to certain Three-dimensional features where repulsion occurs between electron clouds, inflexible chemical bonds or bulky alkyl groups.

RECEPTOR

- Majority of drugs produce their effect through an interaction with some chemical components of the living cell called a receptor. It is a specific macromolecular protein (membrane bound protein or intracellular) which is capable of binding with specific functional groups of the drug or endogenous substance.

- Its structure resembles with the three-dimensional configuration of the drug in the same way as the levers of lock are the three-dimensional mirror images of the grooves of the key with which it opens. Binding of a drug with its receptor results in the formation of drug–receptor (DR) complex which is responsible for triggering the biological response.

$$D + R \rightleftharpoons [DR] \longrightarrow \text{Response}$$

- This binding is usually specific and reversible (when there is formation of hydrogen bonds, van der Waals bonds or electrostatic bonds) but in certain cases irreversible also (e.g.

organophosphorus insecticides bind irreversibly to acetylcholine estrase by forming a covalent bond).

- At times the binding may be stereoselective also, i.e. if the drug has optical isomer, then usually it is levo or dextro form which is active, e.g. levoepinephrine, dextroamphetamine are active while their opposite optical isomers are not.

- Since receptors are broadly speaking macromolecular proteins with which the drug is presumed to interact, there may be several types of receptors, e.g. receptors for hormones, autocoids, growth factor and neurotransmitters; receptors for enzymes governing crucial metabolic and regulatory pathways (e.g. dihydrofolate reductase – the receptor for trimethoprim and for anticancer drug methotrexate); receptors as proteins involved in various transport processes (e.g. $Na^+ - K^+$ ATPase) the membrane receptor for cardiac glycoside used in congestive heart failure; receptors as proteins that serve the structural roles (e.g. tubulin – a receptor for antigout drug colchicines) and receptor as nucleic acids for anticancer drugs.

- Thus the term 'receptor' has been used operationally to denote any cellular macromolecule to which a drug binds to initiate its effect. If the binding of the drug to some chemical components of the cell does not lead to any pharmacological effect (as in the case of drug binding to plasma proteins), then the components is not called as the receptor but is merely referred to as 'acceptor site' or 'non-specific binding site'.

The overall effect is attributed to the two factors— affinity and intrinsic activity or efficacy.

Affinity

This means the capability of a drug to form the complex with its receptor (DR complex), e.g. the key entering the key hole of the lock has got an affinity to its levers.

Intrinsic Activity or Efficacy

Which means an ability of a drug to trigger the pharmacological response after making the drug–receptor complex (to exemplify: if the same key after entering into the key hole of the lock opens it too, it has got intrinsic activity also otherwise only affinity). On the basis of affinity and efficacy, the drugs can be broadly classified as— agonist and antagonist.

Agonist

Which have both, the high affinity as well as high intrinsic activity and therefore can trigger the maximal biological response or mimic the effect of the endogenous substance after combining with the recptor, e.g. methacholine is a cholinomimmetic drug (agonist) which mimics the effect of acetylcholine on cholinergic receptor.

Antagonist

Which have only the affinity but no intrinsic activity. These drugs bind to the receptor but do not mimic, rather block or interfere with, the binding of an endogenous agonist. For example, atropine blocks the effect of acetylcholine on the cholinergic–muscarinic receptors.

When two drugs are binding to the same receptors and at the same site, why it is so that one is acting as an agonist while another is serving as an antagonist? This central question in pharmacodynamics is answered by considering "the concept of dual nature of the receptors" wherein, the molecular forces during, drug–receptor interaction with the agonist only, alter the receptor conformation (antagonists are unable to activate the inactive receptor conformation).

Receptor usually exists in at least two conformations – the active (Ra) and inactive (Ri) (Fig. 3.1).

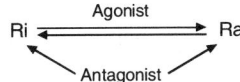

Fig. 3.1: Two state model of the receptor

These Ra and Ri conformation might relate to:

- The open or closed state of any ion channel, or
- To the active or inactive state of protein tyrosine kinase, or
- To the productive or non-productive G-protein, if Ra and Ri conformations are in equilibrium, the extent to which this equilibrium shall be perturbed will be determined by the relative affinity of the drug for these two conformations.

In such a situation, the following features may be manifested:

a. When the drug has a very high affinity for the active conformation (Ra) than inactive inactive (Ri): Such a drug will be an agonist as it will shift the equilibrium towards the active state, i.e. it will activate the receptor.

b. When the drug binds to either of these conformations (Ra and Ri) with equal affinity: Such a drug would not perturb the equilibrium, i.e. would neither activate the receptor nor will shift the equilibrium towards any side.

c. There are some additional subtitles besides these two categories of the drugs:

Partial agonists: These have full affinity to the receptor but with low intrinsic activity and hence these are only partially as effective as an agonist, e.g. pentazocine (a narcotic analgesic) is a partial agonist at the receptor subtype of opioid receptor.

Partial agonists influence the relative distribution of Ra and Ri in a slightly different manner. These have slightly higher affinity for Ra than Ri and hence shift the equilibrium towards Ra to a lesser extent than true agonist. Such drugs therefore display an intermediate effectiveness between the agonist and the antagonist.

Inverse agonists: These have full affinity towards the receptor, but their intrinsic activity ranges between zero to minus one. These drugs have a preferential affinity for the inactive state (Ri) of the receptor and therefore prevent any shift in the equilibrium towards Ra.

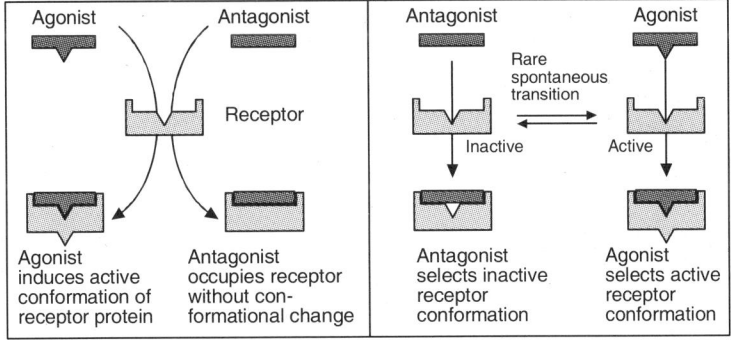

Fig. 3.2: Molecular mechanism of drug–receptor interaction

In other words, they stabilize the receptor from undergoing the productive conformational change. Consequently, they will produce an effect opposite to that of an agonist even in its absence. For example, carboline acts as inverse agonist at benzodiazepine receptor and produces the effects like anxiety awakening and seizure, which are just the opposite to the effects of benzodiazepines (anti-anxiety, sedation and anticonvulsant).

However, if the pre-existing equilibrium lies more towards Ri, negative antagonism may not be evident and shall be difficult to be distinguished from competitive antagonism (Fig. 3.2).

Specific drugs acting at low doses exert their effect by interacting with biomolecules in living cells. The 'primary mechanism' is the formation of a reversible drug–receptor complex. In general, receptors are "proteins that are embedded in a phospholipids layer."

Agents interact specifically with a receptor site on a specialized receptor molecule. Consider a closet in a home; a specific subspace within the domain. It is usually capable of accommodating a human comfortably but not a car. There are several groups of receptors distinguished on the basis of chemical superstructure (Fig. 3.3).

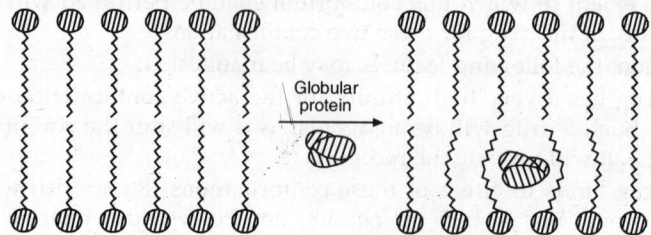

Fig. 3.3: Basic structure of receptor

- **Lipoprotein/glycoprotein:** Most common receptor type. Their environment governs their activity/receptiveness since they are usually membrane bound.
- **Lipids:** Less common as receptors. Consider the lipid bilayer and how certain proteins/large molecules may distort it. A cascade type effect.
- **Pure proteins:** Often recognized as drug receptors. Also known as enzymes. Enzymes are vital to biochemical reactions, regulating countless energy-related, neurotransmitter, metabolism, etc. processes.

    Modification of any of the enzyme mediated processes leads to a response. It is difficult, however, to precisely distinguish between enzyme and receptor in many instances. Consider a drug-receptor and substrate–enzyme combinations.

    A chemical change usually happens to a substrate, whereas nothing needs to "happen" to a drug. In fact, drugs normally dissociate from a receptor unchanged. Receptors, therefore, can transfer a message of the first messenger across a membrane. Next, the receptor is coupled to an 'effector system,' that causes a change in a second messenger, which then activates enzymes or ion channels.

- **Nucleic acids:** A number of antibiotics and anti-tumor agents interfere with DNA replication or transcription, or inhibit translation.

TYPES OF RECEPTORS

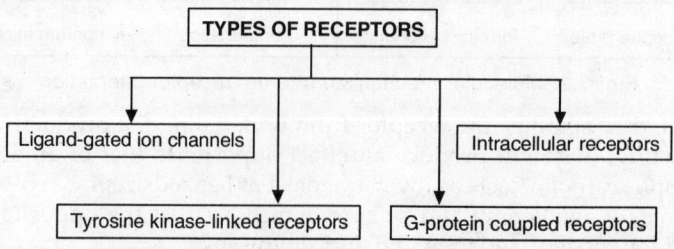

G-Protein Coupled Receptors (Fig. 3.4)

- It consists of an amino acid chain that weaves in and out of the membrane in serpentine fashion. The extramembrane loop regions of the molecule may possess sugar residues at different N-glycosylation sites.
- The seven α-helical membrane-spanning domains probably form a circle around a central pocket that carries the attachment sites for the mediator substance. Binding of the mediator molecule or of a structurally related agonist molecule induces a change in the conformation of the receptor protein, enabling the latter to interact with a G-protein (= guanyl nucleotide binding protein). G-proteins lie at the inner leaf of the plasma-lemma and consist of three subunits designated α, β, and γ.

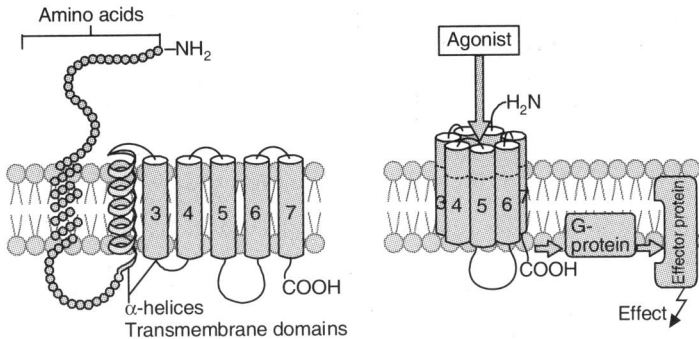

Fig. 3.4: G-protein coupled receptor

- There are various G-proteins that differ mainly with regard to their α-unit. Association with the receptor activates the G-protein, leading in turn to activation of another protein (enzyme, ion channel). A large number of mediator substances act via G-protein-coupled receptors.

Mechanism

- Signal transduction at G-protein coupled receptors uses essentially the same basic mechanisms. Agonist binding to the receptor leads to a change in receptor protein conformation.
- This change propagates to the G-protein: The α-subunit exchanges GDP for GTP, then dissociates from the two other subunits, associates with an effector protein and alters its functional state.
- The α-subunit slowly hydrolyzes bound GTP to GDP. Gα-GDP has no affinity for the effector protein and re-associates with the β and γ subunits. G-proteins can undergo lateral diffusion in the membrane; they are not assigned to individual receptor proteins. However, a relation exists between receptor types and G-protein types.
- Furthermore, the α-subunits of individual G-proteins are distinct in terms of their affinity for different effector proteins, as well as the kind of influence exerted on the effector protein. Gα-GTP of the GS-protein stimulates adenylate cyclase, whereas α-GTP of the Gi-protein is inhibitory.
- The G-protein-coupled receptor family includes muscarinic cholinoceptors, adrenoceptors for norepinephrine and epinephrine, receptors for dopamine, histamine, serotonin, glutamate, GABA, morphine, prostaglandins, leukotrienes, and many other mediators and hormones. Major effector proteins for G-protein-coupled receptors include adenylate cyclase (ATP

intracellular messenger cAMP), phospholipase C (phosphatidyl inositol intracellular messengers inositol trisphosphate and diacylglycerol), as well as ion channel proteins (Fig. 3.5).

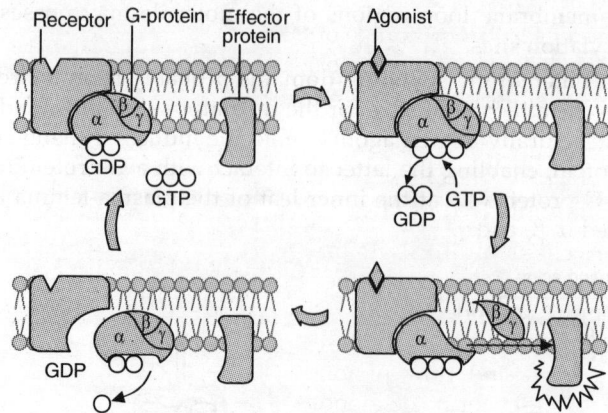

Fig. 3.5: G-protein-mediated effect of agonist

- Numerous cell functions are regulated by cellular cAMP concentration, because cAMP enhances activity of protein kinase A, which catalyzes the transfer of phosphate groups to functional proteins. Elevation of cAMP levels leads to relaxation of smooth muscle tons and enhanced contractility of cardiac muscle as well as increased glycogenolysis and lipolysis.

- Phosphorylation of cardiac calcium-channel proteins increases the probability of channel opening during membrane depolarization. It should be noted that cAMP is inactivated by phosphodiesterase. Inhibitors of this enzyme elevate intracellular cAMP concentration and elicit effects resembling those of epinephrine (Fig. 3.6).

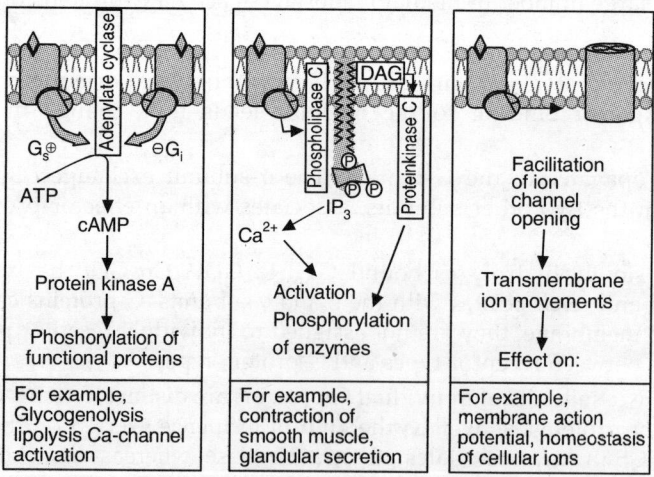

Fig. 3.6: G-protein, cellular messenger substance and effects

- The receptor protein itself may undergo phosphorylation, with a resultant loss of its ability to activate the associated G-protein. This is one of the mechanisms that contributes to a decrease in sensitivity of a cell during prolonged receptor stimulation by an agonist (desensitization). Activation of phospholipase C leads to cleavage of the membrane phospholipids phosphatidylinositol-4,5 diphosphate into inositol trisphosphate (IP_3) and diacylglycerol (DAG).

- IP_3 promotes release of Ca^{2+} from storage organelles, whereby contraction of smooth muscle cells, breakdown of glycogen or exocytosis may be initiated. Diacylglycerol stimulates protein kinase C, which phosphorylates certain serine or threonine containing enzymes.
- The α-subunit of some G-proteins may induce opening of a channel protein. In this manner, K^+ channels can be activated.

Ligand-Gated Ion Channels (Fig. 3.7)

- These receptors are coupled directly to an ion channel. These channels are 'agonist-regulated' opens only when the receptor is occupied by an agonist.
- So that whenever agonist attaches at the receptor site, ion channel get opened and flow of ions trigger the cellular response in the form of depolarization or hyperpolarization of the cell membrane.

Example

Such phenomenon of opening of ion-channel observed into the β cells of pancreas, which is ATP regulated K^+ channel. These β cells secrete insulin in response to hyperglycemic condition. These channels close when intracellular ATP concentration increases and open when falls.

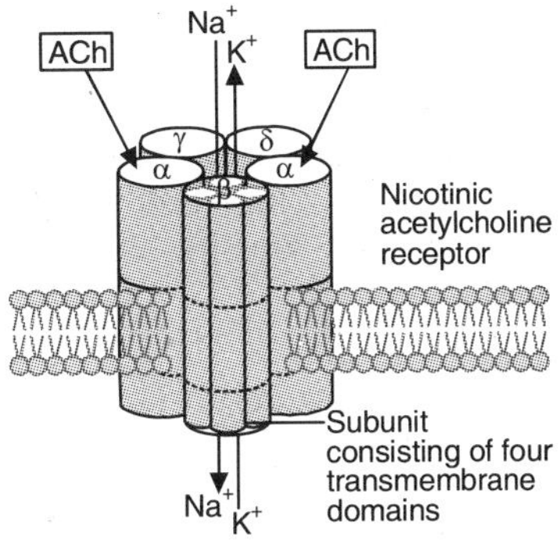

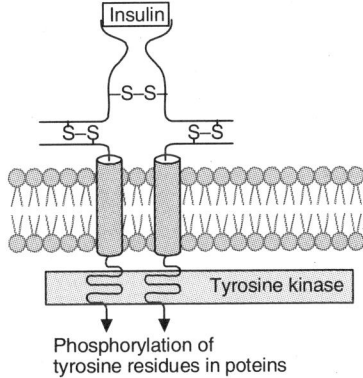

Fig. 3.7: Ligand-gated ion channel

Tyrosine Kinase-linked Receptor (Fig. 3.8)

- Tyrosine kinase is enzymatic protein. It has two domains, one which is present extracellularly and another present intracellularly having tyrosine kinase activity.
- The agonist binding to the extracellular site (domain) of receptor produces the conformational change that results in activation of intracellular enzyme domain.
- Activated intracellular domain (tyrosine kinase) causes autophosphorylation of protein. This autophosphorylated protein is responsible for alteration of function.

Example

Fig. 3.8: Tyrosine kinase-linked receptor

Upon activation, e.g. by ligands like insulin, the receptor is activated and is able to phosphorylate tyrosine residues of other intracellular proteins. Protein phosphorylation is one of the underlying mechanisms of the regulation of protein function.

Intracellular Receptor

Such type of receptor is present intracellularly within the cytoplasm of cell. When agonist (steroidal drug, hormone) penetrates the cell and bind with steroidal binding site of the receptor.

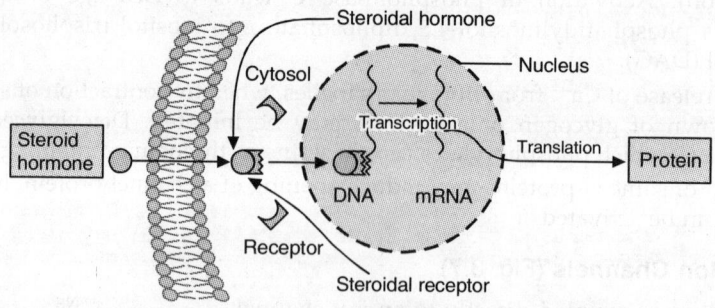

Fig. 3.9: Protein synthesis regulating receptor

This binding of hormone to the steroidal site leads to the exposure of the masked DNA binding site. These complexes entered in nucleus and synthesize mRNA from DNA (transcription). This mRNA is further responsible for protein synthesis (Fig. 3.9).

DRUG–RECEPTOR INTERACTION

Enantioselectivity of Drug Action

- Many drugs are racemates, including β-blockers, non-steroidal anti-inflammatory agents, and anticholinergics. A racemate consists of a molecule and its corresponding mirror image which, like the left and right hand, cannot be superimposed. Such chiral ('handed') pairs of molecules are referred to as enantiomers (Fig. 3.10).

- Usually, chirality is due to a carbon atom (C) linked to four different substituents ('asymmetric center'). Enantiomerism is a special case of stereoisomerism.

- Non-chiral stereoisomers are called diastereomers (e.g. quinidine/quinine). Bond lengths in enantiomers, but not in diastereomers, are the same. Therefore, enantiomers possess similar physicochemical properties (e.g. solubility, melting point) and both forms are usually obtained in equal amounts by chemical synthesis. As a result of enzymatic activity, however, only one of the enantiomers is usually found in nature.

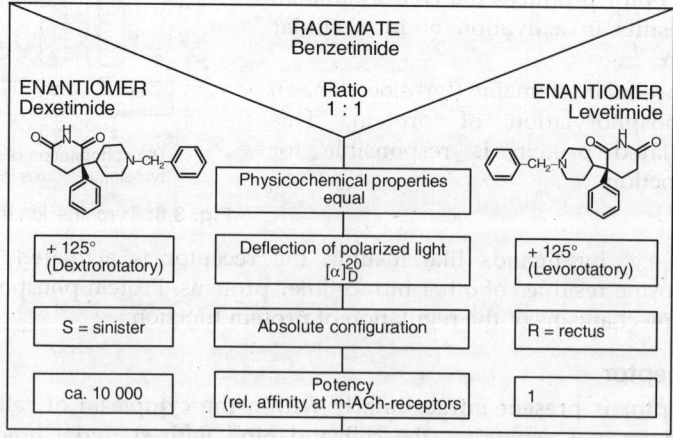

Fig. 3.10: An enantiomeric pair with different affinity for a stereoselective receptor

- In solution, enantiomers rotate the wave plane of linearly polarized light in opposite directions; hence they are referred to as 'dextro' or 'levo-rotatory', designated by the prefixes d or (+) and l or (–), respectively. The direction of rotation gives no clue concerning the spatial structure of enantiomers.

- The absolute configuration, as determined by certain rules, is described by the prefixes S and R. In some compounds, designation as the D- and L-form is possible by reference to the structure of D- and L-glyceraldehyde.For drugs to exert biological actions; contact with reaction partners in the body is required. When the reaction favors one of the enantiomers, enantio-selectivity is observed. In Fig. 3.10 "S" enantiomer of benzetimide is more potent than "R" enantiomer.

Enantioselectivity of Affinity

- If a receptor has sites for three of the substituents (symbolized in Fig. 3.11 by a cone, a sphere, and a cube) on the asymmetric carbon to attach to, only one of the enantiomers will have optimal fit.

- Its affinity will then be higher. Thus, dexetimide displays an affinity at the muscarinic ACh receptors almost 10000 times that of levetimide; and at β-adrenoceptors, S (-)-propranolol has an affinity 100 times that of the R(+)-form.

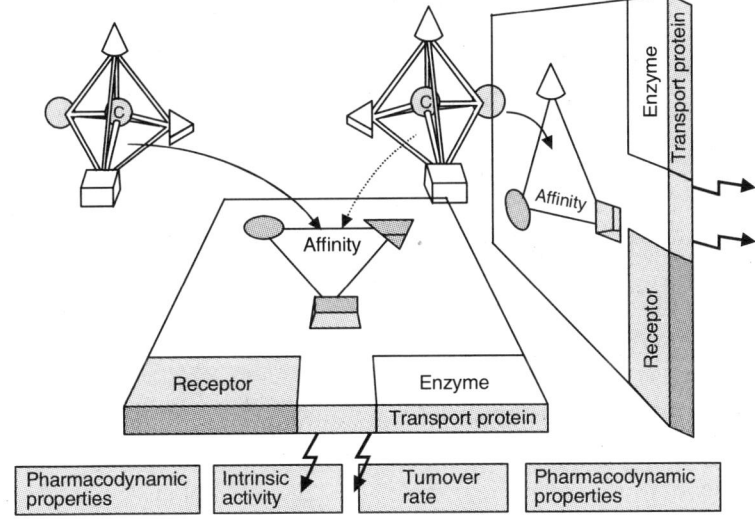

Fig. 3.11: Reason for different pharmacological properties of enantiomer

Enantioselectivity of Intrinsic Activity

- The mode of attachment at the receptor also determines whether an effect is elicited and whether or not a substance has intrinsic activity, i.e. acts as an agonist or antagonist.

- For instance, (-) dobutamine is an agonist at α-adrenoceptors whereas the (+)-enantiomer is an antagonist.

Inverse Enantioselectivity at another Receptor

- An enantiomer may possess an unfavorable configuration at one receptor that may, however, be optimal for interaction with another receptor.

- In the case of dobutamine, the (+)-enantiomer has affinity at α-adrenoceptors 10 times higher than that of the (–)-enantiomer, both having agonist activity. However, the α-adrenoceptors stimulant action is due to the (–)-form.
- As described for receptor interactions, enantioselectivity may also be manifested in drug interactions with enzymes and transport proteins. Enantiomers may display different affinities and reaction velocities.

Conclusion

The enantiomers of a racemate can differ sufficiently in their pharmacodynamic and pharmacokinetic properties to constitute two distinct drugs.

Forces Involved in Drug-receptor Interaction (Fig. 3.12)

- In general, the forces between a drug and receptor are the same that can occur between any organic molecules. Weak interactions can only occur when the molecular surfaces are close since bond strength is distance dependent.
- The formation of a bond between atoms occurs with a decrease in free energy, or ΔG is negative. How can this information be used to understand drug–receptor interactions?
- Remember;

  $\Delta G = -RT (\ln Keq)$ where R = gas constant = 2.0 (in calories) and T = 310 (at physiologic temp $37^{\circ}C$) Keq = binding equilibrium constant for the following equation

  $$\textbf{Drug + Receptor} \; = \; \textbf{Drug–Receptor} \; (\Delta G)$$

- By this expression, a change in free energy of –2 to –3 kcal/mol can have a major effect on secondary binding interactions. Note the following calculation and that the Keq is expressed fractionally and you need to calculate the ratio.

$$\Delta G = -RT (\ln Keq)$$
$$-2700 \text{ cal} = -620 (\ln Keq)$$
$$-0.0043 \text{ kcal} = \ln Keq \;.$$
$$0.013 = Keq$$

- 1.3% in the form of the drug-receptor complex and 98.7% in the form of free drug. A change in free energy of about 2.7 kcal/mol results in a 100-fold change in the equilibrium population.

Seven Major types of Drug–Receptor Interactions

Covalent bonds

- The strongest bond, worth anywhere from –40 to –110 kcal/mol in stability. Not too common in drug–receptor interactions. Bonds in the molecule at right are all covalent even though some are single, double or triple bonds. Not shown are the carbon–hydrogen bonds, which are also covalent.
- Although most drug interactions are non-covalent, phosphorylation of a serine residue on proteases is one example of a covalent bond that is formed during drug action. Alkylation (e.g. of DNA) is another example of covalent bond formation.

Ionic bonds

- At physiologic pH, basic side chains of certain amino acids like arginine, lysine, and in part, histidine are protonated and therefore provide a cationic environment. Acidic groups like aspartic and glutamic acid are deprotonated to give negatively charged groups.

- Therefore, drug and receptor can be mutually attracted by opposite charges on their surfaces, e.g. cationic drug with anionic receptor site. A simple ionic attraction can provide as much as –5.0 kcal/mol and declines as the square of the distance between the charged sites. If an ionic attraction is reinforced by other interactions (H-bonding, etc.) is can provide up to –10.0 kcal/mol.

quaternary amine attracted to glutamate anion

Ion–Dipole and Dipole–Dipole Interactions

- By virtue of varied electronegativity values when compared to carbon certain groups have an asymmetric distribution of electrons that produce dipoles.
- The dipoles in a drug molecule, therefore, can find complementary dipole interactions in the receptor. However, since the net charge on a dipole is less than on a full ion, the interaction is generally weaker (G ranges from –1 to –7 but is usually –1 to –2).

Hydrogen bonds

- A simple variation of a dipole-dipole interaction formed between the proton of a group RX-H (where X = heteroatom) or another electronegative atom or group (Y). In molecules of biological interest, the hydrogen bonds most widely experienced are when X = O, N, S. Hydrogen bonds are usually denoted by a dashed or dotted line as in:

$$R–X——HY-R$$

- What makes hydrogen bonds so unique is that hydrogen is the only atom that can carry a positive charge at physiologic pH while remaining covalently attached to a molecule.
- Further, hydrogen is small enough to permit close approach by another electronegative atom or molecule to accept the hydrogen bond.
- There are two forms of hydrogen bonds — **Intermolecular** (within a single molecule) and **Interamolecular** (between two molecules).
- Hydrogen bonds for example, are important in maintaining the structural integrity of peptides and proteins -helical structure and -sheets derive their structure from hydrogen bonds.
- The ΔG for hydrogen bonding ranges from –1 to –7 kcal/mol but in biosystems is usually between –3 and –5 kcal/mol.

Charge transfer complexes

- This attraction comes about when molecules containing a good electron donor group interact with a molecule that contains an electron-acceptor group. The interaction involves transfer of charge from donor to acceptor.
- Electron donor groups or molecules usually contain a bond (alkenes, alkynes, aromatic moiety) that bears a good electron-donating group (alkyl, methoxy, OR, SR, etc.). Acceptor groups or molecules usually contain a -bond with electron withdrawing groups attached (e.g., cyano, carbonyl, halogen, etc.).

Charge-transfer complex

- The interaction is more rare than H-bonding or ionic and most likely found with the tyrosine residue on certain receptors (as the donor). The ΔG for charge-transfer complexes range from –1 to –7 kcal/mol.

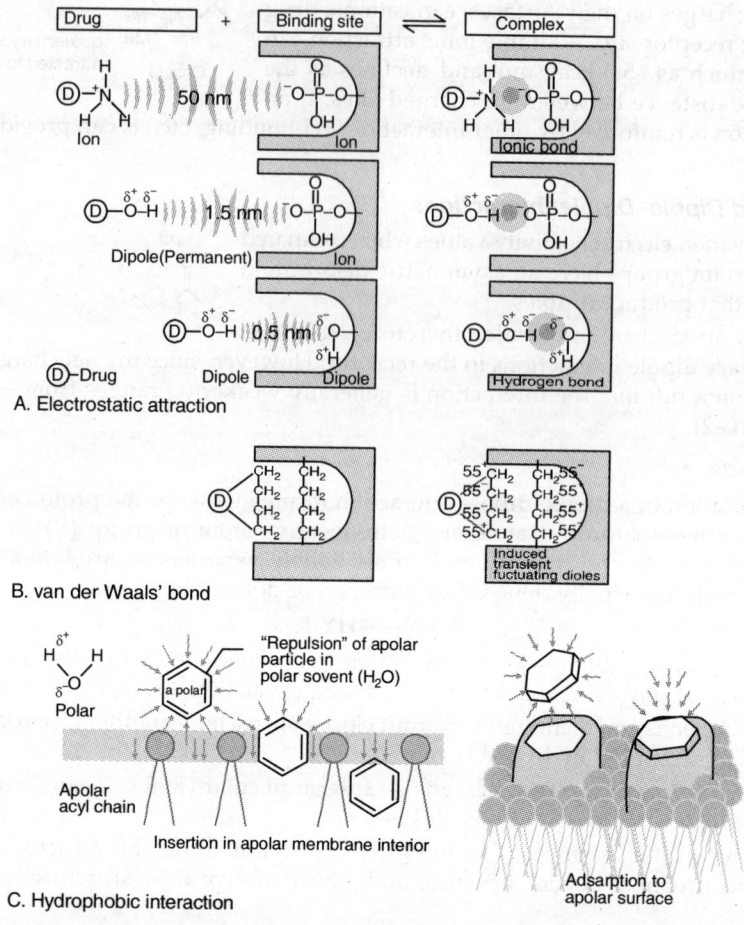

Fig. 3.12: Forces involved in drug–receptor interaction

Hydrophobic Interactions

- Involve a non-polar/non-polar interaction between receptor and drug. Usually alkyl chains are found to stack as in the lipid bilayer except this is for a single interaction.

- It is important to consider in this interaction that each receptor and drug molecule aliphatic chain is surrounded by water molecules, and as the chains approach each water molecule is squeezed out to permit the non-polar chains to align with each other in a 'side by side' position. This orienting results in a drop in the free energy of about 0.1 to 2.0 kcal/mol.

Table 3.1: Drug–receptor bond strength

S.no.	Bond type	Strength kcal/mol	Example
1.	Covalent	40–110	H—C—HN—— Receptor (with H substituents)
2.	Ionic (in solution)	5–10	H_4—O—C Receptors
3.	Hydrogen	1–7	OH ······· O=C Receptor
4.	Dipole–dipole	1–7	R—C ······· N— Receptor
5.	Hydrophobic	1	H—C—H ·········· H—C—H

Van der Waals or London Forces

- Some atoms on mostly non-polar molecules experience or exert a temporary non-symmetric distribution of electrons to cause a dipole.
- As these atoms approach each other in different molecules, the opposite dipoles attract forming an interaction. The ΔG varies greatly and values from –0.1 to –2.0 are reasonable.

Theories of Drug–Receptor Interaction

- Ideas of receptors help medicinal chemists to 'conceptualize' the drug target in simple terms, void of unnecessary factors such as transport, metabolism and excretion. These latter factors are important in understanding a drug profile but do not lend any understanding of the dynamic interaction between drug and event.
- In the 1970s, the concept of receptors was brought to reality by isotopically labeled ligands that bound real receptors to furnish an image of where they reside and how they could be isolated. More importantly, these experiments showed that a receptor actually existed.
- It is generally accepted that there is a 'complementary' fit between an agonist/drug and its receptor site. This suggests a mutual molding and plasticity of the drug and the receptors with the intent to take 'advantage' of the relationship.
- The plasticity of the receptor is important, following interaction with the drug, a conformational change, e.g. indicating fluidity may induce a change in an 'effector' molecule, which then transmits a signal, impulse or charge that elicits the biological response. From this basic understanding, several receptor theories evolved.
  1. Two-state receptor model (Activation-Aggregation Theory).
  2. Occupancy theory.
  3. Rate theory.

4. Induced-fit theory.
5. Macromolecular perturbation theory.
6. Activation-aggregation theory.

Activation-aggregation theory (Two state receptor model)

This theory explains that receptor exist in dynamic equilibrium between an activated form (R1) and inactive form (R2). R1 is responsible for biological response. When agonist bind to the receptor; it shift equillibrium to the R1 active site and elicite the biological response and vice-versa for antagonist.

$$\text{Active site (R1)} \rightleftharpoons \text{(R2) Inactive site}$$

- If two drugs bind the same receptor and have somewhat similar structures, how can one be an agonist and the other produces no effect?
- Consider a receptor that itself constitutes or is capable of interacting with and regulating a specific channel for ions (Ca^{+2}, K^+, etc.) to permeate a cell membrane.
- The ultimate physiologic response of interest is a change in ionic permeability.
- If the channel (receptor) can exist in two conformations that are in equilibrium (open = Ro and closed = Rc) and Rc predominates when no ligand (drug) is present, the drug will affect the opening of the channel, if it binds preferentially to (has affinity for) the open conformation.
- The extent to which the equilibrium Rc and Ro is perturbed (to produce an effect) is determined by the relative ability of the drug for the two different conformations. Thus, if a drug binds to the same site on R but with only slightly greater affinity for Ro than for Rc, the observed effect may be less. This defines a partial agonist.
- It also follows that an agent that has equal affinity for Rc and Ro will not alter the pre-existing equilibrium; hence no activity as an agonist. However, when bound, such compound will act as antagonist because it impairs the ability of an agonist to alter the equilibrium and produces a response.
- A graphic representation of these concepts is presented in Fig. 3.1.

Occupancy theory

- It states that the drug effect is directly proportional to the number of receptors occupied. The effect ceases when the drug–receptor complex dissociates.
- Because not all agonists produce a maximal effect regardless of dose size, this theory does not account for 'partial' effects. Ariens who separated the occupancy theory into two parts forwarded a modification of this theory.
1. **Affinity:** Complexation of the drug with the receptor (capacity of a drug to bind the receptor).
2. **Intrinsic activity:** Initiation of the biological effect (measures, which equals the ability of drug–receptor complex to initiate the biological response).

Rate theory

- It states that the activation of receptors is proportional to the total number of encounters of the drug with its receptor per unit time.
- The rate theory therefore suggests that pharmacological activity is a function of the rate of association and dissociation and not the number of occupied receptors. Again, the rate theory does not account for why different types of compounds exhibit the characteristics that they do.

Induced-fit theory

This theory explains that drug is responsible for inducing conformational changes in the receptor and receptor does not required to change itself according to that of the drug. This theory explain that pharmacological action (intensity) of drug–receptor interaction is depend upon the confirmational changes produced by that of drug.

- Originally used for enzyme–substrate interactions, the induced-fit theory suggests that receptors need not be in the needed conformation to accept the drug, rather, as the drug begins to interact with the receptor, a conformational change is induced which orients the essential binding sites.
- The conformational change that occurs while the drug is being accepted into the binding pocket may initiate the biological effect.

Macromolecular perturbation theory

Belleau argued that in the interaction of a drug with its receptor, two general types of macromolecular perturbations could occur.

A. Specific conformational perturbations— binding of certain molecules that produce an effect. (agonist)

B. Non-specific conformational perturbation— accommodates other types of molecules that do not elicit an effect (antagonists).

METHODS OF RECEPTOR CHARACTERIZATION

A. Affinity methods
   1. Affinity chromatography.
   2. Affinity labeling.

B. Radioisotope and fluorescence methods.

C. Magnetic resonance:
   1. NMR
   2. EPR

D. Data treatment — the Scatchard Plot.

Stereochemistry and Biological Activity

Stereochemistry is the branch of science which deals with the structures in three dimensions. Stereoisomers are the kind of isomers which are different from each other only in the way the atoms are oriented in space and the phenomenon is known as stereoisomerism.

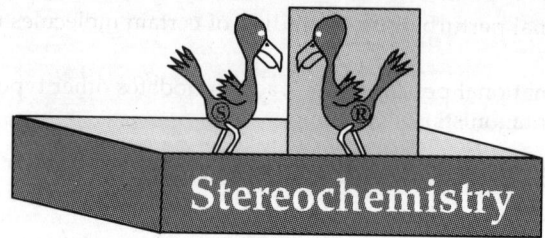

Stereochemistry plays a very vital role in drug–receptor interaction. For interaction of any ligand with receptor, it is essential that ligand and receptor should be present in appropriate conformation.

Following are the steric factors which affect the pharmacological activity of a molecule.
a. Isomerism
b. Conformational isomerism
c. Isosterism
d. Bio-isosterism

ISOMERISM

The compounds having same molecular formula but differs from each other in their physical or chemical properties are known as isomer and phenomenon is known as isomerism. Classification of isomerism is depicted in Flow chart 4.1.

Structural Isomerism

"These are the compounds or isomers having same molecular formula but different structural formula."

This type of isomerism which arises from difference in the arrangement of molecule includes:
1. Positional isomers
2. Chain isomers
3. Functional isomers
4. Tautomer
5. Metamer

Flow chart 4.1: Classification of isomerism

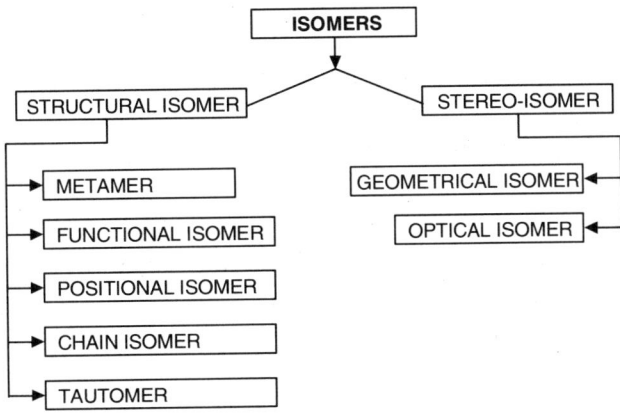

Positional Isomer

The compounds having same molecular formula, only they differ from each other in the position of the substituent or group on the carbon chain. These are called positional isomer and phenomenon is known as positional isomerism. Example:

1 - bromobutane   2 - bromobutane   n - propyl alcohol   Isopropyl alcohol

Effect over biological activity: In case of ter. butyl norepinephrine and terbutalin. Terbutalin is having long duration of action as compare to the initial one.

n - ter.butyl norepinephrine
(Catechol ring)

Terbutalin
(Resorcinol ring)

Chain isomer

The compounds having the same molecular formula but differ in the order in which carbon atoms are bonded to each other. Example:

Effect over biological activity: Phenobarbital and Amobarbital differ only in 5 carbon side chains attached to the barbiturate ring. But phenobarbital is having short duration of action while amobarbital is intermediate in action.

n - butane   Isobutane

Phenobarbital   Amobarbital

Functional isomer

The compound having the same molecular formula but different functional group is known as functional isomer.

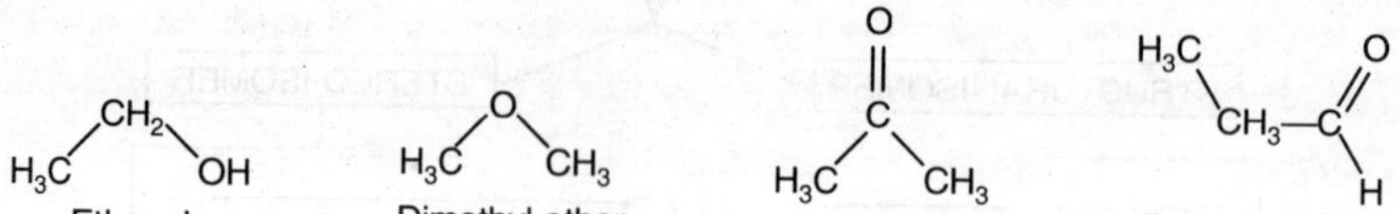

Ethanol · Dimethyl ether · Acetone · Proionaldehyde

Tautomer

It is a special type of functional isomerism in which the isomers are in dynamic equilibrium with each other.

Example: Ethylacetoactate is in equilibrium of the following two forms at room temperature, the mixture contains 93% of keto form plus 6% enol forms.

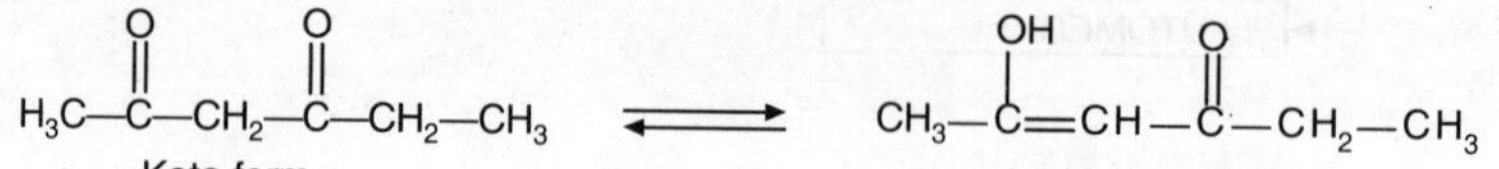

Keto form · Enol form

Metamer

This type of isomerism is due to the unequal distribution of carbon atoms on either side of the functional group. Example:

$H_3C—CH_2—O—CH_2—CH_3$ $H_3C—O—CH_2—CH_2—CH_3$
Diethyl ether   Methyl propyl ether

Stereo-isomerism

"Stereoisomers have same structural formula but they differ from each other in the arrangement of atoms or groups in the space". Stereo-isomers are of two types:

1. Geometrical isomer
2. Optical isomer

Geometrical isomerism

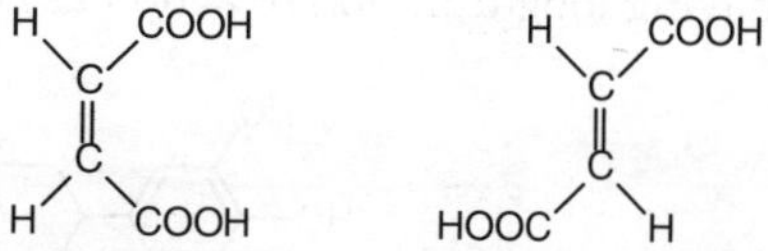

"In this type of isomerism, the isomer possesses the same structural formula containing double bond and differs only in respect to the arrangement of atoms or groups around the double bond". Examples: Maleic acid and Fumaric acid.

Maleic acid · Fumaric acid (trans)

- The carbon atoms of the carbon–carbon double bond are Sp^2 hybridized. The carbon–carbon double bond consists of σ bond and π bond. The σ bond is formed by the overlap of Sp^2 hybrid orbital.
- The π bond is formed by the overlap of the p-orbital. The presence of π-bond locks the molecule in one position. So that rotation around the C=C bond is not possible as that may result in breaking of π bond (Fig. 4.1).

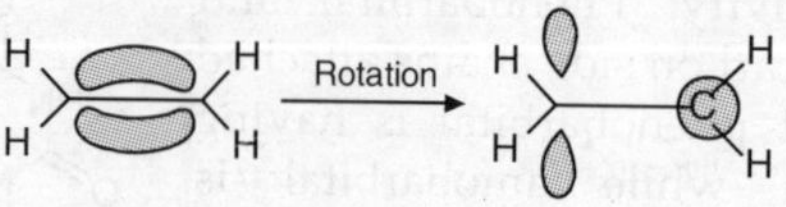

Fig. 4.1: Rotation around the π bond would break π bond

- This restricted rotation about the carbon–carbon bond is responsible for geometric isomerism in alkenes. Due to this restricted, rotation these geometrical isomers exist in two forms.

    1. **Cis isomers:** Cis isomers are those, in which two similar groups are on the same side of double bond.

    2. **Trans isomers:** Trans isomers are those, in which two similar groups are on the opposite side of double bond.

Stability of cis and trans (geometrical isomer): The trans isomer of alkene is usually more stable than its corresponding cis isomer. Consider the cis and trans isomers of the alkene, in which 'A' is bulky group as compare to 'B'. In the cis isomer, the two bulky 'A' groups are very close to each other.

The repulsion due to the overlapping of electron clouds of two bulky 'A' groups will make this isomer less stable than trans isomer in which the bulky 'A' groups are far apart from each other.

Effect over biological activity: As shown in Fig. 4.2, out of the two forms only cis form is active over the receptor than trans. The reason behind this is that cis form is properly oriented over the receptor and vice-versa.

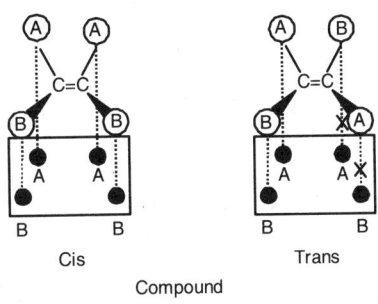

Fig. 4.2: Effect of geometrical isomer over biological activity

Example:

1. *Diethylstilbesterol:* Diethylstilbestrol is used in prostate cancer. Out of the two forms trans form is 14 times more potent than cis form.

2. *Anti-estrogenic effect:* Among the tomoxifen and clomiphen, clomiphen (cis) form is more active.

Tomoxifen

Clomiphen

Optical isomerism

"These are the optically active compound, which rotate the plane of plane polarized light in opposite direction and phenomenon is known as optical isomerism."

Optical activity: It is the ability of the compound to rotate the plane of plane polarized light to right or left hand side, such ability is known as optical activity, while those compounds which possess such activity are known as the optically active compounds.

Polarimeter (Fig. 4.3):

- The polarimeter consists of the light source and two lenses; one is polarizer and another is analyser.

- In between the two lenses, tube is present, which hold the sample. This assembly is so arranged that light passes from one lens (polarizer) which converts natural light to the plane polarized light, which vibrates in only one direction.

- This plane polarized light passes through the sample and then via analyzer to the eye of the observer. If the rotation of plane and hence rotation of the lens is to the right, the substance is dextro rotator and vice-versa.

- With the help of polarimeter, we can conclude about the rotation of the compound, whether it is levo or dextro rotatory.

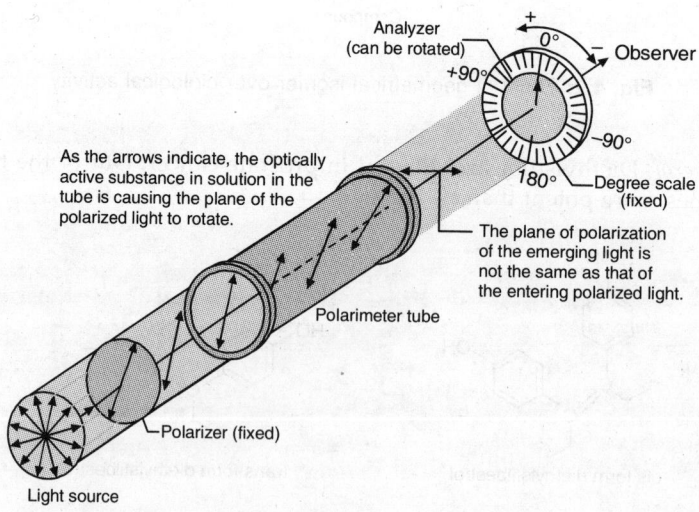

Fig. 4.3: Schematic diagram of polarimeter

1. *Leavo rotatory*: The compound which rotates the plane of plane polarized light to the left (anti-clockwise) is said to be leavo rotatory. This is indicated by (-) sign.
2. *Dextro rotatory*: The compound which rotates the plane of plane polarized light to right (clockwise) is said to be dextro rotation. It is indicated by (+) signs.

Specific rotation: For the measurement of the optical rotation, a new term has been coined.

"It is the number of degree of rotation produced by a solution of length 10 cm, having the concentration 1 gm/ml at given wavelength and temperature"

Mathematically, we can represent this as;

$$[\alpha]_D^T = \frac{\alpha}{l \times c}$$

α : observed rotation
l : sample path length (dm)
c : sample concentration (g/mL)

$$[\alpha]_D^T = \frac{\text{Observed rotation, } \alpha}{\text{Path length, } l(\text{dm}) \times \text{Concentration of sample, } c(\text{g/mL})} = \frac{\alpha}{l \times c}$$

1. The specific rotation depends on the temperature and wavelength of light that is employed.
   a. Sodium D-line : 589.6 nm = 5896Å
   b. Temperature
2. The magnitude of rotation is dependent on the solvent when solution are measured.

(R)-(–)-2-butanol

$[\alpha]_D^{25} = -13.52°$

(S)-(+)-2-butanol

$[\alpha]_D^{25} = +13.52°$

(R)-(+)-2-methyl-1-butanol

$[\alpha]_D^{25} = +5.756°$

(S)-(–)-2-methyl-1-butanol

(S)-(–)-2-methyl-1-butanol

(R)-(–)-1-chloro-2-methylbutane

$[\alpha]_D^{25} = -1.64°$

(S)-(+)-1-chloro-2-methylbutane

$[\alpha]_D^{25} = +1.64°$

Table 4.1: Specific rotation of organic compounds

Compound	$|\alpha|_D$ (degrees)	Compound	$|\alpha|_D$ (degrees)
Camphor	–4.26	Penicillin V	–223
Morphine	–132	Monosodium glutamate	–25.5
Sucrose	–66.47	Benzene	0
Cholesterol	–31.5	Acetic acid	0

Conditions for optical isomerism

1. Assymetric carbon atoms

A carbon atom which is bonded to four different groups is called asymmetric carbon atom.

An asymmetric carbon in formula is usually indicated by the asterisk placed near it.

$$Na^+OOCCHC^*(OH)-\overset{\overset{\displaystyle H}{|}}{\underset{\underset{\displaystyle OH}{|}}{C}}{}^*-COO^+NH_4$$

Sodium ammonium tartrate

$$H_3C-\overset{\overset{\displaystyle H}{|}}{\underset{\underset{\displaystyle OH}{|}}{C}}{}^*-COOH$$

Lactic acid

$$\left(X-\overset{\overset{\displaystyle H}{|}}{\underset{\underset{\displaystyle Y}{|}}{C}}{}^*-Z\right)$$

2. Dissymetric molecule (Symmetry of Molecule)

A plane which divides an object into two symmetric halves is said to be plane of symmetry (Fig. 4.4).

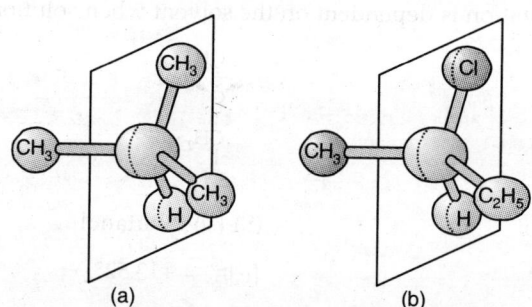

(a)   (b)

Fig. 4.4: (a) 2-chloropropane has a plane of symmetry and chiral
(b) 2-chlorobutane does not possess plane of symmetry and is chiral

An object lacking a plane of symmetry is called dissymmetric. Asymmetric object is referred to as achiral. A dissymmetric object cannot be superimposed on its mirror image.

A left hand, for example, does not possess a plane of symmetry and its mirror image is not another left hand but a right hand. The two are identical, because they cannot be superimposed. If we were to lay one hand on top of the other, the fingers and thumbs would clash.

Optically active compounds should be asymmetric one, i.e. their mirror images should not be superimposed over each others.

3. Non-superimposable mirror images

Optical activity is only produced by those substances which do not superimpose on their mirror images (Figs. 4.5 and 4.6).

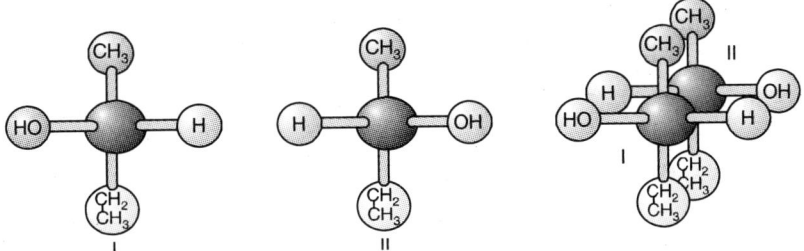

Fig. 4.5: 2-butanol, non-superimposable mirror images of each other

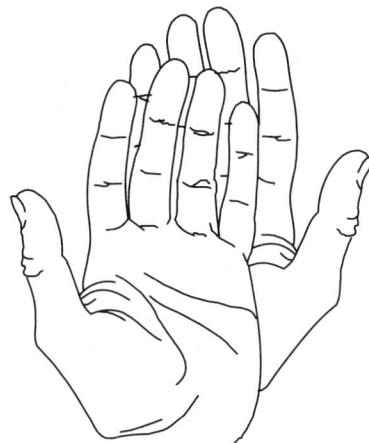

Fig. 4.6: Left and right hands are non-superimposable over each other

4. Chirality

The word chiral is derived from Greek word " cheir" meaning hand, is used for those objects which have right handed and left handed forms, i.e. molecule which have handness and the general property of handness is known as chirality (Fig. 4.7).

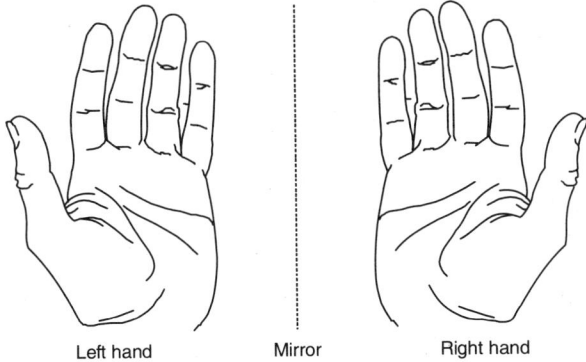

Left hand   Mirror   Right hand

Fig. 4.7: The mirror image of left and right hand showing handness

Criteria for chirality:

1. Non-superimpossable mirror images

2. Asymmetric carbon atom
3. Dissymmetric molecule

Chirality and biological activity:

1. *Limonene*: S-limonene is responsible for the odour of lemon, and the R-limonene for the odour of orange.
2. *Carvone*: S-carvone is responsible for the odour of spearmint and the R-carvone for the odour of carway seed.

Chirality and biological activity

S   Limonene   R
Lemon odor   Orange odor

S   Carvone   R
Sepearmint fragrance   Orange odor

S   Asparagine   R
bitter taste   Sweet taste

S   Dopa (3,4-dihydroxyphenylalanine)   R
Anti-Parkinson's disease   Toxic

S   Epinephrine   R
Toxic   Hormone

S   Thalidomide sedative, hypnotic   R
Teratogenic activity   Causes **NO** deformities

3. *Thalidomide*: Used to alleviate the symptoms of morning sickness in pregnant women before 1963.

a. The S-enantiomer causes birth defect.

b. Under physiological condition, the two enantiomers are interconverted.

c. Thalidomide is approved under highly strict regulation for treatment of serious complication associated with leprosy.

d. Thalidomide's potential use against other condition including AIDS, brain cancer, rheumatide arthritis is under investigation.

4. The origin of biological properties relating to chirality.

a. The fact that the enantiomers of a compound do not smell, the same suggests that the receptor sites in the nose for the compound are chiral, and only the correct enantiomers will fit its particular site (just as a hand requires a glove of the correct chirality for proper fit).

b. The binding specificity for a chiral molecule (like a hand) at a chiral receptor site is only favourable in one way. If either the molecule or the biological receptors site had the wrong handedness, the natural physiological response (e.g. neural impulse, reaction catalyst) will not occur.

c. Because of the tetrahedral stereocenter of the amino acid, three-point binding can occur with proper alignment for only one of the two enantiomers (Fig. 4.8).

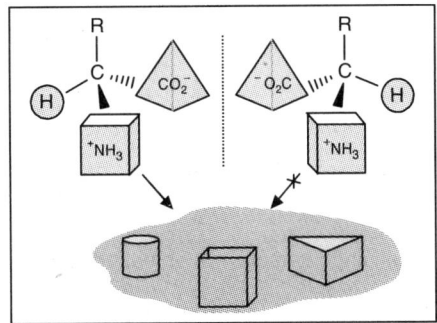

Fig. 4.8: Only one of the two amino acid enantiomers shown can achieve three-point binding with the hypothetical binding site

5. Racemic modification

- A mixture of equal amount of dextro and levo form is known as the racemic mixture. Such mixtures are optically inactive because rotation of dextro is cancelled by levo or vice versa. This is represented by ($\pm$) symbol.

- If particular compound is in equimolar amount forms racemic mixtures, we can say that such compound is optically active.

6. Effect over biological activity

- From above discussion, we come to know that optical isomer exist in two forms, one is (+) dextro rotatory and another (–) leavo rotatory.

- But out of the two forms only one will be active at particular receptor other may be inactive, partial active or showing strong activity. Why this is so happened? To understand this lets have following example (Fig. 4.9).

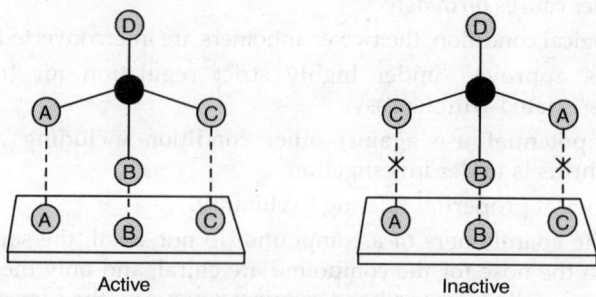

Active   Inactive

Fig. 4.9: Effect of optical isomer on pharmacological activity

- In the compound mentioned above A, B, C and D are the functional group of particular molecule and on corresponding site there is place on receptor for drug molecule.
- It is easily observed that out of the two forms only one is active and another form is inactive, why? Its mere because of orientation of functional group toward the respective site on receptor.

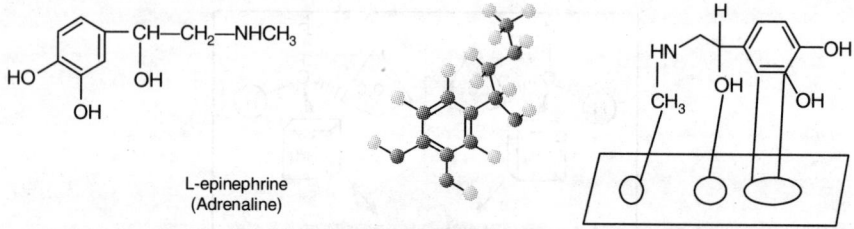

L-epinephrine
(Adrenaline)

Fig. 4.10: Binding interaction of epinephrine with receptor

- In case of epinephrin, levoepinephrine is active only because of proper orientation of the 'OH' functional group. Some time one optical isomer has one activity while other has completely different activity.

Enantiomers (Fig. 4.11)

The optical isomers, that are non-superimposable mirror images of each other is known as enantiomers.

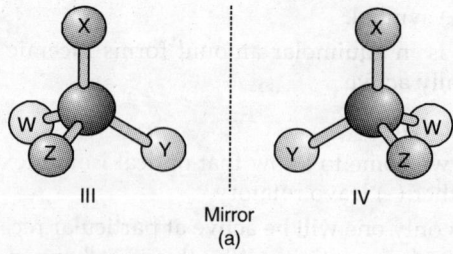

III   IV
Mirror
(a)

Fig.4.11: Enantiomers having non-superimposable mirror images of each other

Example:

Lactic acid   1 - chloro, 1-phenyl ethane

Criteria for enantiomerism: Two conditions are essential for being enantiomer.

1. Asymmetric carbon atom
2. Dissymetricness

Out of these two, if any one is absent then compound does not show the enantiomerism.

Exceptional example: Meso tartaric acid.

- It has asymmetric 'c' atom but does not possess dissymetricness. So it is not showing enantiomerism.

Properties of enantiomers:

1. They have same physical and chemical properties, e.g. melting point, boiling point, refractive index, solubility and density.
2. They, however, differ from each other, in the direction in which they rotate the plane polarized light.
3. A mixture of equal amount of two enantiomers is called as racemic mixture. Such mixtures is optically inactive because the two components rotate the plane of plane polarized light equally opposite direction and cancel one another.

Table 4.2: Physical properties of isomers of 2-butanol

Physical property	(R)-2-butanol	(S)-2-butanol
Boiling point (1 atm)	99.5°C	99.5°C
Density (g mL^{-1} at 20°C)	0.808	0.808
Index of refraction (20°C)	1.397	1.397

Diastereomers

- The optical isomers, which are not mirror images of each other is known as diastereomers.
- Here A is mirror image of B and C is mirror image of D. Now compare A with C, they are not mirror images of each other, nor superimpossable, such isomers are called as diastereomers.
- Generally, if molecule contains one asymmetric carbon atom then number of enantiomer can be calculated by following formula

Diastereomers = 2 (n)

- If two asymmetric carbon atoms are there = 2 (2) = 4

Mesomer

A compound which is optically inactive due to plane of symmetry, even it contains two or more asymmetric carbon atoms. Such compounds are not optically active or enantiomer, since they possess one criterion for optical activity but not the other.

1. They have asymmetric carbon atom
2. But does not possess the dissymetricness

Properties:

1. Optically inactive
2. They possess the asymmetric carbon atoms
3. Plane of symmetry

Epimerization

Epimerization is a change in configuration at one chiral center in a compound, which has more than one such center. It leads to the formation of the diastereomers and not enantiomers of the starting material.

COOH
H₃C—C—OH
- - - - - - - - - - - - - Plane of symmetry
H₃C—C—OH
COOH

Meso-tartaric acid

CHO   CHO
H OH   HO H
C   C
H OH   HO H
H OH   H OH
H OH   H OH
HO   HO
D(+) Glucose   Mannose

5

Physico-chemical Properties and Drug Action

The biological response of a drug molecule is elicited with such bodies as receptors, enzymes, membranes or certain small molecules in biological system. The physico-chemical properties and stereochemical features of a drug greatly affect such interaction by influencing the process of drug transport from the site of action. An adequate knowledge of these aspects is necessary for a medicinal chemist.

FERGUSON PRINCIPLE

- Pharmacologically, active compound can be divided into two major groups:
  1. Structurally specific
  2. Structurally non-specific
- Structurally specific drugs bring their effect by combining with specific receptors.
- On the other hand, structurally non-specific drugs do not act on a specific receptor, instead they penetrate the cell or accumulate in cellular membrane, where they interfere by chemical or physical means with some fundamental processes.

  Example
  1. General anesthetic
  2. Hypnotics
  3. Volatile insecticide
  4. Bactericidal agent

- The biological effect of such drug is more closely corelated with physical properties of the molecule than the chemical structure.

| Cyclopropane | Ether | Chloroform |

Principle

Ferguson explains the potency of structurally non-specific drugs. He measured the potency by determining the 'thermodynamic activity' of such drugs.

Thermodynamic Activity

This quantity is measure of the proportion of the molecules, which are free to react with enzyme systems, nerve membrane and similar biological important site.

The molecules which are not free to act in this way are reacting with one another, with the molecule of the solvent or with molecule of other solute. It follows therefore that, the thermodynamic activity of a drug in a solution is not determined entirely by its concentration.

For example, in case of volatile anesthetic administered with air or oxygen, the thermodynamic activity is proportional to the relative saturation of drug and relative saturation can be given by

$$Relative\ saturation\ =\ Pt/Po\ (for\ volatile)$$

Where,

Pt = Partial pressure of the drug in solution or in the gaseous mixture.

Po = Vapour pressure of the pure drug at the same temperature.

$$Relative\ saturation\ =\ St/So\ (for\ non\text{-}volatile)$$

Where,

St = Molar concentration required to produce the biological effect.

So = Molar solubility of the drug.

Ferguson theory predicts that an aesthetic will show the same degree of biological activity, if their concentration are adjusted so that their thermodynamic activities are equal (or relative saturation value are equal).

Table 5.1: Concentration of gases and vapours producing the same degree of anesthesia in mice.

Anesthetic agent	Saturation pressure at 37°C (Ps) (mmHg)	Activity (Pt/Ps)
Nitrous oxide	59,300	0.01
Acetylene	51,700	0.01
Methyl ether	6,100	0.02
Ethylene oxide	5,900	0.01
Ethyl chloride	1,780	0.02
Diethyl ether	830	0.03
Chloroform	324	0.01

Table 5.2: Bactericidal concentration of miscellaneous organic compounds
Salmonella typhosa

Compound	Bacterial concentration (St)	Solubility (So)	Relative saturation (St/So)
Thymol	0.0022	0.0057	0.38
Propaldehyde	1.08	2.88	0.37
Methyl ethyl ketone	1.25	3.13·	0.40
Acetone	3.89	9.7	0.40
Aniline	0.17	0.40	0.44
Cyclohexanol	0.18	0.38	0.47
Butyraldehyde	0.39	0.51	0.76

CLASSIFICATION OF PHYSICO-CHEMICAL PROPERTIES

Classification of physico-chemical properties is given in Flow charts 5.1.

Flow chart 5.1: Classification of physico-chemical properties

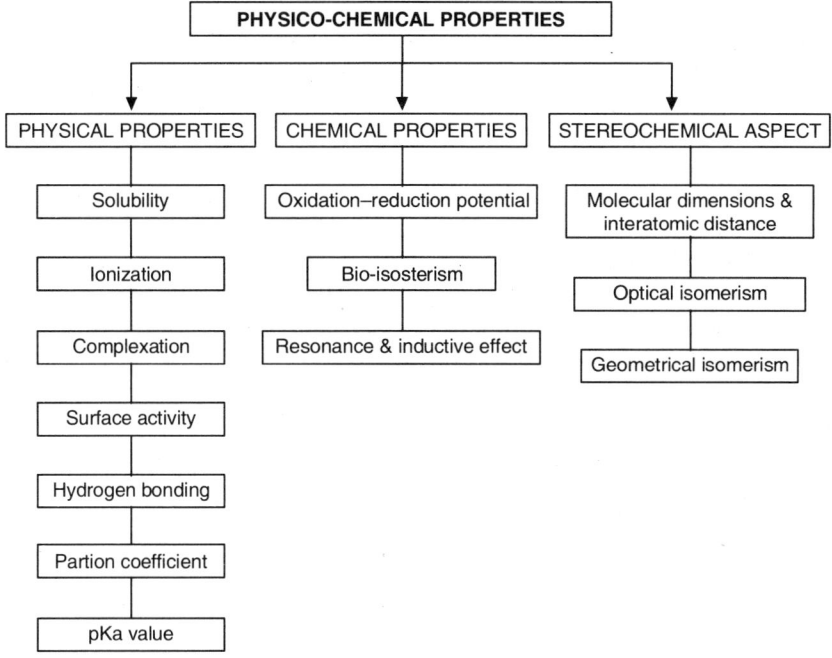

▨ PHYSICAL PROPERTIES

Solubility

- Amount of solid substance that goes into solution per unit time under standard condition of temperature, pH and surface area of solid is called as solubility.
- For making any compound soluble, following forces are involved:
    1. van der Waals force of attraction
    2. Dipole–dipole bonding
    3. Ionic bonding
    4. Hydrogen bonding
- Solubility is important aspect if any drug want to produce its action, since drug have to be dissolve into the biological fluid, then it will penetrate the cell and produce their effect at that site of action.

Methods of improving solubility of drugs

Structural modification:

1. By putting polar groups over the structure, one can enhance the solubility.
2. By modifying the structure of the compound in such a way by which one can increase intermolecular hydrogen bonding and decreasing interamolecular hydrogen bonding.

Use of co-solvent: By adding co-solvents such as propylene glycol, sorbitol and ethanol, one can increase the solubility, since these agents decrease the dielectric constant of the solvent.

Employing surfactant: Surfactants are ampiphilic in nature. At Micelle concentration, they can enhance the solubility of hydrophobic groups since they contain both hydrophilic and lipophilic heads.

Importance of solubility: A drug should be present in solution form before its absorption. Hence for biological effect, solubility is the most important criterion.

Ionization

- Ionized form imparts good water solubility to the drug, which is essential for good binding interaction of drug with its receptor, while non-ionized form helps the drug to cross cell membranes. Hence a good balance of ionized: non-ionized form is essential for better pharmacokinetic and pharmacodynamic features.

- The rate of absorption of a drug which is capable of existing both in ionized and unionized forms is dependent on the concentration of its unionized form, rather than on its total concentration. The unionized form is function of both dissociation constant and pH of environment.

- This can be presented by Henderson-Haselbach equation

$$pH - pKa = \log\left[\frac{[A^-]}{[HA]}\right] \qquad\qquad pH - pKa = \log\left[\frac{[B]}{[HB^+]}\right]$$

| A = Ionised | B = Non-ionised |
| NA = Non-ionised form of acids | HB = Ionised form of base |

Example

1. It can be seen that a solution of weak acid, aspirin (pKa =3.5) in the stomach (pH=1.0) will be more than 99% unionized and since unionized form is lipid soluble, it will get more easily absorbed in the stomach.

2. Quinine having pKa value 8.5 and hence will remain in unionized form in intestine than stomach (Table 5.3).

Table 5.3: pKa values of some drugs

Acids	pKa value
Salicylic acid	3
Aspirin	3
Benzoic acid	4
Sulphadiazine	7

Importance

This provides idea about the site, where drug will absorbed

1. Weak acids........absorbed in stomach.
2. Weak base........absorbed in intestine.

Complexation

- Since complex of drug molecule cannot cross the natural membrane barrier, they render the drug biologically ineffective. The rate of absorption is therefore proportional to the concentration of the free molecule.

- Due to the reversibility of the complexation, they always exist in equilibrium between the free drug and drug complex. Such equilibrium is presented by,

$$\text{Drug + Complexing agent} \rightleftharpoons \text{Drug complex}$$

- Complexation reduces the rate of absorption of the drug but does not affect the total availability of it, because the absorption of the free drug molecule shift the equilibrium to the right, causing the free molecule to released from drug-complex.

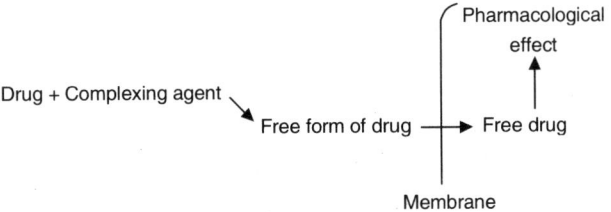

Example

Tetracycline absorption decreases, if taken with calcium, because tetracycline chelate with Ca^{2+}, which is present in milk.

Importance

1. Penicillamine is an effective anti-dote for the treatment of copper poisoning because it forms water soluble chelate with copper and other metal ions.
2. 8-hydroxyquinoline is acting as antimicrobial and antifungal agents by complexing with iron or copper.

Surface Activity

A surfactant is briefly defined as a material that can greatly reduce the surface tension. Surfactants consist of the two portions:

1. Hydrophilic part
2. Hydrophobic part

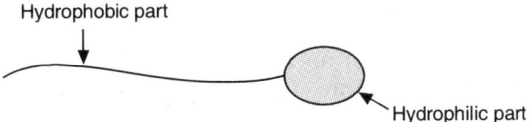

It is evident that in lower concentration the surfactant enhances the rate and at higher concentration reduces the rate. In lower concentration, the surfactants reduce the surface tension and bring about better absorption through better contact of the molecule with the absorbing membrane. But when the concentration crosses the critical micelle concentration (CMC), the surfactant molecules in the bulk of the solution form colloidal aggregate known as Micelle, entrap the molecule in their hydrophobic core, resulting in retardation of absorption.

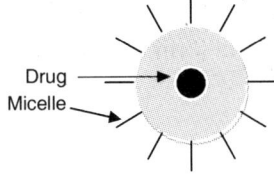

Example

Bile salt solution of approximately physiological concentration greatly enhances the dissolution rate of poorly water-soluble drug like griseofulvin by virtue of solubilization.

Hydrogen Bonding

Atoms which are capable of forming H-bonds are electronegative atoms, these include F, Cl, N, O and S.

Types of hydrogen bonding

1. **Intermolecular H-bonding:** Such kind of hydrogen bonding occurs between two or more than two molecules of the same compound.

$$H—O\cdots H—O\cdots H—O$$
$$\underset{H}{|}\qquad\underset{H}{|}\qquad\underset{H}{|}$$

Hydrogen bonding in water.

2. **Intramolecular H-bonding:** In this type, Hydrogen bonding occurs within two atoms of the same molecule.

Hydrogen bonding in
O-chlorophenol

Importance

1. 1-phenyl 3-methyl-5-pyrazolone shows no analgesic properties, while 1-phenyl-2,3 dimethyl-5-pyrazolone (antipyrine) is a well-known analgesic agent.

Intermolecular H-bonding of 1-phenyl 3-methyl 5-pyrazolone

2. This effect appears to be best explained by the fact that first compound through intermolecular H-bonding forms a linear polymer.

3. On the other hand, antipyrine cannot form H-bonding and has only comparatively weak attraction force between its molecules hence can cross the CNS, producing analgesia.

1 phenyl-2,3-demethyl-5-pyraxolone

4. Salicylic acid has a quite on appreciable antibacterial activity but the paraisomer p-hydroxybenzoic acid is inactive because salicylic acid is orthoisomer that can form intermolecular H-bonding.

Intramolecular
hydrogen bonding

While p-isomer forms intermolecular H-bonding

5. Intermolecular H-bonding of p-isomer enhances water solubility but decreases lipid solubility and vice versa for salicylic acid. Because of lower partition coefficient, p-isomer has low antibacterial activity.

Partition Coefficient

The ratio of concentration of drug in lipid phase to the aqueous phase is known as partition coefficient.

$$\text{Partition coefficient} = \frac{[\text{Drug}]\,\text{lipid}}{[\text{Drug}]\,\text{aqueous}}$$

Measurement of partition coefficient

In vitro, it can be measured using 1-octanol as the lipid phase and phosphate buffer of pH 7.4 as aqueous phase.

Importance

Partition coefficient thoroughly influences drug transport characteristic. Since the blood distributes drug, it must penetrate and travel many cells to reach the site of action. Hence a partition coefficient will determine to which tissue a given compound can reach.

Table 5.4: Partition coefficient of some compounds

Compound	Partition coefficient
Ethanol	0.03
Morphine	0.40
Barbitone	1.40
Phenobarbitone	5.90

Barbiton and phenobarbiton is having higher partition coefficient so that they can cross the CNS.

pKa Value (Dissociation Coefficient)

- The amount of drug that exists in unionized form is a function of dissociation constant (pKa) of the drug and pH of the fluids at the absorption site.
- Lower the pKa of an acidic drug stronger the acid.
- Higher the pKa value of basic drug stronger the base.
- Thus from the knowledge of pKa of drug and pH of the absorption site, we can determine about the percentage of drug, which remain in ionized and non-ionized form.

This pKa can be calculated as follows.

For weak acids

$$\text{pH} = \text{pKa} + \log\frac{[\text{Ionized drug}]}{[\text{Unionized drug}]}$$

For weak bases

$$\text{pH} = \text{pKa} + \log\frac{[\text{Unionized drug}]}{[\text{Ionized drug}]}$$

Importance

1. **Weak acids:** Drugs having pKa 2.5 to 7.5 can be better absorbed from stomach because in acidic condition of stomach maximum drug will be in non-ionized form.
2. **Stronger acid:** pKa < 2.5 ionized in the entire pH of the GIT and therefore poorly absorbed.
3. **Weak bases:** pKa 5 to 11 absorbed in intestine because of basic pH of intestine.
4. **Stronger bases:** pKa > 11 not absorbed because of ionization throughout the GIT.

▨ CHEMICAL PROPERTIES

Oxidation–Reduction Potential

- The tendency of a compound to give or to receive electrons is measured quantitatively by its oxidation–reduction potential or redox potential.
- Since the oxidation–reduction potential applies to a single reversible ionic equilibrium in living organism, the correlation between redox potential and biological activity can only be drawn for the compounds of very similar structure and physical properties.

Importance

1. The optimum bacteriostatic activity in quinines is associated with the redox potential at +0.003 volt, when tested against *Staphylococcus aureus*.
2. The biological activity of riboflavin is due to its ability to accept electrons and is reduced to the dihydro form. This reaction has a potential of E_0 = -0.185 volt. By retaining most of the structural features and altering its redox potential, one may develop compounds antagonistic to riboflavin. Kuhn prepared the analogue in which the two methyl groups of riboflavin were replaced by chlorine and having a potential of E_0 = –0.095 volt. Its antagonistic properties are due to the dichloro-dihydro form being a weaker reducing agent than the dihydro form of riboflavin. It may be absorbed at specific receptor sites but not have a negative enough potential to carry out the biological reduction of riboflavin.

Riboflavin E_0 = –0.185   Riboflavin analogue E_0 = –0.095

3. The optimum anti-helmintic activity in a series of substituted phenothiazine is associated with the Em potential of 0.583 volt (acetic acid-water) which could lead to maximal formation of semiquinone ion (a radical ion) at physiologic pH. (against mixed infestation of *Syphacia obvelata* and *Aspiruculurus tetreptera* in mice). The semiquinone facilitates an essential biological electron transfer reaction, producing a toxic or paralyzing effect.
4. The necessity of free 3 or 7 positions in the phenothiazine nucleus for significant anti-helmintic activity and the inactivity of phenothiazine tranquilizing drugs (2-substituted 10 – dimethyl aminopropyl phenothiazine) is only due to the difficulty of correlating redox potential and activity.

Bio-isosterism (for detail study refer chapter 2)

- In SAR studies and drug design, it is always necessary to compare the formal and three-dimensional structures with the substituent and functional groups of compounds that show a similar spectrum of biological activities. In most instances, one may find similarities in molecular shape and overall chemical function and will base one's explanation of biological similarities on this resemblance. This total complex of analogies that comprises steric, electronic and molecular orbital comparison is called bio-isosterism.

- Bio-isosteric replacement is the principal guide followed by medicinal chemist in developing analogues of the 'lead" compound, whether as agonists or antagonists of biological effects. The parameters being changed are molecular size, steric shape, bond angles, hybridization, electron distribution, lipid solubility, water solubility, pKa the chemical reactivity to cell components, metabolizing enzymes and the capacity to undergo H-bonding (receptor interaction).

- In order to develop a new drug, the structure of the drug is considered to consist of two parts, i.e. critical and non-critical parts.

Critical parts

Any change in this part results in decreased in activity.

Non-critical

The non-critical part allows sufficient changes without considerable changes in the biological activity. The various molecular modifications done on this non-critical part are classified as follows.

Selectophores: Those modifications which confirm selectivity in action of the drug by regulating drug distribution.

Contactophores: The modification which by increasing penetration, helps the drug to reach the receptor site.

Carrier moieties: These moieties increase affinity of a drug. Thus non-critical part of a drug molecule is not involved in drug–receptor interaction but is involved in passive transport of the drug. While any change or modification of critical part of the drug molecule will result in the change of its biological activity, only those groups having similar steric, electronic and solubility characteristic can be interchanged. The study of such groups (bio-isosteres) and their applications in medicinal chemistry is known as Bio-isosterism.

Importance

1. An important compound of catecholamine series is phenylephrine.
2. An alkylsulphonamido group may be substituted for the phenolic hydroxyl group. Some of the resulting compounds have agonist activity whereas others are antagonist.

Phenylephrine

3. While a classical example of rings versus non-cyclic structure is diethylstilbestrol and estradiol.

Diethylstilbestrol   Estradiol

4. Diethylstilbestrol has about the same potency as the naturally occurring estradiol. The central double bond of diethylstilbestrol is highly important for the correct orientation of the phenolic and ethyl groups at the receptor site.

Resonance and Inductive Effects

- Resonance is define as delocalization of π electrons. In other words, the phenomenon in which two or more structures can be written for a compound which involve identical position of atom is called 'resonance'.
- Electron density and electron displacement pattern help to explain a drug reactivity and they also have interference on physicochemical property such as acidity.
- Similarly, inductive effects are readily transmitted through conjugation. This involves delocalization of the σ bond due to the difference in electronegativity, it results in polarity.

Procaine

- The local anesthetic effects of procaine is due to hybrid structure, where a carbonyl function is partially ionic, i.e. the drug should be both in ionized and unionized form. It confirms that the amino group, which has the tendency to displace electron and thereby providing an ionized carbonyl group which is necessary for activity.

▮ STEREOCHEMICAL ASPECT

Molecular Dimensions and Interatomic Distance

- Most of the receptors that interact with drug and produce drug reaction are proteinaceous in nature and are made up of several amino acids which are joint together by peptide bonds. The distance between two consecutive peptide bonds is about 3.6 Å units and the distance between two consecutive turns of coil is about 5.5 Å units.

Carbachol

Diphenhydramie

- Therefore the drugs which have functional groups believe to involve in receptor binding must have the same distances as that of peptide bonds as in multiple of those distances.

Optical Isomerism (given in detail see Chapter 4)

Optical isomers differ from each other in their ability to rotate the plane of polarized light. Dextro-rotatory means, which rotate the plane polarized light to right direction (clockwise) while which rotate to left side chain is called as levo-rotatory.

D-glucose   L-glucose

Importance

- Because of different isomer, it may be possible that one isomer may be more active than other or other may be having any other activity.

- In case of epinephrine, only levo form is active as compared to dextro because of proper orientation of the hydroxyl group of the levo epinephrine over the receptors (Fig. 5.1).

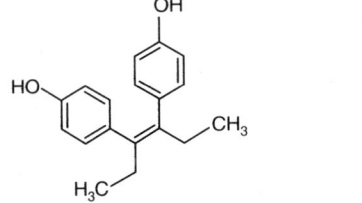

Fig. 5.1: Proper orientation of levo epinephrine over receptor

- In case of amphetamine, levo amphetamine is having sympathomimetic activity while dextro amphetamine is having CNS stimulation.

Geometrical Isomerism (given in detail see Chapter 4)

- These are compounds which differ from each other in arrangement of atoms or groups around the double bond.
- This is further classified according to the arrangement of atoms.

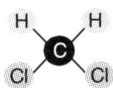 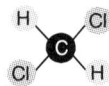

cis isomer   trans isomer

Cis-form: Cis isomers are those in which two similar groups are on the same side chain.

Trans-form: Trans isomers are those in which two similar groups are on opposite side.

Importance

1. In case of diethylstilbestrol, trans form is 14 times more active than cis.

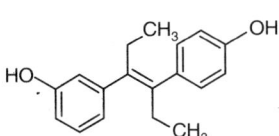

Cis diethylstilbestrol   Trans diethylstilbestrol

2. In the same way, clomiphen is having more anti-estrogenic activity as compared to the tomoxifen.

6

Quantitative Structure–Activity Relationship (QSAR)

We studied the various strategies which can be used in the design of drugs. Several of these strategies involved a changed shape such that the new drug had a better 'fit 'for its receptor. Other strategies involved a change in the physical properties of the drug such that its distribution, metabolism or receptor binding interactions were affected.

- These latter strategies often involved the synthesis of analogues containing arrangement of substituents on aromatic/heteroaromatic rings or accessible functional groups.
- There are an infinite number of possible analogues which can be made, if we were to try and synthesize analogues with every substituent and combination of sub-segments possible. Therefore, it is clearly advantageous, if a rational approach can be followed in deciding which substituents to use. The QSAR (quantitative structure–activity relationship) approach has proved extremely useful in tackling this problem.
- The QSAR approach attempts to identify and quantify the physicochemical properties of a drug and to see whether any of these properties has an effect on the drug's biological activity. If such a relationship holds true, an equation can be drawn up which quantifies the relationship and allows the medicinal chemist to say with some confidence that the property (or properties) has an important role in the distribution or mechanism of the drug.
- It also allows the medicinal chemist some level of prediction. By quantifying physicochemical properties, it should be possible to calculate in advance what the biological activity of a novel analogue might be.
- There are two advantages to this. Firstly, it allows the medicinal chemist to target efforts on analogues which should have improved activity and thus cut down the number of analogues which have to be made. Secondly, if an analogue is discovered which does not in the equation, it implies that some other feature is important and provides a lead for further development.
- What are these physicochemical features which we have mentioned? Essentially, they refer to any structural, physical, or chemical property of a drug. Clearly, any drug will have a large number of such properties and it would be a herculean task to quantify and relate them all to biological activity at the same time.
- A simple, more practical approach is to consider one or two physicochemical properties of the drug and to vary these while attempting to keep other properties constant. This is not as simple as it sounds, since it is not always possible to vary one property without affecting another. Nevertheless, there have been numerous examples where the approach has worked.

▨ GRAPHS AND EQUATIONS

- In the simplest situation, a range of compounds are synthesized in order to vary one physico-chemical property (e.g. log P) and to test how this affects the biological activity (log 1/C) (we will come to the meaning of log 1/C and log P in due course).

- A graph is then drawn to plot the biological activity on the y axis versus the physicochemical feature on the x axis (Fig. 6.1).

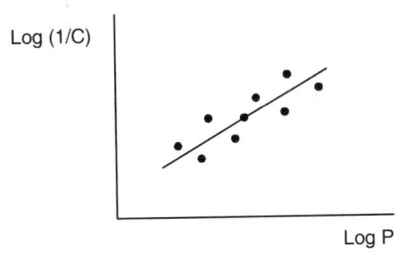

Fig. 6.1: Biological activity versus physico-chemical property

- It is then necessary to draw the best possible line through the data points on the graph. This is done by a procedure known as linear regression analysis by the first squares method'. This is quite a mouthful and can produce a glazed expression on any chemist who is not mathematically orientated. In fact, the principle is quite straight forward.
- If we draw a line through a set of data points, most of the points will be scattered on either side of the line. The best line will be the one closest to the data points. To measure how close the data points are, vertical lines are drawn from each point. These verticals are measured and then squared in order to eliminate the negative values. The squares are then added up to give a total. The best line through the points will be the line where this total is a minimum.
- The equation of the straight line will be $y = k_1x + k_2$ where k_1 and k_2 are constants.

  By varying k_1 and k_2, different equations are obtained until the best line is obtained.

  This whole process can be speedily done by computer programme (Fig. 6.2).

- The next stage in the process is to see whether the relationship is significant. We may have obtained a straight line through points which is so random that it means nothing. The significance of the equation is given by a term known as the regression coefficient (r). This coefficient can again be calculated by computer. For a perfect fit, $r^2 = 1$. Good fits generally have r^2 values of 0.95 or above.

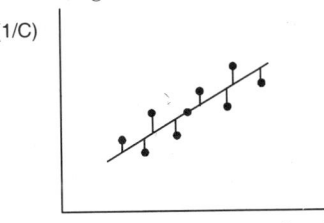

Fig. 6.2: Proximity of data points to line of best it

PHYSICO-CHEMICAL PROPERTIES

- There are many physical, structural, and chemical properties which have been studied by the QSAR approach but the most commonly studied are hydrophobic, electronic, and steric. This is because it is possible to quantify these effects relatively easily.
- In particular, hydrophobic properties can be easily quantized for complete molecules or for individual substituents. On the other hand electronic and steric properties are more difficult to quantify, and quantification is only really feasible for individual substituents.
- Consequently, QSAR studies on a variety of totally different structures are relatively rare and are limited to studies on hydrophobicity. It is more common to QSAR studies being carried out on compounds of the same general structure, where substituents on aromatic rings or accessible functional groups are varied. The QSAR study then considers how the hydrophobic, electronic and steric properties of the substituents affect biological activity.
- The three most studied physicochemical properties will now be considered in some detail.

Hydrophobicity

- The hydrophobic character of a drug is crucial to how easily it crosses cell membranes and may also be important in receptor interactions.
- Changing substituents on a drug may well have significant effects on its hydrophobic character and hence its biological activity. Therefore, it is important to have a means of predicting this quantitatively.

The partition coefficient

- The hydrophobic character of a drug can be measured experimentally by testing the drug's relative distribution in an octanol/water mixture.
- Hydrophobic molecules will prefer to dissolve in the octanol layer of this two-phase system, whereas hydrophilic molecules will prefer the aqueous layer. The relative distribution is known as the partition coefficient (r) and is obtained from the following equation:

$$P = \frac{\text{Concentration of drug in octanol}}{\text{Concentration of drug in aqueous solution}}$$

- Hydrophobic compounds will have a high P value, whereas hydrophilic compounds will have a low P value.
- Varying substituents on the lead compound will produce a series of analogues having different hydrophobicities and therefore different P values. By plotting these P values against the biological activity of these drugs, it is possible to see if there is any relationship between the two properties. The biological activity is normally expressed as $1/C$, where C is the concentration of drug required to achieve a defined level of biological activity (The reciprocal of the concentration ($1/C$) is used, since more active drugs will achieve a defined biological activity at lower concentration.).
- The graph is drawn by plotting $\log (1/C)$ versus log. The scale of numbers involved in measuring C and P usually covers several factors of ten and so the use of logarithms allows the use of more manageable numbers.
- In studies where the range of the log values is restricted to a small range (e.g. $\log P = 1$–4), a straight-line graph is obtained showing that there is a relationship between hydrophobicity and biological activity. Such a line would have the following equation:

$$\log \left(\frac{1}{C} \right) = k_1 \log P + k_2$$

For example, the binding of drugs to serum albumin is determined by their hydrophobicity and a study of 40 compounds resulted in the following equation:

$$\log \left(\frac{1}{C} \right) = 0.75 \log P + 2.30$$

- The equation shows that serum albumin binding increases as log P increases. In other words, hydrophobic drugs bind more strongly to serum albumin than hydrophilic drugs. Knowing how strongly a drug binds to serum albumin can be important in estimating effective dose levels for that drug. When bound to serum albumin, the drug cannot bind to its receptor and so the dose levels for the drug should be based on the amount of unbound drug present in the circulation.

- The equation above allows us to calculate how strongly drugs of similar structure will bind to serum albumin and gives an indication of how 'available' they will be for receptor interactions.
- Despite such factors as serum albumin binding, it is generally found that increasing the hydrophobicity of lead compound results in an increase in biological activity.
- This reflects the fact that drugs have to cross hydrophobic barriers such as cell membranes in order to reach their target. Even if no barriers are to be crossed (e.g. in vitro studies), the drug has to interact with a target system such as an enzyme or receptor where the binding site is usually hydrophobic. Therefore, increasing hydrophobicity aids the drug in crossing hydrophobic barriers or in binding to its target site.
- This might imply that increasing log P should increase the biological activity *ad infinitum*. In fact, this does not happen. There are several reasons for this. For example, the drug may become so hydrophobic that it is poorly soluble in the aqueous phase. Alternatively, it may be trapped in fat depots and never reach the intended site. Finally, hydrophobic drugs are often more susceptible to metabolism and subsequent elimination.
- A straight-line relationship between log P and biological activity is observed in many QSAR studies because the range of log P values studied is often relatively narrow. For example, the study carried out on serum albumin binding was restricted to compounds having log P values in the range 0.78 to 3.82.
- If these studies were to be extended to include compounds with very high log P values then we would see a different picture. The graph would be parabolic. Here, in (1/C) the biological activity increases as log P increases until a maximum value is obtained. The value of log P at the maximum (log P^0) represents the optimum coefficient for biological activity. Beyond that point, an increase in log P results in a decrease in biological activity (Fig. 6.3).

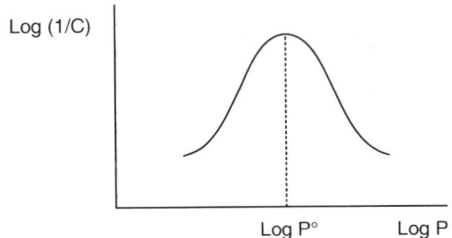

Fig. 6.3: Parabolic log (1/2) vs. log P curve

- In situations where the partition coefficient is the only factor influencing biological activity, the parabolic curve can be expressed by the mathematical equation:

$$\log\left(\frac{1}{C}\right) = -k_1(\log P)^2 + k_2 \log P + k_3$$

- Note that the $(\log P)^2$ term has a negative sign in front of it. When P is small, the $(\log P)^2$ term is very small and the equation is dominated by the log P term. This represents the first part of the graph where activity increases with increasing P.
- When P is large, the $(\log P)^2$ term is more significant and eventually 'overhelms' the log P term. This represents the last part of the graph where activity drops with increasing P. k_1, k_2, and k_3 are constants and can be determined by a suitable computer programme.

- There are relatively few drugs where activity is related to the log P factor alone. Those that do, tend to operate in cell membranes where hydrophobicity is the dominant feature controlling their action. The best examples of drugs which operate in cell membranes are the general anesthetics. These are thought to function by entering the central nervous system and dissolving into cell membranes where they affect membrane structure and nerve function. In such a scenario, there are no special drug–receptor interactions and the mechanism of the drug is controlled purely by its ability to enter cell membranes (i.e. its hydrophobic character).

- The general anesthetic activity of a range of ethers was found to at the parabolic equation:

$$\log\left(\frac{1}{C}\right) = -0.22\,(\log P)^2 + 1.04\,\log P + 2.16$$

- According to the equation, anesthetic activity increases with increasing hydrophobicity (P) as determined by the log P factor. The negative $(\log P)^2$ factor shows that the relationship, township is parabolic and that there is an optimum value for log P ($\log P^0$) beyond which increasing hydrophobicity causes a decrease in anesthetic activity.

- With this equation, it is now possible to predict the anesthetic activity of other ether structures, given their partition coefficients.

- There are limitations to the use of this particular equation. For example, it is derived purely for anesthetic ethers and is not applicable to other structural types of anesthetic. This is generally true in QSAR studies. The procedure works best, if it is applied to a series of compounds which have the same general structure.

- QSAR studies have been carried out on other structural types of general anesthetic and in each case a parabolic curve has been obtained. Although, the constants for each equation are different, it is significant that the optimum hydrophobicity (represented by $\log P^0$) for anesthetic activity is close to 2.3, regardless of the class of anesthetic being studied. This finding suggests that all general anesthetic are operating in a similar fashion, controlled by the hydrophobicity of the structure.

- Since different anesthetics have similar $\log P^0$ values, the log P value of any compound can give some idea of its potential potency as an anesthetic. For example, the log P values of the gaseous anesthetic ether, chloroform, and halothane are 0.98, 1.97, and 2.3 respectively. Their anesthetic activity increases in the same order.

- Since general anesthetics have a simple mechanism of action based on the deficiency with which they enter the central nervous system (CNS). It implies that log P values should give an indication of how easily any compound can enter the CNS.

- In other words, compounds having a log P value close to 2 should be capable of entering the CNS efficiently.

- This is generally found to be true, e.g., the most potent barbiturates for sedative and hypnotic activity are found to have log P values close to 2.

- As a rule of thumb, drugs which are to be targeted for the CNS should have a log P value of approximately 2. Conversely, drugs which are designed to act elsewhere in the body should have log P values significantly different from 2 in order to avoid possible CNS side-effects (e.g. drowsiness).

- As an example of this, the cardiologic agent shown in figure was found to produce 'bright visions' in some patients, which implied that it was entering the CNS.

a) R=OMe
b) R=S(O)Me Sulmazole

Cardiotonic agents

- This was supported by the fact that the log P value of the drug was 2.59. In order to prevent the drug entering the CNS, the 4-OMe group was replaced with a 4-S (O) Me group. This particular group is approximately the same size as the methods group, but more hydrophilic. The log P value of the new drug (sulmazole) was found to be 1.17. The drug was now too hydrophilic to enter the CNS and was free of CNS side effects.

The Substituent Hydrophobicity Constant (π)

- We have seen how the hydrophobicity of a compound can be quantized by using the partition coefficient P. However, in order to get P, we have to measure it experimentally and that means that we have to synthesize the compounds.
- It would be much better, if we could calculate P theoretically and decide in advance whether the compound is worth synthesizing. QSAR would then allow us to target the most promising looking structures. For example, if we were planning to synthesize a range of barbiturate structures, we could calculate log P values for them all and concentrate on the structure had log P values closest to the optimum log P^0 value for barbiturates.
- Fortunately, partition coefficients can be calculated by knowing the contribution that various substituents make to hydrophobicity. This contribution is known as the substituent hydrophobicity constant (π).
- The substituent hydrophobicity constant is a measure of how hydrophobic a substituent is, relative to hydrogen. The value can be obtained as follows. Partition coefficients are measured experimentally for a standard compound with and without a substituent (X). The hydrophobicity constant (π_X) for the substituent (X) is then obtained using the following equation:

$$\pi_X = \log P_X - \log P_H$$

- Where P_H is the partition coefficient for the standard compound, and P_x is the partition coefficient for the standard compound with the substituent.
- A positive value of π indicates that the substituent is more hydrophobic than hydrogen. A negative value indicates that the substituent is less hydrophobic. The π values for a range of substituents are shown in Table 6.1.

Table 6.1: π values for a range of substituents

Group	CH_3	But	OH	OCH_3	CF_3	Cl	Br	F
p (aliphatic substituents)	0.50	1.68	−1.16	0.47	1.07	0.39	0.60	−0.17
p (aromatic substituents)	0.52	1.68	−0.67	−0.02	1.16	0.71	0.86	0.14

- These π values are characteristic for the substituent and can be used to calculate how the partition coefficient of a drug would be affected by adding these substituents. The P value for the lead compound would have to be measured experimentally, but once that is known, the P value for analogues can be calculated quite simply.
- As an example, consider the log P values for benzene (log P = 2.13), chlorobenzene (log P = 2.84), and benzamide (log P = 0.64). Since benzene is the parent compound, the substituent constants for C1 and $CONH_2$ are 0.71 and −1.49, respectively. Having obtained these values, it is now possible to calculate the theoretical log P value for meta-chlorobenzamide

$$\begin{aligned} \log P_{(chlorobenzamide)} &= \log P_{(benzene)} + \pi_{Cl} + \pi_{CONH_2} \\ &= 2.13 + 0.71 + (-1.49) \\ &= 1.35 \end{aligned}$$

- The observed log P value for this compound is 1.51.
- It should be noted that π values for aromatic substituents are different from those used for aliphatic substituents. Furthermore, neither of these sets of π values are in fact true constants and are accurate only for the structures from which they were derived. They can be used as good approximations when studying other structures, but it is possible that the values will have to be adjusted in order to get accurate results.

Benzene
(Log P = 2.13)

Chlorobenzene
(Log P = 2.84)

Benzamide
(Log P = 0.64)

Metachlorobenzamide

P vs π

- QSAR equations relating biological activity to the partition coefficient P have already been described, but there is no reason why the substituent hydrophobicity constant π cannot be used in place of P, if only the substituents are being varied.
- The equation obtained would be just as relevant as a study of how hydrophobicity affects biological activity. That is not to say that P and π are exactly equivalent— different equations would be obtained with different constants.
- Apart from the fact that the constants would be different, the two factors have different emphases. The partition coefficient P is a measure of the drug's overall hydrophobicity and is therefore an important measure of how efficiently a drug is transported to its target site and bound to its receptor. The π factor measures the hydrophobicity of a special region on the drug's skeleton. Thus, any hydrophobic bonding to a receptor involving that region will be more significant to the equation than the overall transport process. If the substituent is involved in hydrophobic bonding to a receptor, then the QSAR equation using the A factor will emphasize that contribution to biological activity more dramatically than the equation using P.
- Most QSAR equations will have a contribution from P or from π or from both. However, there are examples of drugs which have only a slight contribution, e.g. a study on antimalarial drugs showed very little relationship between antimalarial activity and hydrophobic character. This finding lends support to the theory that these drugs are acting in red blood cells, since previous research has shown that the ease with which drugs enter red blood cells is not related to their hydrophobicity.

Electronic Effect

- The electronic effects of various substituents will clearly have an effect on a drug's ionization or polarity. This in turn may have an effect on how easily a drug can pass through cell membranes or how strongly it can bind to a receptor. It is therefore useful to have some measure of the electronic effect a substituent can have on a molecule.
- As far as substituents on an aromatic ring are concerned, the measure used is known as the Hammett substitution constant which is given the symbol σ.
- The Hammett substitution constant (σ) is a measure of the electron withdrawing or electron donating ability of a substituent and has been determined by measuring the dissociation of a series of substituted benzoic acids compared to the dissociation of benzoic acid itself.

- Benzoic acid is a weak acid and only partially ionizes in water.

Ionization of benzoic acid.

- An equilibrium is set up between the ionized and non-ionized forms, where the relative proportion of these species is known as the equilibrium or dissociation constant K_H. (The subscript H signals that there are no substituents on the aromatic ring).

$$K_H = \frac{[PhCO_2^-]}{[PhCO_2H]}$$

- When a substituent is present on the aromatic ring, this equilibrium is affected. Electron withdrawing groups, such as a nitro group, result in the aromatic ring having a stronger electron withdrawing and stabilizing influence on the carboxylate anion.
- The equilibrium will therefore shift more to the ionized form such that the substituted benzoic acid is a stronger acid and has a larger K_X value (X represents the substituent on the aromatic ring).
- If the substituent X is an electron donating group such as an alkyl group, then the aromatic ring is less able to stabilize the carboxylate ion. The equilibrium shifts to the left and a weaker acid is obtained with a smaller K_X value
- The Hammett substituent constant (π_X) for a particular substituent (X) is defined by the following equation:

$$\sigma_X = \log \frac{K_X}{K_H} = \log K_X - \log K_H$$

- Benzoic acids containing electron withdrawing substituents will have larger K_X values than benzoic acid itself K_H and therefore the value of π_X for an electron withdrawing substituent will be positive. Substituents such as C1, CN can have positive σ values.

Electron withdrawing group

Electron withdrawing group

- Benzoic acids containing electron donating substituents will have smaller K_X values than benzoic acid itself and hence the value of σ_X for an electron donating substituent will be negative. Substituents such as Me, Et, and Bu have negative or positive values. The Hammett substituent constant for H will be zero.
- The Hammett constant takes into accounts both resonance and inductive effects. Therefore, the value of π for a particular substituent will depend on whether the substituent is meta or para. This is indicated by the subscript m or p after the π symbol.
- For example, the nitro substituent has $\pi_p = 0.78$ and $\pi_m = 0.71$. In the meta position, the electron withdrawing power is due to the inductive silence of the substituent, whereas at the para position inductive and resonance both play a part and so the π_p value is greater.

Meta nitro group— electronic influence on R is inductive.

Para nitro group— electronic influence on R is due to inductive and resonance effects.

- For the OH group $\pi_m = 0.12$ while $\pi_p = -0.37$. At the meta position, the influence is inductive and electron withdrawing. At the para position, the electron donating silence due to resonance is more significant than the electron withdrawing silence due to induction.
- Most QSAR studies start off by considering σ and if, there is more than one substituent, the π values are summed. However, as more compounds are synthesized, it is possible to refine or finetune the QSAR equation. As mentioned above, σ is a measure of a substituent's inductive and resonance electronic effects. With more detailed studies, the inductive and resonance effects can be considered separately.

Meta Hydroxyl Group — electric influence on R is inductive

Para hydroxy group—electronic influence on R dominated by esonance effects.

- Tables of constants are available which quantify a substituent's inductive effect (F) and its resonance effect (R). In some cases, it might be found that a substituent's effect on activity is due to F rather than R, and vice versa. It might also be found that a substituent has a more significant effect at a particular position on the ring and this can also be included in the equation.
- There are limitations to the electronic constants which we have described so far, e.g. Hammett substituent constants cannot be measured for ortho substituents since such substituents have an important steric, as well as electronic effect.
- There are very few drugs whose activities are solely silenced by a substituent's electronic effect, since hydrophobicity usually has to be considered as well. Those that do are generally operating by a mechanism whereby they do not have to cross any cell membranes.

Alternatively, in vitro studies on isolated enzymes may result in QSAR equations lacking the hydrophobicity factor, since there are no cell membranes to be considered.

- The insecticidal activity of methyl phenyl phosphates is one of the few examples where activity is related to electronic factors alone:

$$\log\left(\frac{1}{C}\right) = 2.282\sigma - 0.348$$

- The equation reveals that substituents with a positive value for π (i.e. electron withdrawing groups) will increase activity.

- The fact that the π parameter is not significant is a good indication that the drugs do not have to pass into or through a cell membrane to have activity. In fact, these drugs are known to act against an enzyme called acetylcholinesterase which is situated on the outside of cell membranes.

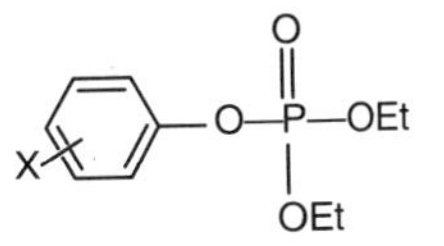

Diethyl phenyl phosphate

- The above constants (π, R, and F) can only be used for aromatic substituents and are therefore only suitable for drugs containing aromatic rings. However, a series of aliphatic electronic substituent constants are available.

- These were obtained by measuring the rates of hydrolysis for a series of aliphatic esters. Methyl ethanoate is the parent ester and it is found that the rate of hydrolysis is affected by the substituent X.

- The extent to which the rate of hydrolysis is affected is a measure of the substituent's electronic effect at the site of reaction (i.e. the ester group). The electronic effect is purely inductive and is given the symbol σ_1. Electron donating groups reduce the rate of hydrolysis and therefore have negative values, e.g. σ_1 values for methyl, ethyl and propyl are –0.04, –0.07, and –0.36, respectively. Electron withdrawing groups increase the rate of hydrolysis and have positive values.

- The σ_1 values for NMe^+_3 and CN are 0.93 and 0.53, respectively.

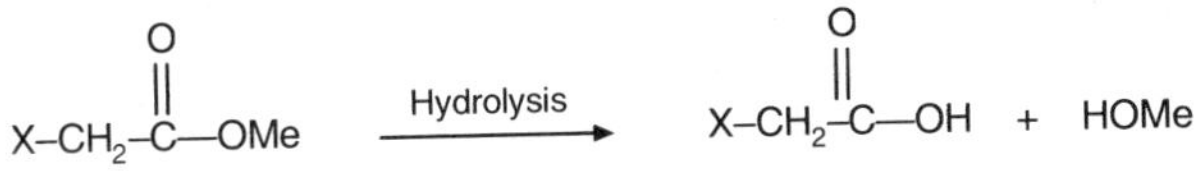

Fig. 6.4: Hydrolysis of an aliphatic ester

- It should be noted that the inductive effect is not the only factor affecting the rate of hydrolysis. The substituent may also have a steric effect, e.g. a bulky substituent may shields the ester from attack and lowers the rate of hydrolysis.

- It is therefore necessary to separate out these two effects. This can be done by measuring hydrolysis rate under basic conditions and also under acidic conditions.

- Under basic conditions, steric and electronic factors are important, whereas under acidic conditions only steric factors are important. By comparing the rates, values for the electronic effect (π_1), and for the steric effect (E_s) (see below) can be determined.

Steric Factors

- In order for a drug to interact with an enzyme or a receptor, it has to approach, then bind to a binding site.

- The bulk, size, and shape of the drug may have an influence on this process, e.g. a bulky substituent may act like a shield and hinder the ideal interaction between drug and receptor.

Alternatively, a bulky substituent may help to orientate a drug properly for maximum receptor binding and increase activity.

- Quantifying steric properties is more difficult than quantifying hydrophobic or electronic properties.

- Several methods have been tried and three are described here. It is highly unlikely that a drug's biological activity will be affected by steric factors alone, but these factors are frequently to be found in Hansch equations.

Taft's factors (E_s)

- Taft's steric factor (E_s); attempts have been made to quantify the steric features of substituents by using Taft's steric factor (E_s).

- The value for E_s can be obtained as described above. However, the number of substituents which can be studied by this method is restricted.

Molar refractivity (MR)

- Molar refractivity (MR); another measure of the steric factor is provided by a parameter known as molar refractivity (MR). This is a measure of the volume occupied by an atom or group of atoms. The molar refractivity is obtained from the following equation:

$$MR = \frac{(n^2 - 1)}{(n^2 + 2)} \times \frac{MW}{d}$$

- Where n is the index of refraction, MW is the molecular weight, and 'd' is the density. The term MW/d defines a volume, while the $(n^2 - 1)/(n^2 + 2)$ term provides a correction factor by defining how easily the substituent can be polarized.

- This is particularly significant, if the substituent has pi electrons or lone pairs of electrons.

Verloop steric parameter

Another approach to measuring the steric factor involves a computer programme called STERIMOL which calculates steric substituent values (Verloop steric parameters) from standard bond argles, van der Waals radii, bond lengths and possible conformations for the substituent. Unlike E_s, the Verloop steric parameter can be measured for any substituent.

Other Physico-chemical Parameters

- The physico-chemical properties most commonly studied by the QSAR approach have been described above, but other properties have also been studied.

- These include dipole moments, hydrogen bonding, conformation, and interatomic distances. However, difficulties in quantifying these properties limit the use of these parameters.

▨ HANSCH EQUATION

- In the above section, we looked at the physico-chemical properties commonly used in QSAR studies and how it is possible to quantify them. In a simple situation where biological activity is related to only one such property, a simple equation can be drawn up.

- However, the biological activity of most drugs is related to a combination of physico-chemical properties. In such cases, simple equations involving only one parameter are relevant only if the other parameters are kept constant. In reality, this is not easy to achieve and equations which relate biological activity to more than one parameter are more common.

- These equations are known as Hansch equations and they usually relate biological activity to the most commonly used physicochemical properties (P and/or π, σ, and a steric factor). If the range of hydrophobicity values is limited to a small range then the equation will be linear as follows:

$$\log\left(\frac{1}{C}\right) = k_1 \log P + k_2 \sigma + k_3 E_s + k_4$$

- If the P values are spread over a large range then the equation will be parabolic for the same reasons described in above section.

$$\log\left(\frac{1}{C}\right) = -k(\log P)^2 + k_2 \log P + k_3 \sigma + k_4 E_s + k_s$$

- The constants k_1–k_5 is determined by computer in order to get the best eating line. Not all the parameters will necessarily be significant, e.g. the adrenergic blocking activity of β-halo-β-aryl amines was related to π and σ and did not include a steric factor:

$$\log\left(\frac{1}{C}\right) = 1.22\pi - 1.59\sigma + 7.89$$

- This equation tells us that biological activity increases, if the substituents have a positive π value and a negative σ value. In other words, the substituents should be hydrophobic and electron donating.
- Since the P value and the π factor are not necessarily correlated, it is possible to have Hansch equations containing both of these factors, e.g. a series of 102 phenanthrene aminocarbinols were tested for antimalarial activity and found to it the following equation:

β-halo-β-aryl amines

Phenanthrene aminocarbinol structure

$$\log\left(\frac{1}{C}\right) = -0.015\,(\log P)^2 + 0.14 \log P + 0.27\Sigma\pi_X + 0.40\Sigma\pi_Y$$
$$+ 0.65\Sigma\sigma_X + 0.88\Sigma\sigma_Y + 2.34$$

- This equation tells us that antimalarial activity increases very slightly as the hydrophobicity of the molecule (P) increases. The constant of 0.14 is low and shows that the increase is slight. The $(\log P)^2$ term shows that there is an optimum P value for average activity.
- The equation also shows that activity increases significantly, if hydrophobic substituents are present on ring X and in particular on ring Y. This could be taken to imply that some forms of hydrophobic interaction are involved at these sites. Electron withdrawing substituents on both rings are also beneficial to activity, more so on ring Y than ring X.
- When carrying out a Hansch analysis, it is important to choose the substituents carefully to ensure that the change in biological activity can be attributed to a particular parameter. There are plenty of traps for the unwary.
- Take, for example, drugs which contain an amine group. One of the most frequently carried out studies on amines is to synthesize analogues containing a homologous series of alkyl substituents on the nitrogen atom (i.e. Me, Et, Prn, Bun).

- If activity increases with the chain length of the substituent, is it due to increasing hydrophobicity or to increasing size or to both? If we look at the σ and MR values of these substituents, both increase in a similar fashion across the series and we would not be able to distinguish between them.

Values for π and MR for a series of substituents

Substituent	H	Me	Et	Prn	Bun	OMe	NHCONH₂	I	CN
p	0.00	0.56	1.02	1.50	2.13	−0.02	−1.30	1.12	−0.57
MR	0.10	0.56	1.03	1.55	1.96	0.79	1.37	1.39	0.63

- In this example, a series of substituents would have to be chosen where π and MR are not related. The substituents H, Me, OMe, NHCOCH₂, I, and CN would be more suitable.

The Craig Plot

Although tables of π and σ factors are readily available for a large range of substituents, it is often easier to visualize the relative properties of different substituents by considering a plot where the y axis is the value of the σ factor and the x axis is the value of the π factor. Such a plot is known as a Craig plot. The example shown in Fig. 6.5.

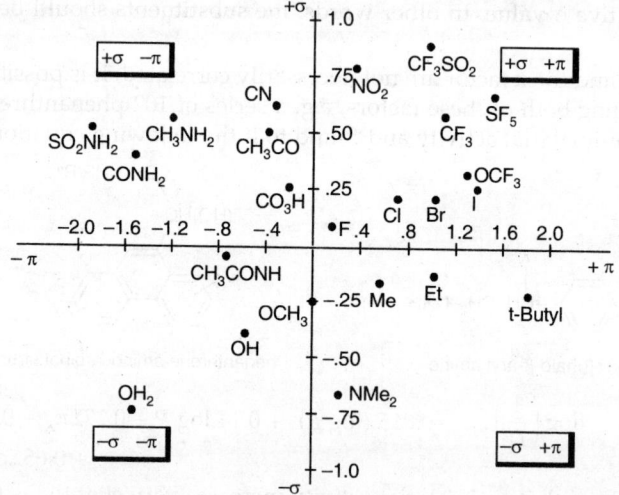

Fig. 6.5: Craig plot

There are several advantages of such a Craig plot.

1. The plot shows clearly that there is no overall relationship between π and σ. The various substituents are scattered around all four quadrants of the plot.

2. It is possible to tell at a glance which substituents have positive π and σ parameters, which substituents have negative π and σ parameters, and which substituents have one positive and one negative parameter.

3. It is easy to see which substituents have similar π values. For example, the ethyl, bromo, trifluromethyl, and trifluoromethylsulfonyl groups are all approximately on the same vertical line on the plot. In theory, these groups could be interchangeable on drugs where the principal factor affecting biological activity is the π factor.

4. Similarly, groups which form a horizontal line can be identified as being isoelectronic or having similar σ values (e.g. CO_2H, Cl, Br, I).

5. The Craig plot is useful in planning which substituents should be used in a QSAR study. In order to derive the most accurate equation involving π and σ, analogues should be synthesized with substituents from each quadrant, e.g. halide substituents are useful representatives of substituents with increased hydrophobicity and electron withdrawing properties (positive π and positive σ), whereas an OH substituent has more hydrophilic and electron donating properties (negative π and negative σ). Alkyl groups are examples of substituents with positive π and negative σ values, whereas acyl groups have negative π and positive σ values.

6. Once the Hansch equation has been derived, it will show whether π or σ should be negative or positive in order to get good biological activity. Further developments would then concentrate on substituents from the relevant quadrant, e.g. if the equation shows that positive π and positive σ values are necessary, then further substituents should only be taken from the top right quadrant.

- Craig plots can also be drawn up to compare other sets of physico-chemical parameters, such as hydrophobicity and MR.

▨ THE TOPLISS SCHEME

- In certain situations, it might not be feasible to make the large range of structures required for a Hansch equation. For example, the synthetic route involved might be difficult and only a few structures can be made in a limited time. In these circumstances, it would be useful to test compounds for biological activity as they are synthesized and to use these results to determine the next analogue to be synthesized.

- A Topliss scheme is a flow diagram' which allows such a procedure to be followed. There are two Topliss schemes, one for aromatic substituents and one for aliphatic side-chain substituents (Fig. 6.6). The schemes were drawn up by considering the hydrophobicity and electronic factors of various substituents and are designed such that the optimum substituent can be found as efficiently as possible.

- However, they are not meant to be a replacement for a full Hansch analysis. Such an analysis would be carried out in due course, once a suitable number of structures have been synthesized.

- The Topliss scheme for aromatic substituents (Fig. 6.7) assumes that the lead compound has been tested for biological activity and contains a monosubstituted aromatic ring. The first analogue in the scheme is the 4-chloro derivative, since this derivative is usually easy to synthesize. The chloro substituent is more hydrophobic and electron withdrawing than hydrogen and therefore, π and σ are positive.

Fig. 6.6: Topliss scheme for aliphatic side chain substituents

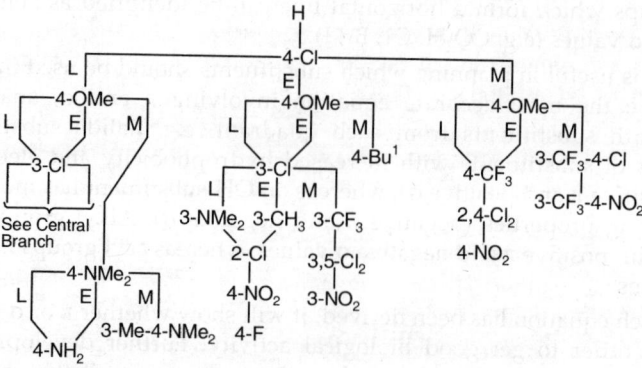

Fig. 6.7: Topliss scheme for aromatic substituents

- Once the chloro analogue has been synthesized, the biological activity is measured. There are three possibilities. The analogue will have less activity (L), equal activity (E), or more activity (M). The type of activity observed will determine which branch of the Topliss scheme is followed next.

- If the biological activity increases, then the (M) branch is followed and the next analogue to be synthesized is the 3,4-dichloro-substituted analogue. If, on the other hand, the activity stays the same, then the (E) branch is followed and the dimethyl analogue is synthesized. Finally, if activity drops, the (L) branch is followed and the next analogue is the 4-methoxy analogue. Biological results from the second analogue now determine the next branch to be followed in the scheme.

What is the Rationale behind this?

- Let us consider the situation where the 4-chloro derivative increases in biological activity. Since the chloro substituent has positive π and σ values, it implies that one or both of these properties are important to biological activity.

- If both are important, then adding a second chloro group should increase biological activity yet further. If it does, substituents are varied to increase the π and σ values even further. If it does not, then an unfavorable steric interaction or excessive hydrophobicity is indicated then test the relative importance of π and steric factors.

- We shall now consider the situation where the 4-chloro analogue drops in activity. This suggests either that negative π and/or σ values are important to activity or that a para substituent is statistically unfavorable. It is assumed that an unfavorable or effect is the most likely reason for the reduced activity and so the next substituent is one with a negative σ factor (i.e. 4-OMe).

- If activity improves, further changes are suggested to test the relative importance of the σ and π factors. If, on the other hand, the 4-OMe group does not improve activity, it is assumed that an unfavorable steric factor is at work and the next substituent is a 3-chloro group. Modifications of this group would then be carried out in the same way.

- The last scenario is where the activity of the 4-chloro analogue is little changed from the lead compound.

- This could arise from the drug requiring a positive π value and a negative σ value. Since both values for the chloro group are positive, the beneficial effect of the positive a value might be cancelled out by the detrimental effects of a positive σ value.

- The next substituent to try in that case is the dimethyl group which has the necessary positive π value and negative σ value. If this still has no sensible effect, then it is assumed that there is an unfavorable steric interaction at the para position and the 3-chloro substituent is chosen next. Further changes continue to vary the relative values of the π and σ factors.
- The validity of the Topliss scheme was tested by looking at structure–activity results for various drugs which had been reported in the literature, e.g. the biological activities of nineteen substituted benzene sulfonamides have been reported. The second most active compound was the nitro-substituted analogue which would have been the fifth compound synthesized, if the Topliss scheme had been followed.
- Another example comes from the anti-inflammatory activities of substituted aryltetrazolylalkanoic acids. Twenty-eight of these were synthesized. Using the Topliss scheme, three out of the four most active structures would have been synthesized from the first eight compounds synthesized.
- The Topliss scheme for aliphatic side-chains was set up following a similar rationale to the aromatic scheme, and is used in the same way for side groups attached to a carbonyl, amino, amide, or similar functional group.
- The scheme only attempts to differentiate between the hydrophobic and electronic effects of substituents and not the steric properties. Thus, the substituents involved have been chosen to try and minimize any steric differences. It is assumed that the lead compound has a methyl group.

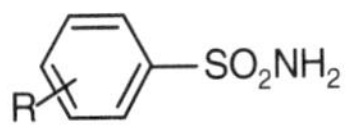

Order of synthesis	R	Biological activity	High potency
1	H	-	
2	4-Cl	M	
3	3,4-Cl$_2$	L	
4	4-Br	E	
5	4-NO$_2$	M	*

R—⟨benzene⟩—SO$_2$NH$_2$

M = More activity
L = Less activity
E = Equal activity

Fig. 6.8: Biological activity of substituted benzene sulfonamides

- The first analogue suggested is the isopropyl analogue. This has an increased σ value and in most cases would be expected to increase activity, since it has been found from experience that the hydrophobicity of most lead compounds are less than the optimum hydrophobicity required for activity.
- Let us concentrate first of all on the situation where activity rises. Following this branch, a cyclopentyl group is now used. A cyclic structure is used since it has a larger σ value, but keeps any increase in steric factor to a minimum.
- If activity rises again, more hydrophobic substituents are tried. If activity does not rise, then there could be two explanations. Either the optimum hydrophobicity has been passed or there is an electronic effect (σ_1) at work. Further substituents are then used to determine which is the correct explanation.
- Let us now look at the situation where the activity of the isopropyl analogue stays much the same. The most likely explanation is that the methyl group and the isopropyl group are on either side of the hydrophobic optimum.

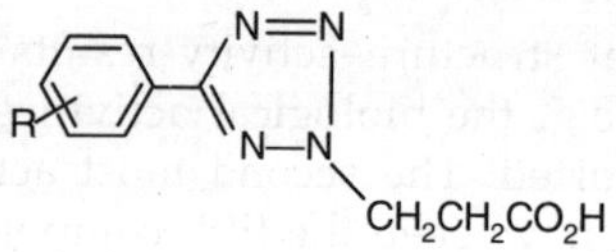

Order of synthesis	R	Biological activity	High potency
1	H	-	
2	4-Cl	L	
3	4-MeO	L	
4	3-Cl	M	*
5	3-CF_3	L	
6	3-Br	M	*
7	3-I	L	*
8	3,5-Cl_2	M	*

M = More activity
L = Less activity
E = Equal activity

Fig. 6.9: Anti-inflammatory activities of substituted aryltetrazolylalkanoic acids

- Therefore, an ethyl group is used next, since it has an intermediate I value. If this does not lead to an improvement, it is possible that there is an unfavorable electronic effect. The groups used have been electron donating, and so electron withdrawing groups with similar σ values are now suggested.

- Finally, we shall look at the case where activity drops for the isopropyl group. In this case, hydrophobic and/or electron donating groups could be bad for activity and the groups suggested are suitable choices for further development.

- The Topliss scheme has proved useful many times, but it will not work in every case, and is not meant to be a replacement for more detailed QSAR studies.

▨ BIOISOSTERES

- Tables of substituent constants are available for various physico-chemical properties. Knowledge of these constants allows the medicinal chemist to identify substituents which may be potential bioisosteres. Thus, the substituents CN, NO_2, and COMe have similar hydrophobic, electronic, and steric factors and might be interchangeable. Such interchangeability was observed in the development of cimetidine. The important thing to notice is that groups can be bioisosteric in some situations, but not others (Fig. 6.10).

Substituent	$\overset{O}{\overset{\|}{-C}}-CH_3$	$\overset{NC}{\underset{}{\searrow}}\overset{CN}{\underset{-C-CH_3}{\swarrow}}$	$\overset{O}{\overset{\|}{-S}}-CH_3$	$\overset{O}{\underset{O}{\overset{\|}{\underset{\|}{-S}}}}-CH_3$	$\overset{O}{\underset{O}{\overset{\|}{\underset{\|}{-S}}}}-NHCH_3$	$\overset{O}{\overset{\|}{-C}}-NMe$
p	−0.55	0.40	−1.58	−1.63	−1.82	−1.51
sp	0.50	0.84	0.49	0.72	0.57	0.36
sm	0.38	0.66	0.52	0.60	0.46	0.35
MR	11.2	21.5	13.7	13.5	16.9	19.2

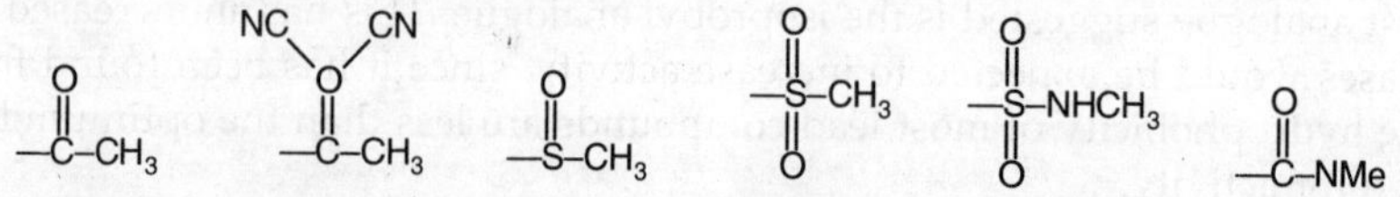

Fig. 6.10: Physico-chemical parameters for 6 substituents

- Figure 6.10 shows some physico-chemical parameters for 6 different substituents. If the most important physico-chemical parameter for biological activity is σp, then the $COCH_3$ group (0.50) would be a reasonable bioisosteres for the $SOCH_3$ group (0.49). If, on the other hand, the dominant parameter is π, then a more suitable bioisosteres for $SOCH_3$ (−1.58) would be SO_2CH_3 (−1.63).

7

Drug Design and Molecular Modeling

Although the phrase computer-aided drug design may seem to imply that drug discovery lies in the hands of the computational scientists who are able to manipulate molecules on their computer screens, the drug designing process is actually a complex and interactive one, involving scientists from many disciplines working together to provide many types of information.

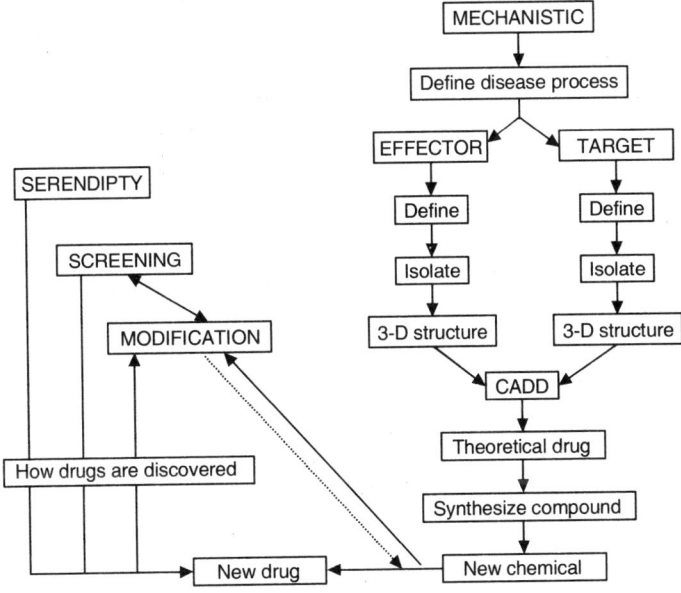

How Drugs are Discovered

- The modern computational and experimental techniques that have been developed in recent years can be used together to provide structural information about the biologically active molecules that are involved in disease processes and in modulating disease processes.

- Occasionally, new drugs are found by accident. More frequently, they are developed as part of an organized effort to discover new ways to treat specific diseases. The discovery of new pharmaceutical agents has gone through an evolution over the years and has been adding new technologies to this increasingly complex process.

SCREENING FOR NEW DRUGS

- The traditional way to discover new drugs has to screen a large number of synthetic chemical compounds or natural products for desirable effects. Although this approach for the development of new pharmaceutical agents has been successful in the past, it is not an ideal one for number of reasons.

- The biggest drawback to the screening process is the requirement for an appropriate screening procedure. Although drugs are ultimately developed in the clinic, it is usually inappropriate to put chemicals of unknown efficacy directly into humans. Initial screens are often *in vitro* tests for some fundamental activity, such as the ability to kill bacteria in solution; however, more applicable *in vivo* screens are needed. This second level of screening is normally carried out using animal model systems for the disease.

- Screens have inherent limitations. Primary screens are used for large numbers of chemicals to choose as which compounds should be further tested with more sophisticated tests. If the primary test does not select for an appropriate activity, an active structure will appear to be inactive and will not be discovered. Secondary screening in animal model systems has additional problems, such as: (1) the animal model may not accurately reflect the human disease; (2) the chemical may be extensively metabolized to a different compound in the animal before it reaches its target; (3) the chemical may not be absorbed or distributed as it is in humans. In each of these cases, the active structure potentially will not be identified.

- Another serious problem with the screening process is its random nature. It is inherently repetitious and time-consuming just to find a chemical entity with the desired activity. Furthermore, chemical compounds discovered by this approach commonly do not have optimal structures for modulating the biological process. This in turn may require administration of larger quantities of the drug and increase the risk of unwanted side effects.

Modification for Improvements

- Once an active (lead) compound has been identified and its chemical structure determined, it is usually possible to improve on this activity and or to reduce side effects by making modifications to the basic chemical structure.

- Modifications to improve performance are often carried out using chemical or bioinformentative means to make changes in the lead structure or its intermediates. Alternatively, for some natural products, the gene itself may be engineered so that the producer organism synthesizes the modified compound directly.

- The process of developing drugs via modification of active lead compounds requires that the structure of the compound be known. One still does not need to know the structure of the target on which the drug works. Likewise, no information about the underlying disease process is required.

- As with screening the process of modification is often based on a primarily trial-and-error approach. Because more information is know, this process can be carried out with much greater probability of success than a purely random process. A prime example of the original first generation cephalosporin has led to second and now third-generation offspring with substantially improved characteristics.

Mechanism-based Drug Design

- As still more information becomes available about the biological basis of a disease, it is possible to begin to design drugs using a mechanistic approach to the disease process. When the disease process is understood at the molecular level and the target molecule (s) are defined, drugs can be designed specifically to interact with the target molecule in such a way as to disrupt the disease.

- Clearly a mechanistic approach to drug design requires a great deal of knowledge. Further processing this knowledge in such a way that a scientist can use the knowledge to develop a new drug. Nonetheless, it is clear that the major breakthrough in drug design in the future are most likely to come via the use of this approach. Because of the massive amount of information that must be harnessed to develop drugs by this technique, it is in this area where computer-aided drug design will have its greatest impact.

Combining Techniques

- In discussing the various techniques for finding new drugs, it is important to remember that drug discovery is both a cumulative and a reiterative process. Potential drugs developed by modifying a lead structure are certain to be sent through selective screening process to confirm activity and select for the best candidate to go on for further development.
- Likewise, drugs developed mechanistically will likely be both screened and later modified in order to produce the best candidate drug. Above figure presents schematically some of the various interactions that can occur in the discovery of a new drug.
- Every new chemical entity that affects the disease process whether found by accident, screening, modification, or mechanistic design provides useful information for developing still better compounds.
- This is true whether the chemical has positive or negative effects on the disease process. Each new chemical increases the data base of information about the disease–target–drug interaction. This in turn is the basis for rational drug design.

▨ THE BASICS OF MECHANISTIC DRUG DESIGN

Clinical manifestations for most diseases affecting man have been identified. Thus we are familiar with medical conditions such as hypertension, cancer, infections, etc. Modern biological techniques now have enabled researchers to study such diseases at molecular level and to identify the processes or molecules responsible for producing the observed clinical effects.

Defining the Disease Process

- The first step in the mechanistic design of drugs to treat diseases is to determine the biochemical basis of the disease process. Ideally, one would know the various steps involved in the physiological pathway that carries out the normal function. In addition, one would know the exact step(s) in the pathway that are altered in the diseased state. Knowledge about the regulation of the pathway is also important. Finally, one would know the three-dimensional structures of the molecules involved in the process.
- Once the biochemical basis of the disease is understood, one can select a target for modulating the disease process. These targets are often macromolecules such as enzymes, receptors, or nucleic acids and are discussed in the next section. In the normal condition the interaction of targets with their effector molecules produces a necessary physiologic function. Although most diseases have not been so fully characterized that all the above information is available, in many instances sufficient information is available to design a rational approach to block or reverse the disease process.

Defining the Target

There is potentially many ways in which biochemical pathways could become abnormal and result in disease. Therefore, knowledge of the molecular basis of the disease is important in order to select a target at which to disrupt the process. Targets for mechanistic drug design usually fall into three categories— enzymes, receptors and nucleic acids.

Enzymes as targets

- Enzymes are frequently the target of choice to fight a disease. If a disease is the result of the overproduction of a certain biocomponent then one or more of the enzymes involved in its synthesis can often be inhibited, resulting in a decrease in production of the respective biocomponent and disruption of the disease process.

- This is the theoretical basis behind the design of both the angiotensin-converting enzyme inhibitors and the rennin inhibitors. Inhibition of either of these enzymes, which are in the same biochemical pathway, decreases the production of angiotensin II and consequently reduces blood pressure.

- In other instances, specific enzymes may be required for pathogenic microorganisms or cancerous cells to live and grow, thereby causing disease. Inhibition of such enzymes would prevent the growth of these microbes or cells and hence reverse the disease. Similarly dihydrofolate reductase can also be blocked to elicit clinical effects.

- Enzymes are preferred targets, as they are relatively small, aqueous-soluble proteins and can be isolated for study. When enough of the enzyme is difficult to obtain from its natural source, genetic engineering techniques are frequently utilized to provide material for conducting X-ray crystallography, NMR spectroscopy and enzyme kinetic studies.

- Ultimately, the data obtained by these techniques allow one to determine the three-dimensional structures of the enzyme molecule in its active conformation. These structures provide a starting point for the design of new effector molecules (i.e. drugs) by computer graphics and molecular modeling techniques.

Receptors as targets

- Sometimes a disease can be modulated by blocking the action of an effector at its cellular receptor. A classic example of this is the well-known inhibition of the gastric histamine-2 receptor by the drug cimetidine, which decreases acid secretion in the stomach and reduces ulcer formation.

- Unlike enzymes, which often circulate in the body and can be isolated and studied outside their biological environment, cellular receptors consist of proteins imbedded in a surface membrane. Consequently, these targets are difficult to isolate and thus it is difficult to determine their structure. Nonetheless, molecular biological techniques are beginning to produce these macromolecules in larger amounts. Structural information will soon be available for many of them, using the same experimental techniques used for determining enzyme structures.

- Receptors that are easily isolated are the most amenable to rational design of effectors. An illustrative use of this concept is in the three-dimensional structural determination of rihnoviruses, which then can serve as a receptor-type target for the design of antiviral drugs.

Nucleic acids as targets

- Preventing the synthesis of undersirable proteins at the nucleic acid level can also potentially block disease. This strategy has frequently been employed in the antimicrobial and antitumor areas, where DNA-blocking drugs are used to prevent the synthesis of critical proteins.

- Since the microorganisms or tumor cells cannot grow and or replicate, the disease process is effectively blocked. Examples include the use of the DNA-intercalating drug actinomycine to treat certain forms of cancer.

Defining the Effector

- Effector molecules are compounds that can occupy an active site of a target molecule. As used in this context, they can be substrates, natural effectors that regulate the target in positive or negative ways, or drugs. Effector molecules and their targets interact with each other via a lock-and-key type of mechanism, in which the target enzyme or receptor is the lock and the effector is the key.

- In reality, the relationship between effector and target is more complex. The natural effector molecule fits into the active site of the enzyme or the binding site of the receptor in a manner that maximizes the complementarity of the two molecules. In addition, this complementarity not only is recognized as a function of shape, but also includes interaction of charged regions, hydrogen bonding, hydrophilic interactions, etc. The best information for designing drugs is obtained when one can determine the three-dimensional structure of both the target and effector molecules.

Designing New Drugs to Effect Targets

- To make a good drug, a compound should exhibit a number of useful characteristics. In addition to producing the desired effect, it should be sufficiently potent that large amounts need not have to be administered. It should have low toxicity and minimal side effects. Drugs that have to be given for chronic conditions should have considerable residence time in the body (half-life) so that continuous administration is not required.

- In the normal condition, natural effectors interact with their targets to carry out a needed physiological function. The natural effector for a target thus often represents an optimal structure for the complex formed. These natural molecules are not often used as drugs, for a number of reasons. The body generally has the ability to produce these effectors whenever they are needed to modulate a biological process.

- Natural effector molecules are often used as the starting point for the development of new drugs, since they generally have selectivity and potency for the desired target. By careful manipulation of the native structure, one can frequently retain the binding characteristics of the effector while designing in other desirable characteristics. Examples of drug design with natural effectors as the starting point include the use of the structure of luteinizing hormone-releasing hormone in the design of LHRH receptor agonists such as the anticancer drug leuprolide and the use of the structure of the enkephalins in the design of opioid receptor agonists as potential analgesics.

- There are other sources for complementary structures for enzyme and receptor targets, which can also be used as a starting point or to provide additional structural information for designing new drugs. If the natural effector is unavailable, similar effectors from different host may be used, e.g. the structure of renin angiotensinogen was used in the development of early human renin inhibitors.

- Synthetic compounds with only a vague resemblance to the effector may also have regions of complementarity and provide useful information. For example, trimethoprim, a unique synthetic compound with little resemblance to folic acid, is an excellent inhibitor of bacterial dihydrofolate reductase and was an important lead structure in the design of inhibitors of DHFR enzymes. In each case, the goal of the drug designer, when modifying the natural or other effectors is to remove those characteristics that confer instability and poor absorption and to add features that improve potency while providing greater specificity.

Overcoming Obstacles in Mechanistic Drug Design

- It is easiest to design new drugs when one has a full understanding of the disease process and reliable structural information about the target and its effectors. Unfortunately, such complete information is not often available.

- Receptor molecules make still more difficult targets, because they are much larger and frequently membrane-associated. In many cases, the receptor has never been isolated in pure form and little about its chemical and structural characteristics is known. In these cases, all the information available about the effector–receptor complex comes from the effectors structure alone.

- Accurate structural information about the complex is made more difficult when the effector molecule is a flexible one with many possible conformations in solution. In such a case, attempts are made to constrain the structure of the effector through cyclization or other chemical modifications.

- These more rigid structures then become useful probes for the macromolecular receptor and are often able to select for specific receptor subtypes. Since the database that supports that knowledge is still developing and is growing at a very rapid rate, it is important for medicinal scientists both to be receptive to new information and to be creative with its use.

▓ IMPORTANT TECHNIQUES FOR DRUG DESIGN

To obtain the structural information about molecules necessary for mechanistic design of drugs, a variety of chemical, physical and theoretical techniques must be used. Different techniques provide complementary types of information, which together can be used to determine how molecules interact.

X-ray Crystallography

X-ray crystallography is often the starting point for gathering information for mechanistic drug design. This technology has the potential to determine total structural information about a molecule.

NMR Spectroscopy

The major limitations of X-ray crystallography are the necessity to obtain good crystals and the fact that three-dimensional data obtained with crystals may not reflect the molecular structure under biological conditions that involve molecules in solution. The best technique for determining structural information on molecules in solution is nuclear magnetic resonance (NMR) spectroscopy.

Advantage of NMR is its ability to examine small molecule–macromolecule complexes, such as an enzyme inhibitor in the active site of the enzyme. Such information can be obtained by X-ray crystallography only after co-crystallization or crystal 'soaking' techniques. In addition, NMR can often be used to gather structural information more rapidly than X-ray crystallography.

▓ MOLECULAR MODELING

One of the most important advances in mechanistic drug design has been the recent development of computerized molecular modeling. Computerized modeling can provide scientists with five major types of information that are important for mechanistic design of drugs.

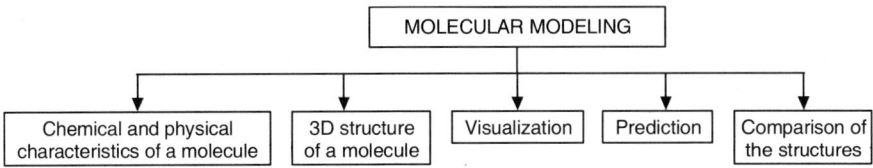

1. The three-dimensional structure of a molecule.
2. The chemical and physical characteristics of a molecule.
3. Comparison of the structure of one molecule with different molecules.
4. Visualization of complexes formed between different molecules.
5. Predictions about how related new molecules might look.

- Model building has been used for many years to approximate structures of biomolecules. Modern computer graphic techniques have enabled the three-dimensional visualization of structures on specialized computer terminals. It has made possible the manipulation of these structures in real time to allow visualization of different parts of the molecule, to change the orientation of specific functions while holding others constant and to take at different feasible conformations.

- Molecular modeling can also present the scientist with a visualization of specific characteristics of a molecule that influence its interactions with other molecules. Examples include structures that show the van der Waals radii of atoms, the electrostatic potential of molecules, solvent accessible surface of molecules, the contour of electron density, etc.

- Molecular modeling also has the ability to compare the structure of one molecule with related molecules to determine areas of similarity and difference. This comparison can include charged regions and other chemical characteristics as well as gross structural features.

- Finally, this technology has the potential power to design theoretically new molecules to satisfy predetermined shapes. An example would be 'finding' a new structure that mimics the shape of an active compound and is therefore able to occupy the active site of an enzyme.

FUTURE PROSPECTS

- Future developments will continue to improve the efficiency of all aspects of drug discovery. Knowledge about the molecular basis of disease is rapidly expanding on all fronts and will be continue.

- Molecular biologists will soon be able to provide quantities of receptor molecules and enzymes that have not yet been available to drug researchers. Improvements in X-ray and NMR techniques will yield needed structural information in shorter times and will give more details of the drug-target complex.

- With these new data will come improvements in computational techniques and their ability to predict the conformational state of a small compound and its macromolecular receptor. In addition, these techniques will be able to depict more clearly the biological molecules under physiological conditions.

- Finally, as more and more drug researchers understand and become familiar with the concepts and methods of mechanistic, computer-aided drug design, new applications of the integration of these techniques will emerge and will have a major impact both on basic since and on discovering new drugs for the future.

8

Drug Metabolism

Drug metabolism may be defined as biochemical modification or degradation of drugs usually through specialized enzymatic systems. Drug metabolism often converts lipophilic chemical compounds into more readily excreted polar products. Its rate is an important determinant of the duration and intensity of the pharmacological action of drugs.

- Drug metabolism can result in toxication or detoxication—the activation or deactivation of the chemical. While both occur, the major metabolites of most drugs are detoxication products (Fig. 8.1).
- Drugs are almost all xenobiotics. Other commonly used organic chemicals are also drugs, and are metabolized by the same enzymes as drugs.
  1. Phase I vs. phase II
  2. Sites
  3. Major enzymes and pathways

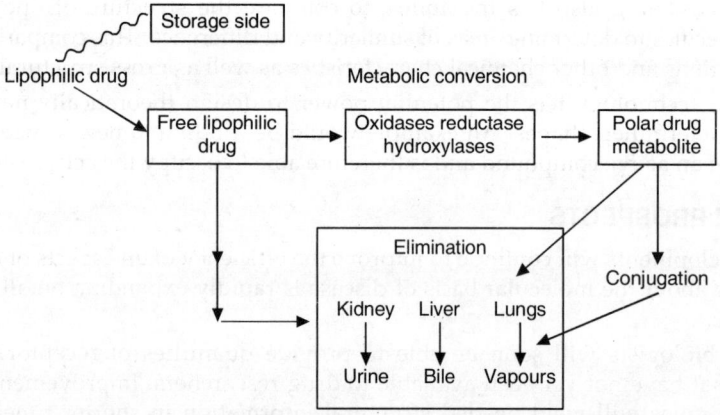

Fig. 8.1: Major enzymes and pathways involved in metabolism of drug

PHASE I Vs PHASE II

- **Phase I and phase II** reactions are biotransformation of chemicals that occur during drug metabolism. Biotransformation of drugs is defined as the conversion from one chemical form to another.
- The term is used synonymously with metabolism. The chemical changes are usually affected enzymatically in the body and thus, the definition excludes chemical instability of a drug within the body, e.g. conversion of penicillin to penicillonic acid by the bacterial

penicillinase and mammalian enzymes is metabolism but its degradation by the stomach acid to penicillenic acid is chemical instability.

- **Phase I reactions** usually precedes phase II, though not necessarily. During these reactions, polar bodies are either introduced or unmasked, which results in (more) polar metabolites of the original chemicals. In the case of pharmaceutical drugs, Phase I reactions can lead either to activation or inactivation of the drug. Phase I reactions (also termed non-synthetic reactions) may occur by oxidation, reduction, hydrolysis, cyclization, and decyclization reactions. Oxidation involves addition of oxygen (forming a negatively charged radical) or removal of hydrogen (forming a positively charged radical).

- The process of oxidation takes place in the presence of mixed function oxidases and mono-oxygenases in the liver. These oxidative reactions typically involve a cytochrome p-450, haemoprotein, NADPH and oxygen. The classes of pharmaceutical drugs that utilize this method for their metabolism include phenothiazines, paracetamol, and steroids. If the metabolites of phase I reactions are sufficiently polar, they may be readily excreted at this point.

- However, many phase I products are not eliminated rapidly and undergo a subsequent reaction in which an endogenous substrate combines with the newly incorporated functional group to form a highly polar conjugate.

- **Phase II reactions** — usually known as conjugation reactions [e.g. with glucuronic acid, sulfonates (commonly known as sulfation), glutathione or amino acids] — are usually detoxication in nature, and involve the interactions of the polar functional groups of phase I metabolites.

SITES OF BIOTRANSFORMATION

- Quantitatively, the smooth endoplasmic reticulum of the liver cell is the principal organ of drug metabolism, although every biological tissue has some ability to metabolize drugs. Factors responsible for the liver's contribution to drug metabolism include that it is a large organ, that it is the first organ perfused by chemicals absorbed in the gut, and that there are very high concentrations of most drug-metabolizing enzyme systems relative to other organs.

- If a drug is taken into the GI tract, where it enters hepatic circulation through the portal vein, it becomes well-metabolized and is said to show the *first pass effect*. Other sites of drug metabolism include epithelial cells of the gastrointestinal tract, lungs, kidneys, and the skin. These sites are usually responsible for localized toxicity reactions.

MAJOR ENZYMES AND PATHWAYS

Several major enzymes and pathways are involved in drug metabolism, and can be divided into phase I and phase II reactions.

Phase I or Fuctionalization Reaction

1. Oxidation
2. Reduction
3. Hydrolysis

Enzyme system involved in the oxidation

1. Cytochrome P-450 monooxygenase system.
2. Flavin-containing monooxygenase system.
3. Alcohol dehydrogenase and aldehyde dehydrogenase.

4. Monoamine oxidase.

5. Co-oxidation by peroxidases.

Role of cytochrome p-450 monooxygenase in biotrasformation

- **CYP450** is a diverse super family of hemoproteins found in bacteria and eukaryotes. Cyt-p-450 uses a plethora of both exogenous and endogenous compounds as substrates in enzymatic reactions.

- Usually they form part of multicomponent electron transfer chains, called p-450-containing systems. The most common reaction catalyzed by cytochrome p-450 is a monooxygenase reaction, i.e. insertion of one atom of oxygen into an organic substrate (RH) while the other oxygen atom is reduced to water:

$$RH + O_2 + 2H^+ + 2e^- \rightarrow ROH + H_2O$$

- CYP enzymes have been identified from all lineages of life, including mammals, birds, fish, insects, worms, sea squirts, sea urchins, plants, fungi, slime molds, bacteria and archaea. More than 6700 distinct CYP sequences are known.

- The name p-450 refers to the "pigment at 450 nm", so named for the characteristic peak formed by absorbance of light at wavelengths near 450 nm when the heme iron is reduced (with sodium dithionite) and complexed to carbon monoxide.

- The active site of cytochrome p-450 contains a heme iron center. The iron is tethered to the p-450 protein via a thiolate ligand derived from a cysteine residue. This cysteine and several flanking residues (RXCXG) are absolutely conserved among all known CYPs. Because of the vast variety of reactions catalyzed by CYPs, activities and properties of the many CYPs differ in many aspects. A general description of the p-450 enzyme properties can be summarized as follows:

  1. The resting state of the protein is as oxidized Fe^{3+}.

  2. Binding of a substrate initiates electron transport and oxygen binding.

  3. Electrons are supplied to the CYP by another protein, either cytochrome p-450 reductase, ferredoxins, or cytochrome b5 to reduce the heme iron.

  4. Molecular oxygen is bound and split by the reduced heme iron.

  5. An iron-bound oxidant, in some cases an iron (IV), oxidizes the substrate to an alcohol or an epoxide, regenerating the resting state of the CYP.

- Because most CYPs require a protein partner to deliver one or more electrons to reduce the iron (and eventually molecular oxygen). CYPs are properly speaking part of p-450-containing systems of proteins. Five general schemes are known.

Mixed Function Oxidases

- Many drug-metabolizing enzymes are located in the lipophilic membranes of the endoplasmic reticulum of the liver and other tissues. When these lamellar membranes are isolated by homogenization and fractionation of the cell, they re-form into vesicles called microsomes. Microsomes retain most of the morphologic and functional characteristics of the intact membranes, including the rough and smooth surface features of the rough (ribosome-studded) and smooth (no ribosomes) endoplasmic reticulum.

- Whereas the rough microsomes tend to be dedicated to protein synthesis, the smooth microsomes are relatively rich in enzymes responsible for oxidative drug metabolism. In particular, they contain the important class of enzymes known as the mixed function oxidases (MFO), or monooxygenases.

- The activity of this enzyme system requires both a reducing agent (NADPH) and molecular oxygen. In a typical reaction, one molecule of oxygen is consumed (reduced) per substrate molecule, with one oxygen atom appearing in the product and the other in the form of water. Two enzymes are important in this process.
- *NADPH-cytochrome p-450 reductase.* One mole of this enzyme (molecular weight of 80,000) contains one mole each of flavin mononucleotide (FMN) and flavin adenine dinucleotide (FAD). Because cytochrome C can serve as an electron acceptor, the enzyme is often referred to as NADPH-cytochrome C reductase.
- *Cytochrome p-450.* The name cytochrome p-450 is derived from the spectral properties of this hemoprotein. In its reduced (ferrous) form, it binds carbon monoxide to give a ferrocarbonyl adduct that absorbs maximally in the visible region of the electromagnetic spectrum at 450 nm. Over half of the heme synthesized in the liver is committed to hepatic cytochrome p-450 formation. The relative abundance in liver of cytochrome p-450, as compared to that of the reductase, makes the reductase the rate-limiting step in hepatic drug oxidations.
- Microsomal drug oxidations require cytochrome p-450, cytochrome p-450 reductase, NADPH, and molecular oxygen. The cycle involves four steps:
  1. Oxidized (Fe^{3+}) cytochrome p-450 combines with a drug substrate to form a binary complex.
  2. NADPH donates an electron to the cytochrome p-450 reductase, which in turn reduces the oxidized cytochrome p-450 drug complex.
  3. A second electron is introduced from NADPH *via* the same cytochrome p-450 reductase, which serves to reduce molecular oxygen and form 'activated oxygen'-cytochrome p-450-substrate complex.
  4. This complex in turn transfers 'activated' oxygen to the drug substrate to form the oxidized product. The potent oxidizing properties of this activated oxygen permit oxidation of a large number of substrates.
- Substrate specificity is very low for this enzyme complex. High solubility in lipids is the only common structural feature of the wide variety of structurally unrelated drugs and chemicals that serve as substrates in this system.

▨ GENERAL SUMMARY OF PHASE-I METABOLIC PATHWAY

Oxidative reaction

1. Oxidation of aromatic moieties.
2. Oxidation of olefins.
3. Oxidation of benzylic, alicyclic carbon atom, and carbon atom α to carbonyl and imines.
4. Oxidation at aliphatic and alicyclic carbon atom.
5. Oxidation involving carbon–heteroatom system.
6. Carbon–nitrogen system (aliphatic and aromatic amines): N-dealkylation, oxidative deamination, N-oxide formation, N-hydroxylation.
7. Carbon–oxygen system (O-dealkylation).
8. Carbon–sulfur system(S-dealkylation,S-oxidation, and desulfuration).
9. Oxidation of alcohol and aldehyde.
10. Miscellaneous oxidation.

1. Oxidation of aromatic moieties
Aromatic hydrocarbons:

1.

2.

Phenytoin

p-hydroxyphenytoin

3.

Phenobarbitone

p-hydroxyphenytoin

4.

Propranolol

2. Oxidation of olefins (oxidation of benzylic, alicyclic carbon atom, and carbon atom a to carbonyl and imines)

Oxidation of benzylic carbon atom:

1.

Imipramine

2.

Amitryptaline

Oxidation at carbon atom α to carbonyles and imines:

1.

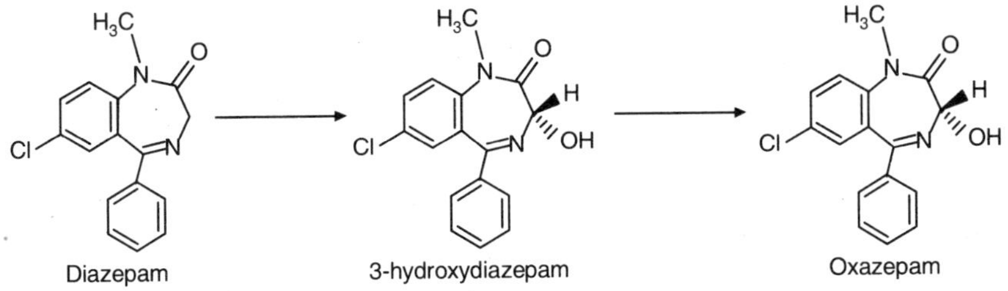

Diazepam   3-hydroxydiazepam   Oxazepam

3. Oxidation at aliphatic and alicyclic carbon atom

1. 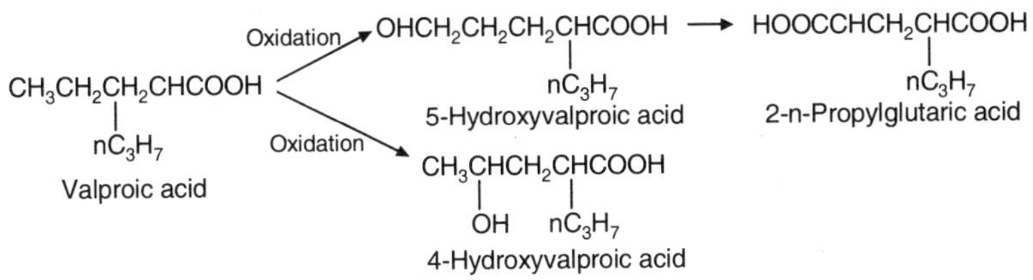 $CH_3CH_2CH_2CHCOOH$

      |

      nC_3H_7

   Valproic acid

Oxidation → $OHCH_2CH_2CH_2CHCOOH$ → $HOOCCHCH_2CHCOOH$

              nC_3H_7 nC_3H_7

      5-Hydroxyvalproic acid   2-n-Propylglutaric acid

Oxidation → $CH_3CHCH_2CHCOOH$

          OH nC_3H_7

    4-Hydroxyvalproic acid

2.

Chlopropamide   2 Hydroxychlopropamide

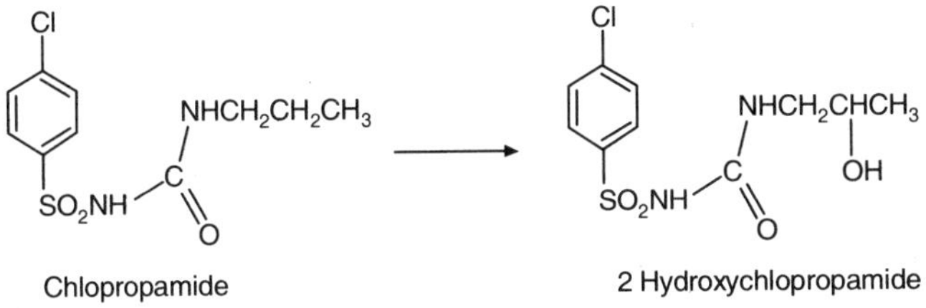

3.

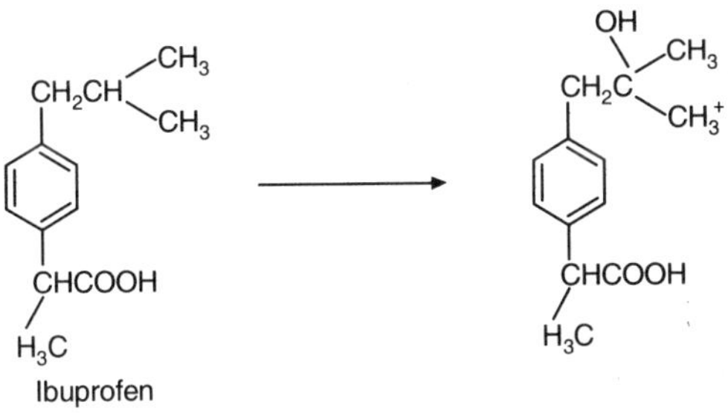

Ibuprofen

4. Oxidation of carbon-heteroatom systems

a. Oxidation of carbon – nitrogen systems:

i. Tertiary amines:

1. 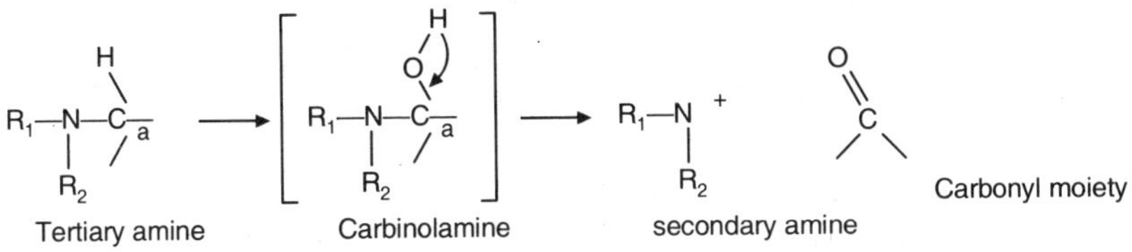 Tertiary amine → Carbinolamine → secondary amine   Carbonyl moiety

2.

Imipramine → Desmethylimipramine → Bisdesmethylimipramine

ii. *Secondary and primary amines:*

1.

Primary amine → Carbinolamine → Carbonyl + NH_3 Ammonia

2.

Phenmetrazine → Carbinolamine intermediate → 3-Oxophenmetrazine

3.

Secondary amine → Hydroxylamine → Nitrone

4.

Amphetamine → carbon hydroxylation → $+ NH_3$

iii. *Aromatic amines and heterocyclic nitrogen compounds:*

1.

Tertiary aromatic amine → N-oxide (N-oxidation), carbon hydroxylation → Carbinolamine

2.

Hydroxylamine → Nitrone → Hydroxylamine

b. Oxidation involving carbon–oxygen systems:

1.
$$R-O-\underset{H}{\overset{H}{\underset{|}{C}}}_a \xrightarrow[\text{Hydroxyaltion}]{-\text{carbon}} \left[R-O-\underset{OH}{\overset{H}{\underset{|}{C}}}_a \right] \longrightarrow R_{OH} + C_{\text{carbonyl moiety}}$$

Ether   Hemiacetal or Hemiketal   phenol

2.

Phenacetin   Acetominophen

c. Oxidation involving carbon–sulphur system:

1.

6-(Methylthio)-purine   6-mercaptopurine

2.

3.

Thiopental   Pentobarbital

5. Oxidation of alcohol and aldehyde

$$RCH_2OH \underset{\text{Primary alcohol}}{\overset{NAD \quad NADH}{\rightleftharpoons}} RCHO \xrightarrow[\text{Aldehyde}]{NAD+ \quad NADH} RCHO$$
Acids

Medazepam   Hydroxy medazepam   Diazepam

▨ REDUCTION

Niro-, azo-, and carbonyl groups are subject to reduction, resulting in the formation of more polar hydroxy and amino groups. There are several reductases in the liver, which depend upon NADH or NADPH, that catalyze such reaction.

Reduction of aldehyde and ketone carbonyl

Aldehyde → Primary alcohol

Ketone → Secondary alcohol

Chloral hydrate ⇌ (H2O / −H2O) Chloral → Trichloroethanol

Chlorpheniramine — bis-n demethylation, Oxidative deamination → Aldehyde metabolism

Reduction → 3-(p-chlorobenzyl)3-(2-pyridyl)-propane-1-ol

Oxidation → 3-(p-chlorobenzyl)3-(2-pyridyl)-propanoic acid

Reduction of nitro and azo compound

Ar—N (Nitro) → Ar—N = O (Nitroso) → Ar—N (Hydroxylamine) → Ar—NH₂ (Amine)

Ar—N (Azo) → Ar—NH (Hydrazo) → Ar—NH₂ + Ar'—NH₂ (Amines)

Sulfasalazine → Sulfipyridine + 5-Amino salicylic acid

Nirazepam → 7-amino metabolite

Miscellaneous reductive reaction

$$CH_3 - \underset{O}{S} - CH_3 \longrightarrow CH_3SCH_3$$

Dimethyl sulfoxide → Dimethyl sulfide

- NADPH-cytochrome P-450 reductase.
- Reduced (ferrous) cytochrome P-450.
- It should be noted that during reduction reactions, a chemical can enter *futile cycling*, in which it gains a free-radical electron, then promptly loses it to <u>oxygen</u> (to form a superoxide anion).

▨ HYDROLYSIS REACTION

- Hydrolysis is a major biotransformation pathway for drugs containing the ester, functionality. Ester and more slowly amide are hydrolysed by enzymes in the blood, liver microsome, kidney and many other tissues.
- Thus, the local anesthetic procaine which is an ester is rapidly inactivated by plasma cholinesterase, where its amide analouge, procainamide is not attacked by this enzyme and thus suitable for systemic use as an anti-dysarrhythemic drug. Main enzyme involved in hydrolysis are:
  1. Esterases and amidases
  2. Epoxide hydrolase

Hydrolysis of ester and amides

Aspirin → Salicylic acid + CH$_3$COOH (Acetic acid)

Procainamide — Slow hydrolysis

Procaine — Fast hydrolysis

Phase II Reaction

- Parent drugs or their phase I metabolites that contain suitable chemical groups often undergo coupling or conjugation reactions with an endogenous substance to yield drug conjugates. In general, conjugates are polar molecules that are readily excreted and often inactive.

- Conjugate formation involves high-energy intermediates and specific transfer enzymes. Such enzymes (transferase) may be located in microsomes or in the cytosol. They catalyze the coupling of an activated endogenous substance (such as the uridine 5'-diphosphate [UDP] derivative of glucuronic acid) with a drug (or endogenous compound), or of an activated drug (such as the S-CoA derivative of benzoic acid) with an endogenous substrate.

- Because the endogenous substrates originate in the diet, nutrition and disease play critical roles in the regulation of drug conjugation.

- Drug conjugations were once believed to represent terminal inactivation events and as such have been viewed as 'true detoxification' reactions. However, this concept must be modified, since it is now known that certain conjugation reactions sulfation of N-hydroxy acetyl amino fluorene and N-acetylation of isoniazid) may lead to the formation of reactive species responsible for the hepatotoxicity of the drug.

Enzyme Involved in the Phase II Reaction

1. Gluocuronic acid conjugation.
2. Glutathione S-transferases.
3. Mercaptouric acid biosynthesis.
4. UDP-glucuronyl transferases.
5. N-acetyltransferases.
6. Amino acid N-acyltransferases.
7. Sulfotransferases.

1. Glucuronic acid conjugation

- The most commonly used conjugation reaction is glucouronide formation and this is the major portion of the metabolite formed in the excreta. Glucuronic acid is an organic acid derived from glucose in which the presence of four extra hydroxyl groups conforms great water solubility.

- Glucuronide formation involves the formation of high energy phosphate compound uridine diphosphate glucuronide acid (UDPGA). From UDPGA, the glucuronic acid part is transferred to an electron rich atom N, S or O on the substrate forming an amide, ester, or thiol bond. The enzyme involved in this reaction is UDP glucuronyl transferase.

Formation of UDPGA and β-glucuronide conjugate:

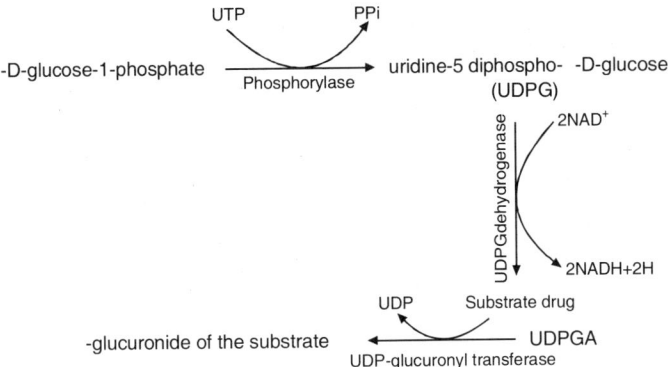

Compound containing OH group:

Acetominophen

Trichloroethanol

p-hydroxyphenytoin

Compound contain carboxyl group:

Salicylic acid

Naproxen

Compound containing aromatic amines:

Desipramine

7-amino-5-nitroindazole

Compound contains sulfahydryl group:

Methimazole

Propyl thiouracil

2. Sulfate conjugation

- Sulfate conjugation is one of the important metabolic reactions in which transfer of the sulfate group to the fuctional group.
- Before transfer, sulfate is activated in the form of 3-phosphoro adenosine-5-phosphosulfate (PAPS). Transfer of sulfate group from PAPS to the fuctional group takes under the influence of a number of sulfokinase enzymes.

Formation of PAPS and sulfate conjugate:

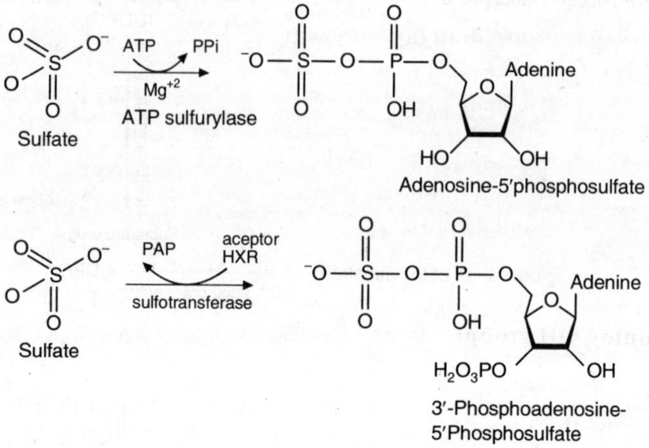

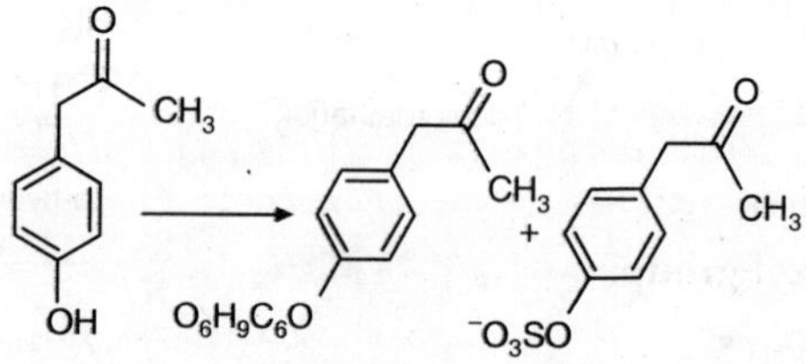

Adenosine-5'phosphosulfate

3'-Phosphoadenosine-
5'Phosphosulfate

3. Formation of glycine and glutamine conjugates of phenylacetic acid

Glycine is the most common amino acid used in phase II conjugation. In this amino acid conjugation, first xenobiotic is activated by coenzyme A in presence of acyl synthatase to form the thioester. The activated thioester reacts with amino acid in presence of transacetylase.

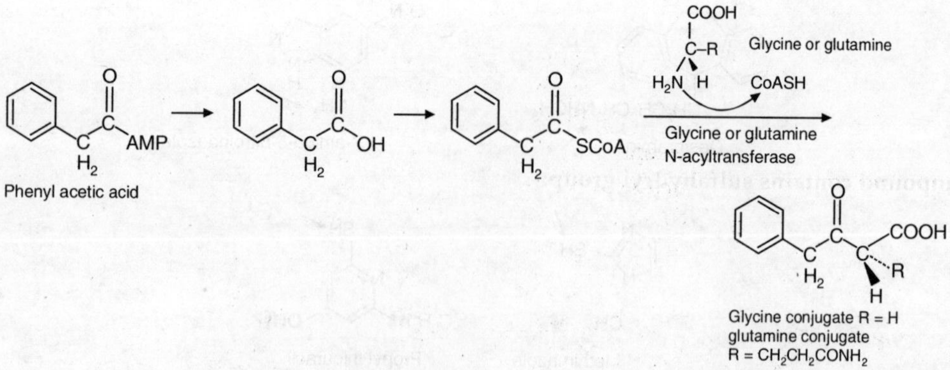

Glycine conjugate R = H
glutamine conjugate
R = $CH_2CH_2CONH_2$

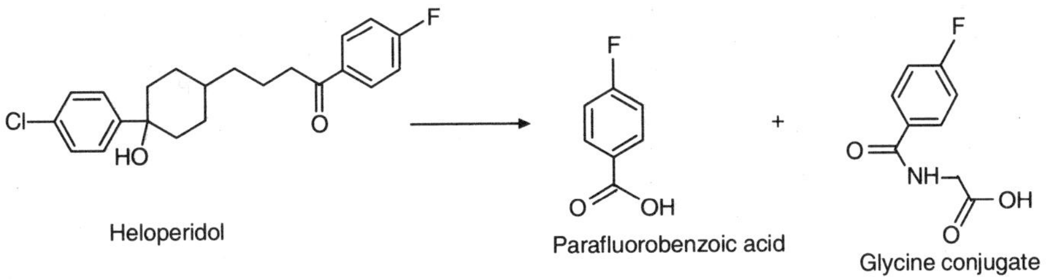

Heloperidol → Parafluorobenzoic acid + Glycine conjugate

4. Glutathione or mercaptouric acid conjugation

- The glutathione S-transferase (GST) family of enzymes comprises a long list of cytosolic, mitochondrial, and microsomal proteins which are capable of multiple reactions with a multitude of substrates, both endogenous and xenobiotic.
- Glutathione (GSH) is a thiol containing tripeptide of great significance in the detoxification and toxification of drugs and other xenobiotics. It reacts in different ways because of nucleophilic property of thiol group in glutathione and its reducing or oxidizing nature.

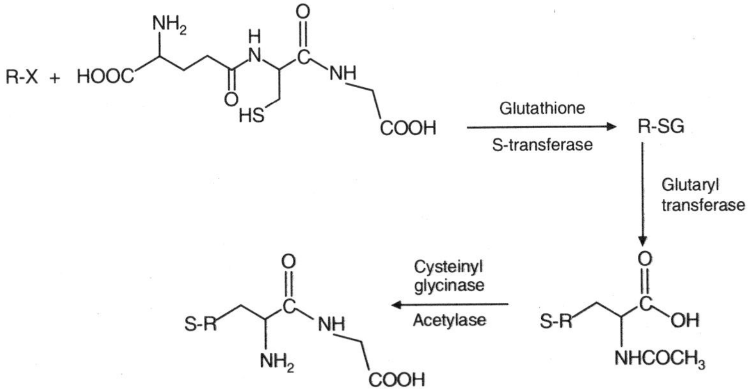

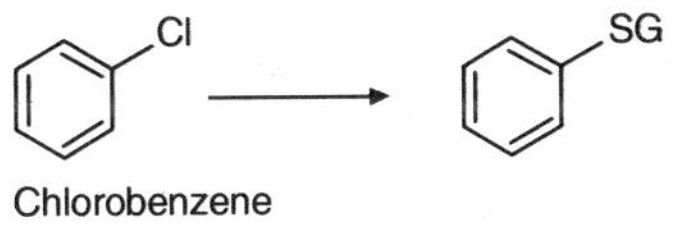

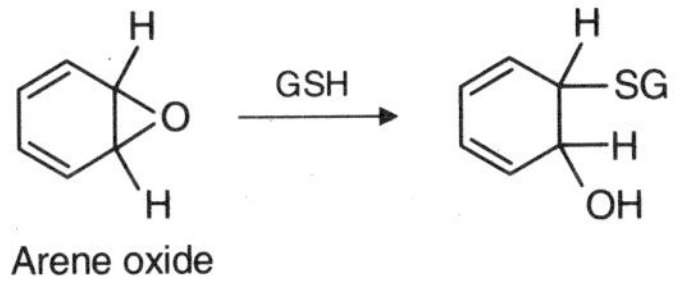

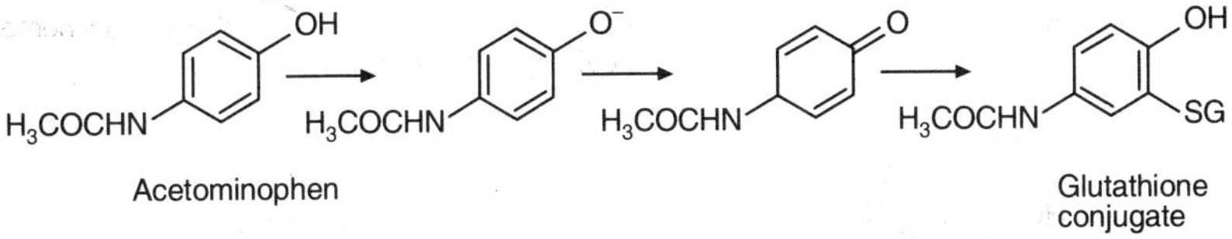

Chlorobenzene

Arene oxide

Acetominophen → Glutathione conjugate

5. Acetylation

- Aromatic and aliphatic amines, e.g. aniline histamine, hydrazine can be acetylated by coenzyme A. Here the acetyl moiety is bound by a thioester linkage. The transfer of acetyl group takes place in presence of N-acetyl transferase.

- In acetylation, although water solubility is not increased, it helps in terminating the pharmacological activity of drug or its amino metabolite.

Examples of different types of compound undergoing N-acetylation. Arrow indicates site of acetylation.

6. Methylation

Methylation with methyl group transfer from S-adenosyl methionine important pathway of metabolism. Amine like catecholamines methylated on phenolic group by catechol-O-methyl transferase (COMT). Methyl group in S-adenosyl methionine is bound to a sulfonium centre, giving it a marked electrophilic character.

FACTORS AFFECTING METABOLISM

The duration and intensity of pharmacological action of most lipophilic drugs are determined by the rate they are metabolized to inactive products. The cytochrome P-450 mono-oxygenase system is the most important pathway in this regard. In general, anything that increases the rate of metabolism (e.g. enzyme induction) of a pharmacologically active metabolite will decrease the duration and intensity of the drug action. The opposite is also true (e.g. enzyme inhibition).

Various *physiological* and *pathological* factors can also affect drug metabolism. Physiological factors that can influence drug metabolism include age, individual variation (e.g. pharmacogenetics), enterohepatic circulation, nutrition, intestinal flora, or sex differences.

1. Age: In general, drugs are metabolized more slowly in fetal, neonatal and elderly humans and animals than in adults. Young males are more prone to sedation from barbiturates than female. Rats show more prolonged effect from nicotine, and strychinine neonates cannot detoxify chloramphenicol.

2. Genetics: Genetic variation (polymorphism) accounts for some of the variability in the effect of drugs. With N-acetyltransferases (involved in phase II reactions), individual variation creates a group of people who acetylate slowly (slow acetylators) and those who acetylate quickly, split roughly 50:50 in the population of Canada. This variation may have dramatic consequences, as the slow acetylators are more prone to dose-dependent toxicity.

Cytochrome P-450 monooxygenase system enzymes can also vary across individuals, with deficiencies occurring in 1–30% of people, depending on their ethnic background.

3. Pathological factors: It can also influence drug metabolism, including liver, kidney, or heart diseases. The half-life and clearance of isoniazid, diazepam, ampicillin and phenobarbiton decreased in case of hepatic disease.

In case of actual viral hepatitis, the half-lives of diazepam, meperidine and Phenobarbiton are decreased. Renal disease results in a considerable impairment of the elimination of water-soluble and or their metabolites. The activity and elimination rate of isoniazid, procaine, and cortisone is showed in case of renal failure.

4. Pharmacodynamic factor: The dose, the route and the frequency of administration of drugs can affect their metabolic profiles. Drugs given too frequently may overload the metabolic system available to it, leading to elevated blood and tissue level of the drug. The effect of protein binding also influences the metabolism.

5. Environmental factor: Diet can influence metabolism, starvation can deplete glycine stores and alter glycine conjugation; circadian rhythm is another factor which influences metabolism. In rats and mice, the rate of hepatic metabolism of some drugs follows a diurnal rhythm. This may be true in humans as well.

6. Enzyme inhibition: Environmental pollutants are capable of inducing cytochrome P-450. For example, exposure to benzo-pyrene, present in tobacco smoke, charcoal-broiled meat, and other organic pyrolysis products, is known to induce cytochrome P-450 and to alter the rates of drug metabolism in both experimental animals and in humans.

Other environmental chemicals known to induce specific cytochrome P-450 isoenzymes include the polychlorinated biphenyls (PCBs), which are used widely in industry as insulating materials and plasticizers, and 2,3,7,8-tetrachlorodibenzo-p-dioxin (dioxin, TCDD), a trace by-product of the chemical synthesis of the defolate 2,4,5-trichlorophenol and the antibacterial compound hexachlorophene.

Other drug substrates may inhibit cytochrome p-450 enzyme activity. A well-known inhibitor is proadifen (SK&F 525-A). This compound binds avidly to the cytochrome p-450 molecule and thereby competitively inhibits the metabolism of potential substrates. Cimetidine is a popular therapeutic agent that has been found to impair the in vivo metabolism of other drugs by the same mechanism.

Some substrates irreversibly inhibit cytochrome p-450 via covalent interaction of a metabolically generated reactive intermediate that may react with either the apoprotein or the heme moiety of the cytochrome. A growing list of such inhibitors includes the steroids ethinyl estradiol, norethindrone, and spironolactone; the anesthetic agent fluroxene; the antimicrobial agent chloramphenicol; the barbiturates secobarbital and allobarbital; the analgesic sedatives allylisopropylacetylurea, diethylpentenamide and ethchlorvynol; the solvent carbon disulfide; and propylthiouracil.

7. Enzyme induction: An interesting feature of some of these chemically dissimilar drug substrates is their ability, on repeated administration, to 'induce' cytochrome p-450 by enhancing the rate of its synthesis or reducing its rate of degradation. Induction results in an acceleration of metabolism and usually in a decrease in the pharmacologic action of the inducer and also of coadministered drugs.

However, in the case of drugs metabolically transformed to reactive intermediates, enzyme induction may exacerbate drug-mediated tissue toxicity.

Various substrates appear to induce distinct forms of cytochrome p-450. The two isoenzymes that have been most extensively studied are cytochrome p-450 IIB 1, which is induced by treatment with phenobarbital; and cytochrome p-450IAI, which is induced by polycyclic aromatic hydrocarbons, of which 3-methylcholanthrene is a prototype.

9

Prodrug Concept

Almost all drugs possess some undesirable physio-chemical and biological properties. Their therapeutic efficacy can be improved by minimizing or removing undesirable properties. This can be possible by three ways:

1. Biological approach.
2. Physical approach.
3. Chemical approach—this is most preferable one. It involves:
   a. Design and development of new drug.
   b. Design of hard and soft drugs.
   c. Prodrug design.

Out of above mentioned approach except first remaining two are mostly used.

Hard Drug

- A hard drug is one, which is resistant to biotransformation and therefore has a longer biological half-life.
- Design of the hard drug involves metabolic stabilization of existing drug by putting certain functional groups, which are stable and does not undergo biotransformation.

Soft Drug

- A soft drug is one, which undergoes rapid biotransformation in predictable manner into non-toxic compound.
- This design is possible by introducing a certain functional group over lead compound, which undergo rapid biotransformation. Replacement of the alkyl side chain of the drug with an ester group.

PRODRUG

- A prodrug is chemically modified inert drug precursor, which upon biotransformation liberates pharmacologically active parent compound.
- Thus, in contrast to soft drug, prodrugs are inactive per se and biotransformed in a predictable manner into active metabolites.
- A prodrug is also called as pro-agent, bioreversible derivative or latentiated drug. The design approach is also referred to as drug latentiation.
- A prodrug is a pharmacological substance (drug) which is administered in an inactive (or significantly less active) form. Once administered, the prodrug is metabolized in vivo into the active compound by virtue of chemical or enzyme attack before or after reaching the site(s) of action.

- Prodrugs occur in nature. One example is proinsulin, which is synthesized in the pancreas and releases its active moiety, insulin, and an inactive peptide. Codeine is another example; it can be regarded as a prodrug of morphine, which is responsible for its analgesic effect.

- Most synthetic prodrugs are prepared by attachment of the active drug through a metabolically labile linkage to another molecule, the 'promoiety'. The promoiety is not necessary for activity but may impart some desirable properties to the drug, such as increased lipid or water solubility or site specificity.

- The primary purpose of the prodrug for oral administration is to increase the absorption through the intestine or to reduce the local side effects in GI tract. However, the prodrug can be bioreversibly changed to the active drug to modify its physicochemical properties. This modification results in better drug transport through the intestinal wall and hence increases the bioavailability of the drug in blood as well as at the site of action.

- Thus the prodrug can be an approach to release the drug in controlled manner. Prodrug can be used for the delivery of both water soluble and water insoluble drugs. In case of the delivery of a water soluble drug, this is converted to a water insoluble prodrug.

- This modification results in the slow dissolution and also release of the drug in aqueous medium. Thus the drug will be available in plasma at a slower controlled rate. Example: Theophylline and its prodrug 7, 7'- succinylditheophylline.

- Alternatively water insoluble drug can be better absorbed in brush border region in the intestine. The water-soluble prodrug complexes after the enzymatic metabolism release the drug at the intestinal membrane and due to high partition coefficient the drug level will increased in the plasma.

Classification of Prodrug

Carrier-linked prodrug (Fig. 9.1)

- Carrier-linked prodrugs are those in which the active drug is covalently linked to an inert carrier or transport moiety. They are generally esters or amides. Such prodrugs have greatly modified lipophilicity due to attached carrier. The active drug is released by hydrolytic cleavage, either chemically or enzymatically.0

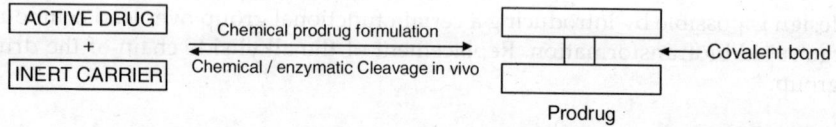

This is further classified as;

A. **Bipartate:** These prodrugs comprised of one carrier attached to the active substance or the drug.

B. **Tripartate:** In these prodrugs, the active drug is linked to the carrier moiety through a spacer or connector group.

C. **Mutual:** It consist of two pharmacologically active agents, in which one act as a carrier, thus might give synergistic action.

- A compound that contains an active drug linked with a transport moiety (promoeity) which is mostly lipophilic in nature and is removed enzymatically.

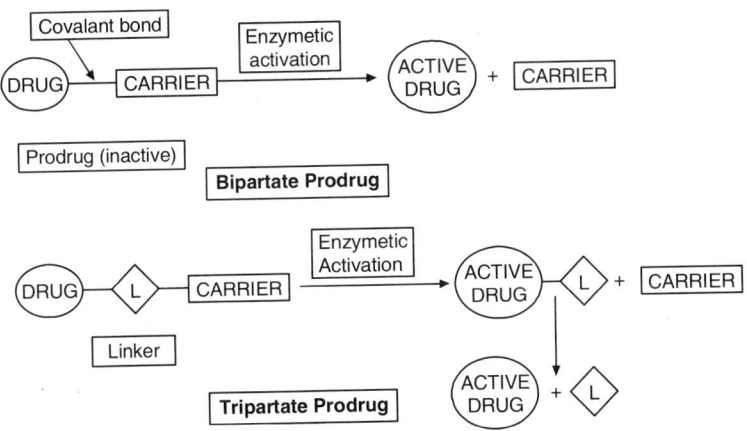

Fig. 9.1: Types of carrier-linked prodrugs

Bioprecursor

- These are inert molecules obtained by chemical modification of the active drug but do not contain a carrier.
- Such a moiety has almost the same lipophilicity as the parent drug and is bioactivated generally by redox biotransformation, only enzymatically, e.g. arylacetic acid NSAID such as fenbufen from aroyl propionic acid precursors.

Mutual prodrug

Prodrug of two active compounds are called as mutual prodrug, here two pharmacologically active compounds are coupled together to form a single molecule such that each acts as the carrier for the other, e.g. benorylate is a mutual prodrug of NSAIDs, aspirin and paracetamol.

Benorylate

Chemical Classification

1. Ester prodrugs
2. Amines prodrugs.
3. Azo prodrugs.
4. Carbonyl prodrugs.

Ester prodrugs

- These compounds comprises of –COOH or –OH due to the presence of a wide variety of esterases in various body tissues. By suitable esterification of molecules containing a carboxylic acid or hydroxyl group, it is possible to attain derivatives with almost any desirable hydrophilicity, lipophilicity, and in vivo liability.
- One should always kept in mind that enzyme catalyzed ester hydrolysis is quite dissimilar from nonenzymatic ester hydrolysis in terms of electronic and steric requirements in the substrates. Enzymatic reactions are more likely influenced by steric rather than electronic effects.

- It should also be kept in mind that there are considerable interspecies variations in the enzyme's expression level and catalytic capacity (Fig. 9.2).

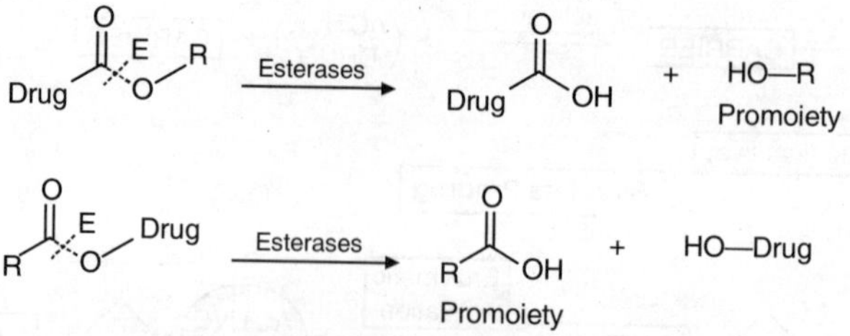

Fig. 9.2: Enzyme-catalyzed ester hydrolysis

- Both the acyl and the alcohol portion surrounding the cleavable ester bond affect the enzyme-catalyzed ester hydrolysis. Sometimes due to steric hindrance in the active drug, a prodrug may not be produced by direct ester formation with the existing functional group that is sufficiently labile in vivo.
- This problem can be overcomed by designing the so-called cascade prodrugs containing double esters using α-acyloxyalkyl, carbonate, or alkoxycarbonyloxyalkyl esters where the terminal ester group is accessible for enzymatic cleavage.
- In these types of prodrugs, a sequence of two or more reactions are required for drug release and activation, usually enhanced by a first enzymatic-catalyzed reaction followed by a spontaneous chemical release/activation step(s). Examples: Several prodrugs of β-lactam antibiotics, corticosteroids, and angiotensin II receptor antagonists.
- The 2-carboxylic acid on the thiazolidine ring of β-lactam antibiotics is required for antibacterial activity, is an active site for attaching a promoiety in the design of ester prodrugs. But due to steric hindrance, simple esters of this carboxylic acid group would oppose enzymatic hydrolysis. Examples of α-acyloxyalkyl ester prodrugs include bacampicillin, pivampicillin, pivmecillinam, cefuroxime axetil, prednicarbate, candesartan cilexetil, etc.

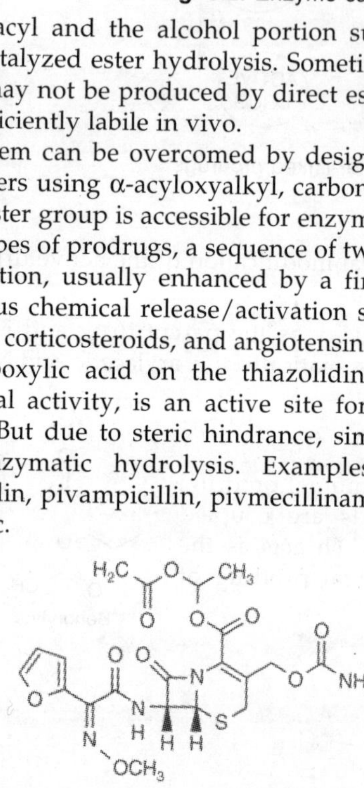

Cefuroxime axetil

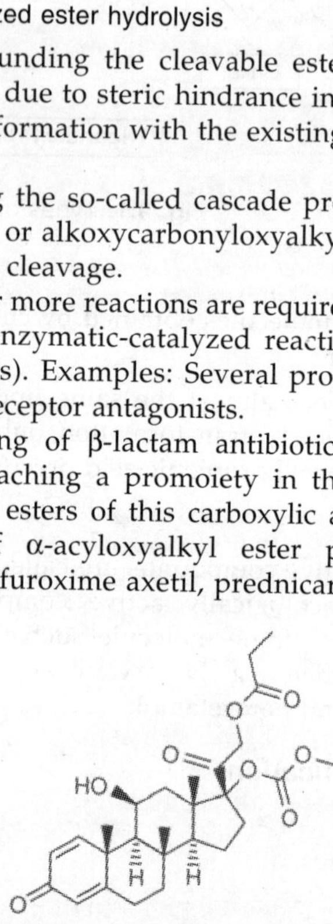

Prednicarbate

Amines prodrugs

Derivatization of amines to give amide has not been widely used as a prodrug because of high chemical stability of amide and lack of amidase enzyme necessary for hydrolysis. A more common approach is to use Mannich base as a prodrug form of amines. Example:

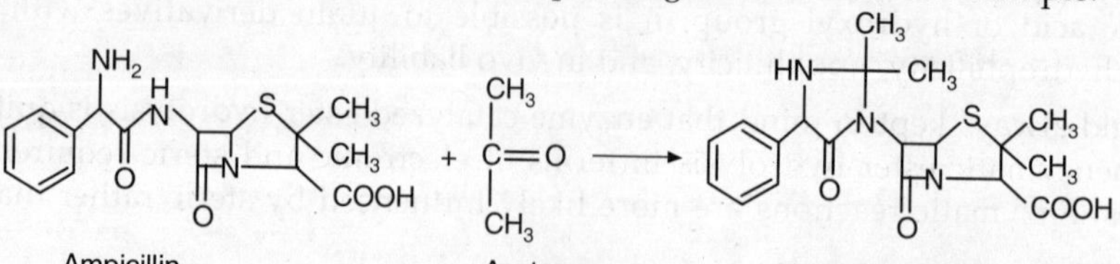

Ampicillin   Acetone   Hetacillin (prodrug)

Azo prodrugs

Amines are derivatized to azo linkage prodrug occasionally. Example:

Carbonyl prodrugs

Carbonyl functionalities such as aldehydes and ketones conversion to prodrug have not found with clinical utility.

Example: Hexamine releases formaldehyde in the urine (acidic pH), which acts as an antibacterial agent.

Prodrug Design Consideration

- Often a situation encountered by medicinal chemists where a structure has adequate pharmacological activity but an inadequate pharmacokinetic profile (i.e. absorption, distribution, metabolism and excretion).
- Usually prodrugs can be designed to improve various physicochemical properties, which result in improvement in pharmacokinetic as well as pharmaceutical properties. In pharmaceutical phase, various parameters should be modified such as:
  1. The physical properties of the drug substance like odor, taste, pain on injection, etc. have to be modified.
  2. Whereas in physicochemical properties include modification such as hydrophilicity–lipophilicity, poor stability, etc.
- The most important requirement in prodrug design is the conversion of the prodrug to the active drug in vivo at the intended compartment. This prodrug-drug conversion may take place before absorption (e.g. in the gastrointestinal system), during absorption (e.g. in the gastrointestinal wall or in the skin), after absorption, or at the specific site of drug action. It is important that the conversion must be essentially completed.
- Prodrugs can be premeditated to use a variety of chemical and enzymatic reactions to attain cleavage to generate their active drug at the desired rate and site of the action. The design is often limited as per the availability of a proper functional group in the active drug for the attachment of a promoiety.
- Rather than using various enzyme systems for the activation of prodrugs, the buffered and relatively constant physiological pH may be used to promote their release. Enzymes considered important to orally administered prodrugs are found in gastrointestinal walls, liver, and blood. In addition, enzyme systems present in the gut microflora may be important in metabolizing prodrugs before they reach the intestinal cells.
- In addition, site-specific delivery can be achieved by exploiting enzymes that are present exclusively or at high concentrations in the targeted tissues relative to non target tissues.

- The process of prodrug development includes three phases– pharmaceutical, pharmacokinetic and pharmacodynamic. Various physical barriers that affect above mentioned parameters are as follows:
  1. Incomplete absorption of the drug through the skin or the blood-brain barrier.
  2. Presystemic metabolism or enzymetic degradation in gastrointestinal lumen, mucosal cell linings and liver may result in incomplete systemic bioavailability.
  3. Rate of absorption or elimination also, onset of action has to be optimized.
  4. Distribution of the drug into the organs other than the target organ may result in local irritation or may be some times toxic.
  5. Poor site-specificity of the drug.
  6. Improved permeability of the drug sometimes may result in avoidance of the first-pass metabolism and may cause side effects.
- The rationale of design of prodrug can be subdivided into 3 steps:
  1. Identification of the drug-delivery problem.
  2. Study of the physicochemical properties of the drug for maximizing the efficacy of the drug delivery.
  3. Selection of the prodrug with desired physicochemical properties so that it can be cleaved in appropriate site of the body.
- Several factors should be considered:
  1. Selection of the functional group on the drug molecule amenable for chemical derivatization.
  2. The mechanism and system of the body required for bioactivation of the prodrug should also be considered.
  3. Synthesis and purification of the prodrug must be simple to proceed.
  4. Stability of the prodrug must be good and prodrug must be compatible with the ingredients used in drug-delivery systems and dosage form.
  5. The prodrug and the promoiety should not be toxic.
  6. The parent drug from the prodrug must be released sufficiently to produce a therapeutic effect in the body.
  7. At last but not least the prodrug should be clinically advantageous than the parent drug.
  8. Evaluation of the biopharmaceutical parameters must be carefully done.

Ideal Characteristics of Prodrug

1. It should not have intrinsic pharmacological activity.
2. It should be rapidly transform, chemically or enzymatically, into the active form where desired.
3. The metabolic fragments, apart from active drug, should be non-toxic.

Advantages of Prodrug

1. Enhancing absorption of drug.
2. Imparting depot activity to the drug.
3. Reducing gastric irritability of a drug.
4. Improving drug stability in vivo and in vitro.
5. Improving site specificity of a drug.

6. Increasing duration of action of drug.
7. Enhancing bioavailability of drug.
8. Diminishing gastrointestinal absorption.
9. Tissue targeting and activation at the site of action.

APPLICATION

1. Pharmaceutical Application

Improvement of taste

- One of the reasons for poor patient compliance, particularly in case of children, is the bitterness, acidity or causticity of the drug.
- Two approaches can be utilized to overcome the bad taste of drug. The first is reduction of drug solubility in saliva and other is to lower the affinity of the drug towards the taste receptors, thus making the bitterness or causticity imperceptible.

Table 9.1: Prodrug with improved taste

Parent drug	Prodrug with improved taste
Chloramphenicol	Palmitate ester
Clindamycin	Palmitate ester
Sulfisoxazole	Acetyl ester
Triamcinolone	Diacetate ester

Improvement of odour

- The odour of a compound depends upon its vapour pressure and hence boliling point; a liquid with high vapour pressure and low boiling point will have strong odour.
- Ethyl mercapten is one of such drug which is a foul smelling liquid of b.p. 35°. The drug useful in the treatment of leprosy is converted into its phthalate ester, which has higher b.p. and is odorless.
- The prodrug is administered by rubbing on the skin. After absorption, the ester is metabolized to parent drug by thioestrases.

Ethyl mercapten → Phthalate ester

Change of physical form of the drug

- Some drugs which are in liquid form are unsuitable for formulation as a tablet especially if their dose is very high.
- The method of converting such liquid drugs into solid prodrugs involves formation of symmetrical molecules having a higher tendency to crystallize, e.g. esters of ethyl mercapten and trichloroethanol.

Ethyl mercapten → Phthalate ester

Trichloroethanol   p - Acetamiddobenzoic acid ester

Reduction of GI irritation

- Several drugs cause irritation and damage to the gastric mucosa through direct contact, increased stimulation of acid secretion or through interference with the protective mucosal layer.
- The NSAIDs especially the salicylates have such a tendency. They lower the gastric pH and induce or aggravate ulceration. Examples of prodrugs designed to overcome such problems of gastric distress are as given in Table 9.2.

Table 9.2: Prodrug that causes little or no gastric distress

Parent drug	Prodrug that cause little/no gastric distress
Salicylic acid	Salsalate, aspirin
Diethylstilbestrol	Fosfestrol
Kanamycin	Kanamycin pamoate
Phenylbutazone	N-methyl piperazine salt
Nicotinic acid	Nicotinic acid hydrazide
Oleandrin	Oleandrin acetate

Reduction of pain on injection

- Intramuscular injection is particularly painful, when the drug precipitates or penetrates into the surrounding cell or when the solution is strongly acidic, alkaline or alcoholic; for example, the low aqueous solubility of clindamycin hydrochloride and the alkaline solution of phenytoin are responsible for pain on injection.
- This can be overcome by use of more water soluble prodrugs of such agents, e.g. the 2 phosphate ester of clindamycin.

Enhancement of solubility and dissolution rate of drug (Table 9.3)

- Hydrophilic or water soluble drugs are desired where dissolution is the rate limiting step in the absorption of poorly aqueous soluble agents or when parental or ophthalmic formulation of such agents are desired.
- Drugs with hydroxyl function can be converted into their hydrophilic forms by use of half-esters such as hemisuccinate, hemiglutarate or hemiphthalates; the other half of these acidic carriers can form sodium, potassium or amine salts and render the moiety water soluble.

Table 9.3: Prodrug with enhanced hydrophilicity

Parent drug	Prodrug with enhanced hydrophilicity
Chloramphenicol	Sodium succinate ester
Tocopherols	Sodium succinate ester
Corticosteroids	21-sodium succinates, 21-phosphate esters
Testosterone	Phosphate ester
Menthol	β-Glucoside
Tetracycline	Glucosyl sulfanilamide
Diazepam	L-lysine ester

- For phenolic drugs and some alcohols as in the case of steroidal drugs such as cortisol, prednisolone and dexmethasone, the sodium succinate salts have poor chemical stability and hence phosphate esters are preferred.
- Glycosidic prodrugs of some agents and L-lysine esters of benzodiazepines are also water soluble. Such hydrophilic promoities when meant for parental use are advantageous over their propylene glycol solutions which are toxic or painful.

Enhancement of chemical stability

- A drug may destabilize either during its shelf-life or in the GIT when used orally. Shelf-life is particularly important in the case of drugs for intravenous use.
- The conventional approach is to lyophilize such a solution into a powder which can be reconstituted before use. The prodrug design of such agents is also a good alternative to improve stability. An example of this is the antineoplastic drug, azacytidine.
- The aqueous solution of this drug is readily hydrolyzed but the bisulfate prodrug is stable to such a degradation at acidic pH and is more water soluble than the parent drug. The prodrug converts into active drug at the physiological pH of 7.4

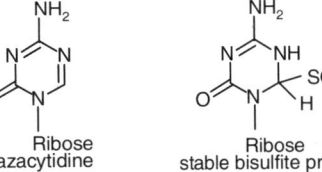

Ribose azacytidine	Ribose stable bisulfite prodrug

- The dry powder of nafate ester of prodrug of cefamandole has improved shelf-life over the parent drug. The prodrugs rapidly convert to the active drug upon reconstitution for the parental administration.
- A class of drugs succeptible to hydrolysis and destabilization in gastric acid is penicillin, carbenicillin, broad-spectrum penicillin, cannot be given orally for the same reason. Its ester prodrugs— carindacillin and carfecillin are however stable at gastric pH. In the intestine, hydrolysis of these agents releases carbenicillin at pH above 7.0. The latter is stable under such a condition and is absorbed intact.

2. Pharmacokinetic Application

Enhancement of Bioavailability

- Most drugs absorbed by passive diffusion for which lipophilicity is an important prerequisite. Two reasons can be attributed to the enhanced oral bioavailability of lipophilic compounds.

Name	R
Ampicillin	H
Becampicillin	
Telecampicillin	
Pivampicillin	

- The lipophilic form of a drug has enhanced membrane/water partition coefficient as compared to the hydrophilic form thus favouring passive diffusion; for example, the pivampicillin, bacampicillin and talampicillin prodrugs of ampicillin are more lipophilic, better absorbed and are rapidly hydrolysed to the parent drug in blood.
- The lipophilic prodrugs, for example, the esters of erythromycin, have poor solubility in gastric fluids and thus greater stability and better absorption
- The dipalmitoyl glycerol ester of NSAID naproxen produces less gastric irritation and higher plasma concentration. The intraocular penetration of polar drugs such as β-blockers and epinephrine, in the treatment of glaucoma, can be promoted by use of lipophilic carrier prodrugs of such agents; for example, the diacetate ester of nadolol is 20 times more lipophilic and 10 times more readily absorbed ocularly. The dipivoloyl ester of epinephrine has good ocular penetrability in comparison to the parent drug.
- A big advantage of increased bioavailability through increased lipophilicity is reduction in drug dosage; e.g. bacampicillin is as effective as ampicillin in just one-third the dose of latter.

Prolongation of duration of action

- Frequent dosing is required for drugs having short biological half-lives; this can be overcome by use of both controlled release and prodrug approaches. The two rate-controlling steps in the enhancement of duration of action are as follows:
  a. The rate of release of prodrug from the site of application or administration in to the systemic circulation
  b. The rate of conversion of prodrug into active drug in the blood.
- The control of either of these two steps would result in prolongation of drug action. The easier approach that of controlling the release rate of prodrug is useful when in vivo conversion of the latter into active drug is rapid. Examples include the *i.m.* depot injection of lipophilic ester prodrug of steroids (testosterone cypionate and propionate, estradiol). Since testosterone and estradiol are natural soft drugs, their lipophilic prodrugs are sometimes called as prodrug-soft drug.
- The second approach of controlled conversion of prodrug to active drug though difficult, was successfully utilized to deliver pilocarpine to eyes in the treatment of glaucoma. The diesters of the drug when applied as ophthalmic solution showed better intraocular penetration due to improved lipophilicity and slow conversion of the ester prodrug to active pilocarpine prolonged the therapeutic effect. The rate of conversion is greatly dependent upon the ester group.

Reduction of toxicity

- An important objective of drug design is to develop one with high activity and low toxicity. Examples of drugs for systemic use with local side effects such as gastric distress with NSAIDs, which can be overcome by prodrug design, have already been discussed.
- Another example of this is the bioprecursor sulindac. As a sulfoxide, it does not cause any gastric irritation and is absorbed better. In blood, it is converted to its active sulfide form.
- The utility of some drugs for local use is limited by the incidence of systemic side effects such as those with timolol and epinephrine which are used in the treatment of glaucoma.
- Therapy of such condition requires instillation of higher concentration of drug since the agents have poor intraocular penetration. But higher doses of such drugs cause irritation to eyes and systemic absorption precipitates undesirable cardiovascular effects. Lipophilic ester prodrugs of such agents on the other hand have better intra-ocular penetration enabling a

reduction in the instilled dose and thus adverse effects are limited; for example the therapeutic index of alkyl ester prodrugs of timolol improved 16 times while that of dipiverfine increased 10 times. The epinephrine prodrug also has improved chemical and biochemical stability.

Site-specific drug delivery

- After its oral administration, the drug is distributed to the various parts of the body including the target site as well as the non-target tissues. Such a distribution pattern has several disadvantages:

  1. The drug may lead to undesirable toxic effects in the non-target tissues.
  2. A smaller fraction of the drug will reach its target site because of dilution due to distribution which may be insufficient to evoke the therapeutic response.
  3. If the target site has a long distribution time, the drug may get eliminated without reaching such site.
  4. Even if the drug reaches the target cells in sufficient amounts, it may not able to penetrate into them.

- This problem can be overcome by targeting the drug to its site of action by altering its deposition characteristics. There are several approaches to drug targeting and prodrug design is one of them.

Selective uptake system

Kidney:

- Dopamine, a neurotransmitter, produces vasodilatation of renal tissues by binding to specific receptors in the kidney and thus can be used to treat renal hypertension. However, the therapeutic index of dopamine is small as it precipates high blood pressure by interaction with the adrenergic receptors.

- This can be overcome by taking advantage of the fact the γ-glutamyl derivatives of amino acids and peptides selectively accumulates in the kidneys.

- Such a derivative of dopamine, on reaching the kidneys, is act upon successively by two enzymes that are present in high concentration in the renal tissues. γ-glutamyl transpeptidase and L-aromatic amino acid decarboxylase to release the active drug dopamine locally. The increase in dopamine levels produces a marked increase in renal blood flow.

Glaucoma:

- Enzymatic activation of the prodrug at the site of action or target is also utilized to deliver epinephrine to eyes in the treatment of glaucoma. The disadvantages of direct ocular administration of adrenaline are known.

Gamma glutamyl DOPA (prodrug)

↓ Gamma glutamyl transpeptidase

DOPA (bioprecursor)   + Glutamic acid

↓ CO_2

Dopamine

↓

Renal vasodilation

- The drug is also known to cause corneal staining. Use of a simple ester prodrug has the disadvantage of being hydrolyzed rapidly because of easy availability of esterases in several tissues.
- Specific delivery to the eyes necessitates presence of a specific ocular enzyme different from esterases that act on a specifc prodrug to activate it.
- The iris-cilliary body of the eyes where the epinephrine acts contains an enzyme ketone reductase in addition to the usual estrases. Hence when a diesters ketone prodrug, di-isovaleryl adrenalone is administered, the sequential reduction-hydrolysis by the two enzymes regenerates adrenaline that shows its pharmacological action at the target site.
- The drug is generated only when reduction preceds hydrolysis. If hydrolysis occurs first, adrenalone formed will not be reduced to epinephrin.

Ulcerative colitis:
- Mesalamine is a drug useful in the treatment of inflammatory bowel disease since it is not absorbed into the systemic circulation. However, following oral administration, the drug is inactivated before reaching the lower intestine, the site of action.

- Covalent binding of this agent to sulfapyridine yields the prodrug sulfasalazine, an azo compound. This prodrug reaches the colon intact where cleavage by the bacterial enzyme azo reductase releases the active mesalamine for local action.

2. Redox system for drug delivery to brain
- The high selectivity and poor permeability of the blood-brain barrier (BBB) limits the delivery of hydrophobic drugs to the brain and thus, therapeutic concentration is difficult to achieve.

- Conversion into their lipophilic forms leads to simultaneous enhancement of transport of drug to other tissues thereby greatly increasing the chances of systemic toxicity. Moreover, to achieve therapeutic levels in the brain, the plasma concentration of the drug has to be very high. Thus, specific delivery of the drug to the brain is very difficult.

- A more recent, novel and smart approach for delivery of drugs to brain is use of dihydropyridine–pyridinium salt redox system. The drug to be delivered to the brain is covalently linked to the lipoidal dihydropyridine carrier group to form a prodrug which will partition across the highly selective BBB. Following administration, the prodrug is rapidly distributed throughout the body as well as in the brain.

- The reduced or the dihydro form of the carrier prodrug is oxidized by NAD-NADH systeme, both, in the brain and the body, to form lipid insoluble, polar quaternary pyridinium salt form (which is inactive).

- Due to high hydrophilicity of such an ionic prodrug, the amount present in the systemic circulation is subjected to rapid renal excretion but the similar polar form present in the brain is prevented from diffusing out of the lipophilic BBB resulting in its lock-in the CNS.

- The drug is slowly released from such an oxidized prodrug into the CSF by chemical/enzymatic process, allowing the therapeutic concentration to be maintained over a prolonged period of time. Thus, the drug is preferentially targeted over a prolonged period of time. Thus, the drug is preferentially targeted to the brain where as its systemic concentration is negligible.

- The choice of the carrier in such a redox system is important; it must be nontoxic, both, when alone and as a conjugate with the drug. The carrier that was used successfully is trigonelline (N-methyl nicotinic acid) the technology holds great potential in treating various condition of brain caused by neurotransmitter disorder such as Parkinsonism as was proved by successful delivery of dopamine to the brain of rats.

- A similar approach was utilizes to treat poisoning with organophosphorus compounds (nerve gas) which are cholinesterase inhibitors.

- The antidote, N-methyl pyridinium-2-carbaldoxime (pralidoxime), a potent reactivator of cholinesterase penetrates the BBB poorly due to its quaternary nitrogen. However, the reduced dihydropyridine form of 2-PAM, called as pro-2-PAM, readily enteres the CNS. Once inside the brain, it is oxidized to polar 2-PAM and thus trapped in the CNS.

3. Site-specific drug delivery in cancer

- Several cancerous tissues and tumors are rich in certain enzymes as compared to those found in normal tissues. Thus, a prodrug can be designed to selectively target such tumor cells where it can be activated to parent antineoplastic agents. The approach protects the normal cells from the cytotoxic effects of the drug.

  1. Prostrate carcinomas are particularly rich in enzymes acid phosphatase. This fact is used to design stilbestrol diphosphate to treat such conditions. The prodrug is activated to yield stilbestrol exclusively in the target organ.

  2. Prostate cancer can also be treated by utilizing the fact that estrogen has strong and specific affinity for such a tissue. Thus, nitrogen mustard linked to estradiol can be used for selective targeting of prostate where hydrolysis of the prodrug will release the cytotoxic mustard to destroy the cancer cells.

  3. Hepatic carcinoma is rich in azo-reductase levels. Azobenzene mustard prodrug can thus be targeted to such a tissue where it is cleaved to release the active drug.

- A novel approach of the above technology in the treatment of cancer is use of antibody directed enzyme prodrug therapy (ADEPT). The method involves conjugating to the antitumor antibody, a specific enzyme that selectively activates the prodrug of a cytotoxic agent.
- When such an enzyme–antibody conjugate is administered, the antibody selectively attaches to tumor cells. Such an antibody that carries the enzyme specifically to the carcinoma/target site is called as homing device.
- Subsequent administration of the prodrug of cytotoxic agents results in its activation only by the enzyme at the target site thus destroying only the tumor cells,. In mice, the ADEPPT technique was found to be more effective than the conventional chemotherapy.
- The forgoing discussion on the several applications of prodrug design suggests that the gain in therapeutic benefits from an approach may either be modest or marked. For well-accepted useful drugs that display some unwanted property which can be ameliorated by prodrug design, the gain is usually modest but real.
- Prodrugs of such agents are called as post-hoc designed. On the other hand, for active compounds that suffer from some severe limitation, e.g. high hydrophilicity restricting bioavailability, prodrug design leads to marked therapeutic gain. Prodrugs of such agents are called as ad-hoc designed.

Limitation of Prodrug Design

One of the biggest problems that can arise in prodrug design is the toxicity, which may be due to:

1. Formation of an unexpected metabolite from the total prodrug that may be toxic.
2. The inert carrier generated following cleavage of prodrug may also transform into toxic metabolite.
3. During its activation stage, the prodrug might consume a vital cell constituent such as glutathione leading to its depletion.
4. An example of generation of reactive intermediates from prodrug is phenacetin. The activity of this agent is due to formation of paracetamol by de-ethylation. Compared to phencetin, paracetamol is relatively safe unless used in high doses. Phenacetin, apart from generating acetaminophen, is also hydrolyzed at the acetamido likage to form p-phenetidine, which is further metabolized to yield products that precipitate methemoglobinemia, hemolysis and renal toxicity. Moreover, the N-hydroxylated metabolites of phenacetin generate reactive intermediate.

Unit II

Drugs Affecting on Autonomic Nervous System

10

General Consideration of Autonomic Nervous System (ANS)

Cellular systems for the transduction of external stimuli into intracellular signals are essential components of the plasma membranes.

- According to the theory of neurohumoral transmission, specific chemical agents are responsible for transmission of nerve impulse across most synapse and neuro-effector junction. These agents are known as neurohumoral transmitters.

- The concept of "chemical neurotransmission" was first proposed by Dale and co-workers, instead of electrical transmission hypothesis. The release of transmitter substance occurs when the nerve impulse elicits the response at smooth, cardiac and skeletal muscles, exocrine glands and postsynaptic neurons.

- These neurotransmitters cross the synapse or the neuro-effector junction to initiate activity in another neuron or in muscle or a gland cell by interacting with the postsynaptic receptors. A clear understanding of the impulse transmission therefore, is essential to study the pharmacology of the drug acting on autonomic nervous system.

NERVOUS SYSTEM

Principally, the nervous system may be described as a device of:

1. Receiving information (i.e. sensory input).
2. Processing information (i.e. integration).
3. Transmitting information (i.e. motor output).

The fundamental unit of nervous system is the neuron or nerve cell (Fig. 10.1). Each neuron consists of a nucleus and a cell body from which, stems an extensive network of branches, the axon – (long process) and the dendrites (short process).

Mechanism of Nerve Transmission

- The surface membrane of a neuron consists of a semipermeable layer of lipoprotein. The composition of salt solution inside the membrane is usually different from that on the outside.

- This is due to difference in the permeability of the membrane to the various ions like Na^+, K^+ Ca^{++} Cl^-, HCO_3^-, etc. In the resting state, the inside of neuronal membrane is more negative than the outside.

- This normal situation is known as resting state or polarized state. When any exogenous stimulus is applied; a change in the electrical activity occurs within the neuron. At the point, where an exogenous stimulus occurs, the inside neuronal membrane becomes positive than the outside.

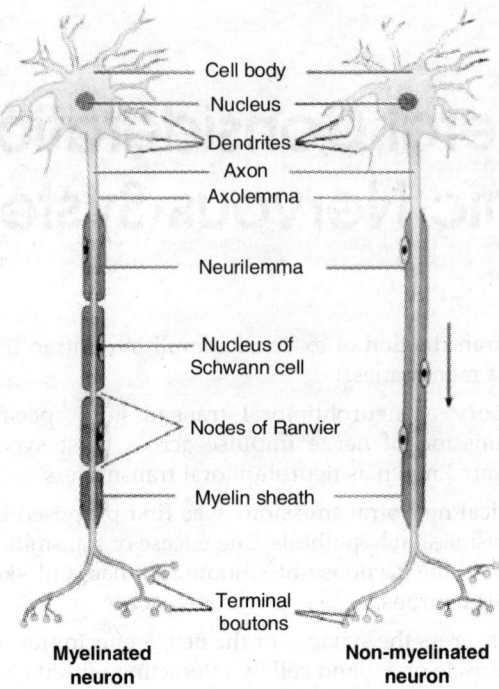

Fig. 10.1: Nerve cell or neuron

- As a result, local action currents are set up, which have the effect of transferring the area of reversed polarization to an adjoining region of the nerve while normal resting conditions are re-established in the previously stimulated area.

- In this way, the path of reversed polarization is transmitted along with nerve. This process is continued until the whole length of the nerve has been visited by the impulse. The nerve impulse, in other words, jumps from one patch to other patch. As soon as this impulse reaches the terminal buttons, it activates the influx of extracellular Ca^{++} ions. These ions, upon their entry in the cytoplasm lead to the release of intracellular Ca^{++} ions from the sacs present on sarcoplasmic reticulum.

- When the cytoplasmic concentration of Ca^{++} ions reaches a threshold value, the storage granules for neurotransmitter get ruptured and a discrete amount of neurotransmitter is discharged from the presynaptic nerve endings into the synaptic cleft. The synaptic cleft or junctional cleft is generally about 200-400A° wide but in some blood vessels, it may be as wide as 10,000A°.

- The transmitter then diffuses across the synaptic space and binds to the receptor sites present on the cell body of post-synaptic neuron. This binding causes conformational changes in these receptors, which in turn, produce a change in ion-permeability of the axon membrane of post-synaptic neuron.

- As a result, local action currents are set up into the post-synaptic neuron. The post-synaptic axon branches many times upon entering the effector tissue forming a plexus among the innervated cells. The release of neurotransmitter from post-synaptic nerve terminals into the neuro-effector space then leads to the biological response in a muscle or a gland cell.

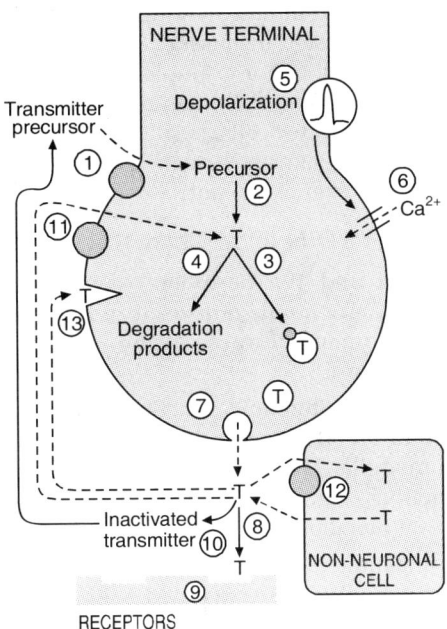

Fig. 10.2: The main processes involved in synthesis, storage and release of amine and amino acid transmitters

1. Uptake of precursors, 2. Synthesis of transmitter, 3. Uptake/transport of transmitter into vesicles, 4. Degradation of surplus transmitter, 5. Depolarization by propagated action potential, 6. Influx of Ca^{2+} in response to depolarization, 7. Release of transmitter by exocytosis, 8. Diffusion to postsynaptic membrane, 9. Interaction with postsynaptic receptors, 10. Inactivation of transmitter, 11. Reuptake of transmitter or degradation products by nerve terminals, 12. Uptake of transmitter by non-neuronal cells and 13. Interaction with presynaptic receptors. The transporters (11 and 12) can release transmitter under certain conditions by working in reverse. These processes are well characterized for many transmitters (e.g. acetylcholine, monoamines, amino acids, ATP). Peptide mediators differ in that they may be synthesized and packaged in the cell body rather than the terminals.

- This synapse between a motor neuron and effector cell is also termed as a neuro-effector junction.
- Once the neurotransmitter has interacted with the receptors, it is either removed by active uptake process back to the terminal buttons of presynaptic neuron or by surrounding glial cells where it is destroyed by metabolic deactivation. (Fig. 10.2)

Neuro-Chemical Transmitter

- Following are the examples of chemical agents that act as neuro-chemical transmitter in nervous system.
  1. Aspartic acid, taurine, glycine, gamma amino butyric acid (GABA) and glutamic acid. These can be grouped as amino acids.
  2. Acetylcholine, dopamine, tyramine, norepinephrine, epinephrine, histamine and serotonin. These can be grouped as amines.
  3. Miscellaneous includes peptide substance P, ATP, cAMP, cGMP, prostaglandin E, enkephallins, etc.

- Neurotransmitters have an ability to initiate the impulse propagation. Certain substances do not initiate the process of the impulse transmission but can be modify it. Such substances are termed as modulators of transmission. For example, most of the autonomic drugs act either by mimicking or modifying the action of the neurotransmitter released by the autonomic fibers at either synaptic cleft or effector cells, besides this, the nerve cell is provided with a number of feedback control systems which regulate the biosynthesis, release and metabolism of the neurotransmitter and thus exercise a control over the biological response.

▨ AUTONOMIC NERVOUS SYSTEM (Flow Chart 10.1)

- The ANS consists of central and the peripheral components. It is evident from the investigation that elicitation of autonomic reflexes (e.g. blood pressure changes, vasomotor response to alteration of body temperature, sweating, constriction of urinary bladder) can occur at the level of the spinal cord.

- However, integration of much autonomic function occurs at supraspinal levels. Thus, regulation of respiration and blood pressure is integrated in medulla. The hypothalamus plays a prominent role in medulla. The hypothalamus plays a prominent role in integration of various autonomic functions, e.g. regulation of blood pressure, sleep, emotions, sexual reflexes carbohydrate and fat metabolism.

- Posterior and lateral hypothalamic nuclei are connected with the sympatho-adrenal system, while anterior and midline nuclei are concerned with parasympathetic functions. The posterior-medial hypothalamus is involved in the modulation of the baroreceptor reflex.

- The other higher centeres involved in the integration of various autonomic functions include the neo-startum, limbic system and cerebral cortex.

- The autonomic nervous system (ANS) controls all involuntary actions aimed to maintain the constancy of the internal environment. It provides a homeostasis for the regulation of all metabolic changes which are essential for life. The ANS is termed as the visceral, vegetative or involuntary nervous system. In the periphery, it functions through, ganglia, plexus and regulates autonomic functions which are not under the conscious control.

Flow chart 10.1: Classification of nervous system

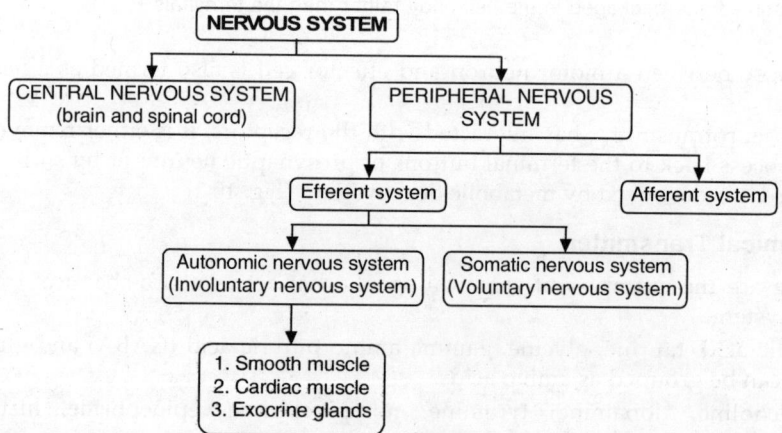

- These include breathing, regulation of the cardiovascular system, glandular secretion, digestion, body temperature and metabolism. Except skeletal muscles, all innervated organs of the body, are supplied with efferent nerves of ANS, while skeletal muscle are provided with somatic nerves.

- Thus, ANS is essentially a motor system. The sensory fibers are numerous than autonomic motor nerves and they pass into the cerebrospinal axis via either somatic nerves or various ramification of ANS without synaptic interruption.
- Hypothalamus is a principle control center for organization and co-ordination of the autonomic nervous system. The cell of the adrenal medulla constitutes an integral part of the ANS, which upon activation, release epinephrine and norepinephrine in to the circulation.

Division of ANS (Fig. 10.3)

- The autonomic nervous system controls tissue, e.g. glands, smooth muscle and cardiac muscle that are under voluntary control. It consists of two main divisions:
  1. Sympathetic nervous system.
  2. Parasympathetic nervous system.
- Both these have essentially opposite action. The sympathetic nervous system is associated with catabolic effects whereas parasympathetic nervous system is characterized by its anabolic effects.

1. The principal neurotransmitter presents in parasympathetic nerves liberates acetylcholine.
2. The preganglionic and post-ganglionic fibers of the parasympathetic nerves liberate acetylcholine.
3. The preganglionic fibers and some post-ganglionic fibers (e.g. salivary glands) of sympathetic nerves liberate acetylcholine.
4. All autonomic ganglia and skeletal muscle end plate region need acetylcholine as a neurotransmitter to evoke biological response. The end plate is a specialized region of the muscle with which the terminal ramification of the motor nerve fiber associated. The ganglionic transmission is a highly complex process and several secondary transmitters or modulators either enhance or diminish the sensitivity of the post-ganglionic cell to acetylcholine.

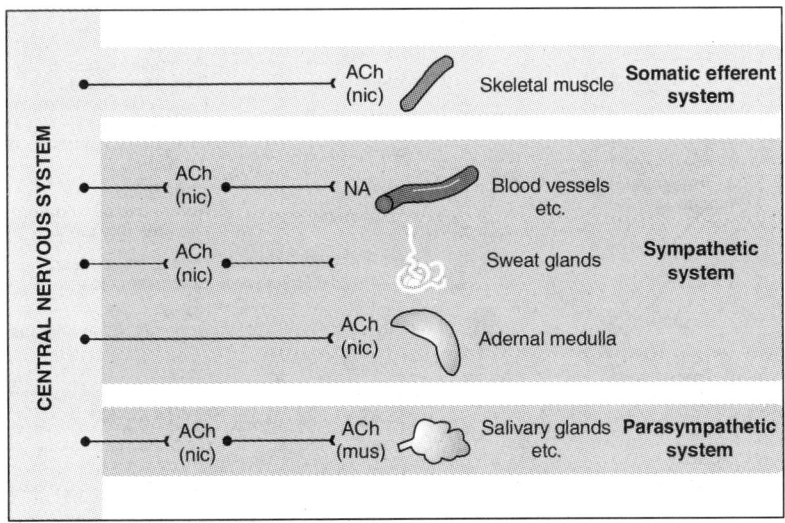

Fig. 10.3: Classification of ANS

Function (Fig. 10.4)

1. Stimulation of parasympathetic nervous system induces the constriction of the pupils, bronchi, decrease in heart activity and an increase in the activity of the digestive system, salivation and GIT secretion are promoted, and the motility of the intestine is increased.

2. Similarly, the principal neurotransmitters present in the sympathetic nervous system include epinephrine (adrenaline) norepinephrine (noradrenaline) and dopamine. The post-ganglionic fibers of the sympathetic nerves with few exceptions bring about their effects by the liberation of norepinephrine.

3. Stimulation of the sympathetic nervous system causes dilation of the pupils, acceleration of rate of (positive chronotropic) and the force of vasoconstriction, glycogenolysis, inhibition of intestinal motility and gastrointestinal secretory activity (except salivary gland).

4. When the transmitter substance reacts with the post-synaptic receptors, it may produce either excitation or inhibition. The action of the transmitter results in selective increase or decrease of ionic permeability of membrane for ions. In inhibition, there is a negligible change in the potential and the fibers remain at near to the resting potential, thereby preventing the fiber to get in an excited position.

5. The transmitter in the neurons is in a state of flux, being continuously biosynthesized, released and metabolized, thus producing profound changes in the activity of the nerves.

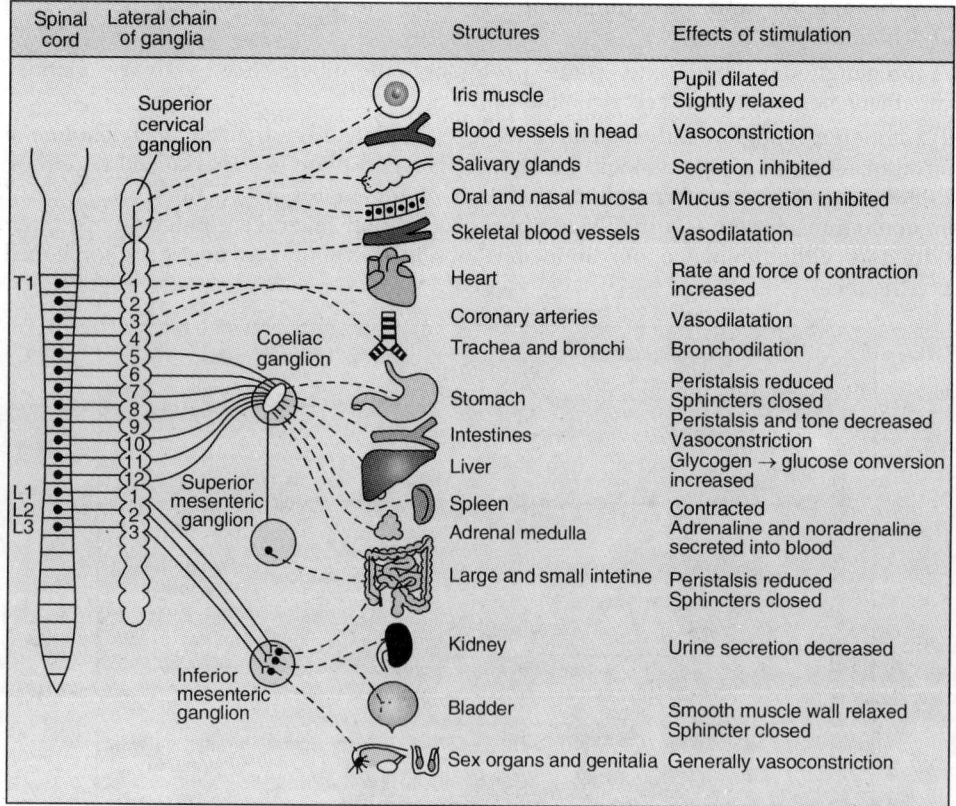

Fig. 10.4: Distribution of ANS nerves and their function

NERVES OF PERIPHERAL SYSTEM

- The nerves in the peripheral nervous system (Fig. 10.5) are classified on the basis of their function into:
  1. Sensory (afferent) neuron.
  2. Motor (efferent) neuron.
  3. Internuncial neuron.
- Sensory neurons transmit impulse from CNS to or towards the muscle or tissues.
- Internuncila neurons are located in CNS and they transmit impulse from sensory to the motor neurons.
- Many neurotransmitter play an important role in the propogation of the nerve impulse in the sensory neurons. These include substance P, Somatostatin, Vasoactive intestinal polypeptides and Cholecytokinin.

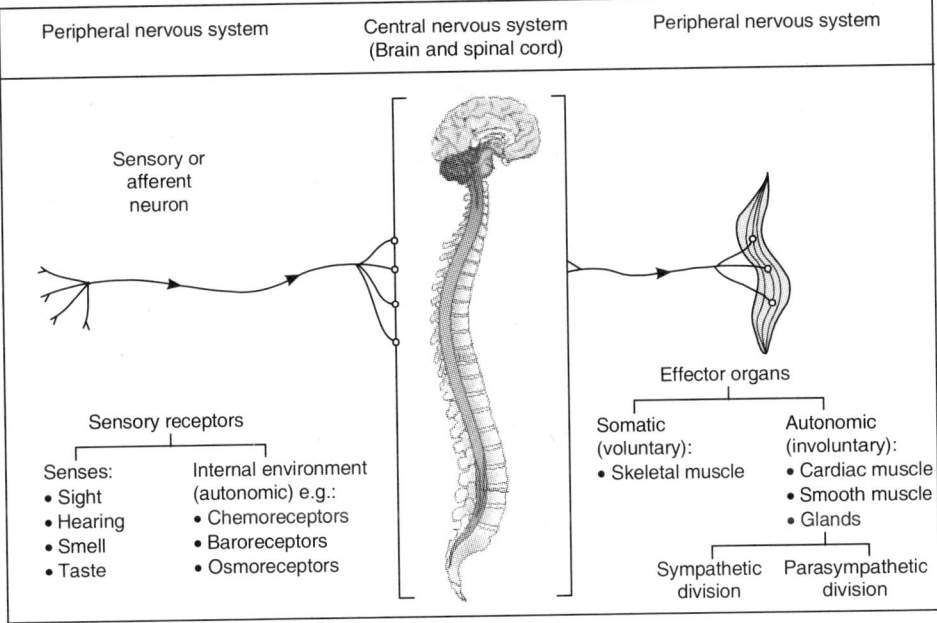

Fig. 10.5: Peripheral nervous system

Efferent Nervous System of ANS (Fig. 10.6)

- The efferent (motor) nervous system of ANS can be broadly categorized into;
  1. Parasympathetic (or craniosacral) division.
  2. Sympathetic (or thoracolumbar) division.
- This classification is mainly based upon the type of neurotransmitters that predominant in each division.
- The cholinergic nervous system consists of preganglionic and post-ganglionic fibers. The preganglionic fibers have their origin in midbrain, medulla oblongata and the sacral part of the spinal cord. Thus, the principal site of control and co-ordination of both sympathetic and para-sympathetic nervous systems is hypothalamus.

- The hypothalamus along with cerebral cortex serves as locus of integration of the entire autonomic nervous system. Hypothalamus also plays an important role in the regulation of gastrointestinal, cardiovascular, sexual, emotional and the functioning of limbic system.

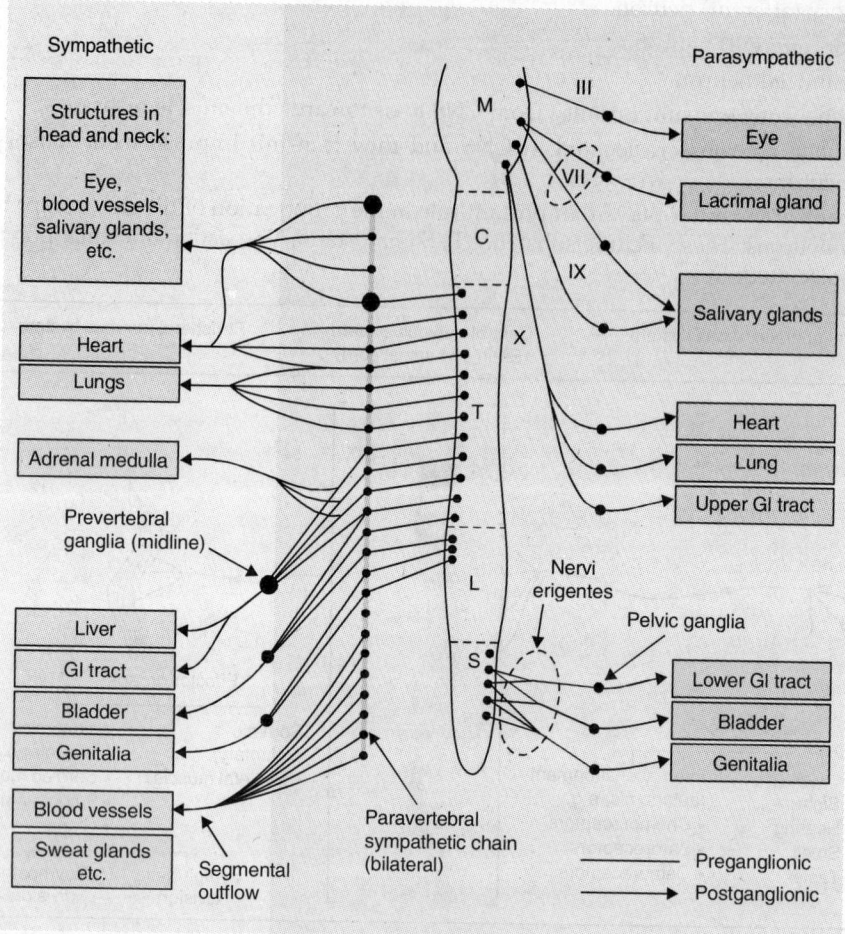

Fig. 10.6: Efferent nervous system of ANS

- In contrast to other cholinergically innervated organs, the cardiac impulse conduction system (i.e. SA node, AV node, Purkunje fiber) has its own activity where the conduction of impulse can be influenced but not initiated by autonomic nervous system. In cardiac cell, cholinergic influences result into inhibitory response due to hyperpolarization. The hyperpolarization results due to the increased permeability of the axon membrane to potassium ions.

- In parasympathetic division, a preganglionic fiber synapses with one or at the most two post-ganglionic neurons. The synapses are located very close to or within the organ innervated.

- Due to the limited distribution, parasympathetic preganglionic neurons can affect only specific organ and do not influence a wide region of the body. In contrast to this, sympathetic synapses are located in the vertebral and prevertbral ganglia.
- Hence, a single sympathetic preganglionic fiber may synapse with 60 to 189 post-ganglionic neurons provided to a widely separated regions of the body. Naturally upon activation, sympathetic nervous system can evoke and influence the biological activities of the whole body.
- The area of functioning of parasympathetic divisions is thus limited and involves accumulation and preservation of body resources. While sympathetic division regulates body compartment of vital importance and prepares the person in condition of stress and emergencies. Its stimulation results in a generalized somatic or mass reflex action.

Parasympathomimetics (Cholinergic Agents)

Cholinergic agents are drugs that either directly or indirectly produce effect similar to those elicited by acetylcholine (ACh).

- Acetylcholine was first synthesized by Bayer in 1867. In general, stimulation of parasympathetic nervous system induces constriction of pupil and bronchi, decrease in heart activity and an increase in the activity of digestive system, i.e. salivation, GIT secretion are promoted and motility of the intestine is also increased.

CHEMICAL FEATURE OF ACETYLCHOLINE

Following are some of the important chemical feature of acetylcholine molecule.

1. Chemically, it is an ester of acetic acid and choline, an amino alcohol.
2. On the structural basis, it offers three sites for molecular modification.
   a. Acetyl group.
   b. Ethylene bridge.
   c. Quaternary ammonium group.

$$H_3C-\overset{\overset{O}{\|}}{C}-O-CH_2-CH_2-N^+\overset{CH_3}{\underset{CH_3}{-CH_3}}$$

Acetyl group | Ethylene bridge | Quaternary ammonium cations

3. The quaternary nitrogen atom bearing a strong positive charge in the center of the so called cationic head and gives acetylcholine (ACh) its basic character. The cationic head fits into a depression in the receptor surface, the anionic site, which bears a negative electrical charge.
4. The alkylamine chain provides a bridge of the correct length between the cationic head and acetyl group of the ACh molecule. Increase or decrease in the length of the alkylamine chain markedly reduces the muscarinic potency.
5. The acetyl group forms the third part of the ACh molecule and bears an overall negative charge. This group is thought to fit into a depression in the receptor surface bearing a positive charge and called esteratic site.
6. Acetylcholine is stable in acidic solution but it is very unstable in alkaline media.
7. Free acetylcholine presents in the tissue fluid and in circulation it is rapidly hydrolysed to acetic acid and choline molecules by cholinesterase enzyme.
8. Acetylcholine exhibits some of its actions via muscarinic receptors while remaining action is propagated through nicotinic receptors.

▨ BIOSYNTHESIS, STORAGE AND RELEASE (FIG. 11.1)

- It is synthesized within the cholinergic neurons by the transfer of an acetyl group from acetyl-coenzyme A to the organic base choline. A specific enzyme choline acetyltransferase is necessary for this reaction.
- Co-enzyme A is widely distributed in the body and choline is an essential dietary constituent, belonging to the B-complex group of vitamins.
- Choline acetyltransferase is synthesized in the cell bodies of cholinergic neurons. ACh is produced throughout the neurons and is stored in synaptic vesicle, which are mainly accumulated at the nerve ending.

In mitochondria:

Step-I

$$\text{Acetate + ATP} \longrightarrow \text{Adenylacetate}$$

In axonal cytoplasm:

Step-II

$$\text{Adenylacetate + Coenzyme A} \xrightarrow{\text{Acetyl kinase}} \text{Acetyl CoA}$$

Step-III

$$\text{Acetyl – CoA + Choline} \xrightarrow{\text{Choline acetylase}} \text{Acetylcholine + CoA}$$

- ACh (acetylcholine), which is produced, is stored in the synaptic vesicle. On the receipt of a stimulus, they combine with the membrane of the nerve ending and discharge their content to the synaptic cleft by a process of exocytosis.

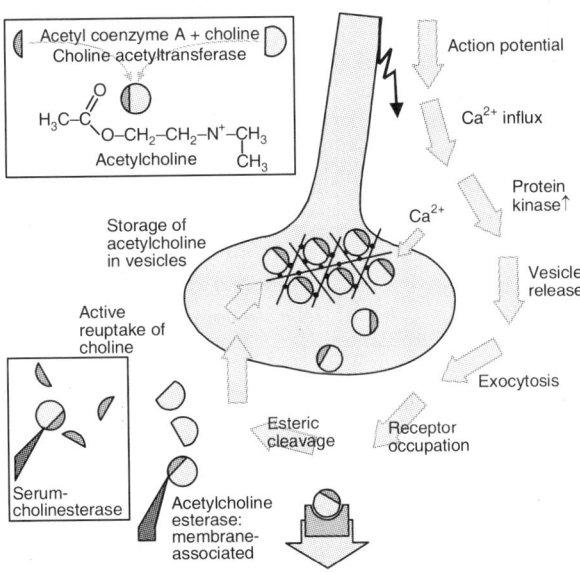

Fig. 11.1: Synthesis, release and hydrolysis of acetylcholine

- Sufficient amount of ACh binds with receptor and produces pharmacological action. Excess of acetylcholine is hydrolysed by that of acetylcholinesterase enzyme.

■ HYDROLYSIS OF ACETYLCHOLINE

At the synaptic cleft ACh (excess amount) is hydrolysed by that of the acetyl cholinesterase enzyme which is present at synaptic cleft. It involves following stages;

Stage-I: Cationic head of ACh is absorbed on the anionic site of the acetylcholinesterase (ACHE) molecule and forms salt. The ester group of ACh is adsorbed on the esteratic site of the ACHE molecule. In this way, ACh forms complex with enzyme.

Stage-II: These steps involve splitting. The substrate enzyme complex reacts to release choline and acetylated enzyme.

Step-III: The third stage of hydrolysis leads to regeneration of the enzyme. The acylated enzyme reacts with water to give acetic acid and liberate enzyme. Thus, the enzyme is regenerated.

■ RECEPTORS

Acetylcholine binds with two receptors and produce respective function. These are :

1. Muscarinic (M) (Table 11.1)
2. Nicotinic (N) (Table 11.2)

Table 11.1: Muscarinic receptors

Muscarinic receptor's subtype	M_1	M_2	M_3
Location and function observed	Autonomic ganglia: Depolarization Gastric glands: Histamine release and acid secretion	SA node : Hyperpolarization, decrease rate of impulse generation AV node: Decrease velocity of conduction Atrium and ventricles: Decrease contractility	Visceral smooth muscle: Contraction Exocrine gland: Secretion Vascular endothelium: Vasodilation

Table 11.2: Nicotinic receptors

Nicotinic receptors subtype	N_M	N_N
Location and function observed	Neuromuscular junction: Contraction of skeletal muscle	Autonomic ganglia: Depolarization Adrenal medulla: Catecholamine release CNS: Site specific excitation or inhibition

▒ PHARMACOLOGICAL ACTION

Depending on the type of receptors through which it is mediated the peripheral action of the ACh may be classified as muscarinic or nicotinic. The central actions are also classifiable and are described separately.

Muscarinic Action (Fig. 11.2)

Heart

- ACh hyperpolarizes the SA nodal cells and decreases the rate of diastolic depolarization. As a result, rate of impulse generation is reduced– bradycardia or even cardiac arrest may occur.
- At the AV node and His–Purkunje fibers, refractory period is increased and conduction is slowed; P-R interval increases and partial to complete AV block may be produced. The force of atrial contraction is markedly reduced and RP of atrial fibers is abbreviated. Due to no uniform vagal innervations, the intensity of effects on RP and conduction of different atrial fibers varies – inducing in homogenecity and predisposing to atrial fibrillation or flutter.
- Ventricular contractility is also decreased but the effects are not marked.

Blood Vessels

- All blood vessels are dilated though only few (skin of face, neck) receive cholinergic innervations.
- Thus, fall in BP and flushing, especially in the blush area occurs. Muscarinic receptors are present on the vascular endothelial cells. Vasodilation is primarily mediated through the release of endothelium dependant relaxing factor (EDRF) which is nitric oxide (NO).
- It may also be due to inhibitory action of ACh on NA release from tonically active vasoconstrictors nerve endings.

Smooth Muscle

- Smooth muscle in most organs is contracted. Tone and peristalsis in the gastrointestinal tract is increased and sphincters relax, abdominal cramps and evacuation of bowel occurs.
- Peristalsis is increased. The detrusor muscle contracts while the bladder trigone and sphinctre relaxes, voiding of bladder.
- Bronchial muscle constrict, asthmatic are highly sensitive, dyspnea, precipitation of an attack of bronchial asthma.

Glands

- Secretion from all parasympathetically innervated glands increased, sweating, salivation, lacrimation, tracheobranchial and gastric secretion increases.
- The effect on pancreatic and intestinal glands is not marked. Secretion of milk and bile is not affected.

Eye

- Contraction of circular muscle of iris, miosis. Contraction of cilliary muscle, spasm of accommodation, increased outflow facility, reduction in intraocular tension (especially in glaucomatous patients).

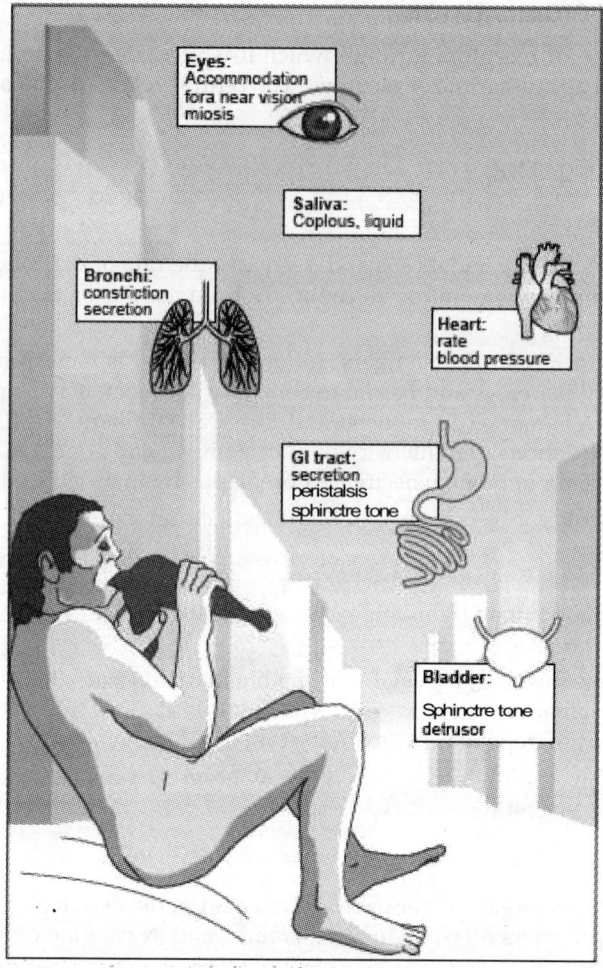

Fig. 11.2: Response to parasympathetic activation

Nicotinic

Autonomic Ganglia

Both sympathetic and parasympathetic ganglia are stimulated. This effect manifested at higher doses. High dose of ACh given after atropine causes tachycardia and rise in BP.

Skeletal Muscle

Iontophoretic application of ACh to muscle end plate causes contraction of the fiber, intra-arterial injection of high dose can cause twitching and fasciculation, but IV injection is generally without any effect (due to rapid hydrolysis of ACh).

CENTRAL NERVOUS SYSTEM

ACh injected IV dose not penetrate blood-brain barrier and no central effects are seen. However, direct injection into the brain of other cholinergic drugs which enter the brain, produce complex pattern of stimulation followed by depression.

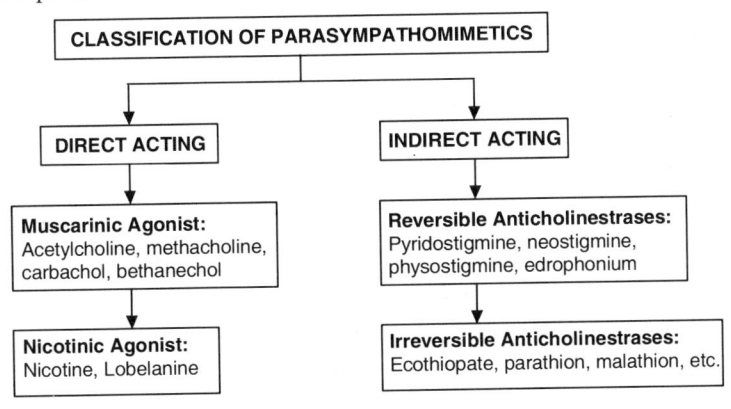

CLASSIFICATION OF PARASYMPATHOMIMETICS

DIRECT ACTING

INDIRECT ACTING

Muscarinic Agonist:
Acetylcholine, methacholine, carbachol, bethanechol

Reversible Anticholinestrases:
Pyridostigmine, neostigmine, physostigmine, edrophonium

Nicotinic Agonist:
Nicotine, Lobelanine

Irreversible Anticholinestrases:
Ecothiopate, parathion, malathion, etc.

Muscarinic Agonist

Carbachol

Methacholine

Pilocarpine

Bethanechol

Oxotremorine

Acetylcholine Chloride

Muscarine

Nicotinic Agonist

Nicotine

Lobeline

Dimethylphenyl piperazinium

Suxamethonium

Decamethonium

Indirectly actinganticholinestrase

A. Reversible anticholinestrase

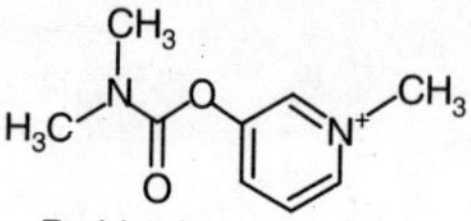

Pyridostigmine

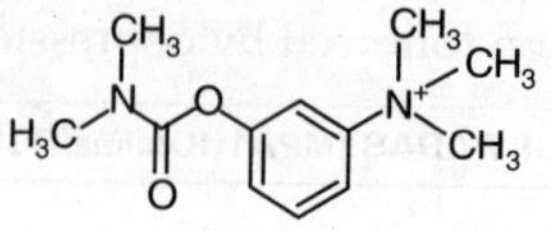

Neostigmine

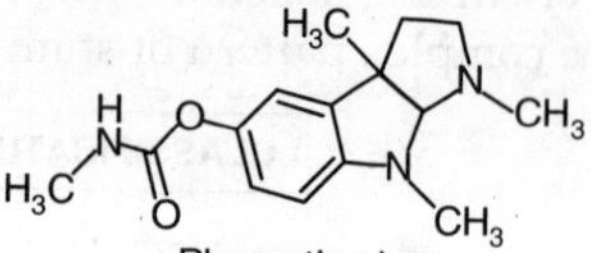

Physostigmine

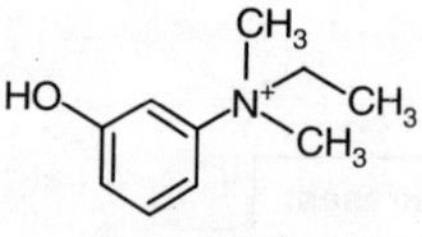

Endrophonium

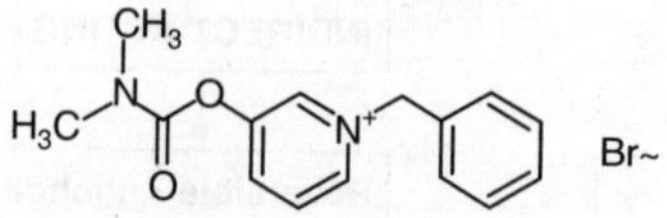

Benzpyrinium bromide

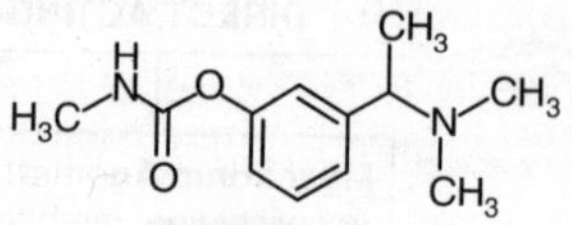

Miotine

B. Irreversible anticholinestrases

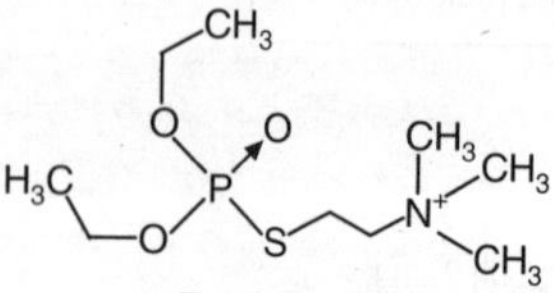

Ecothiopate

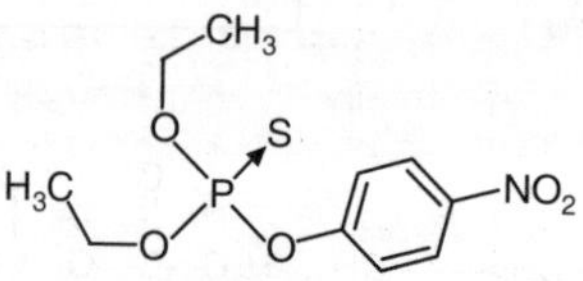

Parathion

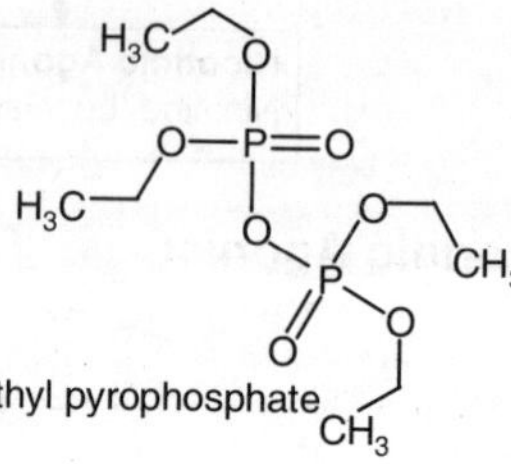

Tetraethyl pyrophosphate

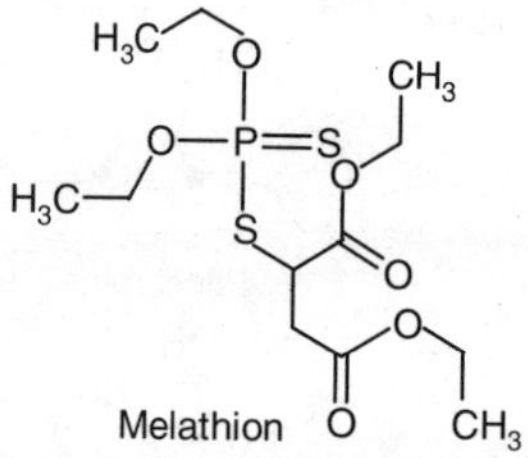

Melathion

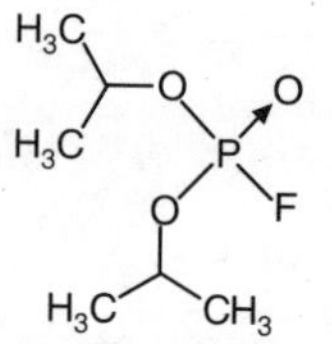

Isoflurophate

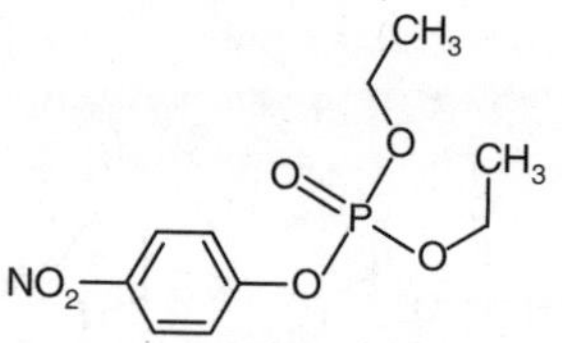

Paraoxon

■ STRUCTURE ACTIVITY RELATIONSHIP

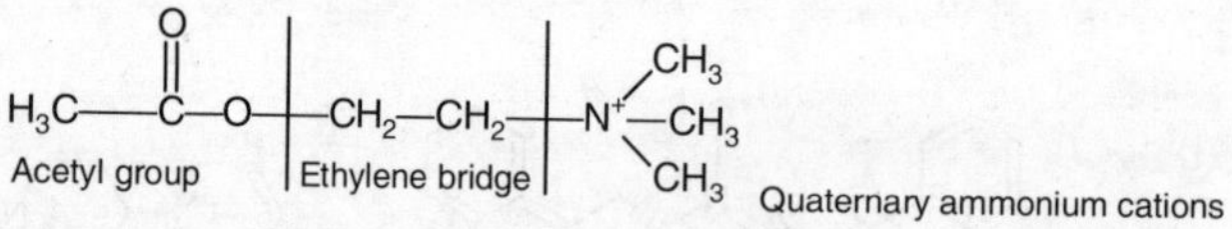

Acetyl group | Ethylene bridge | Quaternary ammonium cations

The Acyloxy Group

1. The higher homologs of methyl group, e.g. propionyl or butyryl are less active than acetylcholine.
2. Esters of aromatic or high molecular weight acids possess cholinergic antagonist activity.
3. The methyl ester is rapidly hydrolysed by cholinesterase.
4. Replacement of ester group with ether or ketone produces chemically more stable and potent compounds. Thus demonstrating that neither the ester functional group nor a carbonyl is required for muscarinic agonistic activity.

5. When the terminal methyl group is replaced by NH_2 group, the resulting compound (the carbamic acid ester), however, is a potent cholinergic with both muscarinic and nicotinic activities.

$$H_2N-\overset{\overset{O}{\|}}{C}-O-CH_2-CH_2-\overset{\overset{CH_3}{|}}{\underset{\underset{CH_3}{|}}{N^{\oplus}}}-CH_3$$

Carbachol

Bethanechol

6. Carbachol is certainly stable to hydrolysis and has the right size to fit the cholinergic receptor. The carbamic acid ester of β -methylcholine is also a stable therapeutic agent. The measured interatomic distances in acetylcholine are 7.0Å ketone oxygen to methyl and 5.3Å ether oxygen to methyl. Obviously, the interprosthetic distances for acetylcholine, methacholine, carbaminoylcholine and urecholine are the same. Apparently, if the interprosthetic distances are optimal, the receptors on the cell do not differentiate between ether, ketone, ester or acetyl oxygen.

7. In carbachol, the terminal methyl group of acetylcholine is replaced by $-NH_2$ group, while size of the molecule remains the same as that of acetylcholine. So it becomes apparent that the size of the molecule may be more important to its activity than the acyl group present. Similarly, the ether oxygen appears to be of primarily importance for higher muscarinic activity. As a result of such reasoning, ethers of choline and alkylamino-ketones were examined for activity.

Choline ethyl ether
(High muscarinic activity)

β-methylcholine ethyl ether
(High muscarinic activity)

8. The reduced biological activity of compound in which oxygen is replaced by sulphur (e.g. thimuscarine) suggests the presence of H-bonding or dipole–dipole interaction between the drug and the receptor because sulphur atom has a less ability to form H-bonds with the receptors.

Thiomuscarine

9. The concept that the ester, i.e. carbonyl or other group is not essential for activity but may enhance it by increasing the affinity of the molecule for the receptor was confined by a study of the muscarinic properties of N-alkyltrimethyl ammonium salts.

N-alkyl trimethyl ammonium salts

10. Compound in this series showed muscarinic activity when n= 1, 2, 3, or 4. Compounds with groups larger than pentyl were partial agonists and those with groups larger than heptyl were antagonists. This appears to belive the hypothesis that size rather than functional group are necessary for intrinsic activity.

11. To reduce the susceptibility of acetylcholine to hydrolysis, acetyl group was replaced with a functional group resistant to hydrolysis. Carbachol were more stable than the acetylcholine because the carbonyl group is less electrophilic. Therefore, carbachol can be administered orally.

Ethylene Bridge

1. As the chain length is increased from 2-carbon to more than 2-carbon atoms, the activity is rapidly reduced.

2. Replacement of the hydrogen atoms of ethylene bridge by methyl groups leads to equal/greater cholinergic activity. Groups larger than methyl lead to decrease in activity.

3. The α or β methyl substituted derivatives affect selectivity. Methacholine (β methyl group) binds selectively on muscarinic receptors. The high selective muscarinic action is due to orientation of methyl group of methacholine in the same position as methylene group in muscarine.

Muscarine   (S)-Methacholine

4. A methyl group alpha to the nitrogen increases nicotinic activity, e.g. acetyl–α-methyl choline is having nicotinic activity.

5. The muscarinic receptors and acetylcholine displays steroselectivity. The S (+) enantiomers of methacholine are equipotent with acetylcholine, while the R (–) enantiomers are about 20-fold less potent.

Quaternary Ammonium Group

1. Quaternary ammonium group is essential for activity.

2. Replacement of nitrogen with sulfur, arsenic or selenium produces less active compounds.

3. Primary, secondary or tertiary amines are less active than acetylcholine.

4. Replacement of methyl groups by ethyl or larger alkyl groups produces inactive compounds.

STEREOCHEMISTRY

1. Acetylcholine can exist in number of conformations. Conformational isomers of ACh derived from rotation around —O—C—C—N axis. Four of these conformations are illustrated by Newman projection below:

Synplaner   Synclinal   Anticlinal   Antiplaner

2. In order to study the conformation requirement of cholinergic activity, rigid analogues of ACh were prepared; cis and trans acetoxy cyclopropyl tri-methyl ammonium (ACTM). Because of cyclopropane ring, the ester and quaternary ammonium functional group cannot change their relative positions by bond rotation.

3. The cis-isomer is similar to the semiplanar conformation of ACh and the trans isomer approximates the anticlinal conformation. The important conclusion drawn from this study was that ACh would most probably interact with muscarinic receptor in its less favored anticlinal conformation.

Cis
Acetoxy cyclopropyl trimethyl ammonium

Trans
Acetoxy cyclopropyl trimethyl ammonium

Binding of the Acetylcholine over Receptors

The hypothetical structure of cholinergic receptor is shown below:

1. The negative charge at the anionic site of the receptor may result from the ionization of a dicarboxylic amino group (i.e. aspartic or glutamic acid) present in the receptor. The quaternary ammonium group forms an electrostatic bond with this anionic site. The ester or other group capable of forming H-bonds interacts at the esteratic site through H-bonding.

2. Since the tissue containing muscarinic receptors are extremely complex, binding studies between acetylcholine analogues and cholinesterases were made. They indicate that the methyl groups present on N-atom along with the terminal methyl group are bound to the receptor by both hydrophobic and van der Waals' forces. This binding assures a close fit of the molecule to the receptor.

Region 1 = Region of hydrophobic binding (van der Waals' force)
Region 2 = Region of hydrogen bonding
Region 3 = Region of ionic bonding

Esteratic site   Anionic site

Pharmacophore of Cholinergic Receptor

1. Beckett proposed that muscarinic receptor contains one anionic and two cationic sites.
2. The anionic site (site 1) accommodates the quaternary nitrogen of muscarine.
3. The site 2 or H-bonding site is for ether oxygen of muscarine or acetylcholine.
4. Site 3 can interact with the carbonyl group of acetylcholine or the ether oxygen of dioxolone or with the alcohol group of muscarine.
5. Although acetylcholine has three reactive sites, only two sites are necessary for the various actions of the compound.

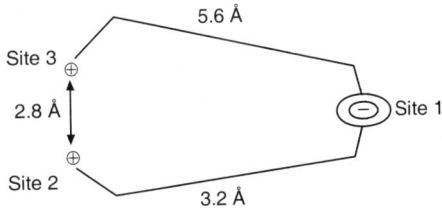

Pharmacophore of acetylcholine at muscarinic receptor site

▨ NICOTINIC AGONISTS (FIG. 11.3)

- These drugs stimulate autonomic ganglia. They selectively act on nicotinic receptors. Nicotinic, lobeline and dimethyl phenylpiperazinium are three drugs that affect ganglionic nicotinic receptors preferentially.

- These substances are of no therapeutic value. Nicotine is important in relation to smoking. Gut motility may be either increased or decreased, though cigarette smoking usually inhibits gastric mobility and diminishes hunger. Secretion of saliva, bronchial mucus and sweat are increased.

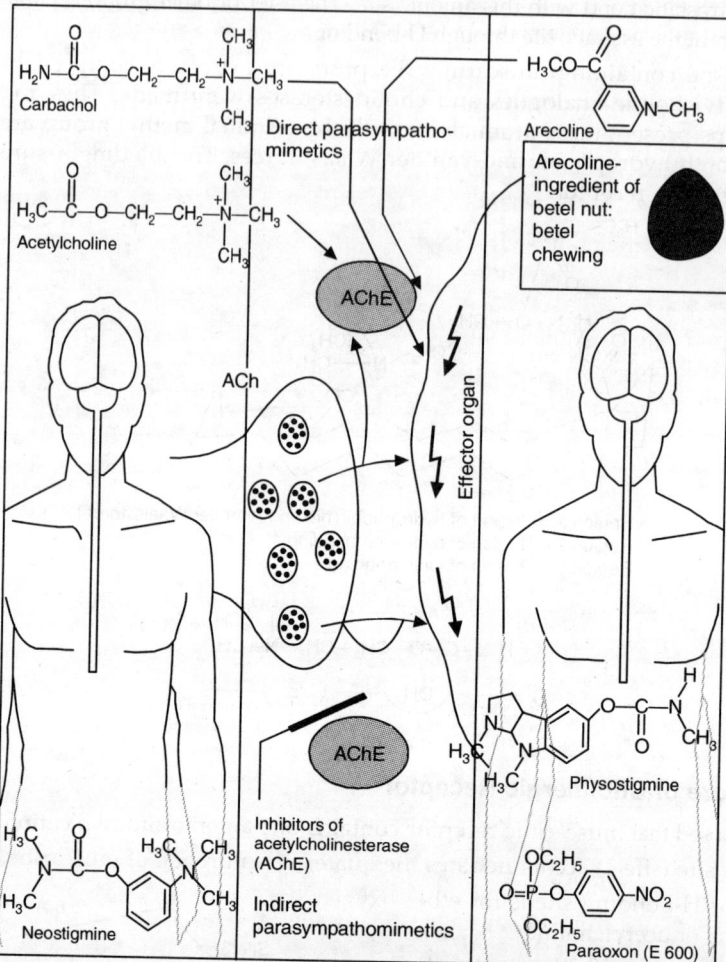

Fig. 11.3: Mode of action of direct and indirect acting drugs

Indirectly Acting Agents

Anticholinesterase

- The cholinesterase enzyme terminates the biological activity of acetylcholine by hydrolyzing acetylcholine into acetic acid and a choline molecule, thus limiting the turnover time of acetylcholine to 150 microseconds. The hydrolysis of acetylcholine occurs through deacetylation reaction which is catalysed by cholinesterase enzyme.
- The cholinesterase present in the human body can be broadly categorised in to;

1. Acetylcholinesterase or true cholinesterase or specific cholinesterase

2. Butyrocholinesterase or pseudocholinesterase or non-specific cholinesterase.

- The specific or acetylcholinesterase is found in RBC in the brain and other nerve tissues. It is present in high concentration on presynaptic sites, postsynaptic membrane sites and at motor nerve end plate regions of cholinergic nervous system.

- At presynaptic sites, its role is to regulate the acetylcholine levels in cholinergic nerve terminals. It is also located in autonomic ganglia and certain cholinergic synapses in CNS. The non-specific or butyrocholinesterase is present in plasma, glial cells, intestine and other organs. The cholinesterases present in the different species or organs sometimes bear basic difference and need not be identical.

- These enzymes are mainly located in the outer basement membrane of the synapse and in the neuromuscular junction cleft. They are also reported to be present in the cisternae of the endoplasmic reticulum. Sometime cholinesterase enzymes have been located in such regions where they cannot claim the role of acetylcholine killer. In such cases, they are supposed to be tied up with some independent activities like;

1. To control membrane permeability.

2. To control the blood level of fatty substances.

- Cholinesterase inhibitors, as the name indicate, increase the concentration of the acetylcholine at the receptor site by inhibiting its metabolism butyrocholinesterases, resulting into prolongation and potentiation of acetylcholine activity at both muscarinic and nicotinic receptors. They do so by competitive antagonism and hence often resemble with acetylcholine in structure.

- The unhydrolysed acetylcholine accumulates and exerts its action. Hence, cholinesterase inhibitors are also termed as indirectly acting cholinomimetic agent.

- The activation of muscarinic receptors results into various muscarinic and nicotinic effects.

Mechanism of Hydrolysis by Cholinesterase (FIG. 11.4)

- The imidazole group of histidine accept a proton from a serine hydroxyl group at the estratic site, creating a strong nucleophiles while OH-from tyrosine just serves as binding site to ether oxygen of the acetoxy group of acetylcholine.

- The anionic site of the enzyme binds with the quaternary nitrogen of the acetylcholine through both ionic and hydrophobic forces. The latter binding force is provided by the presence of three methyl group which are present on the nitrogen. The activated serine, being a strong nucleophile, then attacks on the C atom of carbonyl group of acetylcholine resulting into tetrahedral intermediates. This intermediate is very short-lived and its collapse results into the release of choline molecule, leaving the acetylated serine residue on the enzyme.

- The choline molecule readily dissociate from the anionic site, since it is bound only by van der Waals' forces and hydrophobic forces. The acetyl group, however, forms a covalent bond with the nucleophile group (activated serine residue) of the enzymes. The acylated enzyme then undergoes a conformational change which brings the acetylated serine in close proximity to the second imidazole residue.

- In presence of a water molecule, the imidazole residue catalyzes hydrolysis of acetylated serine to give acetic acid and serine residue. This step is rate limiting step which occurs at very rapid rate and the enzyme is thereby efficiently regenerated back.

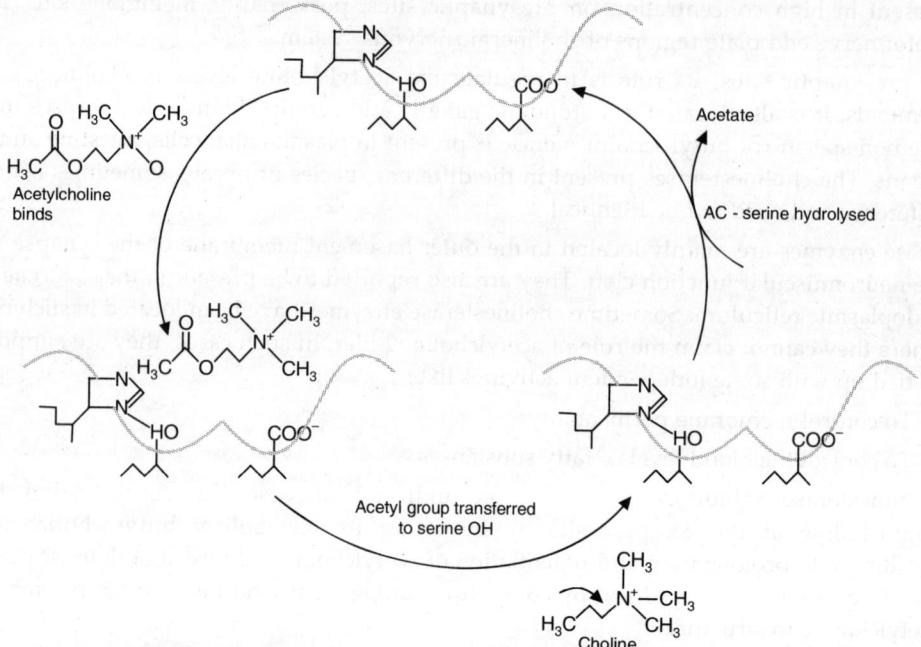

Acetylcholine binds

Acetate

AC - serine hydrolysed

Acetyl group transferred to serine OH

Choline

Fig. 11.4: Mechanism of acetylcholine hydrolysis by acetylcholinesterase

Classification of Anticholinesterase

The anti-cholinesterases are classified in to;

1. Reversible anti-cholinestrases.
2. Irreversible anti-cholinestrases.

1. Reversible Anticholinesterases

- They bear a structural resemblance to acetylcholine, hence capable of combining with the anionic and esteratic sites of cholinesterases and receptor as well.
- They have a great affinity for active sites but no intrinsic activity. This produces the temporary inhibition of the enzyme. In contrast to other reversible cholinesterases, edrophonium forms reversible complex only with the anionic site and hence has a shorter duration of action.
- These can be further divided as:
    1. **Naturally occurring**– physostigmine.
    2. **Synthetic**– neostigmine, pyridostigmine, miotine, demacarium, edrophonium and benzpyrinium.
- In neostigmine, increased stability to hydrolysis is achieved by using a dimethyl carbamate in place of methyl carbamate group. Because of charged nitrogen, neostigmine cannot cross the blood-brain barrier and cause CNS side effects.

SAR:

1. The distance across the ether oxygen and nitrogen atoms approximately same as that between the ether oxygen and nitrogen atoms in acetylcholine.

Pyridostigmine

2. The two heterocyclic rings of physostigmine are not essential for anticholinesterases activity. During hydrolysis, the phenolic fragment of this drug is eliminated, leaving the carbamoyl group attached to the enzyme. The rate of hydrolysis of carbamoyl group is about 60 times less than the rate of hydrolysis of acyl group of acetylcholine.

Physostigmine

2. Irreversible Anticholinesterases

- Organophosphorus compounds combine only with phosphorylated esteratic site. The hydrolysis of this phosphorylated site, however, is extremely slow which produces a long-term inhibition of cholinesterases. In contrast to other organophosphorus compounds, ecothiopate forms complex with both anionic and esteratic sites and hence is much more potent.

Ecothiopate

- A number of phosphate, pyrophosphate and phosphonate esters apparently react irreversibly with cholinesterase by forming phosphate ester with the esteratic site.

- Because the rate of hydrolysis of the phosphorylated enzyme is measured in hours, these compounds have long duration of action. These compounds esterify the serine residue in the cholinesterase enzyme.

- The hydrolysis rate of the phosphorylated serine is extremely slow and hydrolysis to the free enzyme and phosphoric acid derivatives is so limited that the inhibition is considered irreversible.

SAR:

- A general formula for these compounds is as follows:

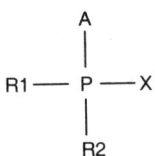

- R1 = Alkoxy group, R2 = Alkoxy, alkyl or tertiary amine X and A are the good leaving group.
  1. A is usually oxygen or sulphur, but may also be selenium. When A is other than oxygen, biological activation is required before compound becomes effective.
  2. X is good leaving group when the molecule reacts with the enzyme.
  3. The R moiety imparts lipophilicity to the molecule and contributes its absorption through skin.
  4. In alkoxy series, compounds which contain fluorine are more active than those containing iodine or other radical.

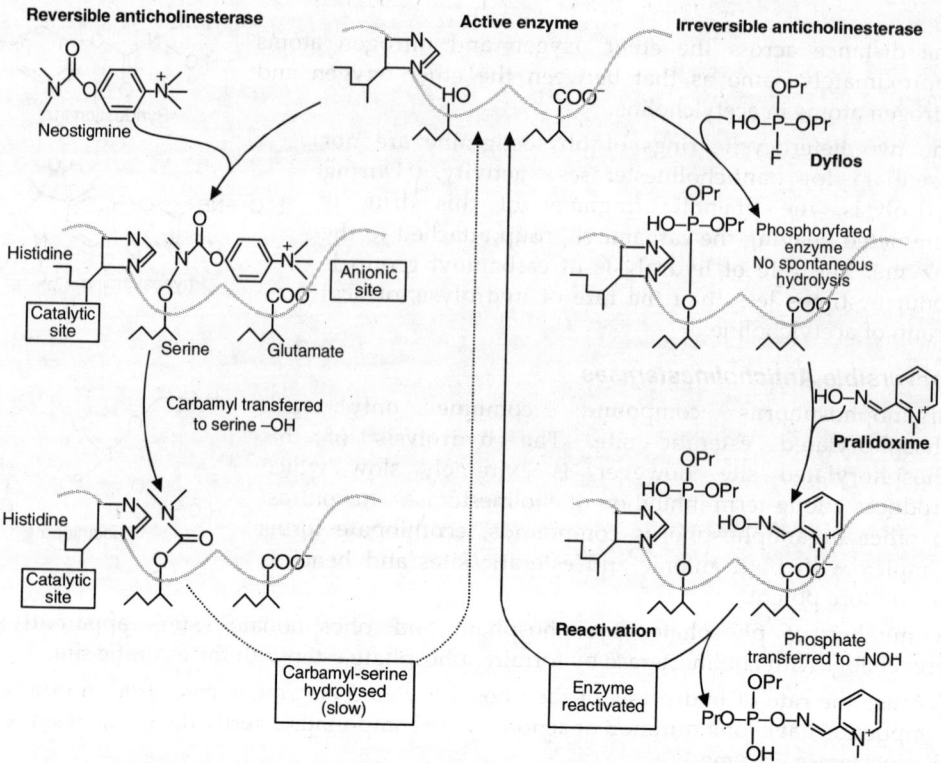

Fig. 11.5: Action of anticholinesterase drugs. Reversible anticholinesterase (neostigmine): Recovery of activity by hydrolysis of the carbamylated enzyme takes many minutes. Irreversible anticholinesterase — reactivation of phosphorylated enzyme by pralidoxime

Acetylcholine chloride

trimethyl-amine (I) + 2-chloroethanol → choline chloride (III) → Acetylcholine chloride

Carbachol

2-chloroethyl chloroformate → 2-chloroethyl carbamate (I)

I + trimethyl-amine → Carbochol

Bethanechol

β-methylcholine chloride   phosgene (I)   Bethanechol chloride

Neostigmine methyl sulfate

3-dimethyl-aminophenol   dimethyl-carbamoyl chloride   3-dimethyl-aminophenol   dimethyl sulfate   Neostigmine methylsulfate

Pyridostigmine

3-hydroxy-pyridine   dimethyl-carbamayl chloride   3-(dimethylamine-carbonyloxy)-pyridine   methyl bromide   Pyridostigmine bromide

Ecothiopate

diethyl phosphochloridate   2-dimethylamino-ethyl mercapton   methyl iodide   Ecothiopate iodide

Parasympatholytic Agents

Anticholinergic agents are also called as parasympatholytic agents, which inhibit the effect of acetylcholine released from post-ganglionic parasympathetic nerve endings. These agents are further divided as follows.

1. **Antimuscarinic agents**: These agents block the action of acetylcholine over the muscarinic receptors. Examples include atropine, scopolamine and pirenzepine.

2. **Nicotinic cholinergic receptor blocking agents:** These agents block the effect of acetylcholine over the nicotinic receptors. These are further classified as:

   a. **Ganglion-blocking agent:** Hexamethonium, trimethaphan.

   b. **Neuromuscular blocking agent:** Suxamethonium, pancuronium.

▨ ANTIMUSCARINIC AGENTS (ANTISPASMODIC DRUGS)

- Acetylcholine is the chemical transmitter at the postganglionic parasympathetic nerve endings, at the sympathetic and parasympathetic ganglia and at the neuromuscular junction in skeletal muscle. Drugs that inhibit the interaction of acetylcholine with the acetylcholine receptors are called as anticholinergics (cholinergic blocking agents; parasympatholytics).

- Anticholinergic drugs which block the somatic neuromuscular junction (neuromuscular blocking agents) and autonomic ganglia (ganglionic blocking agents) are discussed in the second phase of this chapter.

- In the present phase, the drugs which inhibit the action of acetylcholine on autonomic effector innervated by postganglionic cholinergic nerves are discussed. Since the peripheral cholinergic synapses are muscarinic and the anticholinergics acting on them antagonize the muscarinic action of acetylcholine, they are known as antimuscarinic or muscarinic cholinergic blocking agents.

- These agents counteract gastrointestinal and urinary tract spasms, decrease the secretion of saliva and gastric juices, and dilate the pupil of the eye and paralyse accommodation. Consequently, they are used therapeutically for the relief of spasm of gastrointestinal, biliary and urinary tracts, in the treatment of gastric and duodenal ulcers, in ophthalmology and in the treatment of Parkinson's disease.

- Their use as antiparkinsonism drug is based on the cholinergic activity brought about by the loss of central dopaminergic inhibition in parkinsonism

- The solanaceous alkaloids hyoscyamine, its racemates atropine and hyoscine (scopolamine) are the oldest anticholinergics. They became the prototype for the design of a large number of synthetic anticholinergic agents.

Flow chart 12.1: Classification of anti-muscarinic agents

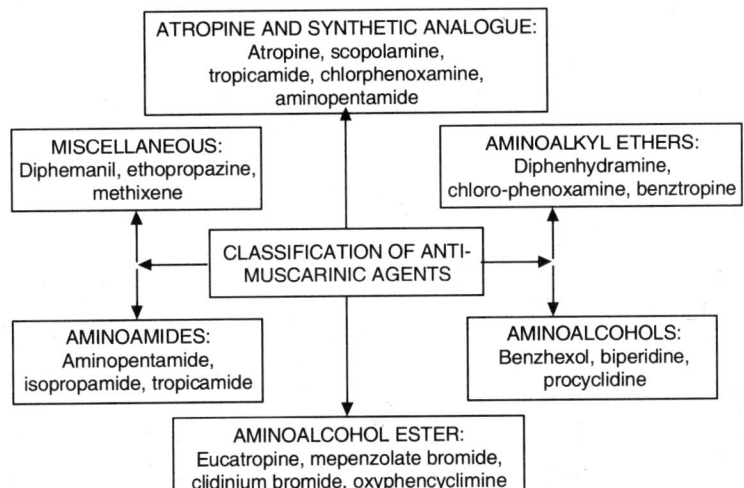

Atropine and Its Synthetic Analouge

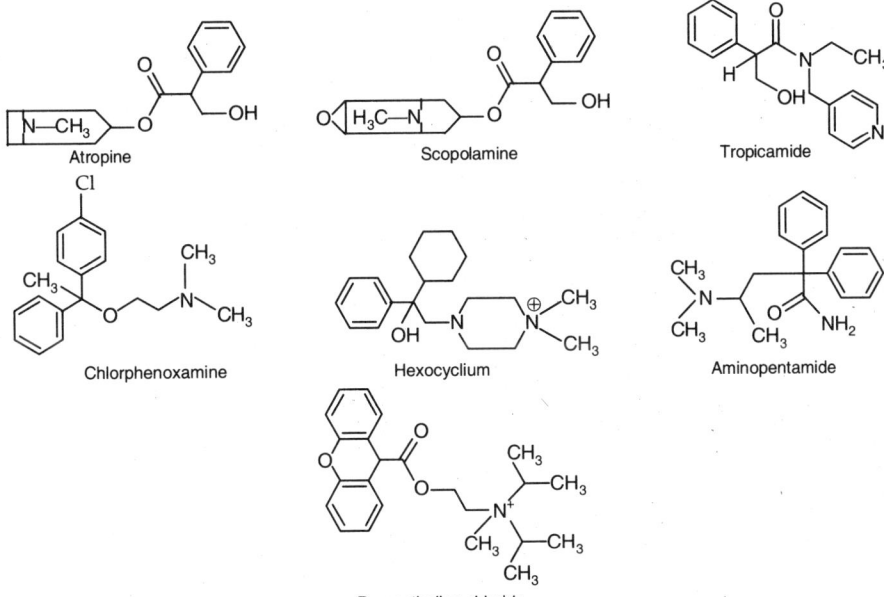

Atropine

Scopolamine

Tropicamide

Chlorphenoxamine

Hexocyclium

Aminopentamide

Propantheline chloride

Aminoalcohol Esters

Eucatropine

Mepenzolate bromide

Clidinium bromide

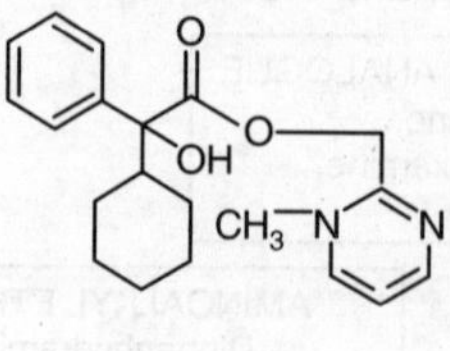

Oxyphencyclimine

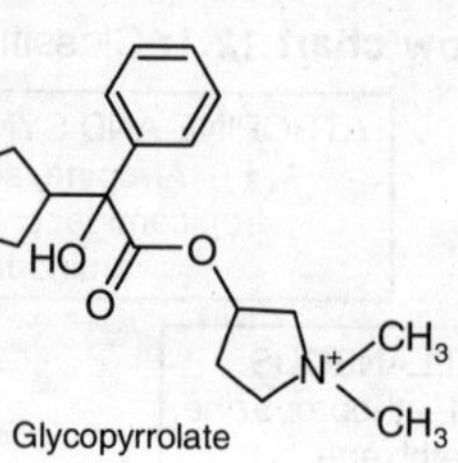

Glycopyrrolate

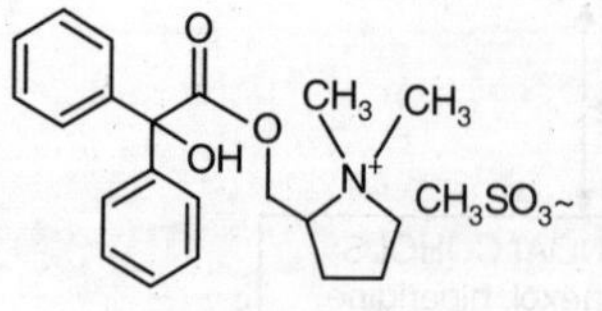

Poldine methylsulphate

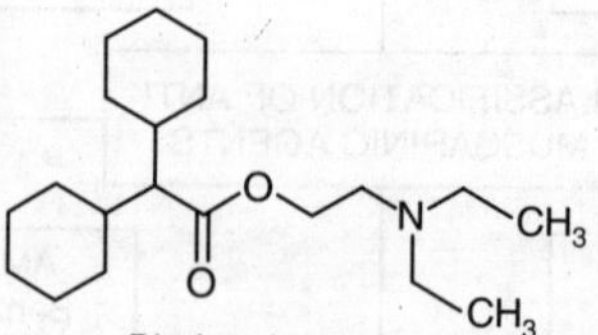

Dicyloamine

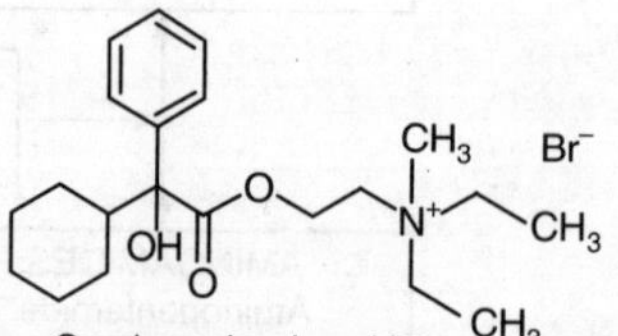

Oxyphenonium bromide

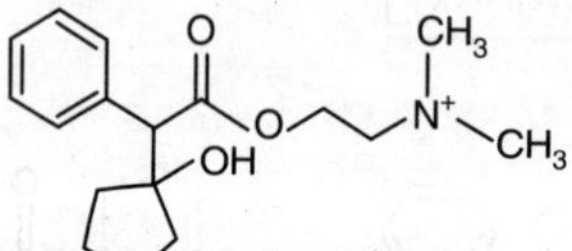

Cyclopentolate

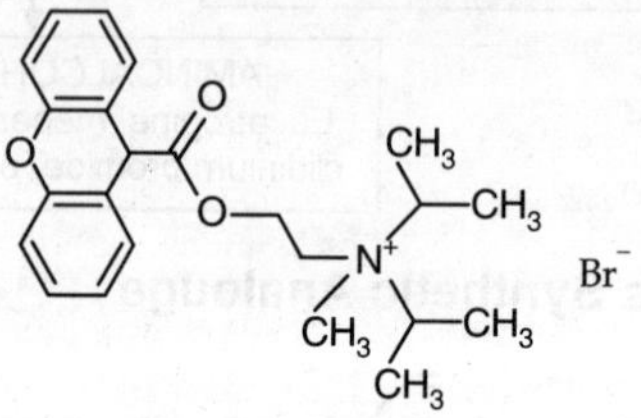

Propantheline bromide

Aminoalkyl Ethers

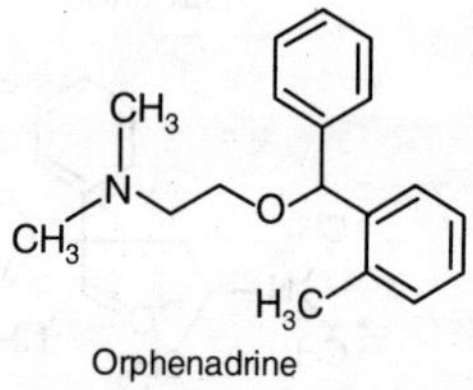

Orphenadrine

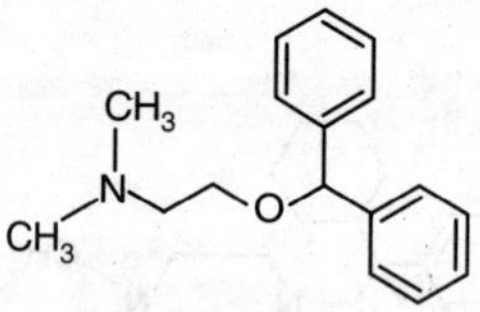

Diphenhydramine

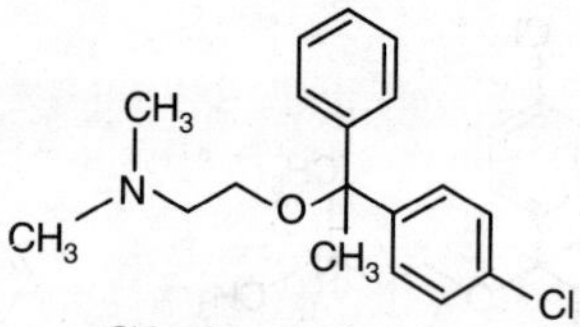

Chlorphenoxamine

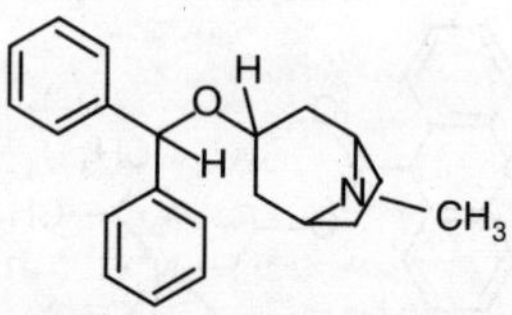

Benztropine

Aminoalcohols

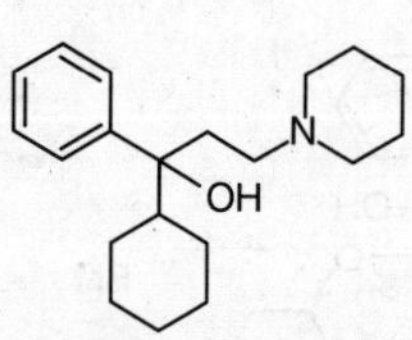

Benzhexol

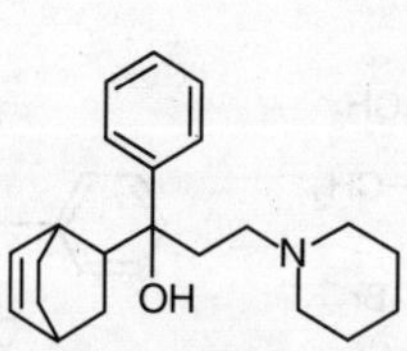

Biperiden

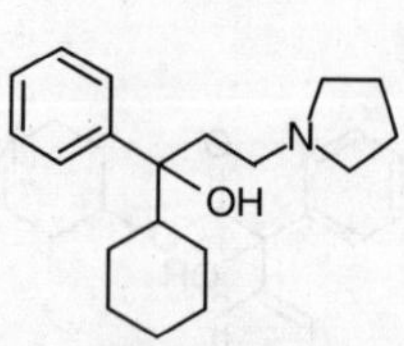

Procyclidine

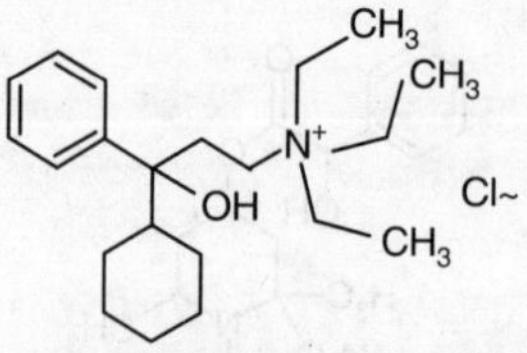

Tridihexethyl chloride

Aminoamides

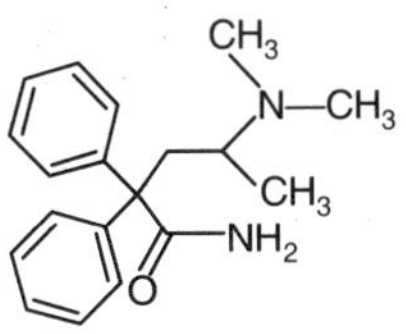

Aminopentamide

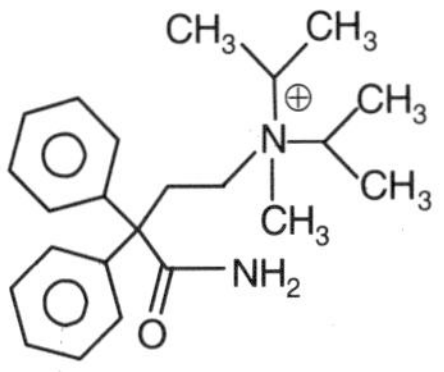

Isopropramide

Miscellaneous

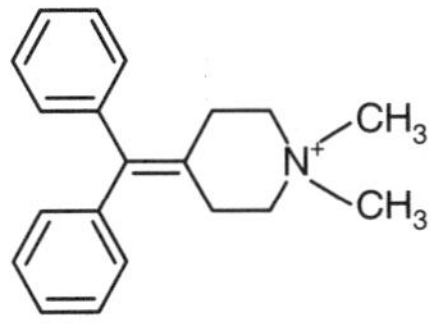

Diphemanil

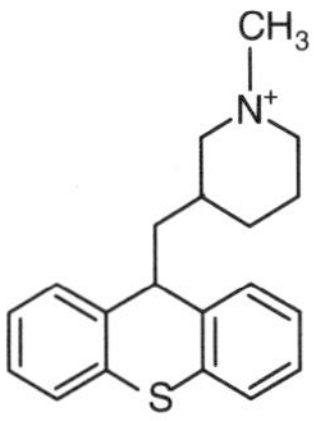

Methixene

Structure–Activity Relationship

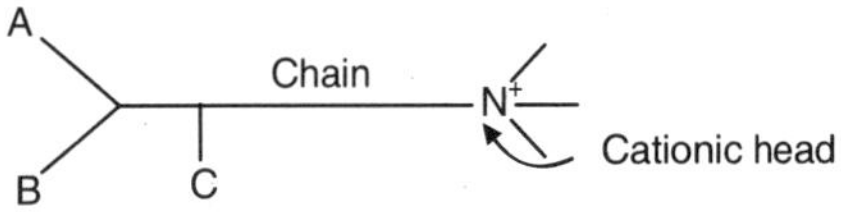

The minimum structure necessary for the antagonistic activity is.

1. In the above general formula, the antagonist may contain larger group than methyl on nitrogen. In general this group should not be greater than butyl, if compound is to be an effective antagonist.

2. The nitrogen atoms in an antagonist need not to be always quaternised. Since the pH of the receptors is acidic, this amino group gets protonated and carries a positive charge that interact with the anionic site of the receptor.

3. The acyl group in an antagonist is always larger than the acyl group in acetylcholine. The larger acyl group ensures the compound is not a partial agonist.

4. The acetylcholine molecule does not cover all the area of the receptors. The area of receptors which is not covered by an acetylcholine molecule appears to be chiefly hydrophobic in nature. Hence hydrophobic substituents increase the affinity of the antagonist by binding to this area.

5. Addition of bulkier group over the carbonyl carbon of ester group resulted in cholinergic blocking activity.

6. This indicates that at least one portion of the molecule should have the space like umbrella, which leads to firm binding at the receptor.

7. Size alone is not sole criteria for potent blocking activity. The compound should have stereochemical features for binding with receptor.

8. The presence of free hydroxyl or carbamide is also important for hydrogen bonding with the receptor.

9. The difference between the hydroxyl group and the quaternary nitrogen is estimated to be between 2 to 3 Å.

10. In place of CH_3 in acetylcholine, if we are putting phenyl, cyclohexyl that results in anticholinergic activity.

Mode of Action

- The main difference in cholinergic and anticholinergic agents appears to be the size of the acyl group.

  In cholinergic compounds R= small group.

  In anticholinergic compound R= large group.

- The large (alkyl or aryl) group may not only increase the affinity of the blocking agent but through an 'umbrella effect' may also block the approach of acetylcholine to the receptor.

Pharmacological Effects

Effects on CNS: Atropine has an overall CNS stimulant action. However, these effects are not appreciable at low doses which produce peripheral effects because of restricted entry into the brain. Hyoscine produces central effect (depressant) even at low doses.

Effects on Eye: The pupil is dilated (mydriasis) by atropine administration.

Effect on GI tract: Gastrointestinal motility is inhibited by atropine; pirenzepine and telenzepine inhibit gastric acid secretion.

Effects on heart rate: The first effect is bradycardia. Slightly larger dose produce tachycardia.

Inhibition of secretion: Salivary, lacrimal, bronchial and scrotal glands secretions are inhibited by very low doses of taropine, producing an uncomfortably dry mouth and skin.

Adverse Effect

1. Adverse effect of the antispasmodic drugs is dose dependant and includes dry mouth and skin, flushing, tachycardia, papillary dilation and blurred vision, cerebral excitement and delirium.
2. The quaternary ammonium compounds may also cause postural hypotension and impotence because of their ganglionic effects.

Uses

1. The anticholinergic drugs have been widely used in the treatment of peptic ulcer disease and irritable bowel and functional disorders, including diarrhea.
2. The main contraindication to anticholinergic drug use is narrow angle glaucoma, pyloric outlet obstruction and reflux oesphagitis.

Tropicamide

Cyclopentolate

Sodium phenyl-acetate + Cyclo-pentanone → (isopropyl bromide, Mg) → α-(1-hydroxy-cyclopentyl)-phenylacetic acid (I) → (2-(dimethyl-amino)ethyl chloride) → Cyclopentolate

Pirenzepine

2-chloro-3-aminopyridine + 2-nitrobenzoyl chloride → → (H₂, Roney–Ni) → (I)

I → (200 °C) → 5, 11-dihydro-6H-pyrido-[2,3-b][1,4]benzo-diazepin-6-one → (chloroacetyl chloride, triethylamine) → (II)

II + 1-methyl-piperazine → Pirenzepine

Dicyclorerine

Benzyl cyanide + 1,5-dibromo-pentane → (NaNH₂) → 1-cyano-1-phenylcyclo-hexane → (H₃C—OH, H₂SO₄) → Ethyl 1-phenyl-cyclohexane-1-carboxylate (I)

I + (II) → (Na) → 2-diethylaminaethyl 1-phenylcyclohexane-1-carboxylate → (H₂, Pto, CH₃COOH) → Dicycloverine

Biperidine

Ocetohenone + (CH₂O)n + Piperidine → 3-piperidino-Propiophenone (I)

I + Bicyclo[2,2-1]-het-5-en-2-yl-magnesium chloride → Biperidene

Atropine methionitrate

Atropine (I) + CH₃–O–NO₂ Methyl nitrote → Atropine methonitrate

Propantheline bromide

Xanthene-9-carboxylic acid →(SoCl₂ thionyl chloride)→ Xanthene-9-carbonyl chloride →(2-(diisopropylamino)-ethanol)→ I

(I) + H₃C—Br methyl bromide → Propantheline bromide

Nicotinic Antagonist (Neuromuscular and Ganglionic Blocking Agents)

These are the drugs which block the action of nicotine and can be classified based on their site of action, mainly into two classes:
1. Ganglionic blocking drugs—hexamethonium, trimethaphan.
2. Neuromuscular blocking drugs—suxamethonium, panacuronium.

Ganglionic Blocking Agents

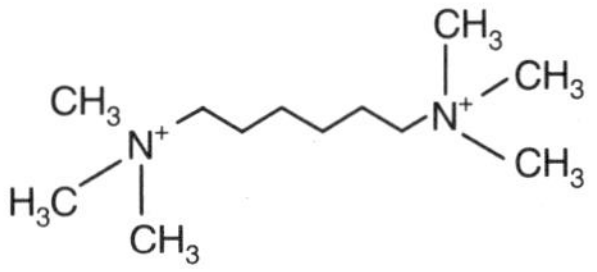

Hexamethonium

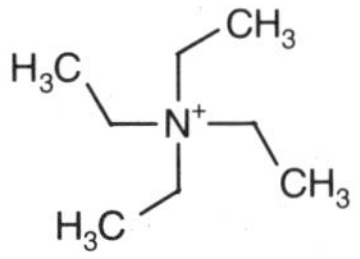

Tetraethyl ammonium

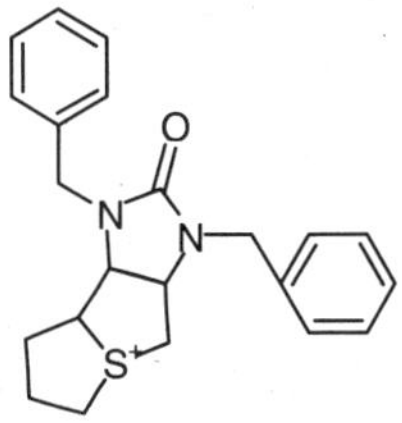

Trimethaphan

Neuromuscular Blocking Agents

A. **Competitive agents**

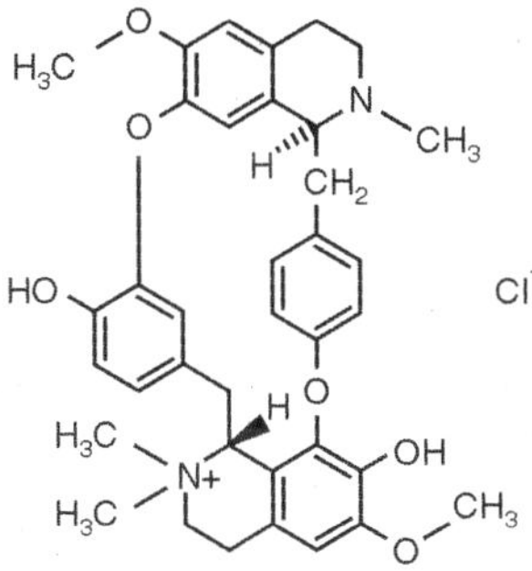

Cl⁻ • HCl • 5H₂O

Tubocurarin chloride

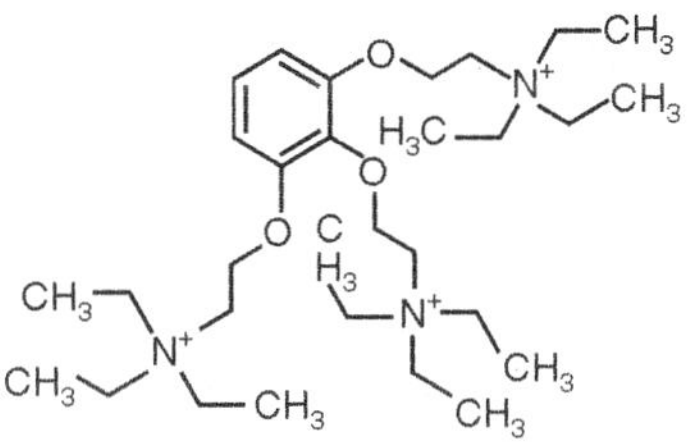

Gallamine

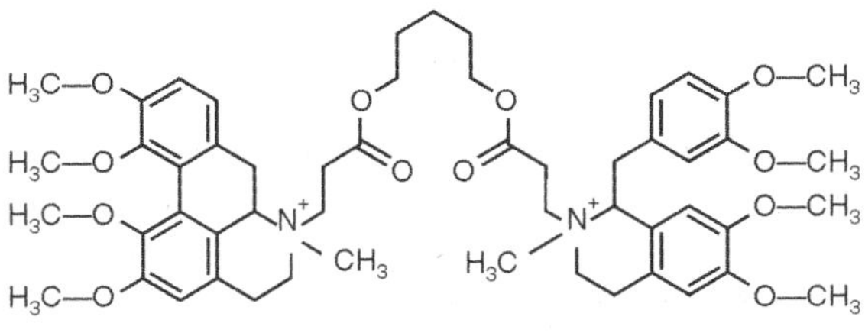

Atracurium

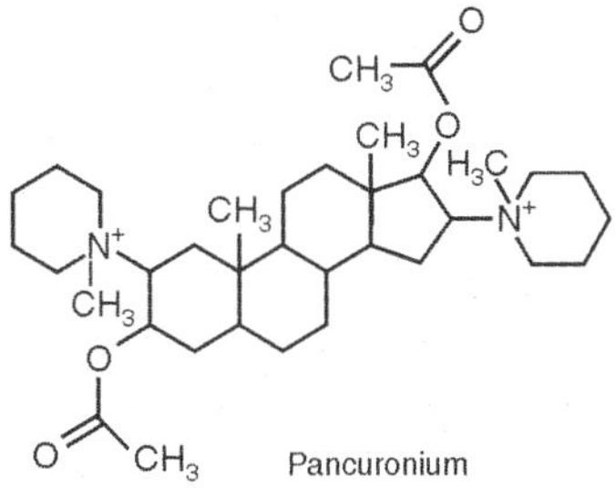

Pancuronium

155

B. **Depolarizing agent**

Succinyl choline

Decamethonium

GANGLION BLOCKING DRUGS

Mechanism of Action

Ganglion blocking can occur by the following mechanism:

1. By interference with acetylcholine release; botulinum toxin, hemicholinium and magnesium ion, are effective in causing block.

2. By interference with the post-synaptic action of acetylcholine. All these drugs act by inhibiting the post-synaptic actions of acetylcholine. The ganglion block is dependent on the length of the polymethylene chain. Compounds with five or six carbon atoms in the methylene chain linking the two quaternary groups produce ganglionic block; when the chain contained nine or ten carbon atoms, they produce neuromuscular block. The only drug of this class in clinical uses is trimethaphan, a short acting drug in anesthesia.

3. By prolonged depolarization, nicotine can block ganglial initial stimulation in this way.

NEUROMUSCULAR BLOCKING DRUGS

- Commands from the central nervous system to the skeletal muscle are transmitted by the skeletomotor system. In this system, a motor neuron originates from a ventral horn of the spinal cord and forms myelinated fiber which continues without interruption to the muscle.

- It then branches in the muscle and forms a neuromuscular end-plate on each muscle fiber. Acetylcholine is the neurotransmitter at the neuromuscular junction.

- The neuromuscular blocking agents, which act by interrupting the transmission of nerve impulse at this junction, are of two types—competitive or non-depolarizing agents and depolarizing agents.

Competitive Agents

- The competitive agents or non-depolarizing agents act by competing with acetylcholine for receptor sites on the motor endplate, thus reducing their response to the neurotransmitter.

- These agents are also called stabilizing agents. Their action is usually reversed by anticholinesterase, such as neostigmine.

- The competitive neuromuscular blocking agents were developed through the study of curare, an arrow poison used by South American Indians for killing wild animals for food. Death of the animals was due to paralysis of skeletal muscle.

- The poison was obtained by the natives from the bark of various species of the genus Strychnos. Depending upon the type of the container used for storage, the curare was named as 'calabash' 'pot' and 'tube' curare.

- Tubocurarine chloride is used intravenously to produce skeletal muscle relaxation during surgical procedures. It blocks the stimulating (nicotinic) action of acetylcholine on skeletal muscle; it exerts little effect on autonomic ganglia, involuntary muscle or glands.

- Considering that the tertiary nitrogen gets protonated at physiological pH and the interonium distance is significant for curare-mimetic action, it has been a basis for the development of other neuromuscular blocking agents.
- Methylation of the free phenolic hydroxyl groups of tubocurarine increases the activity, whereas ethylation or butylation leads to less active or inactive derivatives. A synthetic derivatives metocurine (formerly called as tubocurarine) contains three additional methyl groups. The compound is two to three times more potent than tubocurarine in man. It is used as metocurine iodide.

Depolarizing Agents

- The depolarizing agents block neuromuscular transmission by producing a sustained partial depolarization of the motor end-plate which renders the tissue incapable of responding to acetylcholine.
- Their curarizing action is not reversed by anticholinesterases. The decamethonium halides and suxamethonium halides are typical of this group.

Mechanism of Action

Drugs can block neuromuscular transmission in three main ways.

1. By inhibiting acetylcholine synthesis, e.g. hemicholinium and triethylcholine.
2. By inhibiting acetylcholine release. Agents that inhibit calcium entry have neuromuscular block. These include magnesium ion and various aminoglycoside antibiotics (streptomycin and neomycin). Two potent neurotoxins, namely botulinium toxin produced by the anaerobic bacillus *Clostridium botulinum,* an organism that can multiply in preserved food and cause serious food poisoning and β-bungarotoxin (contained in the venom of various snakes of the cobra family).
3. By interfering with the post-synaptic action of acetylcholine. This category can be further subdivided into:

   a. **Depolarizing blocking agents:** Which are agonists at acetylcholine receptors. Decamethonium and suxamethonium.

   b. **Non-depolarizing agents**: Non-depolarizing agents act as competitive antagonist at the acetylcholine receptors of the end plate and this largely accounts for their action, e.g gallamine, pancuronium, vecuronium and atracurium.

Structure–Activity Relationship

1. All these drugs are quaternary ammonium compounds. The type of alkyl carbon (methyl, ethyl, etc.) determines the charge distribution and binding characteristics of onium compounds.
2. Non-depolarizing drugs are generally bulky and more rigid than depolarizing drugs.
3. As the steric hindrance to receptor increase, the potency decreases. 1-tubocurarine is considerably less potent than d-tubocurarine.
4. The depolarizing agents (e.g. decamethonium) have a more flexible structure that enables bond rotation.
5. While the distance between quaternary groups in the flexible depolarizing agents can vary up to the limit of the maximal bond distance, the distance for the rigid competitive blockers is usually 1.0 nm, when the change is not delocalized.

Duration of Action, Metabolism and Fate

- Neuromuscular-blocking agents are used mainly in anesthesia to produce muscle relaxation. The drugs are given intravenously and act within 30 second. Their duration of action varies considerably. Suxamethonium acts normally for about 3 minute, being hydrolysed by plasma cholinesterase.

- Hydrolysis occurs in two stages to produce products with negligible motor end plate activity. The non-depolarizing blocking agents are with the exception of atracurium, metabolized by the liver and their duration of action varies between about 10 and 60 min.

Unwanted Effects

- The main side effect of tubocurarine is a fall in arterial pressure. Gallamine and pancuronium cause tachycardia and hypertension in man. Other important side effects of tubocurarine include histamine release.

- Pancuronium has also been shown to possess some activity against pseudo-cholinesterase, which may account for the slight miosis shown by most patients.

Gallamine triethiodide

Reagents:
1. Sodium amide
2. 2-diethylamino-ethyl chloride
3. Ethyl Iodide

Pyrogallol → Gallamine tri-ethiodide

Sympathomimetics (Adrenergic Agents)

The substances that produce effects similar to stimulation of sympathetic nervous system are known as sympathomimetic or adrenergic drugs.

- The sympathetic nervous system controls various important systems including cardiovascular, bronchial airway tone, muscular, etc. It prepares the organism against the condition of stress. In addition to epinephrine, a large number of agents can mimic the response obtained as a result of stimulation of adrenergic nerves.
- They bear structural resemblance with neurotransmitter epinephrine. Hence, they can be used to mimic or alter the functioning of sympathetic nervous system in several clinical disorders like hypertension, asthma, arrhythmia and various allergic conditions.

BIOSYNTHESIS (FIG. 14.1)

- The synthesis of noradrenaline is the first step in the process of noradrenergic transmission. Starting material is dietary L-phenyl alanine, which is actively absorbed from gut and oxidized by hepatic 'phenylalanine hydroxylase' to form L-tyrosine.
- This L-tyrosine circulates in bloodstream and is actively transported into the cytoplasm of the noradrenergic neurons. Within the neuronal cytoplasm, L-tyrosine is hydroxylated to form L-DOPA.
- This reaction is catalyzed by cytoplasmic 'tyrosine hydroxylase' and is the rate limiting step in the biosynthesis of noradrenaline, i.e. the activity of tyrosine hydroxylase is governed by the cytoplasmic concentration of noradrenaline and high noradrenaline concentration inhibits the conversion of L-tyrosine to L-DOPA. Further L-DOPA decarboxylase I is the enzyme which converts L-DOPA to dopamine within the neuronal cytoplasm.
- Dopamine is actively transported into the storage vesicles and here it is oxidized by dopamine-beta-hydroxylase to form noradrenaline.
- This endogenous noradrenaline is stored in the synaptic vesicles as complex with ATP and a soluble protein called 'chromogranin'. In cortex part of adrenal gland, noradrenaline is converted into adrenaline.

Release

Two physiological process involved in the release of noradrenaline.

1. When an action potential (impulse) reaches the nerve terminal, the membrane permeability is altered. Na^+, Ca^{++} enter the cell and K^+ leaves the cell. This influx of Ca^{++} triggers the release of noradrenaline into synaptic cleft. The empty vesicles retained within the nerve terminal and refilled with noradrenaline.
2. Some storage vesicle randomly migrates to the terminal and releases their content into the synaptic cleft, which is designated as noradrenaline leak.

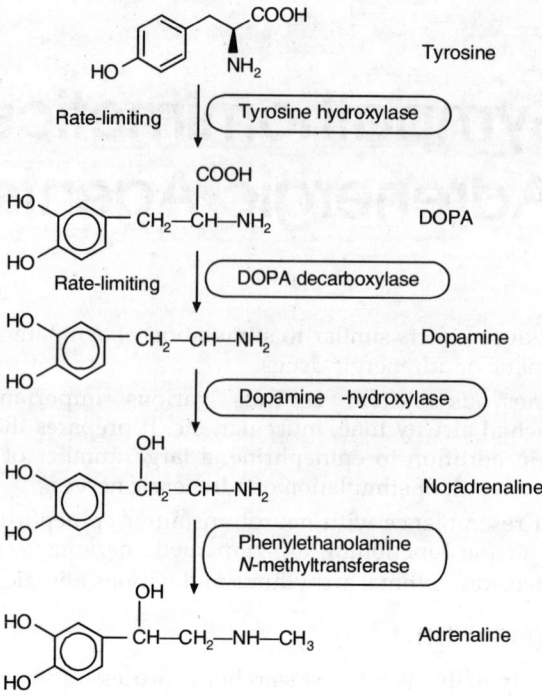

Fig. 14.1: Biosynthesis of adrenaline and noradrenaline

3. The free noradrenaline released into the synaptic cleft is active and attaches itself to the adrenoceptor to produce response. Part of it is washed off in circulation and metabolized by cathecol-o-methyltransferase (COMT) and major remaining part is re-uptaken back to neuron.

Uptake-I (Fig. 14.2)

- This is the major mode of termination of the action of noradrenaline. Here noradrenaline is taken back to the neuron and re-used as neurotransmitter.
- The remaining noradrenaline, which is present in the synaptic cleft is metabolized by MAO and COMT.

Uptake-II (Fig. 14.2)

- This operates only when high amount of noradrenaline is circulating in the blood.
- After transport of noradrenaline back into the neuron by uptake-II, the noradrenaline is not stored but is rapidly metabolized intracellularly by both COMT and MAO.

Metabolism (Fig. 14.3)

- Monoamino oxidase and catechol-o-methyltransferase are the main enzymes which metabolize the sympathomimetic drugs.
- About 60% of the administered dose of epinephrine or norepinephrine in man remains untouched by these main enzymes which then is excreted in its original form or in its conjugated form with sulphuric or glucuronic acid. Conjugation usually occurs at phenolic hydroxyl groups.

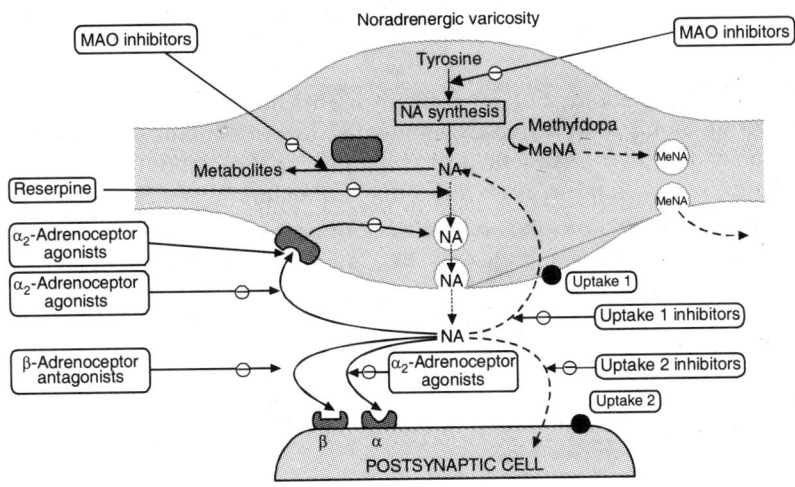

Fig. 14.2: Uptake 1 and 2 and different antiadrenergic drugs

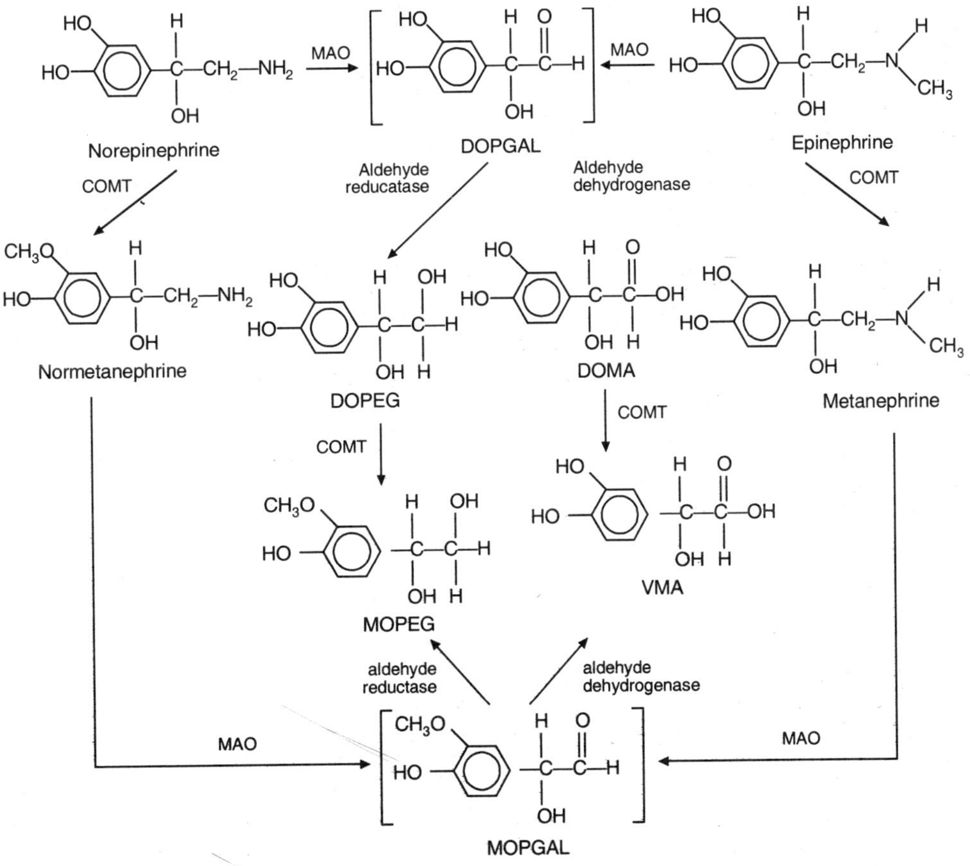

Fig. 14.3: Metabolism of epinephrine and norepinephrine

- The major fraction of natural catecholamine is attacked by MAO and/or COMT. At periphery, they are preferentially oxidised to the acid and in the CNS, they are reduced to glycol.
- Thus the principal metabolites of norepinephrine ((MPOGAL, MOMA and MOPEG) are excreted in urine along with a free or conjugated form of unaltered nor-epinephrine. Of these, 3-methoxy-4-hydroxymandelic acid is the principal metabolite and the estimation of its content in urine can be taken as an index of catecholamine metabolism.
- On an average, about 70% of metabolized dose of epinephrine or norepinephrine follows metabolism by COMT enzymes while only 20% favors the attack by MAO enzymes.
- By using drugs, which inhibit these metabolizing enzymes, the duration and intensity of effects can be raised.
- For example, some agents can specifically block the MAO enzymes and are in clinical use under the name of MAO inhibitors, while only few agents can block the activity of COMT enzymes on circulating catecholamine and did not find clinical applicability. These include pyrogallol and tropolone derivatives.

ADRENERGIC RECEPTORS

- Adrenergic receptors are membrane bound G-protein-coupled receptors, which primarily act by increasing or decreasing the intracellular production of second messenger cAMP or IP_3/DAG.
- In some cases, the activated G-protein itself operates K^+ or Ca^{++} channels or increase prostaglandin production.
- Adrenergic receptors are classified into two types α and β. Details of receptors are given in Tables 14.1 to 14.3.

Table 14.1: Order of potency of α and β receptors

Rank of order of potency of agonists	α-receptors	β-receptors
	Adr > NA > Iso	Iso > Adr > NA

Table 14.2: Subtypes of α-receptors.

	α_1-receptors	α_2-receptors
Location blood vessels	Postjunctional on effector organ	Prejunctional on nerve endings, also post–junctionally in brain, pancreatic β-cells, Platelets and extrajunctional in certain
Function observed	Smooth muscle—contracrion Gland—secretion Gut—relaxation Heart—arrhythmia	Inhibition of transmitter release Vasoconstriction Decreased central sympathetic flow Decreased insulin release Platelet aggregation
Selective agonist	Phenylpherine, Methoxamine	Clonidine
Selective antagonist	Prazosin	Yohimbine

Table 14.3: Subtypes of β-receptors

	β_1	β_2	β_3
Location	Heart Juxtaglomerular cell in kidney	Bronchi Blood vessels, uterus, GIT urinary tract, eye	Adipose tissue
Selective agonist	Dobutamine	salbutamol, terbutaline	

Classification of Sympathomimetics

Classification of sympathomimetics is given in flow chart 14.1.

Flow Chart 14.1: Classification of sympathomimetics

CLASSIFICATION OF SYMPATHOMIMETICS

DEPENDING UPON MECHANISM OF ACTION

SELECTIVITY OF RECEPTOR

THERAPEUTIC USES

Directly acting: Nor-epinephrine, epinephrine, phenylpherine, metarminol

Indirectly acitng: Amphetamine, tyramine

Mixed acting: Ephederine, phenylpropanolamine

α_1 **Receptor agonist:** Phenylephrine, methoxamine

α_2 **Receptor agonist:** Clonidine

β_1 **Receptor agonist:** Metoprolol, atenolol

β_2 **Receptor agonist:** Salbutamol, terbutalin

Pressor agents: Phenylephrine, ephederine, dopamine

Cardiac stimulant: Adrenaline, dobutamine

Bronchodilators: Salbutamol, salmeterol

Nasal decongestant: Naphazoline, xylometazoline

CNS stimulant: Amphetamine, methamphetamine

Anorectics: Fenfluramine, sibutramine

Uterine relaxant: Ritordine

Based on Mechanism of Action

A. Direct acting

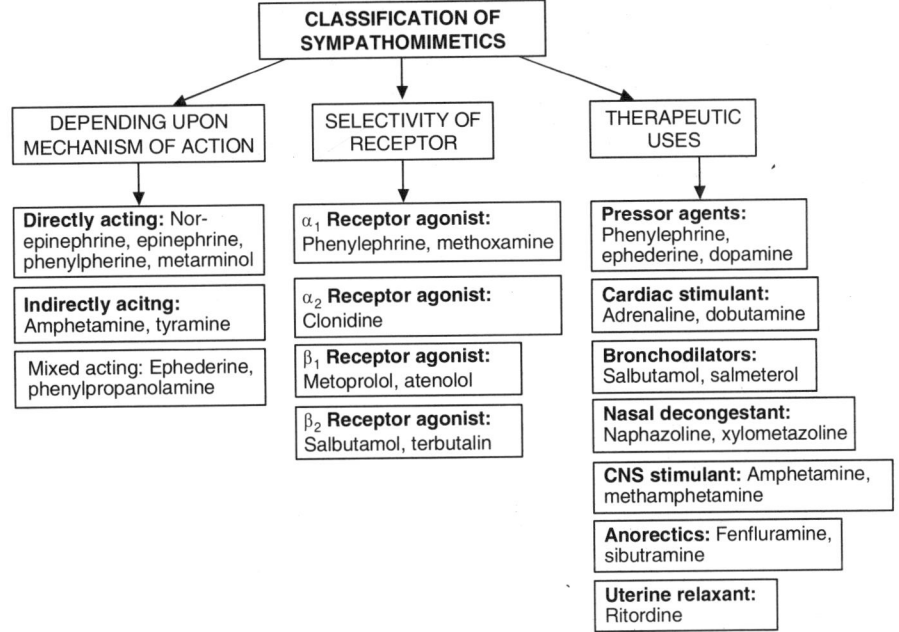

Nor-adrenaline

Adrenaline

Phenylephrine

Isoproterenol

Isoetharine

Metarminol

B. Indirect acting

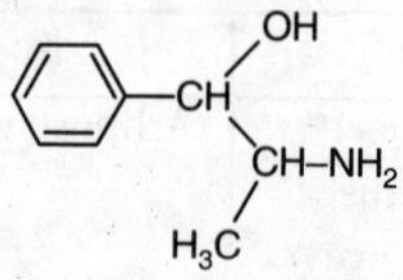

Phenylpropanolamine

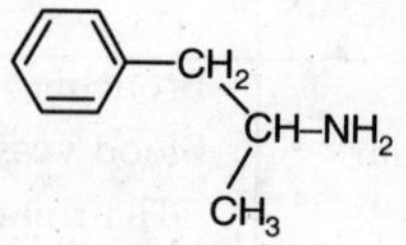

Amphetamine

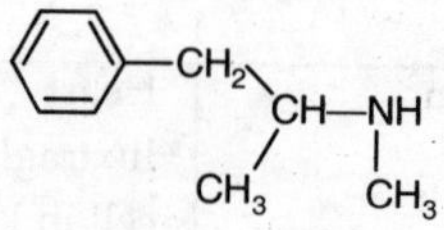

Methamphetamine

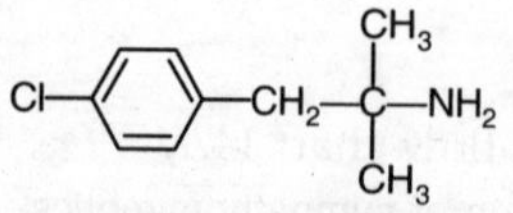

Chlorphentermine

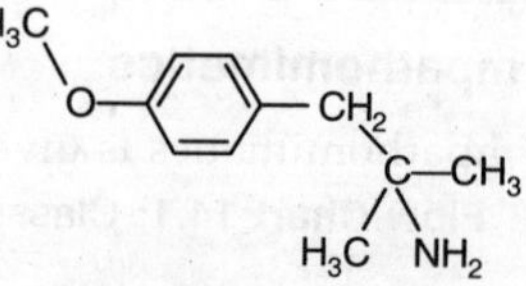

Methoxyphentermine

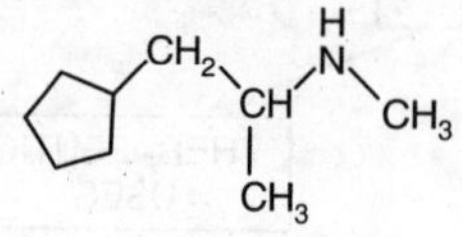

Cyclopentamine

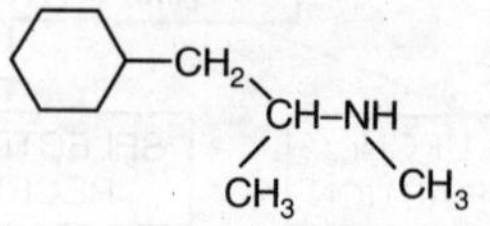

Propylhexedrine

C. Mixed acting

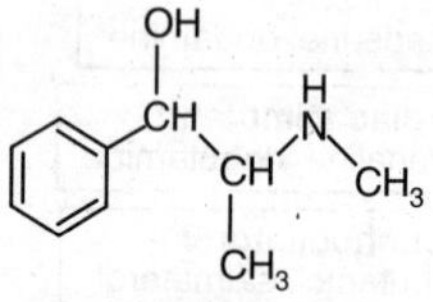

Ephedrine

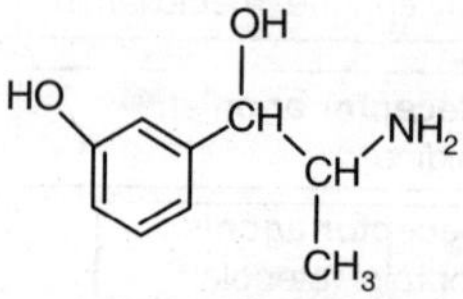

Metarminol

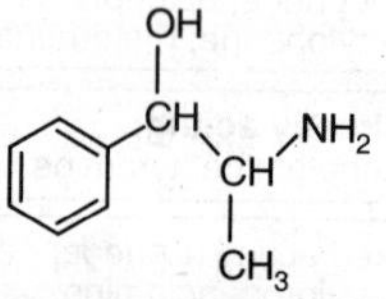

Phenylpropanolamine

Based on Selectivity of Receptor

A. Selective β_1 agonist

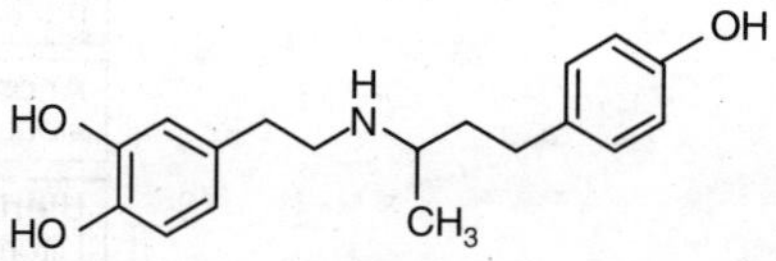

Dobutamine

B. Selective β_2 agonist

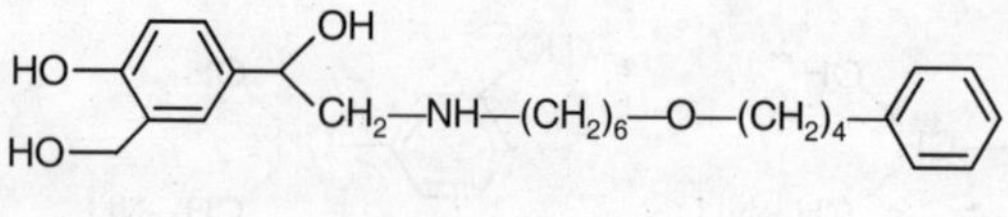

Salmeterol

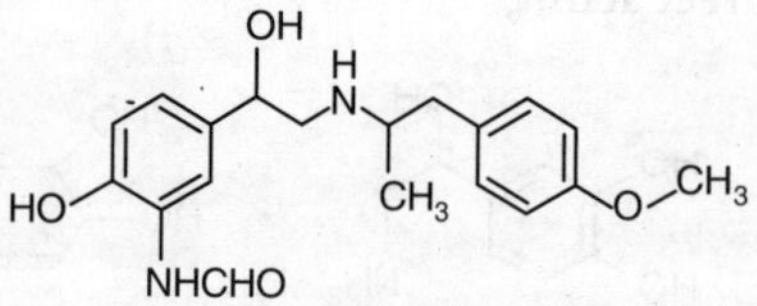

Formoterol

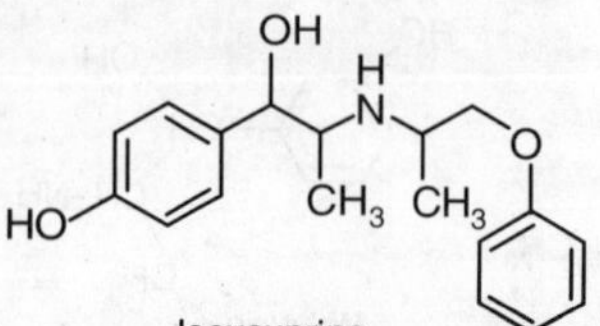

Isoxsuprine

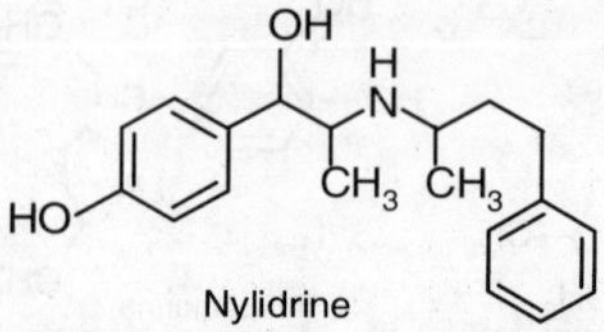

Nylidrine

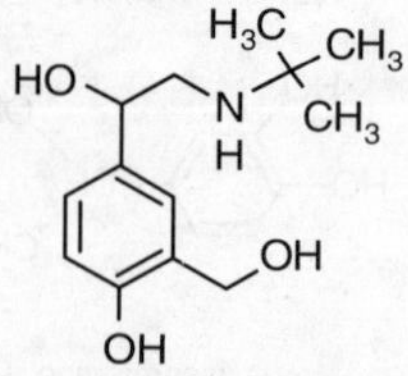

Salbutamol

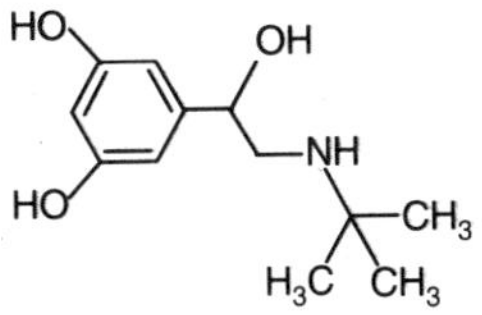

Terbutaline

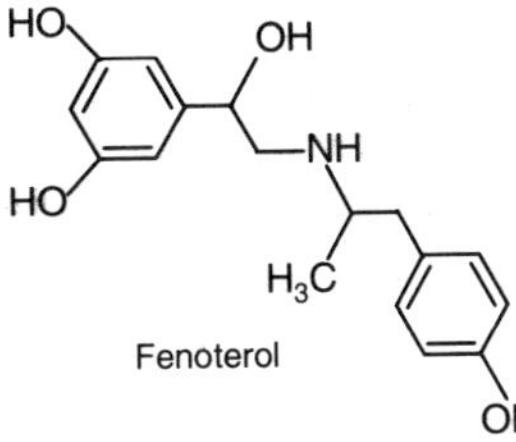

Fenoterol

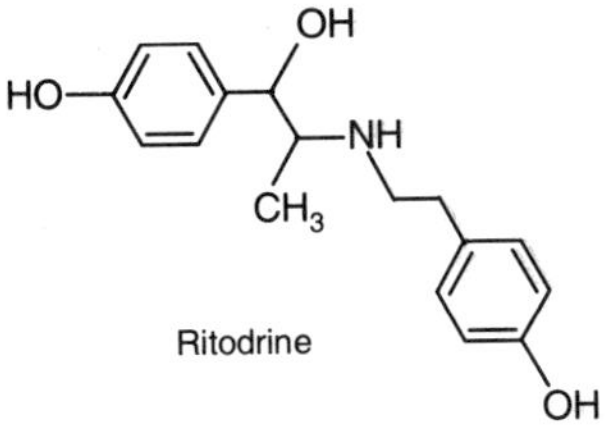

Ritodrine

C. Selective α₁ agonist

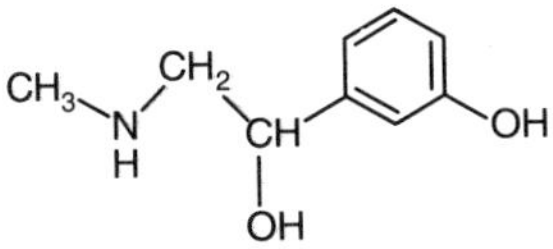

Phenylphrine

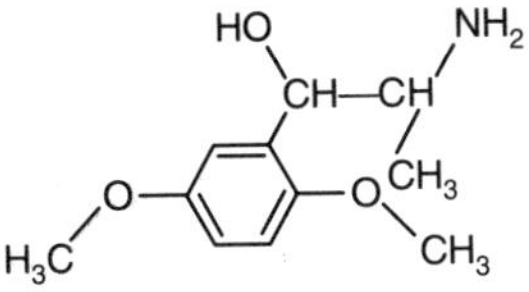

Methoxamine

D. Selective α₂ agonist

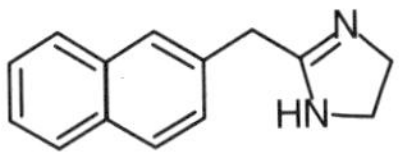

Naphazoline

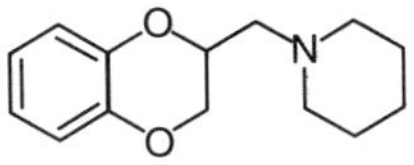

Piperoxan

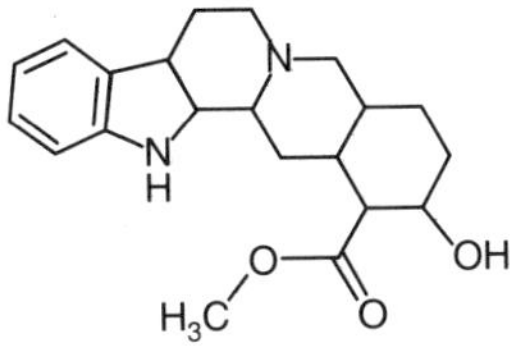

Yohimbine

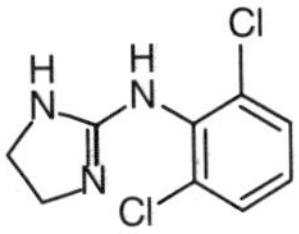

Clonidine

Based on Therapeutic Uses

A. Pressor agent

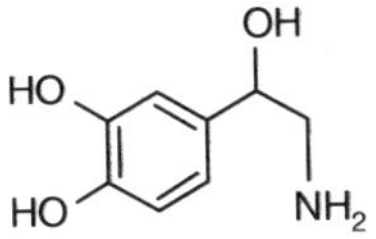

Nor-adrenaline

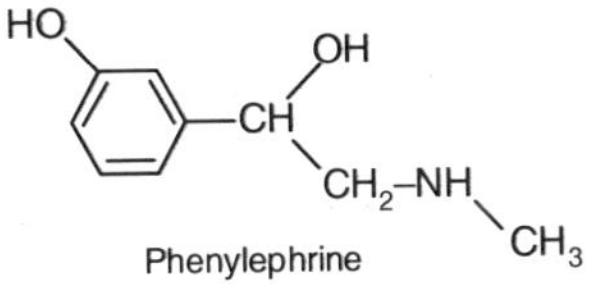

Phenylephrine

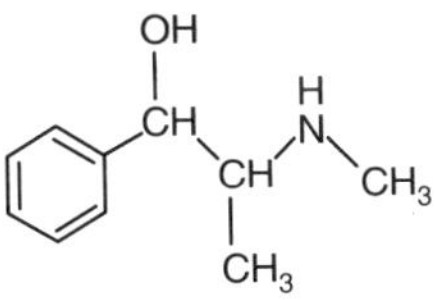

Ephedrine

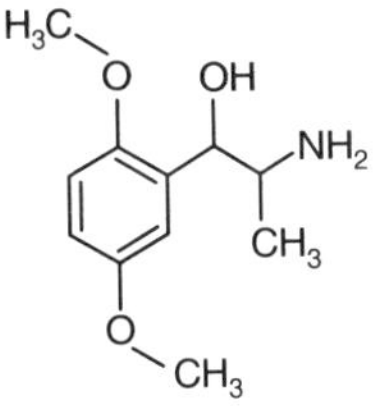

Methoxamine

B. Cardiac stimulant

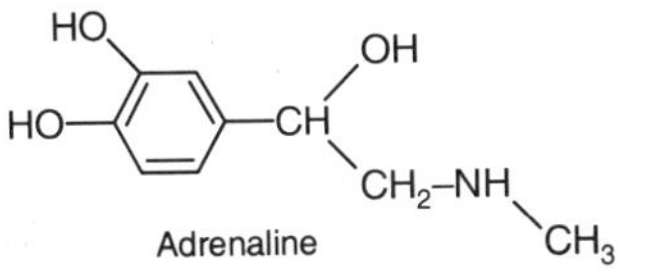

Adrenaline

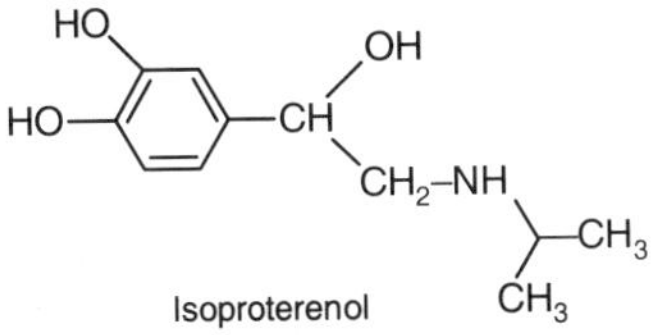

Isoproterenol

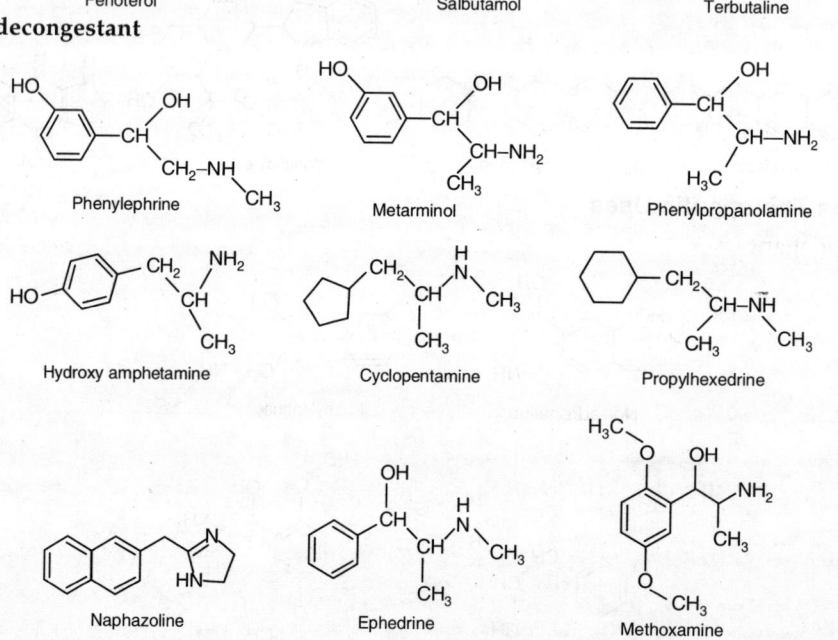

Dobutamine

C. Bronchodilators

Adrenaline

Isoproterenol

Fenoterol

Salbutamol

Terbutaline

D. Nasal decongestant

Phenylephrine

Metarminol

Phenylpropanolamine

Hydroxy amphetamine

Cyclopentamine

Propylhexedrine

Naphazoline

Ephedrine

Methoxamine

E. CNS stimulant

Methamphetamine

Amphetamine

F. Uterine relaxant

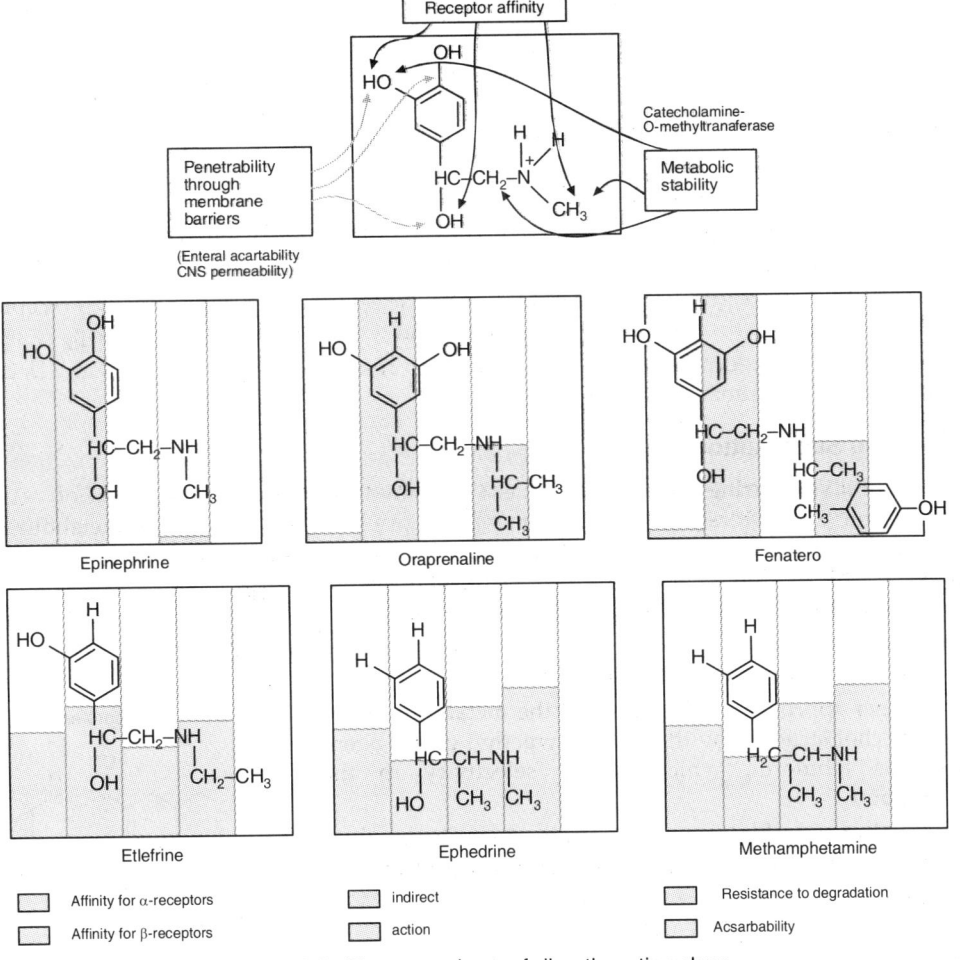

Ritodrine

STRUCTURE ACTIVITY RELATIONSHIP OF DIRECTLY ACTING DRUGS (FIG. 14.4)

Substitution on Nitrogen

1. The presence of amino group in phenylethylamine is important for direct agonist activity.

Fig. 14.4: Pharmacophore of directly acting drug

2. The amino group should be separated from the aromatic ring by two carbon atoms for optimal activity.

3. Both primary and secondary amines are found among the potent direct acting agonist but tertiary or quaternary amines tend to be poor direct agonists.

4. In general, as the bulk of the nitrogen substituent increases, α-receptor agonist activity decreases and β-adrenoceptor activity increases.

5. Above two examples are potent β_1/β_2 agonists because of bulkier group present on nitrogen.

6. In several examples, it has been found that ter.butyl group on nitrogen enhances β_2 selectivity.

   For example, N-ter.butyl norepinephrin is 10 times potent β_2 selective in action.

7. Large substituent on the amino group also protects the amino group from undergoing oxidative de-amination by MAO.

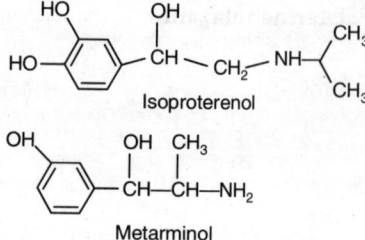

Isoproterenol

Metarminol

N-tertiary butyl norepinephrine

Substitution on Carbon in the Side Chain

1. Methyl or ethyl substitution on the α-carbon of the ethylamine side chain reduces direct receptor agonist activity at both α and β receptors.

2. α-alkyl group (alkyl group on α-carbon atom) increases duration of action of phenylethylamine agonist by making the compound resistant to metabolic deamination by MAO.

3. α-substitution also significantly affects the receptor selectivity, e.g. in case of β-receptor α-methyl or ethyl substitution result in the compound with selectivity toward the β_2-receptors.

4. While in case of α-receptors, α-methyl substitution result in the compounds with selectivity toward the α_2 receptors.

Phenyl Ring Substitution

1. The naturally occurring noradrenaline has 3′, 4′-dihydroxy benzene ring (catechol) active at both α and β receptors. But it has poor oral activity because it is rapidly metabolized by COMT, change in substitution pattern to 3′, 5′-dihydroxy as is in metaprolol gives good oral activity. This is due to its resistance to metabolism by COMT. It also provides selectivity for β_2-receptors.

2. Replacement of catechol ring with resorcinol increases selective β_2-receptors agonistic activity.

3. In another approach, replacement of the metahydroxyl of the catechol structure with a hydroxymethyl group agent such as albuterol, which shows selectivity to the β_2-receptor.

4. Removal of para-hydroxy group from epinephrine gives phenylephrine, which is selective for the α_1-adrenergic receptors.

Metoproterenol

Albuterol

Phenylephrin

Stereochemistry

The highly critical factor in the interaction of adrenergic agonists with their receptor is that of stereo-selectivity for epinephrine, norepinephrin and related compounds, the more potent enantiomer has the R(-) configuration.

Indirectly Acting Drugs

Amphetamine and Tyramine

MOA: These drugs do not act directly on the adrenoceptor. They simply enhance the release of endogenously noradrenaline.

Structure Activity Relationship

1. A phenyl group may be replaced by cycloalkyl and alkyl moieties.
2. They lack phenolic hydroxyl group at the 3 and 4 positions. This enhances absorption of these drugs on oral administration and their penetration into the central nervous system.
3. It does not contain hydroxyl group on the benzene ring, which decreases its polarity and increases lipid solubility thus penetrating blood-brain barrier very easily.

Mixed Acting Drugs

Ephedrine, Phenylpropanolamine

Mode of action: Many sympathomimetic drugs exert their action by acting directly on the receptor sites and partly by their effects on the norepinephrine release.

Mechanism of Action of Sympathomimetics (*Fig. 14.5*)

1. Direct acting agents (open triangle) mimic norepinephrine as agonist at adrenergic receptor without interacting with presynaptic neurons. The chemical structure determines its subclass only.
2. Indirect sympathomimetics force epinephrine release from the presynaptic terminal. Thus the agent enhances the action of endogenous norepinephrine.

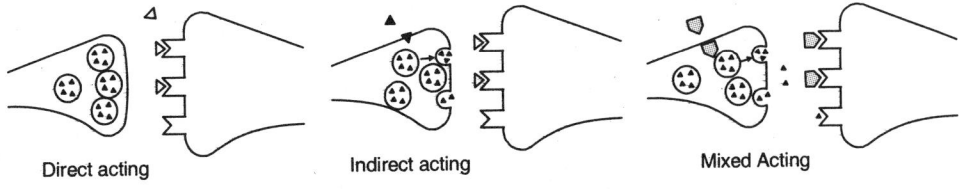

| Direct acting | Indirect acting | Mixed Acting |

Fig. 14.5: Mechanism of action of sympathomimetic agents

3. Mixed sympathomimetics induce the release of norepinephrine and also bind to adrenergic receptors. Sympathetic neuro-transmission is also enhanced by inhibition of the degradative enzymes, monoamine oxidase.

Metarminol

(−)-1-hydroxy-1-
(3-hydroxyphenyl)-
acetone   (I)

Metarminol

Clonidine

ethylene-
diamine

Clonidine

Sympatholytics (Antiadrenergic Agents)

Sympatholytics are the agents which inhibit or prevent the response of the sympathomimetic amine (neurotransmitter) by blocking their action on adrenoreceptors.

- These drugs antagonize the receptor action of adrenaline and related drugs. They are competitive antagonists at adrenergic receptors and differ in important ways from the "adrenergic neuron blocking agents", which act by interfering with the release of adrenergic transmitter on nerve stimulation.

- Since catecholamines play a role in a variety of physiological and pathophysiological responses, drugs that block adrenoceptors have important effects, some of which are of great clinical value.

- Adrenergic antagonists, antiadrenergic agents, also called as adrenergic blocking agent, selectively inhibit certain responses of sympathetic stimulation or block the effects produced by sympathomimetic agents.

CLASSIFICATION OF SYMPATHOLYTICS

Classification of sympatholytics is given in Flow chart 15.1.

Flow chart 15.1: Classification of sympatholytics

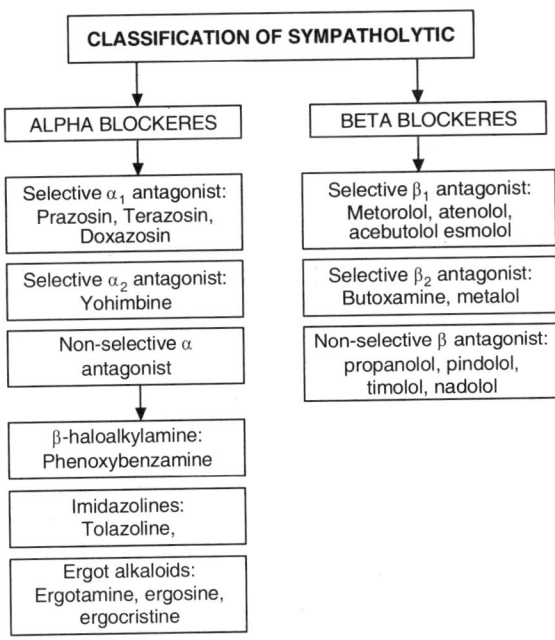

171

- These effects vary dramatically according to the drug's selectivity for receptors. In contrast, blockade of central nervous system dopamine receptors is very important.
- Non-selective antagonists have been used in the treatment of pheochromocytoma (tumors that secrete catecholamines), and 1-selective antagonists are used in primary hypertension and benign prostatic hyperplasia.
- Beta-receptor antagonist drugs have been found useful in a much wider variety of clinical conditions and are firmly established in the treatment of hypertension, ischemic heart disease, arrhythmias, endocrinological and neurologic disorders, and other conditions.

Non-selective α-Blockers

A. β-haloalkylamine derivatives

Phenoxybenzamine

B. Imidazoline

Phentolamine   Tolazoline

C. Ergot alkaloids

Ergosine   Ergocristine

Ergotamine

Selective α₁ Blocker

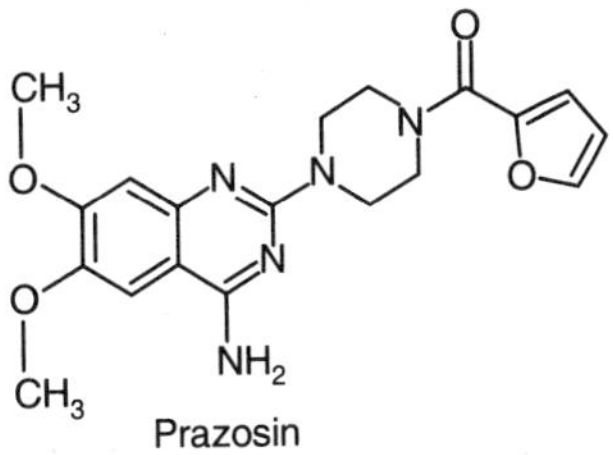

Prazosin

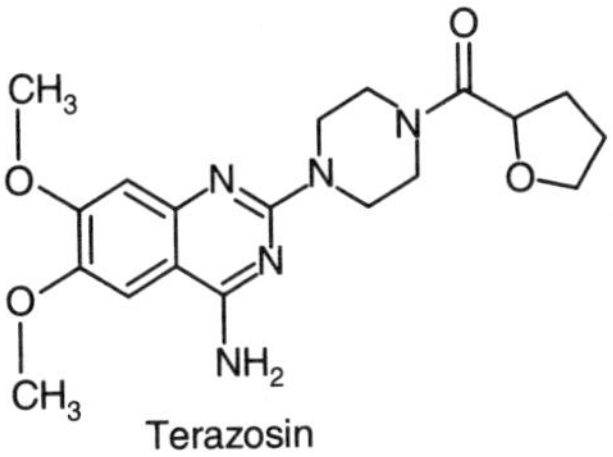

Terazosin

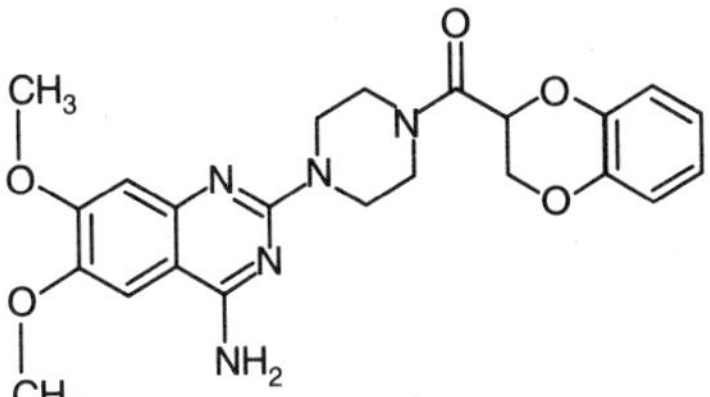

Doaxazocin

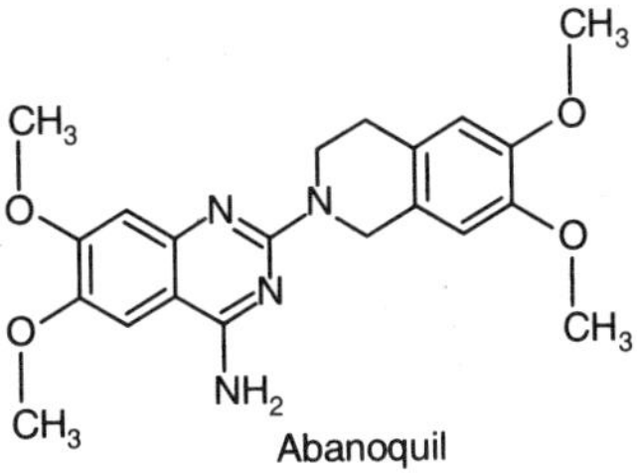

Abanoquil

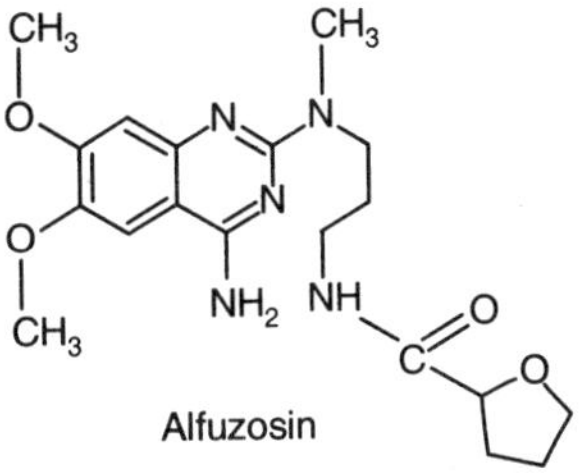

Alfuzosin

Selective α₂ Blocker

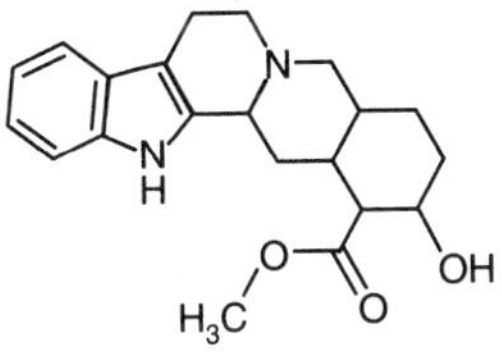

Yohimbine

Non-Selective β-Blocker

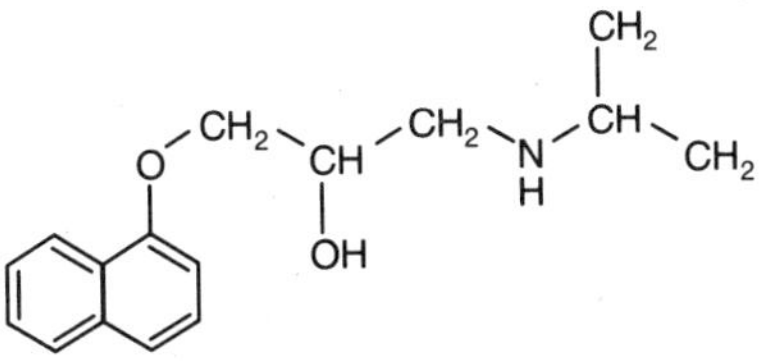

Propanolol

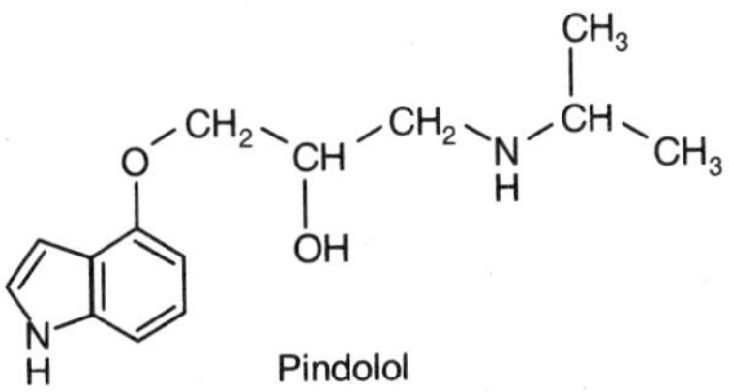

Pindolol

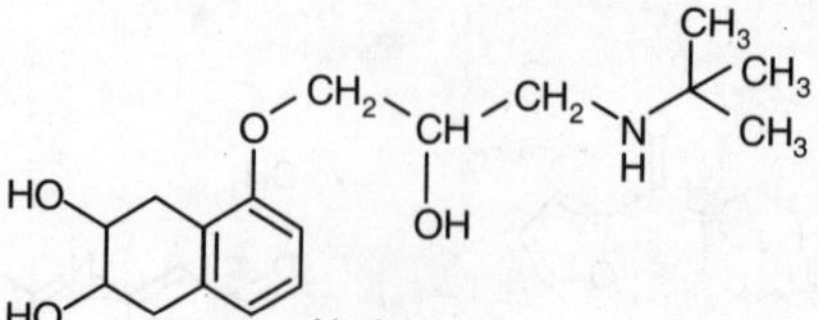

Nadolol

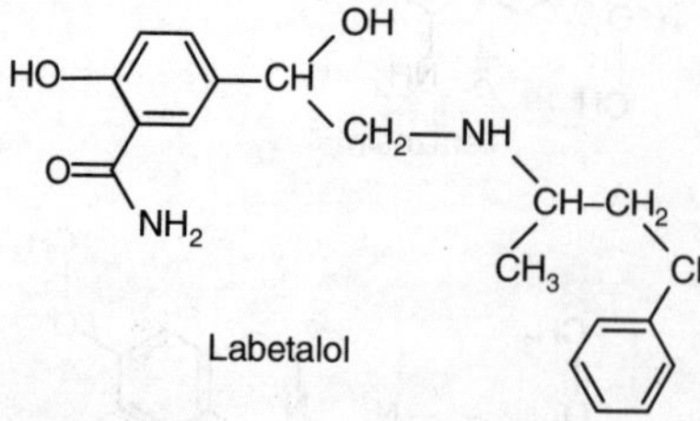

Labetalol

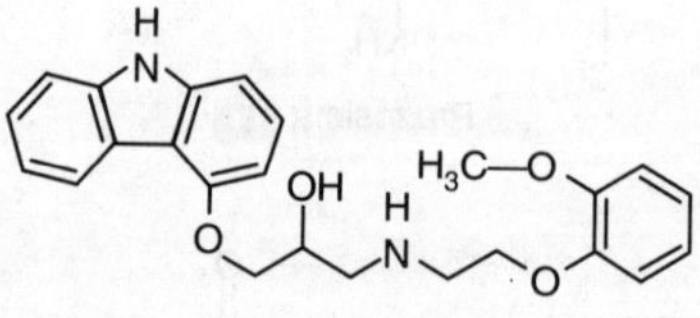

Carvedilol

Selective β₁-Blocker

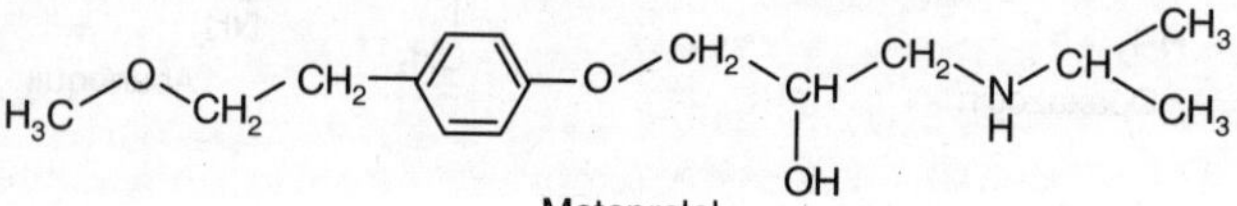

Metoprolol

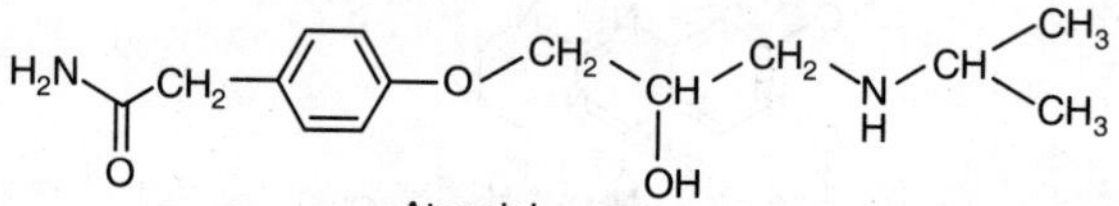

Atenolol

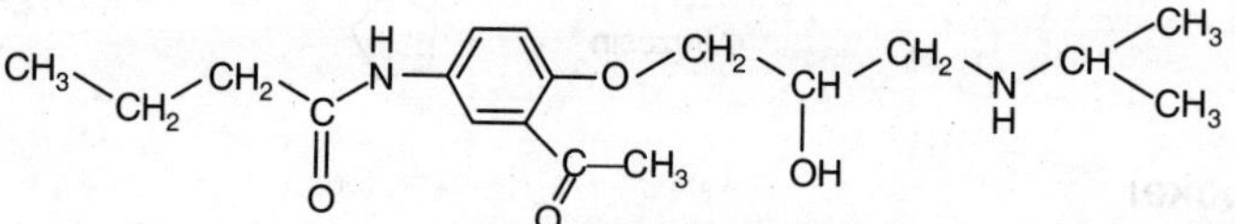

Acebutolol

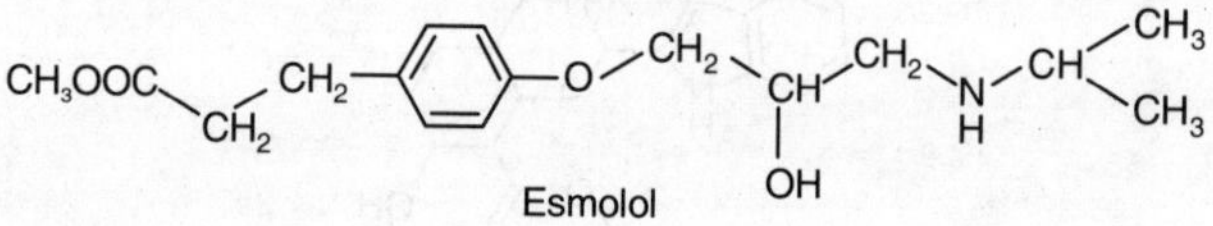

Esmolol

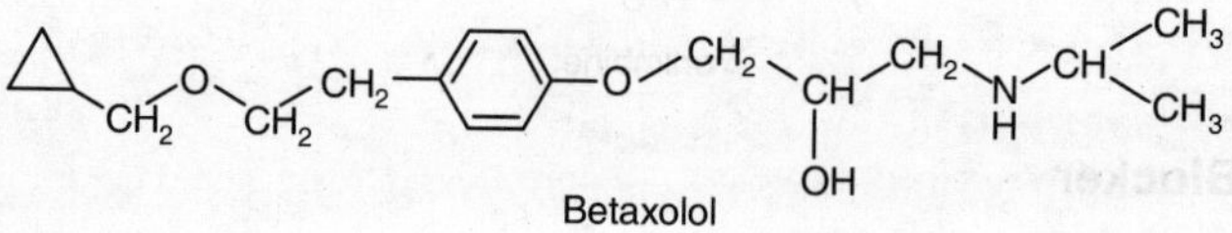

Betaxolol

Selective β₂-Blocker

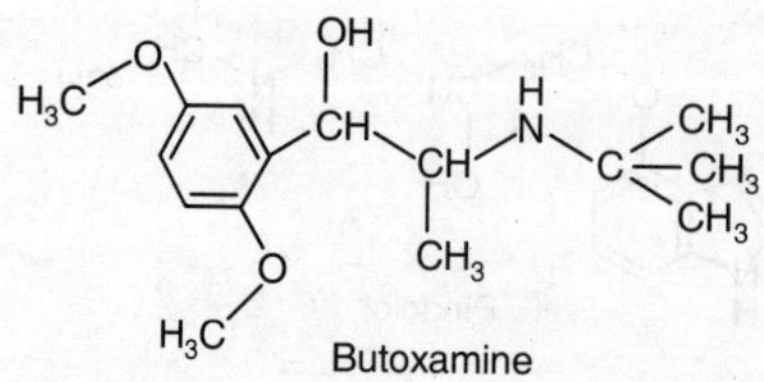

Butoxamine

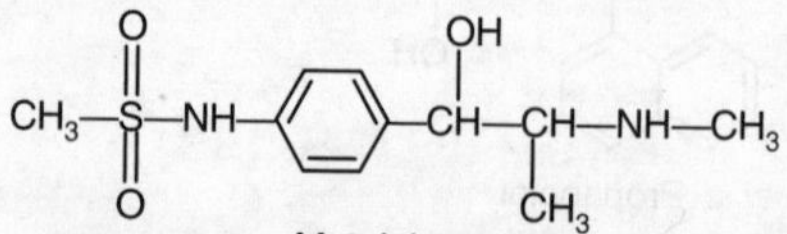

Metalol

Miscellaneous

Alpha methyl tyrosine

Methyl DOPA

Sulfiram

ALPHA BLOCKERS

Non-selective Alpha Blockers

1. **Beta Haloalkylamine**

Phenoxybenzamine

Mechanism of Action

- The beta haloalkylamines through the formation of an ammonium ion interact with a nucleophilic group present in the alpha receptor forming reversible covalent bond.

2. **Ergot alkaloids:** Ergot was recognized as alpha adrenergic agent in 1906. The parent compound is lysergic acid. Ergocristine, ergocryptine, ergocomine and ergonovine which are the derivatives of lysergic acid are found to possess adrenergic blocking action. A number of other amides of lysergic acid have been prepared of which methylegonovine and methylsergide are employed clinically.

3. **Imidazolines:** Tolazoline and phentolamine are the examples of clinically useful agent, which is used in the management of the hypertension.

α_1 Selective Antagonist (Fig. 15.1)

Quinazolines

These are highly selective α_1-receptor antagonists. Structurally, these contain three components:

1. Quinazoline ring.
2. Piperazine ring.
3. Acyl moity.

Structure-Activity Relationship

1. 4-amino group on quinazoline is very essential for the activity.
2. Piperazine ring can be replaced by that of other heterocyclic ring without affecting activity.
3. The nature of acyl group has significant role in pharmacokinetic properties.

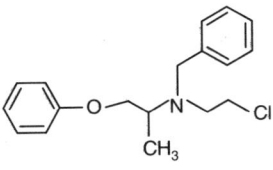

α_2 Selective Antagonist (Fig. 15.1)

Yohimbine is the selective α_2 antagonist.

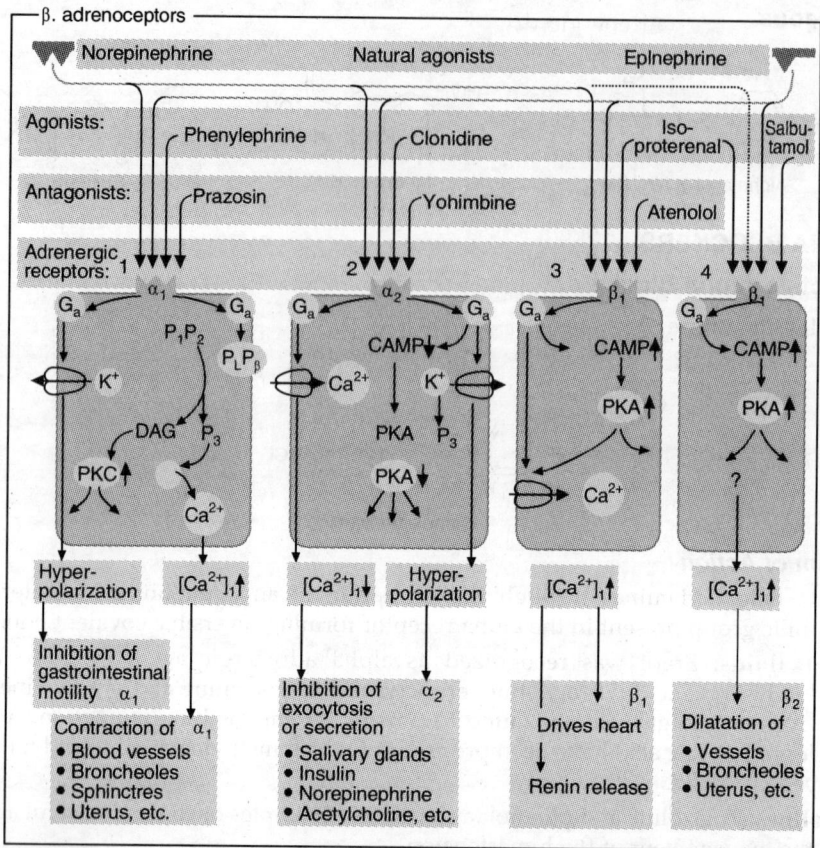

Fig. 15.1: Mode of action of sympatholytic agents

■ BETA BLOCKER

Structure-Activity Relationship

1. The aryloxypropanolamines are more potent than arylethanolamines.
2. Replacement of the ethereal oxygen in aryloxypropanolamine with S, CH_2 or NCH_3 is detrimental to the activity.
3. The most effective amine substituent is isopropyl and tertiary butyl.
4. The beta adrenergic receptor affinity resides chiefly in the D (-) absolute configuration.
5. Introduction of 4-OH group on naphthyl ring of the propanolol, results into a very potent beta antagonist.

$$Ar-O-CH_2-\underset{\underset{OH}{|}}{CH}-CH_2-NH-R\underset{CH_2}{\overset{CH_2}{<}}$$

4- Hydroxypropanolol

6. The catechol ring of (adrenergic drugs) can be replaced by a great variety of other ring system varying from.
   1. Phenylether.................Oxprenolon
   2. Sulphonamide..............Sotalol
   3. Amide......................Labetalol
   4. Indoles....................Pindolol
   5. Naphthalene...............Propanolol

7. Substitution of CH_3, Cl or NO_2 groups on the phenyl ring was most favoured at 2 and 3 positions and least favoured at 4-position.

8. Alkenyl and alkenyloxy groups in the ortho position on phenyl ring provided good activity.

Oxprenolol

Alprenolol

9. Larger alkyl chains are less effective but isopropyl or t-butyl, which gives an optimal basicity or nucleophilicity to the amino group for receptor affinity are most preferred.

10. A major clinical problem with propanolol was its high lipid solubility, which allowed it to penetrate nerve tissue and exert undesirable cardio-depressant effect in addition to its beta blocking action. To solve this problem methane sulphonamide was considered and resulting compound practolol is devoid of this side effect.

Practolol

11. Replacement of catechol hydroxyl groups with chlorine to give dichloroisoproterenol. A classic beta blocker.

Dichloro-isoproterenol

12. Replacement of the electron rich hydroxyl groups with an electron rich phenyl at 3, 4 positions gives pronethol, which is having good beta blocking activity.

13. Converting the aromatic portion to phenanthrene or anthracene was disadvantageous.

N-substitution

1. N, N-disubstituted compounds are inactive.
2. Alpha methyl group decreases activity.
3. Methoxyphenyl ethyl groups are added to amine part of the molecule.
4. Cyclic alkyl substituents are better than corresponding open chain substituent at nitrogen atoms of amine.
5. Chain length may extend to a total of four atoms.

Unwanted Effects

The main side effects of β-receptor antagonists result from their receptor-blocking action includes:

Bronchoconstriction:

- This is of little importance in the absence of airways disease, but in asthmatic patients the effect can be dramatic and life-threatening.
- It is also of clinical importance in patients with other forms of obstructive lung disease (e.g. chronic bronchitis, emphysema).

Cardiac depression: Cardiac depression can occur, leading to signs of heart failure, particularly in elderly people. Patients suffering from heart failure who are treated with β-receptor antagonists (see above) often deteriorate in the first few weeks before the beneficial effect develops.

Bradycardia: This side effect can lead to life-threatening heart block and can occur in patients with coronary disease, particularly if they are being treated with antiarrhythmic drugs that impair cardiac conduction.

Hypoglycemia:

- Glucose release in response to adrenaline is a safety device that may be important to diabetic patients and to other individuals prone to hypoglycemic attacks.
- The sympathetic response to hypoglycemia produces symptoms (especially tachycardia) that warn patients of the urgent need for carbohydrate (usually in the form of a sugary drink). β-receptor antagonists reduce these symptoms, so incipient hypoglycemia is more likely to go unnoticed by the patient.
- The use of β-receptor antagonists is generally to be avoided in patients with poorly controlled diabetes. There is a theoretical advantage in using β_1-selective agents, because glucose release from the liver is controlled by β_2-receptors.

Fatigue: This is probably due to reduced cardiac output and reduced muscle perfusion in exercise. It is a frequent complaint of patients taking β-receptor-blocking drugs.

Cold extremities:

- These are presumably due to a loss of β-receptor-mediated vasodilatation in cutaneous vessels, and are a common side effect.
- Theoretically, β_1-selective drugs are less likely to produce this effect, but it is not clear that this is so in practice.

▦ MISCELLANEOUS

α-Methyl Tyrosine (Fig. 15.2)

MOA: This inhibits the synthesis of tyrosine hydroxylase enzyme in the synthesis of nor-adrenaline, which converts tyrosine to L- DOPA.

Methyldopa (Fig. 15.2)

MOA: It inhibits DOPA-decarboxylase enzyme, which converts L-DOPA to dopamine.

Sulfiram (Fig. 15.2)

MOA: It inhibits Dopamine hydroxylase enzyme, which converts dopamine to noradrenaline

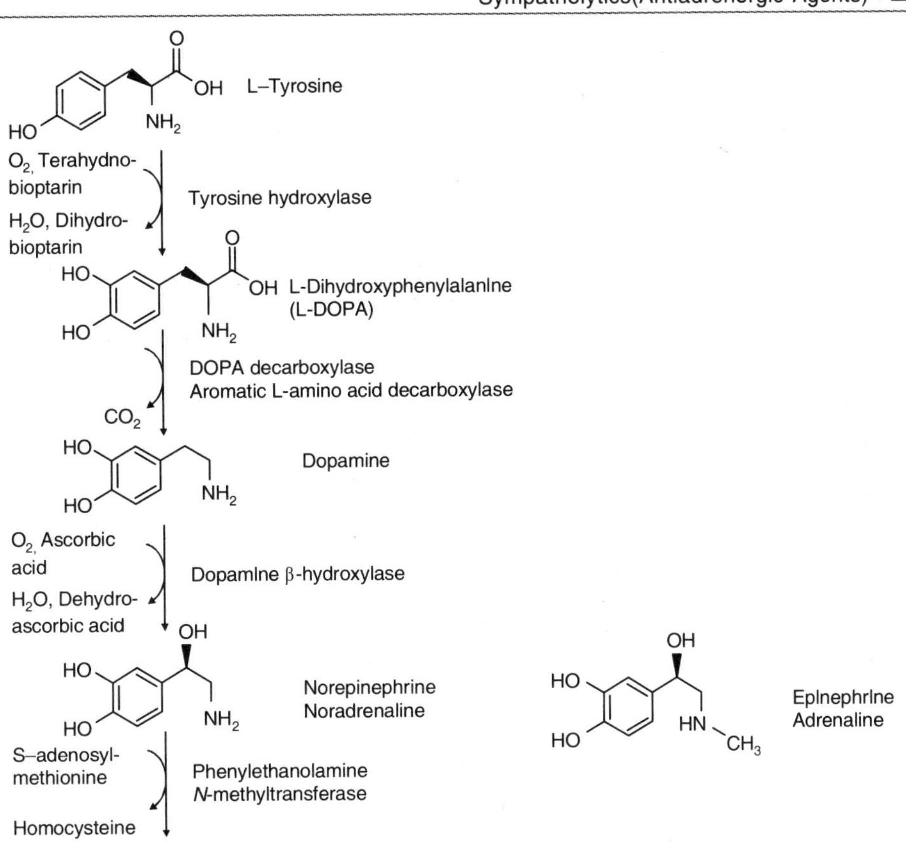

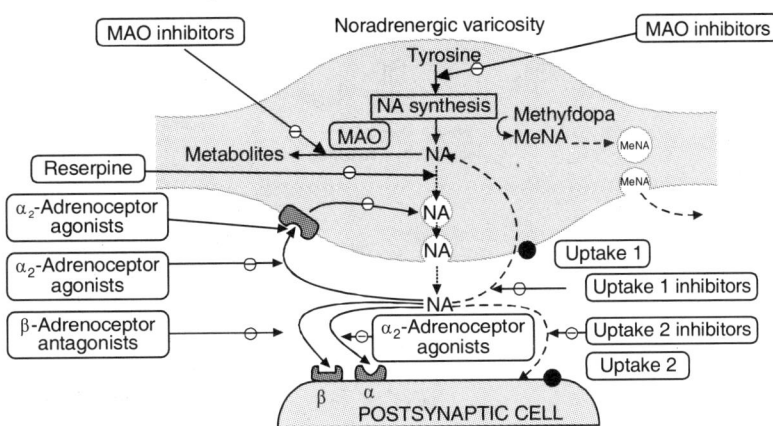

Fig. 15.2: Synthesis of adrenaline and noradrenaline

MECHANISM OF ACTION OF SYMPATHOLYTICS

The main sites of action of drugs that affect adrenergic transmission are depicted in Fig. 15.3.

Fig. 15.3: Generalized diagram of a noradrenergic nerve terminal, showing sites of drug action. MAO, monoamine oxidase; MeNA; methylnoradrenaline; NA, noradrenaline.

Phenoxybenzamine

Phenol + Propylene oxide → 1-phenoxy-2-propanolol → (SOCl₂ thionyl chloride) → 1-phenoxy-2-propyl chloride (I)

I + Ethanolamine → N-(1-methyl-2-phenoxyethyl)-ethanolamine → (benzyl chloride) → II

N-benzyl-N-(1-methyl-2-phenoxyethyl) ethanolamine (II) → (SOCl₂ Thionyl chloride) → Phenoxybenzamine

Phentolamine

Resorcinol + 4-methyl-aniline → 3-(4-methyl-anilino)phenol → (2-chloromethyl-Δ²-imidazoline hydrochloride) → Phentolamine

Tolazoline

Benzyl cyanide + ethonol → (HCl) → ethyl 2-phenyl imidate hydrochloride + HCl → (ethylene-diamine) → Toazoline

Pindolol

4-hydroxy-indole + Epichloro-hydrin → 3-chloro-1-(4-indolyloxy)-2-propanol → Pindolol

Timolol

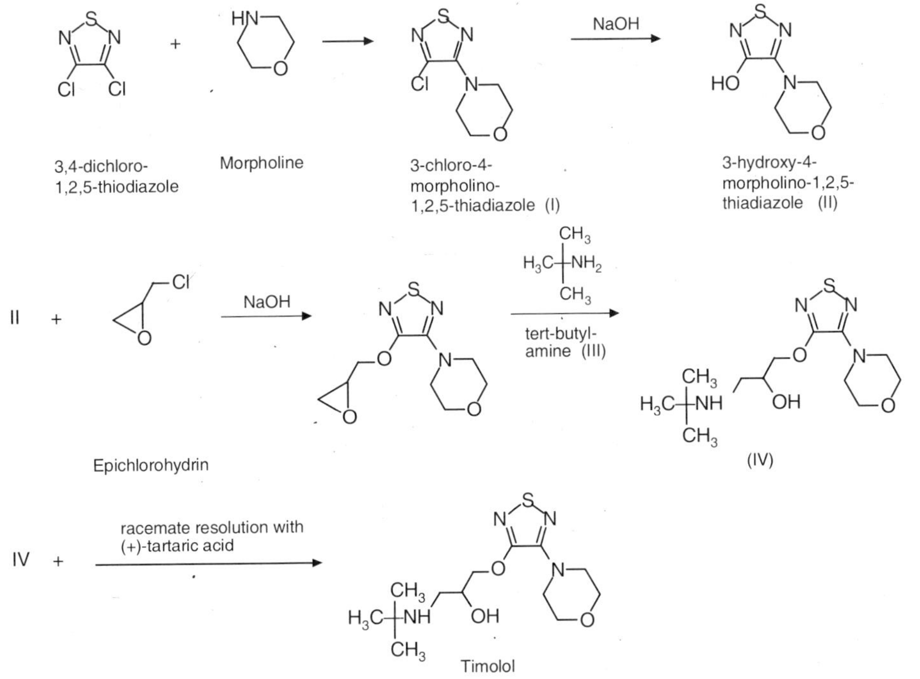
3,4-dichloro-
1,2,5-thiodiazole
Morpholine
3-chloro-4-
morpholino-
1,2,5-thiadiazole (I)
NaOH
3-hydroxy-4-
morpholino-1,2,5-
thiadiazole (II)
II +
Epichlorohydrin
NaOH
tert-butyl-
amine (III)
(IV)
IV +
racemate resolution with
(+)-tartaric acid
Timolol

Nadolol

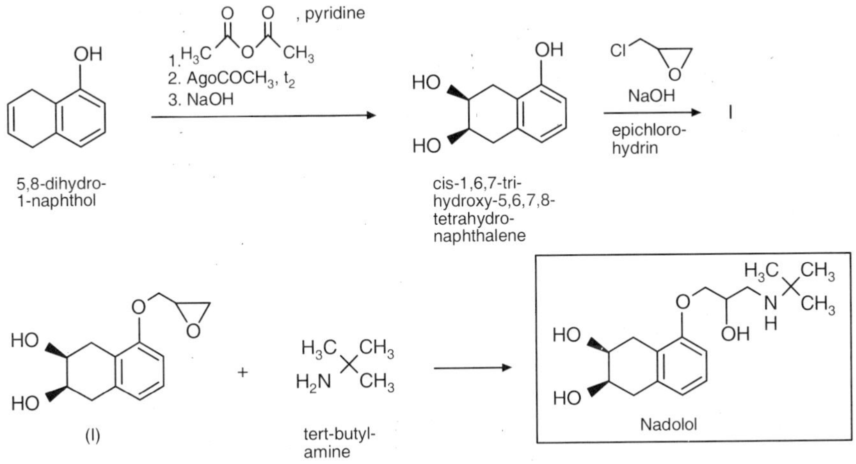
, pyridine
1.
2. AgoCOCH3, t2
3. NaOH
5,8-dihydro-
1-naphthol
cis-1,6,7-tri-
hydroxy-5,6,7,8-
tetrahydro-
naphthalene
NaOH
epichloro-
hydrin
I
(I)
tert-butyl-
amine
Nadolol

Propranolol

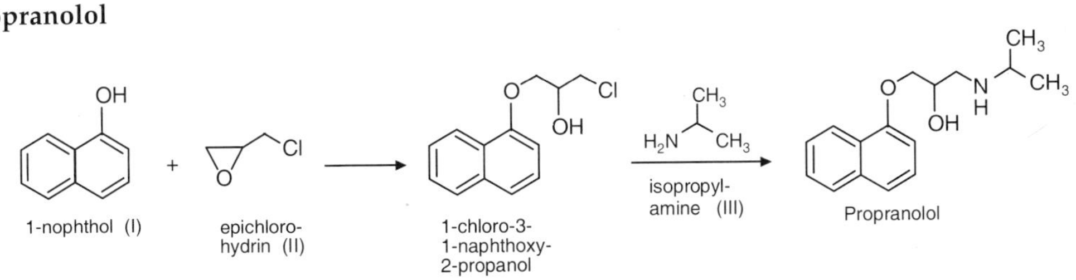
1-nophthol (I)
epichloro-
hydrin (II)
1-chloro-3-
1-naphthoxy-
2-propanol
isopropyl-
amine (III)
Propranolol

Labetalol

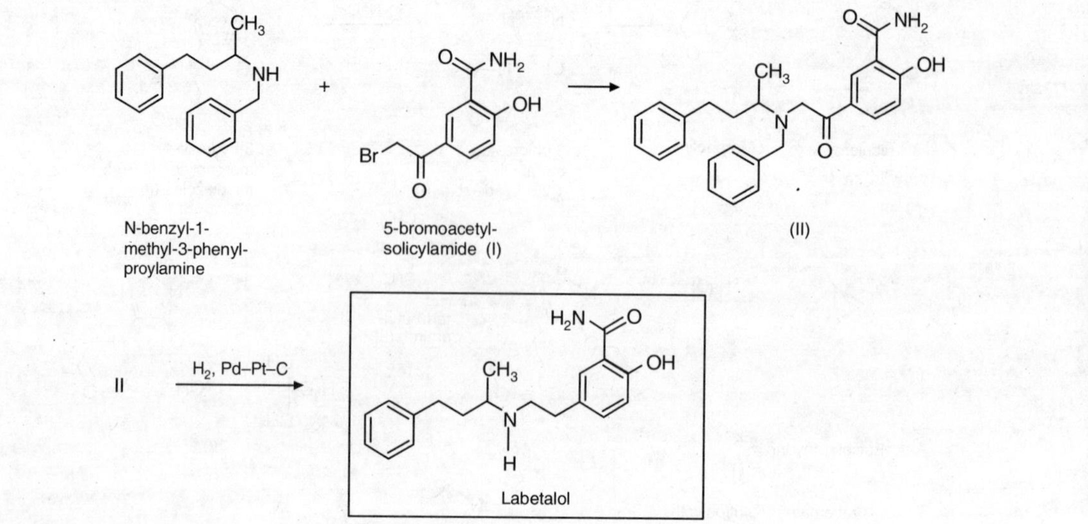

N-benzyl-1-
methyl-3-phenyl-
proylamine

5-bromoacetyl-
solicylamide (I)

(II)

II → H₂, Pd–Pt–C

Labetalol

Metoprolol

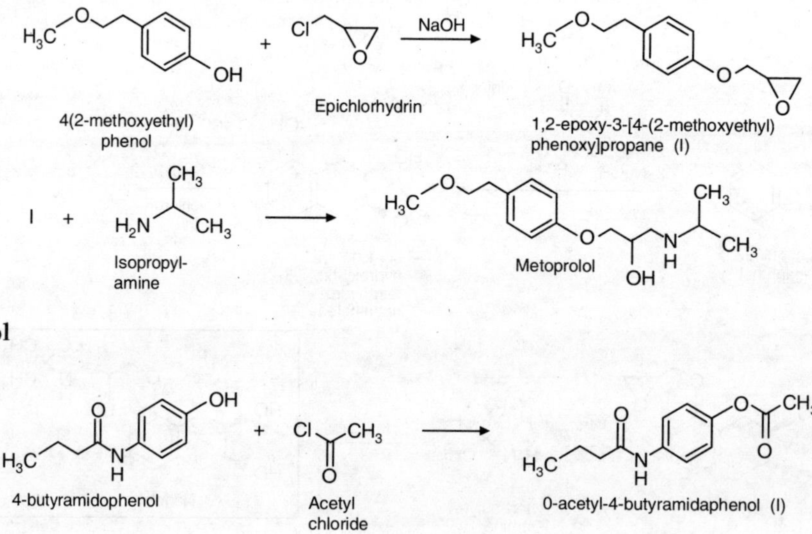

4(2-methoxyethyl)
phenol

Epichlorhydrin

1,2-epoxy-3-[4-(2-methoxyethyl)
phenoxy]propane (I)

I + Isopropyl-
amine

Metoprolol

Acebutolol

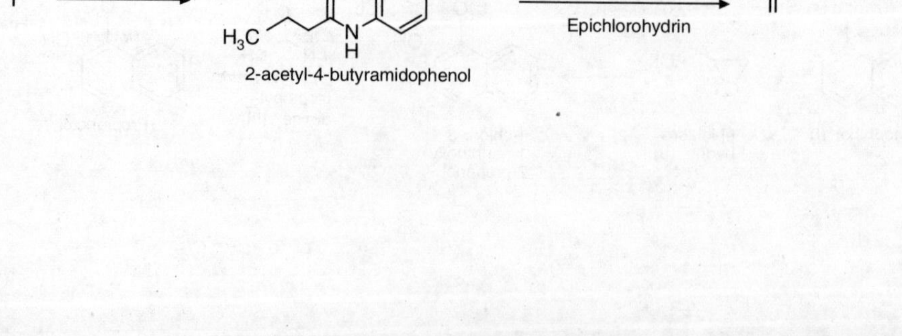

4-butyramidophenol

Acetyl
chloride

0-acetyl-4-butyramidaphenol (I)

I → AlCl₃, 140°C

2-acetyl-4-butyramidophenol

→ Epichlorohydrin , NaOC₂H₅ → II

0-(2-oxironylmethyl)-
2-acetyl-4-butyromidophenol (II)

Acebutolol

Esmolol

Methyl 3-(4-hydroxy-
phenyl)proplonate

Epichloro-
hydrin

Methyl 3-[4-(2,3-eoxy-
propoxy)phenyl]propionate (I)

Isopropylamine

Esmolol

Esmolol

Unit III

Drugs Affecting on Central Nervous System

General Anesthetics

INTRODUCTION

General anesthetics are known to be depressant drug that produces partial or total reversible loss of sense of pain, loss of consciousness.

- This state of insensibility is known as anesthesia. It causes descending depression of the CNS, start from cerebral cortex to basal ganglia then to cerebellum and finally spinal cord. General anesthesia is essential to surgical practice, because it renders patients analgesic, amnesic, and unconscious, while causing muscle relaxation and suppression of undesirable reflexes.
- No single drug is capable of achieving these effects both rapidly and safely. Rather, several different categories of drugs are utilized to produce optimal anesthesia. Potent general anesthetics are delivered via inhalation or intravenous injection.
- With the exception of nitrous oxide, modern inhaled anesthetics are all volatile, halogenated hydrocarbons that derive from early research and clinical experience with diethylether and chloroform. On the other hand, intravenous general anesthetics consist of a number of chemically unrelated drug types that are commonly used for the rapid induction of anesthesia.

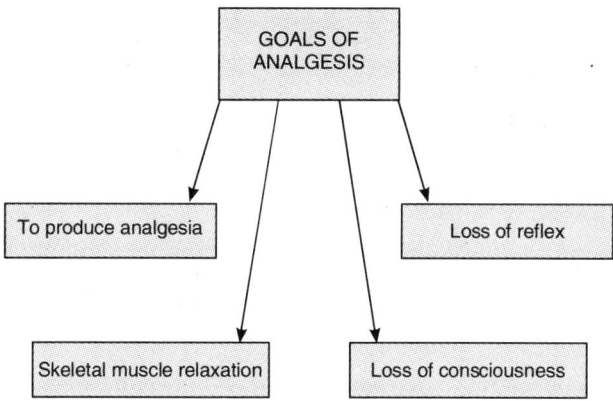

MINIMUM ALVEOLAR CONCENTRATION

- The minimum alveolar concentration (MAC) is defined as the concentration at 1 atmosphere of anesthetic in the alveoli required to produce immobility in 50% of adult patients subjected to a surgical incision.

STAGES OF ANESTHESIA (Fig. 16.1)

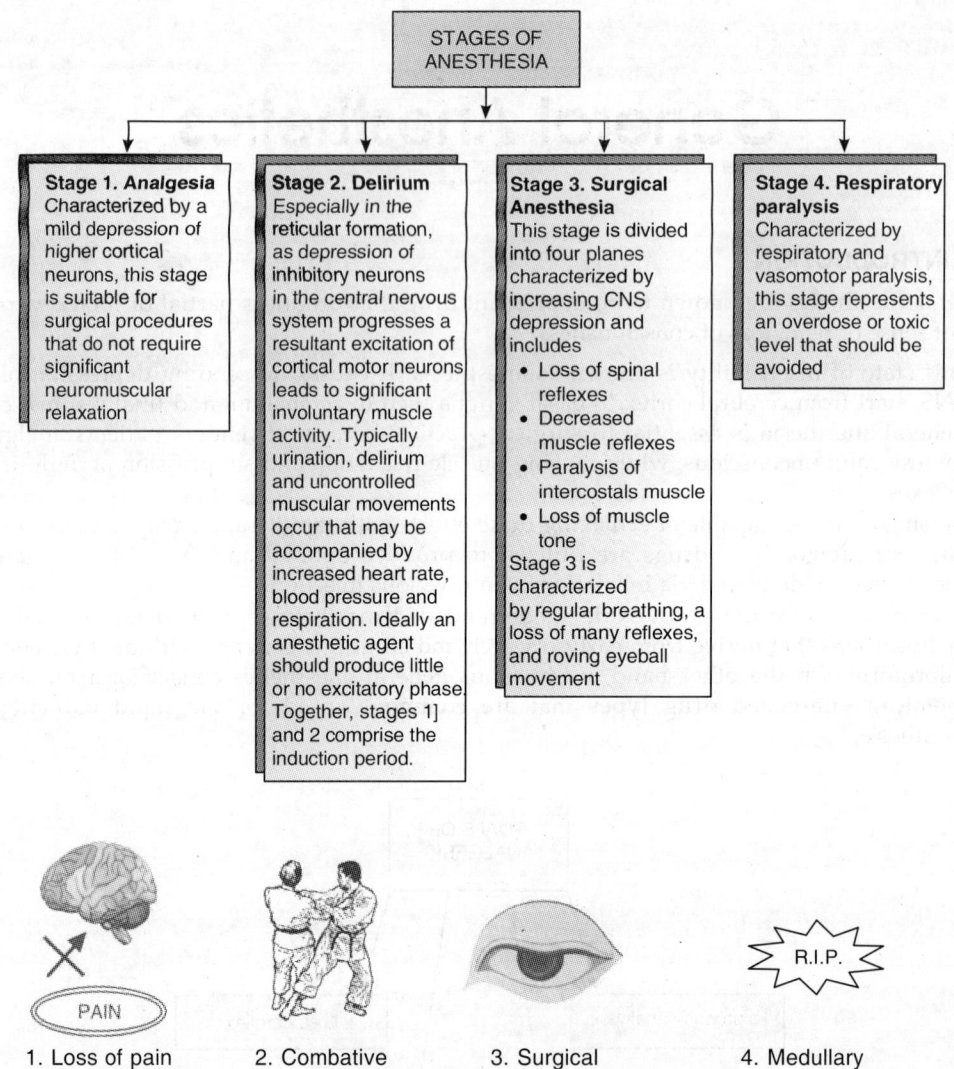

Fig. 16.1: Stages of anesthesia

- At equilibrium, the concentration (or partial pressure) of an anesthetic in the alveoli is equal to that in the brain, and it is this concentration in the brain that probably most closely reflects the concentration at the site responsible for the anesthetic actions.

- Thus, the MAC is often used as a measure of the potency of individual anesthetic agents. The MAC of many of the volatile and gaseous anesthetics in use today. When used in combinations, the MACs for inhaled anesthetics are additive.

- The combination of two anesthetics is, a very common practice as these techniques allows for a reduction in the exposure to the patient of anyone of the individual agents, thereby decreasing the likelihood of adverse reactions.

IDEAL CHARACTERISTIC OF ANESTHETICS

1. Rapid and pleasant withdrawal from anesthesia.
2. Adequate relaxation of skeletal muscles.
3. Potent enough to permit adequate oxygen supply in mixture.
4. Wide margin of safety.
5. Non-toxic.
6. Rapid and pleasant induction of surgical anesthesia.
7. Absence of adverse effects.
8. Noninflammable/non-explosive.
9. Chemically compatible with anesthetic devices.
10. Non-reactive.

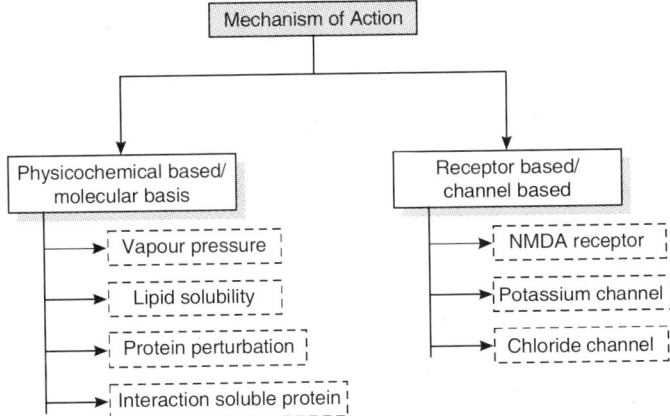

Generally mechanism of action of general anesthetic agents cannot explained by single mechanism of action, because of they are, nonspecific in action, useful in high concentration, distributed in all area of organism and diversity. Mechanisms of action are as follows.

Based on Vapour Pressure

- According to Ferguson (1959), the thermodynamic activity at anesthesia of a volatile anesthetic is defined by the equation.

$$\bullet\ A_{50} = P_{50}/P^0 = EC_{50}/Csat$$

- A_{50} is the thermodynamic activity at the anesthetic partial pressure P_{50} at which half the subjects are anesthetized, and $P°$ is the saturated vapor pressure of the pure liquid anesthetic.
- In aqueous concentration, EC_{50} is the corresponding anesthetic concentration and C_{sat} is the saturated concentration of the anesthetic. Correlation between anesthetic partial pressure and ideal solubility theory because $(1/P°)$ is the ideal solubility predicted by Raoult's law.

- This model predicts that anesthesia "occurs when a certain molar concentration is attained in the lipids of the cell." This theory did not account fully the anesthetic property of fully halogenated hydrocarbon.

Based on Lipid Solubility

- In the early 1900s, Hans Meyer and Charles Overton suggested that the potency of a substance as an anesthetic was directly related to its lipid solubility, or oil:gas partition coefficient. They used olive oil, octanol and other 'membrane-like' lipids to determine the lipid solubility of the agents available at the time.
- Compounds with high-lipid solubility required lower concentrations (i.e. lower MAC) to produce anesthesia. It was postulated that the interaction of the anesthetic molecules with a hydrophobic portion of the membrane caused a distortion of the membrane near the channels that conducted sodium ions, those that mediated the fast action potentials and neuronal cell firing.
- The presence of this critical volume of anesthetic dissolved within the membrane caused the membrane to 'bloat' and 'squeeze' on the channel to interfere with sodium conductance and normal neuronal depolarization.

Protein Perturbation Theory

- According to Meyer-Overton, it was postulated that the interaction of the anesthetic molecules with a hydrophobic portion of the membrane caused a distortion of the membrane near the channels that conducted sodium ions, those that mediated the fast action potentials and neuronal cell firing.
- The presence of this critical volume of anesthetic dissolved within the membrane caused the membrane to 'bloat' and 'squeeze' in on the channel to interfere with sodium conductance and normal neuronal depolarization.

Interaction with the Soluble Protein

- At the molecular level, anesthetics probably exert their effect by direct interaction with proteins rather than by disturbing the lipid-bilayer matrix, as earlier proposed. They may bind directly with hydrophobic region, clefts or poechs of proteins.
- This binding produces disturbances in channel function. Halothane has been found to interact with muscle adenylate kinase resulting in competitive inhibition of the production of ADP.
- Halothane binds deep within the interior of the protein within a hydrophobic pocket lined with eleven amino acids, eight of which have hydrophobic side chains and the remainder has polar ones.

NMDA Receptor Theory

- N-methyl-D-aspartate (NMDA) receptor, which is usually activated by the excitatory amino acid neurotransmitter, glutamate to increase the conductance to sodium.
- Compounds known to stimulate NMDA receptors are typically capable of increasing alertness and acting as convulsants, while pharmacologic agents that act as antagonists at this site are usually sedatives, anticonvulsants and dissociative anesthetics (e.g. ketamine).

Chloride Channel

- These agents depress the function of inotropic glutamate receptor (excitatory), which may contribute to overall anesthetic effect. Halothane has been demonstrated to specifically antagonize the glutamate-stimulated depolarization of neurons, while isoflurane has been shown to decrease glutamate release and enhance its removal from the synaptic cleft.
- Channel that has received the most investigative attention is that for chloride. GABA receptors are linked to chloride channels and normally mediate inhibitory responses within the central nervous system.
- Halothane, isoflurane and other general anesthetics are capable of inhibiting the synaptic destruction of GABA, thereby increasing the GABA-ergic neuro-transmission, which is typically inhibitory in nature.
- Additionally, studies have demonstrated the ability of these anesthetics to enhance the binding of GABA or other allosteric modulators within the GABA-receptor complex.
- At therapeutic concentrations just about all of the general anesthetics are capable of enhancing GABA-nergic function, while at considerably higher concentrations many act directly as GABA-mimetics.
- Most of these agents also potentiate the actions of glycine, the other important inhibitory amino acid neurotransmitter. The combination of GABA-nergic and glycinergic potentiation by the general anesthetics probably accounts for much of their observed activity.

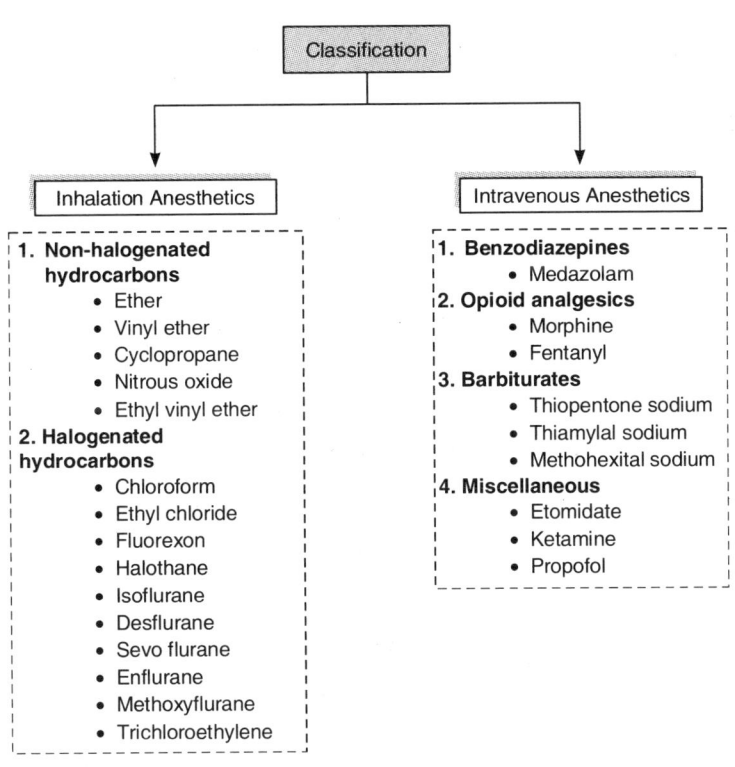

▓▓ POTASSIUM CHANNEL

- Potassium channels have also been suggested as a site for general anesthetic agents. Increasing K^+ conductance normally functions to maintain the polarized state of neu-rons and to assist in the repolarizing of neurons following their stimulation-induced depolarization.
- Thus, enhancing the activity of certain K^+ channels would be expected to result in a decreased likelihood of neuronal excitation. Certain α_2-adrenoceptor agonists (e.g. dexmedetomidine) produce an anesthetic state that is mediated by a G protein-coupled receptor that allosterically modulates K^+ channels.

Inhalation Anesthetics

Non-halogenated hydrocarbons

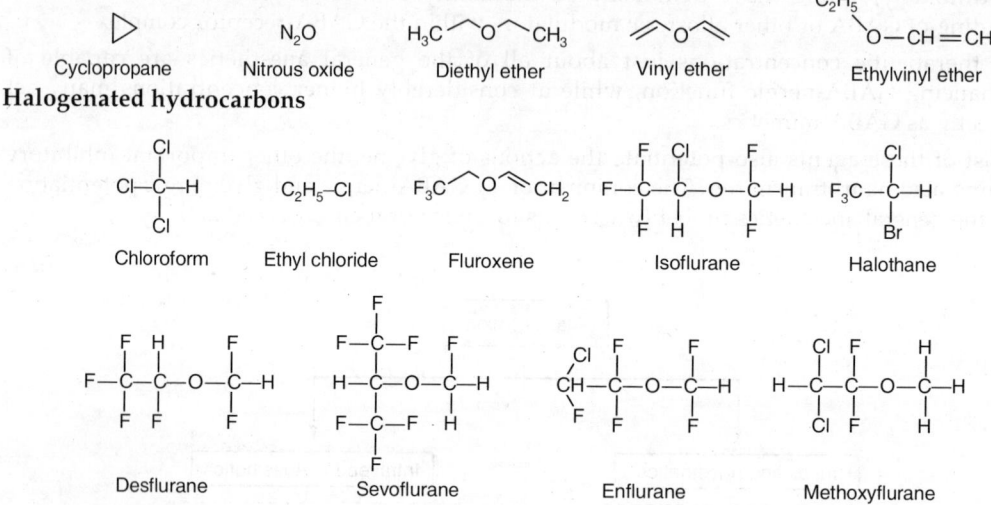

Halogenated hydrocarbons

Intravenous Anesthetics

a. Barbiturates

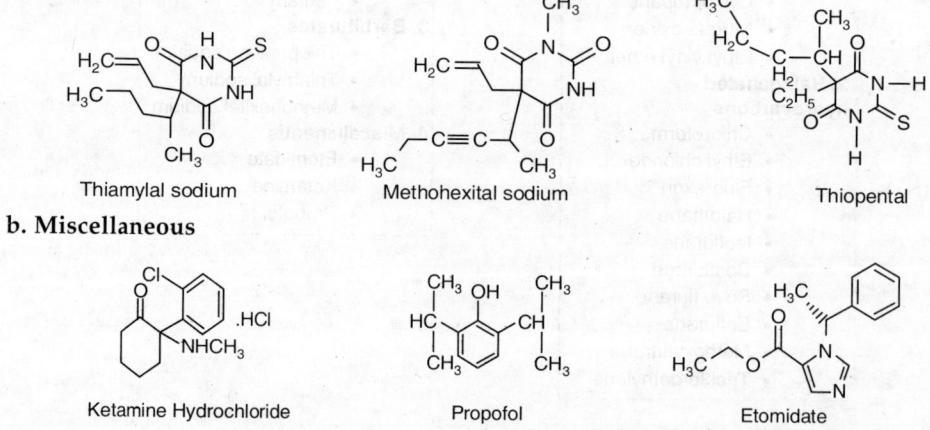

b. Miscellaneous

Synthesis

Halothane

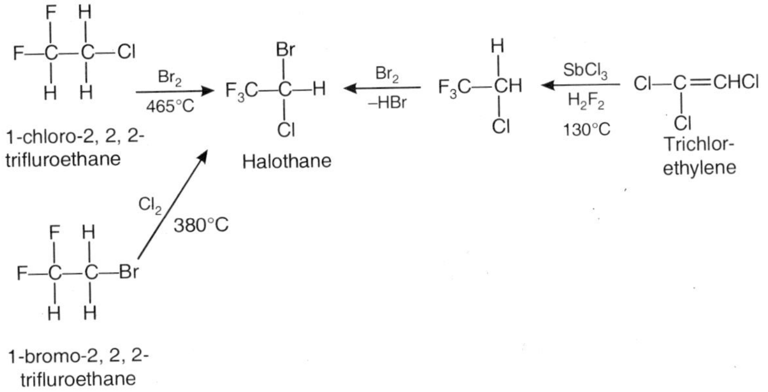
Br$_2$
465°C
Br$_2$
–HBr
SbCl$_3$
H$_2$F$_2$
130°C
1-chloro-2, 2, 2-trifluroethane
Halothane
Trichlor-ethylene
Cl$_2$
380°C
1-bromo-2, 2, 2-trifluroethane

Fluorexone

$$F3C—CH_2OH + HC\equiv CH \longrightarrow F_3CH_2C—O—HC=CH_2$$

2, 2, 2-Trifluoroethyl vinylether (fluorexone)

Ketamine hydrochloride

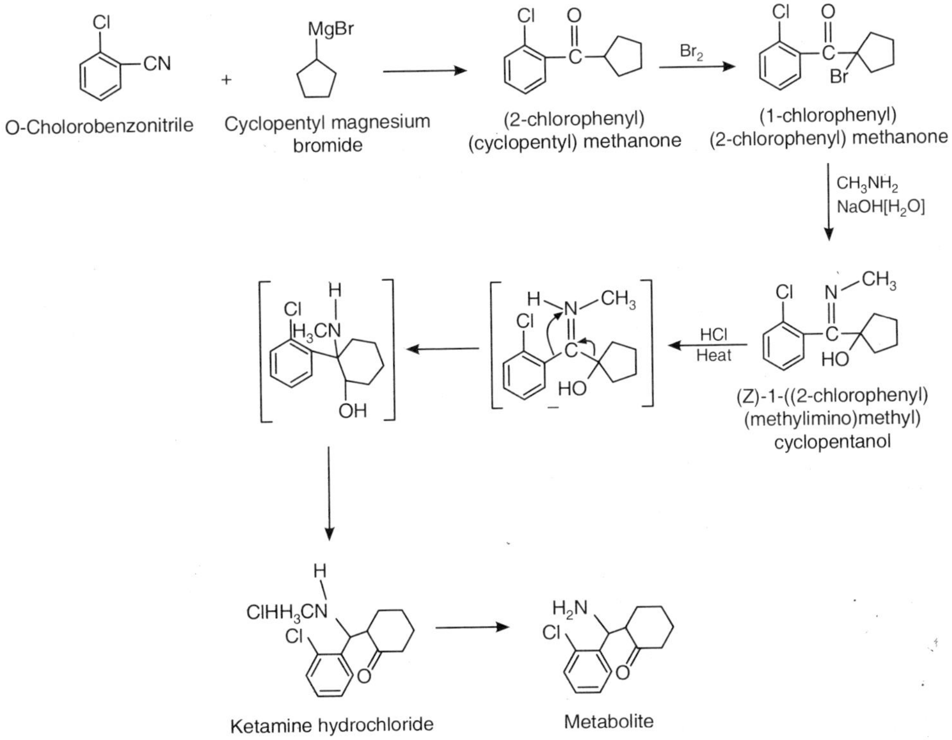
O-Cholorobenzonitrile
Cyclopentyl magnesium bromide
(2-chlorophenyl) (cyclopentyl) methanone
Br$_2$
(1-chlorophenyl) (2-chlorophenyl) methanone
CH$_3$NH$_2$
NaOH[H$_2$O]
HCl
Heat
(Z)-1-((2-chlorophenyl) (methylimino)methyl) cyclopentanol
Ketamine hydrochloride
Metabolite

Methohexital sodium

Thiomylal sodium

Thiopental sodium

Diethyl malonate   2-bromopentane

Thiopental sodium

Local Anesthetics

Local anesthetics are the agents which block both sensory and motor nerve conduction to produce temporary loss of sensation without loss of consciousness. These agents reversibly block the generation and the conduction of impulses along a nerve fiber. They are used to abolish the pain sensation in restricted areas of the body when progressively increasing the concentration of a local anesthetic is applied to nerve fiber, the threshold for excitation increases, the impulse conduction slows, the rate of rise of the action potential declines. The action potential amplitude decreases, and finally, the ability to generate an electrical potential is abolished. All these effects result from the binding of local anesthetic to sodium channels, thus binding results in blockade of the sodium current. If the sodium current is blocked over a critical portion of nerve, the propagation of an impulse over the blockade are no longer is possible.

HISTORY

- The leaves of the coca plant were traditionally used as a stimulant in Peru. It is believed that the local anesthetic effect of coca was also known and used for medical purposes. Cocaine was isolated in 1860 and first used as a local anesthetic in 1884.

- The turn of the century was a tremendous time of scientific progress, and the new discipline of organic chemistry enabled the synthesis of the first analog of cocaine in 1905. (An analog of a chemical molecule is one in which the original molecule is progressively modified to retain and enhance certain holistic characteristics of the original substance while ridding it of other unwanted characteristics.) The first synthetic local anesthetic was procaine, better remembered today by its trade name, 'novocain'. Novocain was not without its problems. It took a very long time to set (i.e. to produce the desired anesthetic result), wore off too quickly and was not nearly as potent as cocaine. On top of that, it is classified as an ester. Esters have a very high potential to cause allergic reactions. It is estimated that about one-third of all persons who received it developed at least minor allergic reactions to it.

- Faced with the legal and ethical difficulties associated with the use of cocaine as a local anesthetic, and with the inefficiencies and allergenicity associated with the use of procaine, it is not surprising that most dentists of the day worked without any local anesthetic at all. (Nitrous oxide gas was available during this period.)

- Today, procaine is not even available for dental procedures. The search for a less toxic and less addictive substitute led to the development of the aminoester local anesthetic procaine in 1904. Since then, several synthetic local anesthetic drugs have been developed and put into clinical use, notably lidocaine in 1940, bupivacaine in 1957 and prilocaine in 1959.

$$\text{Lidocaine}$$

Lidocaine

- The first modern local anesthetic agent was lidocaine (trade name Xylocaine®). It was invented in the 1940s. Lidocaine is in a broad class of chemicals called amides, and unlike ester-based anesthetics, amides are hypoallergenic. It sets quickly and when combined with a small amount of epinephrine (adrenalin), it produces profound anesthesia for several hours. Lidocaine is still shortly after the first use of cocaine for topical anesthesia, blocks on peripheral nerves were described. Brachial plexus anesthesia by percutaneous injection through axillary and supraclavicular approaches was developed in the early 20th century. The search for the most effective and least traumatic approach for plexus anesthesia and peripheral nerve blocks continues to this day.

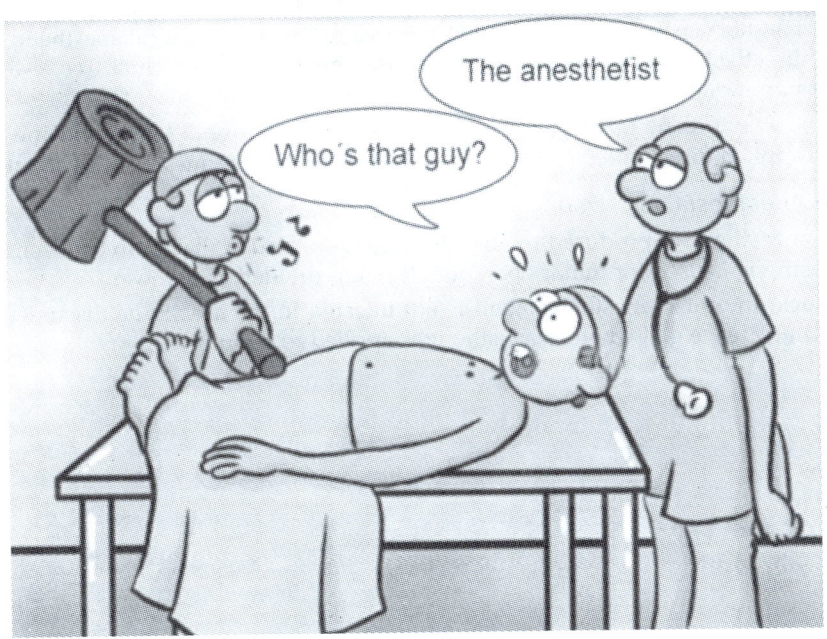

- In recent decades, continuous regional anesthesia using catheters and automatic pumps has evolved as a method of pain therapy. Intravenous regional anesthesia was first described by August Bier in 1908. This technique is still in use and is remarkably safe when drugs of low systemic toxicity such as prilocaine are used.
- Spinal anesthesia was first used in 1885 but not introduced into clinical practice until 1899, when August Bier subjected himself to a clinical experiment in which he observed the anesthetic effect, but also the typical side effect of postpunctural headache.
- Within few years, spinal anesthesia became widely used for surgical anesthesia and was accepted as a safe and effective technique. Although atraumatic (non-cutting-tip) cannulas and modern drugs are used today, the technique has otherwise changed very little over many decades.

- Epidural anesthesia by a caudal approach had been known in the early 20th century, but a well-defined technique using lumbar injection was not developed until the 1930s. With the advent of thin flexible catheters, continuous infusion and repeated injections have become possible, making epidural anesthesia a highly successful technique to this day.
- Beside its many uses for surgery, epidural anesthesia is particularly popular in obstetrics for the treatment of labour pain. The most widely used local anesthetic in America today.
- Over the next 30 years, a number of other amide local anesthetics were invented, most not differing significantly from lidocaine.

■ VARIOUS TECHNIQUES OF LOCAL ANESTHETICS

Local anesthetics vary in their pharmacological properties and they are used in various techniques of local anesthesia as given below.

Surface Anesthesia

- Application of local anesthetic spray, solution or cream to the skin or a mucous membrane. The effect is short lasting and is limited to the area of contact. The local anesthetic solution is applied directly to the mucosal surface as nose and mouth, bronchial tree, esophagus or genitourinary tract.
- It must be able to penetrate tissue readily. Recently, a mixture of lignocaine and prilocaine has been applied directly to the skin and can produce complete anesthesia in about one hour.

Infiltration Anesthesia (Fig. 17.1)

Infiltration aneasthesia is produced by injecting agent, to render all area to be insensitive. This form of anesthesia is used for minor operation. It is sub-divided as follows:

1. **Field block:** In which anesthetic agent is not injected in the area to be discussed, but into surrounding area, e.g Field block anesthesia is applied to scalp.

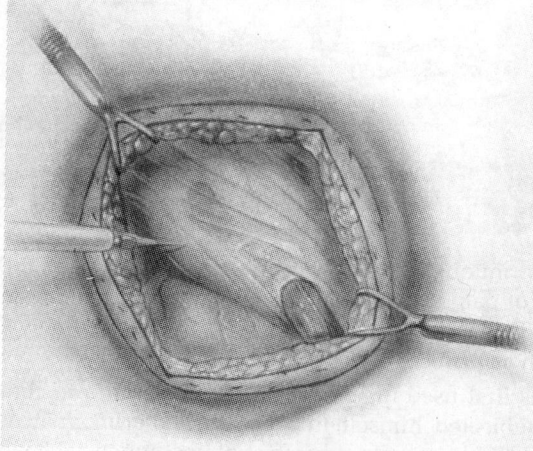

Fig. 17.1: Infiltration anesthesia

2. **Peripheral nerve blocks:** Injection of local anesthetic is deposited close to mix nerve to anesthetize that nerve's area of innervations.

Plexus Anesthesia (*Fig. 17.2*)

Injection of local anesthetic in the vicinity of a nerve plexus, often inside a tissue compartment that limits the diffusion of the drug away from the intended site of action. The anesthetic effect extends to the innervation areas of several or all nerves stemming from the plexus.

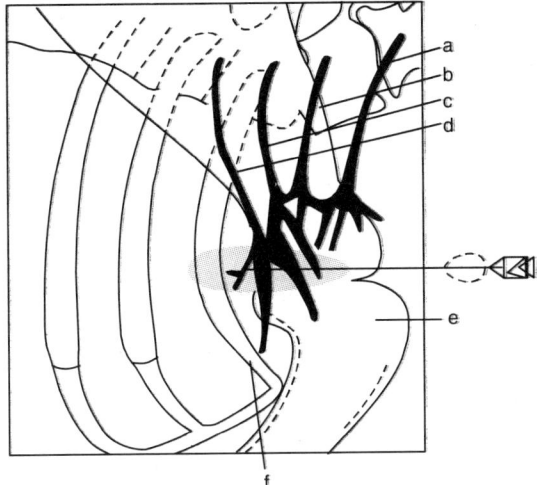

Fig. 17.2: Plexus anesthesia

Epidural Anesthesia (*Fig. 17.3*)

A local anesthetic is injected into the epidural space where it acts primarily on the spinal nerve roots. Depending on the site of injection and the volume injected, the anesthetized area varies from limited areas of the abdomen or chest to large regions of the body.

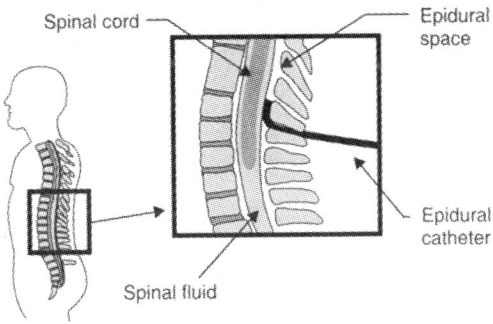

Fig. 17.3: Epidural anesthesia

Spinal Anesthesia (*Fig. 17.4*)

A local anesthetic is injected into the cerebrospinal fluid, usually at the lumbar spine (in the lower back), where it acts on spinal nerve roots and part of the spinal cord. The resulting anesthesia usually extends from the legs to the abdomen or chest.

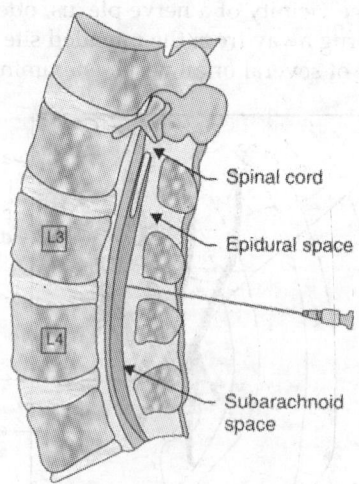

Fig. 17.4: Spinal anesthesia

Intravenous Regional Anesthesia (Bier's Block) (Fig. 17.5)

- Blood circulation of a limb is interrupted using a tourniquet (a device similar to a blood pressure cuff), then a large volume of local anesthetic is injected into a peripheral vein. The drug fills the limb's venous system and diffuses into tissues where peripheral nerves and nerve endings are anesthetized.
- The anesthetic effect is limited to the area that is excluded from blood circulation and resolves quickly once circulation is restored.

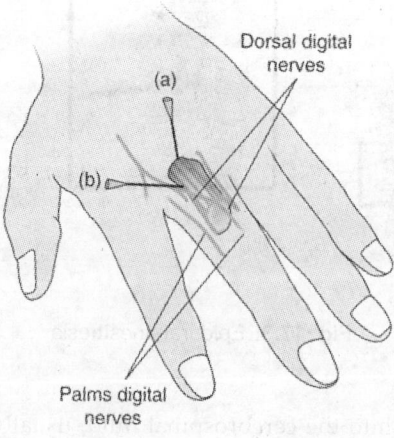

Fig. 17.5: Intravenous anesthesia

CLASSIFICATION OF LOCAL ANESTHETICS

Classification of local anesthetics is depicted in Flow chart 17.1.

Flow chart 17.1: Classification of LA

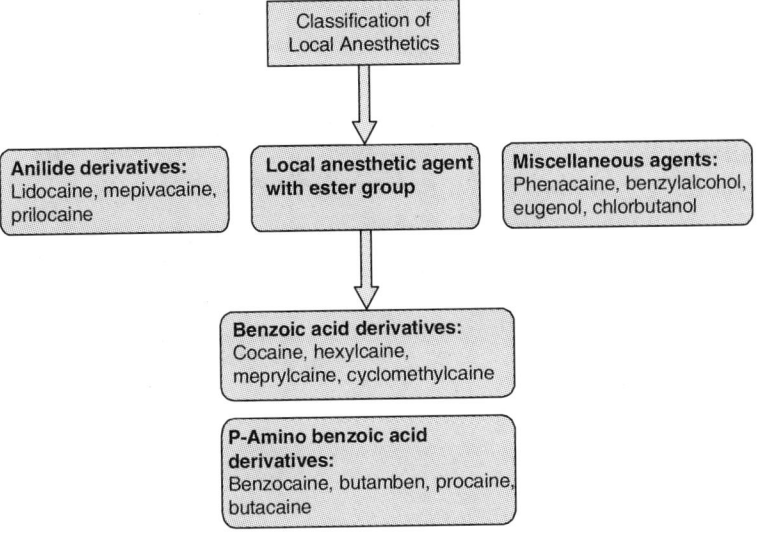

Local Anesthetic Agents with Ester Group

Benzoic Acid Derivatives

Cocaine

Hexylcaine

Meprylcaine

Cyclomethylcaine

Isobucaine

Piperocaine

p-Aminobenzoic Acid Derivatives

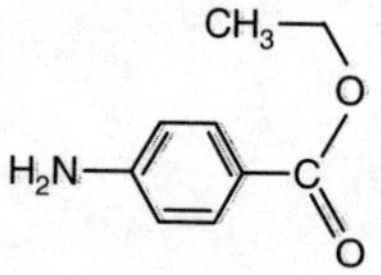

Benzocaine

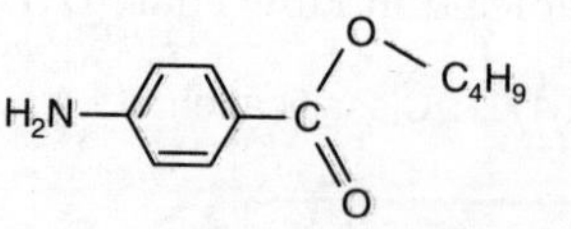

Butamben

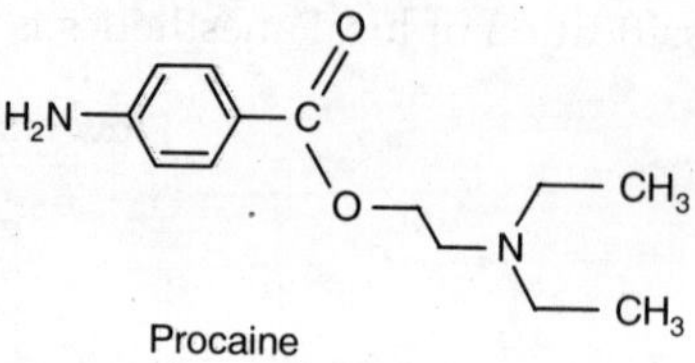

Procaine

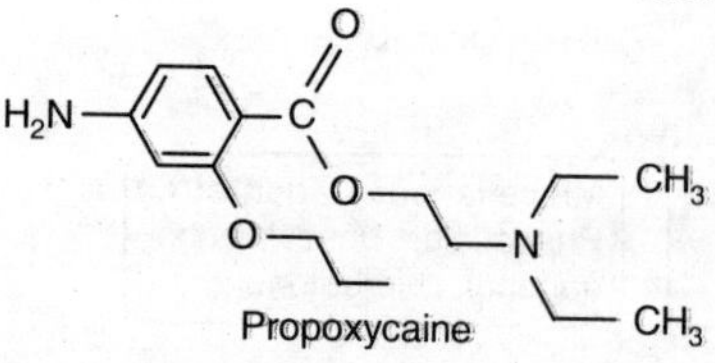

Propoxycaine

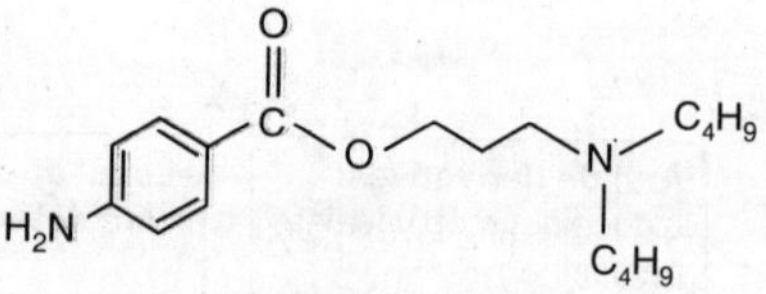

Butacaine

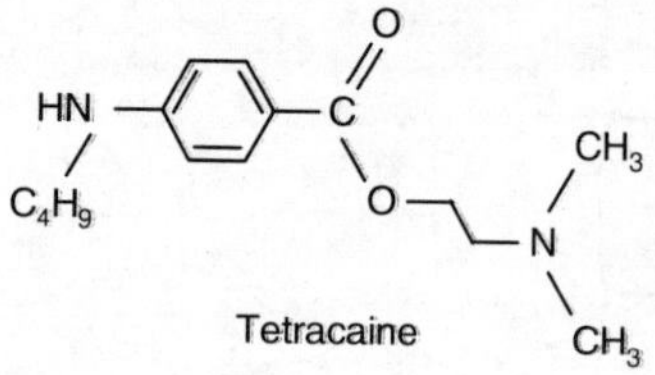

Tetracaine

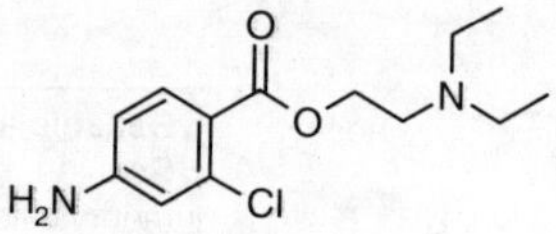

Chlorprocaine

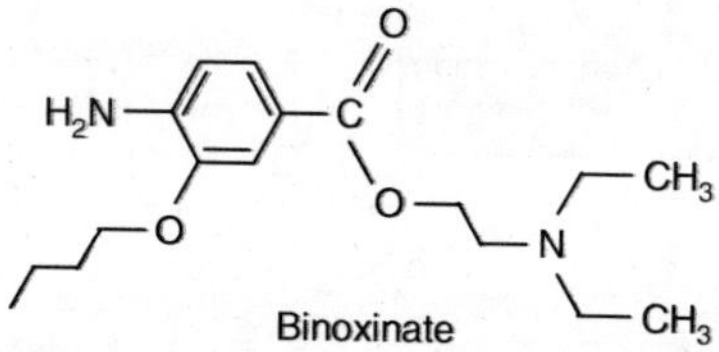

Binoxinate

Anilide Derivatives

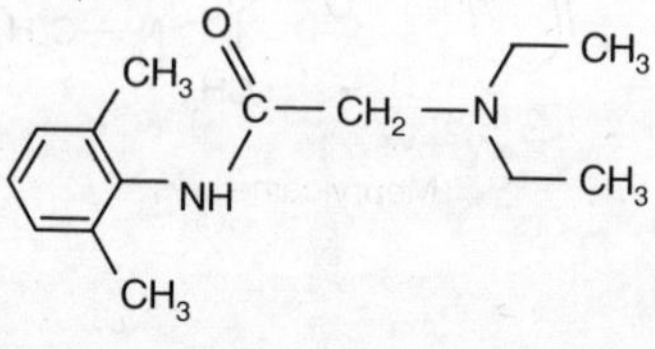

Lidocaine

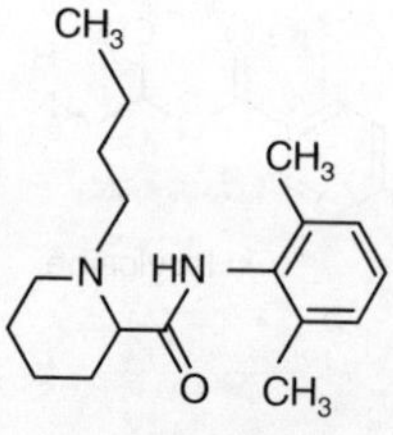

Bupivacaine

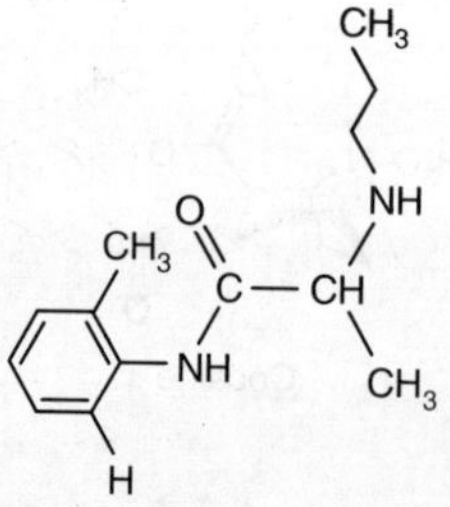

Prilocaine

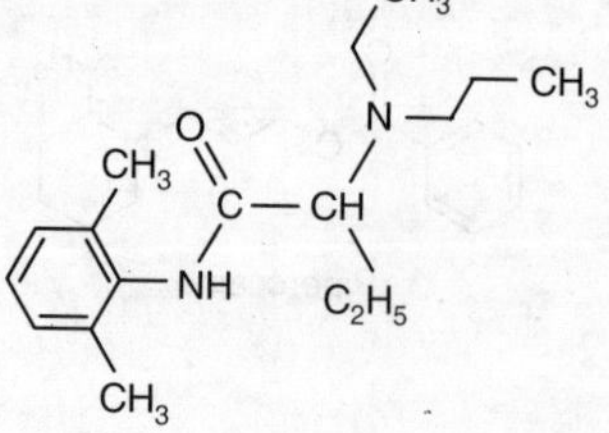

Etidocaine

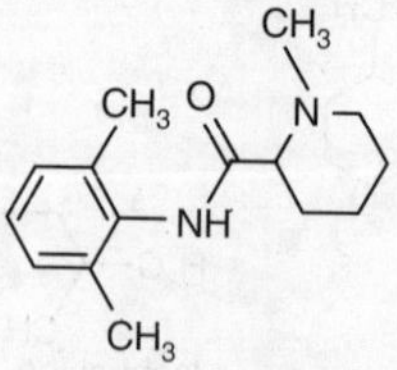

Mepivacaine

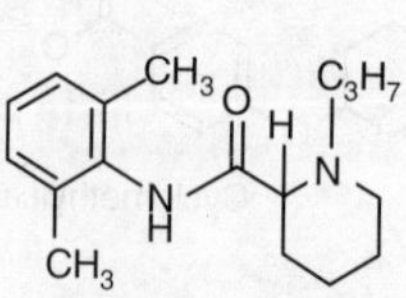

Ropivacaine

Miscellaneous

H₃C

Phenacaine

MECHANISM OF ACTION

How Nerves Conduct an Impulse?

- If you think of a nerve bundle as an electrical cable, the blue axons represent the 'wires' that carry the impulse from the tooth to the ganglion at the other end. The rest of the tissue surrounding the axons represents the 'insulation' which separates the various wires in the cable from each other.

- At this point, the analogy breaks down because, while the insulation in an electrical cable is a passive material that serves only to separate the wires from each other to prevent short circuits, the insulation in a nerve bundle is an active participant in the conduction of the impulse (Fig. 17.6).

- The connective tissue that is associated with each neuron is composed of a special material called myelin, which is itself made up of the cell bodies of specialized cells called Schwann cells. The myelin sheath is almost continuous along the entire axon.

- There are, however, tiny breaks in the continuity of the myelin sheath between each succeeding Schwann cell. These breaks are called 'nodes of Ranvier'. These nodes are quite important in the conduction of an impulse along a nerve axon on its way to the cell body in the ganglion, mostly because their presence along the way speeds the impulse quite a bit.

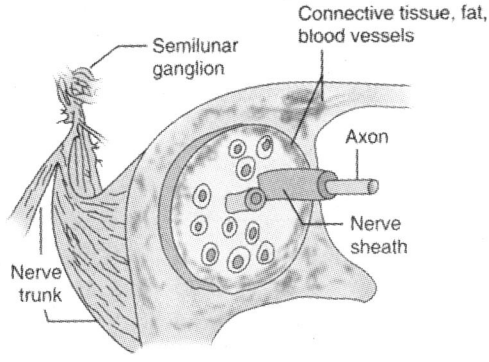

Fig. 17.6: Impulse conduction through nerve

A Nerve Fiber Transmits an Impulse (Fig. 17.7)

- Nerves are not like electrical wires with electrons traveling their length to transfer information from one end to the other. They are actually complex electrochemical structures, which utilize the electrical potential difference between the fluid inside of the axon, and the fluid that surrounds the axon.

- The fluid inside the axon (called cytoplasm) contains a high concentration of potassium ions, while the fluid outside contains a high concentration of sodium ions. There is no real difference in electrical potential between a potassium ion and a sodium ion, however, the fact that they exist in different concentrations on either side of the cell membrane sets up an electrochemical pressure gradient between the two.

- Sodium ions want to flow into the nerve cytoplasm, while the potassium ions want to flow out, but both are prevented from doing so by the presence of the nerve cell membrane. When a nerve is stimulated, this sets up a chain reaction in which sodium ions begin to penetrate through the nerve cell membrane and flow into the axon, while potassium ions begin to flow out. This activity happens at the nodes of Ranvier. This process is called depolarization of the nerve membrane.

- The imbalance in the chemical makeup of the extracellular fluid then causes an imbalance in the concentration of sodium ions at the adjacent node, which stimulates an identical depolarization at this node as well. This process proceeds from node to node until the impulse reaches the cell body of the nerve in the ganglion where it stimulates a similar cascade in a network of other neurons, which make contact with it.

- You might think that once all the potassium and sodium ions have exchanged places, the nerve would no longer be able to conduct impulses. The nerve, however, is a living entity and can regenerate the original concentrations of ions using energy from the food you eat in almost the same way that muscle cells use that same energy to cause muscle movement. It does this using proteins embedded in the cell membrane which act as 'ion pumps'.

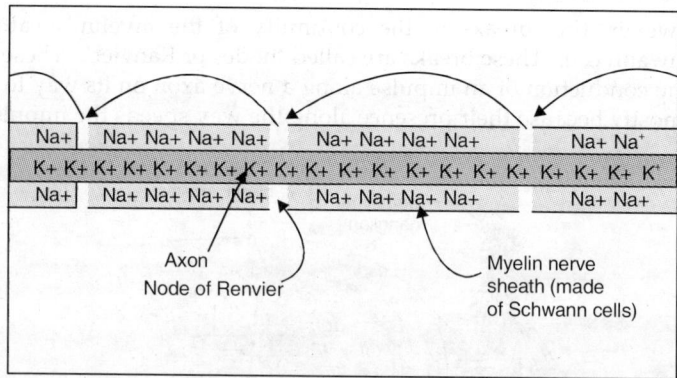

Fig. 17.7: Transmission of impulse in nerve fiber

How Local Anesthesia Interrupts this Process?

- Local anesthetic drugs act mainly by inhibiting sodium influx through sodium-specific ion channels in the neuronal cell membrane, in particular the so-called voltage-gated sodium channels. When the influx of sodium is interrupted, then the potassium ions cannot flow out, thus inhibiting the depolarization of the nerve.

- If this process can be inhibited for just a few nodes of Ranvier along the way, then nerve impulses generated downstream from the blocked nodes cannot propagate to the ganglion. In order to accomplish this feat, the anesthetic molecules must actually enter through the cell membrane of the nerve.

- Herein lies the differences in the potency, time of onset and duration of the various local anesthetics, an action potential cannot arise and signal conduction is inhibited. The receptor site is thought to be located at the cytoplasmic (inner) portion of the sodium channel. Local anesthetic drugs bind more readily to 'open' sodium channels, thus onset of neuronal blockade is faster in neurons that are rapidly firing. This is referred to as state dependent blockade.

- Local anesthetics are weak bases and are usually formulated as the hydrochloride salt to render them water-soluble. At physiologic pH, the protonated (ionized) and unprotonated (unionized) forms of the molecules exist in equilibrium but only the unprotonated molecule diffuses readily across cell membranes.

- Once inside the cell, the lower pH results in the molecule being protonated, thus inhibiting its passage back out of the cell. This is referred to as 'ion-trapping'. In the protonated form, the molecule binds to the local anesthetic binding site on the inside of the ion channel near the cytoplasmic end.

- Acidosis such as caused by inflammation at a wound partly reduces the action of local anesthetics. This is partly because most of the anesthetic is ionised and therefore unable to cross the cell membrane to reach its cytoplasmic-facing site of action on the sodium.

STRUCTURE–ACTIVITY RELATIONSHIP

General SAR

Amino ester

Amino amide

- The diagrams above show the essential structures of the two major types of local anesthetic agents; the molecule shown in the left diagram represents the structure of procaine (novocain). The chain that connects the benzene·ring on the left with the amide tail on the right is an 'ester linkage'. The diagram to the right represents lidocaine and its analogs. The connecting chain in this case is called an 'amide linkage'. The amide linkage contains an extra nitrogen to the left of the C=O (carboxyl) group.

- All local anesthetics are weak bases. They all contain:

  a. An **aromatic group** (the benzene ring seen on the left side of both structures above);

  b. An intermediate chain, either an **ester** or an **amide**; and

  c. An **amine** group seen on the right side of both molecular structures above.

1. The characteristics of any given anesthetic are determined by the exact structure and relationship of each of these three components. The aromatic ring structure is soluble in lipids. (The nerve cell membrane is made of a lipid bilayer and thus the aromatic ring is important in making it possible for the anesthetic molecule to penetrate through the nerve membrane).

2. The amino structure (seen on the right side of the molecules diagramed above) is soluble in water which is what makes it possible for the anesthetic molecule to dissolve in the water in which it is delivered from the dentist's syringe into the patient's tissue. It is also responsible for allowing it to remain in solution on either side of the nerve membrane. The trick that the anesthetic molecule must play is getting from one side of the membrane to the other.

3. The local anesthetic activity and its duration is very much dependent upon the stability of these two structures. The main factor governing the stability of these two derivatives is the hydrolysis of ester and amides. The mechanism of hydrolysis of esters and amides is dependent on the fuctional group. Xylidide ion is a poor leaving group than the diethylamino-ethyloxide group, which is responsible for slower hydrolysis of the lidocaine amide bond, resulting in more stable and longer duration of action.

4. Introduction of electron withdrawing chloro group in procaine makes the ester bond more susceptible to hydrolysis. Therefore, chloroprocaine has shorter duration of action.

5. On the other hand, introduction of electron releasing o-propoxy group as in propoxycaine, makes the ester hydrolysis difficult as compared to procaine and propoxycaine is having longer duration of action.

SAR of Ester Derivatives

The general structure may be represented by:

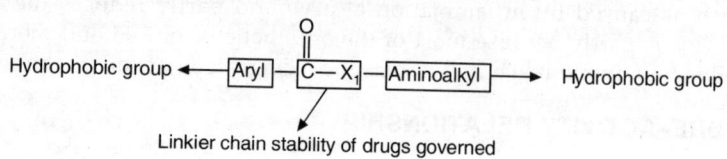

1. Chloroprocaine has a chloro substituent in the 2-position. The electron-withdrawing chlorine atom destabilizes the ester group to hydrolysis. Chloroprocaine is hydrolysed by plasma more than four times faster than procaine. It is more rapid in onset of action than procaine.

2. The presence of a non-polar n-butyl group on the aromatic nitrogen atom probably accounts for the greater lipid solubility of tetracaine, which is one of the most easily absorbed drugs.

3. The presence of 3-butoxy group appears to stabilize the molecule to hydrolysis as in benoxinate.

Aryl Group

1. The aromatic ring structure is soluble in lipids. The nerve cell membrane is made of a lipid bilayer and thus the aromatic ring is important in making it possible for the anesthetic molecule to penetrate through the nerve membrane.

2. The aryl group is attached directly to the carbonyl group. Substitutions of the aryl moiety with substituents that increase the electron density of the carbonyl oxygen enhance activity. Favourable substituents include alkoxy, amino and alkylamino groups in the para or ortho-positions. However, these substituents also alter the liposolubility of the molecule.

3. Arylaliphatic radicals, which contain an alkylene group between the aryl radical and carbonyl group result in inactive compounds. In these compounds, the mesomeric effect of the aryl radical does extend to the carbonyl group.

Bridge X

1. The bridge X may be carbon, oxygen, nitrogen, or sulfur. In an isosteric procaine series, conduction-anesthetic potency decreases in the order; sulfur, oxygen, carbon and nitrogen. These modifications affect duration of action and relative toxicity. In general, amides (X=N) are most resistant to metabolic hydrolysis than esters (X=O). Thio ester (X=S) may cause dermatitis.

Aminoalkyl Group

1. The amino function is considered to be the hydrophilic part of the local anesthetic molecule. Tertiary amines appear to produce longer action but they are more irritating; primary amines are not very active and cause irritation.
2. Alkyl groups, including the intermediate chain linked to X, primarily influence the relative lipid solubility.

SAR of Amide Derivatives

- Lidocaine derivatives are essentially anilide progenesis of isogramine with the following general structural characteristics.

$$\text{Aryl} - \text{NH} - \overset{\overset{\textstyle X}{\|}}{\text{C}} - \text{AMINOALKYL}$$

1. Phenyl group is attached to the SP^2 carbon atom through a nitrogen bridge. Substitution of the phenyl with a methyl group in 2- or 6-position enhances the activity.
2. The amide bond is more stable to hydrolysis than the ester bond. In addition, the methyl substituent provides steric hinderance to the hydrolysis of the amide bond and increases the coefficient of distribution.

Substituent X

X may be carbon (isogramine), oxygen (lidocaine) or nitrogen (phenacaine). Lidocaine (X= 0) has provided useful products.

Aminoalkyl Group

It is hydrophilic portion of the molecule and undergoes salt formation. Tertiary amines are more useful clinically because primary and secondary amines are more irritating.

▓ COEIFFICIENT OF DISTRIBUTION

Nerve membranes consist primarily of lipids. Increasing the lipid solubility of a series of compounds should result in facilitated penetration of nerve membranes. The potency of local anesthetics is directly proportional to distribution coefficients in vitro.

1. Substitution of the aryl radical by alkyl, alkoxy and alkylamino groups leads to homologous series in which partition coefficient increases with increasing number of melhylene ($-CH_2-$) groups; maximum activity as shown by C4, C5 or C6.
2. Branching of N-alkyl groups is often accompanied by an intensification of activity. The aminoalkyl group may be part of an aliphatic heterocyclic ring.
3. The tertiary amino group may be diethylamino, piperidino, or pyrrolidino, with same degree of activity. More hydrophilic morphilino group usually leads to diminished potency.
4. Clinically useful agents exhibit pKa values in the range of 8.00 to 9.5, because the compounds with higher pKa values are ionized 100% at physiological pH and so have difficulty in reaching the biophase.
5. In few cases, the effect of optical isomerism on local anesthetic activity has been studied. Only when structural rigidity is imposed on the molecule. The optical antipodes show significant different blocking properties as has been observed in spirotetraline succinimides.

6. Steric requirements are necessary for effective interaction between a local anesthetic agent and specific sites on or in the nerve membrane. S-isomer of dexivacaine has been found to show longer effect as compared to mepivacaine.

■ THE EFFECT OF pH ON LOCAL ANESTHETIC ACTION (FIG. 17.8)

- This section is quite conceptually difficult because it involves some essential chemistry, but it makes for very rewarding reading because it will enable the reader to understand the differences between the common local anesthetic solutions. It will help to explain the reasons that some anesthetics take longer to set than others, and why some cause more prolonged anesthesia than others.

- Synthetic anesthetics are prepared as weak bases and during manufacture, precipitate as powdered solids. These solids are unstable in air and poorly soluble in water. They are therefore combined with an acid to form a salt which can be combined with sterile water or saline. The salt dissolves to produce a stable solution which is injectable. The pH (the acid/base balance) of the solution is adjusted to complement the specific molecular structure of the anesthesia in question. Remember that the lower the pH, the more acidic the solution is, and the higher the pH, the more alkaline (basic) it is.

- In any given solution of anesthetic, the molecular structure shifts between two forms; an uncharged base molecule (RN) and a positively charged cation (RNH^+). These two forms of the anesthetic molecule exist in an equilibrium dependent upon the exact PH of the solution:

$$RNH^+ \longleftrightarrow RN + H^+$$

- If the surrounding medium becomes more acidic (lower pH), by definition, the concentration of hydrogen ions increases. These positively charged ions combine with the uncharged anesthetic radical (molecule) shifting the above equation to the left, and producing a higher proportion of charged cationic structures. If the pH rises, (i.e. the solution becomes more alkaline) there are fewer positively charged hydrogen ions.

- Thus the charged radicals release their hydrogen ions into solution and the equation shifts to the right producing more of the uncharged base.

- The pH that produces an equal number of uncharged basic molecules (RN) and charged cationic forms (RNH^+) is called the pKa(also called the dissociation constant). This is important because the molecular form of the anesthetic that is able to diffuse through the lipid membrane of the nerve cell is the uncharged (RN) form, while once inside the neuron, the active form that inhibits sodium influx is the charged cationic (RNH^+) form.

- As more and more of the uncharged base diffuses through the membrane, the concentration of the uncharged base outside the membrane decreases and the formula re-equilibrates forming more of the uncharged base from the newly higher concentration of positive cations. This continues until all the base eventually diffuses from the outside of the cell membrane to the inside.

- Once inside the cell membrane, the formula shifts to the left in an attempt to recreate the original concentrations of cations and neutral base molecules. But the positively charged base molecules inside the cell now tend to bind to sodium channel proteins and are removed from the dynamic balance.

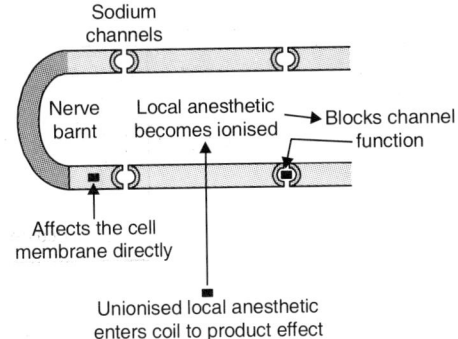

Fig. 17.8: Effect of pH on adsorption of local anesthetic

- This creates a sort of 'vacuum' which keeps drawing more and more neutral base molecules from the outside of the cell. It is the binding of the base cations to cellular sodium channel proteins which is the mechanism that limits nerve conduction and creates numbness.
- Since the pH of normal body tissue is 7.4, the ideal pKa of an anesthetic would also be 7.4. This would mean that 50% of all the molecular structures outside the nerve

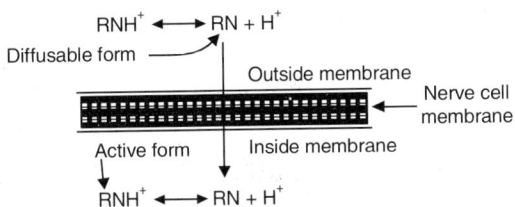

cell bodies would be in the form of the uncharged base, and quick diffusion of the anesthetic into the cell bodies would occur. Unfortunately, all local anesthetics have pKa values above 7.4. The higher the pKa, the lower the concentration of uncharged base, and the slower the diffusion into the nerve cells. Thus, the higher the pKa, the longer it will take for that anesthetic to set.

- The pH of normal body tissue is 7.4. In situations in which there is an active infection present, the tissue pH can be considerably lower, in the vicinity of 5 or 6. This very reduced pH shifts the equation (outside of the nerve cell) to the left reducing the number of neutral (RN) radicals available to diffuse through the nerve cell membrane.
- This accounts for the difficulty in anesthetizing such an area. The relative difference between the pKa of the anesthetic and the pH of the body tissue can make quite a large difference in the percentage of anesthetic that is available to diffuse immediately through the nerve membrane, and thus on the amount of time it takes for the anesthetic effect to be felt.

Hexylcaine

Benzocaine

Ethyl 4-nitro-benzoate → Fe, H⁺, H₂O → Benzocaine

Procaine

Ethyl 4-amino-benzoate + 2-diethylamino-ethanol (I) → NaOC₂H₅ → Procaine

Chloroprocaine

4-amino-2-chlorobenzoic acid → SOCl₂ → 4-amino-2-chlorobenzoyl chloride hydrochloride + 2-diethylamino-ethanal hydrochloride → Chloroprocaine

Lidocaine

Chloroacetyl chloride + 2, 6-dimethyl aniline → α-chloro-2, 6-dimethyl-acetanilide + diethyl-amino → Lidocaine

Bupivocaine

Pyridine-2-carbonyl chloride + 2, 6-dimethyl-aniline → 2, 6-picolino xylidide (II) → butyl bromide (II) → III

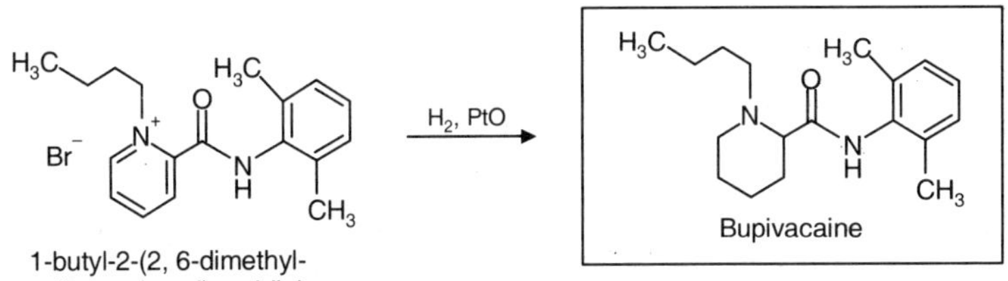

1-butyl-2-(2, 6-dimethyl-
anilinocarbonyl) pyridinium
bromide (III)

Bupivacaine

Prilocaine

o-toluidine

2-bromopropionyl
bromide

propylamine

Prilocaine

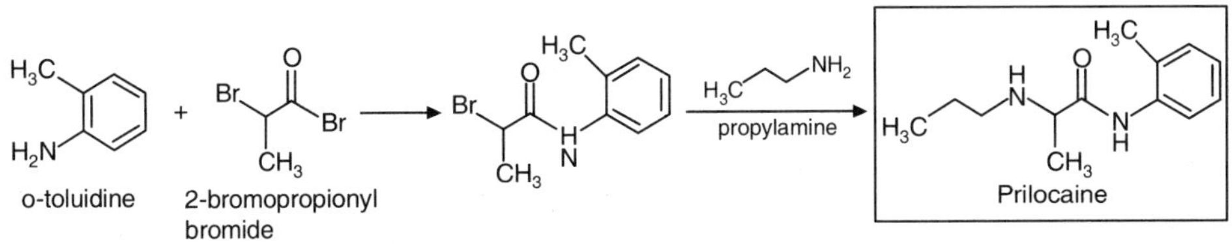

Sedatives and Hypnotics

Sedatives are drugs which exert a quieting effect accompanied by relaxation and rest but do not necessarily induce sleep on the other hand hypnotics induce the drowsiness, compelling the patient to sleep by depressing CNS, particularly the reticular activity which characterizes wakefulness.

- Hypnotics and sedatives are non-selective or general depressants of the central nervous system. They are used to reduce restlessness and emotional tension and to induce either sleep or sedation. The condition that depicts unsatisfactory or insufficient sleep is called insomnia. The three major types of insomnia are as follows.

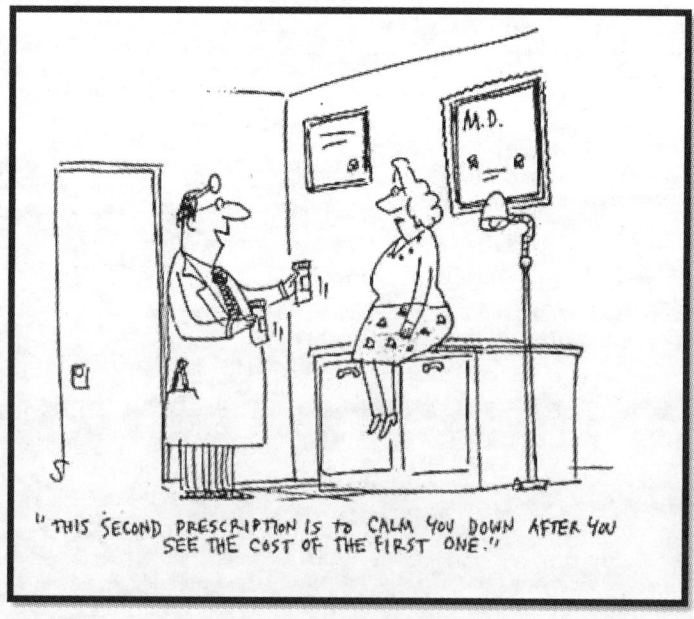

" THIS SECOND PRESCRIPTION IS TO CALM YOU DOWN AFTER YOU SEE THE COST OF THE FIRST ONE."

1. **Transient insomnia:** This is caused by acute stress or stressful situation in people who usually have no problems with sleep.
2. **Short-term insomnia:** This may be precipated by situational stress of a finite duration. It is often due to conflict situation, anxiety and mood disorder.
3. **Long-term insomnia:** This is most often caused by psychopathological factors, psychiatric illness.

Ideal Characteristic of Hypnotics

1. Promotes a sleep state identical to natural sleep.
2. Induce sleep promptly after administration.
3. Does not cause day time sedation or drowsiness.
4. Does not lead to dependence.
5. Does not cause 'rebound insomnia' when suddenly discontinued.
6. Causes no drug interaction.
7. It should not be harmful, if over dosage is taken.
8. It should be economical.

Sleep and Its Stages

The duration and pattern of sleep varies considerably among individuals. Age has an important effect on quantity and depth of sleep. After intensive and extensive study it has been recognized that sleep is an architecture cyclic process. The different phases of sleep and their characteristics are as follows.

Stage 0 (Awake): From lying down to falling asleep and occasional nocturnal awakening; constitutes 1-2 % of sleep time. EEG shows α activity when eyes are closed and β activity when eyes are open. Eye movements are irregular or slowly rolling.

Stage 1 (dozing): α activity is interspersed with waves. Eye movement is reduced but there may be bursts of rolling. Neck muscle relaxes. Occupies 3-6% of sleep time.

Stage 2 (unequivocal sleep): θ waves with interspersed spindles, K complex can be evoked on sensory stimulation; subjects are easily arousable. This comprises 40-50% of sleep time.

Stage 3 (deep sleep transition): EEG shows θ, δ and spindle activity, K complex can be evoked with strong stimuli only. Eye movements are few; subjects are not easily arosable; comprises 5-8% of sleep time.

Stage 4 (cerebral sleep): δ activity predominates in EEG, K complex cannot be evoked. Eyes are practically fixed; subjects are difficult to arouse. Night terror may occur at this time. It comprises 10-20% of sleep time.

During stage 2, 3 and 4 heart rate, BP and respiration are steady and muscles are relaxed. Stages 3 and 4 together are called slow wave sleep.

REM Sleep (Paradoxical Sleep)

- EEG has waves of all frequencies; K complexes cannot be elicited. There are marked, irregular and dating eye movements; dreams and nightmares occur which may be recalled if the subject is aroused. Heart rate and BP fluctuate; respiration is irregular.
- Muscles are fully relaxed, but irregular body movements occur occasionally. Erection occurs in males. About 20-30 % of sleep time is spent in REM.
- Normally, stages 0-4 and REM occur in succession over a period of 80-100 min. Then stages 1-4 REM are repeated cyclically.
- The EEG waves have been divided in to;
  A: High amplitude 8-14 c.p.s.
  β: Low amplitude 15-35 c.p.s.
  θ: Low amplitude 4-7 c.p.s.
  δ: High amplitude 0.5-3 c.p.s.

CLASSIFICATION OF SEDATIVE AND HYPNOTICS

Ciassification of hypnotics and sedatives are given in flow chart 18.1.

Flow chart 18.1: Classification of sedative and hypnotics

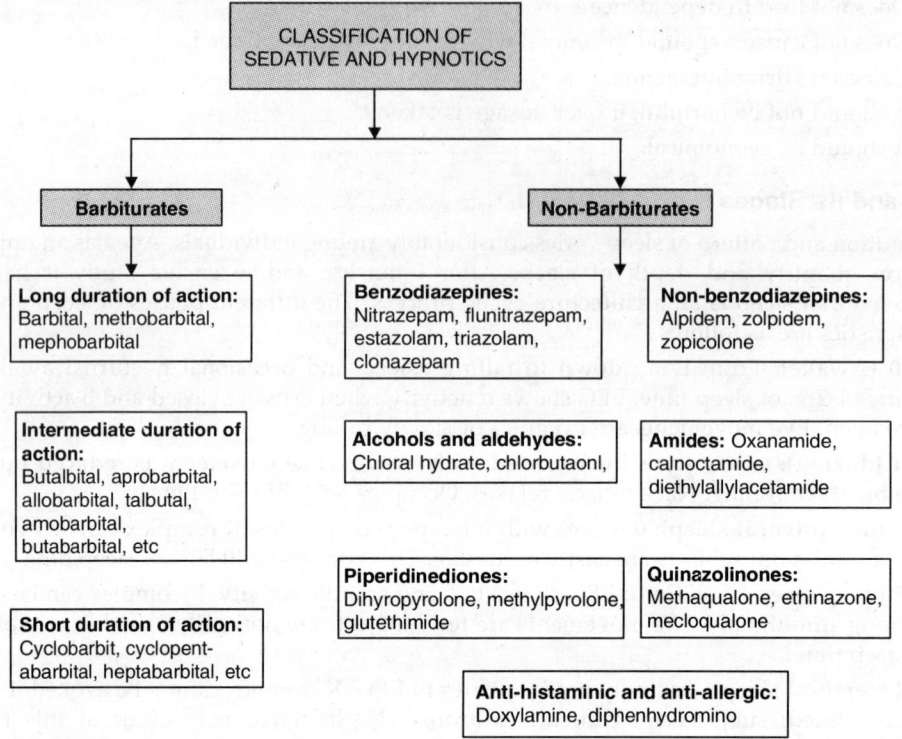

Barbiturates

Long duration of action

Barbital   Mephobarbital   Methobarbital

Intermediate duration of action

Aprobarbital   Allobarbital   Talbutal   Amobarbital

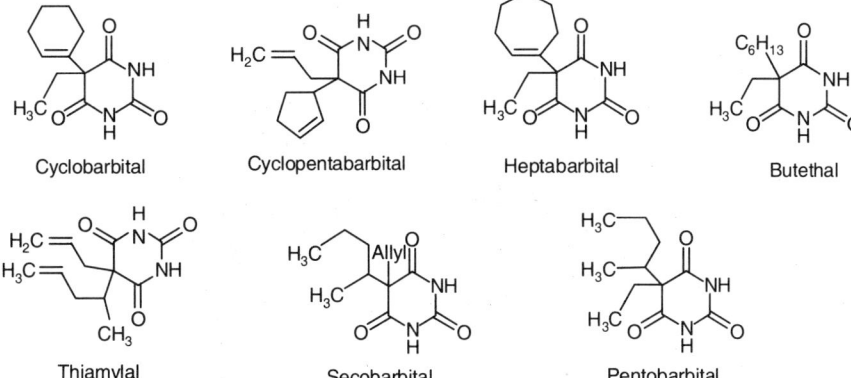

Butethal   Butabarbital   Probarbital

Short duration of action

Cyclobarbital   Cyclopentabarbital   Heptabarbital   Butethal

Thiamylal   Secobarbital   Pentobarbital

Ultra short duration of action

Thiopental   Hexobarbital

Non-Barbiturates

Benzodiazepines

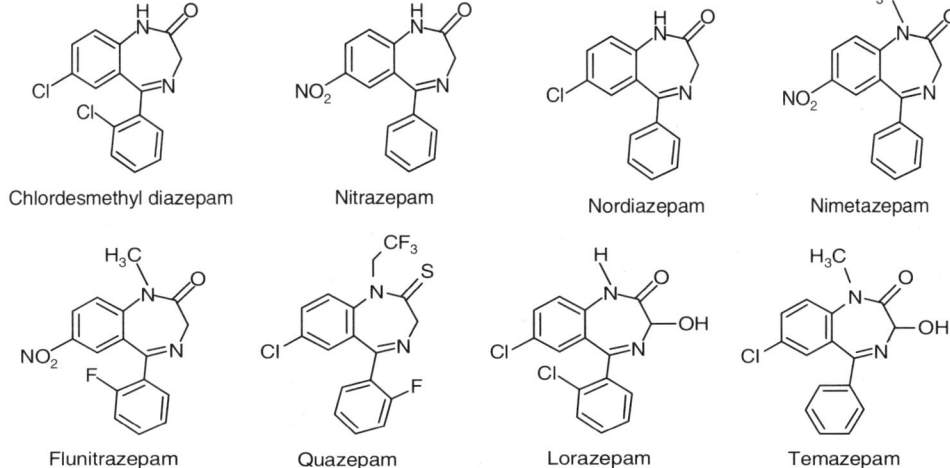

Chlordesmethyl diazepam   Nitrazepam   Nordiazepam   Nimetazepam

Flunitrazepam   Quazepam   Lorazepam   Temazepam

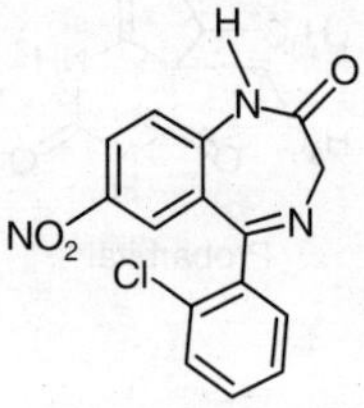

Clonazepam

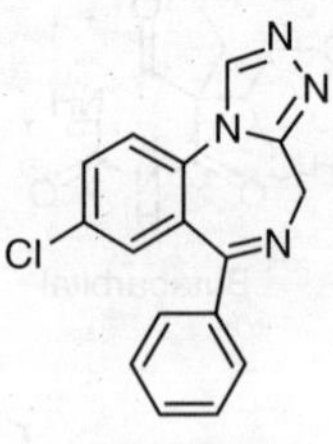

Estazolam

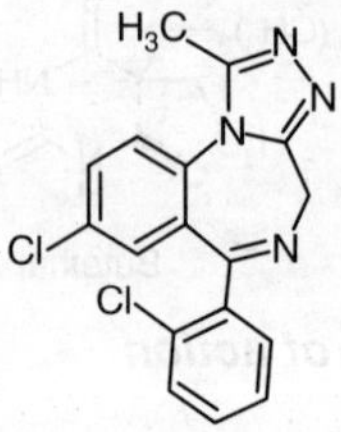

Triazolam

Non-benzodiazepines

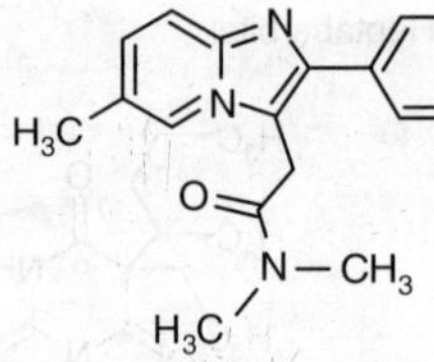

Zolpidem

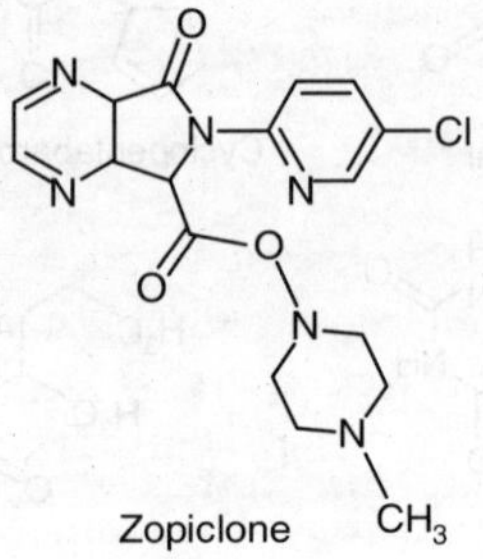

Zopiclone

Carbamate derivatives

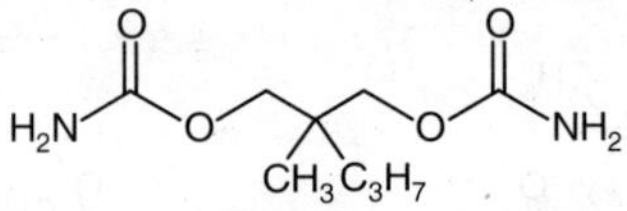

Meprobamate

Amide derivatives

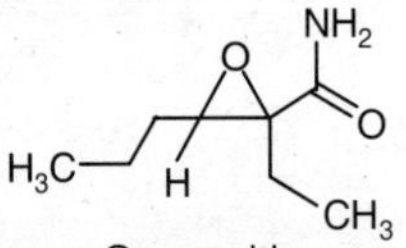

Oxanamide

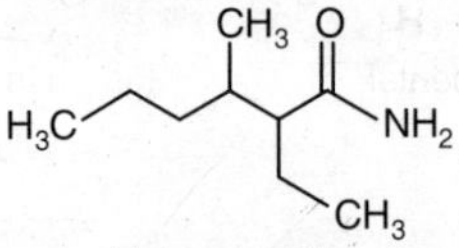

Valnoctamide

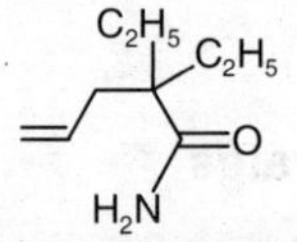

Diethyl allyl acetamide

Piperidinediones

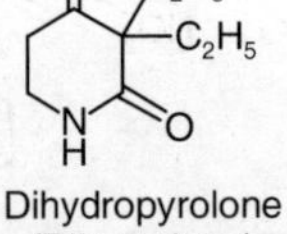

Dihydropyrolone
(Dihyprylone)

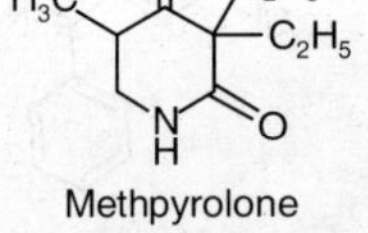

Methpyrolone

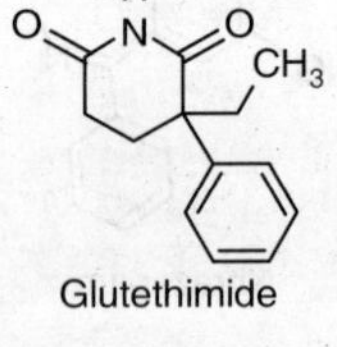

Glutethimide

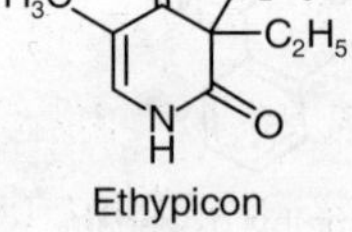

Ethypicon

Quinazolinones

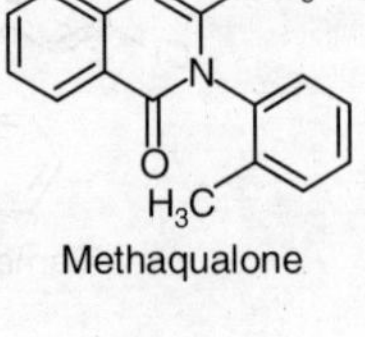

Methaqualone

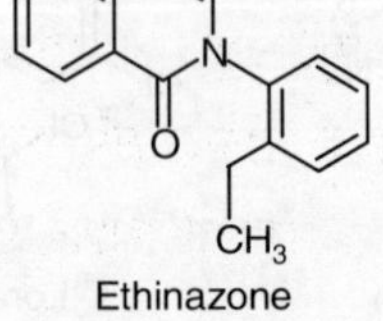

Ethinazone

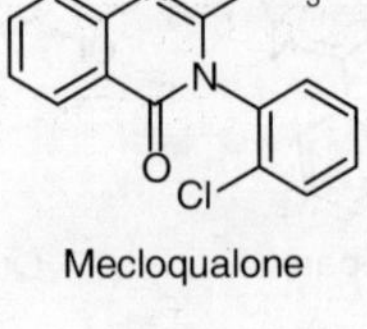

Mecloqualone

Alcohols and aldehydes

| Amylene hydrate | Chlorbutanol | Methylpentynol | Chloral hydrate |

Antihistaminic and anticholinergics

| Doxylamine | Diphenhydramine | Pyrilamine |

BARBITURATES

Structure Activity Relationship

1. The polar portion of the molecule is one of the most water-soulblizing of the non-ionic functional groups. These include, with their Hansch value as measures of polar character, the unsubstituted barbituric acid nucleus (–CCONH= – 1.35) amides (–CONH$_2$ = –1.6). These polar groups are attached to a non-polar moiety, usually alkyl, aryl or halo alkyl, so that the partition coefficient is close to 100 (log p=2).

2. It appears that these molecules have proper solubility characteristics to be absorbed from the gastrointestinal tract and transported in the aqueous body fluids. These characteristics are to be sufficiently lipophilic so that they readily penetrate the central nervous system, where their non-ionic surfactant characteristics may serve to distort essential lipoproteins matrics, thus depressing the function.

3. The sum of the carbon atom of both substituents at carbon 5 should be between 6 and 10 in order to attain optimal hypnotic activity. This is also an index of duration of action Table 18.1).

Table 18.1: Relation between sum value and duration of action

Sum value	Duration of action
7-9	Rapid onset and shortest duration of action.
5-7	Intermediate duration of action.
4	Slowest onset and longest duration of action.

4. The branched chain isomer has greater lipid solubility and hypnotic activity but has shorter duration of action.

5. Within the same series, the unsaturation (i.e. allyl, alkenyl, cycloalkenyl analogues) may result in greater potency than the saturated analogues with the same number of carbon atoms.

6. Alicyclic or aromatic substituted analogues are more potent than analogues with aliphatic substituents with the same number of carbon atoms.

7. Introduction of a halogen atom into the 5-alkyl substituent increases potency.

8. The greater the branching more potent will be the drug, e.g. pentobarbital is more potent than amobarbital.

9. Introduction of a polar subistuents (OH, NH_2, COOH, CO, RNH, and SO_3H) into the aromatic group at C-5 results in decreased lipid solubility and potency.

10. Alkylation at 1 or 3 position may results in compound having shorter onset and duration of action since N-methyl group reduce acid value.

11. Introduction of more sulphur atoms (at C-4 and C-6) decrease the hypnotic activity.

12. Both the hydrogen atoms in position-5 of barbituric acid must be replaced for maximal activity. This is likely due to the susceptability to rapid metabolic attack and to the high acidity and ionization of C-H bonds in such a position.

13. Increasing the length of an alkyl chain in position-5 enhances the potency up to 5-6 carbon atoms; beyond that depressant action decrease and convulusant action may result. This is probably due to the excess over the ideal lipophilic character.

14. Branched, cyclic or an unsaturated chain in position-5 generally produce a short duration of action than does the normal saturated chain containing the same number of carbon atoms. This appears to be due to a combination of decreased lipophilic character and increased ease of metabolic conversion to a more polar, inactive metabolite.

15. Compounds with alkyl groups in the 1 or 3 position may have a shorter onset and duration of action. The N-Me group results in a barbiturate which is a weaker acid compared with that N-Me substituent. The weaker acid exists largely in the non-ionic lipid-soluble form, which readily enters CNS and rapidly equilibrates into peripheral fatty stores.

16. Replacement of oxygen by sulfur on carbon-2 shortens the onset and duration of action. Thiobarbiturates are much more lipid soluble in the non-ionized form than the corresponding oxygen analogue. Rapid movement into and out of CNS, as well as ease of metabolic attack, account for the rapid onset and short duration of action.

Mechanism of Action (Fig. 18.1)

- At low doses, barbiturates either have a γ-amino butyric acid (GABA) like action or enhance the effect of GABA, an inhibitory neurotransmitter. It has been suggested that the effects of barbiturates on synaptic transmission are caused by an alteration in the postsynaptic sensitivity of the neurons to excitory and inhibitory transmitter. Barbiturates activate GABA receptors in high concentration, thereby enhancing pre- and post-synaptic inhibition.

- When GABA receptors are activated, chloride channels open. Chloride enters the cell, hyperpolarizes it, and produces decreased excitation. GABA receptors are part of a supramolecular complex that also includes the benzodiazepine receptor and a picrotoxin site. Barbiturates bind to picrotoxin site and decrease chloride ion flux and produce an increased chloride concentration. The greater the affinity of a barbiturate for the picrotoxin binding site, the greater is the potency.

- In addition to barbiturates and benzodiazepines, ethanol appears to produce depression of central nervous system function, in part by enhancing the ability of GABA to bind to the GABA-A receptor. This may explain why these three classes of drugs potentiate each others' effects and why tolerance to one results in cross-tolerance to another.

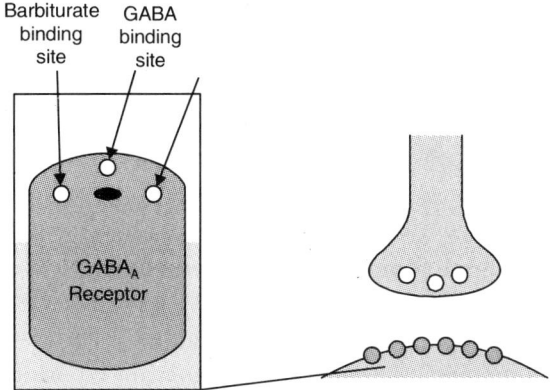

Fig. 18.1: Mode of action of barbiturates

Adverse Effect

1. Physiologic as well as psychological dependence can occur. Withdrawal of a barbiturate may result in grand mal seizures.
2. Skin eruption and porphyria can occur.
3. An overdose can result in coma, diminished reflexes, severe respiratory depression, hypotension leading to cardiovascular collapse and renal failure.

Therapeutic Uses

1. IV anesthesia: Thiopental (Pentothal) and methohexital (Brevital).
2. Convulsions: Emergency treatment (eclampsia, tetanus, status epilepticus), but benzodiazepines are preferable.
3. Epilepsy.
4. Rarely used as a sedative due to the availability of safer benzodiazepine agents.

BENZODIAZEPINES

Benzodiazepines

Structure–Activity Relationship

Ring A

1. In ring A, an electron withdrawing group such as Cl, Br, NO_2, or CF_3 or CN at position C-7 is essential for the activity.

2. Replacement of the benzene ring by hetero atom ring resulted in compound with interesting activity, e.g. ripazepam.

Ripazepam

Ring B

1. A methyl group is attached to the nitrogen atom in 1 position in ring B. However, substitutions at position 1 that are metabolically removed are still clinically useful.

2. Replacement of the carbonyl function with two hydrogens in the 2-position gives medazepam, less potent than diazepam. Replacement of one of the hydrogen with OH group on 3 position lowers activity on the one hand and aids elimination on the other.

3. Introduction of a carboxyl function in the 3 position increases the duration of action and also favours formation of water soluble salts.

4. A phenyl substitution at the 5 position, α-Pyridyl derivative and cycloalkyl substituents at 5 positions give potent compounds.

5. Derivatives with additional rings joining the diazepine nucleus at the 1 and 2 positions are generally more active than the corresponding 1- methylbenzodiazepines.

6. The position of a triazole ring on the α-face of the 1, 4-benzodiazepines nucleus, in place of the amide moiety of the benzodiazepinones, enhances its biological activity.

7. Saturation of the 4, 5-double bond reduces potency, as does a shift of the unsaturation into the 3, 4-position.

Ring C

1. Activity is increased by putting substituents such as Cl or F at the ortho position and disubstitution in both ortho positions in ring C.

Mechanism of Action (Fig. 18.2)

- It is suppose to augment the action of GABA (gamma amino butyric acid), an inhibitory neurotransmitter. The pharmacological effects of GABA were confined to GABA receptors in the central nervous system, which produce an increased chloride conductance. Benzodiazepines do not open chloride channels by themselves but they act allosterically to increase the affinity of the receptor for GABA. Therefore, benzodiazepines produce no effects on chloride conductance in the absence of GABA.

- The targets for benzodiazepines action are the γ-amino butyric acid (GABA) receptors. These receptors are composed of α,β,γ subunit families of which combination of five or more span the postsynaptic membrane. Depending on the types, number of subunit and brain region localization, the activation of the receptor results in different pharmacological effects. Benzodiazepines modulate the GABA effects by binding to a specific, high affinity site located at the interface of the α subunit and γ-2 subunit.

- These binding sides are sometimes labeled benzodiazepines receptor, which are designated as BZ_1 or BZ_2, depending on their affinity for a particular α subunit. The benzodiazepines receptor location in the CNS parallels those of the GABA neuron. Binding of GABA to its receptor triggers an opening of chloride channel, which lead to increase in chloride conductance.
- Benzodiazepines increase of the channel opening produced by GABA. The influx of chloride ion causes a small hyperpolarization that moves the postsynaptic potential away from its firing threshold and thus, inhibits the formation action potential.

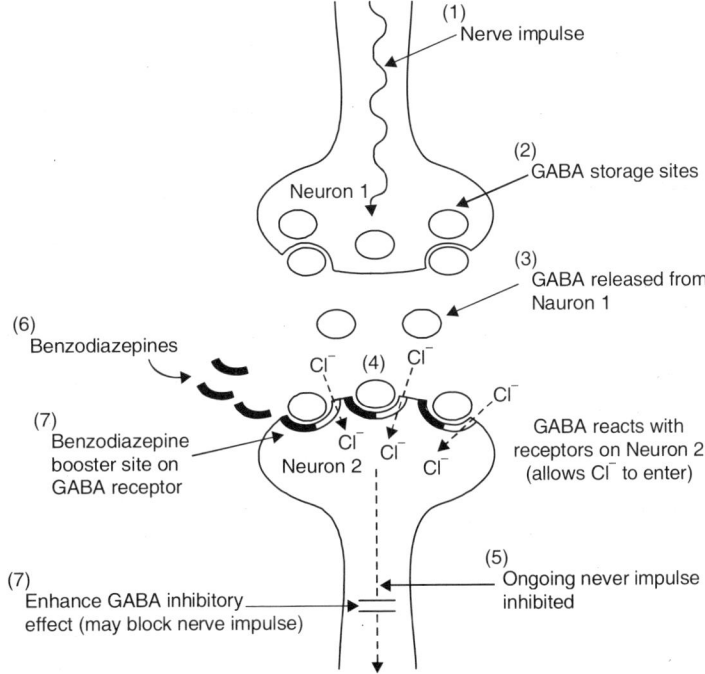

Fig. 18.2: Mode of action of benzodiazepines

- The clinical effects of various benzodiazepines correlate well with each drugs binding affinity for the GABA receptor chloride ion channel complex.

Pharmacokinetics

- The pharmacokinetic parameter is useful for selecting a benzodiazepine for its therapeutic action. For quick onset of action, the benzodiazepines must dissolve completely in the stomach and cross the stomach mucosa into the systemic circulation.
- After this, it must also cross the blood-brain barrier in order to enter the CNS. Therefore, the lipophilicity of the benzodiazepine is important. Most benzodiazepines are highly lipophilic except the 3-OH substituted benzodiazepines being the list lipophilic.
- Benzodiazepines are metabolized primarily by microsomal oxidation and glucouronide conjugation. They vary greatly in duration of action. The duration of action of

benzodiazepines is dependent upon formation of active metabolite, which has much longer plasma elimination half-lives than their parent compounds.

• Diazepam and chlorazepate are metabolized to active metabolite such as N-desmethyl diazepam. The half-life of this compound is about 60 hrs, and this accounts for the tendency of many benzodiazepines to produce cumulative effects and long hangovers. The short acting compounds are those that are metabolized directly by conjugation with glucuronide.

• The first stage of metabolism is the removal of methyl group at one position to give nordiazepam an active metabolite. The second phase of metabolism involves hydroxylation at position 3 and usually yields an active derivative.

Toxicity

• Benzodiazepines in acute overdose are considerably less dangerous than the other anxiolytic drugs, e.g. barbiturates. The availability of an effective antagonist, flumazenil, is useful in counteracting the effect of benzodiazepines. The main side effect is drowsiness, confusion and impaired motor conduction.

NON-BENZODIAZEPINE

MOA: It binds to the Omega-I site of GABA receptors and produces anxiolytic action by opening chlorine channels.

Carbamates

MOA: It is used primarily as centrally acting muscle relaxant and anti-anxiety drug. In larger doses, it is sometimes used as a hypnotic. It is less toxic but exhibits some degree of addiction as that of barbiturates.

Amides

MOA: The agents from this class are marketed as tranquilizers and muscle relaxants having good sedative properties.

Piperidinediones

MOA: As compared to the barbiturates, agents from this class are less active but better tolerated sedative-hypnotics. Glutethimide does not offer any advantage over barbiturates. More potent than any other non-barbiturate hypnotics, other properties remain same as that of methyl pyrolone.

Quinazolinones

MOA: It is similar with barbiturates in hypnotic activity; it is also potent anti-tussive agent.

ANTIHISTAMINIC AND ANTICHOLINERGIC

MOA: Histamine is responsible for the anxiety. Antihistaminics block its effect and produce calmness in the patient.

Phenobarbital

Benzyl cyanide (I) + Ethanol $\xrightarrow{H_2SO_4}$ Phenylacetic acid ethylester (II)

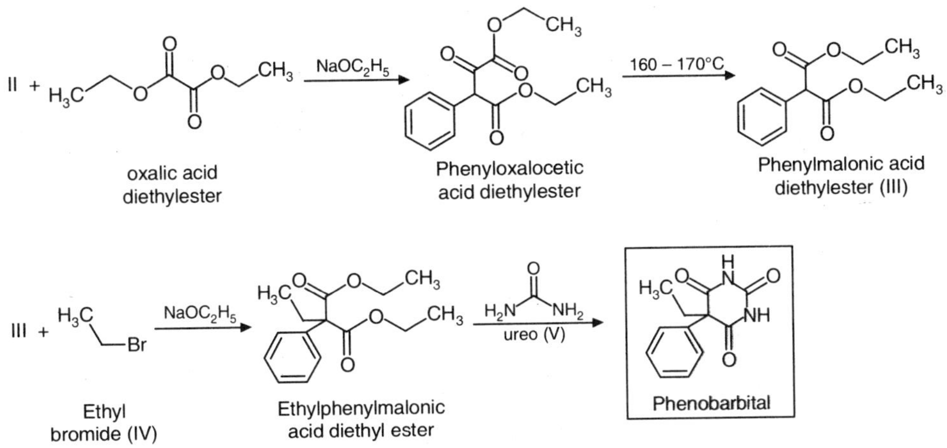

II +
NaOC2H5
160 – 170°C
oxalic acid diethylester
Phenyloxalocetic acid diethylester
Phenylmalonic acid diethylester (III)
III +
Br
NaOC2H5
ureo (V)
Ethyl bromide (IV)
Ethylphenylmalonic acid diethyl ester
Phenobarbital

Amylobarbitone

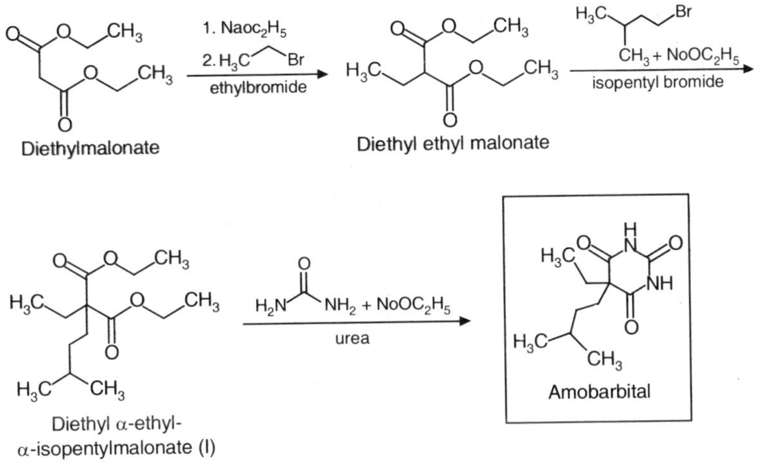

1. Naoc2H5
2. H3C Br
ethylbromide
Diethylmalonate
Diethyl ethyl malonate
CH3 + NoOC2H5
isopentyl bromide
NH2 + NoOC2H5
urea
Diethyl α-ethyl-α-isopentylmalonate (I)
Amobarbital

Cyclobarbital

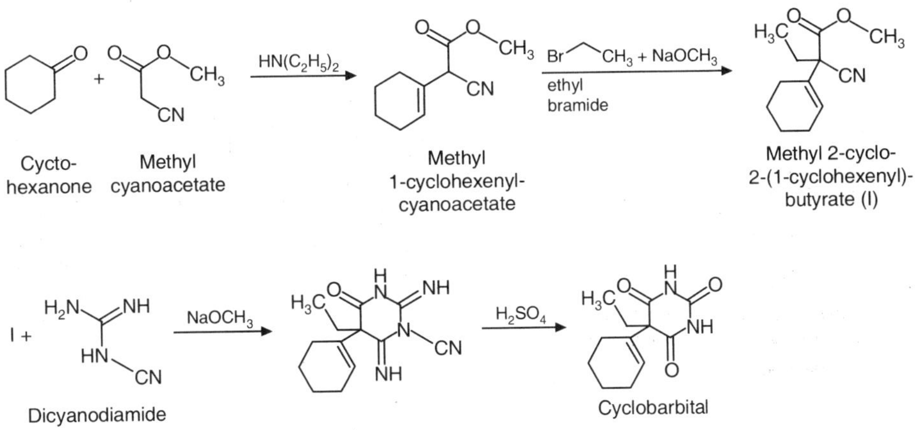

HN(C2H5)2
Br CH3 + NaOCH3
ethyl bramide
Cycto-hexanone
Methyl cyanoacetate
Methyl 1-cyclohexenyl-cyanoacetate
Methyl 2-cyclo-2-(1-cyclohexenyl)-butyrate (I)
I +
NaOCH3
H2SO4
Dicyanodiamide
Cyclobarbital

Hexobarbital

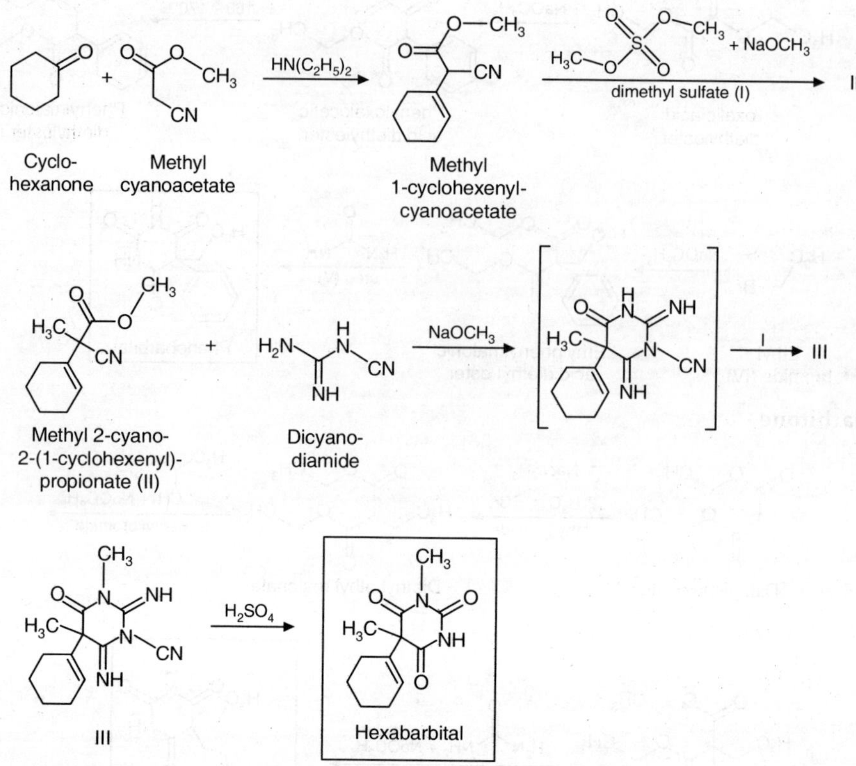

HN(C2H5)2
dimethyl sulfate (I)
+ NaOCH3
Cyclohexanone
Methyl cyanoacetate
Methyl 1-cyclohexenyl-cyanoacetate
II
NaOCH3
Methyl 2-cyano-2-(1-cyclohexenyl)-propionate (II)
Dicyanodiamide
I
III
H2SO4
Hexabarbital

Flurazepam

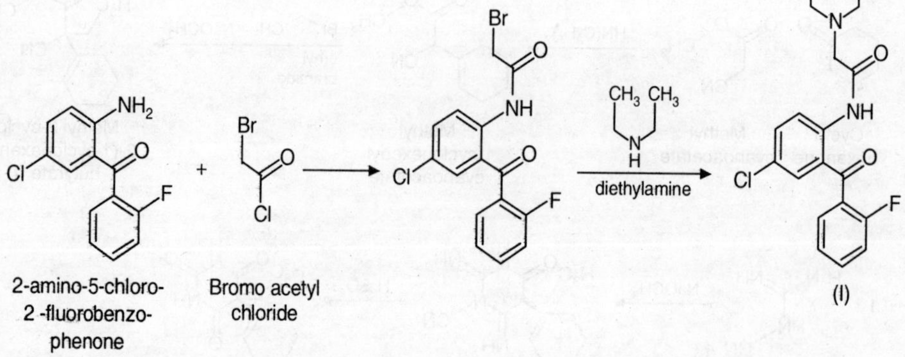

diethylamine
2-amino-5-chloro-2 -fluorobenzophenone
Bromo acetyl chloride
(I)

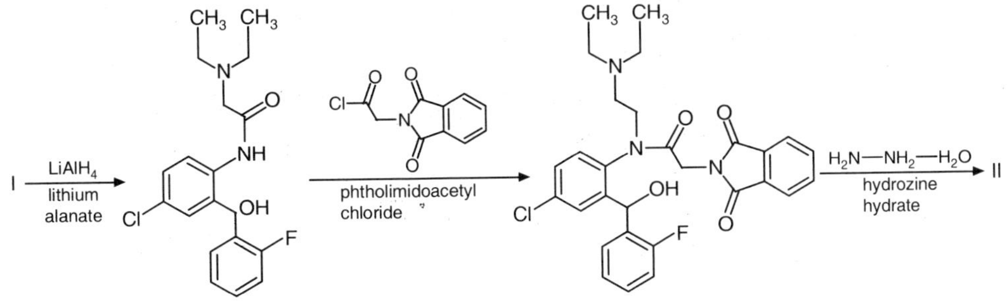

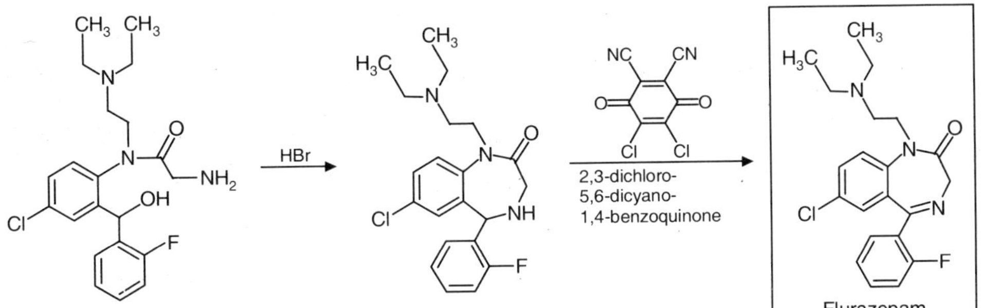

Flurazepam

Temazepam

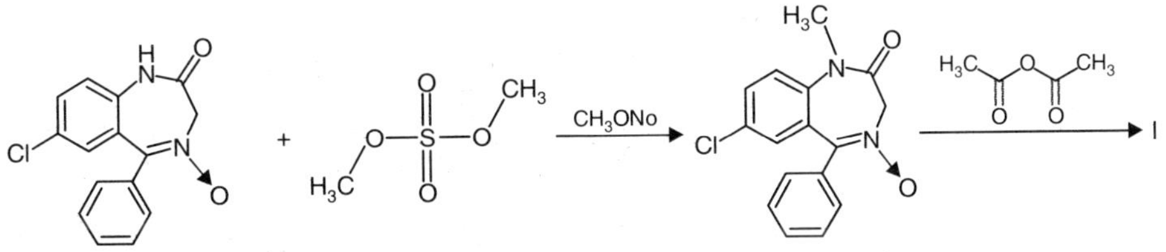

7-chloro-5-phenyl-
2-oxo-1, 3-dihydro-
2H-1, 4-benzodiazepine
4-oxide

Dimethyl
sulfate

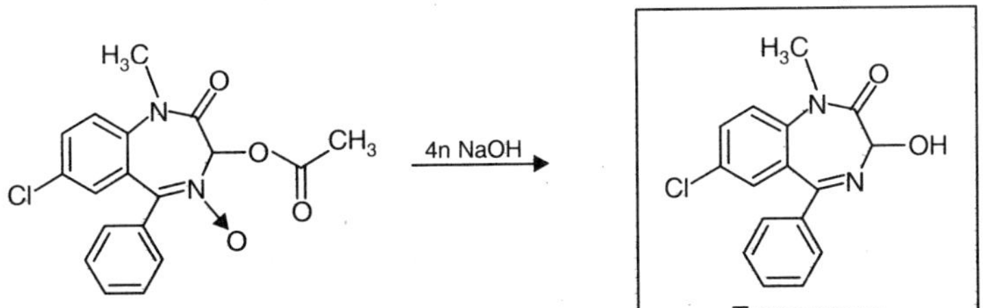

3-acetoxy-7-chloro-1-
methyl-5phenyl-2-oxo-
1, 3-dihydro-2H-1, 4-
benzodiazepine (1)

Temazepam

Triazolam

2-amino-2, 5-dichlorobenzophenone

Glycine ethyl ester hydrochloride

7-chloro-5-(2-chlorophenyl)-2-oxo-2, 3-dihydro-1H-1, 4-benzodiazepine

7-chloro-5-(2-chlorophenyl)-2-thioxo-2, 3-dihydro-1H-1, 4-benzodiazepine (I)

Acetyl-hydrozine

Triazolam

Zolpidem

2-amino-5-methylpyridine

Bromomethyl 4-methylphenyl ketone

2-(4-methylphenyl)-6-methylimidozo[1, 2-a]-pyridine

dimethyl-amine (I)

1. CH$_3$I
2. NoCN

1. methyl iodide
2. sodium cyanide

1. HCl, CH$_3$COOH
2. POCl$_3$
3. I
2. phosphoryl chloride

Zolpidem

Zopiclone

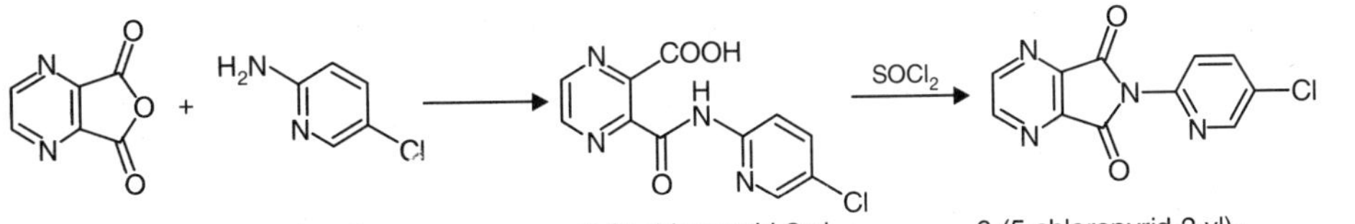

Pyrazine-2, 3-
dicarboxylic
anhydride

2-amino-5-
chloropyridine

3-(5-chloropyrid-2-yl-
carbamoyl) pyrazine-2-
corboxylic acid

6-(5-chloropyrid-2-yl)-
5, 7-dioxo-6, 7-dihydro-
5H-pyrrolo[3, 4-b] pyrazine (I)

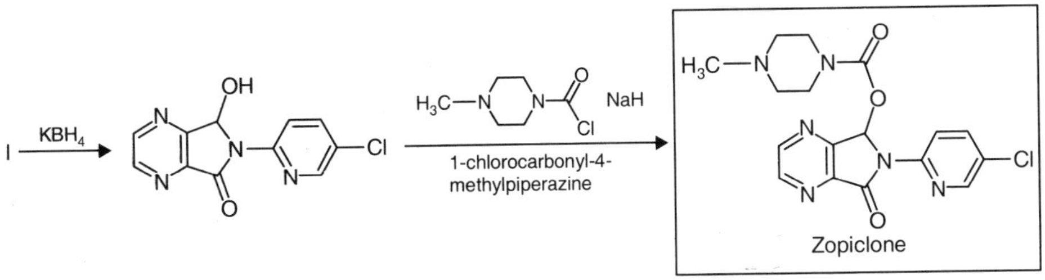

1-chlorocarbonyl-4-
methylpiperazine

Zopiclone

19

Anxiolytic Agents

Anxiety is an emotional state, unpleasant in nature associated with uneasiness, discomfort and concern or fear about some defined or undefined future threat. The anti-anxiety agents or anxiolytic drugs are the chemical agents which are used to control the effects of stress and the feeling of discomfort, tension, fearful anticipation of untoward events and dysphoria in patients with neuroses and mild depressive states. In addition to the disturbance of mood, hyperanxiety usually involves changes in sleep, GIT and automatic nervous system.

BIOCHEMICAL BASIS OF THE ANXIETY (FIG. 19.1)

- The limbic system of the brain located in the most primitive part of the cortex and in the hypothalamus, is the seat of emotion. This system have a balance of complex excitory and inhibitory components (excitory component = different neurotransmitters and inhibitory component = GABA). In anxiety, excitory component is increased than the inhibitory one. This imbalance is solely responsible for the anxiety.

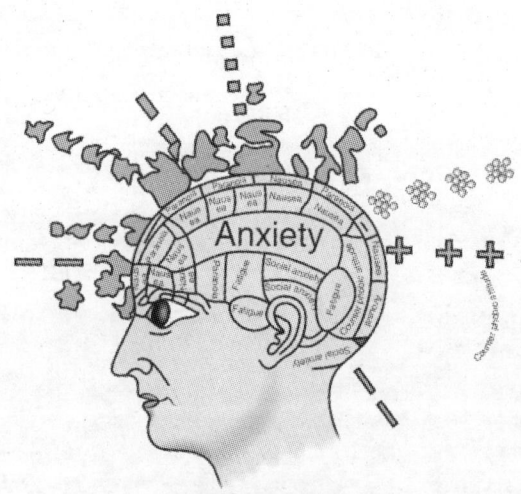

- Anxiolytics inhibit the spontaneous increased activity of limbic neurons by interacting with GABA receptors, resulting into the presynaptic inhibition of different excitory neurotransmitter.

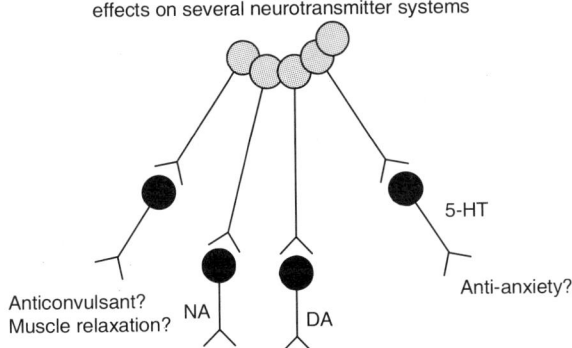

Fig. 19.1: Biochemical basis of anxiety

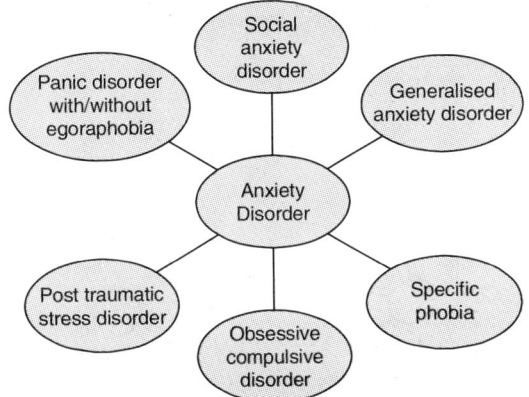

Fig. 19.2: Types of anxiety

CLASSIFICATION OF ANXIOLYTICS

Classification of anxiolytics is given in Flow chart 19.1.

Flow chart 19.1: Classification of anxiolytics

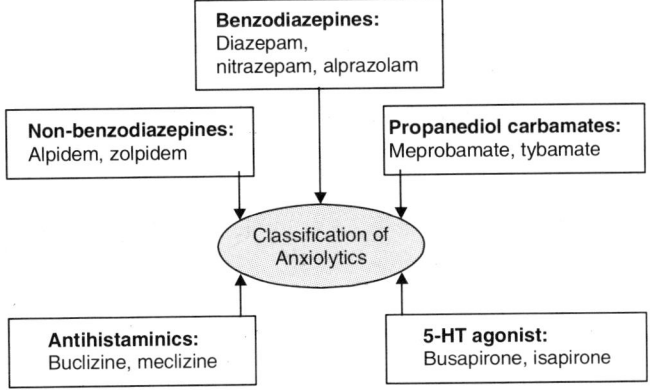

Benzodiazepines

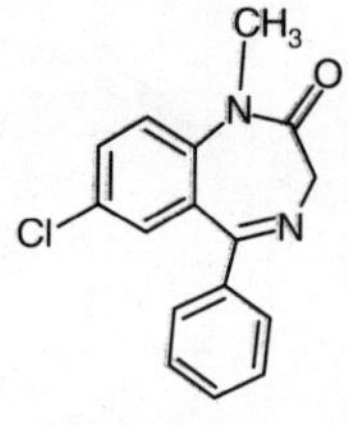

Diazepam

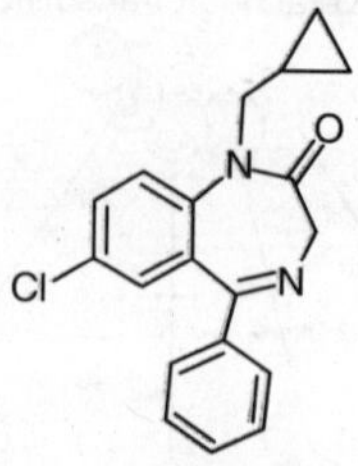

Prazepam

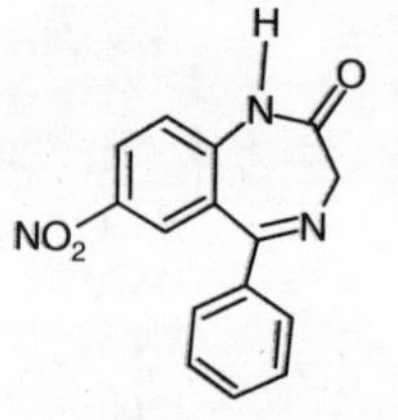

Nitrazepam

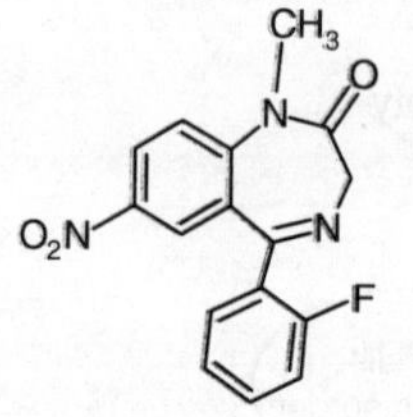

Flunitrazepam

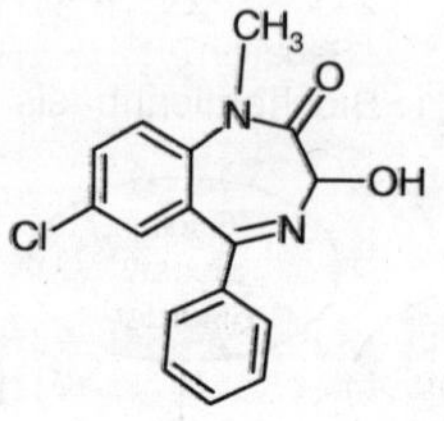

Temazepam

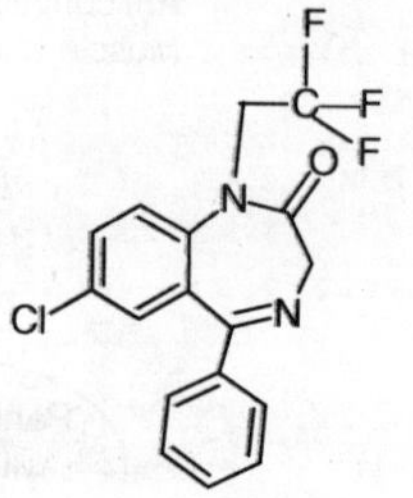

Halazepam

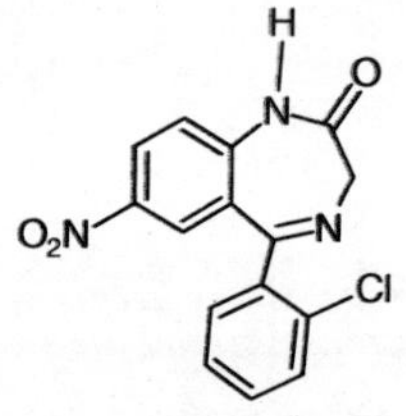

Clonazepam

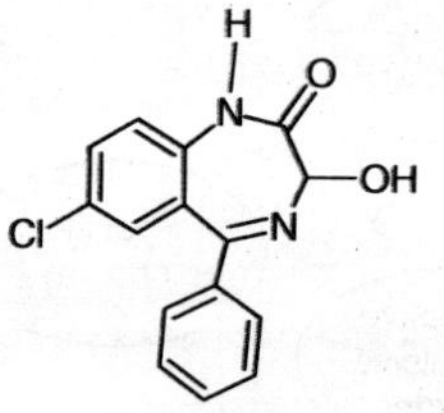

Oxazepam

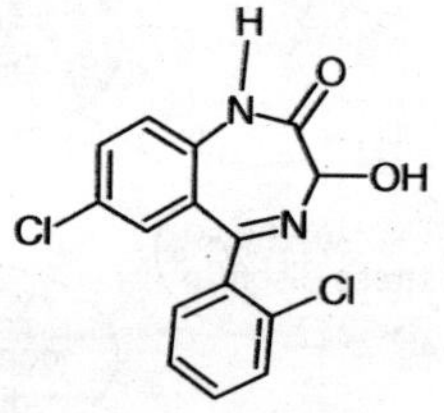

Lorazepam

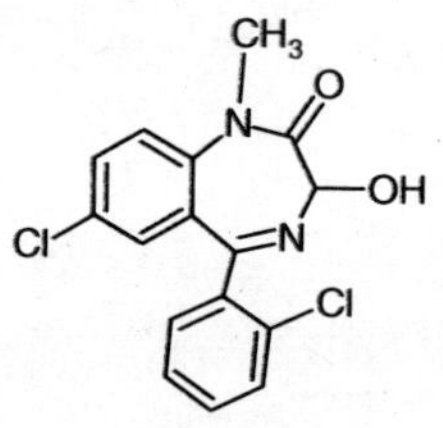

Lormetazepam

Newer benzodiazepines

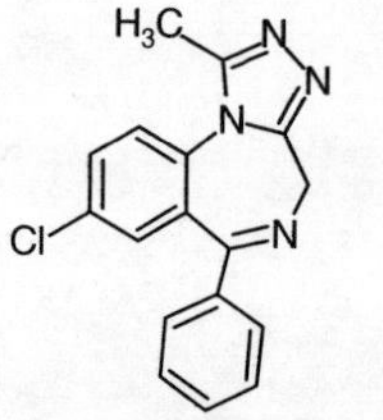

Alprazolam

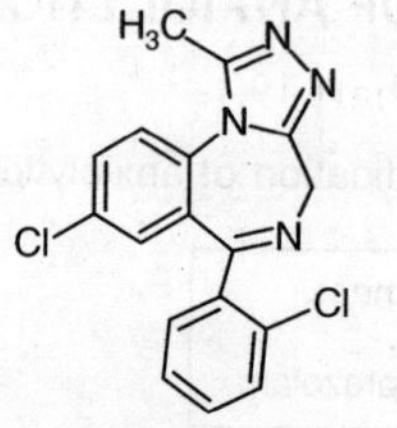

Triazolam

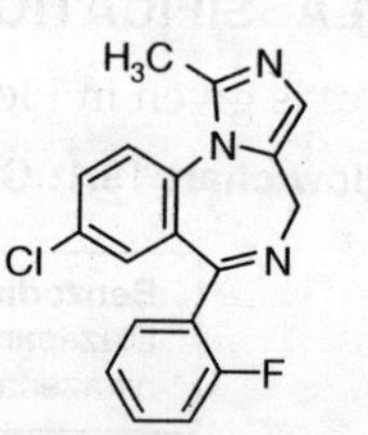

Midazolam

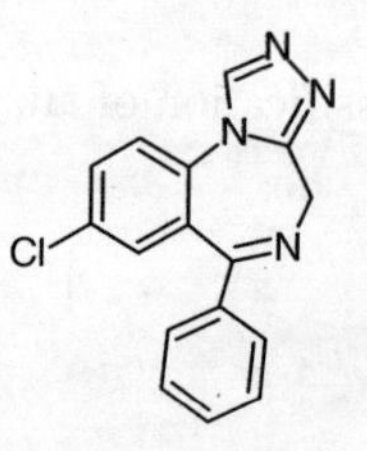

Estazolam

Non-benzodiazepines

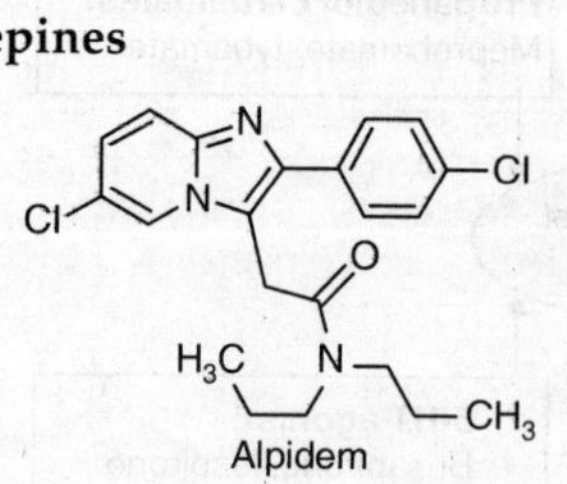

Alpidem

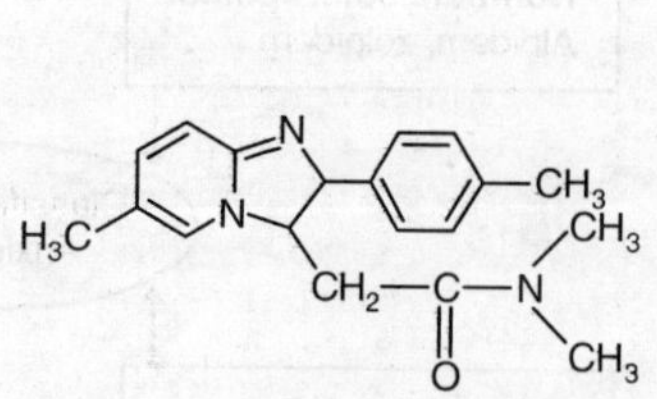

Zolpidem

Carbamate derivatives

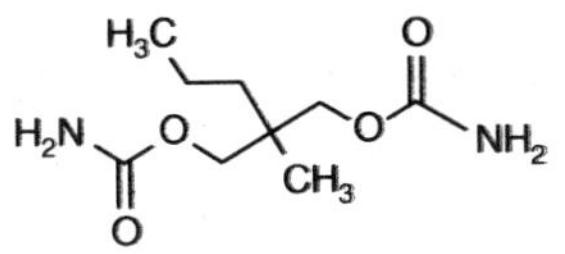

Meprobamate

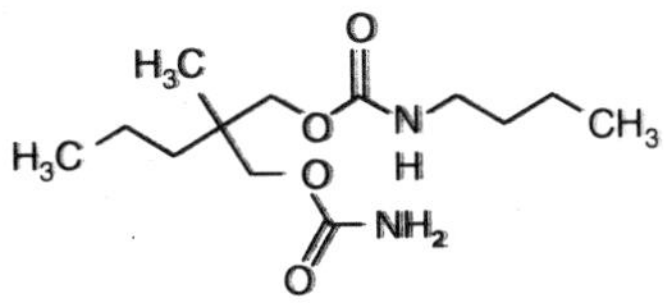

Tybamate

Anti-histaminic

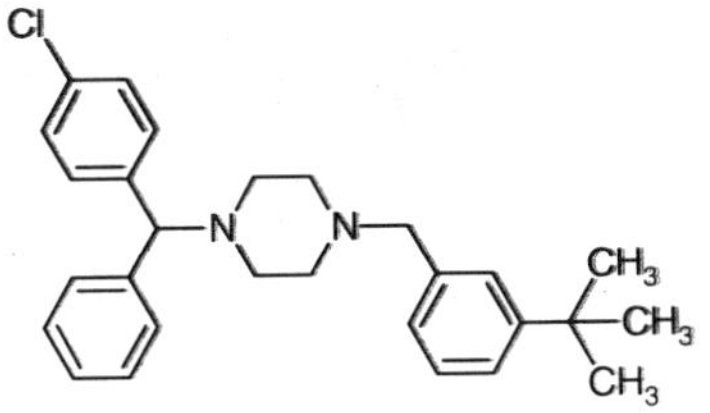

Buclizine

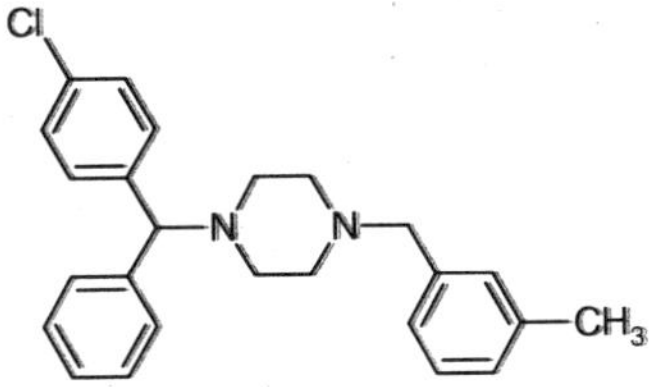

Meclizine

5-HT antagonist

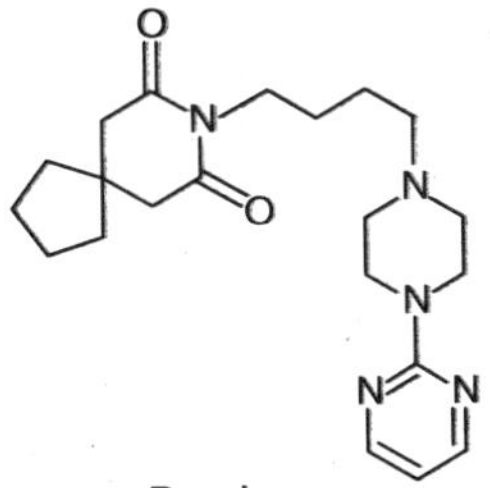

Buspirone

■ **BENZODIAZEPINES** (For details refer Chapter 18)

■ **NON-BENZODIAZEPINE**

MOA: It binds to the Omega-I site of GABA receptors and produce anxiolytic action by opening chloride channels.

Carbamates

MOA: It acts at the N-methyl-D-aspartate (NMDA) receptor and remains effective against intracerebroventricular NMDA-induced against clonus in mice. It also modulates Na-channel conductance.

Anti-Histaminics

MOA: Histamine is responsible for the anxiety. Anti-histamines block its effect and produce calmness in the patient.

5-HT Agonist

MOA: Busapirone is agonist at 5-HT_{1A} presynaptic receptor, stimulation of which results in decrease in release of serotonin, which is one of the excitory neurotransmitter responsible for anxiety.

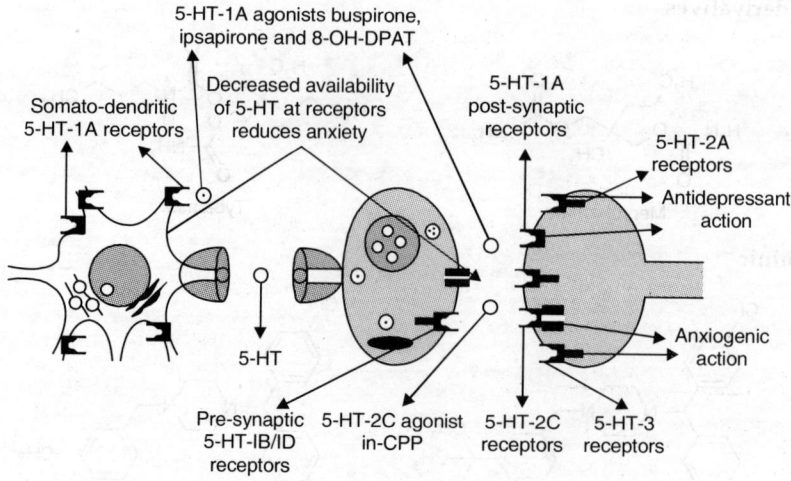

Fig. 19.3: Mode of action of different anti-anxiety agents

Diazepam

2-amino-2, 5-dihlorobanzo-phenone + Glycine ethyl ester hydrochloride (II) → (Pyridine) 7-chloro-2-oxo-5-phenyl-2, 3-dihydro-1H-1, 4-benzodiazepine → (NaOCH₃, dimethyl sulfate (III)) Diazepam

2-amino-2 , 5-dihlorobanzo-phenone

Glycine ethyl ester hydrochloride (II)

7-chloro-2-oxo-5-phenyl-2, 3-di-hydro-1H-1, 4-benzodiazepine

Diazepam

Oxazepam

6-chloro-2-chloromethyl-4-phenylquinozoline 3-oxide → (NaOH) **7-chloro-5-phenyl-2-oxo-1, 3-dihydro-2H-1, 4-benzodiaze-pine 4-oxide** → (ocetic onhydride) **7-chloro-5-phenyl-2-oxo-1, 3-acetoxy-1, 3-dihydro-2H-1, 4-benzodiazepine (I)**

→ (C₂H₅OH, NaOH) **Oxazepam**

Nitrazepam

2-amino-benzophenone	Glycine ethyl ester hydrochloride (I)		2-oxo-5-phenyl-2, 3-dihydro-1H-1, 4-benzodiazepine (II)	Nitrazepam

Flunitrazepam

4-chloroaniline   2-fluorobenzoyl chloride   2-amino-5-chloro-2′-fluorobenzophenone   2-omino-2′-fluore-benzophenone (I)

Bromoacetyl bromide   5-(2-fluorophenyl)-1, 3-dihdro-2H-1, 4-benzodiazepine-2-one (II)

5-(2-fluorophenyl)-7-nitro-1, 3-dihydro-2H-1, 4-benzodiozepine-2-one   Methyl iodide   Flunitrazepam

Lorazepam

2-amino-2 , 5-dichloro-benzophenone   chloroocetyl chloride

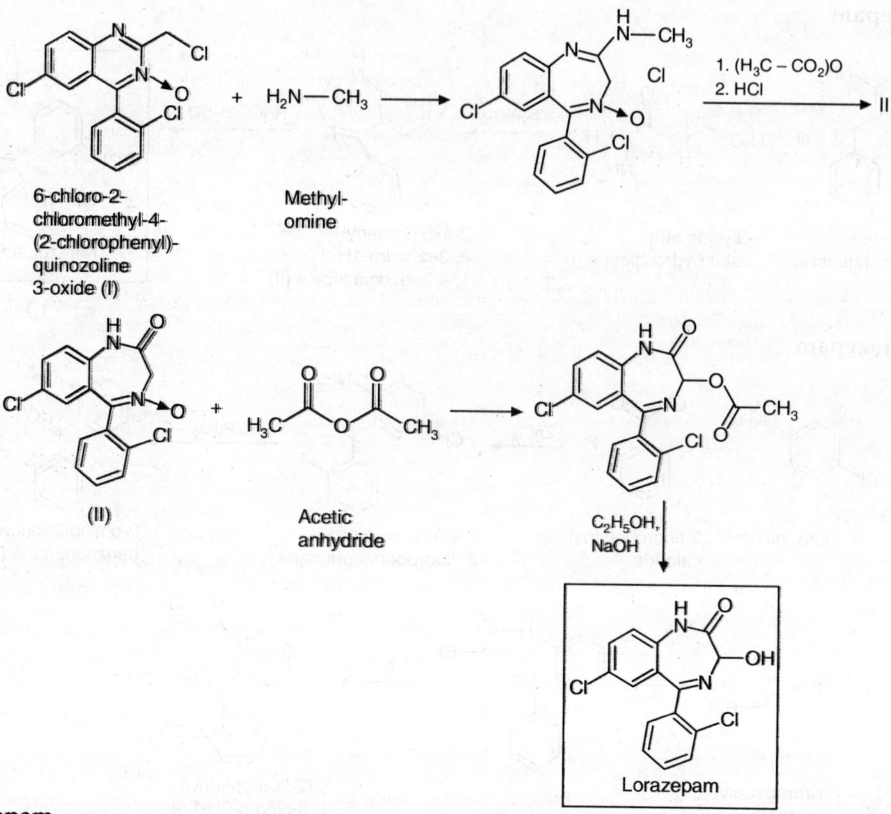

6-chloro-2-chloromethyl-4-(2-chlorophenyl)-quinozoline 3-oxide (I)

Methyl-omine

1. (H₃C – CO₂)O
2. HCl

II

(II)

Acetic anhydride

C₂H₅OH, NaOH

Lorazepam

Medazepam

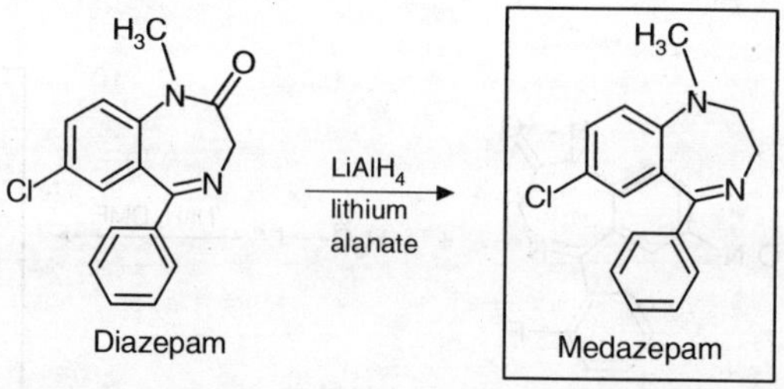

Diazepam

LiAlH₄ lithium alanate

Medazepam

Temazepam

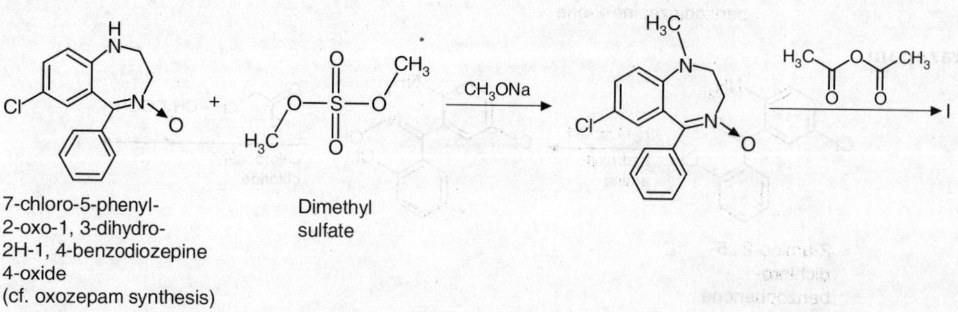

7-chloro-5-phenyl-2-oxo-1, 3-dihydro-2H-1, 4-benzodiozepine 4-oxide
(cf. oxozepam synthesis)

Dimethyl sulfate

CH₃ONa

I

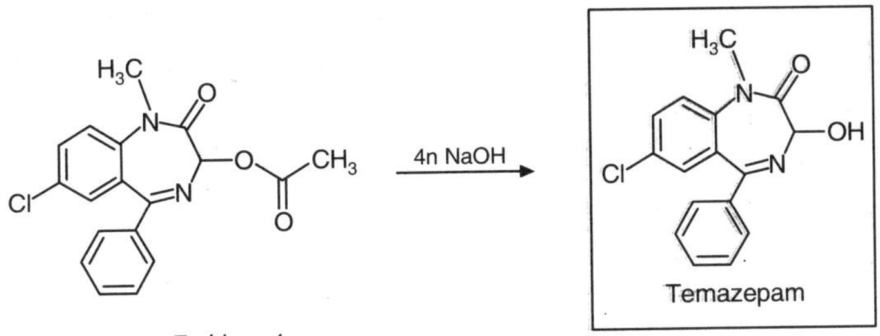

3-ocetoxy-7-chloro-1-
methyl-5-phenyl-2-oxo-
1, 3-dhydro-2H-1, 4-
benzodiazepine

Temazepam

Bromazepam

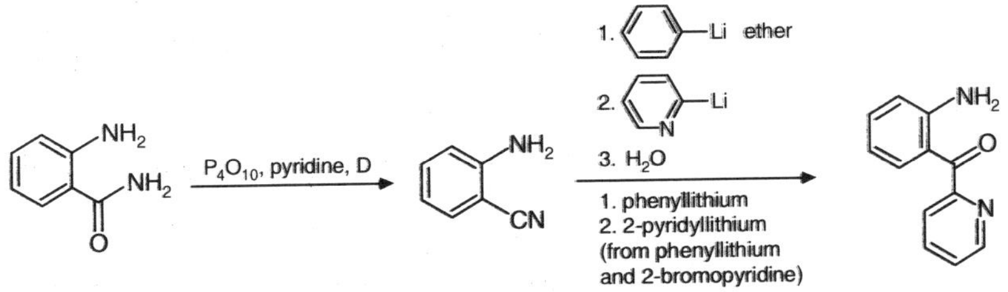

anthranilamide

anthranilonitrile

2-(2-aminobenzoyl)-
pyridine (I)

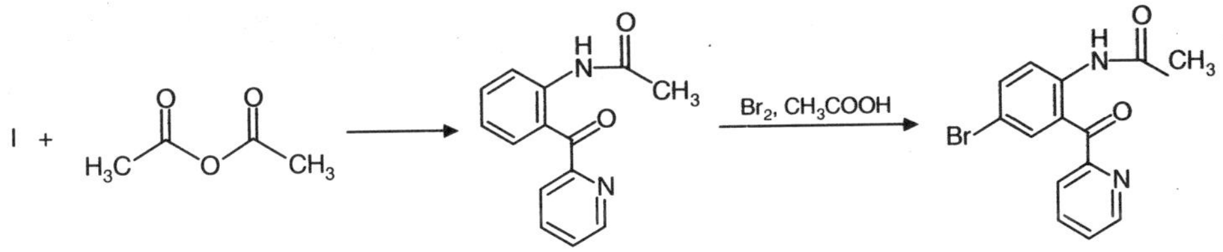

Acetic anhydride

2-(acetamido-
benzoyl)pyridine

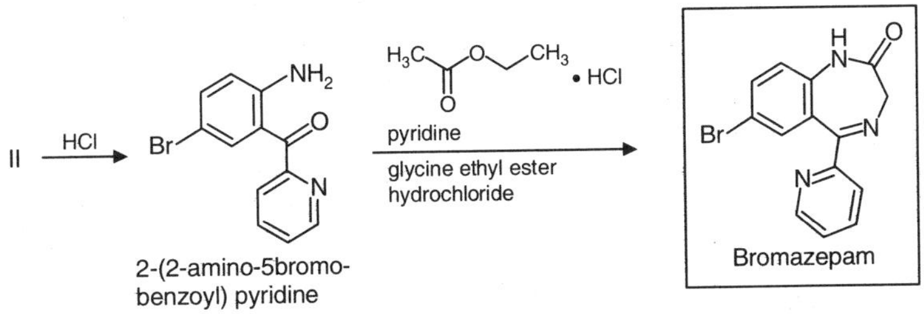

2-(2-amino-5bromo-
benzoyl) pyridine

Bromazepam

Alprazolam

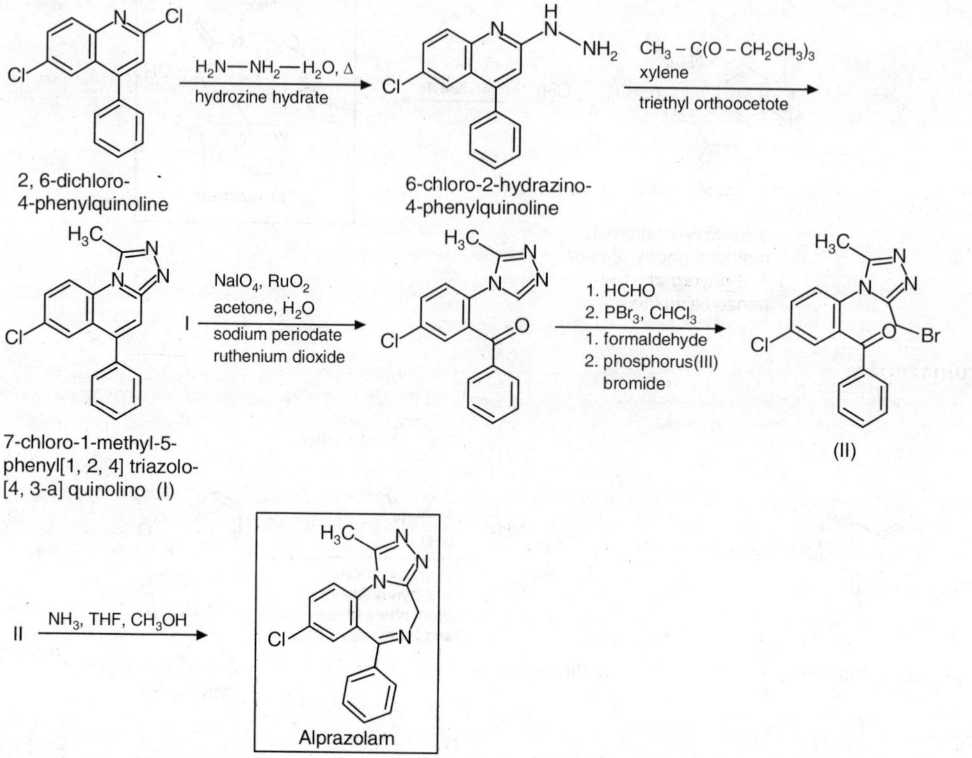
Cl
Cl
$H_2N—NH_2—H_2O$, Δ
hydrozine hydrate
H
N
NH2
Cl
$CH_3 – C(O – CH_2CH_3)_3$
xylene
triethyl orthoocetote
2, 6-dichloro-
4-phenylquinoline
6-chloro-2-hydrazino-
4-phenylquinoline
H3C
N
N
Cl
$NaIO_4$, RuO_2
acetone, H_2O
sodium periodate
ruthenium dioxide
I
O
1. HCHO
2. PBr_3, $CHCl_3$
1. formaldehyde
2. phosphorus(III)
bromide
Br
7-chloro-1-methyl-5-
phenyl[1, 2, 4] triazolo-
[4, 3-a] quinolino (I)
(II)
II
NH_3, THF, CH_3OH
Alprazolam

Trizolam

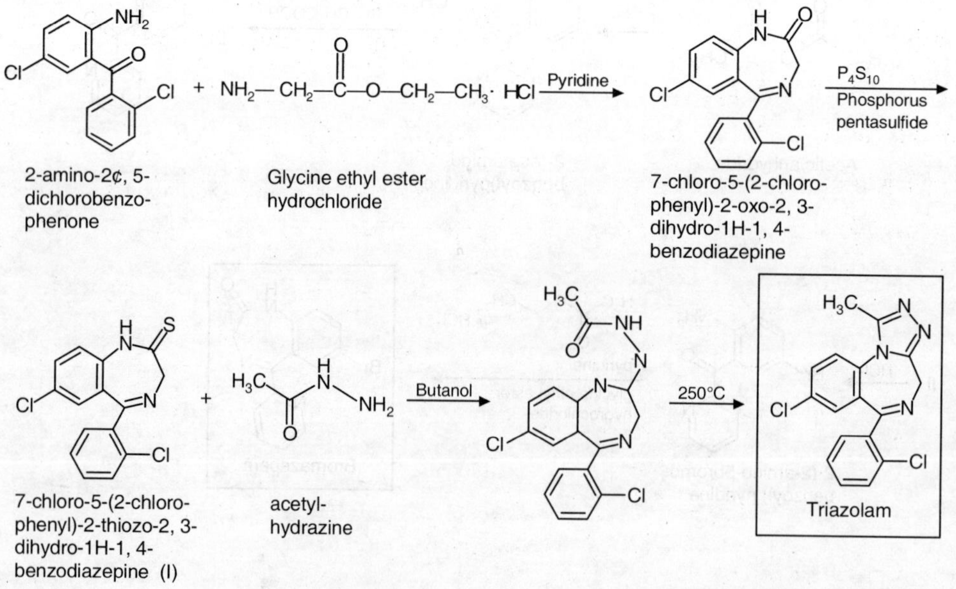
NH_2
O
Cl
Cl
+ $NH_2—CH_2—C(=O)—O—CH_2—CH_3 \cdot HCl$
Pyridine
H
O
N
P_4S_{10}
Phosphorus
pentasulfide
I
2-amino-2¢, 5-
dichlorobenzo-
phenone
Glycine ethyl ester
hydrochloride
7-chloro-5-(2-chloro-
phenyl)-2-oxo-2, 3-
dihydro-1H-1, 4-
benzodiazepine
H
S
+
H3C
NH2
Butanol
NH
250°C
Triazolam
7-chloro-5-(2-chloro-
phenyl)-2-thiozo-2, 3-
dihydro-1H-1, 4-
benzodiazepine (I)
acetyl-
hydrazine

Estazolam

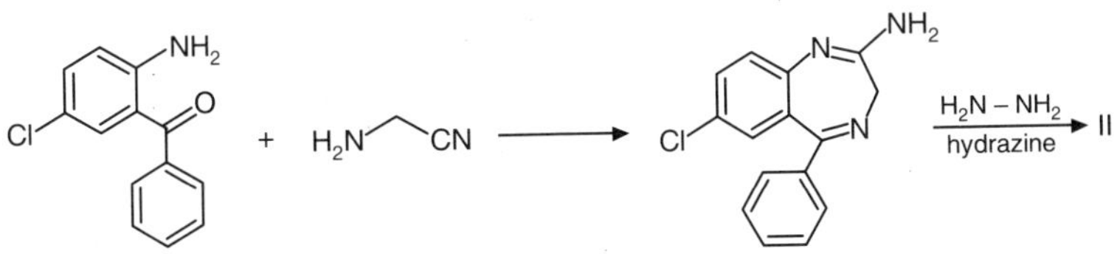

2-amino-5-chloro-
benzophenons (I)

Aminoacetonitrile

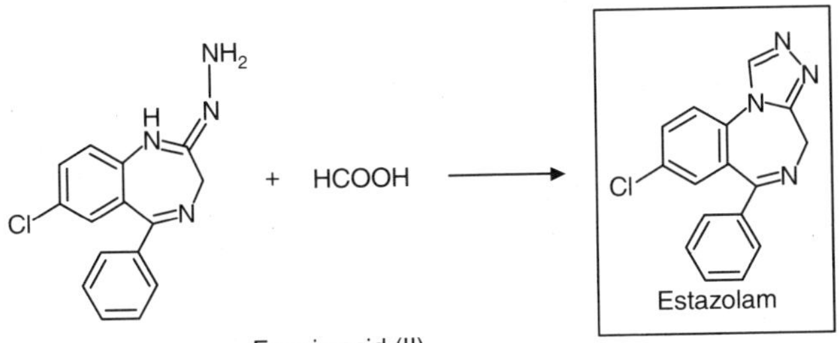

(II)   Formic acid (II)

Estazolam

Loprazolam

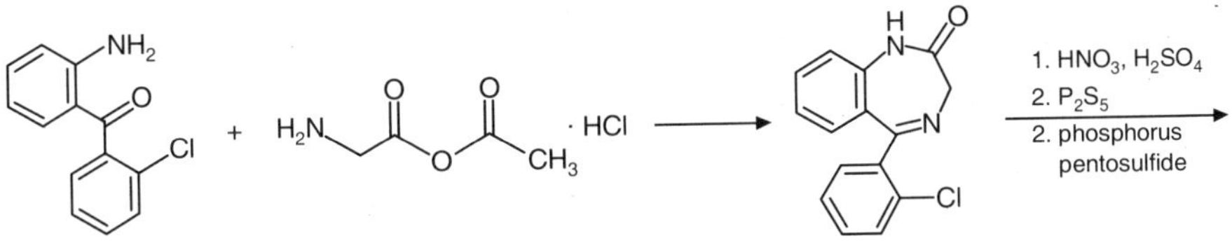

2-amino-2¢-
chlorobenzo-
phenone

Glycine ethyl ester
hydrochloride

1, 3-dihydro-5-
(2-chlorophenyl)-
2H-1, 4-benzo-
diazepine-2-one

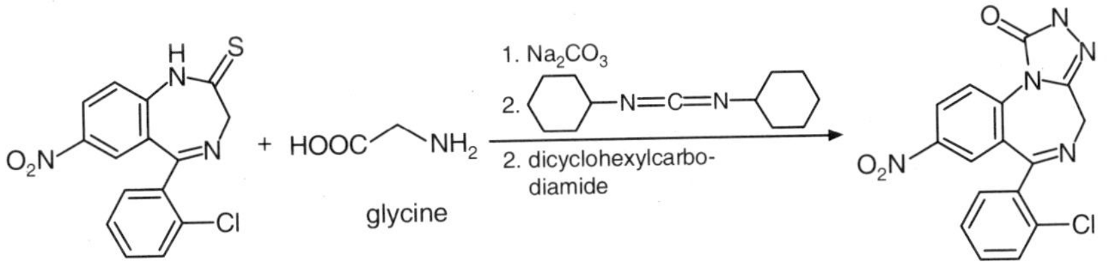

1. HNO₃, H₂SO₄
2. P₂S₅
2. phosphorus
   pentosulfide

(I)

+ glycine

1. Na₂CO₃
2. dicyclohexylcarbo-
   diamide

dimethyl-
Formamide
diethyl acetal

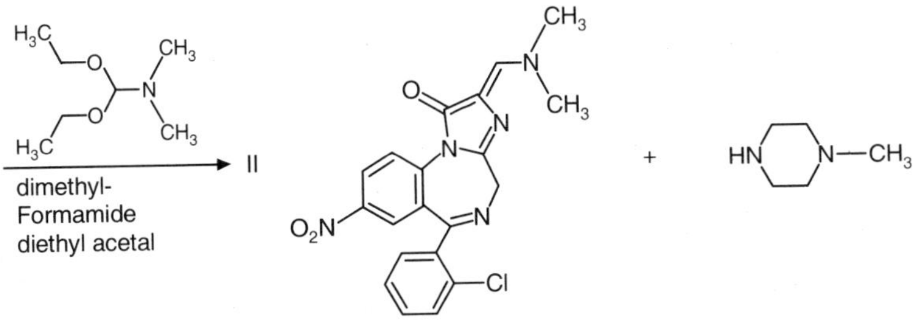

(II)

+ N-methyl piperazine

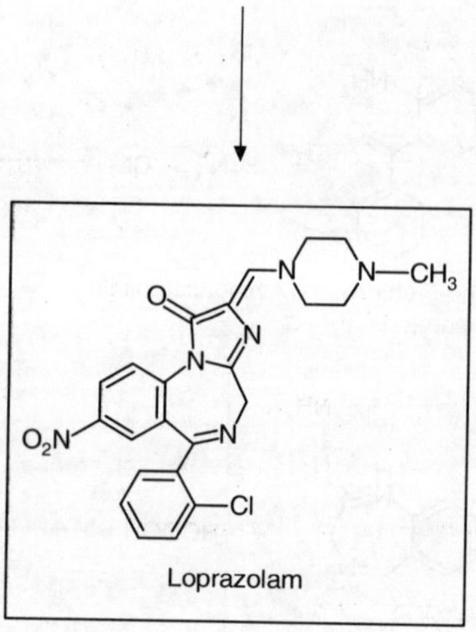

Loprazolam

Alpidem

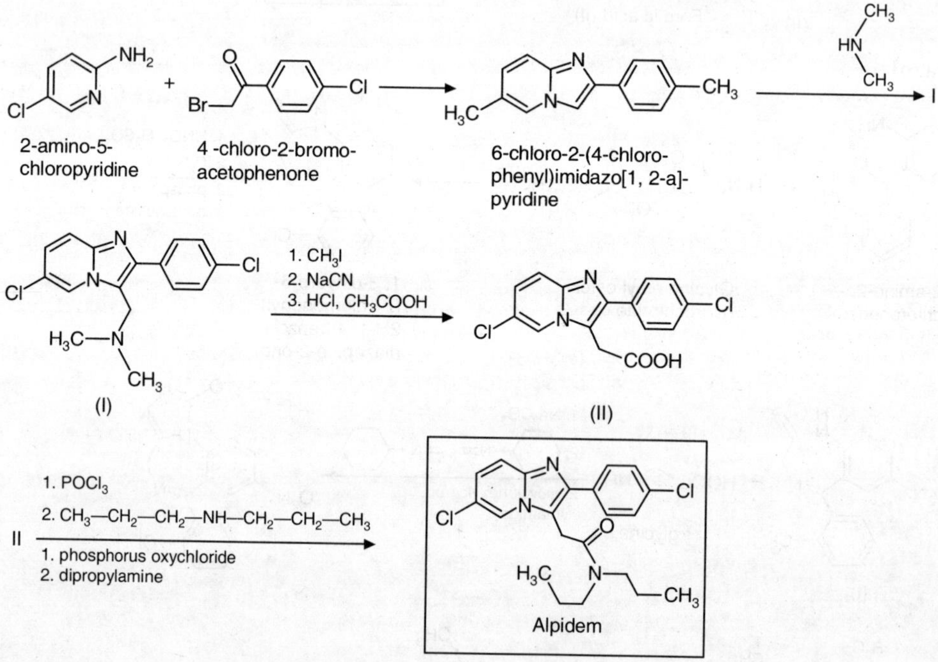

2-amino-5-
chloropyridine
+
4-chloro-2-bromo-
acetophenone
→
6-chloro-2-(4-chloro-
phenyl)imidazo[1, 2-a]-
pyridine

(I)

1. CH₃I
2. NaCN
3. HCl, CH₃COOH

→

(II)

1. POCl₃
2. CH₃—CH₂—CH₂—NH—CH₂—CH₂—CH₃

II

1. phosphorus oxychloride
2. dipropylamine

Alpidem

Zolpidem

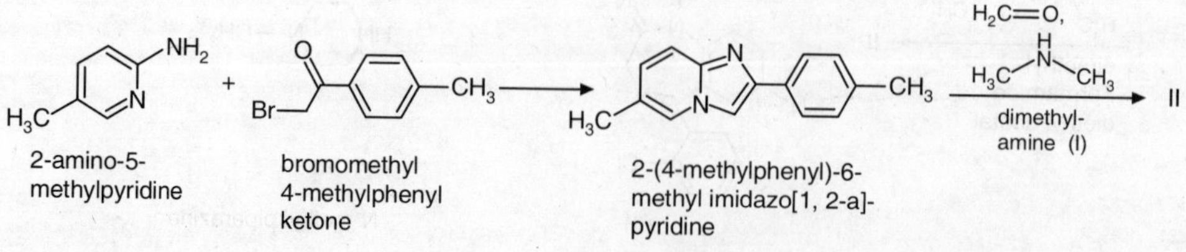

2-amino-5-
methylpyridine
+
bromomethyl
4-methylphenyl
ketone
→
2-(4-methylphenyl)-6-
methyl imidazo[1, 2-a]-
pyridine

H₂C=O,
dimethyl-
amine (I)

II

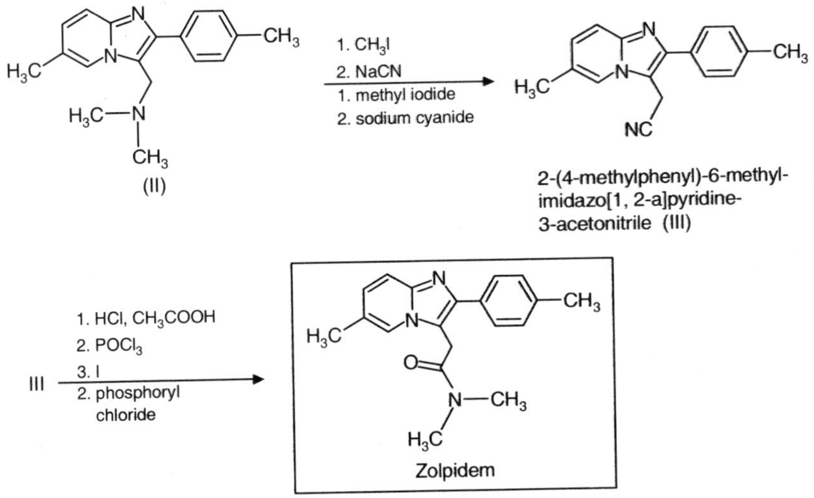

H_3C
N
N
CH_3
$H_3C—N$
CH_3
(II)
1. CH_3I
2. NaCN
1. methyl iodide
2. sodium cyanide
NC
2-(4-methylphenyl)-6-methyl-
imidazo[1, 2-a]pyridine-
3-acetonitrile (III)
III
1. HCl, CH_3COOH
2. $POCl_3$
3. I
2. phosphoryl
chloride
O
$N—CH_3$
Zolpidem

Buclizine

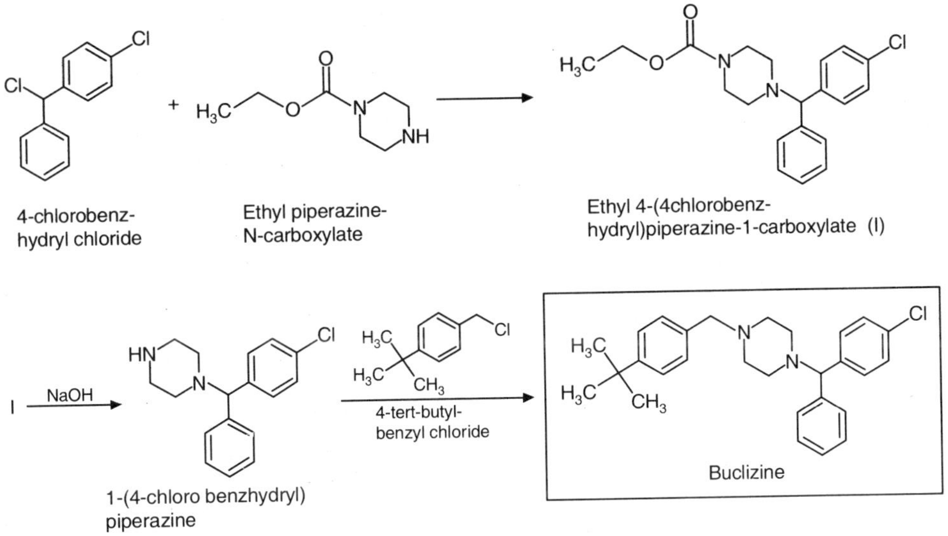

Cl
Cl
+
H_3C
O
N
NH
4-chlorobenz-
hydryl chloride
Ethyl piperazine-
N-carboxylate
Ethyl 4-(4chlorobenz-
hydryl)piperazine-1-carboxylate (I)
I
NaOH
HN
1-(4-chloro benzhydryl)
piperazine
CH_3
4-tert-butyl-
benzyl chloride
Buclizine

Meclizine

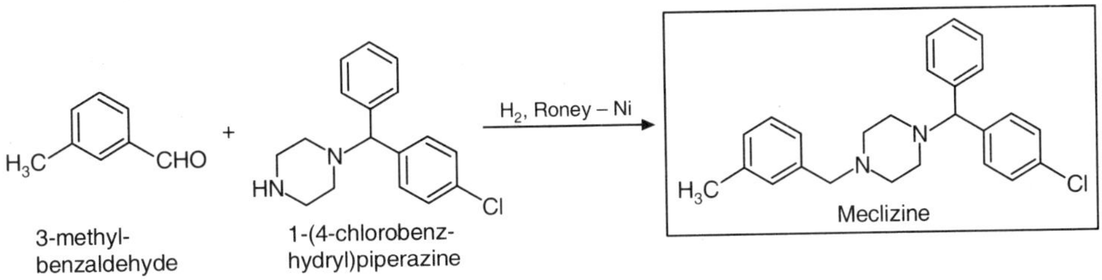

H_3C
CHO
+
HN
N
Cl
H_2, Roney – Ni
3-methyl-
benzaldehyde
1-(4-chlorobenz-
hydryl)piperazine
Meclizine

Meprobamate

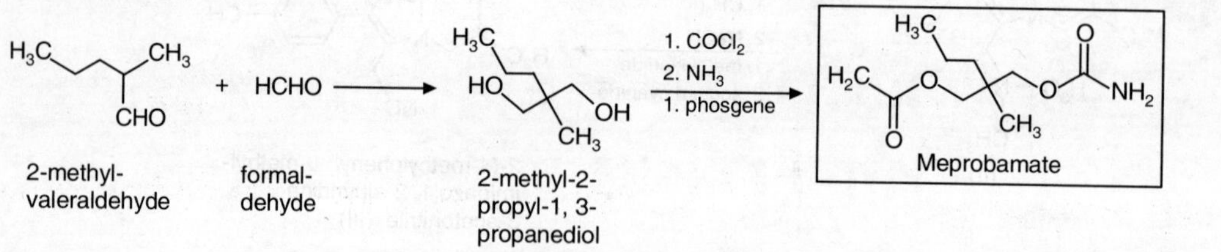
H3C
CH3
CHO
+ HCHO
H3C
HO
OH
CH3
1. COCl2
2. NH3
1. phosgene
H3C
H2C
O
O
O
NH2
CH3
O
Meprobamate
2-methyl-
valeraldehyde
formal-
dehyde
2-methyl-2-
propyl-1, 3-
propanediol

20

Anticonvulsant Agents (Anti-Epileptic Agents)

Epilepsy is a chronic neurological condition characterized by recurrent spontaneous seizures not caused by active cerebral disease. Seizures are sudden, involuntary, time-limited alterations in behavior associated with excessive discharges of cerebral neurons. In other words, it is also defined as, it is a group of disorder of CNS characterized by cerebral dysarrhythmia, manifesting in the brief episodes of loss or disturbance of consciousness with or without characteristic body movement.

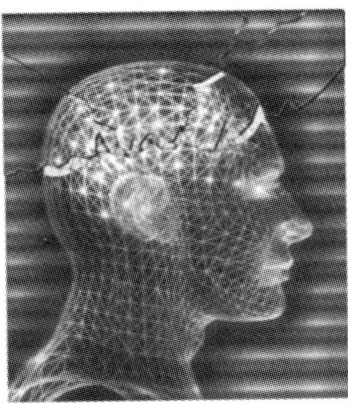

- Epileptic disorders can be primary or secondary. Primary disorders are presumed to result from a genetic disturbance; secondary disorders are presumed to result from a brain injury, such as penetrating head trauma or cerebral infarction. Seizures associated with sleep deprivation, abrupt withdrawal of alcohol or sedative drugs, fever, or uses of convulsive drugs are not reflective of a chronic epileptic disorder.
- Epileptic seizures can be characterized by specific EEG patterns and behavioral events during the seizures. The classification of seizures is of clinical relevance since many antiepileptic drugs are effective only in certain seizure types and are contraindicated for others.
- The most widely used classification system is the International Classification of Epileptic Seizures (ICES) introduced in 1981 by the International League against Epilepsy. According to the ICES system, seizures are classified as either partial or generalized. Partial seizures originate in one cerebral hemisphere; generalized seizures originate in both. When partial seizures evolve to generalized seizures, they are referred to as secondarily generalize seizures.

■ BIOCHEMICAL BASIS OF EPILEPSY

- All forms of epilepsy have their origin in the brain. Epilepsy results when many neurons in the union under a high excited stage, deliver massive discharges abolishing a finely organized pattern of the integrative activity of the brain.

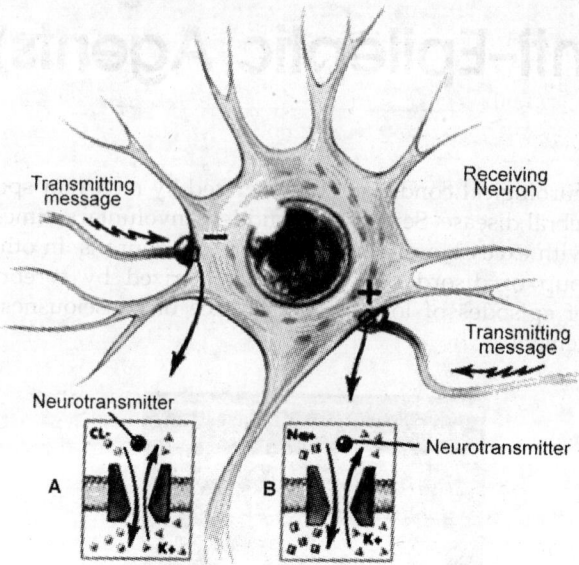

Fig. 20.1: Normal way of signal transmission by opening of Ca^{2+} and Na^+ channels.

- John Jackson proposed that these seizurs are caused by occasional, sudden, excessive, rapid and local discharges of grey matter and once initiated by the abnormal focus, the seizures attack the neighboring normal brain resulting into generalized convulsions. (Figs 20.1 and 20.2)

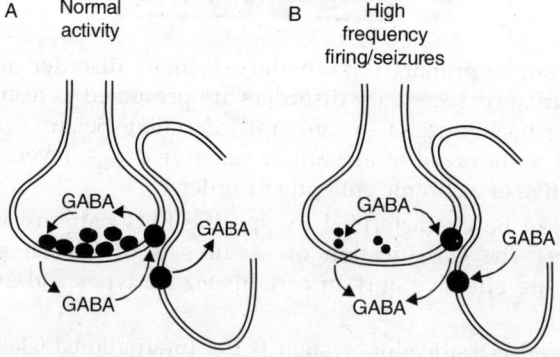

Fig. 20.2: Overfiring of neurotransmitter in epilepsy

- This abnormal focus may originate as a result of local biochemical changes, ischemia or the loss of vulnerable cell inhibitory systems. The normal inhibitory mechanism generally restricts the spread of convulsive activity to the neighboring normal cells. Hence a seizure focus in man may remain normal over long period of time and may not cause signs and symptoms of epilepsy. However, certain physiological changes may trigger the focus and thus facilitate the spread of abnormal electrical activity to normal tissue.

- Such factors include;

1. Changes in blood glucose concentration.
2. Blood gas tension.
3. Plasma pH.
4. Total osmotic pressure and electrolyte composition of the extracellular fluid.
5. Fatigue.
6. Emotional stress.
7. Nutritional deficiency.
8. Trauma, infection, meningitis, brain tumors, cerebrovascular disease or metabolic abnormalities.

- Seizure in fact is nothing but electrical explosions of the brain. Once initiated, a seizure is maintained by re-entry of excitory impulses in a closed feedback fashion which may not include the original seizure focus. Complete depletion of neurotransmitter, metabolic factors (like accumulation of CO_2 and adenosine, depletion of O_2 and high energy phosphate intermediates) may contribute to self-control of intensity and duration of seizures.

- In summary, excessive discharge of the neurotransmitter is the cause of epilepsy. This excessive discharge results due to decreased or hypofunctioning of GABA.

- There are the three ways, by which we can solve this problem.

1. By decreasing the overfiring of the neurotransmitter.
2. By increasing the concentration of GABA, by giving GABA mimetic or facillator.
3. By inhibiting the GABA metabolism, by inhibiting GABA-transaminase, which metabolises GABA to succinic acid.

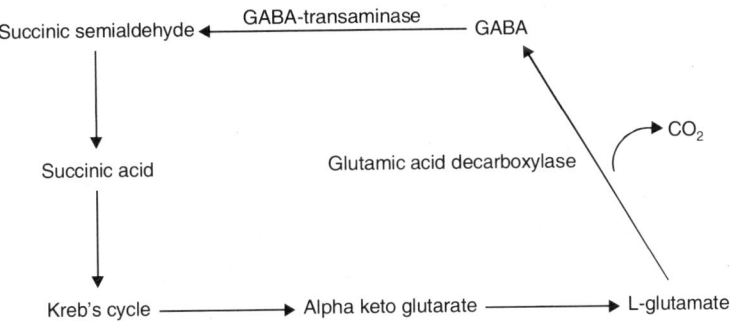

CLASSIFICATION OF EPILEPSY (FLOW CHART 20.1)

- Vitamin B_6 is the precursor in the formation of coenzyme pyridoxal-5- phosphate which is responsible for the decarboxylation of glutamic acid to form GABA and since hydrazine derivatives can inactive the coenzyme, pyridoxal-5-phosphate via hydrazone formation, these facts confirm the fundamental role of GABA in the arrest of convulsions.

Flow chart 20.1: Classification of epilepsy

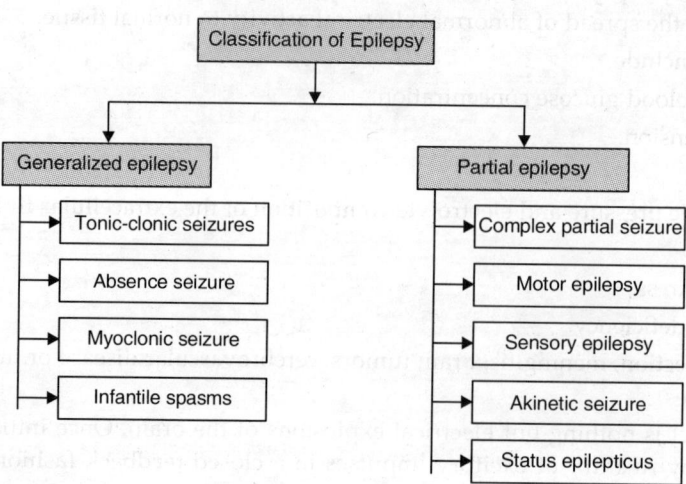

Generalized Epilepsy

- Once initiated, it spreads quickly into the entire or at least the greater part of the brain.

Tonic-clonic seizure (Grand mal)

- It has a close resemblance with electrically induced convulsions where the mass stimulation of cortical neurons occurs. As the name indicates, initially there is a generalized tonic activity followed by a clonic phase. It results due to a potent cerebral excitation and is also known as major seizures.
- Its onset is preintimated to the patient by a warming sensation that is known as major seizures. Patient may become cyanotic. Heart rate and blood pressure increase and dilation of pupils also occur. These signs are characteristics of sympathetic nervous system stimulation. The total attack lasts for several minutes. After the attack, sleep prevails due to neuronal store-exhaustation.

Absence or minor seizures (Petit mal)

- It is reported to occur mainly in young children between the age of 6 to 14. Seizures frequently disappear spontaneously after adolescence.
- Seizures are usually of brief duration accompanied by a momentary loss of consciousness and originate due to synchronization of both, excitory and inhibitory neurons within the brainstem and mesial reticular activating system.

Myoclonic seizures

The attack is characterized by the jerky muscular movements of head, limbs or body as such. The duration of attack remains near about 1 second and it reappears at about 5 seconds intervals for a period of a minute. The etiology of attack is not clear and is supposed to be due to brain damage.

Infantile spasms

The attack sometimes begins with a cry and is often associated with momentary unconsciousness. The structural or functional brain abnormalities or pyridoxine deficiencies are some recognized causes responsible for infantile spasms.

Partial or focal Epilepsy

In this type, the initial neuronal discharge originates from a specific, limited cortical area.

Complex partial seizure

It is usually originates in the mesial anterior temporal lobe and is characterized by hallucination, fear, hate or other emotional and behavioral abnormalities. Symptoms are extremely complex and varied and may sometimes be confused with psychotic disorder.

Motor epilepsy

Only one entire side of the body is affected. Consciousness is usually not lost. In severe cases, motor epilepsy is transformed into grand mal followed by paralysis of the hyperactive side of the body. Motor epilepsy is mainly witnessed in the childhood and is due to more limited cortical abnormalities.

Sensory epilepsy

This is similar to motor epilepsy except the fact that it arises in the sensory cortex. Simultaneous attack of both, motor and sensory epilepsy in the patient is also reported.

Akinetic seizures

Superficially no convulsions are seen. Patient may suddenly fall down on the ground without loss of consciousness.

Status epilepticus

- It is the condition in which one attack follows another without patients regaining consciousness. The attack may be of grand mal, petit mal or partial seizures.

- If it remains untreated, it may be fatal. Status epilepticus originates due to failure of the patient to follow therapeutic regimen prescribed for him. Diazepam, clonazepam, thiopentone or lignocaine may be administered intravenously to control this condition treatment fails, general anesthesia may be required.

CLASSIFICATION OF ANTICONVULSANTS

Classification of anticonvulsants is depicted in Flow chart 20.2.

Flow chart 20.2: Classification of anticonvulsants

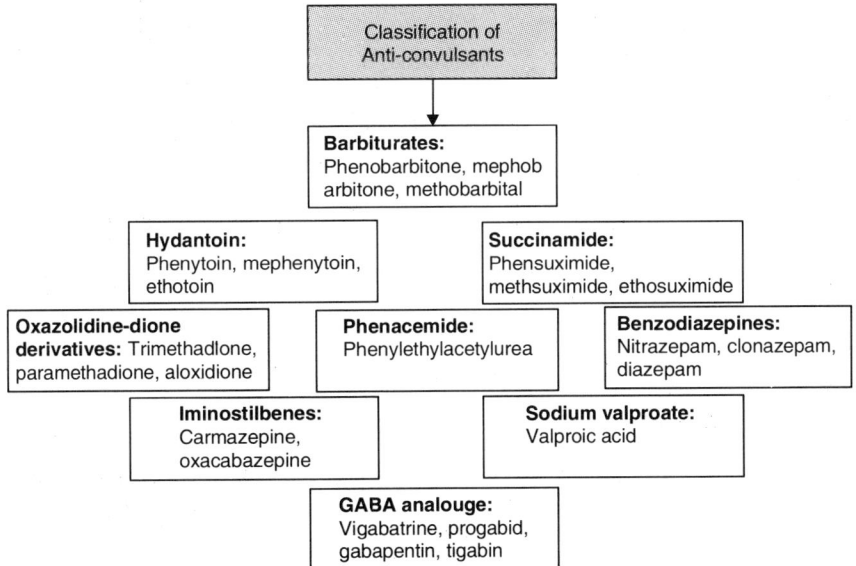

Barbiturates

Phenobarbital   Mephobarbital   Methobarbital

Hydantoin

Phenytoin   Ethotoin   Fosphenytoin sodium   Mephenytoin

Succinamide

Phensuximide   Methsuximide   Ethosuximide

Oxazolidine-dione derivatives

Aloxidione   Trimethadione   Paramethadione

Phenacemide

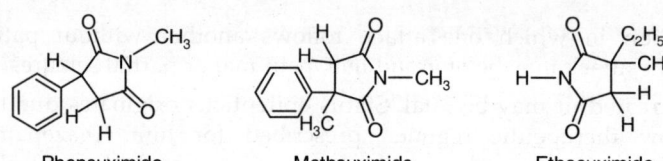

Phenacemide   Phenylethylacetylurea

Benzodiazepines

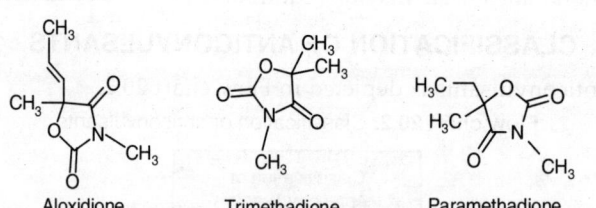

Diazepam   Clonazepam   lorazepam   Midazolam

Iminostilbenes

Carbamazepine   Carbamazepine epoxide   Oxcarbazepine

Sodium valproate

Valproic acid

GABA analouge

Gabapentin   Vigabatrine

Progabid   Tigabin

▨ BARBITURATES

Although sedative hypnotic barbiturates commonly display anticonvulsant properties, only phenobarbital and mephobarbital display adequate anticonvulsant selectivity for use as anticonvulsants.

Barbiturate

Structure–Activity Relationship (SAR)

At C-5

1. Both hydrogens in position C-5 of barbituric acid must be replaced for maximal activity. This is likely due to susceptibility to rapid metabolic attack on this side.

2. The sum of the carbon atoms of both substituent at carbon C-5 should be between 6-to10 to obtain optimal activity.

3. Increasing length of an alkyl chain position at C-5 enhance the potency up to 5-6 carbon atom. But beyond that depressant action decreases.

4. Introduction of a halogen atom into the alkyl substituent at C-5 increases the activity.

5. Introduction of a polar substituent such as OH, COOH RNH, etc. at C-5 results in decrease in lipid solubility and potency.

6. Branched, cyclic or an unsaturated chain in position C-5 generally produce a short duration of action than does the normal saturated chain, containing the same number of carbon atoms.

7. Because of the presence of both polar and non-polar groups, it has coefficient close to 100 (log p= 2). This character is sufficiently lipophilic so that they readily penetrate nervous system.

At C-4 and 6

Introduction of more sulphur atoms at C-4 and 6 decreases the hypnotic activity.

At C-1 and C-3

Compound with alkyl group in 1 or 3 position may have a shorter duration of action and onset of action.

At C-2

Replacement of oxygen by sulfur on carbon-2 shortens the onset and duration of action. Thiobarbiturates are much more lipid soluble in the non-ionized form than the corresponding oxygen analogue.

Mechanism of Action

• These drugs are GABA-mimetic. GABA is inhibitory neurotransmitter. At low doses, barbiturates either have γ-aminobutyric acid like action or enhance the effects of GABA, an inhibitory neurotransmitter.

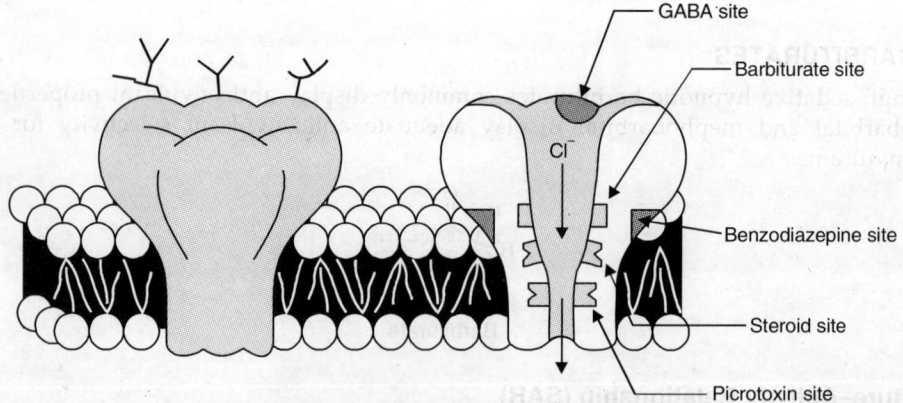

Fig. 20.3: Diagram of the GABA receptor

• It has been suggested that the effects of barbiturates on synaptic transmission are caused by an alteration in the postsynaptic sensitivity of the neurons to excitory and inhibitory transmitters. Barbiturates activate GABA receptors (Fig. 20.3) in high concentration, thereby enhancing pre- and post-synaptic inhibition. When GABA receptors are activated, chloride channels open, chloride enters the cell, hyperpolarize it, and produce decreased excitation.

- GABA receptors are part of supra-molecular complex that also include the benzodiazepine receptor and a picrotoxin site. Barbiturates bind to picrotoxin site and decrease chloride ion flux and produce an increased chloride concentration. The greater the affinity of a barbiturate for the picrotoxin binding site the greater is its potency.

HYDANTOIN

Hydantoin

Structure–Activity Relationship

1. 5-phenyl and other aromatic substituents are essential for the activity.
2. Alkyl substitution at position C-5 may contribute to sedation, a property absent in phenytoin.
3. Among other hydantoin like thiohydantoin and 1, 3 disubstituted hydantoin exhibit activity against chemically induced convulsion.

Mechanism of Action (Fig. 20.4)

- Epileptic seizures cause an accumulation of Na^+ ions within the cerebral neurons, which initiates enhanced synaptic transmission following rapid, repetitive presynaptic stimulation.

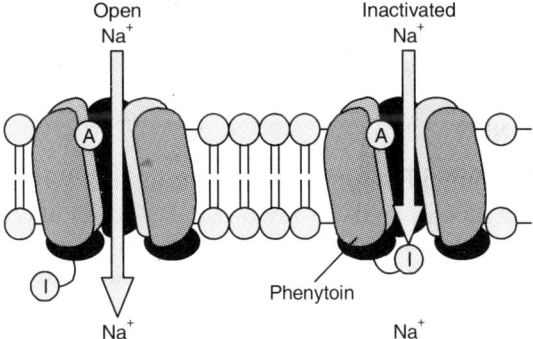

Fig. 20.4: Mechanism of action of hydantoins

- Phenytoin decreases the intracellular Na^+ ion concentration by prolonging the inactivated state Na^+ channel. As a result, high frequency discharge of neurotransmitter is inhibited.

SUCCINAMIDE

Structure–Activity Relationship

1. Methosuximide and phensuximide have phenyl substituent which makes them active against electrically induced convulsion.

2. N-methylation decreases activity against electroshock seizure and impart more activity against chemically induced convulsions.

3. A-methylalkoxyphenyl succinamides and alkoxybenzyl succinamide were active anticonvulsant. The length of the alkoxy group determines the activity.

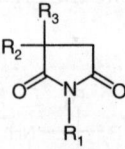

Succinamide

Mechanism of Action (Fig. 20.5)

• It suppose to inhibit 'T' type of Ca^{2+} current, resulting into decreased in neuron flux.

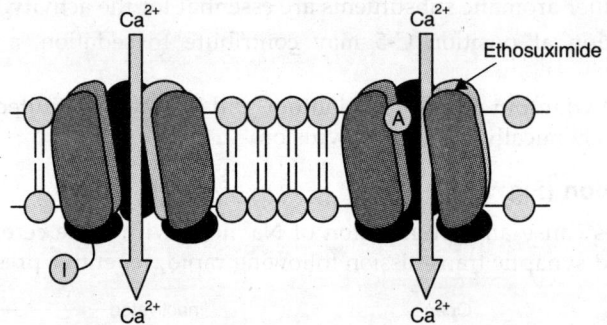

Fig. 20.5: Mechanism of action of ethosuximide

OXAZOLIDINEDIONES

Structure–Activity Relationship

1. The nature of the substituents on C-5 is important, e.g. lower alkyl substituent tend toword antipetitmal activity while aryl substituents towards antigrandmal activity, e.g. malidione active against petitmal epilepsy while 5, 5-diphenyloxazolidine-2,4-dione active against grandmal epilepsy.

Malidione

5, 5-diphenyloxazolidine-2, 4dione

2. The N-alkyl substituent does not affect the activity since all clinically used agents from this class undergo N-dealkylation in metabolism. The anticonvulsant activity of trimethadione is due to mainly its N-demethylated metabolite.

Trimethadione

N-demethylation

Dimethadione

3. Alkylation of imido-nitrogen could serve two functions first to increase the partition coefficient and second to prevent the dissociation of the imido-hydrogen. In both the case favouring the more distribution of the drug to the central nervous system.

Mechanism of Action

- It suppose to inhibit 'T' type Ca^{2+} current, resulting into decreased in neuron flux. Other assumption includes that it may increase the threshold for production of petit-mal seizure of the thalamic centers and thus prevents the spread of electrical activity to the thalamus.
- It also decreases synaptic transmission by increasing the duration of the refractory period in the neurons through which repetitive discharges occur.

PHENACEMIDE

Structure–Activity Relationship

1. Among the aliphatic acetylureas, the highest anticonvulsant activity is found in those, which are derived from branched chain acids of about seven carbon atoms.
2. With a further increase in molecular weight, the anticonvulsant activity gradually terminates and hypnotic effect predominates.
3. Phenacemide is most active agent amongst the aromatic ureas.

Phenacemide

4. Any substitution on the nitrogen of phenacemide does not increase further anticonvulsant activity.
5. Activity decrease with aromatic substitution of phenacemide with a gradual increase in hypnotic activity.
6. Diphenyl urea is inactive.

Mechanism of Action

It stabilize presynaptic membranes by blocking voltage dependant Na^+ channel, thereby preventing the release of excitory neurotransmitter, particularly glutamate and aspartate.

▨ BENZODIAZEPINES

Structure–Activity Relationship

- Refer antianxiety chapter.

Mechanism of Action (Fig. 20.6)

These drugs are GABA mimetic as well as GABA facillator in nature. It suppose to increase the affinity of GABA for receptor sites in brain membranes. It also facilitate the release of GABA at synaptic systems.

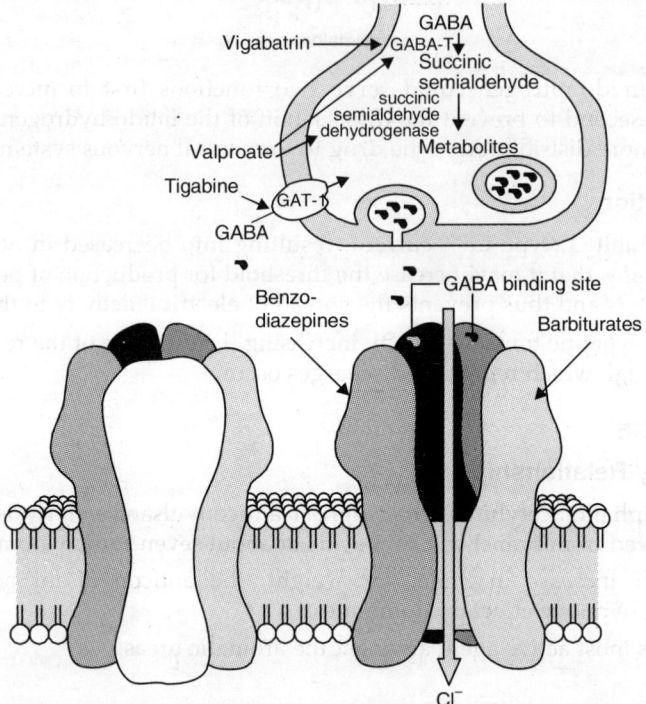

Fig. 20.6: Mechanism of action of benzodiazepines and other drugs

Metabolic Studies

Clonazepam is principally metabolized to inactive 7-amino derivatives. Diazepam metabolises to the N-dimethyl analogue and oxazepam, both are biologically active.

Toxicity

Drowsiness and fatigue are among the most common symptoms. Muscular inco-ordination, behavioural disturbances and increased salivary and bronchial secretion constitute less frequent side-effects.

▨ SODIUM VALPROATE

SAR

1. The anticonvulsant activity increases with increased chain length.
2. Introduction of double bond decreases the activity.

H₃C⎯⎯⎯CH₃

HO⎯O

Valproic acid

3. Introduction of a secondary or tertiary hydroxyl group or replacement of carboxyl by hydroxyl group has no effect.

MOA *(Fig. 20.7)*

1. This is suppose to facilitate the GABA.
2. Valproic acid inhibits GABA deactivating enzyme like transaminase.
3. Valproic acid causes phenytoin like frequency dependant prolongation of Na^+ channel inactivation.

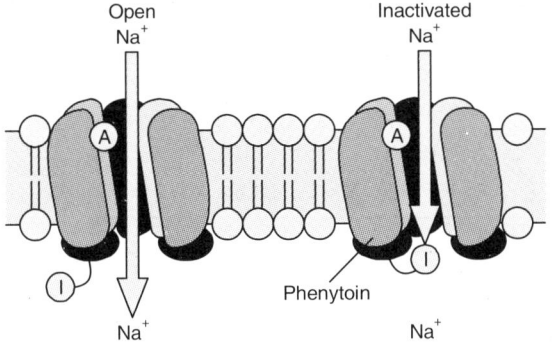

Fig. 20.7: Mode of action of sodium valproate

IMINOSTILBENES

MOA

This is suppose to increase the availability of adenosine, which is a natural anticonvulsant or convulsions modulator.

GABA ANALOUGE

Vigabatrine

MOA

This is inhibitor of GABA-transaminase enzyme, which degrade GABA.

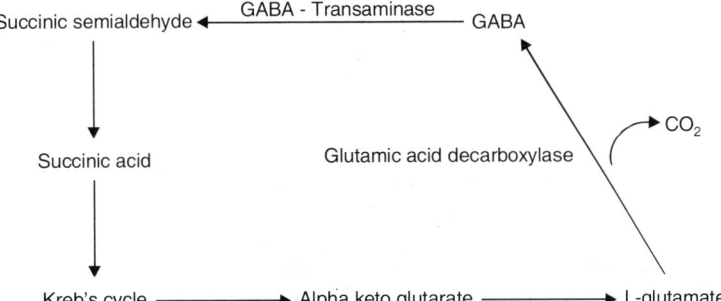

Progabid

MOA

This is GABA mimetic in nature.

Gaba Pentin and Tigabin

MOA

GABA-facilator in nature.

■ ISOSTERISM IN ANTICONVULSANT DRUG

Isoster

- These are group of atom, which impart some biological activity to a compound because of its similarity in electronic configuration and stereochemical aspect is known as isoster.

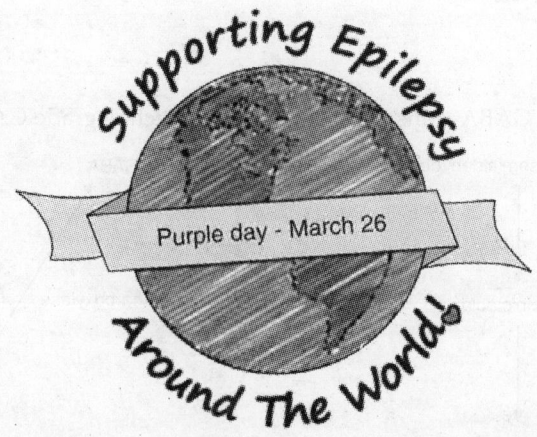

$Y = C, N, O; n = 1, 2$

Class	Y
Barbiturates	—NH— with C=O
Hydantoin	—NH—
Oxazolidinedione	—O—
Succinamide	—CH$_2$—

- From above discussion, we can say that all anticonvulsant possess isosterism having same biological activity with different structure.

Supporting Epilepsy

Purple day - March 26

Around The World!

Phenytoin

Benzil + Urea → Phenytoin

Ethotoin

Benzaldehyde + Sodium cyanide → Mandelo-nitrile → (I)

5-phenyl-hydantoin → ethyl iodide → Ethotoin

Trimethadione

Ethyl α-hydroxy-isobutyrate + urea → 5,5-dimethyl-2,4-oxozolidine-dione → Trimethadione

Mephenytoin

Benzyl cyanide + Diethyl carbonate → Ethyl-α-phenyl-cyanoacetate → (I)

I + Ethyl-bromide → 2-cyano-2phenyl-butyramide → 5-ethyl-5-phenylhydantoin (II)

II + Dimethyl sulfate (III) → Mephenytoin

Dimethyl sulfate (III)

Mephenytoin

Paramethadione

Methyl ethyl ketone $\xrightarrow[\text{sodium cyanide}]{\text{NaCN}}$ 2-hydroxy-2-methyl-butyronitrile $\xrightarrow[\text{ethanol}]{\text{H}_3\text{C} \text{OH, HCl}}$ 2-hydroxy-2-methyl-butyric acid ethyl ester (I)

Methyl ethyl ketone

2-hydroxy-2-methyl-butyronitrile

2-hydroxy-2-methyl-butyric acid ethyl ester (I)

I $\xrightarrow{\text{urea}}$ 5-ethyl-5-methyl-2, 4-oxazalidinedione $\xrightarrow[\text{dimethyl sulfate}]{\text{, NaOCH}_3}$ Paramethadione

5-ethyl-5-methyl-2, 4-oxazalidinedione

Paramethadione

Carbamazepine

5H-dibenz-[b, f] azepine (I) + Phosgene → $\xrightarrow{\text{NH}_3, \text{C}_2\text{H}_5\text{OH}}$ Carbamazepine

5H-dibenz-[b, f] azepine (I)

Phosgene

Carbamazepine

Ethosuximide

Ethyl cyano-acetate + Butanone $\xrightarrow{\text{Piperidine}}$ $\xrightarrow{\text{NaCN}}$ (I)

Ethyl cyano-acetate

Butanone

(I)

[I] $\xrightarrow{\text{H}_2\text{SO}_4}$ 2-ethyl-2-methyl-succinic acid $\xrightarrow{\text{NH}_3}$ $\xrightarrow{\Delta}$ Ethosuximide

2-ethyl-2-methyl-succinic acid

Ethosuximide

Primidone

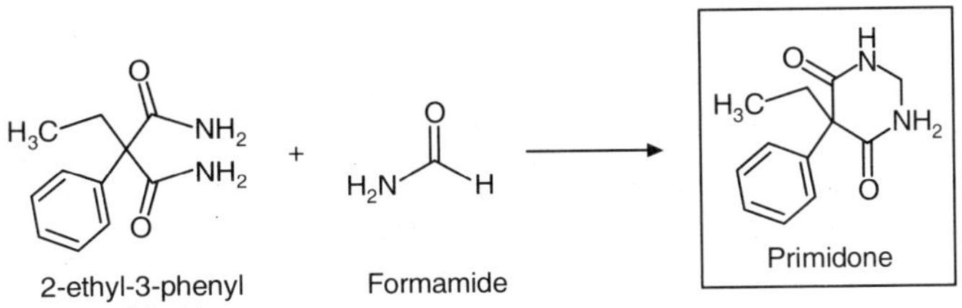

2-ethyl-3-phenyl
succinimide

Formamide

Primidone

Valproic acid

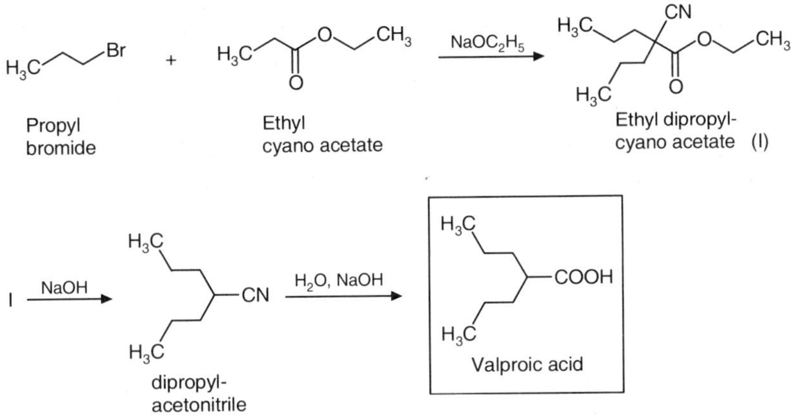

Propyl
bromide

Ethyl
cyano acetate

Ethyl dipropyl-
cyano acetate (I)

dipropyl-
acetonitrile

Valproic acid

Clonazepam

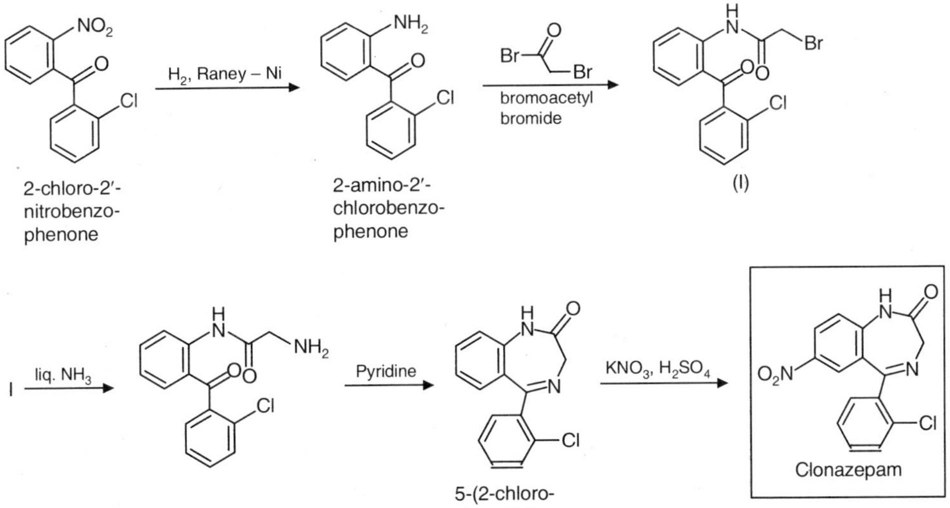

2-chloro-2'-
nitrobenzo-
phenone

2-amino-2'-
chlorobenzo-
phenone

bromoacetyl
bromide

(I)

5-(2-chloro-
phenyl)-2-oxo-
2, 3-dihydro-
1H-1, 4-benzo-
diazepine

Clonazepam

Phensuximide

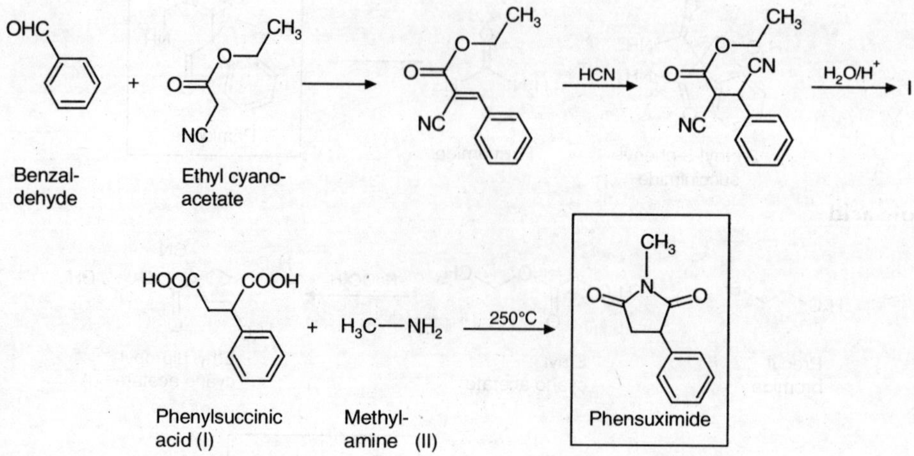
OHC
CH3
O
NC
O
CH3
O
O
NC
HCN
CH3
O
CN
O
NC
H2O/H+
I
Benzal-
dehyde
Ethyl cyano-
acetate
HOOC
COOH
H3C—NH2
250°C
CH3
N
O
O
Phenylsuccinic
acid (I)
Methyl-
amine (II)
Phensuximide

Vigabatrin

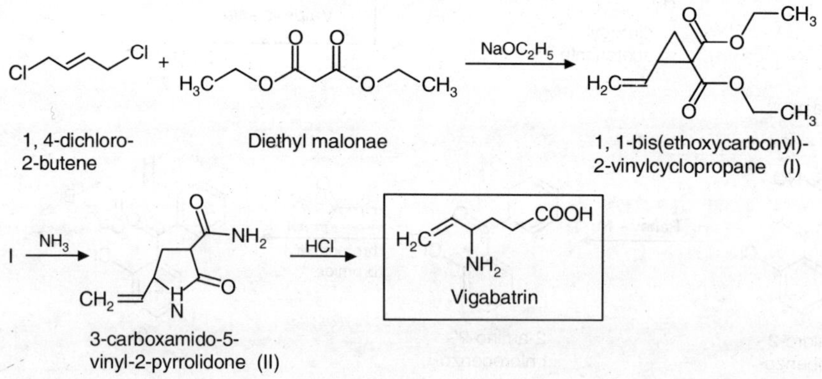
Cl
Cl
O
O
H3C
O
O
CH3
NaOC2H5
O
O
CH3
H2C
O
O
CH3
1, 4-dichloro-
2-butene
Diethyl malonae
1, 1-bis(ethoxycarbonyl)-
2-vinylcyclopropane (I)
I
NH3
O
NH2
CH2
H
N
O
HCl
COOH
H2C
NH2
Vigabatrin
3-carboxamido-5-
vinyl-2-pyrrolidone (II)

Progabide

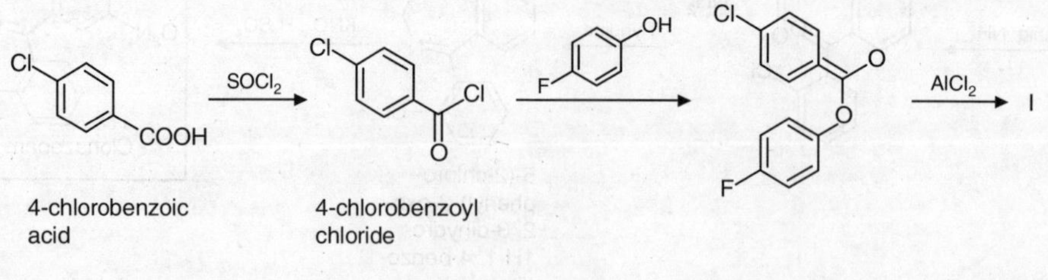
Cl
COOH
SOCl2
Cl
Cl
O
F
OH
Cl
O
O
F
AlCl3
I
4-chlorobenzoic
acid
4-chlorobenzoyl
chloride

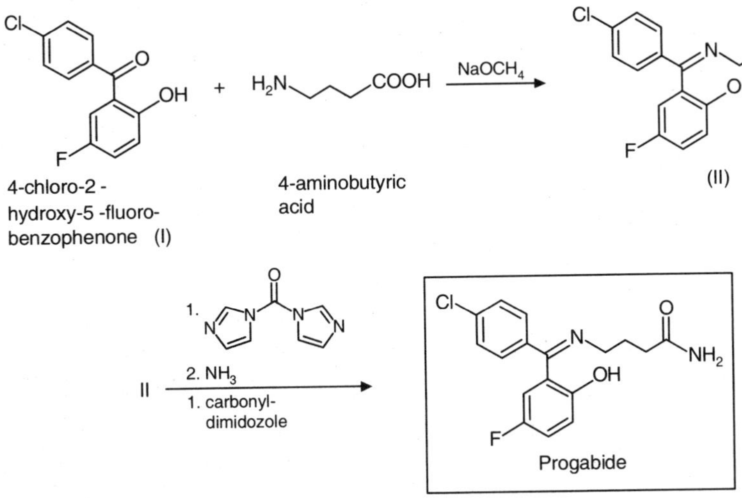
Cl
OH
4-chloro-2 -
hydroxy-5 -fluoro-
benzophenone (I)
H2N
COOH
4-aminobutyric
acid
NaOCH4
(II)
II
1.
2. NH3
1. carbonyl-
dimidozole
NH2
Progabide

Opioid Analgesics

Pain is a designation for a spectrum of sensations of highly divergent character and intensity ranging from unpleasant to intolerable. Pain stimuli are detected by physiological receptors (sensors, nociceptors) least differentiated morphologically, viz. free nerve endings.

- The body of the bipolar afferent first-order neuron lies in a dorsal root ganglion. Nociceptive impulses are conducted via unmyelinated (C-fibers, conduction velocity 0.2-2.0 m/s) and myelinated axons (δ-fibers, 5-30 m/s).

- The free endings of δ fibers respond to intense pressure or heat, those of C-fibers respond to chemical stimuli (H^+, K^+, histamine, bradykinin, etc.) arising from tissue trauma. Irrespective of whether a chemical, mechanical, or thermal stimulus is involved, they become significantly more effective in presence of prostaglandins.

- Chemical stimuli also underlie pain secondary to inflammation or ischemia(angina pectoris, myocardial infarction), or the intense pain that occurs during over distention or spasmodic contraction of smooth muscle abdominal organs, and that may be maintained by local anoxemia developing in the area of spasm (visceral pain).

- A δ and C-fibers enter the spinal cord via the dorsal root, ascend in the dorsolateral funiculus, and then synapse on second-order neurons in the dorsal horn. The axons of the second order neurons cross the midline and ascend to the brain as the anterolateral pathway or spinothalamic tract. Based on phylogenetic age, neo- and paleospinothalamic tracts are distinguished.

- Thalamic nuclei receiving neospinothalamic input project to circumscribed areas of the postcentral gyrus. Stimuli conveyed via this path are experienced as sharp, clearly localizable pain.

- The nuclear regions receiving paleospinothalamic input project to the postcentral gyrus as well as the frontal, limbic cortex and most likely represent the pathway subserving pain of a dull, aching, or burning character, i.e. pain that can be localized only poorly.

- Impulse traffic in the neo- and paleospinothalamic pathways is subject to modulation by descending projections that originate from the reticular formation and terminate at second-order neurons, at their synapses with first-order neurons, or at spinal segmental inter-neurons (descending antinociceptive system). This system can inhibit impulse transmission from first- to second-order neurons via release of opiopeptides (enkephalins) or monoamines (norepinephrine, serotonin).

- Pain sensation can be influenced or modified as follows:

  (a) elimination of the cause of pain lowering of the sensitivity of nociceptors (antipyretic analgesics, local anesthetics)

  (b) interrupting nociceptive conduction in sensory nerves (local anesthetics)

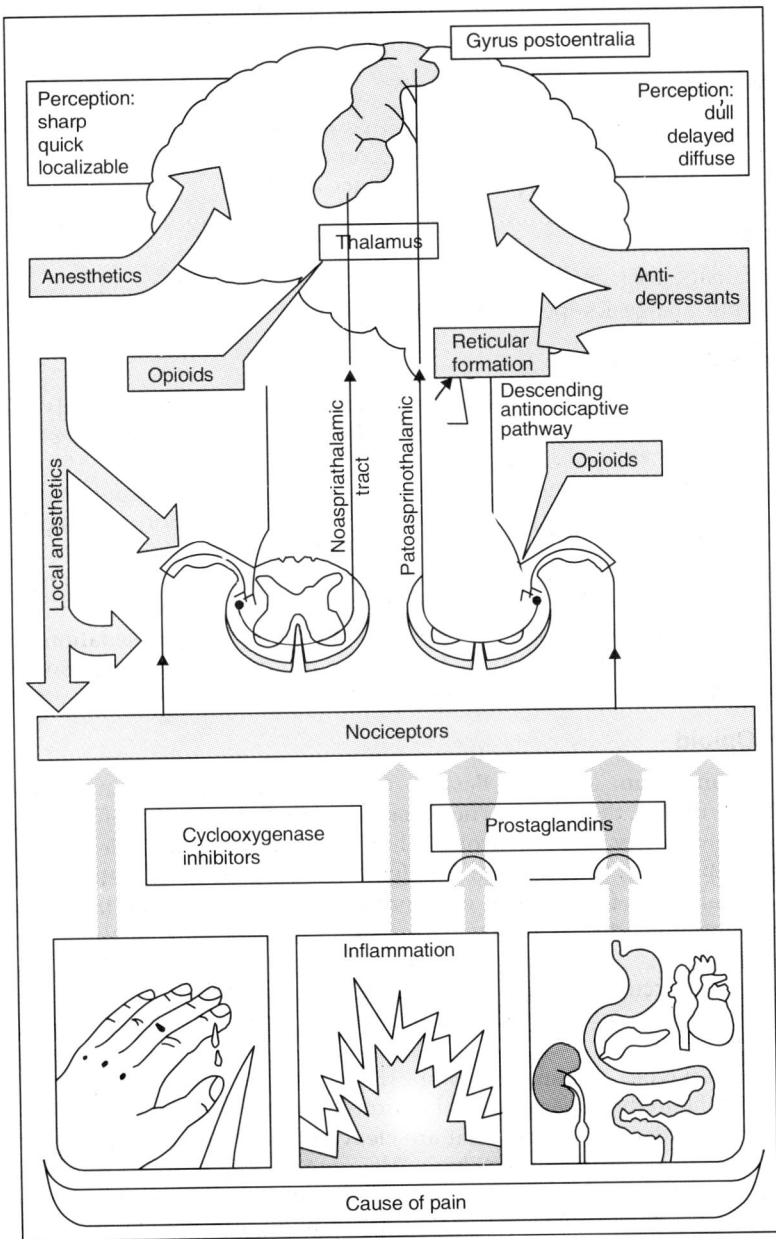

Fig. 21.1: Pain mechanism and pathway

(c) suppression of transmission of nociceptive impulses in the spinal medulla (opioid)

(d) inhibition of pain perception (opioid, general anesthetics)

(e) alter in emotional responses to pain, i.e. pain behavior.

▒ ANALGESICS

Analgesia may be defined as a state of relative insensitivity to pain, where the capacity to tolerate pain is increased without the loss of consciousness. The term 'analgesic' is generally applied to the agents or action required to produce analgesia.

Classification

1. Narcotic analgesics (centrally acting drugs).
2. Non-narcotic analgesics (peripherally acting drugs).

1. Narcotic Analgesics

- Sertuner, in 1805, isolated and discovered the potent analgesic activity of morphine, an alkaloid isolated from the juice of unriped seed capsules of the poppy plant, *Papaver somniferum* (Fig. 21.2).
- The term opioid is used generally to designate collectively the drugs (natural or synthetic) which bind specifically to any of subspecies of receptors of morphine like action. They are often known as the narcotic analgesics due to their ability to produce drug dependence. With the development of many analgesics which are morphine derivatives with little tendency to produce physical dependence, the term narcotic is no longer useful.
- Other actions which are associated with narcotic analgesics are sedation and constipation (useful in the control of diarrhea). In therapeutic doses, morphine sometime produces nausea or vomiting. The related compound, apomorphine is a powerful emetic agent.

Sources of Opioid

- *Morphine* is an opium alkaloid. Besides morphine, opium contains alkaloids devoid of analgesic activity, e.g. the spasmolytic papaverine, that are also classified as opium alkaloids.
- All semisynthetic derivatives (hydromorphone) and fully synthetic derivatives (pentazocine, pethidine, meperidine, l-methadone, and fentanyl) are collectively referred as *opioids*.
- The high analgesic effectiveness of xenobiotic opioids derives from their affinity for receptors normally acted upon by endogenous opioids (enkephalins, β-endorphin, and dynorphins).
- Opioid receptors occur in nerve cells. They are found in various brain regions and the spinal medulla, as well as in intramural nerve plexuses that regulate the motility of the alimentary and urogenital tracts.
- There are several types of opioid receptors, designated μ, δ, κ that mediate the various opioid effects; all belong to the super family of G-protein-coupled receptors.
- Endogenous opioids are peptides that are cleaved from the precursors proenkephalin, pro-opiomelanocortin, and prodynorphin. All contain the amino acid sequence of the pentapeptides [Met]- or [Leu]-enkephalin. The effects of the opioid can be abolished by antagonists (e.g. naloxone; A), with the exception of buprenorphine.

Mode of Action of Opioids (Fig. 21.3)

- Most neurons react to opioids with hyperpolarization, reflecting an increase in K^+ conductance. Ca^{2+} influx into nerve terminals during excitation is decreased, leading to a decreased release of excitatory transmitters and decreased synaptic activity.

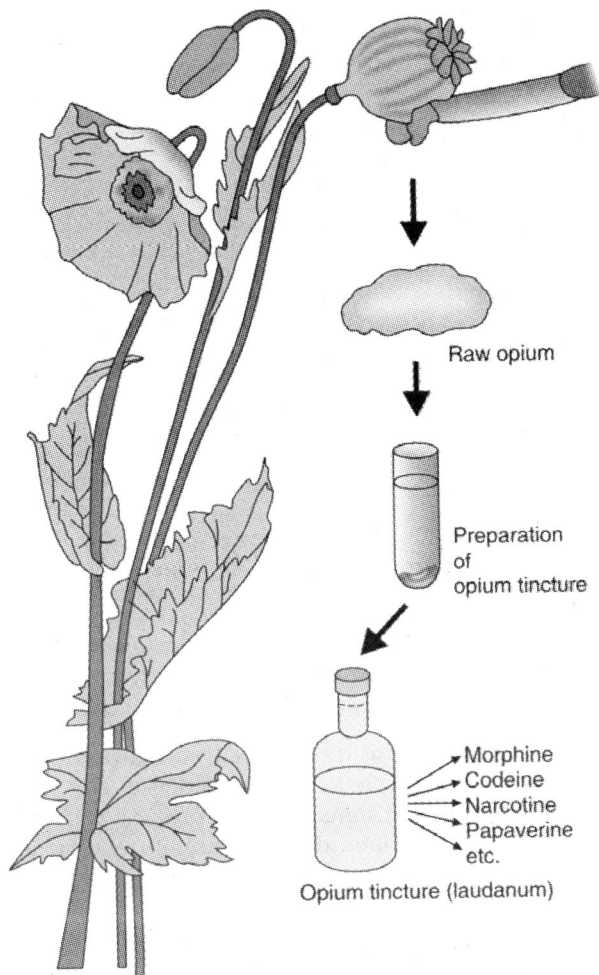

Raw opium

Preparation
of
opium tincture

Morphine
Codeine
Narcotine
Papaverine
etc.

Opium tincture (laudanum)

Fig. 21.2: Papaver somniferum

- Depending on the cell population affected; this synaptic inhibition translates into a depressant or excitant effect.

Effects of Opioids (Fig. 21.4)

- The analgesic effect results from actions at the level of the spinal cord (inhibition of nociceptive impulse transmission) and the brain (attenuation of impulse spread, inhibition of pain perception).
- Attention and ability to concentrate are impaired. There is a mood change, the direction of which depends on the initial condition.
- Beside from the relief associated with the abatement of strong pain, there is a feeling of detachment (floating sensation) and sense of well-being (euphoria), particularly after intravenous injection and, hence, rapid buildup of drug levels in the brain.

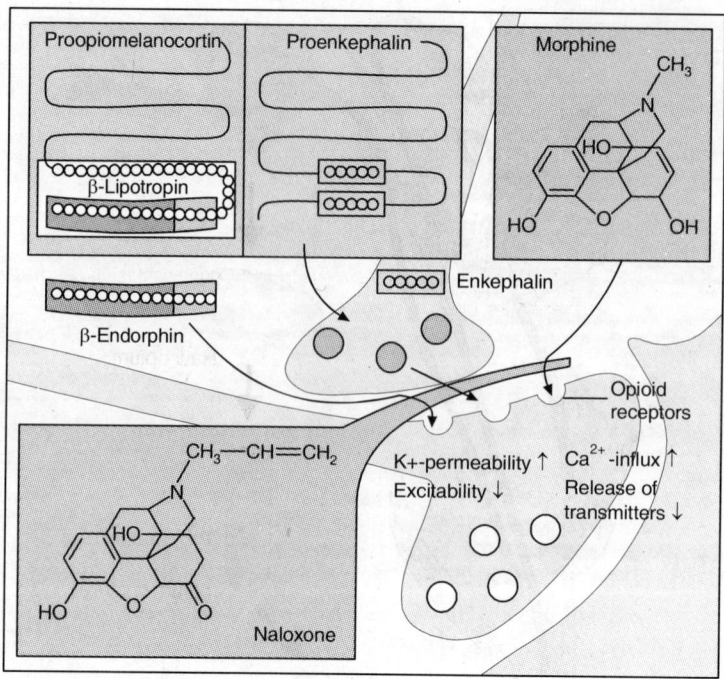

Fig. 21.3: Mode of action of morphine and others

- The desire to re-experience this state by renewed administration of drug may become overpowering— development of psychological dependence. The atttempt to quit repeated use of the drug results in withdrawal signs of both a physical (cardiovascular disturbances) and psychological (restlessness, anxiety, depression) nature. Opioids meet the criteria of 'addictive' agents, namely, psychological and physiological dependence as well as a compulsion to increase the dose.

- For these reasons, prescription of opioids is subject to special rules. Regulations specify, among other things, maximum dosage (permissible single dose, daily maximal dose, and maximal amount per single prescription). Prescriptions need to be issued on special forms the completion of which is rigorously monitored. Certain opioid analgesics, such as codeine and tramadol, may be prescribed in the usual manner, because of their lesser potential for abuse and development of dependence.

Metabolism (Fig. 21.5)

- Like other opioids bearing a hydroxyl group, morphine is conjugated to glucuronic acid and eliminated renally.

- Glucuronidation of the OH-group at position 6, unlike that at position 3, does not affect affinity.

- The extent to which the 6-glucuronide contributes to the analgesic action remains uncertain at present. At any rate, the activity of this polar metabolite needs to be taken into account in renal insufficiency (lower dosage or longer dosing interval).

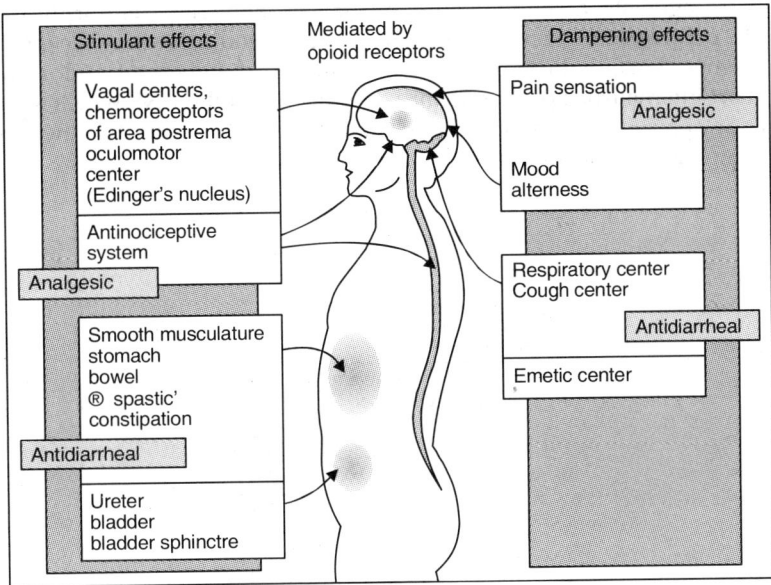

Fig. 21.4: Pharmacological effect of morphine

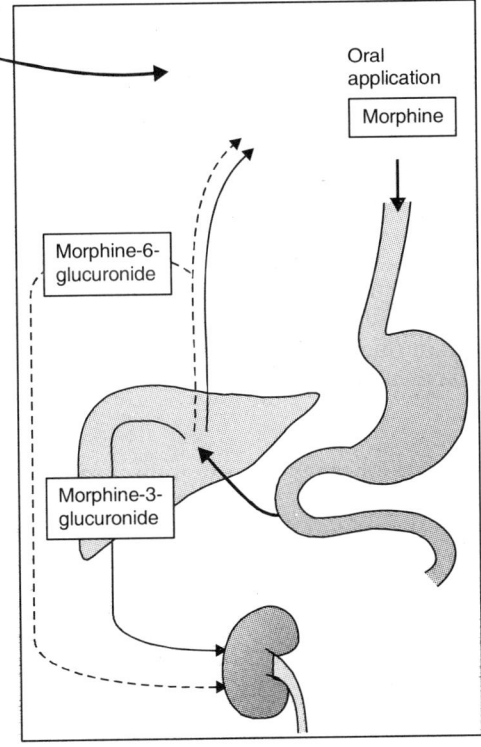

Fig. 21.5: Metabolism of morphine

- Opioids act as agonists of endogenous substances known as endorphins (a group of morphine like peptides), interacting with stereospecific binding sites or receptors in the brain and other tissues. Enkephalins represent the simplest members of endorphins. They are located in short interneurons predominantly in the areas of the CNS which are related to the perception of pain, movement, mood and behavior and to the regulation of neuroendocrinological functions.

```
┌─────────────────┐
│ Opioid analgesics │
└─────────────────┘
          │
          ▼
   ┌──────────────────┐
   │ Morphine and     │
   │ related opioids  │
   └──────────────────┘
      ┌──────────────────┐
      │ Meperidine and   │
      │ congener         │
      └──────────────────┘
         ┌──────────────────┐
         │ Methadone and    │
         │ congener         │
         └──────────────────┘
            ┌────────────────────┐
            │ Opioid receptor    │
            │ antagonist and     │
            │ partial antagonist │
            └────────────────────┘
```

- Opioid-mediated inhibition of transmitter release in various mammalian cells has been reported to involve either a reduction in the influx of Ca^{2+} through activation of κ-receptors or an increased outward K^+ conductance through Ca^{2+} activated K^+ channels following activation of either μ or σ receptors. The inflow of potassium ions hyperpolarizes the membrane potential. This results in decrease in neuron excitability.
- Opioids have been shown to inhibit either basal or neurotransmitter stimulated increase in adenyl cyclase activity in several areas of the mammalian CNS. The mechanism for opioid inhibition of adenylate cyclase appears to involve stimulation of a high affinity membrane associated GIPase, reflecting an activation of the guanine nucleotide regulatory binding protein G.
- Thus under the influence of enkephalin, presynaptic terminals fail to release neurotransmitter in the synaptic cleft and pain impulse is not received by post-synaptic neuron. The opioid mediated fall in cyclic AMP levels also contributes to produce analgesia.
- It is assumed that all opioid (morphine like drugs) produce their effects by mimicking the action of endogenous enkephalins.

Opioid Receptors

- Although it has been assumed for many years that there are analgesic receptors, information about them has only been gained relatively recently (1973).
- The present knowledge on the subject is that there are at least four different receptors with which morphine can interact, three of which are analgesic receptors.
- The initial theory on receptor binding assumed a single receptor site, but this does not invalidate many of the proposals which were made. Therefore, it is informative to look at the just theory—the Beckett-Casy hypothesis.

Beckett-Casy hypothesis (Fig. 21.6)

- In this theory, it is assumed that there is a rigid receptor site and in that morphine and its analogues fit in a classic lock-and-key analogy.

- Based on the results already described, the following features were proposed as being essential, if an analgesic is to interact with its receptor.
- There must be a basic centre (nitrogen) which can be ionized at physiological pH to form a positively charged group. This group then forms an ionic bond with a comparable anionic group in the receptor. As a consequence of this, analgesics have to have a pKa of 7.8-8.9 such that there is an approximately equal chance of the amine being ionized or un-ionized at physiological pH. This is necessary since the analgesic has to cross the blood-brain barrier as the free base, but once cross has to be ionized in order to interact with the receptor.

Morphine and Related Opioids

Phenanthrenes

Morphine   Codeine   Heroine

Nalorphine   Dihydrocodeine   Hydromorphone   Oxymorphone

Hydrocodone   Naloxone   Naltrexone   Oxycodone

Benzylisoquinolines

Papaverine   Noscapine

1. The pKa values of useful analgesics all match this prediction.

2. The aromatic ring in morphine has to be properly orientated with respect to the nitrogen atom to allow a van der Waals interaction with a suitable hydrophobic location on the receptor. The nature of this interaction suggests that there has to be a close spatial relationship between the aromatic ring and the surface of the receptor.

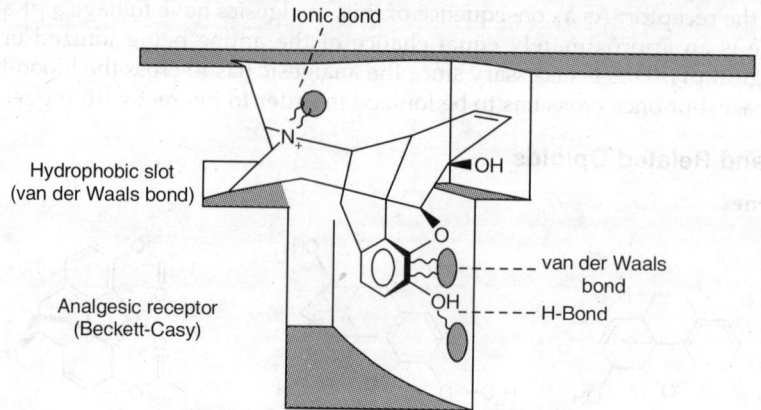

Fig. 21.6: Beckett-Casy hypothesis

3. The phenol group is probably hydrogen-bonded to a suitable residue at the receptor site.
4. There might be a (hole just large enough for the ethylene bridge of carbons 15 and 16 to fit. Such a fit would help to align the molecule end enhance the overall fit.

- This was the theory proposed and sated in well with the majority of results.
- There can be no doubt that the aromatic ring, phenol, and the nitrogen groups are all important, but there is some doubt as to whether the ethylene bridge is important, since there are several analgesics which lack it (e.g. fentanyl).
- The theory also fails to include the extra binding site which was discovered by drug extension. This fact can easily be sated into the theory, but other anomalies exist which have already been discussed (e.g. the different results obtained for meperidine compared to morphine when a substituent such as the allyl group is attached to nitrogen).
- Another anomaly was described earlier where the pethidine analogue containing a cinnamic acid residue is 30 times more active than pyridine itself, whereas the same group on morphine eliminates activity. Such results strongly suggest that a simple one-receptor theory is not applicable.

Multiple Analgesic Receptors

- The previous theory tried to explain analgesic results based on a single analgesic receptor. It is now known that there are several different analgesic receptors which are associated with different types of side effects. It is also known that several analgesics show preference for some of these receptors over others. This helps to explain the anomalies resulting from the previous Beckett-Casy hypothesis.
- It is important to appreciate that the main points of the original theory still apply for each of the analgesic receptors now to be described. The important binding groups for each receptor are the phenol, the aromatic ring, and the ionized nitrogen centre.
- However, there are subtle differences between each receptor which can distinguish between finer details of different analgesic molecules. As a result, same analgesics show preference for one analgesic receptor over another or interact in different ways.

- There are three analgesic receptors to which the morphine molecule itself can bind and switch on. These receptors have been tabbed with Greek letters.

1. The Mu (µ) Receptor

- Morphine binds strongly to this receptor and produces analgesia. Receptor binding also leads to the undesired side effects of respiratory depression, euphoria, and addiction.
- We can now see why it is so difficult to remove the side effects of morphine and its analogues, since the receptor with which they bind most strongly is also inherently involved with these side effects.

Mechanism

- As shown in Fig. 21.7 morphine binds to mu receptor induces a change in shape. This change in conformation opens up an ion channel in the cell membrane and as a result, potassium ions can now out of the cell. This now hyperpolarizes the membrane potential and makes it more difficult for an active potential to be reached.
- Therefore, the frequency of action potential is decreased, which results in a decrease in neuron excitability.

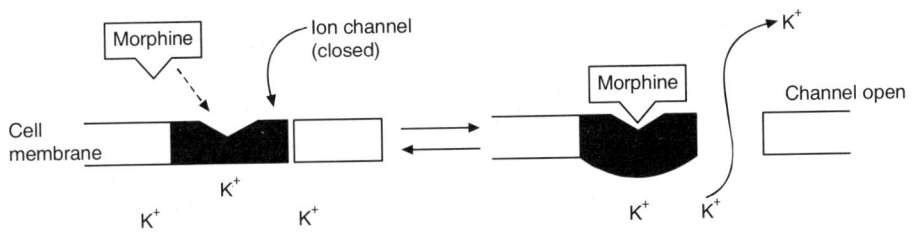

Fig. 21.7: Morphine binding to µ receptor

- This increase in potassium permeability has an indirect effect, since it also decreases the input of calcium ions into the nerve terminal and this in turn reduces neurotransmitter release. Both effects, therefore, shut down' the nerve and block the pain messages.
- Unfortunately, this receptor is also associated with the hazardous side effects of narcotic analgesics. There is still a search to see if there are possibly two slightly different mu receptors, one which is solely due to analgesia and one responsible for the side effects.

2. The Kappa (κ) Receptor

- This is a different analgesic receptor to which morphine can bind and activate. However, the strength of binding is less than to the µ receptor. The biological response is analgesia with sedation and none of the hazardous side effects. It is this receptor which provides the best hope for the ultimate safe analgesic.
- The earlier results obtained from nalorphine, pentazocine, and buprenorphine can now be explained. Nalorphine acts as an antagonist at the µ receptor, thus blocking morphine from acting there.
- However, it acts as a weak agonist at the κ receptor (as does morphine) and so the slight analgesia observed with nalorphine is due to the partial activation of the κ receptor. Unfortunately, nalorphine has hallucinogenic side effects. This is caused by nalorphine also binding to a completely different, non-analgesic receptor in the brain called the sigma (σ) receptor where it acts as an agonist.

- Pentazocine interacts with the μ and κ receptors in the same way, but is able to switch on' the κ receptor more strongly. It too suffers the drawback that it switches on' the σ receptor. Buprenorphine is slightly different.
- It binds strongly to all three analgesic receptors and act as an antagonist at the Δ (see below) and κ receptors, but acts as a partial agonist at the μ receptor to produce its analgesic effect. This might suggest that buprenorphine should suffer the same side effects as morphine. The fact that it does not related in same way to the rate at which buprenorphine interacts with the receptor. It is slow to bind, but once it has bound, it is slow to leave.

Mechanism

- The κ receptor is directly associated with a calcium channel. When an agonist binds to the κ receptor, the receptor changes conformation and the calcium channel (normally open when the nerve is bring and passing on pain messages) is closed. Calcium is required for the production of the nerves neurotransmitters and therefore the nerve is shut down and cannot pass on pain messages (Fig. 21.8).

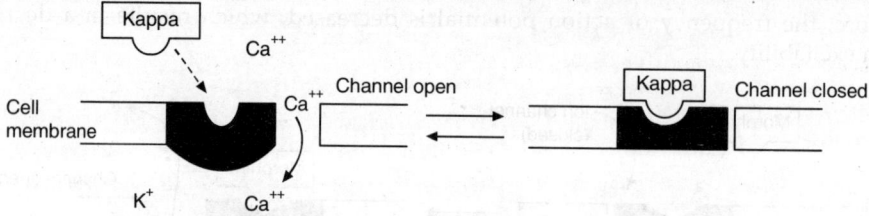

Fig. 21.8: The association of κ receptor with calcium channel

- The nerves affected by the κ mechanism are those related to pain induced by non- thermal stimuli. This is not the case with the μ receptor where all pain messages are inhibited. This suggests a different distribution of κ receptors from μ receptors.

3. The Delta (Δ) Receptor

- The Δ receptor is the brain's natural pain killers (the enkephalins) interact. Morphine can also bind quite strongly to this receptor.
- Table 21.1 shows the relative activities of morphine, nalorphine, pentazocine, enkephalins, pethidine, and naloxone. A minus sign indicates the compound is acting as an agonist. A minus sign means it ants as an antagonist. A zero sign means there is no activity or minor activity.

Table 21.1. Relative activities of morphine, nalorphine, pentazocine, enkephalins, pethidine and naloxone

		Morphine	Nalorphine	Pentazocine	Enkephalins	Pethidine	Naloxone
Mu	Analgesia respiratory depression euphoria addiction	+ + +	–	–	+	+ + +	– – –
Kappa	Analgesia	+	+	+	+	+	–
Sigma	Psychotomimetic	0	+	+ +	0	0	0
Delta	Analgesia	+ +	–	–	+ + +	+	–

+, Compounds acting as agonists; –, as antagonists. 0, No activity or minor activity.

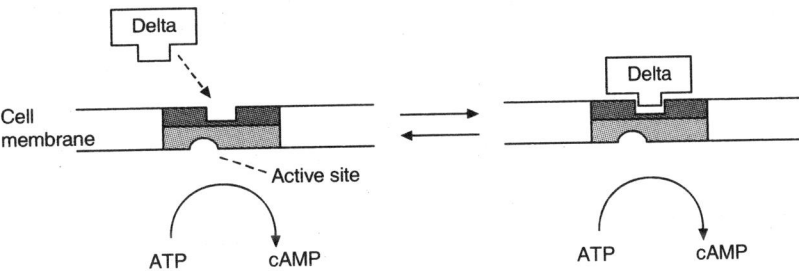

Nalbuphine
(same activity as morphine)
Low addiction liability
No psychotomimetic activity
Not orally active

Butorphanol
(not orally active)

Fig. 21.9: Relative activities of analgesic

- There is now a search going on for orally active opiate structures which can act as antagonists at the receptor, agonists at the κ receptor, and have no activity at the or receptor. Same success has been obtained, especially with the compounds shown in Fig. 21.9, but even these compounds still suffer from certain side effects, or lack the desired oral activity.

Mechanism

- Like the μ receptor, the nerves containing the Δ receptor do not discriminate between pain from different sources.
- In this case, there are no ion channels involved. The substrate molecule binds to the Δ receptor and, in some way, the message is transmitted through the cell.

Fig. 21.10: The delta receptor

- Membrane to a second membrane bound protein. This protein then acts as an enzyme for the formation of cyclic AMP. Normally, the active site is open when the nerve is receiving pain message, such that cyclic AMP acts as a secondary messenger and passes on the pain messages.

- However, when the Δ receptor is activated it probably changes shape and as a result leads to a change in the shape of the cyclase enzyme to close down the active site by which it can make cyclic AMP.

cAMP

The Sigma (σ) Receptor

- This receptor is not an analgesic receptor, but we have seen that it can be activated by certain opiate molecules such as nalorphine. When activated, it produces hallucinogenic effects.

- The σ receptor may be the one associated with the hallucinogenic and psychotomimetic effects of phencyclidine (PCP), otherwise known as angel dust.

The phencyclidine or angel dust

Structure–Activity Relationship

- The story of how morphine's secrets were uncovered is presented here in a logical step-by-step fashion. However, in reality this was not how the problem was tackled at the time. Different compounds were made in a random fashion depending on the ease of synthesis, and the logical pattern followed on from the results obtained.
- By presenting the development of morphine in the following manner, we are distorting history, but we do get a better idea of the general strategies and the logical approach to drug development as a whole.
- The easiest morphine analogues which can be made are those involving peripheral medications of the molecule (that is, changes which do not affect the basic skeleton of the molecule). In this approach, we are looking at the different functional groups and discovering whether they needed or not.
- We now look at each of these functional groups in turn.

The phenolic OH

- Codeine is the methyl ether of morphine and is also present in opium. It is used for treating moderate pain, coughs, and diarrhea.
- By methylating the phenolic OH, the analgesic activity drops drastically and codeine is only 0.1% as active as morphine. This drop in activity is observed in other analogues containing a masked phenolic group. Clearly, a free phenolic group is crucial for analgesic activity.

R = Me	CODEINE	Analgesic
R = Et	ETHYLMORPHINE	Activity
R = Acetyl	3-ACETYLMORPHINE	

- However, the above result refers to isolated receptors in laboratory experiments. If codeine is administered to patients, its analgesic effect is 20% that of morphine—much better than expected. Why is this so?
- The answer lies in the fact that codeine can be metabolized in the liver to give morphine. The methyl ether is removed to give the free phenolic group. Thus, codeine can be viewed as a prodrug for morphine. Further evidence supporting this is provided by the fact that codeine has no analgesic effect at all if it is injected directly into the brain. By doing this, codeine is injected directly into the CNS and does not pass through the liver. As a result, demethylation does not take place.
- In all the following examples, the test procedures were carried out on animals or humans and so it must be remembered that there are several possible ways in which a change of activity could have resulted.

The 6-Alcohol

- The results show that masking or the complete loss of the alcohol group does not decrease analgesic activity and, in fact, often has the opposite effect. Again, it has to be emphasized that the testing of analgesics has generally been done in vivo and that there are many ways in which improved activity can be achieved.

- In these examples, the improvement in activity is due to the pharmacodynamic properties of these drugs rather than their activity for the analgesic receptor. In other words, it rejects how much of the drug can reach the receptor rather than how well it binds to it.

- There are a number of factors which can be responsible for affecting how much of a drug reaches its target. For example, the active compound might be metabolized to an inactive compound before it reaches the receptor. Alternatively, it might be distributed more efficiently to one part of the body than another.

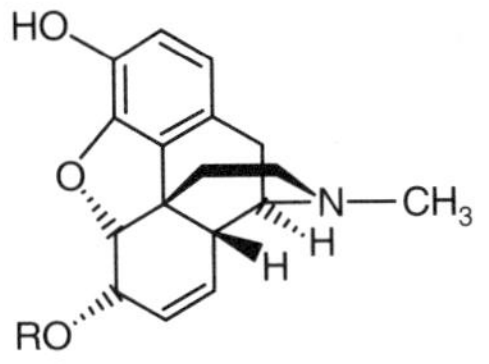

R	Analgesia with respect to morphine	
Me	Heterocodeine	5x
Et	6-Ethylmorphine	greater
Acetyl	6-Acetylmorphine	4x

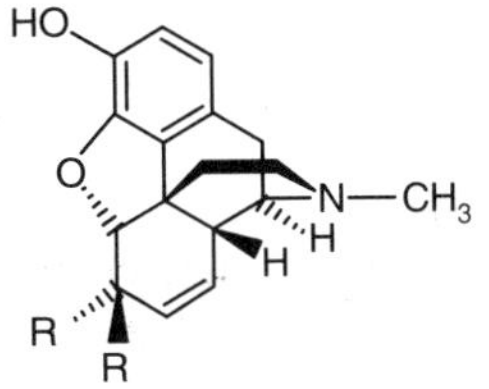

R	R	Analgesia with respect to morphine
H	OH	Increased
H	H	or
Ketone	Ketone	similar

Fig. 21.11: Effect of loss of alcohol group on analgesic activity

- In this case, the morphine analogues shown (Fig. 21.11) are able to reach the analgesic receptor far more efficiently than morphine itself. This is because the analgesic receptors are located in the brain and in order to reach the brain, the drugs have to cross a barrier called the blood-brain barrier. The capillaries which supply the brain are lined by a series of fatty membranes which overlap more closely than in any other part of the body. In order to enter the brain, drugs have to negotiate this barrier. Since the barrier is fatty, highly polar compounds are prevented from crossing. Thus, the more polar groups a molecule has, the more difficulty in reaching the brain. Morphine has three polar groups (phenol, alcohol, and an amine), whereas the analogues above have either lost the polar alcohol group or have it masked by an alkyl or acyl group.

- Therefore, they enter the brain more easily and accumulate at the receptor sites in greater concentrations; hence, the better analgesic activity.

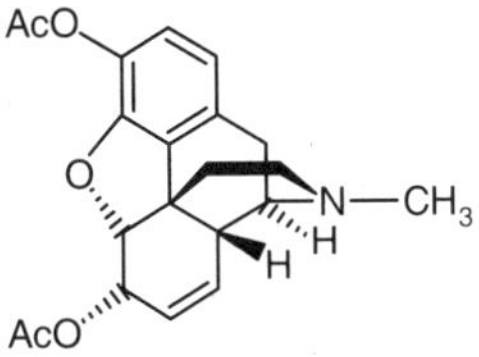

Diamorphine

- It is interesting to compare the activities of morphine, 6-acetylmorphine, and diamorphine (heroin). The most active (and the most dangerous) compound of the three is 6-acetylmorphine. It is four times more active than morphine.

- Heroin is also more active than morphine by a factor of two, but less active than 6-acetyl morphine. How do we explain this? 6-acetylmorphine, as we have seen already, is less polar than morphine and will enter the brain more quickly and in greater concentrations. The phenolic group is free and therefore it will interact immediately with the analgesic receptors.

- Heroin has two polar groups which are masked and is therefore the most efficient compound of the three to cross the blood-brain barrier.

- However, before it can act at the receptor, the acetyl group on the phenolic group has to be removed by esterases in the brain. Therefore, it is more powerful than morphine because it enters the brain more easily, but it is less powerful than 6-acetylmorphine because the dactyl group has to be removed before it can act.

- Heroin and 6-acetylmorphine are both more potent analgesics than morphine. Unfortunately; they also have greater side-effects and have severe tolerance and dependence characteristics. Heroin is still used to treat terminally ill patients, such as that dying of cancer, but 6-acetylmorphine is so dangerous that its synthesis is banned in many countries.
- To conclude, the hydroxyl group is not required for analgesic activity and its removal can be beneficial to analgesic activity.

The double bond at 7-8

- Several analogues including dihydromorphine have shown that the double bond is not necessary for analgesic activity.

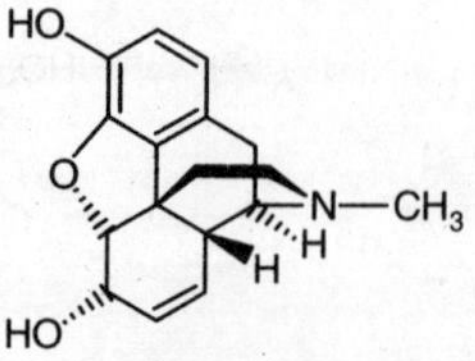

Dihydromorphine

The N-methyl Group

- The N-oxide and the N-methyl quaternary salts of morphine are both inactive, which might suggest that the introduction of charge destroys analgesic activity.
- However, we have to remember that these experiments were done on animals and it is hardly surprising that no analgesia is observed, since a charged molecule has very little chance of crossing the blood-brain barrier (Figure 21.12).

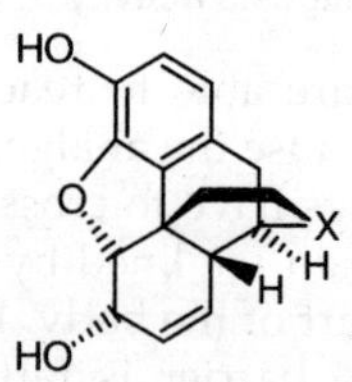

X		Analgesic activity with respect to morphine
NH	Normorphine	25%
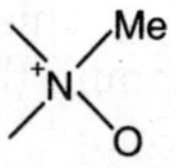 +N with Me, O	N-Oxide	0%
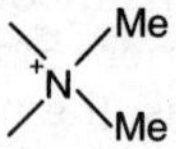 +N with Me, Me	Quaternary salt	0%

Fig. 21.12: Effect of introduction of charge group on analgesic activity

- If these same compounds are injected directly into the brain, a totally different result is obtained and both these compounds are found to have similar analgesic activity to morphine. This fact, allied with the fact that neither compound can lose its charge, shows that the nitrogen atom of morphine is ionized when it binds to the receptor.
- The replacement of the N-methyl group with a proton reduces activity but does not eliminate it. The secondary NH group is more polar than the tertiary N-methyl group and therefore it is more difficult to cross the blood-brain barrier, leading to a drop in activity. The fact that significant activity is retained despite this shows that the methyl substituent is not essential to activity.
- However, the nitrogen itself is crucial. If it is removed completely, all analgesic activity is lost. To conclude, the nitrogen atom is essential to analgesic activity and interacts with the analgesic receptor in the ionized form.

The aromatic ring

The aromatic ring is essential. Compounds lacking it show no analgesic activity.

The ether bridge

As we shall see later, the ether bridge is not required for analgesic activity. If we summarize the SAR, we can say that:

1. Masking the phenolic 3-OH group by etherification to methyl ether (codeine) and ethyl ether (ethyl morphine) results in about one-tenth the analgesic activity of morphine. The phenolic OH may augment through hydrogen bonding the binding of the opiate pharmacophore to its receptor binding site. The ethers are not easily hydrolysed to OH group.

2. Esterification of 3-OH group gives compound more active than morphine.

3. Blockade of the alcoholic 6-OH by acetylation on its conversion to carbonyl function, gives compounds several times more active. Inversion of 6-OH group and its removal altogether gave compound with enhanced analgesic potency.

4. Introduction of 14-OH substituent gave compounds several times more potent as analgesics as compared to parent drugs.

5. Replacement of N-CH$_3$ by -N-C$_2$H$_5$ resulted in only a slight fall in analgesic response. More hydrophobic group such as propyl, pentyl, hexyl and phenylethyl gave an increase in activity. N-allyl morphine has powerful antagonist activity.

6. Breaking of the ether bridge and opening of piperidine ring cause decrease in activity.

7. Hydrogenation of the C7-C8 double bond produces compounds with equal or superior analgesic action.

8. Substitution other than 3 position in the aromatic ring results in reduction of opioid actions.

Stereochemistry

- At this stage, it is worth making same observations on stereochemistry. Morphine is an asymmetric molecule containing several chiral centers, and exists naturally as a single enantiomer.

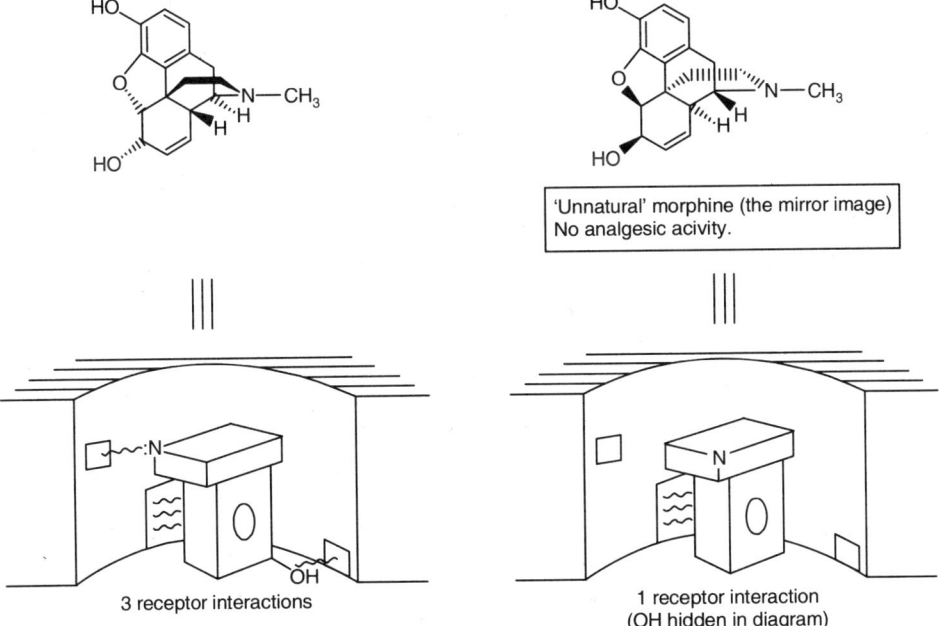

'Unnatural' morphine (the mirror image)
No analgesic acivity.

3 receptor interactions

1 receptor interaction
(OH hidden in diagram)

Fig. 21.13: Morphine and unnatural morphine

- When morphine was east synthesized, it was made as a racemic mixture of the naturally occurring enantiomer plus its mirror image. These were separated and the unnatural mirror image was tested for analgesic activity. It turned out to have no activity whatsoever.
- This is not particularly surprising If' we consider the interactions which must take place between morphine and its receptor. We have identifier that there are at least three important interactions involving the phenol, the aromatic ring and the amine on morphine.
- Let us consider a diagrammatic representation of morphine as a T-shaped block with the three groups marked as shown in Fig. 21.13. The receptor has complementary binding groups placed in such a way that they can interact with all three groups. If we now consider the mirror image of morphine, then we can see that it can interact with only one binding site at any one time.
- Epimerization of a single chiral center (Fig. 21.14) such as the composition is not beneficial either, since changing the stereochemistry at even one chiral centre can result in a drastic change of shape, making it impossible for the molecule to bind to the analgesic receptors.

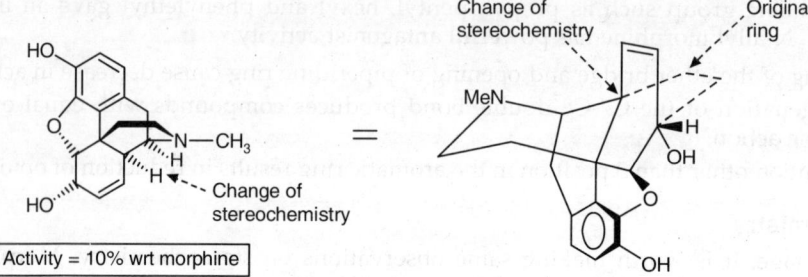

Fig. 21.14: Epimerization of a single chiral center

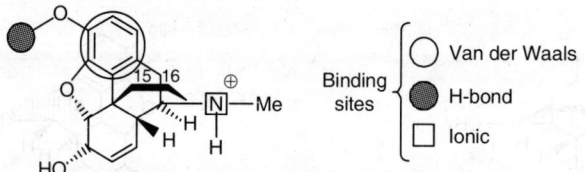

Fig. 21.15: Important functional group essential for analgesic activity

DEVELOPMENT OF MORPHINE ANALOGUE

We now move on to consider the development of morphine analogues. As mentioned, there are several strategies used in drug development. We shall consider the following strategies in the development of morphine analogues.

Variation of Substituents (Fig. 21.15)

- A series of alkyl chains on the phenolic group give compounds which are inactive or poorly active. We have already idea that the phenol group must be free for analgesic activity.
- The removal of the N-methyl group to give nor-morphine allows a series of alkyl chains to be built on the basic center.

Drug Extension (Fig. 21.16)

- Drug extension is a strategy by which the molecule is extended by the addition of extra abiding groups'. The reasoning behind such a tactic is to probe for further binding sites which might be available on the receptor surface and which might improve the interaction between the drug and the receptor.

- This is a reasonable assumption since it is highly unlikely that a compound such as morphine (which is produced in a plant) would be the perfect binding substrate for a receptor in the human brain.

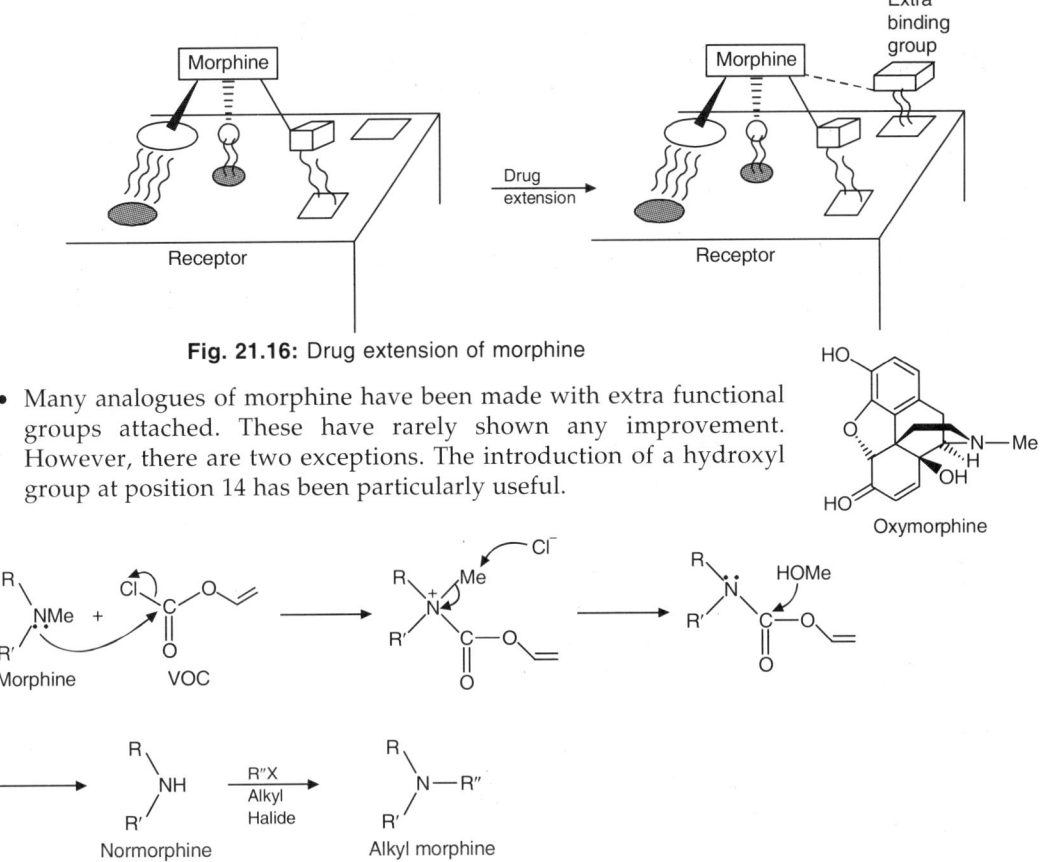

Fig. 21.16: Drug extension of morphine

- Many analogues of morphine have been made with extra functional groups attached. These have rarely shown any improvement. However, there are two exceptions. The introduction of a hydroxyl group at position 14 has been particularly useful.

Oxymorphine

Fig. 21.17: Demethylation and alkylation of the basic center

- This might be taken to suggest that there is a possible hydrogen bond interaction taking place between the 14-OH group and a stable amino acid residue on the receptor. The easiest position to add substituents (and the most advantageous) has been the nitrogen atom. The synthesis is easily achieved by removing the N-methyl group from morphine to give normorphine, then alkylating the amino group with an alkyl halide (Fig. 21.17).

R =	Me	Et	Pr	Bu	Amyl, Hexyl	CH₂CH₂Ph
	Agonism decreases Antagonism increases			Zero activity	Agonists	14 x activity with respect to morphine

Fig. 21.18: Change in activity with respect to alkyl group size

- Degradation with cyanogen bromide, but is now more conveniently carried out using a chloroforming reagent such as vinyloxycarbonyl chloride. The alkylation step can sometimes be replaced by a two-step process involving an actuation to give an amide, followed by reduction.

- The results obtained from the alkylation studies are quite dramatic. As the alkyl group is increased in size from a methyl to a butyl group, the activity drops to zero. However, with a larger group such as an amyl or a hexyl group, activity recovers slightly (Fig. 21.18).

- None of this is particularly exciting, but when a phenethyl group is attached the activity increases 14 fold—a strong indication that a hydrophobic binding site has been located which interacts favorably with the new aromatic ring.

- To conclude, the size and nature of the group on the nitrogen is important to the activity spectrum. Drug extension can lead to better binding by making use of additional binding interaction (Fig. 21.19).

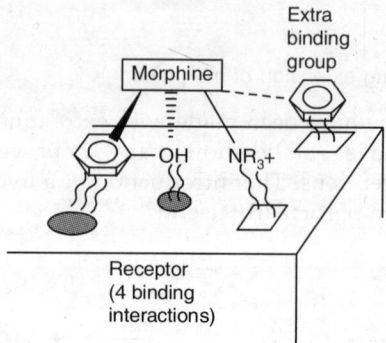

Fig. 21.19: Indication of fourth binding site

- Before leaving this subject, it is worth describing another series of important results arising from substituents on the nitrogen atom. Spectacular results were obtained when an allyl group or a cyclopropyl methylene group were attached. No increase in analgesic activity was observed.

- Naloxone, for example, has no analgesic activity at all, whilst nalorphine retains only weak analgesic activity. However, the important feature about these molecules is that they act as antagonists to morphine.

- They do this by binding to the analgesic receptors without switching them on'. Once they have bound to the receptors, they block morphine from binding. As a result, morphine can no longer act as an analgesic. One might be hard pushed to see an advantage in this and with good reason. If we are just considering analgesia, there is none.

- However, the fact that morphine is blocked from all its receptors means that none of its side effects are produced either, and the blocking of these effects which make antagonists extremely useful.

$$R = \quad -CH_2-CH{=}CH_2 \quad -CH_2-\triangleleft$$

Allyl

Antagonists

HO   HO

Nalorphine   Naloxone

- In particular, accident victims have sometimes been given an overdose of morphine. If this is not treated, then the casualty may die of suffocation. By administering nalorphine, the antagonist displaces morphine from the receptor and binds more strongly, thus preventing morphine from continuing its action.
- There is, however, a far more important observation arising from the biological results of these antagonists. For many years, chemists had been trying to synthesize a morphine analogue with analgesic properties, but without the depressant effects on breathing, or the withdrawal symptoms. There had been so little success that many workers believed that the two properties were directly related, perhaps through the same receptor. The fact that the antagonist naloxone blocked morphine analgesia and side effects at the same time did nothing to change that view.
- However, the properties of nalorphine offered a glimmer of hope. Nalorphine is a strong antagonist and blocks morphine from its receptors. Therefore, no analgesic activity should be observed. However, a very weak analgesic activity is observed and what is more, this analgesia appears to be free of the undesired side effects. This was the first sign that a non-addictive, safe analgesic might be possible.
- But how can this be? How can a compound be an antagonist of morphine but also act as an agonist and produce analgesia? If it is acting as an agonist, why is the activity so weak and why is it free of the side effects? As we shall see later, there is not one single type of analgesic receptor, but several. Multiple receptors are common.
- In the same way, there are at least three types of analgesic receptor. The differences between them are slight such that morphine cannot distinguish between them and activates them all, but in theory it should be possible to add compounds which would be selective for one type of analgesic receptor over another. However, this is not the way that nalorphine works.
- Nalorphine binds to all three types of analgesic receptor and therefore blocks morphine from all three. Nalorphine itself is unable to switch on two of the receptors and is therefore a true antagonist at these receptors. However, at the third type of receptor, nalorphine is acting as a weak or partial agonist. In other words, it has activated the receptor, but only weakly. We could imagine how this might occur, if the third receptor is controlling same thing like an ion channel.
- Morphine is a strong agonist and interacts strongly with this receptor leading to a change in receptor conformation which fully opens the ion channel. Ions now in or out of the cell, resulting in the activation or deactivation of enzymes. Naloxone is a pure antagonist. It binds strongly, but does not produce a change in the receptor conformation. Therefore, the ion channel remains closed. Nalorphine binds to the third receptor and changes the tertiary structure of the receptor very slightly, leading to a slight opening of the ion channel. It is therefore a weak agonist at this receptor, but it is also an antagonist since it blocks morphine from fully switching on' the receptor.
- The results observed with nalorphine show that activation of this third type of analgesic receptor leads to analgesia without the undesirable side effects associated with the other two analgesic receptors.
- Unfortunately, nalorphine has hallucinogenic side effects resulting from the activation of a non-analgesic receptor, and is therefore unsuitable as an analgesic, but for the first time a certain amount of analgesia had been obtained without the side effects of respiratory depression and tolerance (Fig. 21.20).

Simplification or Drug Dissection

- We turn now to more drastic alterations of the morphine structure and ask whether the complete carbon skeleton is really necessary. After all, if we could simplify the molecule, it would be easier to make in the laboratory.

- This in turn would allow the chemist to make analogues much more easily, and any useful compounds could be made more efficiently and cheaply.
- There are five rings present in the structure of morphine and analogues were made to see which rings could be removed.

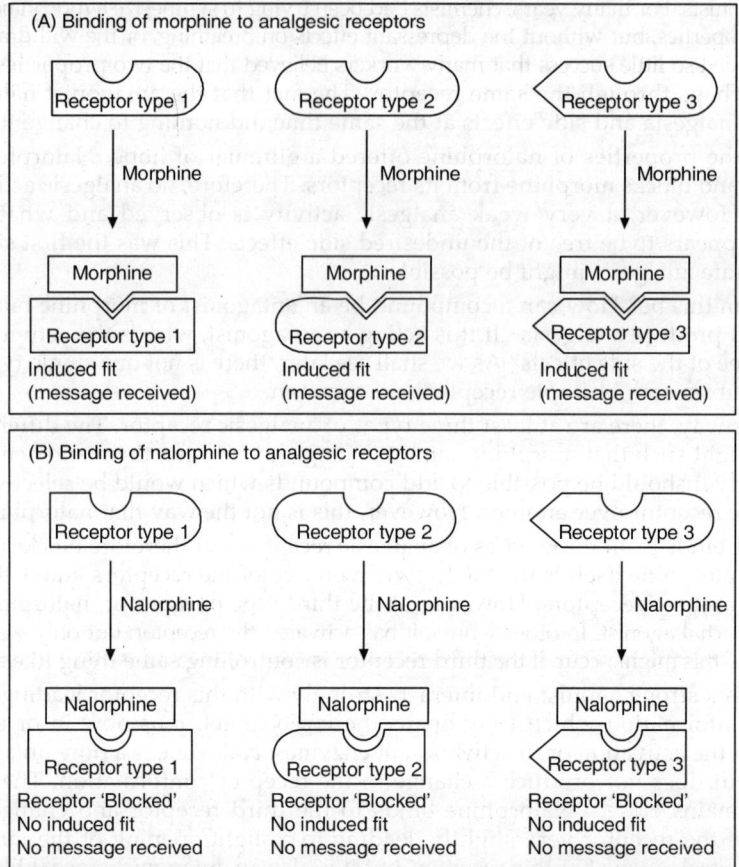

Fig. 21.20: Action of morphine and nalorphine at analgesic receptor

Removing ring E
Removing ring E leads to a complete loss of activity. This result emphasizes the importance of the basic nitrogen to analgesic activity.

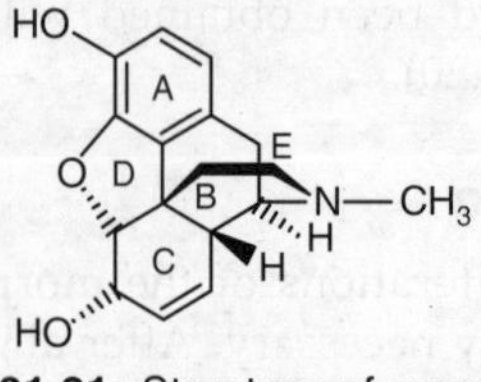

Fig. 21.21: Structure of morphine

Removing ring D

- Removing the oxygen bridge gives a series of compounds called the morphinans which have useful analgesic activity. This demonstrates that the oxygen bridge is not essential.

| N-methyl morphinan (20% activity of morphine) | Levorphanol (5x more potent than morphine) | Levallorphan (Antagonist 5x more potent than nalorphine) | (15x more potent than morphine) |

- N-methyl morphines were the just such compound tested and are only 20% active as morphine, but since the phenolic group is missing, this is not surprising. The more relevant levorphanol structure is five times more active than morphine and, although side effects are also increased, levorphanol has a massive advantage over morphine in that it can be taken orally and lasts much longer in the body. This is because levorphanol is not metabolized in the liver to the same extent as morphine.
- As might be expected, the mirror image of levorphanol (dextrorphan) has insignificant analgesic activity.
- The same strategy of drug extension already described for the morphine structures was also tried on the morphinans with similar results. For example, adding an allyl substituent on the nitrogen gives antagonists. Adding a phenethyl group to the nitrogen greatly increases potency. Adding a 14-OH group also increases activity.

Conclusions:

- Morphinans are more potent and longer acting than their morphine counterparts, but they also have higher toxicity and comparable dependence characteristics.
- The medications carried out on morphine, when carried out on the morphinans, lead to the same biological results. This implies that both types of molecule are reacting with the same receptors in the same way.
- The morphinans are easier to synthesize since they are simpler molecules.

Removing rings C and D

- Opening both rings C and D gives an interesting group of compounds called the benzomorphans which are found to retain analgesic activity. One of the simplest of these structures is metazocine which has the same analgesic activity as morphine.
- Notice that the two methyl groups in metazocine are cis with respect to each other and represent the stumps of the C ring.
- If the same types of chemical medications are carried out on the benzomomhans as were described for the morphinans and morphine, then the same biological effects are observed. This suggests that the benzomorphans (Fig. 21.22) interact with the same receptors as the morphinans and morphine analogues.
- For example, replacing the N-methyl group of metazocine with a phenethyl group gives phenazocine which is four times more active than morphine and the first compound to have a useful level of analgesia without dependence properties.
- Further developments led to pentazocine which has proved to be a useful long-term analgesic with a very low risk of addiction. A newer compound (bremazocine) has a longer

duration, is 200 times the activity of morphine, appears to have no addictive properties, and does not depress breathing.

- These compounds appear to be similar in their action to nalorphine in that they act as antagonists at two of the three types of analgesic receptor, but act as an agonist at the third. The big difference between nalorphine and compounds like pentazocine is that the latter are far stronger agonists, resulting in a more useful level of analgesia.
- Unfortunately, many of these compounds have hallucinogenic side effects due to interactions with a non-analgesic receptor.

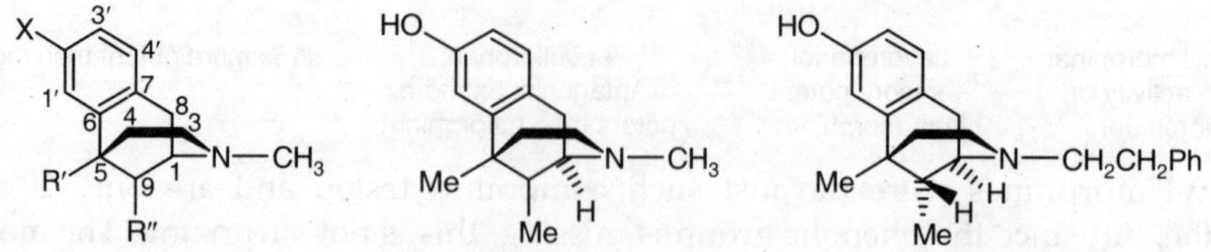

Metazocene
(same potency as morphine)

Phenazocene
(4x more potent than morphine)

Fig. 21.22: Benzomorphans

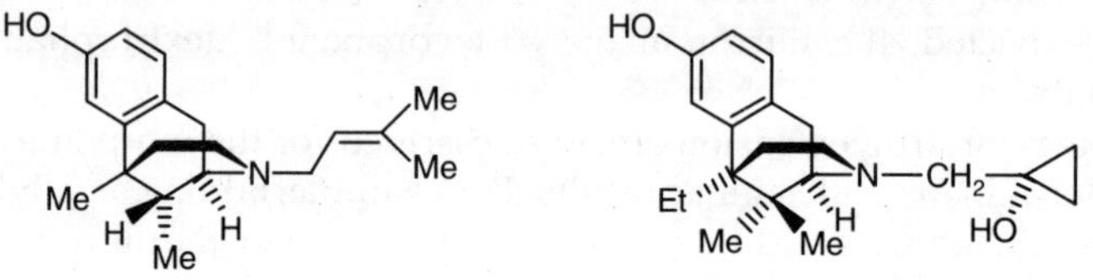

Pentazocine
(33% activity of morphine,
short duration, low
addiction liability)

Bremazocine

Fig. 21.23: Benzomorphans with low rate of dependency

- We shall come back to the interaction of benzomorphans with analgesic receptors later. For the moment, we can make the following conclusions about benzomorphans.
  1. Rings C and D are not essential to analgesic activity.
  2. Analgesia and addiction are not necessarily coexistent.
  3. 6,7-Benzomorphans are clinically useful compounds with reasonable analgesic activity, less addictive liability, and less tolerance (Fig. 21.23).
  4. Benzomorphans are simpler to synthesize.

Removing rings B, C and D

- Removing rings B, C and D gives a series of compounds known as 4-phenylpiperidines (Fig. 21.24).
- The analgesic activity of these compounds was discovered by chance in the 1940s, when chemists were studying analogues of cocaine for antispasmodic properties.
- Their structural relationship to morphine was only identifier when they were found to be analgesics, and is evident if the structure is drawn. Activity can be increased six-fold by introducing the phenolic group and altering the ester to a ketone to give ketobemidone.
- Meperidine (pethidine) is not as strong an analgesic as morphine and also shares the same undesirable side effects. However, it has a rapid onset and a shorter duration and as a result

has been used as an analgesic for difficult childbirths. The rapid onset and short duration of meperidine mean that there is less chance of it depressing the baby's breathing.

- The piperidines are more easily synthesized than any of the above groups and a large number of analogues have been studied. There is some doubt as to whether they act in the same way as morphine at analgesic receptors since same of the chemical adaptations we have already described do not lead to comparable biological results.

- For example, adding allyl or cyclopropyl groups does not give antagonists. The replacement of the methyl group of meperidine with a cannabic acid residue increases the activity by 30 times, whereas putting the same group on morphine eliminates activity (Fig. 21.25).

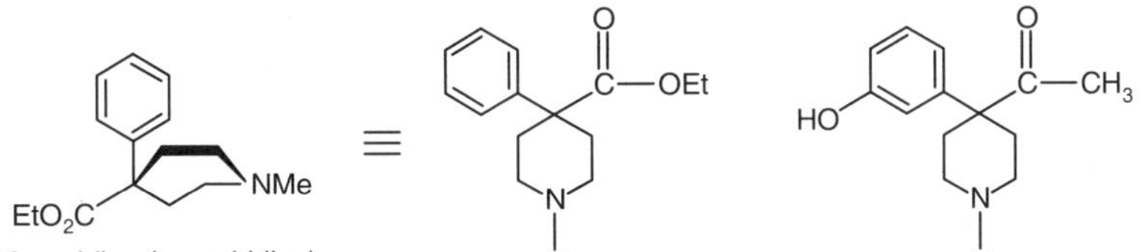

Meperidine (or pethidine)
(20% activity of morphine)

Me

Me

Ketobemidone

Fig. 21.24: Phenyl piperidines

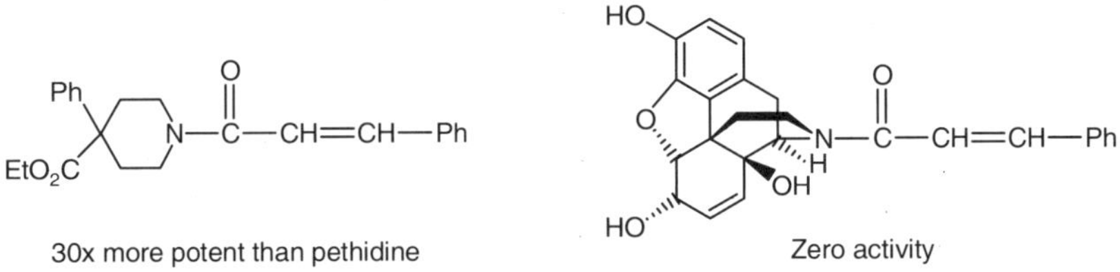

30x more potent than pethidine

Zero activity

Fig. 21.25: Effect of addition of cinnamic acid residue on meperidine and morphine

- These results might have samething to do with the fact that the piperidines are far more legible molecules than the previous structures and are thus more likely to interact with receptors in different ways.

- One of the most successful piperidine derivatives is fentanyl which is up to 100 times more active than morphine. The drug lacks a phenolic group, but is very lipophilic. As a result, it can cross the blood-brain barrier efficiently.

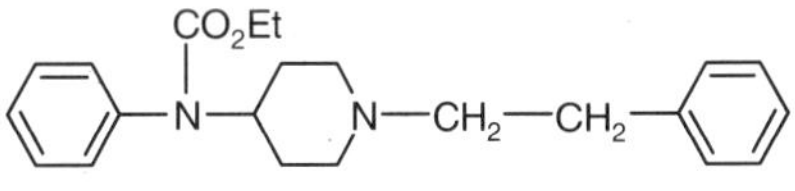

Fentanyl

Conclusion:

1. Rings C, D, and E are not essential for analgesic activity.
2. Piperidines retain side effects such as addiction and depression of the respiratory centre.
3. Piperidine analgesics are faster acting and have shorter duration.
4. The quaternary centre present in piperidines is usually necessary (fentanyl is an exception).
5. The aromatic ring and basic nitrogen are essential to activity, but the phenol group is not.
6. Piperidine analgesics appear to interact with analgesic receptors in a different manner to previous groups.

Removing rings B, C, D and E

- The analgesic methadone was discovered in Germany during the second World War and has proved to be a useful agent comparable in activity to morphine.

- Unfortunately, methadone retains morphine-like side effects. However, it is orally active and has less severe emetic and constipation affects. Side effects such as sedation, euphoria, and withdrawal are also less severe and therefore the compound has been given to drug addicts as a substitute for morphine (or heroin) in order to wean them off these drugs.

Methadone

- This is not a complete cure since it merely swaps an addiction to heroin for an addiction to methadone. However, this is considered less dangerous.

- The molecule has a single choral centre and when the molecule is drawn in the same manner as morphine, we would expect the R enantiomer to be the more active enantiomer. This proves to be the case with the R enantiomer being twice as powerful as morphine, whereas the S enantiomer is inactive. This is quite a dramatic difference. Since the R and S enantiomers have identical physical progenies and lipid solubility, they should both reach the receptor site to the same extent, and so the difference in activity is most probably due to receptor–substrate interactions.

- Many analogues of methadone have been synthesized, but with little improvement over the parent drug.

Rigidification

- Up till now, we have considered minor adjustments of functional groups on the periphery of the morphine skeleton or drastic supplication of the morphine skeleton.

- A completely different seated is to make the molecule more complicated or more rigid. This state is usually employed in an attempt to remove the side effects of a drug or to increase activity.

- It is usually assumed that the side effects of a drug are due to interactions with additional receptors other than the one we are interested in. These interactions are probably due to the molecule taking up different conformations or shapes.

- If we make the molecule more rigid so that it takes up fewer conformations, we might eliminate the conjugations which are recognized by undesirable receptors, and thus restrict the molecule to the specie conformation which fits the desired receptor. In this way, we would hope to eliminate such side effects as dependence and respiratory depression. We might also expect increased activity since the molecule is more likely to be in the correct conformation to interact with the receptor.

- The best example of this tactic in the analgesic sold is provided by a group of compounds known as the oripavines (Fig. 21.26). These structures often show remarkably high activity.

- The oripavines are made from an alkaloid which we have not described so far- thebaine. Thebaine can be extracted from opium along with codeine and is very similar in structure to both these compounds. However, unlike morphine and codeine, thebaine has no analgesic activity. There is a diene group present in ring C of febrile and when febrile is reacted with methyl vinyl ketone, a Diels-Alder reaction takes place to give an extra ring and increased rigidity to the structure.

- A comparison with morphine shows that the extra ring sticks out from what used to be the crossbars of the T-shaped structure (Fig. 21.27).

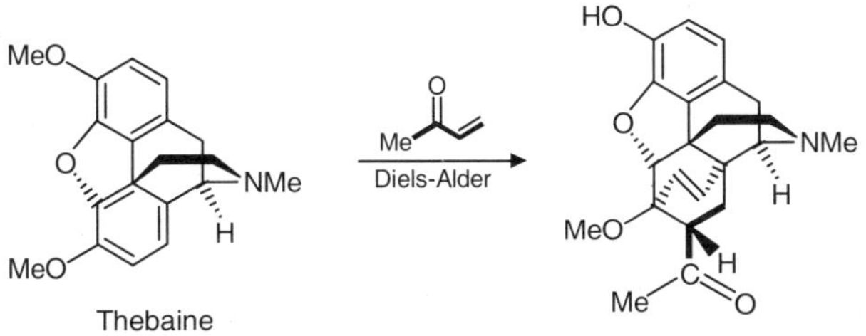

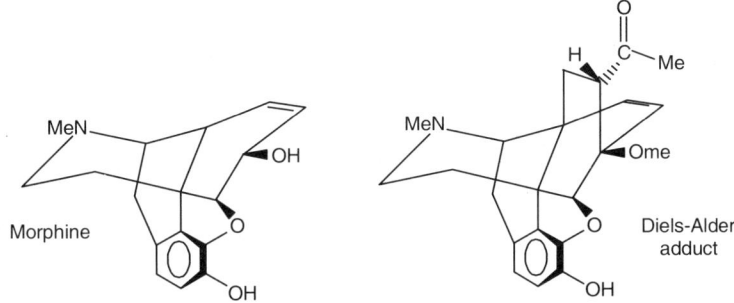

Fig. 21.26: Formation of oripavines

Fig. 21.27: Comparison of morphine and oripavine

- Since a ketone group has been introduced, it is now possible to try the strategy of drug extension (Fig. 21.28), this time by adding various groups to the ketone via a Grignard reaction.
- It is noteworthy that the Grignard reaction is stereospecific. The Grignard reagent complexes to both the 6-methoxy group and the ketone, and is then delivered to the less-hindered face of the ketone to give an asymmetric center (Fig. 21.29).
- By varying the groups added by the Grignard reaction, same remarkably powerful compounds have been obtained. Etorphine, for example, is 10 000 times more potent than morphine. This is a combination of the fact that it is a very hydrophobic molecule and can cross the blood-brain barrier 300 times more easily.

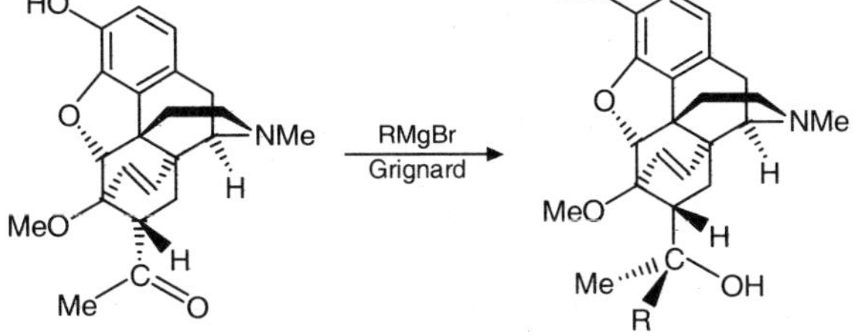

Fig. 21.28: Drug extension

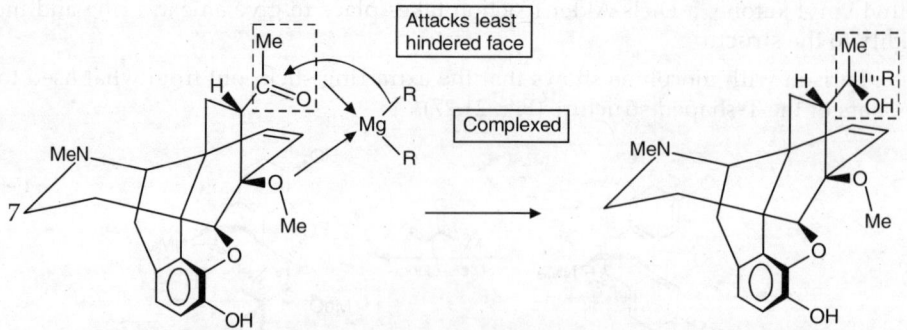

Fig. 21.29: Grignard reaction leads to asymmetric center

- Than morphine, as well as the fact that it has 20 times more affinity for the analgesic receptor site due to better binding interactions. At slightly higher doses than those required for analgesia, it can act as a knockouts drug or sedative.

- The compound has a considerable margin of safety and is used to immobilize large animals such as elephants. Since the compound is so active, only very small doses are required and these can be dissolved in such small volumes (1 ml) that they can be placed in crossbow darts and fires into the hide of animal.

- The addition of lipophilic groups (R) is found to improve activity dramatically, indicating the presence of a hydrophobic binding region close by on the 1. The group best able to interact with this region is a phenethyl substituent receptor and the product containing this group is even more active than etorphine.

Etorphine

- As one might imagine, these highly active compounds have to be handled very carefully in the laboratory.

- Because of their rigid structures, these compounds are highly selective agents for the analgesic receptors. Unfortunately, the increased analgesic activity is also accompanied by unacceptable side effects. It was therefore decided to see if putting substituents on the nitrogen, such as an allyl or cyclopropyl group, would give antagonists as found in the morphine, and benzomorphan series of compounds. If so, it might be possible to obtain an oripavine equivalent of a pentazocine or a nalorphine—an antagonist with same agonist activity and with reduced side effects.

- Putting on a cyclopropyl group gives a very powerful antagonist called diprenorphine , which is 100 times more potent than nalorphine and can be used to reverse the immobilizing effects of etorphine (see above). Diprenorphine has no analgesic activity.

Diprenorphine   Buprenorphine (1968)

- Replacing the methyl group derived from the Grignard reagent with a l-butyl group gives buprenorphine which has similar properties to drugs like nalorphine and pentazocine, in that it has analgesic activity with a very low risk of addiction. This feature appears to be related to the slow onset and removal of buprenorphine from the analgesic receptors. Since these effects are so gradual, the receptor system is not subjected to sudden changes in transmitter levels.

- Buprenorphine is the most lipophilic compound in the oripavine series of compounds and therefore enters the brain very easily. Usually, such a drug would react quickly with its receptor. The fact that it does not interact with the receptor rather than the ease with which it can reach the receptor. It is 100 times more active than morphine as an agonist and four times more active than nalorphine as an antagonist. It is a particularly safe drug since it has very little effect on respiration and what little effect it does have actually decreases at high doses.

- Buprenorphine has been used in hospitals to treat patients suffering from cancer and also following surgery. Its drawbacks include side effects such as nausea and vomiting as well as the fact that it cannot be taken orally. A further use for buprenorphine is as an alternative means to methadone for weaning addicts off heroin.

- Buprenorphine binds slowly to analgesic receptors, but once it does bind, it binds very strongly. As a result, less buprenorphine is required to interact with a certain percentage of analgesic receptors than morphine.

- On the other hand, buprenorphine is only a partial agonist. In other words, it is not very efficient at switching the analgesic receptor on. This means that it is unable to reach the maximum level of analgesia which can be acquired by morphine.

- Overall, buprenorphine stronger amenity for analgesic receptors outweighs its relatively weak action such that a lower dose of buprenorphine can produce analgesia, compared to morphine. However, if pain levels are high, buprenorphine is unable to counteract the pain and morphine has to be used.

- Nevertheless, buprenorphine provides another example of an opiate analogue where analgesia has been separated from dangerous side effects.

- It is time to look more closely at the receptor theories relevant to the analgesics.

MEPERIDINE SERIES

- The 1930s saw many new antispasmodics of general formula $ArCO_2 (CH_2)_2NR_2$, Ar_2CHCO_2-$(CH_2) NR_2$ and similar structure. The rules of isosterism emerging at that time emphasized that reversed esters could be a good variation to improve anticholinergics activity. This leads to synthesis of meperidine by Eisleb in 1930.

- It had lived up to its expectations and had moderate antispasmodic as well as sedative properties. When Schaumann tested it in the cat, he was surprised by an exhibition of Straub's tail, a phenomenon (test for analgesic activity) associated with morphine. Further studies indicated that meperidine had 10-20% of overall activity of morphine. Schaumann succeeded to spot the segment in morphine structure similar to meperidine as a result of molecular dissection.

- The discovery of analgesic properties of meperidine opened new avenues for the search of simpler, relatively small, structurally uncomplicated analgesics.

- Meperidine was not designed by molecular dissection. It was of 'reversed' antispasmodic structure and its analgesic properties were observed during pharmacological workup.

- The various modifications of meperidine are as follows.

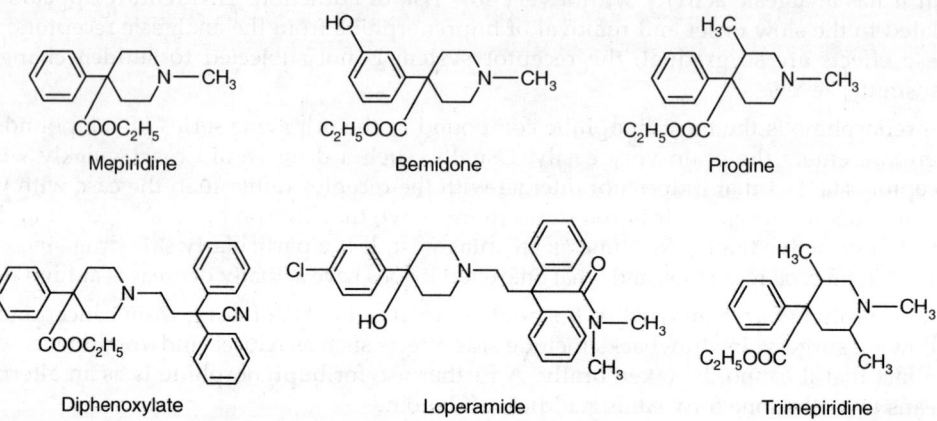

| Mepiridine | Bemidone | Prodine |

| Diphenoxylate | Loperamide | Trimepiridine |

Structure–Activity Relationship

1. Replacement of 4-phenyl group by hydrogen, alkyl, aroalkyl or heterocyclic group results in reduced activity.
2. Many N-substituted analogues of meperidine have been prepared. Anileridine is employed clinically.

Anileridine   Pheneridine

3. Replacement of carbethoxyl group (-COOC₂H₅) by acyloxy group (OCOC₂H₅) results in better analgesic activity.
4. The replacement of N-methyl group by various aralkyl groups can increase the analgesic property markedly.
5. Series of compounds were prepared where piperidine is enlarged to 7-membered azepine ring.

Piminodine

6. Proheptazine is among the more active analgesic agents in higher ring homologue of meperidine.

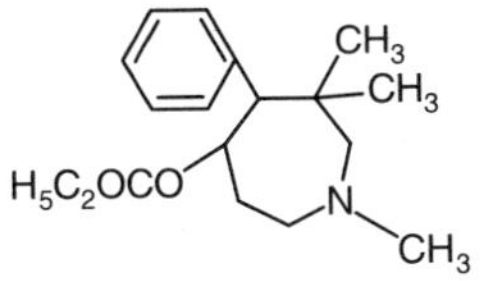

3, 3-Dimethyl-4-phenyl-
4-propionoxy hexahydroazepine
(proheptazine)

7. Substitution of the piperidine ring with 5-membered pyrrolidine ring is also successful.
8. The presence of m-hydroxyl group in the phenyl ring resembles that of C3 phenolic hydroxyl group in the morphine. Bemidone represents this class.
9. Replacement of the ester moiety by a ketone function in the bemidone, yielded a new series of compounds, ketobemidone.
10. Prodines are the reversed esters of meperidine. Here the ester of meperidine $(COOC_2H_5)$ is replaced by $(OCOC_2H_5)$ propionoxy function.

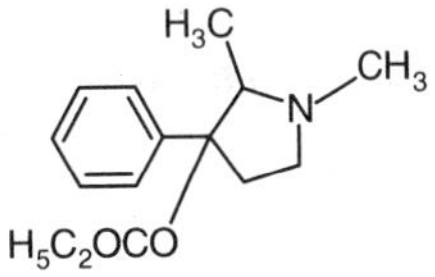

Prodilidene

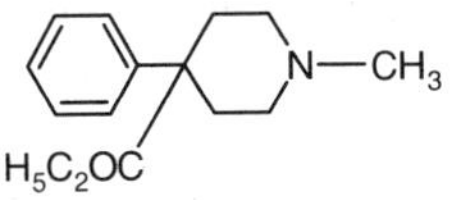

Bemidone

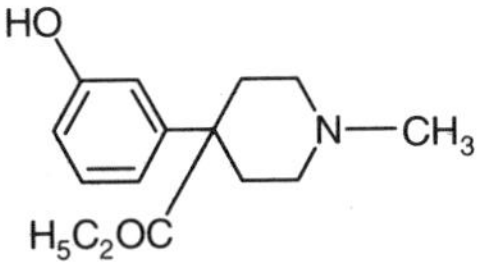

Ketobemidone

11. In all the above structures, phenyl ring and acyl group are directly attached to the piperidine ring. In fentanyl series, phenyl ring and acyl group are separated from the ring by nitrogen.

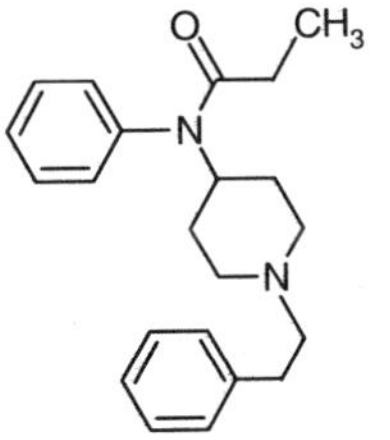

Fentanyl

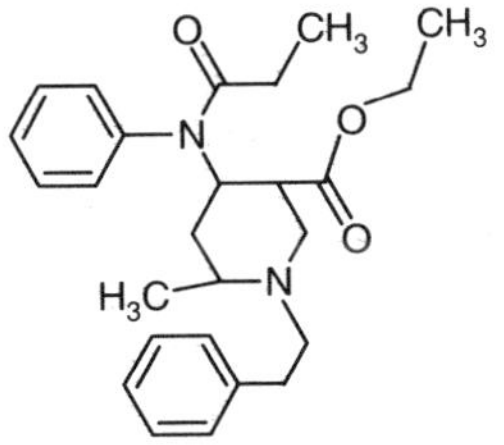

Lofentanyl

12. Sufentanil is a recent example from fentanyl series.

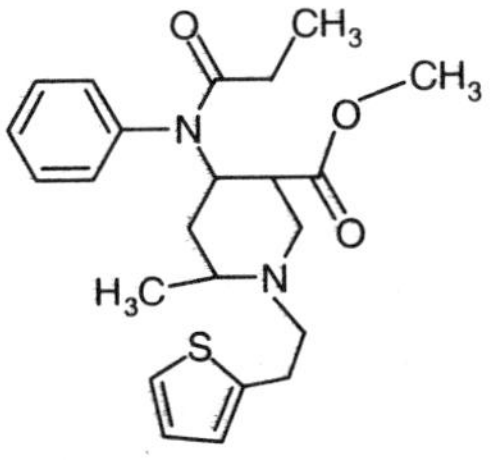

Sufentanil

13. Fentanyl is about 500 times as potent as pethidine. Some of the 4, 4 - disubstituted piperidines, alfetanyl, sulfentanyl and carfentanyl are even more potent. The latter two

have a much longer duration of analgesia and respiratory depression and indicate a different therapeutics use, e.g. anesthesia.

■ METHADONE SERIES

The further simplification of morphine nucleus by opening of the nitrogen ring resulted into methadone series of compounds. Methadone itself possesses analgesic as well as spasmolytic properties. The resemblance of methadone structure with meperidine structure can easily be seen.

Structure–Activity Relationship

1. Unlike meperidine or bemidone series, the insertion of m-hydroxyl group in one of the phenyl rings of methadone causes a marked decrease in analgesic activity.

2. The methadone derivatives are generally more potent analgesics (and also more toxic) than the isomethadone analogues.

3. The replacement of propionyl group by hydrogen, hydroxyl or acetyloxy, led to decrease in activity.

\4. Similarly attempts were also made to replace propionyl group by amide functions, e.g. racemoramide; it is more active than methadone.

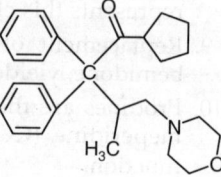

Racemoramide

5. Removal of any of the two phenyl rings results into decreased activity.

6. The dimethylamino group is replaced by heterocyclic rings like morpholone and piperidine. The clinically employed agents from this class are– phenadoxone and dipanone.

Phenadoxone

Dipanone

7. The following are N-demethylated derivatives which are metabolites of methadone analogues in man and are found to retain the analgesic activity.

Metabolite of alpha acetylmethadol

Metabolite of methadone

8. Molecular modification of methadone include: homologation and cyclization of di CH$_3$-amino group, reduction of CO to - CHOH, removal and relocation of CH$_3$ branching, isosteric replacement of one or both phenyls by thienyl, etc. Examples: Replacement of the keto group by an amide group results into dextromoramide. Insertion of ester oxygen between blocking groups and carbonyl (as well as a benzyl instead of one phenyl) gave dextropropoxyphene rings converge on an amine chain and instead of an electron rich carbonyl group, a double bond is introduced.

Thiambutene

Methadone Derivatives

Methadone

Dextromoramide

Isomethadone

Normethadone

Propoxyphene

Dipanone

MORPHINAN SERIES

Various compounds belonging to morphinan and benzomorphan series have been synthesized and tested clinically. These compounds lack the ether bridge between the carbon atoms 4 and 5.

N-methylmoprphinan

Structure–Activity Relationship

1. The levo form of morphinan possesses the analgesic activity while the dextro form (dextromethorphan) is having cough suppressant activity.
2. Introduction of a hydroxyl group at C 3 enhances the analgesic activity.
3. The ethers and acylated derivatives of the 3-hydroxyl form also have considerable analgesic activity.
4. The 14-hydroxylation results in potent derivatives with both agonist and antagonist properties, e.g.

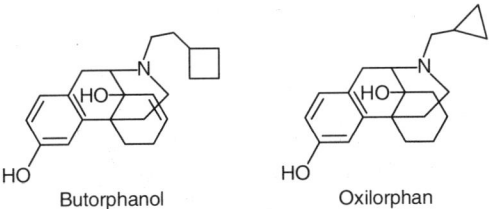

Butorphanol

Oxilorphan

5. N-substitution may result into either agonist or antagonist depending upon the nature of substituent, e.g. the N-phenylethyl or N-p-amino phenylethyl derivatives of levorphanol

are potent analgesics. The N-furylethyl and N-acetophenone analogues are also potent analgesics. While N-allyl derivatives (cyclorphan) possess antagonistic properties.

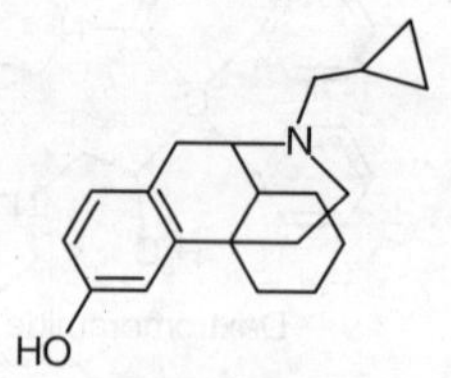

Cyclorphan

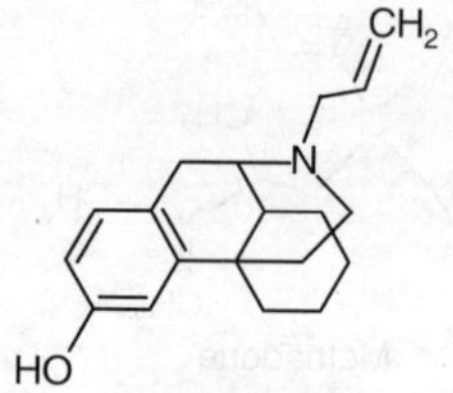

Levallorphan

AGONIST AND ANTAGONIST

Depending upon the activity, drugs can be classified as follows:

1. Pure antagonist— naloxone.
2. Partial antagonist— nalorphin, levallorphan and cyclazocine
3. Partial agonists of morphine— propiram and propafol.

- We return now to look at a particularly interesting problem regarding the agonist/antagonist properties of morphine analogues. Why should such a small change as replacing an N-methyl group with an allyl group result in such a dramatic change in biological activity such that an agonist becomes an antagonist? Why should a molecule such as nalorphine act as an agonist at one analgesic receptor and an antagonist at another? How can different receptors distinguish between such subtle changes in a molecule? We shall consider one theory which attempts to explain how these distinctions might take place, but it is important to realize that there are alternative theories.

- In this particular theory, it is suggested that there are two accessory hydrophobic binding sites present in an analgesic receptor.

- It is then proposed that a structure will act as an agonist or as an antagonist depending on which of these extra binding sites is used. In other words, one of the hydrophobic binding sites is an agonist binding site, whereas the other is an antagonist binding site.

Morphine Agonist and Antagonist

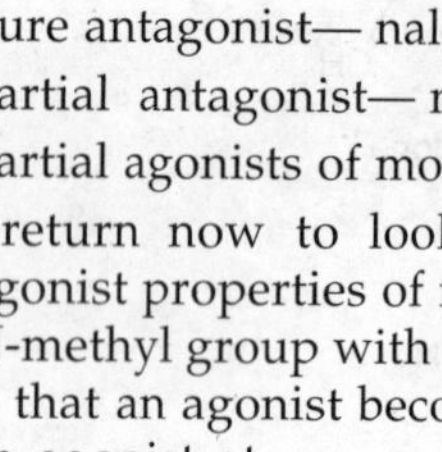

Nalorphine

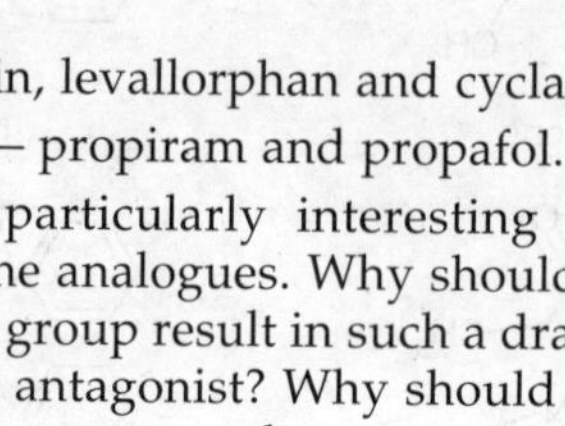

Buprenorphine

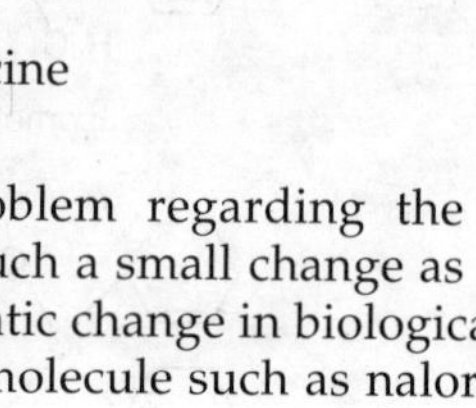

Butraphanol

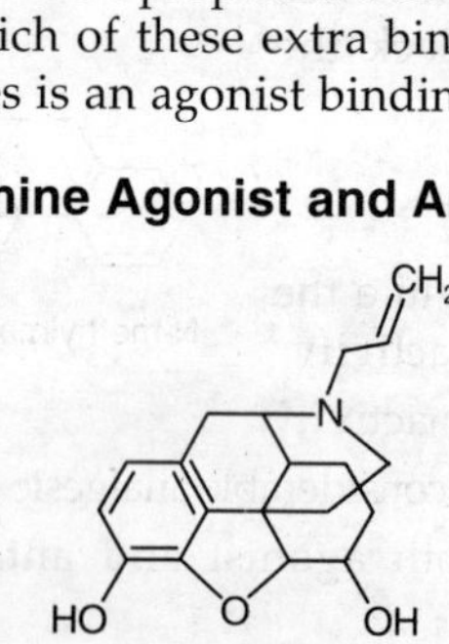

Naloxone

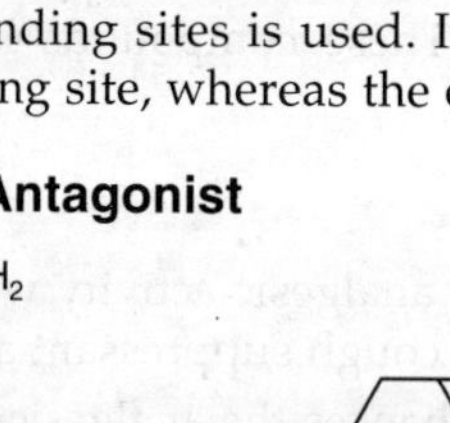

Naltrexone

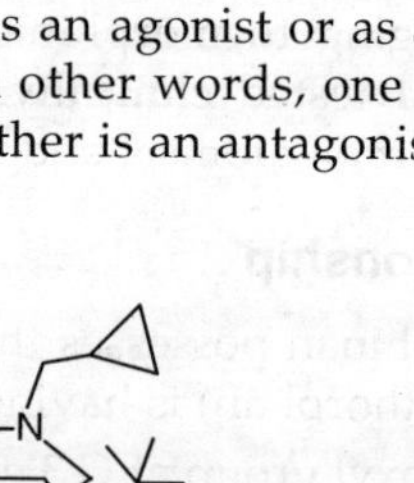

Pentazocine

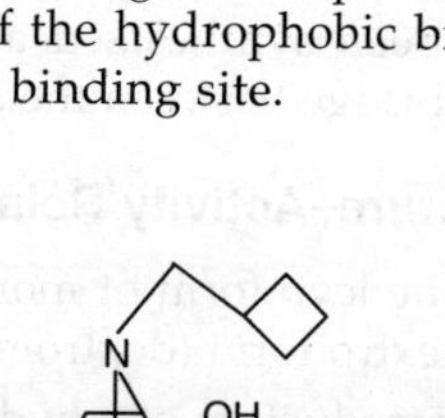

Nalbuphine

- The model was proposed by Snyder and coworkers and is shown in Fig. In the model, the agonist binding site is further away from the nitrogen and positioned axially with respect to it. The antagonist site is closer and positioned equationally.
- Let us now consider the morphine analogue containing a phenethyl substituent on the nitrogen. It is proposed that this structure binds as already described, such that the phenol, aromatic ring, and basic center are interacting with their respective binding sites. If the phenethyl group is in the axial position, the aromatic ring is in the correct position to interact with agonist binding site.
- However, if the phenethyl group is in the equatorial position, the aromatic ring is placed beyond the antagonist binding site and cannot bind. The overall result is increased activity.
- Let us now consider what happens if the phenethyl group is replaced with an allyl group (Fig. 21.31). In the equatorial position, the allyl group is able to bind strongly to the antagonist binding site, whereas in the axial position it barely reaches the agonist binding site, resulting in a weak interaction.

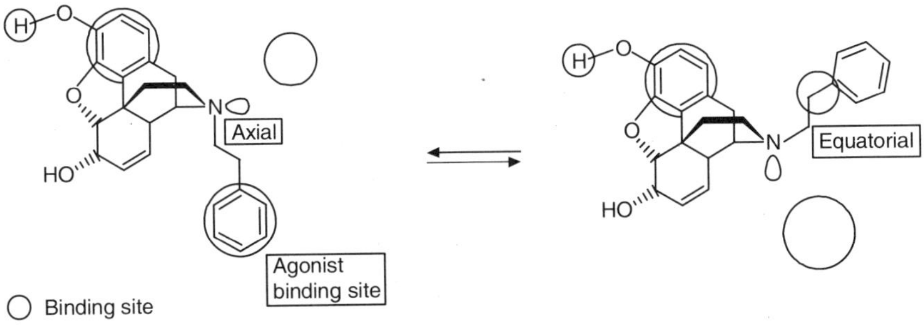

Fig. 21.30: Morphine analogue containing phenethyl substituent on nitrogen

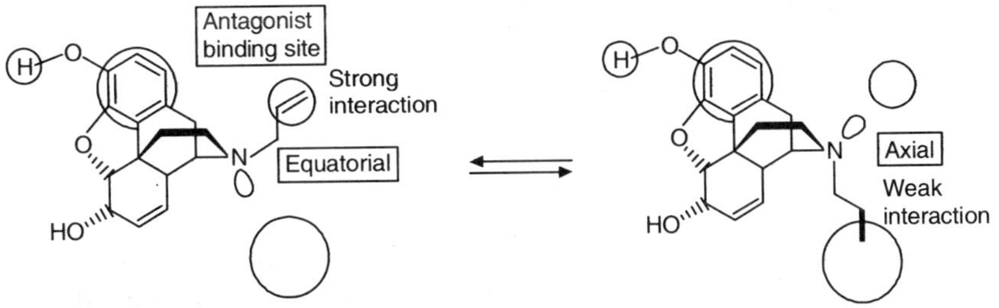

Fig. 21.31: Morphine analogue containing an allyl substituent

- In this theory, it is proposed that a molecule such as phenazocine (with a phenethyl group) acts as an agonist since it can only bind to the agonist binding site. A molecule such as nalorphine (with an allyl group) can bind to both agonist and antagonist sites and therefore acts as an agonist at one receptor and an antagonist at another.
- The ratio of these effects would depend on the relative equilibrium ratio of the axial and equatorial substituted isomers.

- A compound which is a pure antagonist would be forced to have a suitable substituent in the equatorial position. It is believed that the presence of a 14-OH group stereochemically hinders the isomer with the axial substituent, and forces the substituent to remain equatorial.

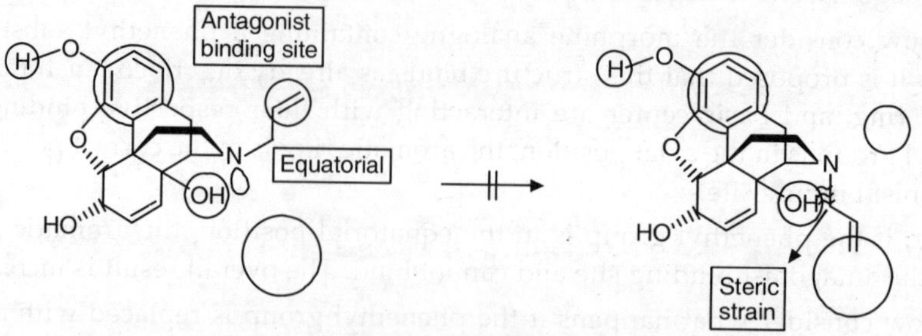

Fig. 21.32: Influence of 14-OH on binding

NATURALLY OCCURRING ENKEPHALINS AND ENDORPHINS

- Morphine, as we have already discussed, is an alkaloid which relieves pain and acts in the CNS. There are two conclusions which can be drawn from this. First conclusion is that there must be analgesic receptors in the CNS.
- The second conclusion is that there must be chemicals produced in the body which interact with these receptors. Morphine itself is not produced by humans and therefore the body must be using a different chemical as its natural pain killer.
- The search for this natural analgesic took many years, but ultimately led to the discovery of the enkephalins and the endorphins. The CST enkephalins to be discovered were the pentapeptides Met-enkephalin and Leu-enkephalin.

H—Tyr—Gly—Gly—Phe—Met—OH   H—Tyr—Gly—Gly—Phe—Leu—OH

- At least 15 endogenous reptiles have now been discovered, varying in length from 5 to 33 amino acids (the enkephalins and the endorphins).
- These compounds are thought to be neurotransmitters or neurohormones in the brain and operate as the body's natural pain killers as well as having a number of other roles. They are derived from three inactive precursor proteins—proenkephalin, prodynorphin, or pro-opiomelanocortin .

Proenkephalin
Prodynorphin
Pro-opiomelanocortin } ⟶ Endorphins + Enkephalins

- All 15 compounds are found to have either the Met- or the Leu-enkephalin skeleton at their N-terminus, which emphasizes the importance of this pentapeptides structure towards analgesic activity. It has also been shown conclusively that the tyrosine part of these molecules is essential for activity and much has been made of the fact that there is a tyrosine skeleton in the morphine skeleton.
- Enkephalins are thought to be responsible for the analgesia resulting from acupuncture.

Analogues of Enkephalins

- SAR studies on the enkephalins have shown the importance of the tyrosine phenol ring and the tyrosine amino group. Without either, activity is lost.

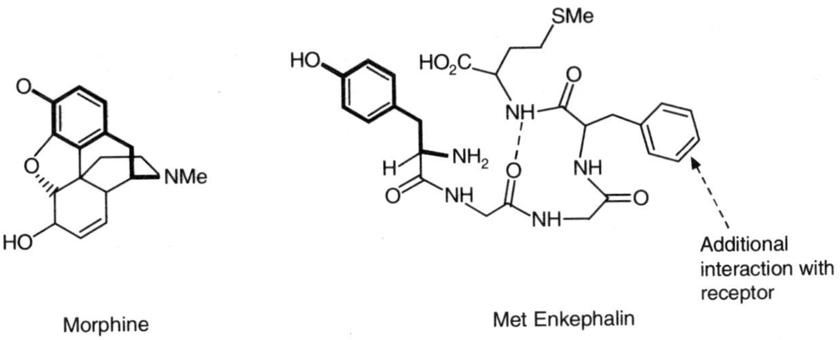

Fig. 21.33: The tyrosine section is very essential for activity

- If tyrosine is replaced with another amino acid, then activity is also lost (the only exception being D-serine). It has also been found that the enkephalins are easily inactivated by peptidase enzyme in vivo. The most labile peptide bond in the enkephalins is that between the tyrosine and glycine residues.
- Much work has been done therefore, to try and stabilize this bond towards hydrolysis.
- It is possible to replace the amino acid glycine with an unnatural D-amino acid such as D-alanine. Since D-amino acids are not naturally occurring, peptidases do not recognize the structure and the peptide bond is not attacked. The alternative tactic of replacing L-tyrosine with D-tyrosine is not possible, since this completely alters the relative orientation of the tyrosine aromatic ring with respect to the rest of the molecule (Fig. 21.34).
- As a result, the analogue is unable to bind to the analgesic receptor and is inactive.
- Putting a methyl group on to the amide nitrogen can also block hydrolysis by peptidases. Another tactic is to use unusual amino acids which are either not recognized by peptidases or prevent the molecule from eating the peptidase active site.
- Unfortunately, the enkephalins also have some activity at the mu receptor and so the search for selective agents continues.

H—L-Tyr—Gly—Gly—L-Phe—L-Met—OH	Delta agonist + a little mu activity
H—L-Tyr—D-AA—Gly—NMe-L-Phe—L-Met—OH	Resistant to peptidase. Orally active.
N, N-Diallyl-L-Tyr—aib—aib—L-Phe—L-Leu—OH	Antagonist to delta receptor. (aib = alpha-aminobutyric acid)
Longer enkaphalins/endorphins	Increase in kappa activity Slight increase in mu activity

Fig. 21.34: Tactics to stabilize the bond between tyrosine and glycine

Therapeutic Uses of Opioid Antagonists

1. In the treatment of opioid-induced respiratory depression.
2. Chronic administration of nalorphine along with morphine prevents or minimizes the development of dependence on morphine.
3. Therapeutic agents in the treatment of compulsive users of opioids.
4. Reduce the intensity of various untoward effects of opioids, e.g. euphoria, drowsiness, vomiting and muscular incoordination.

5. An abstinence syndrome characterized by abnormal pain, irritability, cold sweats, diarrhea, nausea and vomiting. These effects usually last 4–10 weeks. Nalorphine precipates the withdrawal symptoms in patients addicted to heroin and methadone. In acute poisoning due to morphine and related compounds.

Fentanyl

1-benzyl-4-piperidone   aniline

4-aniline-1-benzylpiperidine (I)   propionic anhydride

N-(4-piperidyl)-
propionanilide (II)   2-phenylethyl
chloride   Fentanyl

Methadone

diphenyl-
acetonitrile   2-dimethylamino-
1-methylethyl
chloride   4-dimethlamino-
2, 2-diphenyl-
voleronitrile (I)

Ethylmagnesium
bromide   (±)-Methadone   (–)-Methadone

Naloxone

Oxycodone → Oxymorphone → (I)

14-hydroxydihydro-normorphinone → Naloxone

Nalorphine

Morphine + → Diamorphine → I

(I) → Nalorphine

Naltrexone

oxymorphone (I) + Cyclopropylmethyl bromide → Naltrexone

Nalbuphine

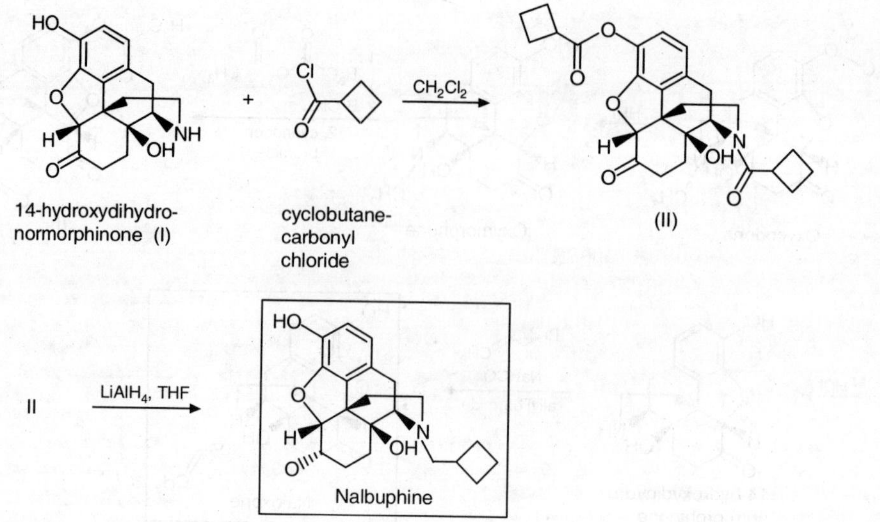

14-hydroxydihydro-
normorphinone (I)

cyclobutane-
carbonyl
chloride

(II)

II → LiAlH$_4$, THF →

Nalbuphine

Pentazocine

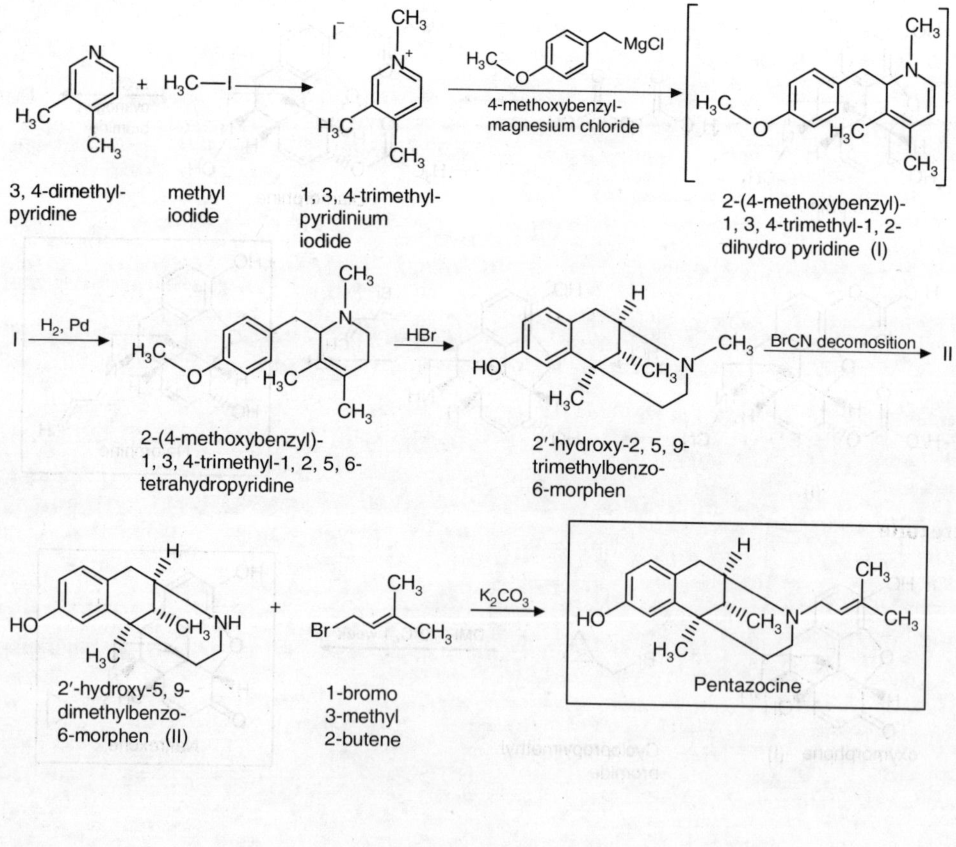

3, 4-dimethyl-
pyridine

methyl
iodide

1, 3, 4-trimethyl-
pyridinium
iodide

2-(4-methoxybenzyl)-
1, 3, 4-trimethyl-1, 2-
dihydro pyridine (I)

I → H$_2$, Pd →

2-(4-methoxybenzyl)-
1, 3, 4-trimethyl-1, 2, 5, 6-
tetrahydropyridine

HBr →

2'-hydroxy-2, 5, 9-
trimethylbenzo-
6-morphen

BrCN decomosition → II

2'-hydroxy-5, 9-
dimethylbenzo-
6-morphen (II)

1-bromo
3-methyl
2-butene

K$_2$CO$_3$ →

Pentazocine

22

CNS Stimulants

The drugs having the main effect (note side effect) to increase the activity of various portion of the central nervous system are collectively called as central nervous stimulant.

- Drugs that have a predominantly stimulant effect on the central nervous system fall into three broad categories.
    1. Convulsant and respiratory stimulant.
    2. Psychomotor stimulant.
    3. Psychotomimetic drugs.

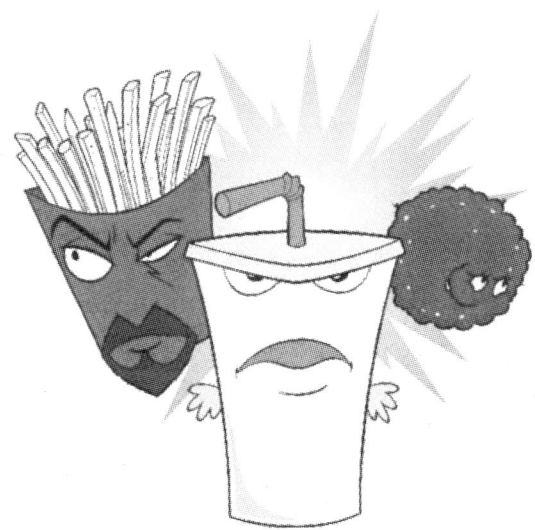

- Drugs in the first category (e.g. doxapram, nikethamide, leptazol) have relatively little effect on mental function and appear to act mainly on the brainstem and spinal cord, producing exaggerated reflux excitability, and increase in the activity of the respiratory vasomotor center, and with higher doses convulsion.
- Drugs in the second category (e.g. amphetamine, caffeine and cocaine) have a marked effect on the mental function and behavior, producing excitement and euphoria, reduced sensation of fatigue and an increase in the motor activity.
- Drugs in third category (lysergic acid diethylamide, phencyclidine and cannabis) mainly affect through pattern, perception and mood, producing effect that superficially resemble the changes seen in schizophrenia.

CLASSIFICATION OF CNS STIMULANTS

Classification of CNS stimulants is depicted in Flow chart 22.1.

Flow chart 22.1: Classification of CNS stimulants

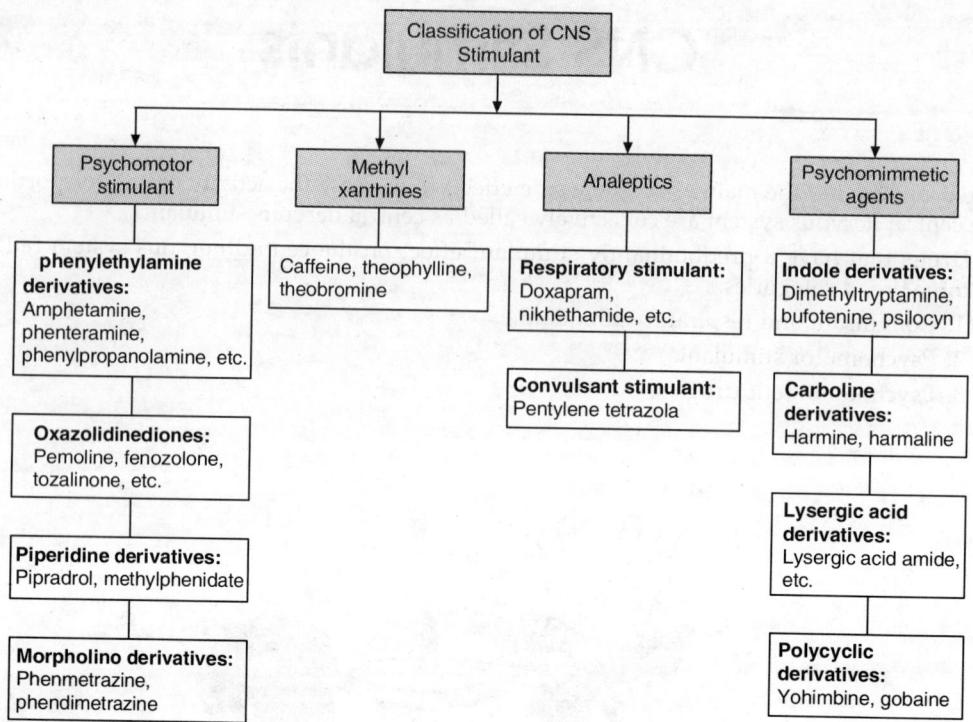

Analeptics

[A] Respiratory stimulant

Doxapram

Nikethamide

Ethamivan

Bemigride

Strychnine

[B] Convulsant stimulant

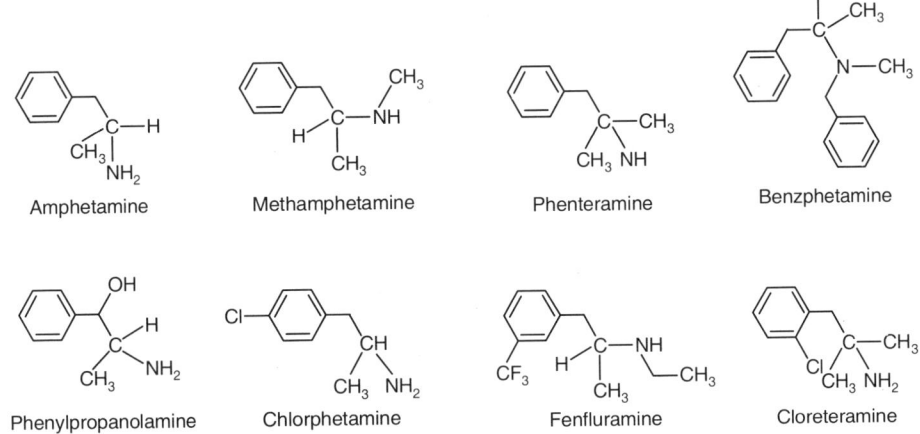

Pentylene tertrazole

Psychomotor Stimulant

[A] β-phenylethlamine derivatives

Amphetamine

Methamphetamine

Phenteramine

Benzphetamine

Phenylpropanolamine

Chlorphetamine

Fenfluramine

Cloreteramine

[B] Oxazolidinedione derivatives

Fenozolone

Pemoline

Tozalione

[C] Morpholino derivatives

Phenmetrazine

Phendimetrazine

[D] Piperidine derivatives

Pipradrol

Methyl phenidate

Methylxanthines

Caffeine

Theophylline

Theobromine

Etofylline

Proxyphylline

Pentoxyphylline

Psychomimetic Agents

[A] Indole derivatives and carboline derivatives

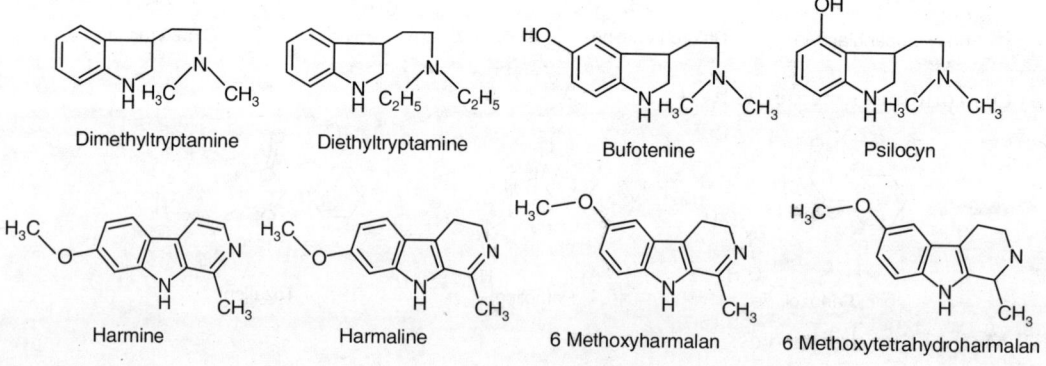

Dimethyltryptamine

Diethyltryptamine

Bufotenine

Psilocyn

Harmine

Harmaline

6 Methoxyharmalan

6 Methoxytetrahydroharmalan

[B] Lysergic acid derivatives

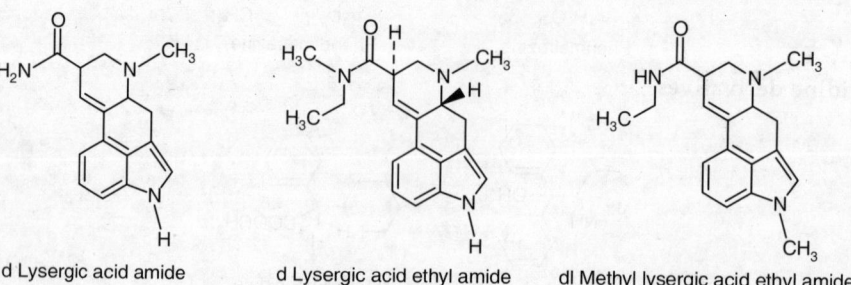

d Lysergic acid amide

d Lysergic acid ethyl amide

dl Methyl lysergic acid ethyl amide

dl Acetyl lysergic acid ethyl amide   d Lysergic acid dimethyl amide   d Lysergic acid diethyl amide

dl Methyl lysergic acid diethyl amide   dl Acetyl lysergic acid diethyl amide

[C] Polycyclic derivatives

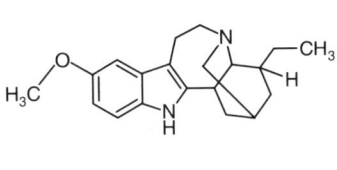

Yohimbine   Ibogaine

Analeptics

Mechanism of action

- Both inspiratory and expiratory centers are located in the reticular formation of the medulla and together are responsible for spontaneous respiration. Many physiological factors like, temperature blood flow, irritation of respiratory passages, vomiting, swallowing, joint movement, etc. alter the rate and depth of respiration.

- Analeptics stimulate the entire nervous system particularly medulla, thereby counteracting the respiratory depression resulting from overdose of depressant drugs. These agents act as competitive antagonist of the inhibitory transmitter at post-synaptic inhibitory sites.

- These agents may produce convulsion due to their ability to stimulate all parts of the brain and hence these agents act as an analeptics (rather than convulsant), better in the presence of slight depression. An additional benefit is gained due to adrenal catecholamine release resulting in bronchodilation which helps to improve air flow in the lung. Since in the light of current knowledge, the term analeptics and convulsant are virtually synonymous, the respiratory depression is best treated by other supportive measures like artificial respiration, oxygen administration, peritoneal dialysis and forced diuresis for the treatment of patients poisoned by depressant drugs.

Other possible mechanism of action

1. Blockage of post-synaptic inhibition, e.g. strychnine.
2. Blockage of pre-synaptic inhibition, e.g. picrotoxin.
3. Cholinergic augmentation, e.g. pentylenetetrazole, nikethamide, strychnine.
4. Decreased energy levels, e.g. pentylenetetrazole.
5. Prostaglandin release, e.g. picrotoxin, pentylenetetrazole, strychnine.
6. Low surface activity, e.g. picrotoxin, bemegride, pentylenetetrazole.

Contraindication

- Analeptic agents are contraindicated in epilepsy, hypertension, cardiac disease and hyperthyroidism.

Sympathomimetics/Psychomotor Stimulant

β-Phenyl ethylamine derivatives:

Structure–activity relationship

1. The branched methyl group or similar substitution, e.g. incorporation of the nitrogen in ring system (morpholine or piperidine) is very crucial, the O-methyl group prevent the oxidation of the amino group by MAO, providing to enzymatic inactivation by estric protection amino group.
2. The dextro isomers are 10-20 time more stimulating than the levo isomer.
3. Any decrease in distance between the aromatic ring and side chain nitrogen decrease the activity.
4. Hydrophilic substitution decrease stimulant activity.
5. Reduction of the aromatic ring or its replacement with alkyl group, produce loss of the CNS stimulant activity.

Morpholine series: In the morpholine series, substitution on the aromatic ring, as well as aromatic replacement by heterocyclic groups substantially decreases potency.

Piperidine series: Activity in the piperidine series is maximized at the methyl ester.

Mechanism of action

1. Inhibition of reuptake mechanism for several biogenic amines.
2. Enhancement of neuronal release of catecholamines.
3. Direct α-adrenergic receptor stimulation.
4. Inhibition of monoamine oxidase in higher concentration.

Side effect

- Amphetamine congeners, causes insomnia and restlessness due to its CNS stimulation properties.
- Other effects include nervousness, irritability, anorexia and possibility of cardiac irregularities.

Methyl Xanthines

Mechanism of Action

There are many theories to explain the various actions of methyl xanthines.

1. Inhibition of phosphodiestrases, the enzyme that inactivates cyclic AMP.

2. Translocation of intracellular calcium for explaining the capacity of caffeine for muscular work.
3. Blockade of receptor for adenosine— this is the most accepted mode of action of xanthines. Methyl xanthines are potent competitive antagonists of adenosine, a putative neurotransmitter that exhibits sedative, cardiac depressant and Na^+ retaining activities. They antagonize adenosine at A1 receptors.
4. Potentiation of inhibitors of prostaglandin synthesis.

Psychomimetics

Psychomimetics are the agents which induce temporarily changes in mood, perception or behavior that may results into vivid dreams, hallucination or nightmares.

These agents are classified mainly in two classes:
1. True psychomimetics
2. Psychodelics

True Psychomimetics
- Example includes phenyl ethylamines, indole ethylamines and miscellaneous compounds.

Psychodelics
- These agents are highly effective in altering the mood and perception and are used illegally for this purpose, e.g. lysergic acid, diethylamide, etc.
- There is a state of heightened awareness of sensory input but a diminished control over what is experienced. The person feels that one part of self seems to be passive observer of the events and happenings while another part of the self participates and receives the vivid and unusual sensory experience. The surrounding environment seems to be beautiful and harmonious. Commonly there is a diminished capacity to differentiate the boundaries of one object from another and to the self from the environment. These effects are better represented by the term 'mind expanding' drugs.

Mechanism of action
1. Signs of sympathetic stimulation occur after the administration of lysergid which suggests that it may accelerate or induce production of hallucinogenic metabolites from noradrenaline.
2. These agents may cause changes in cerebral blood flow and permeability of cerebral capillaries.
3. Alteration in levels of adrenal, corticoidal and thyroid hormones.
4. Changes in synthesis or metabolism of serotonine, norepinephrine, acetylcholine or other potential transmitter. Since serotonin is an inhibitory neurotransmitter, the removal of its inhibition could lead to behavioral changes. But it is not yet possible to find out the ways which disturb monoaminergic function that manifests itself as a hallucinatory experience.
5. Cerebral function is extremely dependant on the utilization of energy in the form of ATP. Psychomimetics may disrupt cerebral energy, production or utilization in such a fashion that it alters the behavior.

Side effects
These include psychic toxicity, paranoia, confusion and tolerance. Tolerance necessitates the use of increasingly larger doses to achieve the desired level of action which if exceeds the fatal overdose, results into a death of the patient due to respiratory depression.

Doxapram

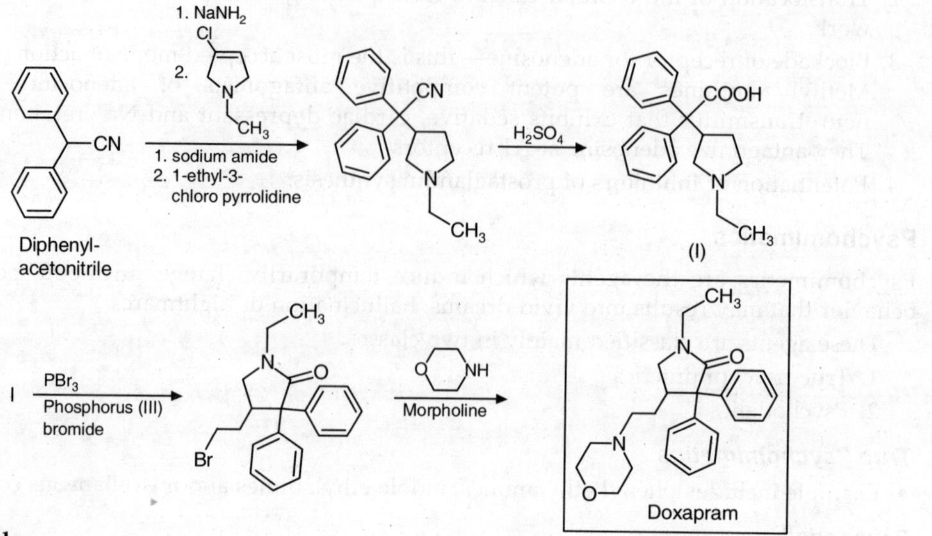

Diphenyl-
acetonitrile

1. NaNH₂
2. 1-ethyl-3-chloro pyrrolidine

1. sodium amide
2. 1-ethyl-3-chloro pyrrolidine

(I)

I

PBr₃
Phosphorus (III) bromide

Morpholine

Doxapram

Nikethamide

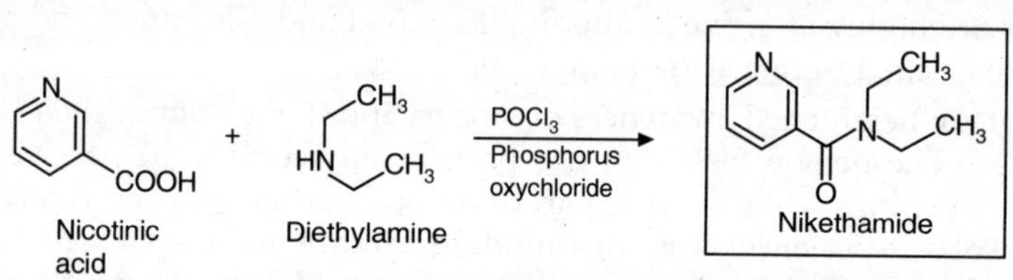

Nicotinic
acid

+

Diethylamine

POCl₃
Phosphorus oxychloride

Nikethamide

Fenfluramine

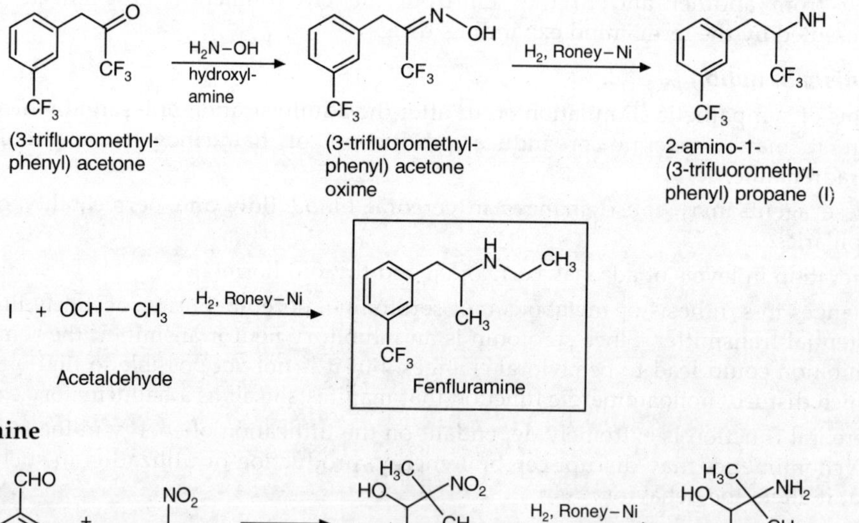

(3-trifluoromethyl-phenyl) acetone

H₂N—OH
hydroxyl-amine

(3-trifluoromethyl-phenyl) acetone oxime

H₂, Roney–Ni

2-amino-1-(3-trifluoromethyl-phenyl) propane (I)

I + OCH—CH₃

Acetaldehyde

H₂, Roney–Ni

Fenfluramine

Phentermine

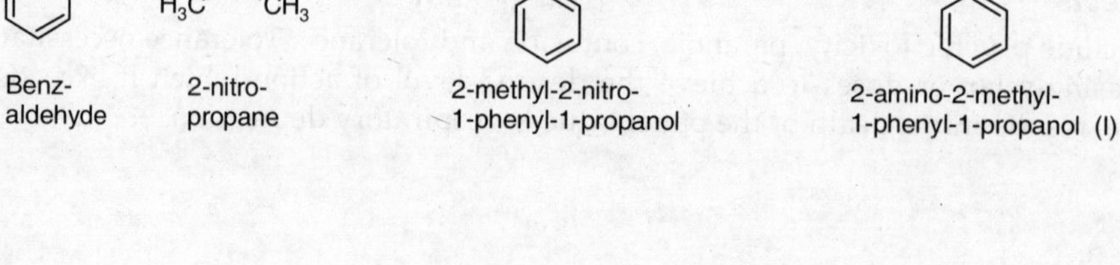

Benz-aldehyde

+

2-nitro-propane

2-methyl-2-nitro-1-phenyl-1-propanol

H₂, Roney–Ni

2-amino-2-methyl-1-phenyl-1-propanol (I)

I $\xrightarrow[\text{thionyl}\\ \text{chloride}]{\text{SOCl}_2}$

2-amino-2-methyl-
1-phenylpropyl
chloride hydrochloride • HCl $\xrightarrow{\text{H}_2,\text{ Pd}-\text{CaCO}_3}$

Phentermine

Phenmetrazine

Propiophenone $\xrightarrow[\text{Bromine}]{\text{Br}_2}$ α-bromopropio-
phenone $\xrightarrow[\text{ethanol}]{\text{2-benzylamino-}}$ α-[benzyl(2-hydroxyethyl)-
amino] propiophenone (I)

I $\xrightarrow{\text{H}_2,\text{ Pd}-\text{C}}$ 2-(2-hydroxyethyl-
amino)-1-phenyl-1-
propanol $\xrightarrow{\text{conc. H}_2\text{SO}_4}$ Phenmetrazine

Pemoline

Mandelic acid
ethyl ester + Guanidine $\longrightarrow$ Pemoline

Caffeine

Theophylline + Dimethyl sulfate $\longrightarrow$ Caffeine

23

Antipsychotics (Neurolepitcs)

Antipsychotic agents, also been called major tranquilizers, neuroleptics, produce calm or neurosedation in severely disturbed patients. However, contrary to the effect caused by hypnotics and sedatives, they do not cloud consciousness or depress vital centers. Therefore, they are widely used for prolonged treatment of acute and chronic schizophrenia. These drugs have in common the pharmacological property of antagonizing the action of dopamine and this is responsible for most of their effects on the nervous system.

SCHIZOPHERNIA

Not an easy question to answer, but one thing it certainly is not that is 'split personality'. This confusion probably arises due to the meaning of the word itself 'split mind,' but in fact schizophrenia is not a disorder of personality at all. It is probably best described as a detachment from reality in which the sufferer experiences hallucinations, delusions and a possible host of other symptoms.

Symptoms of Schizophrenia

- The symptoms are so varied that it is useful to categories them in one of a number of ways: Schneider (1959) described what he termed 'first rank symptoms' (Table 23.1). To be diagnosed with schizophrenia, one or more of these needs to be present:

  1. Thought disturbance.

  2. Hallucinations.

  3. Delusions.

- Similarly the DSM-IV (categorization system used by the American Psychiatric Association) believe that a schizophrenic has to be suffering one or more of the following symptoms:

  1. Control of thoughts.

  2. Hallucinatory voices.

  3. Delusions of control.

  4. Other persistent delusions.

Major symptoms

1. Thought disorder in which there are breaks in the train of thought and the person appears to make illogical jumps from one topic to another (loose association). Words may become confused and sentences incoherent (so called 'word salad').

2. Psychomotor disturbances (or catatonic behavior): Here the patient may adopt strange postures or engage in repetitive movements such as pacing or rocking (which I witnessed in one Victorian-style asylum I visited… as a student!). Catatonic refers to the tendency of some patients to hold a particular position for an extended length of time (in extreme cases several years).

Table 23.1: First rank symptoms of schizophrenia

Symptom	Variations	Description
Thought disturbance or control of thought	Insertion	Thoughts are being placed in the mind by external forces
	Withdrawal	Thoughts are being removed from the mind by external forces
	Broadcasting	Thoughts are being broadcast to others, e.g. over the radio or through the TV
Hallucinations	Auditory	The most common symptom of schizophrenia. Voices telling the person what to do
	Other senses	For example touch or visual. The schizophrenic might see Elvis or feel people touching them.
Delusions	Grandeur	Thinking himself Napoleon really is quite common amongst schizophrenics.
	Persecution	A worrying one in which they think people are out to get them. (Also common in sleep deprivation studies).
	Reference	The person believes those characters in a book, songs or in films is actually referring to them.

3. Lack of volition: In which, a person becomes totally apathetic and sits around waiting for things to happen. They engage in no self-motivated behavior. Their get up and go has got up and gone.

4. Disturbances of effect were the patient may show little in the way of emotional response or in some situations may exhibit inappropriate emotional responses:

- Blunting: Show few signs of emotional sensitivity (e.g. on the death of a friend)

- Flattened effect: More general loss of emotional expression.

- Inappropriate effect: Laugh at bad news or at a funeral (think of the 'giggle-loop' in coupling).

- First rank symptoms appear to be describing the 'core' characteristics of schizophrenia and the ones that most people find most concerning. Slater and Roth on the other hand see these so called 'first rank' symptoms as being secondary manifestations of other underlying processes.

- There is one other, particularly useful, way in which the symptoms can be broken down:

1. **Positive symptoms:** These refer to the characteristics that appear in addition to existing behavior, e.g. hallucinations, delusions and thought disturbances such as thought insertion.

2. **Negative symptoms:** Refer to those symptoms that an impairment of usual behaviors such as psychomotor disturbances, lack of volition, disturbances of mood and thought disorders.

Types of Schizophrenia

• The validity of schizophrenia has a single disorder is questioned by many. This is a useful point to emphasize in any essay on the disorder. The symptoms are so diverse and the possible causes so varied that it seems likely that we are in fact dealing with many different psychological disorders.

• One way round this problem is to consider different types of schizophrenia. Below are the main five subdivisions which just a brief description of each.

Paranoid schizophrenia

• Characterized by type I or positive symptoms. Typically the paranoid schizophrenic experiences delusions of persecution or grandeur that are very detailed and complex.

• Sometimes they are seeking money but often want to give advice on how to run the country or on impending disaster. This category is odd in that patients do not have any of the negative symptoms and other than their strange beliefs show no outward signs of their condition.

Disorganised schizophrenia (formerly hebephrenic)

• Hebephrenic means 'silly mind.' The characteristics of this disorder are silly and incoherent behaviour such as giggling and inane laughter and a tendency to talk about meaningless topics for hours. Negative symptoms such as disorganized behaviour and incoherent language are common.

Catonic schizophrenia

Characterised by impairment of body movement. This may involve wild and uncontrolled movements that put themselves or others in danger or may be simply holding one particular posture for long periods of time.

• 'Waxy flexibility' may also result, when someone attempts to move them they simply freeze in the new position instead. The movements may coincide with hallucinations, often about death and catastrophe.

Simple schizophrenia

Characterised by a withdrawal from reality resulting in declining academic performance, loss of friends and extreme apathy or loss of volition.

Note: Simple schizophrenia is not recognized by all categorizations of the disorder.

Other neurological problems are mentioned below.

Phobias

These are the fearful reaction to leaving home, entering shops, crowds and public places.

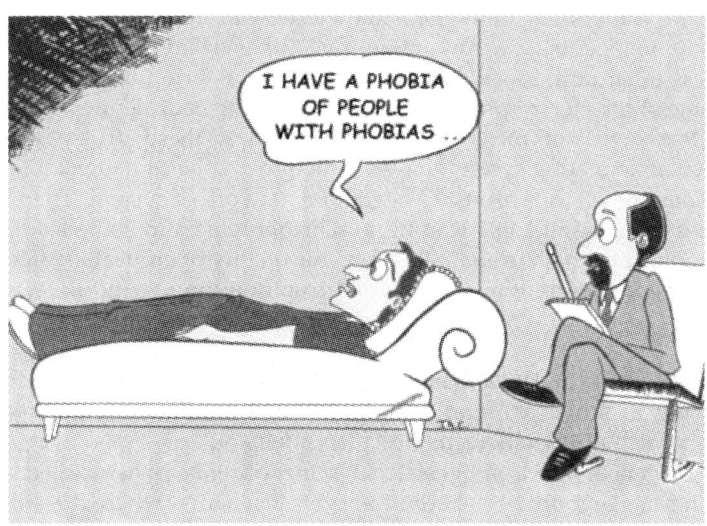

OBSESSIVE COMPULSIVE DISORDER

- It is characterized by recurrent obsessional thoughts or compulsive acts. Obsession thoughts are ideas, images or impulses that enter the patient's mind again and again in a stereotyped form.
- They are almost invariably distressing and the patient often tries unsuccessfully to resist them. Compulsive acts or rituals are stereotyped behaviors that are repeated again and again. Anxiety is almost invariably present. If compulsive acts are restricted, anxiety gets worse.

Dissociative Disorder

A partial or complete loss of normal integration between memories of past, awareness of identity and immediate sensation and control of bodily movements are the characteristic features. They tend to remit after weeks or months particularly if their onset is associated with the traumatic life events.

Mental Retardation

- It is composed arrested or incomplete development of the mind, which is especially characterized by the impairment of skills manifested during the development period that contribute to the overall level of intelligence, i.e. cognitive, language, motor and social abilities. Retardation can occur with or without other mental or physical condition.
- The psychological dysfunction mediating the schizophrenic process is to be found in the information.
- Processing sequence— the sensory attentional, perceptual, cognitive processes and is probably linked to impairment in arousal mechanism. Many schizophrenic patients, either hyperactive or inactive-retarded types, are in a state of over arousal.
- The neural organization usually considered to be involved in regulating the level of arousal are the brainstem and thalamic system that make up the 'classical' ascending reticular

activating or arousal system. Behavioral and electro-physiological observation suggests that the antipsychotic agents, by an action on this system decreases sensory input or responsiveness to stimuli, lower arousal level and thus bring about clinical improvement. However, some of the electro-physiological effects of the neuroleptics may merely reflect the 'sedative' effects and not the antipsychotic action of these drugs. The arousal system includes reticular activating system, limbic structure and basal ganglia.

- There may be more than one arousal system or a network of system. Therefore there may be many varieties of 'arousal' some leading to schizophrenia and some leading to other forms of psychopathology or to none at all. Possibly, the quality of arousal in affective disorder, e.g. manic depression, is different from that in schizophrenia.

Biochemical Basis

- In our body, dopamine and acetylcholine both are present appropriately in CNS for normal functioning. But in schizophrenia, the concentration of dopamine increases greater than acetylcholine, which ultimately leads to schizophrenia.
- There is an evidence which suggests that schizophrenia is associated with presence of greater than normal amount of dopamine at central synapse, where it results in overfiring of neurons.
- Blocking dopamine receptors causes depletion of dopaminergic neurons. This result in an increase in concentration of excitory component (acetylcholine) and decreasing the concentration of inhibitory component (dopamine).
- Antipsychotic drugs shift the balance in favor of acetylcholine, this difference between the concentration of dopamine and acetylcholine leads to an increase in extra pyramidal effects (posture and the involuntary aspect of movement). Hence all anti-psychotic drugs are always associated with a varying degree of extra pyramidal effect.

Mechanism of Action (Fig. 23.1)

- It has been postulated that neurotransmitter agents interfere with central dopaminergic mechanism. They block the post-synaptic dopamine receptor. Antagonism of dopamine-mediated synaptic neurotransmission is an important action of neuroleptic drug. Almost all of the clinically effective antipsychotic agent have characteristically high affinity for D1-D2 receptor site.
- Drugs like chlorpromazine increases metabolic rate of dopamine. Blocking of D2 receptor and reserpine like drug which causes depletion of dopaminergic neuron. This results in increase in concentration of excitatory component. (ACh) and decreasing the concentration of inhibitory component (dopamine). There is an evidence of direct quantitative correlation between the antipsychotic activity of various neuroleptic drugs and their ability to block H-dopamine in the neostraital slices. The entire antipsychotic drug increases the turnover of dopamine in the brain.
- All antipsychotic drugs tend to block D2 receptors in the dopamine pathways of the brain. This means that dopamine released in these pathways has less effect. Excess release of dopamine in the mesolimbic pathway has been linked to psychotic experiences. It is the blockade of dopamine receptors in this pathway which is thought to control psychotic experiences.
- Typical antipsychotics are not particularly selective and also block dopamine receptors in the mesocortical pathway, tuberoinfundibular pathway and the nigrostriatal pathway. Blocking D2 receptors in these other pathways is thought to produce some of the unwanted side effects that the typical antipsychotics can produce. They were commonly classified on a

spectrum of low potency to high potency, where potency referred to the ability of the drug to bind to dopamine receptors, and not to the effectiveness of the drug. High potency antipsychotics such as haloperidol typically have doses of a few milligrams and cause less sleepiness and calming effects than low potency antipsychotics such as chlorpromazine and thioridazine, which have dosages of several hundred milligrams. The latter have a greater degree of anticholinergic and antihistaminergic activity which can counteract dopamine-related side effects.

- Atypical antipsychotic drugs have a similar blocking effect on D2 receptors. Some also block or partially block serotonin receptors (particularly 5HT2A, and 5HT1A receptors): Ranging from risperidone which acts overwhelmingly on serotonin receptors, to amisulpride which has no serotonergic activity. The additional effects on serotonin receptors may be why some of them can benefit the 'negative symptoms' of schizophrenia.

Dopamine

- The brain neurotransmitter most frequently linked with schizophrenia is dopamine. Initially the dopamine receptors were divided into D1 and D2. This division is based on the ligand binding properties and coupling with second messenger system. Both are located predominantly postsynaptically in the brain region. D2 receptors are also located presynaptically where they function to regulate dopamine synthesis and release. D1 receptors have positive coupling with adenylate cyclase activity.

- Most neuroleptic agents show preference for D2 receptors over D1 receptors. Newer agents show greater selectivity in receptor. Sulpiride showed selectivity for D2 receptors and clozapine for D1 receptors.

- Recently by cloning technique new subtype, of dopamine receptors, D3, D4 and D5 have been identified. The D3 and D4 subtype couple to Gi proteins to inhibit adenyl cyclase. These finding have added to the complexity of selectivity of receptors. The overall distribution pattern of D3 receptor indicates its role in emotional functioning and thus provides a potential important target for antipsychotic drug therapy.

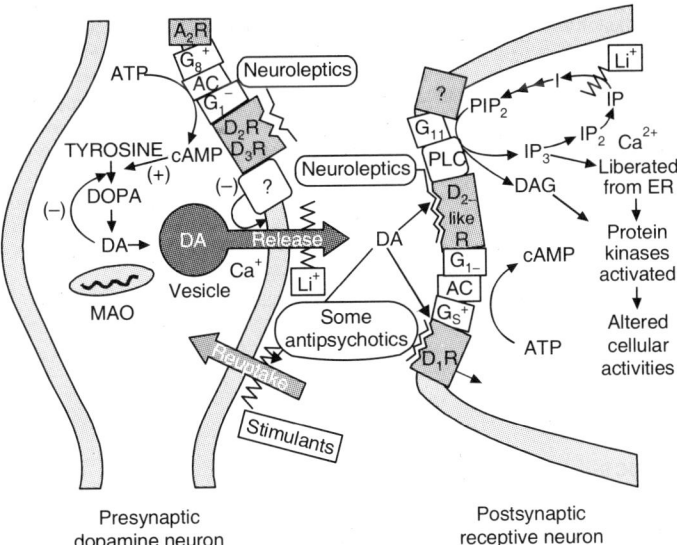

Fig. 23.1: Mode of action of antipsychotic drugs

Serotonin

- Interest in a possible role of 5-HT in schizophrenia has been due to the fact that many atypical neuroleptics have 5-HT antagonist properties. Seven major classes of 5-HT receptors, designated 5-HT1 through 5-HT1 have been identified.
- These are all G-protein-coupled neuronal membrane receptors (except 5-HT3). Ritanserine a more selective 5-HT2 antagonist was shown to improve psychotic symptoms. Clozapine has also been shown to bind to 5-HT3 receptors. Thus clozapine shows mixed 5-HT2/D2 antagonist activity. One such agent with mixed activity in clinical use is risperidone.

Norepinephrine

- Disease state dependency of alteration in norepinephrine turnover in schizophrenia has been proposed. Adrenergic antagonism (α2) may contribute to therapeutic effectiveness of clozapine. The (α2)-adrenergic antagonist, idozoxan affected significant reduction in schizo-affective disorder. Distinction between typical and atypical group is not clearly defined. It has been done on the basis of extrapyramidal side effects and partly on the basis of receptor specificity. Among them such side effects are minimum in 'atypical neuroleptics'.

CLASSIFICATION OF NEUROLEPTICS

Flow chart 23.1 depicts classification of neuroleptics.

Flow chart 23.1: Classification of neuroleptics

```
                    ┌──────────────────────────────┐
                    │ Classification of Neuroleptics│
                    └──────────────────────────────┘
        ┌───────────────────┬──────────────────┬───────────────────┐
   ┌─────────────┐   ┌─────────────┐    ┌─────────────┐
   │   Typical   │   │Phenothiazines│    │  Atypical   │
   │ neuroleptics│   │             │    │ neuroleptics│
   └─────────────┘   └─────────────┘    └─────────────┘
```

Typical neuroleptics:

Rauwolfia alkaloids
Reserpine, deserpidine, rescinnamine

Thioxanthene derivatives
Chlorprothixene, thiothixene, flupenthixol

Flurobutyrphenones
Haloperidol, trifluperidol

Diphenylmethane derivatives
Hydroxyzine, benactyzine

Phenothiazines:

Propyl dialkylamino side chains
Chlorpromazine, promazine, triflupromazine

Propyl piperazine side chains
Prochlorperazine, perphenazine, trifluperazine

Alkyl piperidyl side chain
Thioridazine, mesoridazine

Atypical neuroleptics:

Bnzamide derivatives
Sulpiride

Diphenylbutyl piperidines
Pimozide, penfluridol, fluspirilene

Dibenzyldiazepine
Clozapine, olanzapine

Typical Neuroleptics

A. Phenothiazines

Propyl Dialkylamino Side Chain

Promazine

Chlorpromazine

Triflupromazine

Propyl Piperazine Side Chain

Prochlorperazine

Perphenazine

Trifluperazine

Fluphenazine

Acetophenazine

Carphenazine

Butaperazine

Thioethylperazine

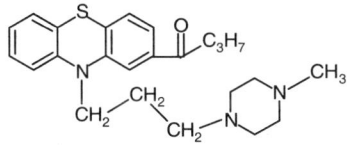

Thiopropazate

Alkyl Piperidyl Side Chain

Thioridazine

Mesoridazine

B. Thioxanthene Derivatives

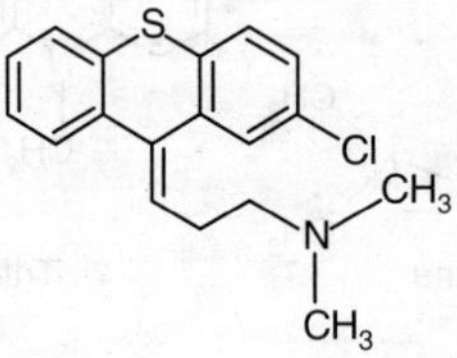

Chlorprothixene

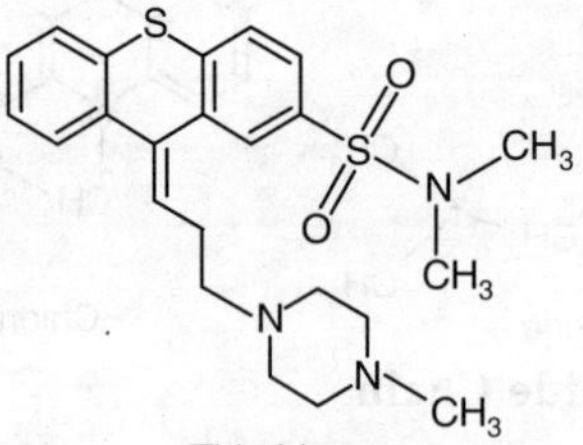

Thiothixene

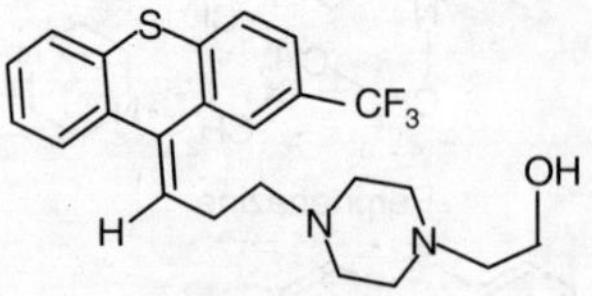

Flupenthixol

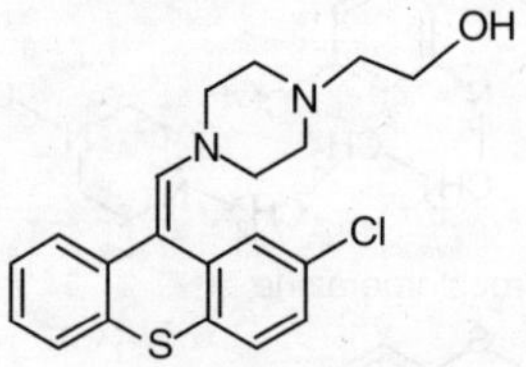

Clopenthixol

D. Rauwolfia Alkaloids

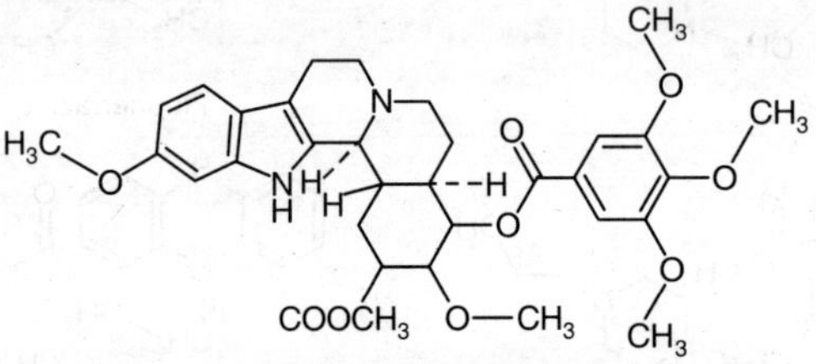

Reserpine

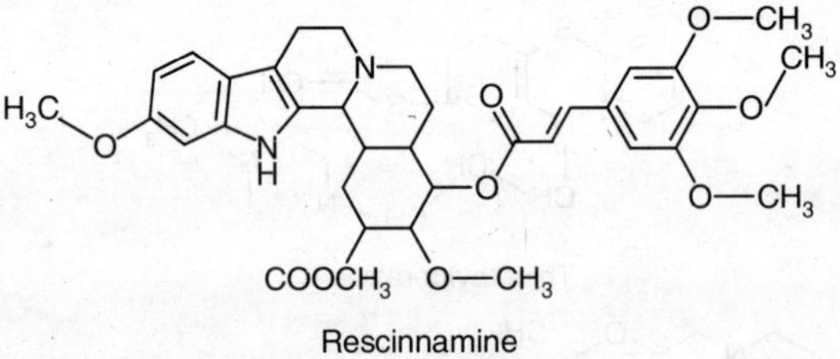

Rescinnamine

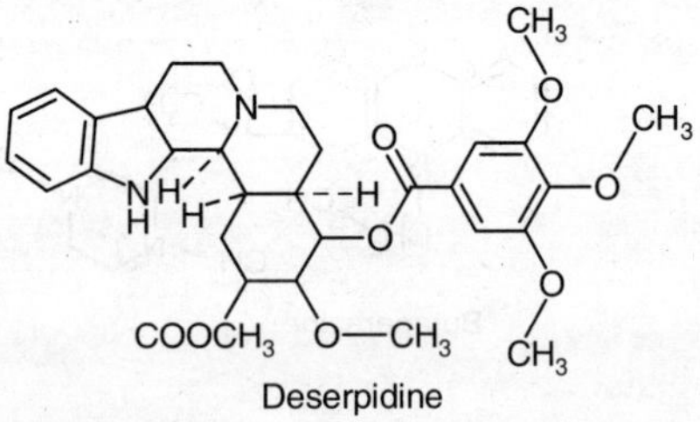

Deserpidine

E. Flurobutyrphenone Derivatives

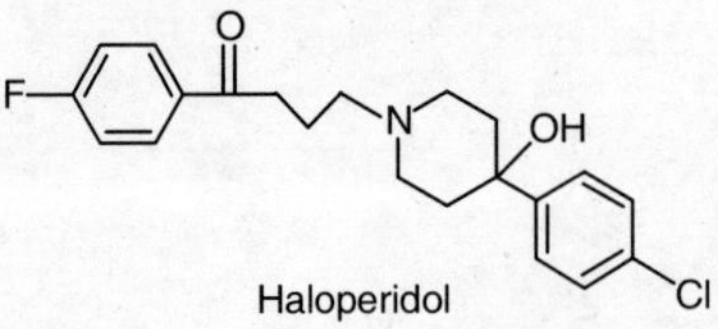

Haloperidol

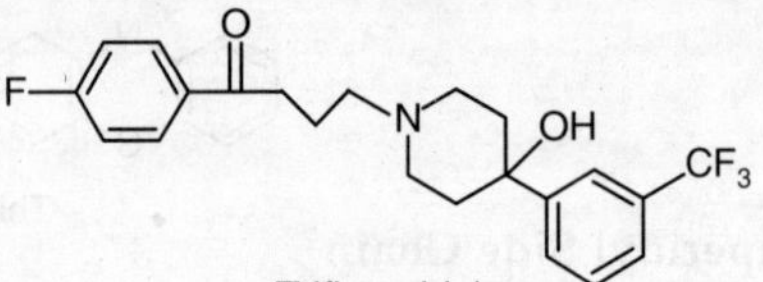

Trifluperidol

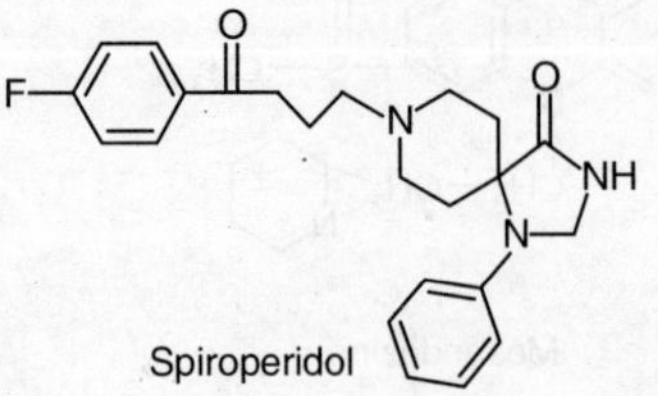

Spiroperidol

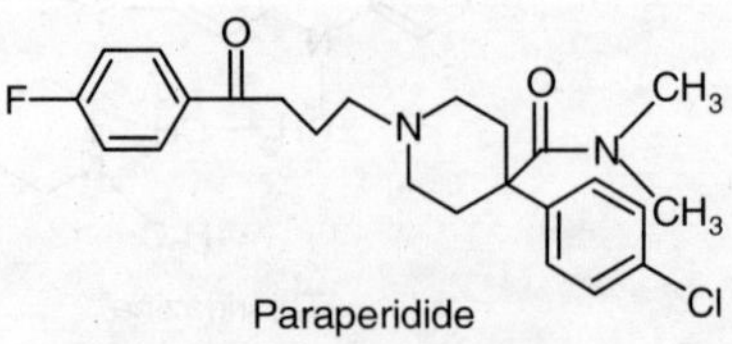

Paraperidide

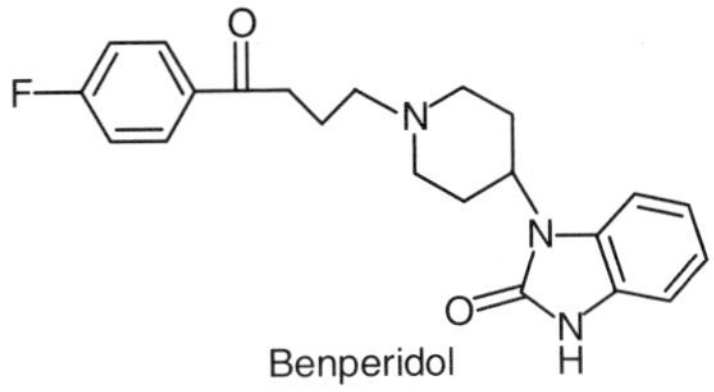

Benperidol

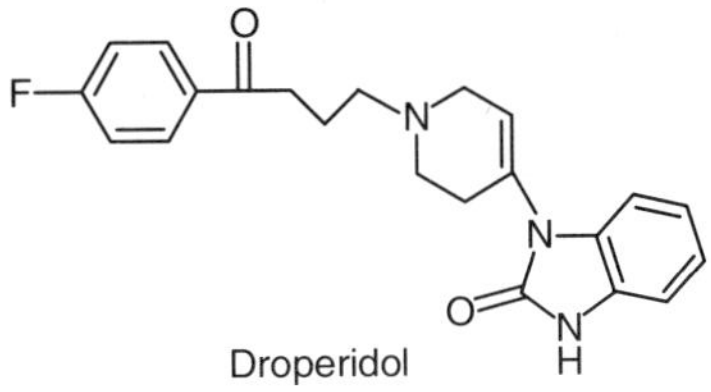

Droperidol

F. Diphenylmethane Derivatives

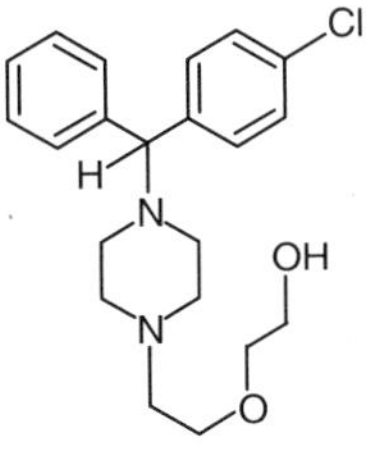

Hydroxyzine

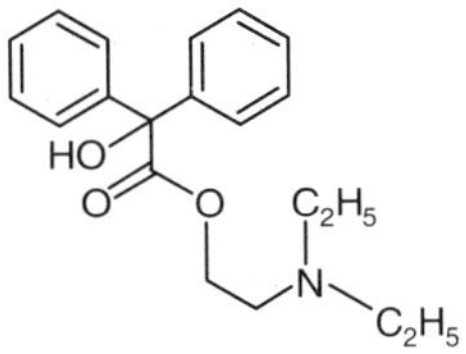

Benactyzine

Atypical Neroleptics

A. Benzamide Derivatives

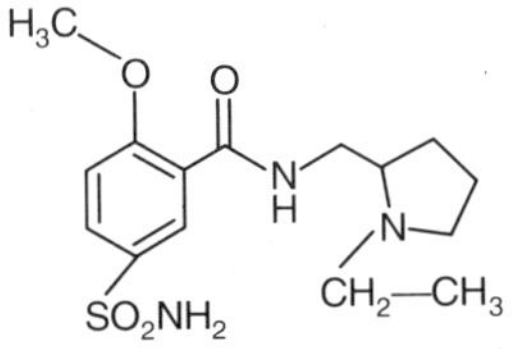

Sulpiride

B. Diphenylbutylpiperidines

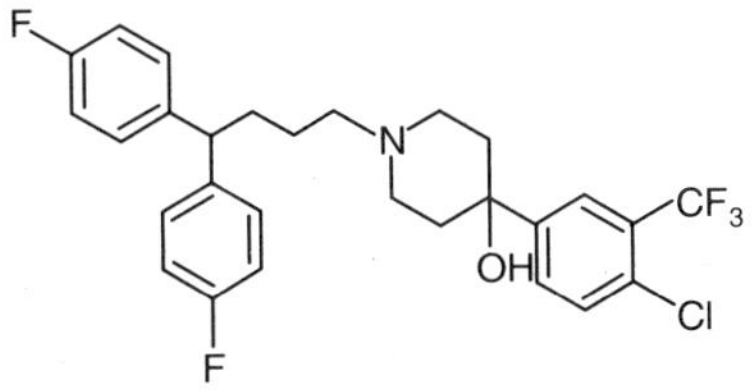

Penfluridol

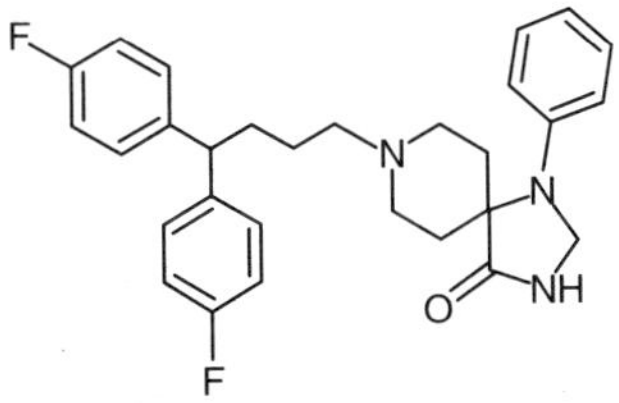

Fluspirilene

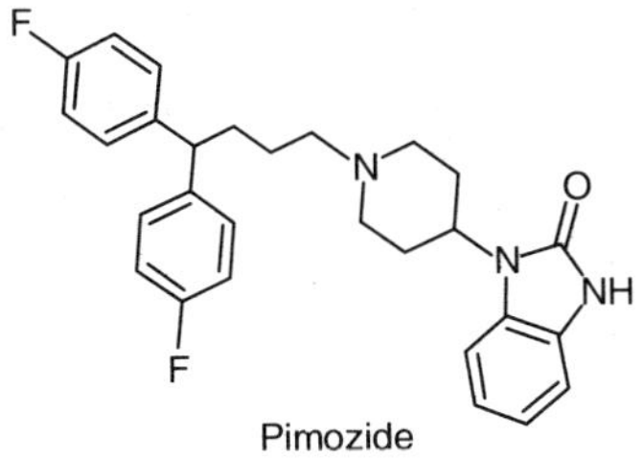

Pimozide

C. Dibenzyldiazepines

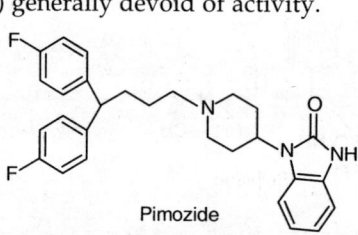

Olanzapine

Clozapine

PHENOTHIAZINE DERIVATIVES

Structure–Activity Relationship

Tricyclic system

1. Most of these compounds have either a six-membered central ring or seven-membered central ring.
2. Compounds having larger central ring are usually devoid of significant anti-psychotic activity.
3. Compounds with a five-membered central ring, e.g. carbazole, also lack anti-psychotic activity and produce only antidepressant effects.
4. Analogs of tricyclic compounds that lack a central ring are (with some exception) generally devoid of activity.

Imipramine

Carbazole

Pimozide

Modification of the Basic Amino Group

1. Maximum neuroleptic potency is retained in compounds having tertiary amino group. In compounds with secondary or primary amino group, activity is either reduced or abolished.
2. In general, alkylation of the basic amino groups larger than methyl, decreases neuroleptic activity.
3. In pharmacological screening, potency is found to be decreased by replacement of dimethylamino group of chlorpromazine with pyrrolidinyl, morphinyl or thiomorphinyl groups.
4. Activity is retained or increased, if the amino group is incorporated in cyclic systems like piperidyl or piperazine, e.g. carphenazine.
5. Bridged piperidine derivatives though are bulky; still retain a high degree of neuroleptic property.

Carfenazine

6. Introduction of hydroxyl, methyl, hydroxymethyl groups at position 4 of piperidine and piperazine moieties result in increase in potency.

7. Piperazine phenothiazine may be esterified with long chain fatty acid to produce slowly absorbed, long acting, lipophilic prodrug.

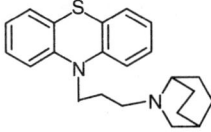

Bridged piperidine derivatives

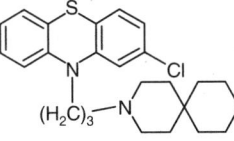

Esteres of piperazino phenothiazine

8. Significant activity is retained when N-4 piperazine substituent are as larger as phenylmethyl or p-aminophenylethyl.

9. In the series of 4,4-disubstituted piperidinyl propyl phenothiazinesazaspirone, is clinically effective anti-psychotic.

10. Replacement of terminal N, N-diethylamino group by piperidino exploits the decreasing valency angle at 30-nitrogen of the latter so that access of the basic group to anionic sites might be decreased.

Azaspirones

Modification of the Alkyl Side Chain

1. Maximum potency is observed for antipsychotic activity, when the nitrogen of phenothiazines ring and the more basic side chain nitrogen is connected by a 3-carbons side chain.

2. Branching at the β-position of the side chain with a small methyl group results in decrease in activity. This is perhaps due to steric repulsion between the methyl group at the β-position and the 1, 9-perihydrogen of phenothiazine rings, resulting in the coplanirity of the benzene ring.

3. Introduction of a methyl group into 2 or 3 position of the 3-aminopropyl side chain has only minor or little influence on activity.

4. Bridging of position 3 of the side chain to position 1 of the phenothiazine significantly reduces neuroleptic activity.

Phenothiazine Ring Substitution

1. With some exception, substitution at position 2 is optimal for neuroleptic potency. In general, potency increases in the following order of ring position 1<4<3<2.

2. 2-substitution of the phenothiazine nucleus increases neuroleptic potency in the following order OH<H<CH$_3$<Cl<CF$_3$.

3. In general disubstitution has a little effect on potency.

4. Oxidation of sulfur at 5-position in antipsychotic phenothiazine decreases neuroleptic activity.

▓ BUTYROPHENONE

- Next to phenothiazine the most active group of the antipsychotic agents are butyrophenones. Haloperidol is the prototype in this series.

- The structures of butyrophenones are different from the phenothiazines but they have same pharmacological property. Haloperidol is used as standard antipsychotic agent and several other agents are also in clinical use.

Structure–Activity Relationship

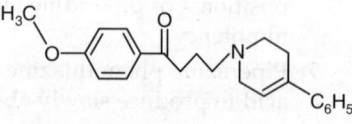

Butyrophenone

1. The potent compound have 4-flurorophenyl group, except, anisoperidone which has methoxy group in the para position of phenyl ring.
2. Reduction of the carbonyl group to CHOH as well as replacement by oxygen or sulfur decreases neuroleptic potency, whereas replacement of the ketone by a sulfones results in a loss of activity.
3. As a rule, lengthening, shortening, or branching of the propylene chain of 4-aminobutyrophenone decrease neuroleptic potency.
4. Considerable variation is possible in the tertiary amino group with retention of neuroleptic activity. The basic nitrogen could be part of a six-membered ring,(piperidine,1,2,3,6-tetrahydropyridyl or piperzinyl). Replacement of six-membered basic heterocycle by larger or smaller or uncyclized amines diminishes neuroleptic potency.
5. Neuroleptic potency is generally associated with 4, 4-disubstituted piperidines. Substitution of 2 or 3 position of piperidines markedly decrease potency. The decrease in basicity of piperidine nitrogen by amide formation or quarternization abolishes activity.
6. High neuroleptic potency among derivative of 4-piperazinyl butyrophenone requires an aromatic substitution in position of the piperazine ring.
7. Modification of the butyrophenone side chain by replacement of the keto function with a 4-flourophenylmethane moiety produced the diphenylbutylpiperidine derivative. These agents are inherently long acting.

Azabuperone

Mechanism of Action

- The diversity of the structure of antipsychotic agents presents a problem for a unfield theory to explain their mode of action. It has been postulated that neuroleptic agents interfere with central dopaminergic mechanisms.
- They block the post-synaptic dopamine receptors. A very good correlation has been found between average clinical dose and blockade of dopamine release. Antagonism of dopamine mediated synaptic neurotransmission is an important action of neuroleptic drug. Almost all of the clinically effective antipsychotic agents have characteristically high affinity for D_1-D_2 receptor sites. Although thioxanthenes have high affinity for dopamine D_1 receptors.
- Clozapine is a potent α_1-adrenergic antagonist, also it has a unique profile to block D_1 receptors; M_1 muscarinic antagonist activity, effects on $5HT_1C$ receptors and inhibition of mesolimbic DA release. Involvement of 5HT, sigma ligands in drug therapy of schizophrenia cannot be ruled out.

Chlorpromazine

2-chloro-
phenothiazine

+

3-dimethylamino-
propylchloride

NaNH₂
sodium
amide

Chlorpromazine

Prochlorperazine

2-chloro-10-(3-chloro-
propyl) phenothiazine

+

1-methyl-
piperazine

→

Prochlorperazine

Fluphenazine

1-(3-hydroxy propyl
piperazine)

+

methyl
formate

→

4-(3-hydroxypropyl)-
piperazine-1-carbox-
aldehyde

$\xrightarrow[\text{thionyl chloride}]{SOCl_2}$ I

4-(3-chloropropyl)-
piperazine-1-
carbox-aldehyde

+

2-trifluoromethyl-
phenothiazine

$\xrightarrow[\text{sodium amide}]{NaNH_2}$

$\xrightarrow{NaOH}$ II

10-[3-(1-piperazinyl) propyl)]-
2-trifluoromethyl-
phenothiazine (II)

1. 2-bromethyl acetate
2. aq. HCl

Fluphenazine

Thioridazine

2-chloro-
benzoic acid

+

3-methylthio-
aniline

$\xrightarrow{K_2CO_3,\ Cu}$

N-(3-methylthiophenyl)-
anthranilic acid

$\xrightarrow{\Delta}$ I

3-methylthiodi-
phenylamine (I)

$\xrightarrow{S,\ I_2}$

2-methylthio-
phenothiazine

1. sodium amide
2. 2-(2-chloroethyl)-
1-methylpiperidine

1. NaNH₂
2.

Thioridazine

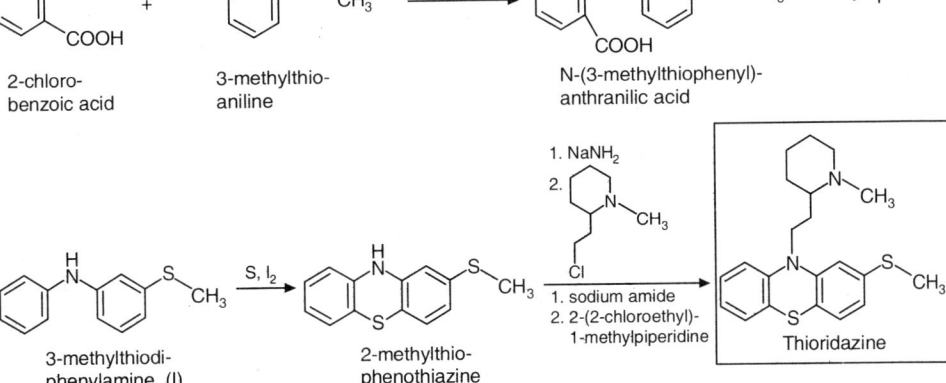

Mesoridazine

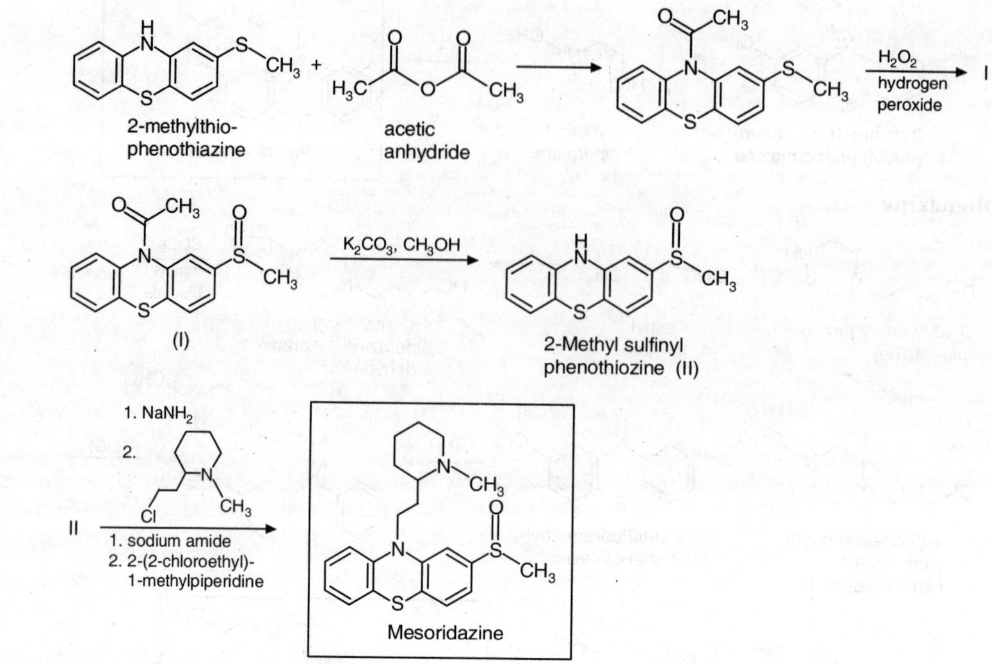

2-methylthio-
phenothiazine

acetic
anhydride

H₂O₂
hydrogen
peroxide
→ I

(I)

K₂CO₃, CH₃OH

2-Methyl sulfinyl
phenothiozine (II)

1. NaNH₂
2.

II

1. sodium amide
2. 2-(2-chloroethyl)-
1-methylpiperidine
→

Mesoridazine

Haloperidol

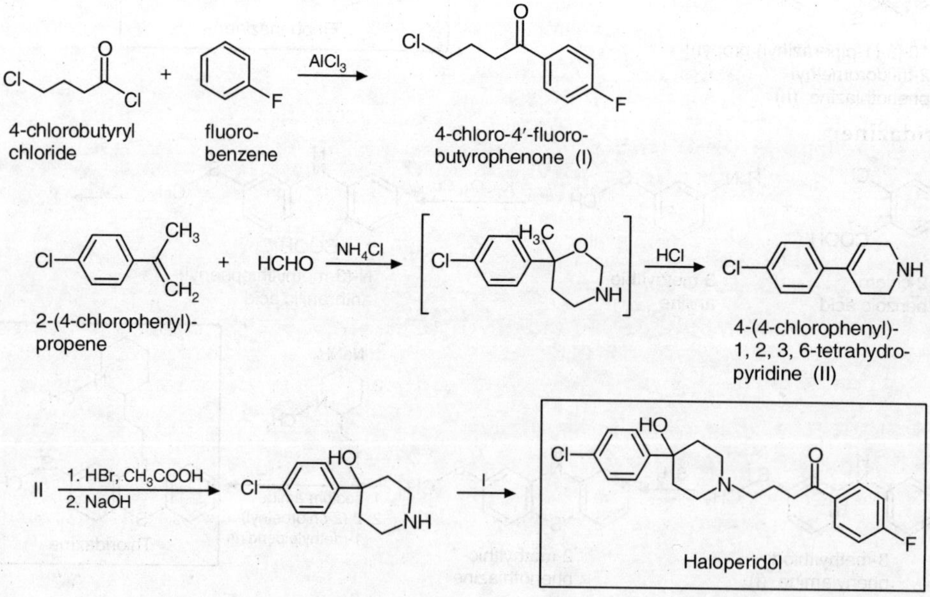

4-chlorobutyryl
chloride

fluoro-
benzene

AlCl₃

4-chloro-4'-fluoro-
butyrophenone (I)

2-(4-chlorophenyl)-
propene

+ HCHO

NH₄Cl

HCl

4-(4-chlorophenyl)-
1, 2, 3, 6-tetrahydro-
pyridine (II)

II

1. HBr, CH₃COOH
2. NaOH

I

Haloperidol

Droperidol

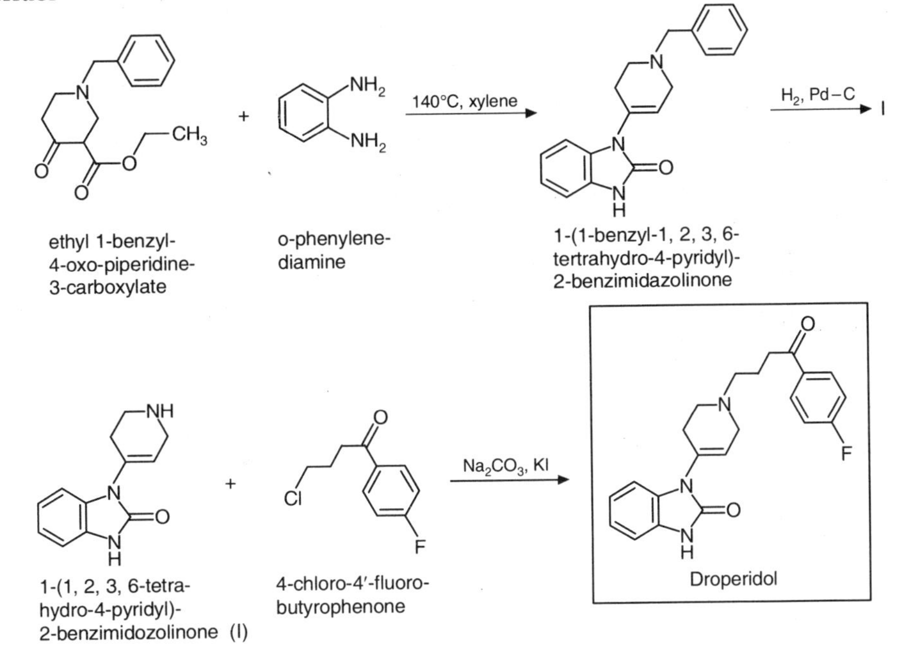

ethyl 1-benzyl-
4-oxo-piperidine-
3-carboxylate

o-phenylene-
diamine

140°C, xylene

1-(1-benzyl-1, 2, 3, 6-
tertrahydro-4-pyridyl)-
2-benzimidazolinone

H_2, Pd–C

I

1-(1, 2, 3, 6-tetra-
hydro-4-pyridyl)-
2-benzimidozolinone (I)

4-chloro-4'-fluoro-
butyrophenone

Na_2CO_3, KI

Droperidol

Hydroxyzine

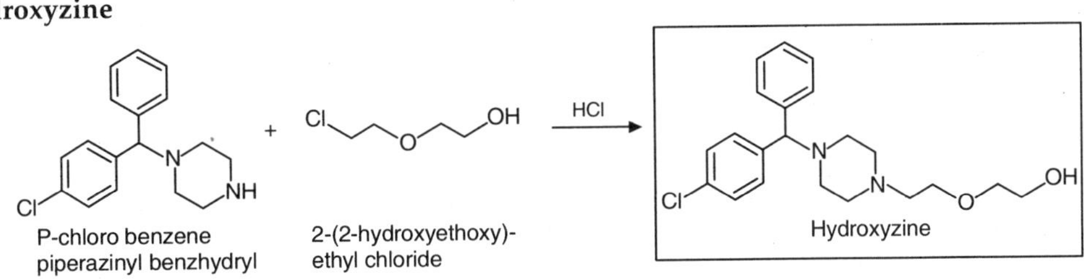

P-chloro benzene
piperazinyl benzhydryl

2-(2-hydroxyethoxy)-
ethyl chloride

HCl

Hydroxyzine

Penfluridol

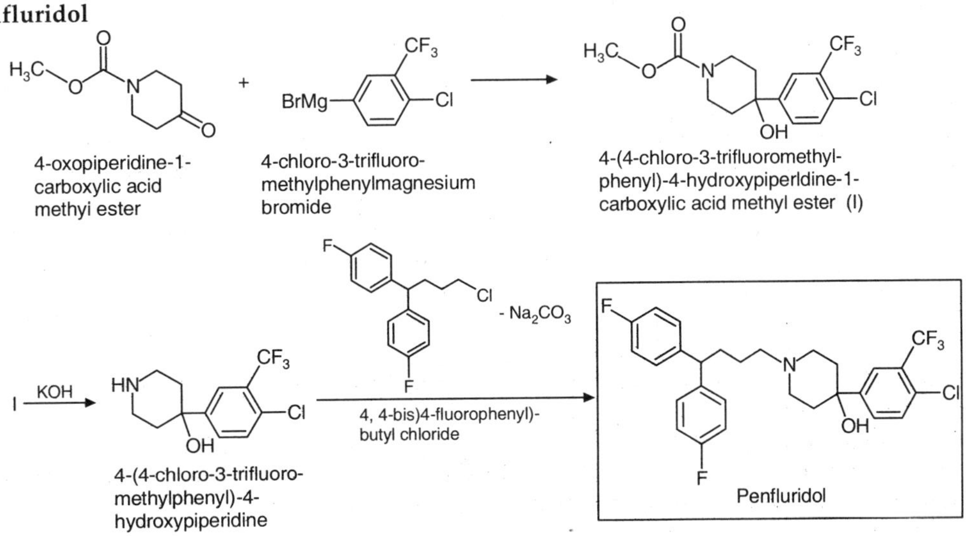

4-oxopiperidine-1-
carboxylic acid
methyi ester

4-chloro-3-trifluoro-
methylphenylmagnesium
bromide

4-(4-chloro-3-trifluoromethyl-
phenyl)-4-hydroxypiperldine-1-
carboxylic acid methyl ester (I)

I

KOH

4-(4-chloro-3-trifluoro-
methylphenyl)-4-
hydroxypiperidine

4, 4-bis)4-fluorophenyl)-
butyl chloride

- Na_2CO_3

Penfluridol

24

Antidepressant Agents

DEPRESSION

Depression is an intense normal response but usually a relatively brief duration of loss and disappointment. It is a prominent feature of several mood disorders (affective disorders).

Symptoms

1. A general feeling of missing, apathy and hopelessness.
2. Preoccupation with guilt, inadequacy and ugliness.
3. Loss of appetite.
4. Slowing of movements.
5. Indecisiveness.

Types

1. Bipolar depression: Here mood and behavior oscillate between depression and mania.

2. Unipolar depression: This depression develops earlier in life and tends to be inherited, it may have feature in common with schizophrenia and more often related to adverse circumstances. Unipolar depression, is more common than bipolar depression and more often related to adverse circumstances, it is common to later in life and is often associated with features of anxiety and aggression.

Biochemical Basis of Depression (Fig. 24.1)

- Many studies have sought to test the amine hypothesis by looking for biochemical abnormalities in cerebrospinal fluid (CSF), blood or urine, or in postmortem brain tissue, from depressed or manic patients.
- They have included studies of monoamine metabolites, receptors, enzymes and transporters, largely with negative results. The major metabolites of noradrenaline and 5-HT, respectively, are 3-methoxy-4-hydroxyphenylglycol (MHPG) and 5-hydroxyindoleacetic acid (5-HIAA) respectively. These appear in the CSF, blood and urine. There are two fundamental problems in relating changes in the concentration of these metabolites in body fluids to changes in transmitter function in the brain. One is that many secondary factors can affect their concentration, such as diet; transport between CSF, blood and urine; or release of monoamines from non-cerebral sites.
- The second is that many patients receive drug treatment, which affects the metabolite concentrations markedly.
- Studies of urinary MHPG excretion in normal and depressed subjects have shown convincingly that the level is reduced in bipolar depressive patients and is lower during the depressive than during the manic phase.

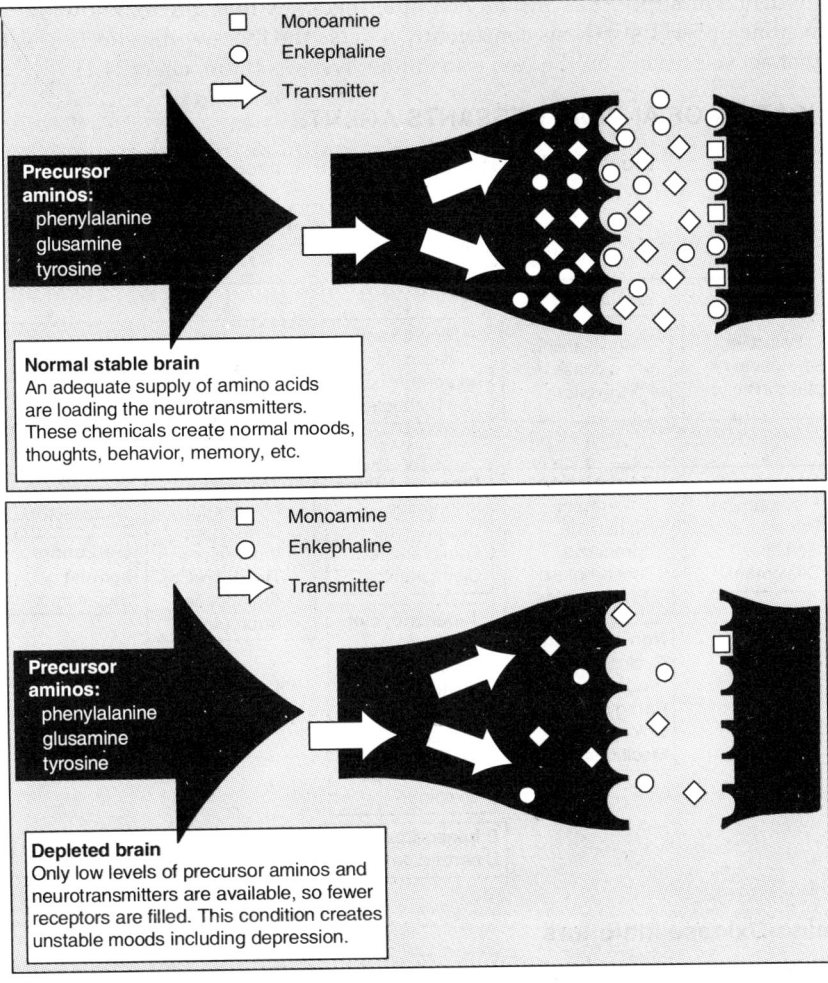

Fig. 24.1: Biochemical basis of depression

- In unipolar depression, however, MHPG excretion, though highly variable between patients, is not significantly lower than in controls, so support for the monoamine theory is at best equivocal. Plasma noradrenaline actually tends to be higher in depressed than in normal subjects, possibly because it reflects peripheral sympathetic activity, which increases with the anxiety that often accompanies depression. It too shows a cyclic variation in bipolar depressive patients.
- Results pertaining to altered 5-HT metabolism are also highly variable.
- Studies of 5-HIAA in CSF and urine have generally failed to find any clear correlation with depression. Low levels of 5-HIAA occur in the brain and CSF of suicide victims but could be associated with violent behavior rather than with depression.
- More consistent changes have been reported in the plasma concentration of L-tryptophan (TRP, the precursor of 5-HT). Though the resting levels are not significantly different in depressed patients, the rise in plasma TRP following an intravenous or oral dose is reduced, implying lower 'TRP availability'.

- Other evidence in support of the monoamine theory is that agents known to block either noradrenaline or 5-HT synthesis consistently reverse the therapeutic effects of antidepressant drugs that act selectively on the two transmitter systems (Flow chart 24.1).

CLASSIFICATION OF ANTIDEPRESSANTS AGENTS

Flow chart 24.1: Classification of antidepressants

```
                          ┌────────────────────┐
                          │   Antidepressant   │
                          └────────────────────┘
```

Selective serotonine re-uptake inhibitors	Mono-amino oxidase Inhibitors	Tricyclic anti-depressant (noradrenaline and 5-HT reuptake	Atypical anti-depressant	Miscellaneous

| Fluoxetine Fluvoxamine Paroxetine Sertaline Citalopram | **Hydralazines** Phenelzine Nialamide Iproniazid Isocarboxazid Pheniprazine | **Dibenzazepines** Imipramine Desipramine Trimipramine Clomipramine | Trazodone Minaserine Mirtazapine Venlafaxine Tianeptine Amineptine Bupropione | **Benzodiazepines** Alurazolam |

Non-hydrazines
Cyclopropylamine
Propargylamines
Paragyline
Chlorgyline
Meclobemide

Dibenzocycloh-eptanes
Amitriptyline
Nortriptyline
Protriptyline
Minaserine

Dibenzoxepine
Oxepine

Dibenzodiazepines
Dibenzepine

β-adrenoreceptor agonist
Salbutamol

Mono-Amino-Oxidase Inhibitors

A. Hydralazines

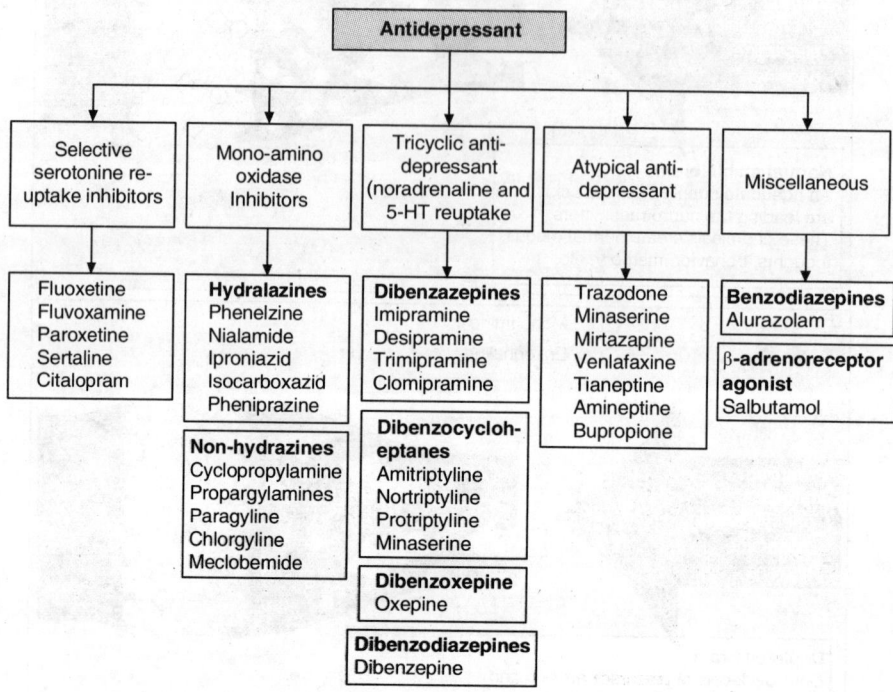

Iproniazid   Isocarboxazid   Phenelzine   Pheniprazine

B. Non-hydrazines

Tranylcypromine   Pargyline   Chlorgyline

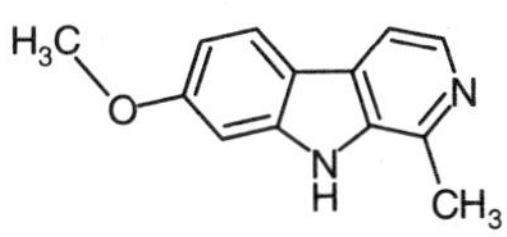

Harmine

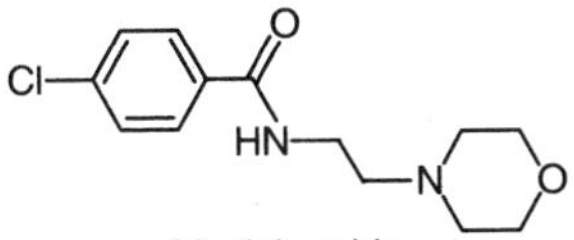

Meclobemide

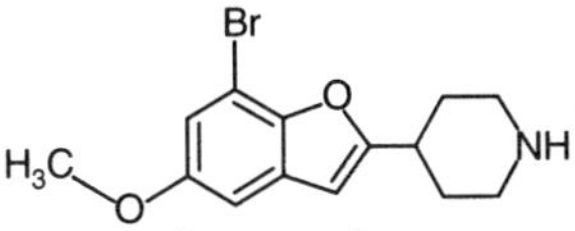

Bromaromine

Tricyclic Antidepressants

A. Dibenzazepines

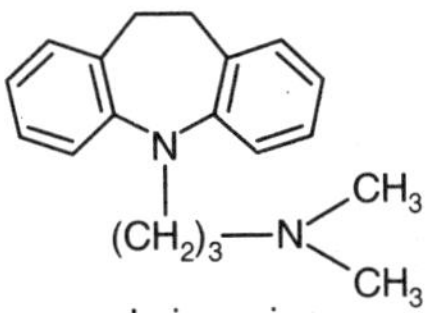

Imipramine

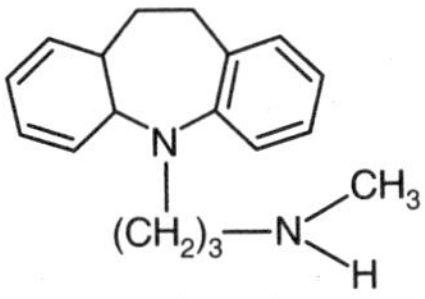

Desipramine

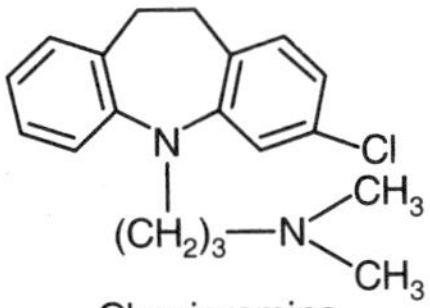

Clomipramine

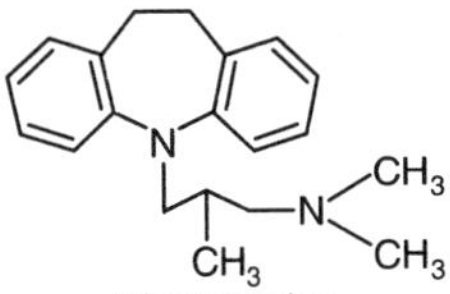

Trimipramine

B. Dibenzocycloheptanes

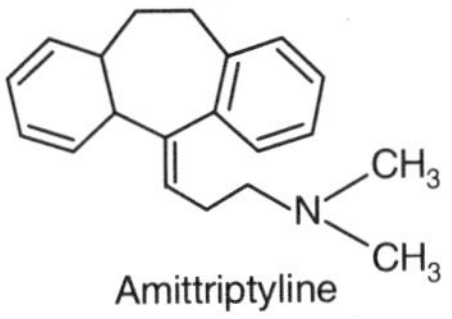

Amittriptyline

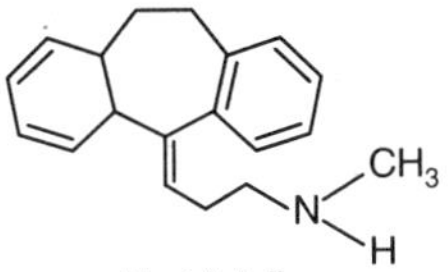

Nortriptyline

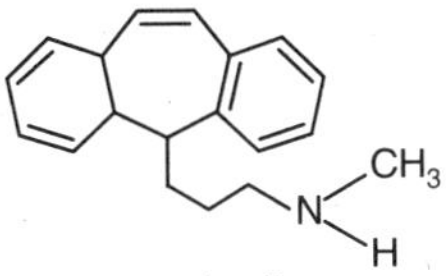

Protriptyline

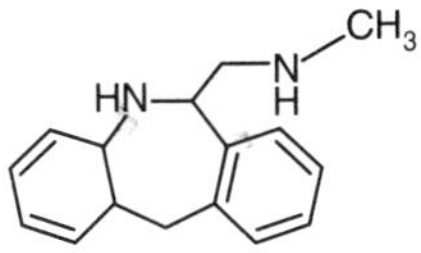

Minaserine

C. Diabezodiazepine Derivatives

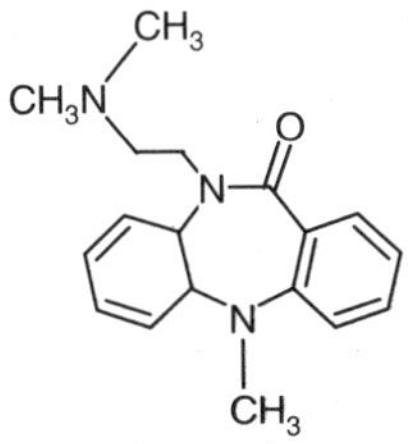

Dibenzepine

D. Dibenzoxepine Derivatives

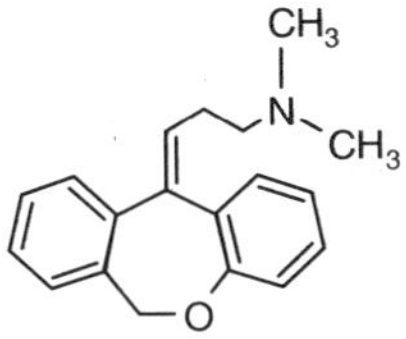

Doxepin

Serotonine Specific Reuptake Inhibitors

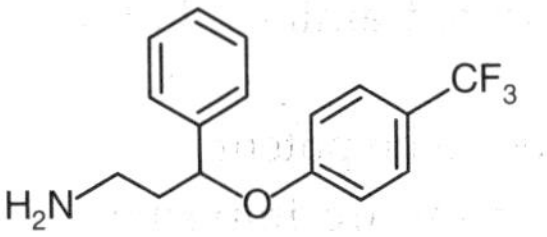

Norfluoxetine

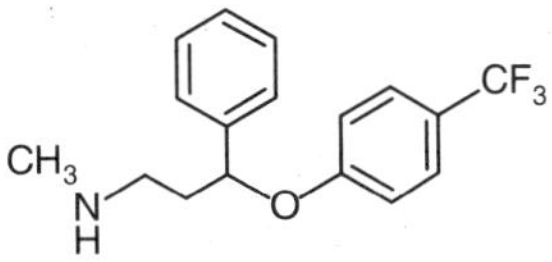

Fluoxetine

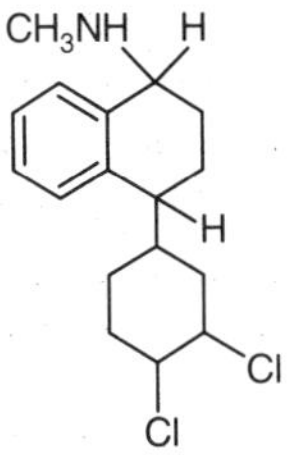

Sertaline

Paroxetine

Atypical Antidepressant

Trazodone

Nefazodone

Bupropione

Venlafaxine

▓ TRICYCLIC ANTIDEPRESSANT

Tricyclic Antidepressant

Structure–Activity Relationship

Variation in side chain

1. Maximum potency of antidepressant dihydrobenzodiazepines occurs when the basic nitrogen is separated from the tricyclic nucleolus by a propylene bridge.

2. Branching of the propylene chain, e.g. trimipramine, has little effect on anti-depressant activity.

3. Analogs bearing a carbonyl functionally in position 1 of the propyl side chain of imipramine have antidepressant-like activity.

4. Activity is confined to methyl substituted or unsubstituted amines. Larger alkyl group abolish activity and introduce toxicity.

5. Side chains with quinaclidine, morpholine nuclei claimed to be potent.

6. The tertiary amine and secondary amine in the side chain are important because they significantly affect both the monoamine reuptake activity as well as interaction with other receptors. For example, tertiary amine is more potent inhibitors of 5-HT reuptake while secondary amines are more potent in their inhibition of NE reuptake. Tertiary amines also have more potent activity to α1-adrenergic, muscarinic and histaminergic receptors.

Variation in ring substitution

1. Introduction of substituent at 3-position has little effect. 3-chloroimipramine is similar to imipramine. However, chlomipramine is more potent inhibitor of 5-HT reuptake and less of NE reuptake than imipramine.
2. 10-keto or methyl derivative is equipotent with desipramine.
3. 2, 8 dimethyl or 3, 7-dichloro are inactive.

Variation in ring system

1. The ring nitrogen of desipramine can be replaced by carbon to give active compounds.
2. Introduction of 10, 11-double bond and protriptyline enhances antidepressant activity.
3. Nortriptyline with exocyclic double bond and protriptyline with indocyclic double bond differ in their metabolism pattern. Protriptyline is less metabolized in vitro leading to prolonged half-life and lower dose requirements.
4. Several amitriptyline analogs with replacement of C-11 with O, S, SO, SO_2, NH, NCH_3 are clinically effective antidepressants.
5. The tricyclic compounds exhibit a lack of coplanirity of aromatic rings and differ in the degree of twisting.
6. In the higher ring homologue, the dibenzo cyclo-octane is more effective.

dibenzo cyclo-octane analouges

7. Several novel bridged ring ether derivatives of amitriptyline are found to possess very powerful antidepressant activity.

amitriptyline analouges

8. Several amitriptyline analogs with the following structures are clinically effective antidepressants.

amitriptyline analouges

The alkene linkage introduces the possibility of cis–trans isomerism into the structure where in some instances one form is more active than the other.

a. X= O→ Doxepine.
b. X= S→ Prothiadine.
c. X= SO→ Potent antihistaminic.

Mode of Action (Fig. 24.2)

- Tricyclic antidepressant inhibits the amine pump on the presynaptic nerve endings. This results in the inhibition of reuptake of the amines in the synaptic cleft which were released during nerve impulse transmission.

- The TCAs block reuptake of both NE and -HT neurotransmitters. One of the properties which distinguishes the TCAs is the specificity with which they block the reuptake of these neurotransmitters.
- For example, desipramine is the most selective NE reuptake inhibitor and clomipramine the most selective for 5-HT reuptake inhibition. Amoxapine is a potent inhibitor of NE reuptake and relatively weak for 5-HT reuptake. Both amoxapine and its metabolites inhibit dopamine receptors.
- Mianserin has considerably affinity for α2 adrenergic presynaptic receptors, thus inhibiting the negative feedback loop which results in an increase in release of NE. Meprotiline is relatively specific for the inhibition of NE reuptake and has little effect on 5-HT or dopamine reuptake.

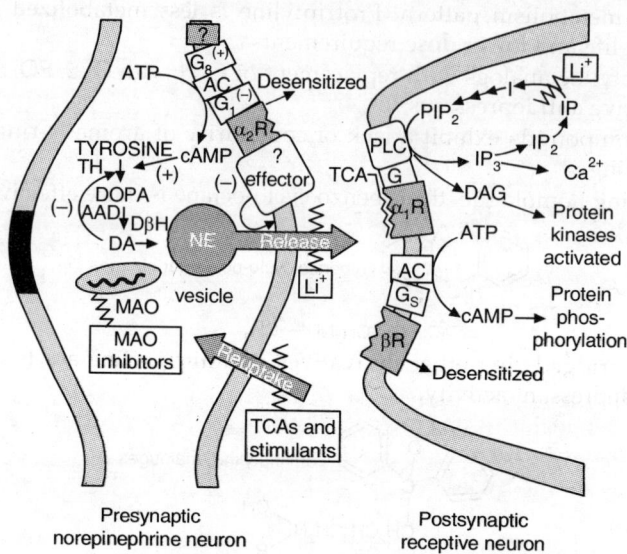

Presynaptic
norepinephrine neuron

Postsynaptic
receptive neuron

Fig. 24.2: Mode of action of TCA

- Among the conventional TCA, there is little selectivity between NE and 5-HT uptake.
- In addition to their effects on amine uptake, most TCAs affect one or more types of neurotransmitter receptors, including muscarinic ACh receptors and histamine receptors. Anticholinergics action of TCA cause dryness of mouth, blurred vision and constipation.

Pharmacokinetics

- The tricyclic antidepressants are well absorbed after oral administration. Peak plasma levels are reached in 2-6 hours after ingestion.
- The mean half-life is about 24 hours allowing for once a day dosing. Imipramine has the shortest half-life of about 12 hours and maprotiline has a half-life of 43 hours. TCAs are up to 90% protein bound.
- TCAs are extensively metabolized in the liver by two main routes, namely N-demethylation, whereby tertiary amines are converted to secondary amines e.g. imipramine to desmethylimipramine, amitriptyline to nortriptyline and ring hydroxylation. Both the desmethyl and the hydroxylated metabolites are biochemically active. Inactivation of drugs occurs by glucuronide conjugation of the hydroxylated metabolites.

Side Effects

- Antidepressant drugs most commonly TCAs are now one of the most frequently used methods for attempted suicide. The initial effects of TCA overdose is to cause excitement and delirium which may be accompanied by convulsions. This is followed by coma and respiratory depression, cardiac dysarrhythmia are common usually arterial or ventricular extra systoles, and sudden death may occur from ventricular fibrillation.
- Tertiary amine tricyclics tend to have more anticholinergic side effects than the secondary amines. This includes impaired memory, confusion, dry mouth, and blur-red vision. Blockade of histamine and possibly α-adrenergic and cholinergic blockade leads to sedation, weight gain, and sexual dysfunction has been associated with tricyclic use and also peripheral edema.

▓ MONO-AMINO OXIDASE INHIBITORS

Hydrazine derivatives

Phenelzine

Structure–Activity Relationship

1. Although hydrazine (NH_2NH_2) lacks significant MAO inhibitors properties. Alkyl substitutions may confer strong activity.
2. Among a series of alkyl substituted hydrazines, maximum effectiveness is observed with ethyl hydrazine. Increasing the size of the alkyl group beyond ethyl decrease the activity. Similarly isopropyl hydrazine is more effective than n-propylhydrazine.
3. In general, cycloalkyl substituted hydrazines are about equipotent with the corresponding n-alkyl hydrazines.
4. A hydrogen atom on the hydrazine nitrogen bearing the alkyl group is essential for MAO inhibitory action.
5. Asymmetrical dialkyl substituted hydrazines ($R_1R_2NNH_2$) are devoid of significant activity. Symmetrical dialkyl substituted hydrazines R_1NHNHR_2 are generally less effective than the corresponding monoalkyl derivatives.
6. Hydroxyalkylhydrazines are usually less effective MAO inhibitors than the corresponding alkylhydrazines.
7. Aromatic ring substituents with polar groups generally decrease the activity.

Isocarboxazid

Hydrazide derivatives

Structure–Activity Relationship

1. Unsubstituted hydrazides ($RCONHNH_2$) do not significantly inhibit MAO.
2. Monosubstituted hydrazides ($RCONHNHR_1$) may enhance the MAO inhibitory activity.

3. In compounds having general formula, RCONR$_2$NHCH (CH$_3$)$_2$, the main function of alkyl group appears to be that of a carrier.

Mechanism of Action (Figs. 24.3 and 24.4)

- According to the current concept, norepinephrine is synthesized within the nerve cells and stored in intraneuronal granules at presynaptic nerve endings from which, it is released by nerve impulse into the synaptic cleft where it interacts with the post-synaptic receptors. The released norepinephrine is inactivated mainly through following ways.
  1. Its reuptake by the neuron.
  2. Its conversion to normetanephrine (metabolite) by the enzyme, catechol-o-methyl- transferase.
- Norepinephrine released intraneuronally, either spontaneously or by interference with the binding mechanism by reserpine like drugs, appears to be inactivated by mono-amine oxidase enzymes. The MAO is a family of enzymes located primarily in the outer membranes of mitochondria. These enzymes inactivate biogenic amines such as norepinephrine, dopamine, serotonin, tryptamine and tyramine by conversion to aldehydes and by subsequent oxidation or reduction to an acid or alcohol.

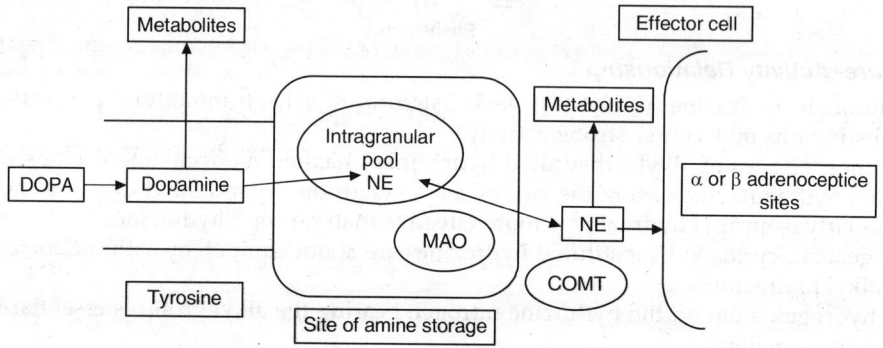

Fig. 24.3: Mechanism of action of MAO inhibitors

- Monoamino-oxidase is a family of flavin-containing enzymes located primarily in the outer membranes of mitochondria. These enzymes inactivate the biogenic amines.
- This process proceeds through enzymatic abstraction of a proton from the α-carbon of the amine. A lysine amino group of the enzyme forms a Schiff's base at the α-carbon of the substrate displacing the amino group from the substrate molecule. This also provides the second hydrogen to complete reduction of the enzyme. Hydrolysis of the Schiff base produces the aldehyde metabolite and the free lysylamine function.
- Certain compounds irreversibly inhibit flavin linked MAO through covalent attachment to flavin. Two forms or isoenzymes have been identified. MAO-A and MAO-B. Both enzymes are found in the central nervous systems as well as in some peripheral organs.
- MAO-A can be found concentrated in dopamine and NE neurons. MAO-B located more so in serotogenic neurons. Inhibition of MAO-A reduces the deamination of NE and to a small degree, 5-HT. This causes an increase in the concentration of NE, 5-HT. This is associated with antidepressant activity of MAOIs.

Pharmacokinetics

After oral administration, the non-specific MAOIs undergo significant first-pass metabolism in the liver. The hydrazine is metabolized via acetylation. Meclobemide and brofaromine are metabolized, the later by O-demethylation and O-glucuronide formation. The half-life of meclobemide and brofaromine is about 12 hours.

Side Effects

- One of the most well-known side effects of MAOIs is the hypertensive crisis. The symptoms include palpitation, chill, sweating, neck stiffness, etc. MAOIs have other side effects, headache, dry mouth, weight gain and blurred vision. Meclobemide and brofaromine have favorable side effect profile.
- Another concern is their interaction with other drugs especially coughs preparation, decongestant and cold preparation containing ephedrine. Concomitants use of MAOIs and SSRIs is contraindicated.

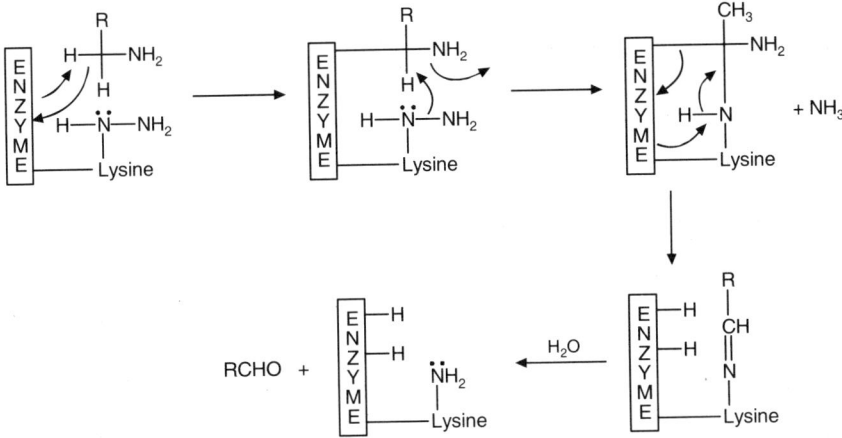

Fig. 24.4: Structural mechanism of MAO inhibitors

SELECTIVE SEROTONIN REUPTAKE INHIBITORS (SSRIs)

Mechanism of Action (Fig. 24.5)

- 5-HT uptake into presynaptic nerve terminals results in its inactivation. The SSRIs selectively inhibit neuronal uptake of serotonin.
- This effect leads to an acute enhancement of serotogenic neurotransmission by allowing serotonin to act at synaptic binding sites for an extended period. Thus the action of SSRIs is dependent on nerve transmission and the release of serotonin.

Adeverse Effect

- Nervousness, restlessness, insomnia, anorexia, dyskinesia, headache and diarrhea are associated with them, but patient acceptability is good.
- Increased incidence of epistaxis and ecchymosis has been reported, probably due to impairment of platelet function. Gastric blood loss due to NSAIDs may be increased by SSRIs.

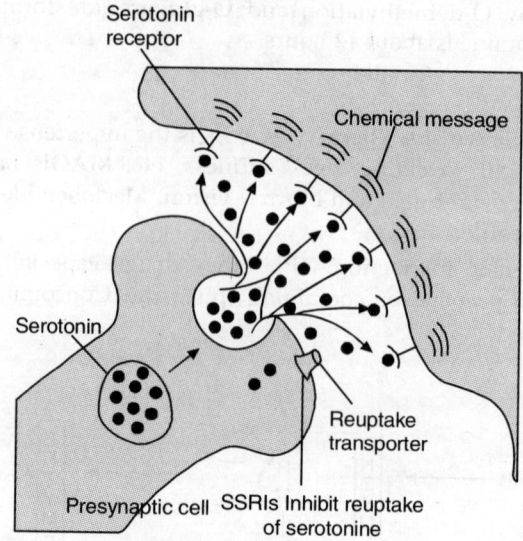

Fig. 24.5: Mode of action of SSRIs

■ ATYPICAL ANTIDEPRESSANT

Traxzodone: It is the first atypical antidepressant; selectively but less efficiently blocks 5-HT uptake and has prominent α blocking as well as weak 5-HT$_2$ antagonistic action.

Venlafazine: A novel antidepressant referred to as serotonin and noradrenaline reuptake inhibitor, because it inhibits the uptake of both these amines.

Bupropion:

- The inhibitor of dopamine and noradrenaline uptake has excitant rather than sedative property. It is metabolized into an amphetamine like compound.
- It has been recently marketed in a sustained release formulation as an aid to smoking cessation.

Imipramine

10, 11-dihydro-5H-dibenz[b, f] ozepine

1. NaNH$_2$
2. 3-dimethylamino-propyl chloride

1. sodium amide
2. 3-dimethylamino-propyl chloride

Imipramine

Desipramine

10, 11-dihydro-5H-dibenz[b, f] azepine (I)

1. NaNH$_2$
2. 1-bromo-3-chloro-propane

1. sodium amide
2. 1-bromo-3-chloropropane

5-(3-chloropropyl)-10, 11-dihydro-5H-dibenz [b, f] azepine

H$_3$C—NH$_2$
methylamine

Desipramine

Trimipramine

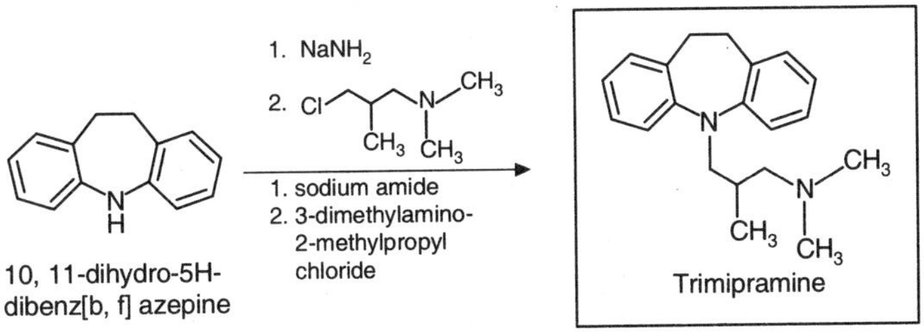

1. NaNH$_2$
2. Cl—CH$_2$—CH(CH$_3$)—CH$_2$—N(CH$_3$)$_2$

1. sodium amide
2. 3-dimethylamino-2-methylpropyl chloride

10, 11-dihydro-5H-dibenz[b, f] azepine

Trimipramine

Clomipramine

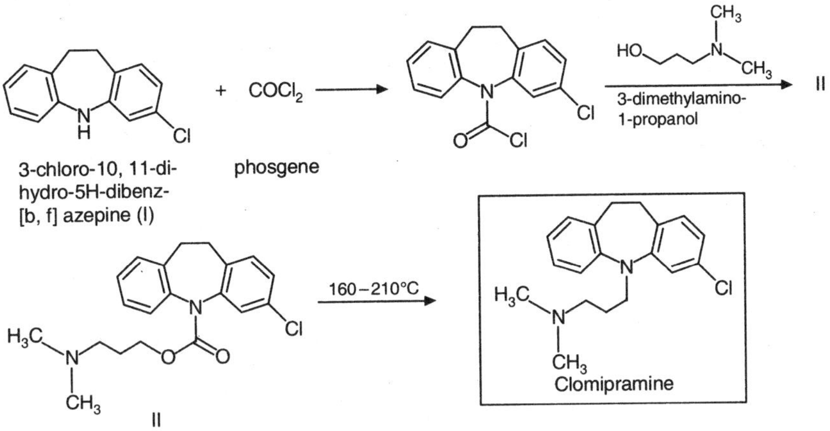

3-chloro-10, 11-dihydro-5H-dibenz-[b, f] azepine (I)   +   COCl$_2$ phosgene

3-dimethylamino-1-propanol

II

160–210°C

Clomipramine

Nortriptyline

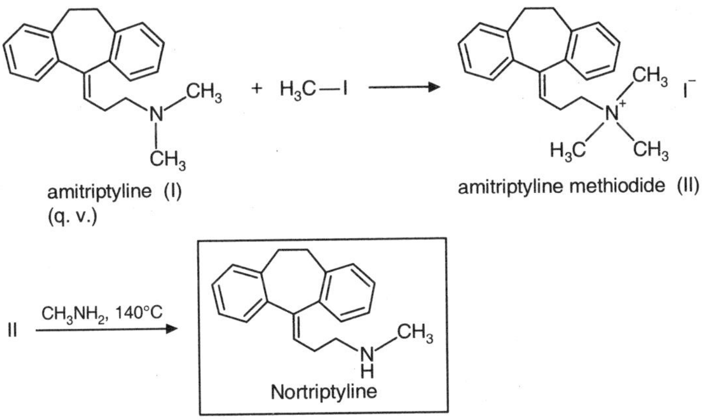

amitriptyline (I)
(q. v.)   +   H$_3$C—I

amitriptyline methiodide (II)

II   CH$_3$NH$_2$, 140°C

Nortriptyline

Phenelzine

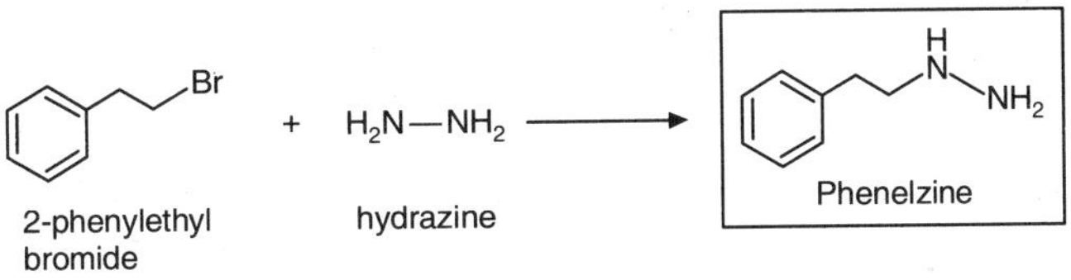

2-phenylethyl bromide   +   H$_2$N—NH$_2$
hydrazine

Phenelzine

Protriptyline

3-methylamino-1-propanol + form-amide → 3-(n-formyl-N-methylamino)-1-propanol → (SOCl₃ thionyl chloride) → 3-(N-formyl-N-methylamino)-propyl chloride (I)

I + 5H-dibenzo[a, d]-cycloheptane → (KNH₂ potassium amide) → → (KOH) → Protriptyline

Mianserin

Styrene oxide + 2-methylamino ethanol → → (SOCl₃, CHCl₃) → I

(I) + 2-amino-benzyl alcohol → (DMF) → → (PPA polyphos-phoric acid) → Mianserin

Iproniazid

Isoniazid + Acetone → → (H₂, Pt) → Iproniazid

Dibenzazepine

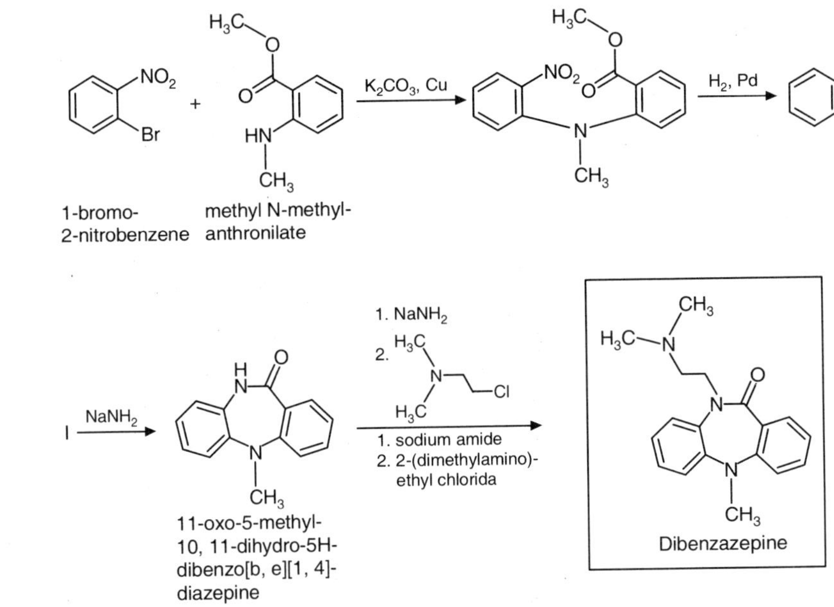

NO2
Br
H3C
O
HN
CH3
1-bromo-2-nitrobenzene
methyl N-methyl-anthronilate
K2CO3, Cu
NO2
N
CH3
H2, Pd
NH2
(I)
I
NaNH2
H
N
11-oxo-5-methyl-10, 11-dihydro-5H-dibenzo[b, e][1, 4]-diazepine
1. NaNH2
2. H3C N Cl H3C
1. sodium amide
2. 2-(dimethylamino)-ethyl chlorida
Dibenzazepine

Doxepin

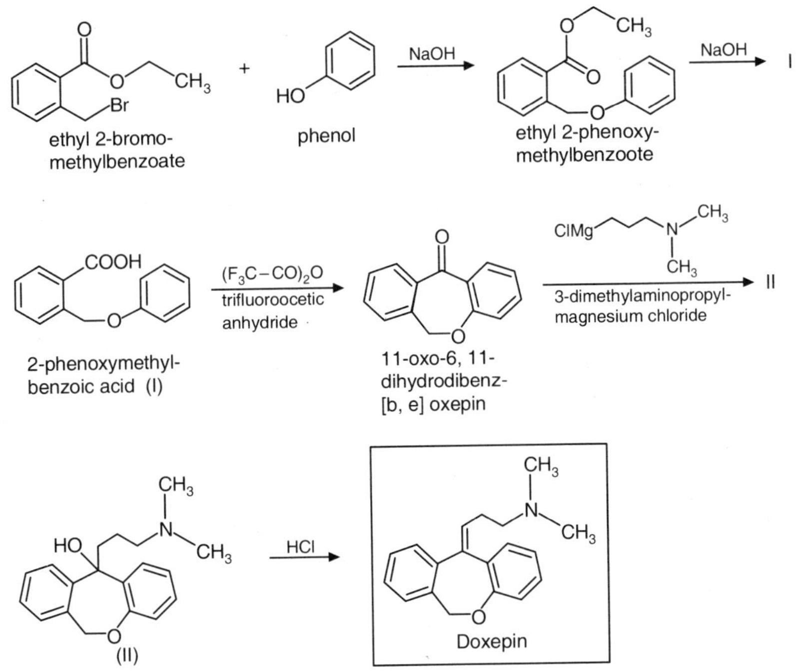

O
CH3
Br
ethyl 2-bromo-methylbenzoate
HO
phenol
NaOH
ethyl 2-phenoxy-methylbenzoote
NaOH
I
COOH
2-phenoxymethyl-benzoic acid (I)
(F3C–CO)2O
trifluoroocetic anhydride
11-oxo-6, 11-dihydrodibenz-[b, e] oxepin
ClMg
N
CH3
3-dimethylaminopropyl-magnesium chloride
II
HO
(II)
HCl
Doxepin

Isocarboxazid

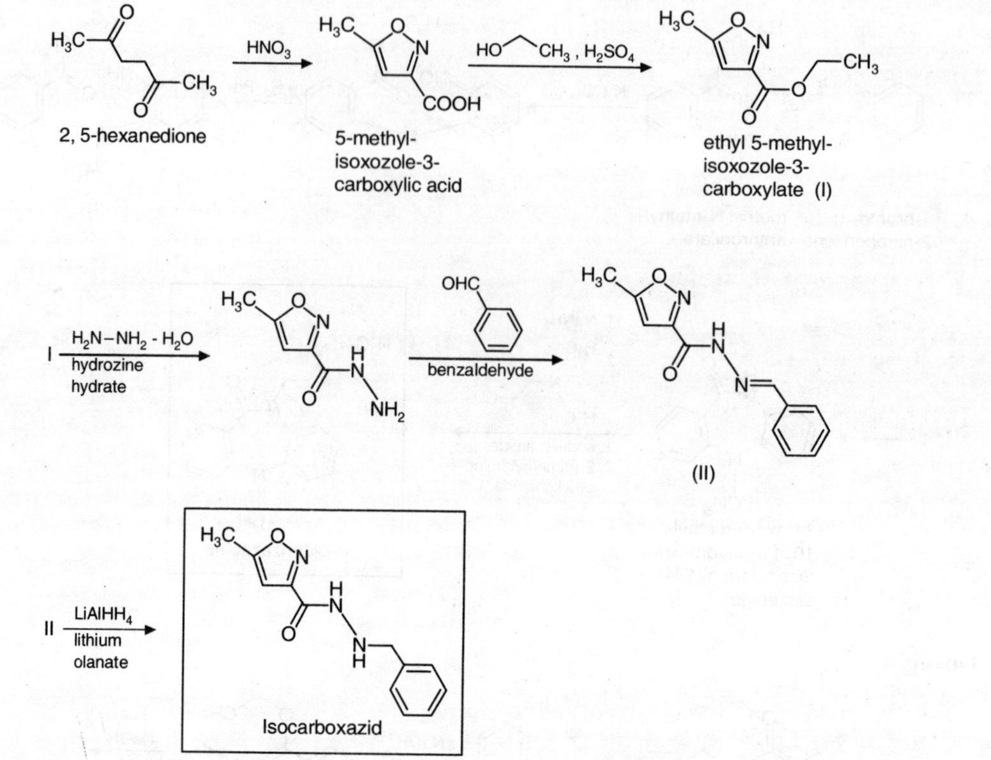

H_3C
CH_3
2, 5-hexanedione
HNO_3
5-methyl-isoxozole-3-carboxylic acid
COOH
HO CH$_3$, H_2SO_4
ethyl 5-methyl-isoxozole-3-carboxylate (I)
I
$H_2N-NH_2 - H_2O$
hydrozine hydrate
NH_2
OHC
benzaldehyde
(II)
II
$LiAlHH_4$
lithium olanate
Isocarboxazid

Tranylcypromine

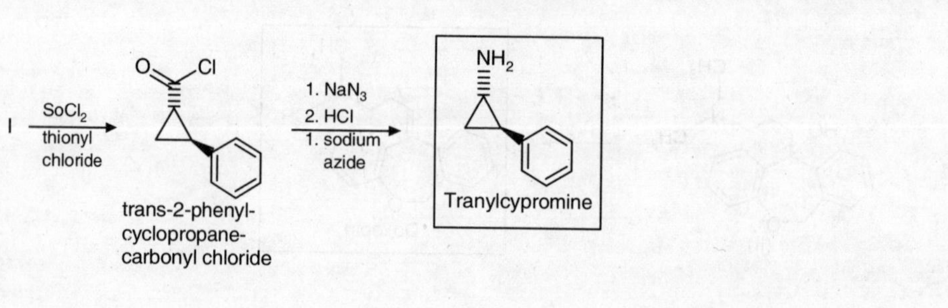

H_2C
Styrene
N_2
Ethyl diazoacetate
CH_3
Ethyl 2-phenyl-cyclopropane-carboxylate
NaOH, C_2H_5OH
COOH
trans-2-phenyl-cyclopropane-carboxyloic acid (I)
I
$SoCl_2$
thionyl chloride
Cl
trans-2-phenyl-cyclopropane-carbonyl chloride
1. NaN_3
2. HCl
1. sodium azide
NH_2
Tranylcypromine

Trazodone

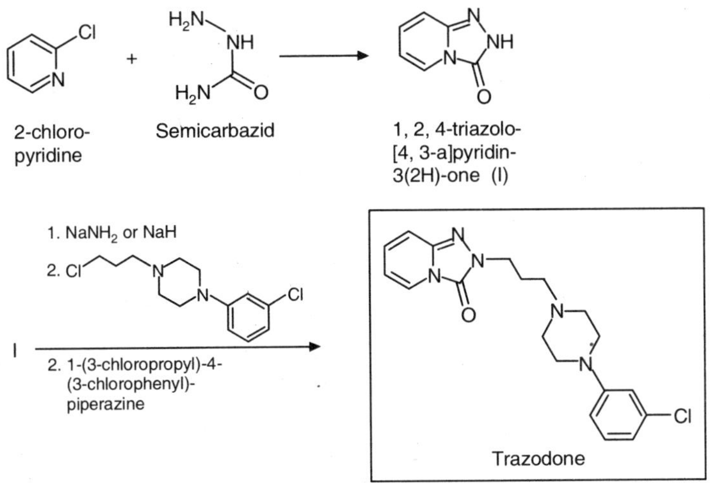

2-chloro-
pyridine

Semicarbazid

1, 2, 4-triazolo-
[4, 3-a]pyridin-
3(2H)-one (I)

1. NaNH$_2$ or NaH

2. Cl

I

2. 1-(3-chloropropyl)-4-
(3-chlorophenyl)-
piperazine

Trazodone

Venlafaxine

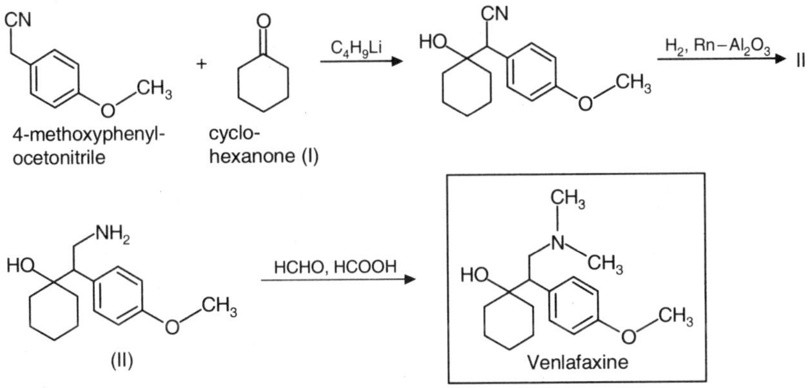

4-methoxyphenyl-
ocetonitrile

cyclo-
hexanone (I)

C$_4$H$_9$Li

H$_2$, Rn−Al$_2$O$_3$

II

HCHO, HCOOH

(II)

Venlafaxine

Fluoxetine

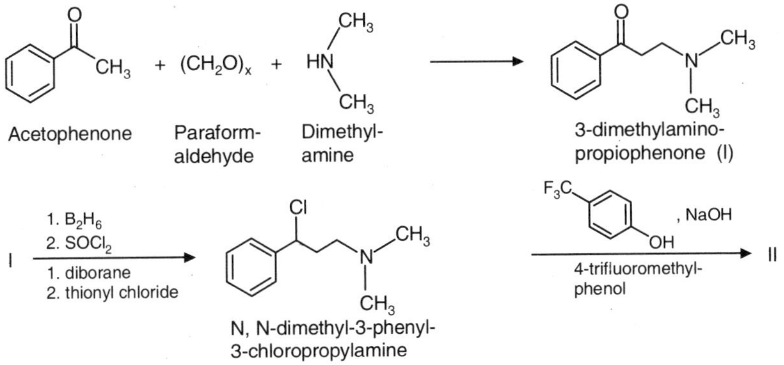

Acetophenone

Paraform-
aldehyde

Dimethyl-
amine

3-dimethylamino-
propiophenone (I)

1. B$_2$H$_6$
2. SOCl$_2$

I

1. diborane
2. thionyl chloride

N, N-dimethyl-3-phenyl-
3-chloropropylamine

F$_3$C

, NaOH

OH

4-trifluoromethyl-
phenol

II

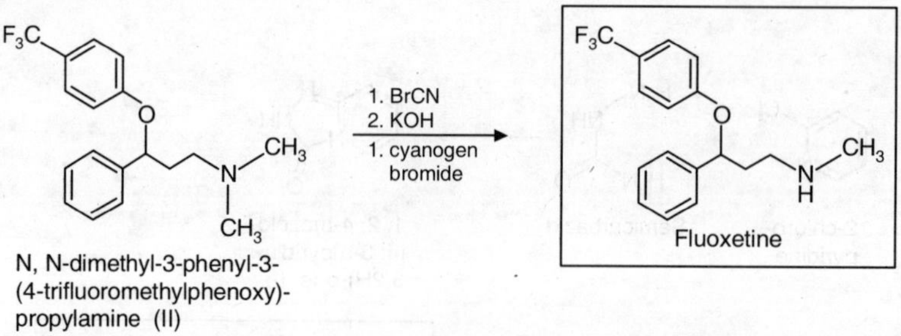

N, N-dimethyl-3-phenyl-3-
(4-trifluoromethylphenoxy)-
propylamine (II)

1. BrCN
2. KOH
1. cyanogen
bromide

Fluoxetine

Fluvoxamine

4'-trifluoromethyl-5-
methoxyvolerophenone (I)

O-(2-aminoethyl)-
hydroxylamine

Fluvoxamine

Paroxetine

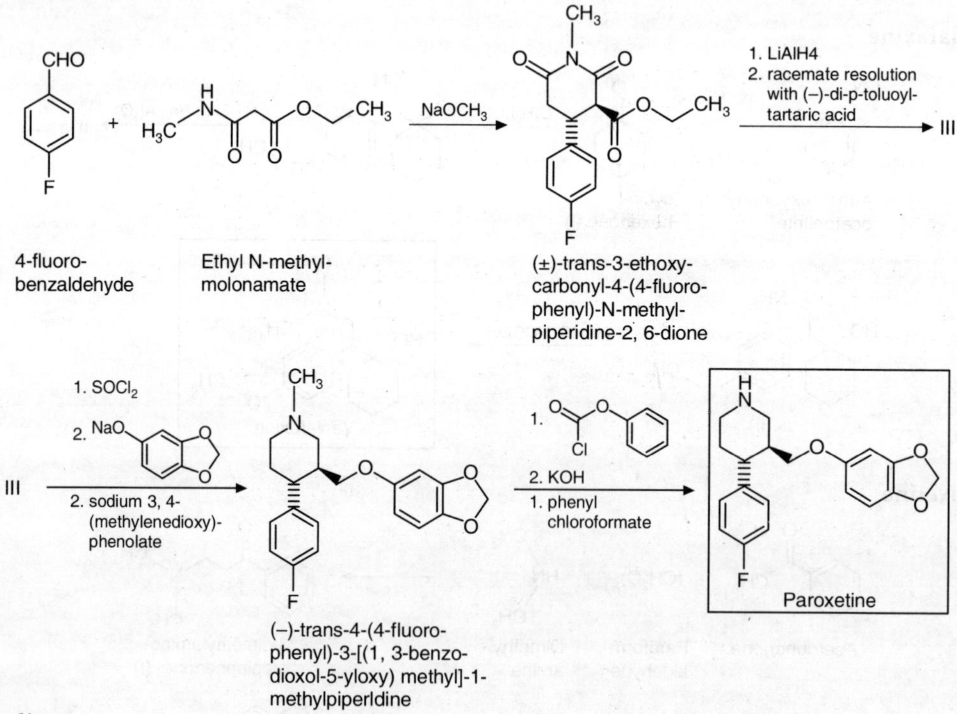

4-fluoro-
benzaldehyde

Ethyl N-methyl-
molonamate

NaOCH₃

(±)-trans-3-ethoxy-
carbonyl-4-(4-fluoro-
phenyl)-N-methyl-
piperidine-2, 6-dione

1. LiAlH4
2. racemate resolution
with (−)-di-p-toluoyl-
tartaric acid

III

III

1. SOCl₂
2. NaO
2. sodium 3, 4-
(methylenedioxy)-
phenolate

(−)-trans-4-(4-fluoro-
phenyl)-3-[(1, 3-benzo-
dioxol-5-yloxy) methyl]-1-
methylpiperldine

1.
2. KOH
1. phenyl
chloroformate

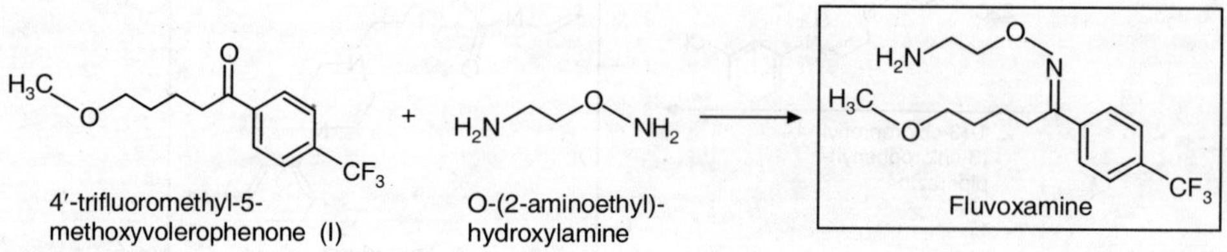

Paroxetine

Pargyline

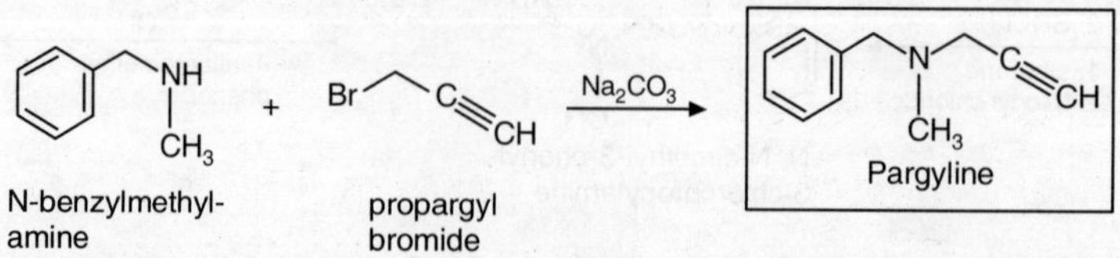

N-benzylmethyl-
amine

propargyl
bromide

Na₂CO₃

Pargyline

Anti-Parkinsonian Agents

Parkinsonism disease (or paralysis agitans) is a chronic progressive disorder of the CNS, which is the result of damage to cell located in basal ganglia of the brain. Parkinsonism is an extrapyramidal motor disorder characterized by rigidity, tremor and hypokinesia (akinesis) with secondary manifestation like defective posture and gait, mask-like face and sialorrhea; dementia may accompany. If untreated, the symptoms progress over several years to end stage disease in which the patient is rigid, unable to move, unable to breath properly; succumbs mostly to chest infection/embolism.

- It is characterized as:
  1. **Akinesis:** This is a lack or difficulty in initiating voluntary muscle movement and in advanced stages is characterized by frozen muscle resulting in a mask-like face, impaired postural reflexes and inability to care oneself.
  2. **Rigidity:** This usually of the plastics or cogwheel type i.e. it gives way in a series of jerk.
  3. **Tremor:** Coarse (3-6 cycle\sec) repetitive muscle activity, usually worse when the patient is at rest, is commonly manifested as 'Pill rolling motion of hands and bobbing of head'.
- In addition, patient may show disturbances in gait, impaired speech, muscle weakness, and autonomic hyperactivity like salivation and sialorrhea.

NEUROCHEMICAL BASIS OF PARKINSONISM (FIG. 25.1)

- Dopamine acts mainly as an inhibitory transmitter and acetylcholine as an excitatory transmitter within nigrostratial pathway of extrapyramidal motor system. A proper balance between the two neurotransmitters is essential for normal function. The selective degeneration of dopaminergic neurons the balance becomes tipped towards cholinergic predominance (increase in ACh). Correction of this imbalance is the basis of drug therapy of Parkinsonism.
- The biochemical basis of Parkinsonism disease is a deficiency of the neurotransmitter dopamine in basal ganglia due to loss of pigmented cells in subtantia nigra of the midbrain. This results in deficiency of dopamine in the striatum which controls muscle tone and co-ordinate movement. An imbalance between dopaminergic (inhibitory) and cholinergic (excitory) system in the striatum occurs giving rise to the motor defect. Though the cholinergic system is not primarily affected, its suppression by anticholinergics tends to restore the balance.
- The cause of selective degeneration of nigrostratial neurons is not precisely known, but appears to be multifactorial. Oxidation of DA by MAO-B and aldehyde dehydrogenase generates hydroxyl free radicals in the presence of ferrous iron (basal ganglia are rich in iron). Normally, these free radicals are quenched by glutathione and other protective mechanisms.

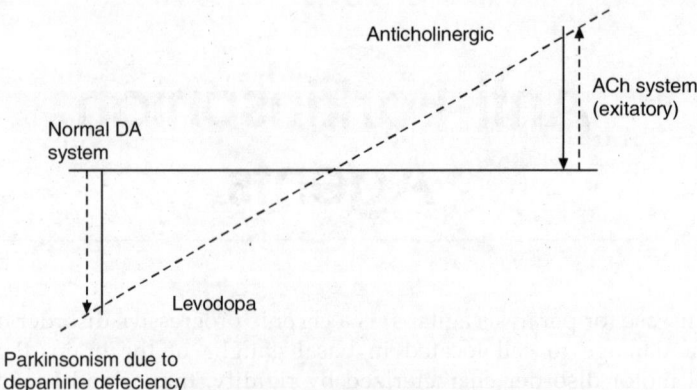

Fig. 25.1: Etiology of Parkinson's disease

$$H_2O_2 + Fe^{2+} \xrightarrow[\text{Reaction}]{\text{Fenton}} OH + OH^- + Fe^{3+}$$

Age-related and/or otherwise acquired defect in protective mechanisms allows the free radicals to damage lipid membranes and DNA resulting in neuronal degeneration. Genetic predisposition may contribute to high vulnerability of substantia nigra neurons.

- Ageing induces defects in mitochondrial electron transport chain. Environmental toxins and/or genetic factors may accentuate these defects in specific areas. A synthetic toxin N-methyl-4-phenyl tetrahydropyridines (MPTP), which occurred as a contaminant of some illicit drugs, produces nigrostriatal degeneration and manifestation similar to Parkinson's disease. It gets converted to the reactive species. It has been proposed that MPTP like chemicals may be present in environment, small quantities of which accelerate age-related or otherwise predisposed neuronal degeneration of Parkinsonism, but there is no proof.

- Dopamine is an inhibitory neurotransmitter, which is liberated from nerve ending in the striatum by neural impulses, and maintains balance with acetylcholine, the excitatory neurotransmitter.

Molecular Level
- There are two types of receptor for dopamine D_1 and D_2.
  1. D_1 — stimulate adenyl cyclase activity.
  2. D_2 — inhibit adenyl cyclase (unlinked). It is in majority with about 60% in the area of substantia nigra and striatum.
- D_1, D_2, D_3, D_4, D_5 all are G-protein-coupled receptors are grouped into two families:
  (1) D_1 like (D_1 and D_5): They are excitatory act by increasing cAMP formation and PIP_2 hydrolysis there by mobilizing intracellular Ca^{2+} and activating protein kinase C through IP_3 and DAG.

(2) D_2 like (D_2, D_3, D_4): They are inhibitory and act by inhibiting adenyl cyclase or opening K^+ channels or depressing voltage sensitive Ca^{2+} channels.

- Both D_1 and D_2 receptors are present in striatum and are involved in the therapeutic response to levodopa. They respectively regulate the activity of two pathways having opposite effects on the thalamic infect to the motor cortex. Thus, stimulation of excitatory D_1 as well as inhibitory D_2 receptors in the striatum achieves the same net effect of smoothening movements and reduces muscle tone.

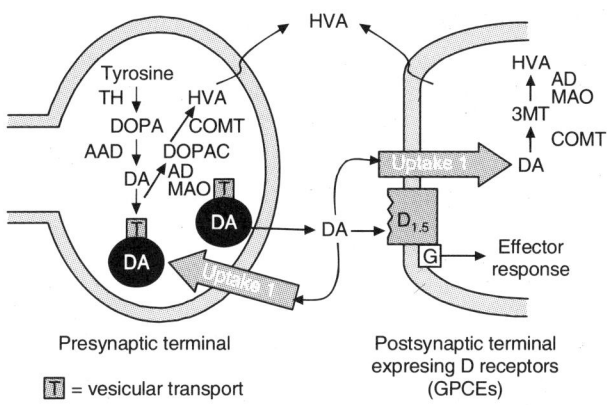

Fig. 25.2: Synthesis and metabolism of dopamine

CLASSIFICATION OF ANTI-PARKINSONISM

Classification of anti-parkinsonism agents is given in Flow chart 25.1.

Flow chart 25.1: Classification of anti-parkinsonism

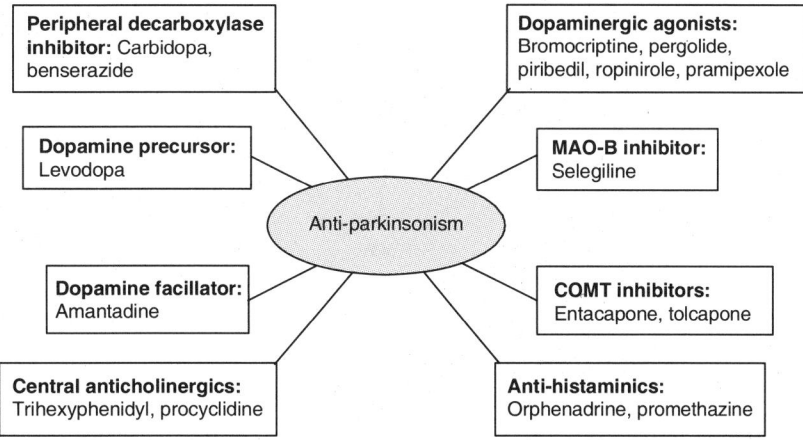

Dopamine precursor

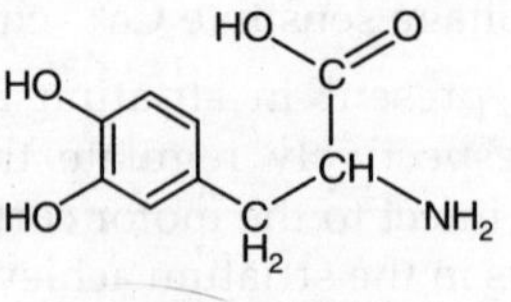

(L-tyrosine, 3-hydroxy)
Levodopa

Peripheral decarboxylase inhibitors

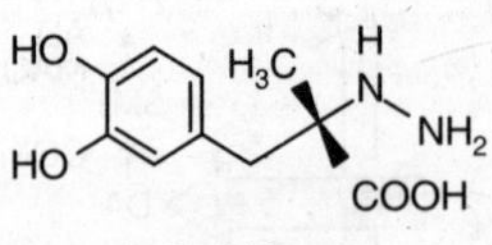

Carbidopa

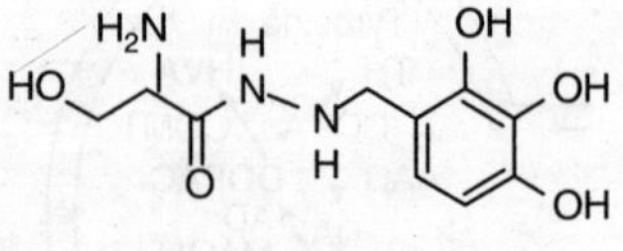

Benserazide

Dopaminergic agonists

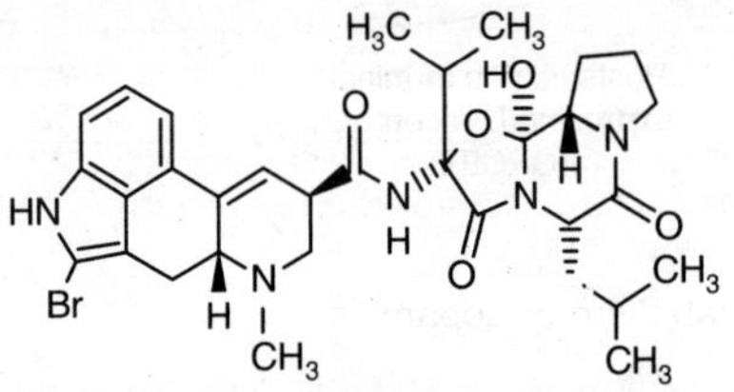

Bromocriptine

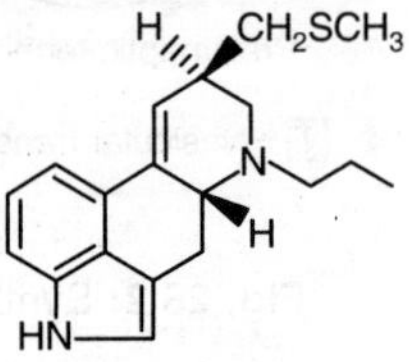

Pergolide

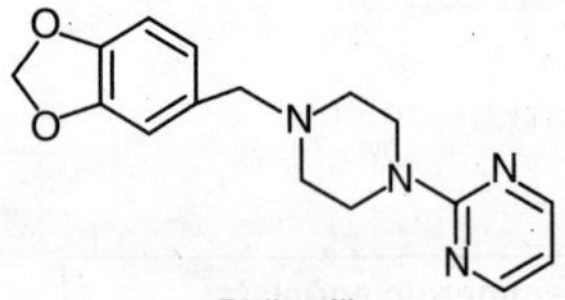

Piribedil

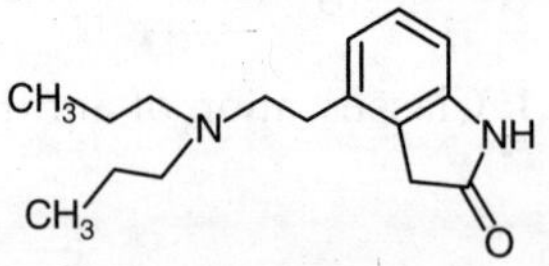

Ropinirole

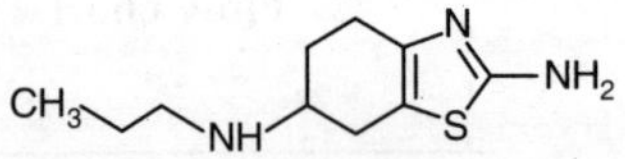

Pramipexole

MAO-B inhibitors

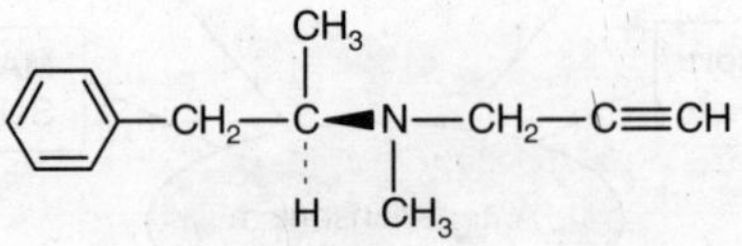

$$CH_2-C-N-CH_2-C\equiv CH$$

Selegiline

COMT inhibitors

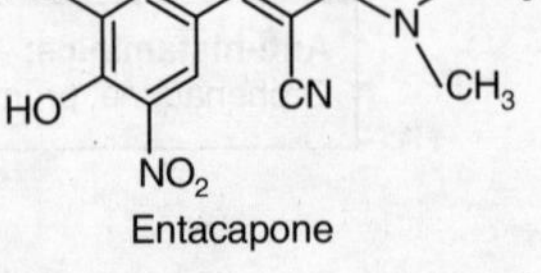

Entacapone

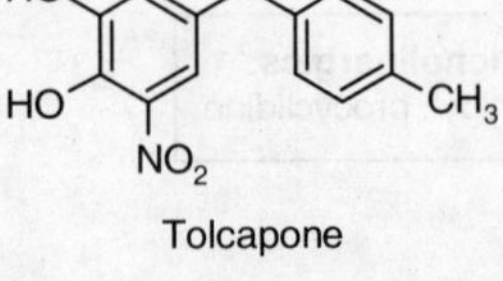

Tolcapone

Dopamine facillator

Amantadine

Central anticholinergics

Trihexyphenidyl

Biperidene

Procyclidine

Benzotropine mesylate

Antihistaminics

Orphenadrine

Miscellaneous

Ethoproprazine

Cycrimine HCl

Structure-activity relationship

1. N-methyl β-phenethylamine analog of dopamine equipotent to dopamine, e.g. epimine.
2. α-methyl analogue of dopamine less potent dopamine agonist.
3. Compound with catechol ring and amino group fused in rigid conformation bind the dopamine receptor, e.g. apomorphine.
4. Apomorphine can pass the BBB but dopamine cannot.
5. The maximum requirement for interatomic distances between two catechol oxygen and nitrogen atom is 7.78 and 6.480A

Dopamine Precursor

Levodopa

6. The β-rotameric conformation of n-methyl was inactive, e.g. isomorphine.
7. Zero isomer of apomorphine has dopamine like activity.

Mechanism of action

- As dopamine does not cross the BBB when administered systematically, it has not therapeutic effect in Parkinsonism. L-dopa is a precursor of dopamine that readily passes the BBB where it is decarboxylated to dopamine. Large doses must be given to increase the concentration of dopamine.
- This increased formation of dopamine in the motor regulatory area of the CNS restores depleted dopamine levels and improves the symptoms of Parkinsonism.
- L-dopa is most effective in controlling rigidity and tremor.

Peripheral Decarboxylase Inhibitors

Carbidopa and benserazide

Mechanism of action

- These are extracerebal dopadecarboxylase enzyme converts the levodopa to dopamine before entering into the brain thus reduces the efficacy of the levodopa. Inhibitors such as carbidopa and levodopa inhibit the dopadecarboxylase enzyme and stops peripheral metabolism of levodopa.
- They do not penetrate BBB and do not inhibit conversion of levodopa to dopamine in brain. Administered along with L-dopa to increase half-life and cross BBB to reach its site of action, by reducing the peripheral conversion of levodopa to dopamine.

Dopaminergic Agonists

Mechanism of action

The dopamine agonist can act on straital dopamine receptors in patient who have largely lost the capacity to synthesize, store and release dopamine from levodopa. Morover, they can be longer acting, exert subtype selective activation of dopamine receptors involved in Parkinsonism and not share the concern expressed about levodopa of contributing to dopaminergic neuronal damage by oxidative metabolism.

MAO-B Inhibitor

Mechanism of action

These are selective MAO-B inhibitors. Two isoenzymes form of MAO, termed as MAO-A and MAO-B both present in peripheral adrenergic structure and intestinal mucosa; MAO-B predominates in brain and blood platelets and is responsible for most of oxidative metabolism of dopamine in the brain. At low doses, selegiline is a selective inhibitor of MAO-B leading to irreversible inhibition of enzyme. Selegiline does not interfere in peripheral metabolism of catecholamines; thus levodopa can be taken safely.

COMT Inhibitors

Mechanism of Action

Potent reversible COMT inhibitors and act as adjuvant to L-dopa, carbidopa for advanced Parkinsonism diseases. When peripheral decarboxylation of L-dopa is blocked by carbidopa or benesezide, it is mainly metabolized by COMT (catechol O-methyl transferase) to 3-O-methyldopa. Blockade of this pathway by entacapone or tolacapone prolongs the half-life of levodopa and allows large fraction of administered dose to cross the BBB. Since COMT inhibitors preserve dopamine formed in the striatum and supplements the peripheral effect.

Dopamine Facilitator

Mechanism of Action

It causes release of dopamine from presynaptic nerve ending and blocks its presynaptic reuptake. Its effectiveness is greatly reduced in the absence of functional dopaminergic neurons in corpus striatum. Action on glutamate receptor through which the straital dopaminergic system exerts its influence has also been suggested.

Central Anticholinergics

Mechanism of Action

- In Parkinson's disease, there is imbalance between the concentration of dopamine and acetylcholine, decreased dopamine and increased acetylcholine concentration has been observed.
- These agents exhibit post-synaptic blocking effect on central cholinergic excitatory pathways which in Parkinsonism become predominant, especially due to lack of fictional dopamine in corpus striatum. Central anticholinergics also related the reuptake of dopamine into presynaptic nerve ending, there by blocking its in-activation.

Antihistaminics

Mechanism of Action

This drug is observed to minimize voluntary muscle spasm by a central effect. It exerts its action by relaxing directly the tense skeletal muscle. It has peripheral atropine-like action and minimizes voluntary muscle spasm by virtue of its central inhibitory activity on the cerebral motor areas.

Levodopa

L-tyrosine (I) → enzymatic hydroxylation → Levodopa

Carbidopa

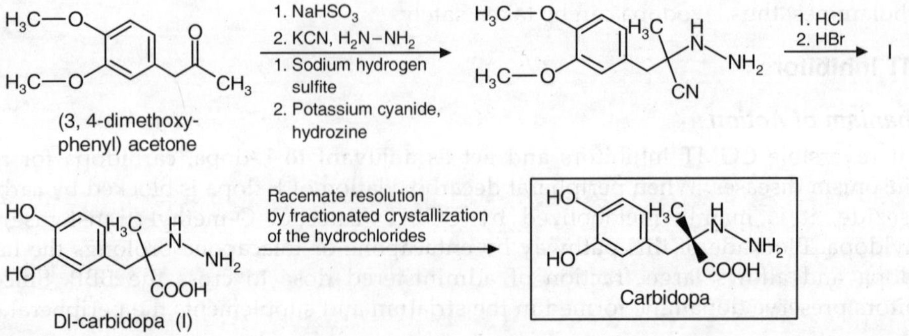

(3, 4-dimethoxy-
phenyl) acetone

1. NaHSO₃
2. KCN, H₂N–NH₂
1. Sodium hydrogen
   sulfite
2. Potassium cyanide,
   hydrozine

1. HCl
2. HBr

Dl-carbidopa (I)

Racemate resolution
by fractionated crystallization
of the hydrochlorides

Carbidopa

Benserazide

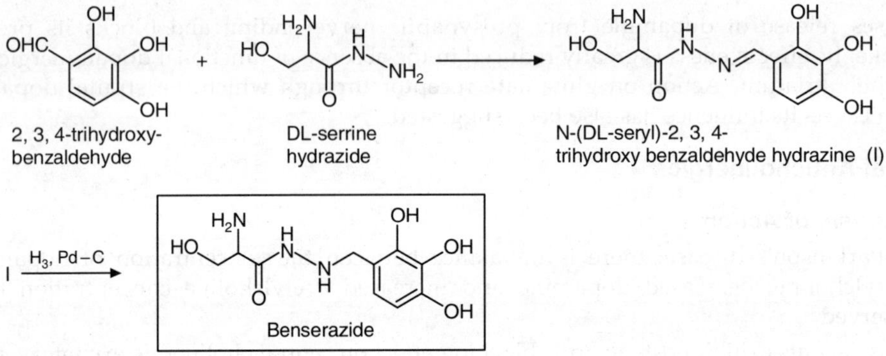

2, 3, 4-trihydroxy-
benzaldehyde

+

DL-serrine
hydrazide

N-(DL-seryl)-2, 3, 4-
trihydroxy benzaldehyde hydrazine (I)

I $\xrightarrow{H_3, Pd-C}$

Benserazide

Amantadine

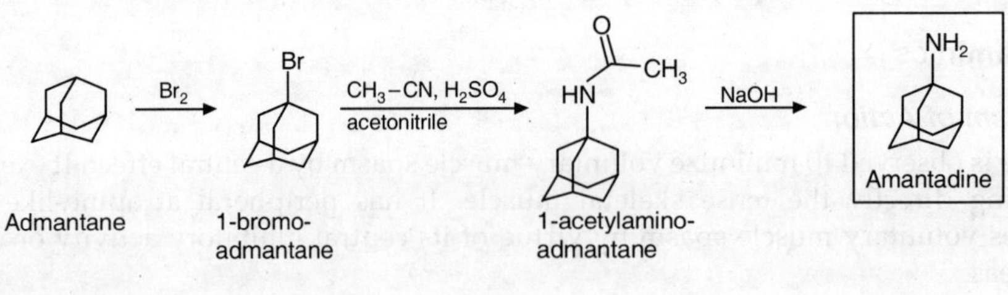

Admantane

$\xrightarrow{Br_2}$

1-bromo-
admantane

$\xrightarrow{CH_3-CN, H_2SO_4}$
acetonitrile

1-acetylamino-
admantane

$\xrightarrow{NaOH}$

Amantadine

Selegiline

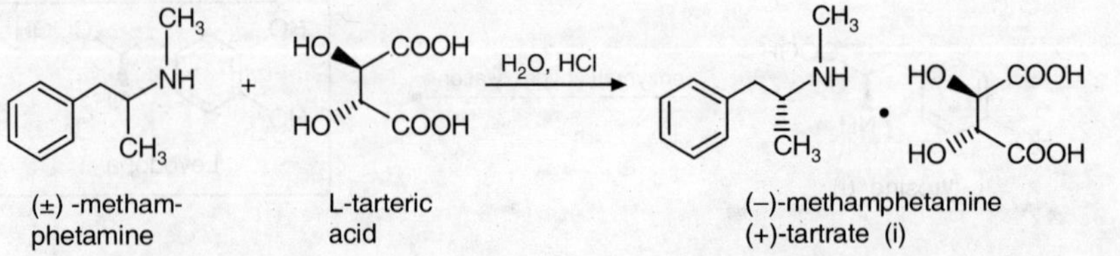

(±) -metham-
phetamine

+

L-tarteric
acid

$\xrightarrow{H_2O, HCl}$

(–)-methamphetamine
(+)-tartrate (i)

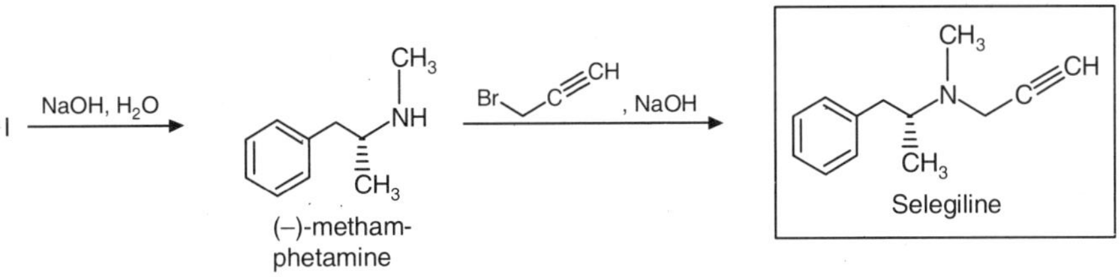
I
NaOH, H2O
CH3
NH
CH3
(–)-metham-
phetamine
Br
C
CH
, NaOH
CH3
N
C
CH
CH3
Selegiline

Bipiridine

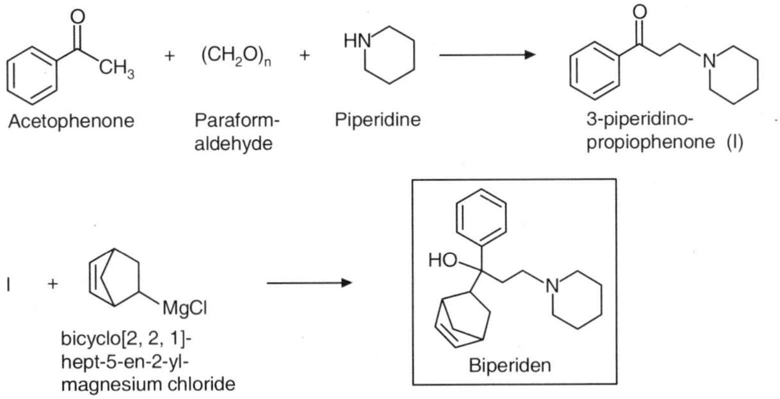
O
CH3
+
(CH2O)n
+
HN
O
N
Acetophenone
Paraform-
aldehyde
Piperidine
3-piperidino-
propiophenone (I)
I
+
MgCl
bicyclo[2, 2, 1]-
hept-5-en-2-yl-
magnesium chloride
HO
N
Biperiden

Procyclidine

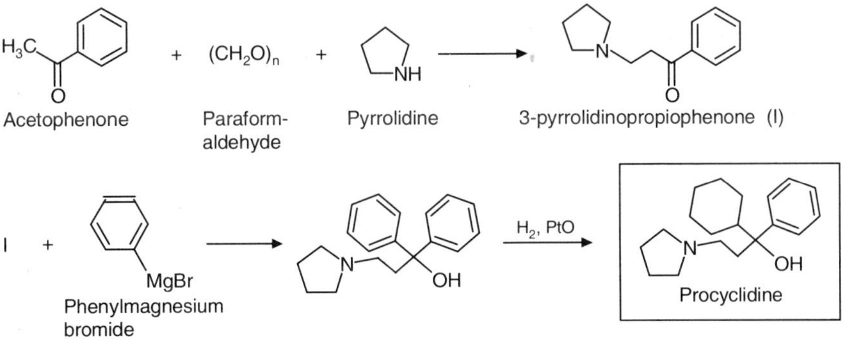
H3C
O
+
(CH2O)n
+
NH
N
O
Acetophenone
Paraform-
aldehyde
Pyrrolidine
3-pyrrolidinopropiophenone (I)
I
+
MgBr
Phenylmagnesium
bromide
N
OH
H2, PtO
N
OH
Procyclidine

Diphenhydramine

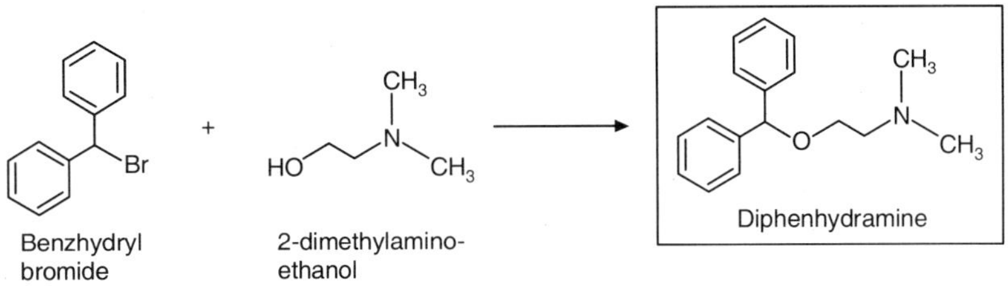
Br
+
CH3
HO
N
CH3
O
CH3
N
CH3
Benzhydryl
bromide
2-dimethylamino-
ethanol
Diphenhydramine

Unit IV

Drugs Affecting the Cardiovascular System

26

Cardiac Glycoside

Cardiac glycosides are having cardiac inotropoic property. They increase myocardial contractility and output in hypodynamic heart without a proportionate increase in O_2 consumption. Thus efficacy of failing heart is increased. In contrast, cardiac stimulants increase the O_2 consumption rather disproportionally and tend to decrease myocardial efficacy i.e. increase in O_2 consumption is more than increase in contractility. Further, cardiac stimulant also increased heart rate and have short lived action, while cardiac glycosides do not increase heart rate and have a prolonged action.

PATHOPHYSIOLOGY OF HEART FAILURE

- Cardiac failure can be described as the inability of the heart to pump blood effectively at a rate that meets the needs of the metabolizing tissues. This occurs when the muscles that perform contraction and force the blood out of heart are performing weakly. Thus cardiac failures primarily arise from the reduced contractility of heart muscles, especially the ventricles. Reduced contraction of heart leads to reduced heart output but new blood keeps coming in resulting in the increase in heart blood volume. The heart feels congested. Hence the term congestive heart failure. Congested heart leads to lowered blood pressure and poor renal blood flow. This results in the development of edema in the lower extremities and the lung (pulmonary edema) as well as renal failure.

- According to the Frank-Starling mechanism, the degree of force of heart muscle contraction is governed by the extent of ventricular muscle stretching. It does not apply to all degree of muscle stretch. If the myocardial fiber is stretched beyond critical length, instead of an increase in force of contraction, a fall in contraction forces results.

- A failing heart does not pump blood efficiently enough to meet the body's needs for oxygen and nutrients due to reduced power of contraction. Blood starts accumulating in the heart due to poor efficiency of the heart. The resulting progressive increase in end-diastolic volume leads to gradual increase in heart failure. The body's compensatory mechanism get activated to cause increased sympathetic tone, elevation of plasma antidiuretic hormone activity.

- The manifestations of failing heart include:

1. Stimulation of sympathetic nervous system, innervated to SA node resulting into vasoconstriction, tachycardia and sweating. These are largely the compensatory body mechanism to counterbalance the effect of inefficient and poorly pumping heart.

2. As a consequence, salt and water retention result into peripheral and pulmonary edema.

3. Secondary symptoms include easy fatiguability, breathlessness and hypertrophy of myocardium.

- The main pharmacodynamic property of digitalis is its ability to increase the force of myocardial contraction. The first proof regarding cardiotonic activity of digitalis was given in 1938 by Cattell and Gold. The beneficial effects of the drug in patients with heart failure include increased cardiac output, decreased pre-load, decreased heart size and venous return, increased renal flow and diuresis; all these effects lead to relief of edema and normal heart rate.

- The decreased heart size brings the heart under the range of operation of Frank-Starling mechanisms. Renal flow allows the drainage of retained edema fluid. The renal sodium ion excretion is increased due to competitive antagonism at mineralocorticoidal receptor because of structural resemblance.

CHEMISTRY OF THE CARDIAC GLYCOSIDES

- Cardiac glycosides are composed of two structural features— the sugar (glycoside) and the non-sugar (aglycone - steroid) moieties (Fig. 26.1)

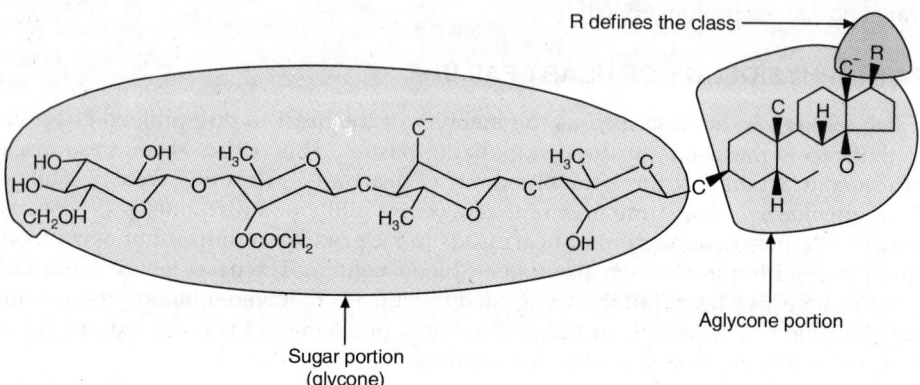

Fig. 26.1: Glycone and aglycone portion of cardiac glycoside.

- The R group at the 17-position defines the class of cardiac glycoside. Two classes have been observed in nature— the cardenolides and the bufadienolides (Fig. 26.1). The cardenolides have an unsaturated butyrolactone ring while the bufadienolides have a-pyrone ring.

Nomenclature

- The cardiac glycosides occur mainly in plants from which the names have been derived. *Digitalis purpurea, Digitalis lanata, Strophanthus gratus,* and *Strophanthus kombe* are the major sources of the cardiac glycosides.

- The term 'genin' at the end refers to only the aglycone portion (without the sugar). Thus the word digitoxin refers to an agent consisting of digitoxigenin (aglycone) and sugar moieties (three). The aglycone portion (Fig. 26.2) of cardiac glycosides are more important than the glycone portion.

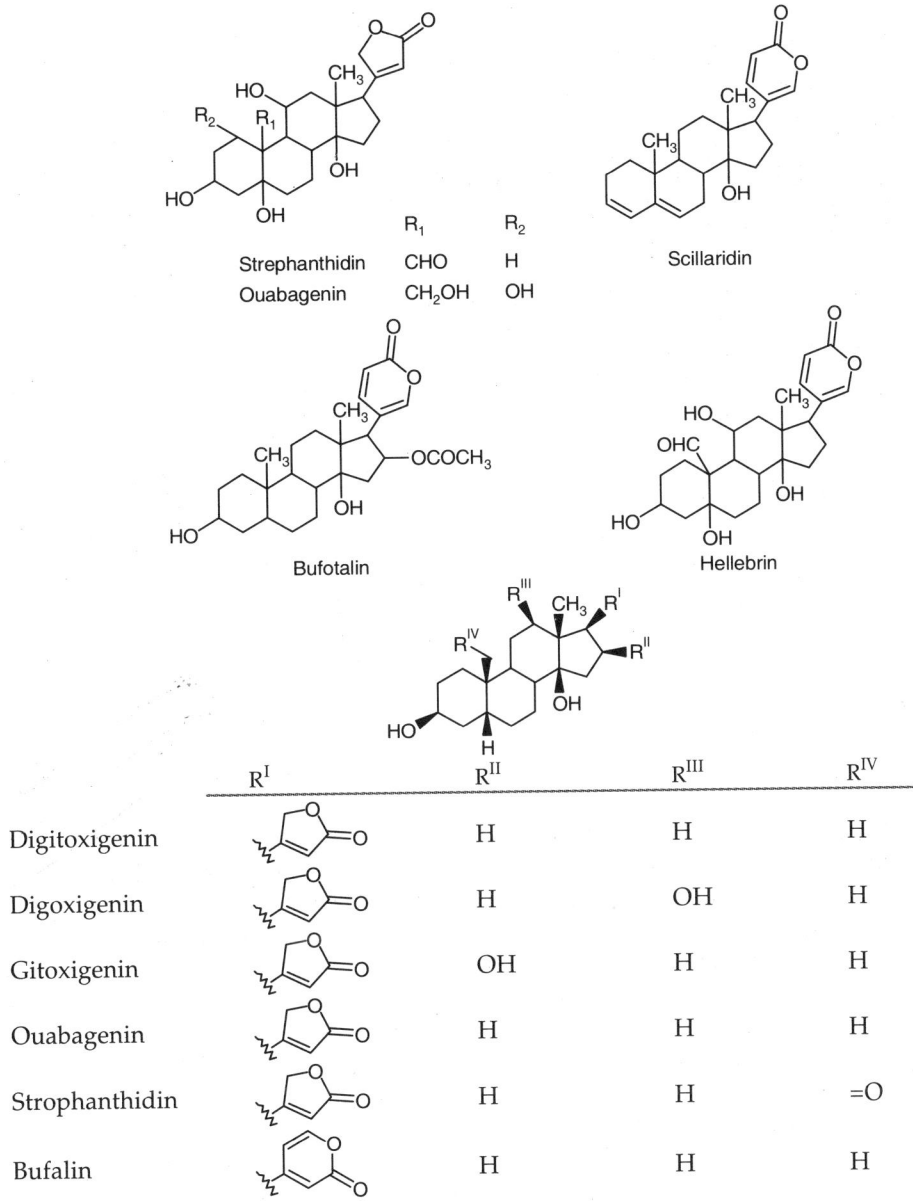

Fig. 26.2: Examples of some aglycones

- Let us discuss some of the important characteristics of each structural feature.

The Aglycone Moiety

- The steroid nucleus has a unique set of fused ring system that makes the aglycone moiety structurally distinct from the other more common steroid ring systems. Rings A/B and C/D are cis fused while rings B/C are trans fused. Such ring fusion gives the aglycone nucleus of cardiac glycosides the characteristic 'U' shape as shown below.

Aglycone moiety

- The steroid nucleus has hydroxyls at 3- and 14-positions of which the sugar attachment uses the 3-OH group. 14-OH is normally unsubstituted. Many genins have OH groups at 12- and 16-positions. These additional hydroxyl groups influence the partitioning of the cardiac glycosides into the aqueous media and greatly affect the duration of action.
- The lactones moiety at C-17 position is an important structural feature. The size and degree of unsaturation varies with the source of the glycoside. Normally plant sources provide a 5-membered unsaturated lactone while animal sources give a 6-membered unsaturated lactone.
- The lactone ring is not essential. The coplanar side-chains instead of a ring have even higher activity.
- The activity of a compound depends to a great extent on the position of the 23rd-carbonyl oxygen, which is held quite rigidly by ring D and the double bond.
- Removal of the sugar portion allows epimerization of this 3β-OH group, with a decrease in activity and an increase in toxicity due to changes in polarity.

Sugar Moiety

- The hydroxyl group at C-3 of the aglycone portion is usually conjugated to monosaccharide or a polysaccharide with β-1,4 glucosidic linkages. One to 4 sugars are found to be present in most cardiac glycosides commonly used include L-rhamnose, D-glucose, D-digitoxose, D-digitalose, D-digginose, D-sarmentose, L-vallarose, and D-fructose.
- These sugars predominantly exist in the cardiac glycosides in the β-conformation. The presence of acetyl group on the sugar affects the lipophilic character and the kinetics of the entire glycoside.
- Because the order of sugars appears to have little to do with biological activity. Nature has synthesized a numerous cardiac glycosides with differing sugar skeleton but relatively few aglycone structures.

β-D-Digitoxose   β-D-glucose   β-L-Rhamnose   -β-D-Cymarose

Structure–Activity Relationship

1. The sugar moiety appears to be important only for the partitioning and kinetics of action. It possesses no biological activity, e.g. elimination of the aglycone moiety eliminates the activity of alleviating symptoms associated with cardiac failure.

2. The 'backbone' U shape of the steroid nucleus appears to be very important. Structures with C/D *trans* fusion are inactive.

3. Conversion to A/B *trans* system leads to a marked drop in activity. Thus although not mandatory A/B *cis* fusion is important.

4. The 14 β-OH group is now believed to be dispensible. A skeleton without 14 β-OH group but retaining the C/D *cis* rings fusion was found to retain activity.

5. Lactones alone, when not attached to the steroid skeleton, are not active. Thus the activity rests in the steroid skeleton.

6. The unsaturated 17-lactone plays an important role in receptor binding. Saturation of the lactone ring dramatically reduced the biological activity.

7. The lactone ring is not absolutely required, e.g. using α, β-unsaturated nitrile (C=C-CN group) the lactone could be replaced with little or no loss in biological activity.

Mechanism of Action

- The mechanism whereby cardiac glycosides cause a positive inotropic effect and electrophysiological changes is still not completely clear. Several mechanisms have been proposed, but the most widely accepted involves the ability of cardiac glycosides to inhibit the membrane bound Na^+ –K^+–ATPase pump responsible for Na^+ – K^+ exchange.
- The process of muscle contraction can be pictured as shown in Fig. 26.3.

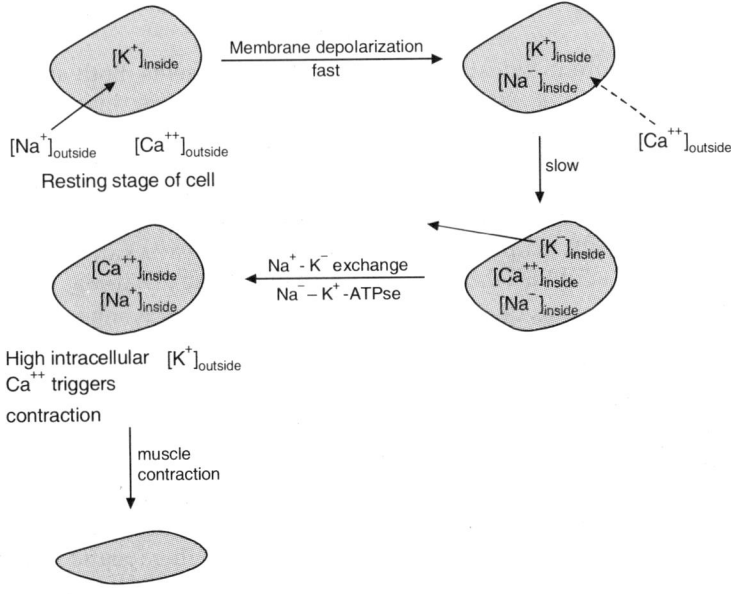

Fig. 26.3: Mode of action of cardiac glycoside

- The process of membrane depolarization/repolarization is controlled by the movement of three captions, Na^+, Ca^{2+}, and K^+, in and out of the cell. At the resting stage, the concentration of Na^+ is high on the outside. On membrane depolarization, sodium fluxes-in leading to an immediate elevation of the action potential. Elevated intracellular Na^+ triggers the influx of free of Ca^{++} that occurs more slowly. The higher intracellular $[Ca^{2+}]$ results in the efflux of K^+. The re-establishment of the action potential occurs later by the reverse of the Na^+–K^+ exchange. The Na^+/K^+ exchange requires energy which is provided by an enzyme Na^+–K^+–ATPase.

- Cardiac glycosides are proposed to inhibit this enzyme with a net result of reduced sodium exchange with potassium that leaves increased intracellular Na^+. This results in increased intracellular (Ca^{2+}). Elevated intracellular calcium concentration triggers a series of intracellular biochemical events that ultimately result in an increase in the force of the myocardial contraction or a positive inotropoic effect.

- Cardiac glycosides work by inhibiting the Na^+/K^+ pump. This causes an increase in the level of sodium ions in the myocytes, which then leads to a rise in the level of calcium ions.

- This inhibition increases the amount of Ca^{2+} ions available for contraction of the heart muscle, improves cardiac output and reduces distention of the heart.

- They do this by stabilizing the E2-P transition state of the Na^+/K^+ pump. The proposed mechanism is the following: inhibition of the Na^+/K^+ pump leads to increased Na^+ levels, which in turn slows down the extrusion of Ca^{2+} via the Na^+/Ca^{2+} exchange pump. Increased amounts of Ca^{2+} are then stored in the sarcoplasmic reticulum and released by each action potential.

- They have an antiarrhythmic effect by prolonging the refractory period of the AV node (atrioventricular node), reducing the number of impulses reaching the ventricles. Cardiac output is restored but atrial fibrillation or atrial flutters are not abolished.

Pharmacokinetics

- Digoxin and digitoxin are the most commonly prescribed agents. Both are readily absorbed from GIT. However, to a considerable extent, digoxin is inactivated to form 2-hydroxydigoxin by intestinal microflora while digitoxin is extensively absorbed. Certain drugs like, kaolin, antacids may interfere with the absorption. These glycosides possess relatively large volume of distribution. This accounts for their slow distribution in the body compartments. Digitoxin is extensively bound to the plasma proteins while digoxin is also significantly bound to plasma proteins. Skeletal muscles, heart, kidneys and RBCs are the body tissues where most of the administered doses of cardiac glycosides get concentrated.

- Digoxin has fairly rapid onset of action when administered intravenously while digitoxin is usually not given by IV route due to its slow onset of action. If used orally, intramuscular route is not preferred for the administration of these drugs due to the induction of severe pain and muscle necrosis.

- The half-life of digoxin is estimated to be about 35-40 hours. It readily crosses placenta. Its metabolites are primarily eliminated in urine. The rate of elimination of cardiac glycosides is very slow which, if not taken into consideration may result into drug intoxication due to its accumulation. Hence, the cardiac glycosides are usually administered orally in two stages. The patient is treated with an initial dose of the drug to get therapeutic response. This dose administration is known as initial digitalization or loading dose. The therapeutic response obtained through digitalization is further maintained by low dose schedule which is known as maintenance dose.

Therapeutic Uses

Congestive cardiac failure

The positive inotropic effect of these glycosides causes the heart to contact more strongly and efficiently. The beneficial effects of these drugs in patients with heart failure include; increased cardiac output, decreased heart size and venous pressure, diuresis and relief of edema. The reduction in myocardial oxygen demand decreases the intensity of compensatory sympathetic nervous system which results in a decrease in systemic arterial resistance and venous tone. However, digitalis treatment is not effective when:

1. Heart failure is associated with very high preload or after load. In such cases, the use of diuretics or vasodilator is given.

2. Chronic treatment is required. This is due to loss in therapeutic efficacy through development of significant tolerance to drug action. In such case, vasodilator and/or inhibitors of angiotensin converting enzyme are the drug of choice used along with digitalis or a diuretics.

Atrial arrhythmias

- At therapeutic doses, cardiac glycosides have a protective action on the ventricles. This action is exerted by increasing the vagal tone and by a direct depressant action on AV conduction. This results into an increased 'filtering' of the impulses which are generated at relatively higher rate during arterial arrhythmias. The reduction in conduction velocity and an increase in refractory period protect the ventricular muscle from excessive stimulation. Atrial arrhythmias where digitalis finds clinical use, include—atrial flutter, atrial fibrillation and proxymal atrial tachycardia.

- However, the glycosides are contraindicated in patients having hypokalemia, hypercalcemia, impaired renal function or ventricular tachycardia or procainamides are better drugs to treat ventricular tachycardia.

Adverse Effect

- The cardiac glycosides have a low therapeutic safety margine. Consequently, the adverse reactions are quite frequent and can be severe in toxic doses. These adverse reactions are many due to:

1. An increased parasympathomimetic tone.

2. A loss of intracellular Ca^{2+} concentration. The cardiac effects of digitalis glycosides are much complicated due to unusual combination.

3. A loss of intracellular potassium.

4. Increased abnormal or ectopic automaticity due to direct drug effect.

- Digitalis glycosides are used to treat a diseased heart. Due to the combination of above two effects. Such a diseased heart easily gets attacked by arrhythmias or AV block occurred due to an exaggeration of depressant action on conduction.

- Digitalis in high dose is likely to induce the development of almost every known cardiac arrhythmia. The infracted myocardium serves as a site to develop ectopic foci which is responsible for the occurrence of both atrial and ventricular tachycardias. It is better to discontinue drug therapy under such condition.

Digitalis Intoxication

- The large volume of distribution and low rate of elimination, the concurrent effect of glycosides on ANS and the peripheral vascular smooth muscles and hypokalemia are the factors that provoke the sensitivity of the patient towards the digitalis intoxication.

- The low therapeutic index of these drugs necessitates careful clinical observation of the patient during the period of initial digitalization. Hence, extreme caution is to be observed when they are given intravenously. Both hypokalemia and hypercalcemia sensitizes myocardium to the glycoside action. In such a condition, a decline in resting membrane potential brings the cell quite near to their threshold value for generating impulse.

- This explains the basis of digitalis-induced extrasystoles during the therapy. An adequate potassium intake should always be maintained in the therapy when hypokalemia is reported. The hypokalemia, if remained uncorrected, may lead to the tachyarrhythmia in digitalis overdose. Hence if needed diuretics are given in patient receiving digitalises then potassium sparing diuretics are to be used.

- However, in toxicity signs due to conduction impairments, potassium intake may provoke the digitalis toxicity. Hence, it is contraindicated in cases of AV blocks. Under such condition, vagolytic agents are used.

- An enhancement of automaticity by digitalis is the probable reason behind the drug induced arterial arrhythmias. Any antiarrhythmic drug can be used to suppress atrial arrhythmias due to digitalis toxicity.

- A considerable fraction of orally administered digoxin is inactivated by intestinal microflora. Hence in the patient receiving digoxin along with an antibiotic, the extent of absorption of active drug suddenly increases. This leads to appearance of toxic effects of digoxin in therapeutic dose level.

Treatment of Intoxication

- Digitalis glycosides have very poor therapeutic index. In case of digitalis intoxication, the therapy should be immediately discontinued so as to lower down the plasma concentration of the drug.

- The patients should be evaluated to trace out hypokalemia, if diuretics are concurrently administered. The plasma potassium level may be maintained in the upper normal level by giving potassium either orally or intravenously. The increasing extracellular K^+ ion concentration may produce the stimulatory effect on Na^+–K^+–ATPase pump, thereby decreasing the binding of digitalis with the pump system. The suppression of ectopic beats and abnormal rhythms are other beneficial effects of potassium intake. However, its administration is contraindicated in the presence of diminished cardiac conduction. In such condition, atropine-like drugs may improve the functioning of heart by suppressing the underlying cause.

- Digitalis increases the automaticity and excitability of myocardial fibers. In toxic doses, digitalis may induce severe atrial arrhythmias. Many anti-arrhythmic agents, e.g. propranolol, phenytoin, lidocaine along with potassium salts can be used in suppressing digitalis induced atrial arrhythmias.

- In severe life-threatening digitalis intoxication (accidental or attempted suicides) above treatment may not be effective to get immediate response. In such cases, specific glycoside antibodies administration leads to rapid recovery of the heart functioning. Digitalis specific fab antibody fragments were first evaluated for their use is accompanied by emergence of allergic reaction in sensitive patients. This limits their use in patients with pre-allergic history.

Alternatives to Digitalis Therapy

- The low margine of safety and inherent toxicities associated with the use of digitalis glycosides, led to the search for development of group of agents having positive inotropic effect.

- There was an increasing tendency to use vasodilators (hydralazine, prazosin, nitrates), diuretics or cardiac stimulant to reduce the preload or after load of the failing heart. However, adrenergic drugs have a shorter duration of action while vasodilators may not be the primary drugs of choice in all the cases.
- Of the available alternatives to digitalis, bipyridine derivatives are of special interest due to the combination of both positive inotropic property and vasodilatory effect in one compound. Examples are amrinone and milrinone.

Amrinone and Milrinone

Both these agents can be used orally as well as intravenously. Milrinone is considerably more potent but has relatively shorter duration of action than amrinone. Their use in congestive heart failure is mainly due to their positive inotropic and vasodilatory effects.

Mechanism of action

- The mechanism of the positive inotropic effects of amrinone differs from that of conventional positive inotropic agents. Since their efficacy is not decreased by the use of adrenergic blockers, the direct activation of adrenergic receptor is not their mechanism of action.
- Probably the mechanism may be related to an increase in intracellular concentration of cAMP by inhibition of phosphodiestrase enzymes.
- The increase in cAMP then lowers the rate of influx of Ca^{2+} ions resulting into vasodilation. The positive inotropic effects make these agents useful in the treatment of congestive cardiac failure, where their inotropic effects are additive to that of cardiac glycosides.

Amrinone   Milrinone

Pharmacokinetics

- Liver serves as the potential site for the metabolism. About six metabolites of amrinone have been identified. Its use in the chronic treatment is not advisable due to serious adverse effects.
- Amrinone during long-term use may induce immunological abnormality. This along with long-term inhibition of phophodiestrases enzyme may contribute for the appearance of side effect.
- On the other hand, milrinone is quite safe drug. Its use is not associated with most of the adverse effects seen in amrinone.

Antiarrhythmic Agents

The pumping action of the heart involves three principal electrical events.
1. The generation of a electrical signal.
2. The conduction or propagation of the signal.
3. The fading away of the signal.
When one or more of these events are disrupted, result into cardiac arrhythmias.

PATHOPHYSIOLOGY

Disorders in the Generation of Electrical Signals

- In normal heart, cells located in the right atrium, referred to as the SA node or pacemaker cells, initiate a cardiac impulse. The spontaneous electrical depolarization of the SA pacemaker cells is independent of the nervous system; however, these cells are innervated by both sympathetic and parasympathetic fibers, which can cause increases or decreases in heart rate as a result of nervous system stimulation.
- Other special cells in the heart also possess the ability to generate an impulse, and may influence cardiac rhythm, but are normally surpassed by the dominant signal generation of SA pacemaker cells.
- When normal pacemaker function is suppressed—caused by pathological changes occurring from infarction, digitalis toxicity, or excessive vagal tone or when excessive release of catecholamines from sympathomimetic nerve fibers occurs, these other automatic cells (including special atrial cells, certain AV node cells, the bundle of His, and Purkinje fibers) have the potential to become ectopic pacemakers, which can dominant cardiac rhythm and consequently lead to arrhythmias.

Disorders in the Conduction of the Electrical Signal

- Disorders in the transmission of the electrical impulse can lead to conduction block and re-entry phenomenon. Conduction block may be complete (no impulses pass through the block), partial (some impulses pass through the block), and bi-directional or unidirectional.
- During bidirectional block, an impulse is blocked regardless of the direction of entry; a unidirectional block occurs when an impulse from one direction is completely blocked, while impulses from the opposite direction are propagated (although usually at a slower than normal rate).

Heart Block (The Fading Away of the Signal)

- Heart block occurs when the impulse signal from the SA node is not transmitted through either the AV node or lower electrical pathways properly.
- Heart block is classified by degree of severity.

1. First degree heart block, all impulses moving through the AV node are conducted, but at a slower than normal rate.

2. Second degree heart block, some impulses fully transit the AV node, whereas others are blocked (as a result, the ventricles fail to beat at the proper moment).

3. Third degree heart block, no impulses reach the ventricles (automatic cells in the ventricles initiate impulses, but at a slower rate, and as a result the atria and ventricles beat at somewhat independent rates). Pulses reach the ventricles (automatic cells in the ventricles initiate impulses, but at a slower rate, and as a result the atria and ventricles beat at somewhat independent rates).

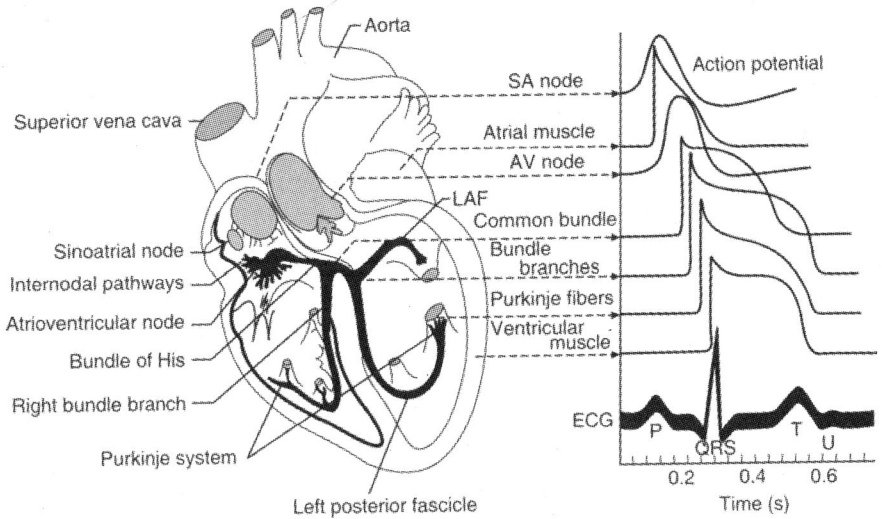

Fig. 27.1: Action potentials and the conducting system of the heart

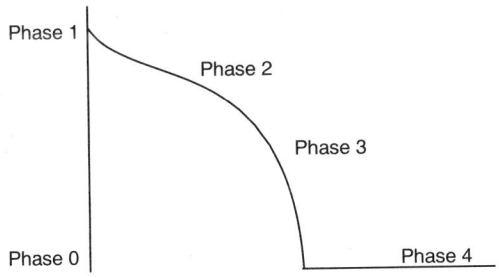

Phase 0

- Upstroke.
- Due to opening of fast Na^+ channels when the threshold potential (~ -70 mV) is reached.
- There is a massive influx of Na^+ into the muscle cell, causing a rapid depolarization.

Phase 1

- Partial repolarization.
- Due to closure of the Na^+ channels.

Phase 2
- Plateau phase.
- Due to opening of slow Ca^{2+} channels.

Phase 3
- Repolarization.
- Due to closure of the Ca^{2+} channels and opening of the K^+ channels, causing a massive loss of K^+ out of the cell.

Phase 4 (Fig. 27.2)
- Pacemaker potential.
- This phase is unimportant in non-conducting heart tissues.
- In conducting tissues (SA and AV nodes), the pacemaker potential gradually depolarizes during diastole to reach the threshold potential, resulting in a spike.
- Conducting tissues always fire action potentials, at varying frequencies (they have intrinsic firing capacity). The SA node fires the fastest and so assumes the role of the pacemaker.
- Non-conducting tissues need a 'jump start' impulse from the conducting tissues in order to depolarise (i.e. they are not capable of intrinsically firing, unless under pathological conditions).
- In conducting tissues, the opening of Na^+ channels is less important. The upstroke is largely due to the slow entry of Ca^{2+}.

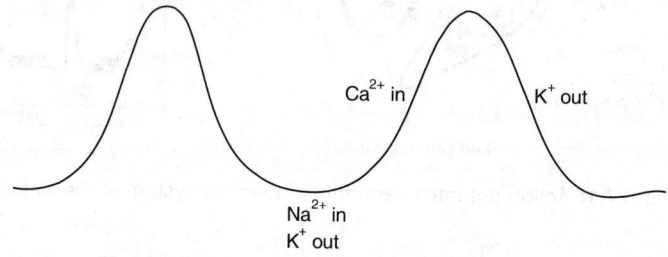

Fig. 27.2: Action potential in conducting tissues

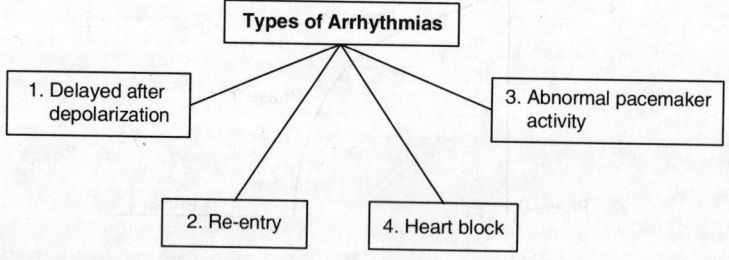

1. Delayed after depolarization
- Non-pacemaker cells (non-conducting fibers) normally have a quiescent phase 4 (i.e. they do not fire unless they receive a signal from the pacemakers).
- In this condition, non-conducting cells have a slow, rising phase 4, which allows them to fire without a signal from the pacemaker.
- It is due to an increase in intracellular Ca^{2+} which increases the pacemaker potential
- Conditions which can lead to an increased intracellular Ca^{2+} are:

✓ Cardiac glycosides.

✓ The actions of cardiac glycosides will be discussed in a later chapter.

✓ Increased sympathetic tone (adrenergic stress).

✓ Myocardial ischemia.

2. Re-entry

- Re-entry occurs when a heart muscle fiber is made to contract immediately after its refractory period, by the same impulse which caused its contraction in the first place.

- Normally, this does not occur because the muscle fiber is still in the refractory phase, and so is not sensitive to any stimulation.

- The best example of re-entry is when there are 2 different pathways for an action potential (Fig. 27.3).

- As the action potential separates to depolarise the 2 different pathways, it meets again (Fig. 27.4).

- Re-entry occurs when there is a blockage of one of these pathways. The action potential which passes through the unblocked pathway can circle back and depolarise part of the blocked pathway, *provided that the time it takes the action potential to circle back is greater than the refractory period of the muscle fiber which has already depolarised.* If this is not the case, re-entry does not occur.

- Re-entry causes the muscle fibers to beat at an excessive rate. Therefore, drugs which prolong the refractory period (e.g. class III drugs) are effective at preventing re-entry.

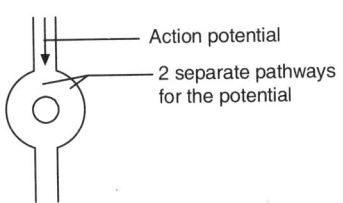

Fig. 27.3: Propagation of action potential

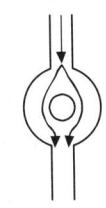

Fig. 27.4: Re-entery phenomenon of action potential leading to arrhythmia

3. Abnormal pacemaker activity

- The pacemaker is the tissue which has the fastest rate of firing. Normally, this is the SA node.
- Sometimes, other tissues in the heart can assume the role of pacemaker.
- The main predisposing factors are similar to those in delayed after depolarization:

A. β adrenoceptor stimulation: Causes increase in Ca^{2+} levels.

B. Myocardial ischemia:

✓ There is a reflex increase in sympathetic tone as a result of poor perfusion. This increase in sympathetic tone increases Ca^{2+} levels.

✓ Also, ischemia affects the Na^+ pump which requires ATP to extrude Na^+ out of the cell, against its concentration gradient. If this pump fails to work (due to lack of ATP) Na^+ concentrations increase in the cell, resulting in depolarization.

4. Heart block

- Damage to nodal tissue (e.g. during a myocardial infarct), prevents conduction of the signal to the parts of the heart.
- The areas of the heart which normally rely on this signal start to beat independently, under the action their own pacemakers.
- A myocardial infarct damages nodal tissue by:

✓ Causing fibrosis.

✓ Causing ischemia in the area of conduction tissue.

- Clinically, arrhythmias are classified according to:
  - ✓ Their site of origin (atrial or ventricular).
  - ✓ Whether they cause bradycardia or tachycardia.

CLASSIFICATION OF ANTIARRHYTHMIC DRUGS

Classification of antiarrhythmic drugs is given in Flow chart 27.1.

Flow chart 27.1: Classification of antiarrhythmic drugs

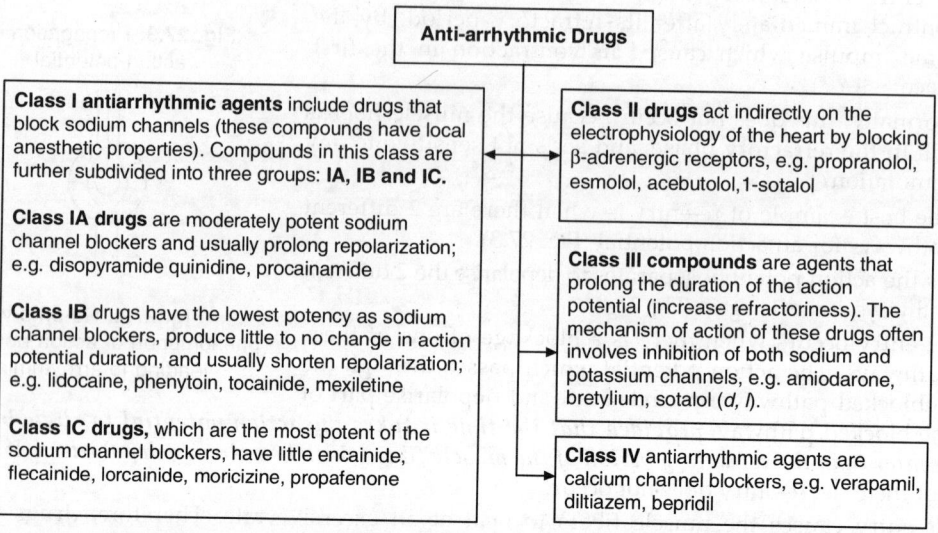

Anti-arrhythmic Drugs

Class I antiarrhythmic agents include drugs that block sodium channels (these compounds have local anesthetic properties). Compounds in this class are further subdivided into three groups: **IA, IB and IC.**

Class IA drugs are moderately potent sodium channel blockers and usually prolong repolarization; e.g. disopyramide quinidine, procainamide

Class IB drugs have the lowest potency as sodium channel blockers, produce little to no change in action potential duration, and usually shorten repolarization; e.g. lidocaine, phenytoin, tocainide, mexiletine

Class IC drugs, which are the most potent of the sodium channel blockers, have little encainide, flecainide, lorcainide, moricizine, propafenone

Class II drugs act indirectly on the electrophysiology of the heart by blocking β-adrenergic receptors, e.g. propranolol, esmolol, acebutolol, 1-sotalol

Class III compounds are agents that prolong the duration of the action potential (increase refractoriness). The mechanism of action of these drugs often involves inhibition of both sodium and potassium channels, e.g. amiodarone, bretylium, sotalol (*d, l*).

Class IV antiarrhythmic agents are calcium channel blockers, e.g. verapamil, diltiazem, bepridil

Rationale for the Selection of Drugs Used as Antiarrhythmic Agents

Arrhythmias arise from 3 general mechanisms:

1. Increased sympathetic tone ⟶ results in increased Ca^{2+} entry.
2. Myocardial infarct ⟶ results in increased Ca^{2+} entry.
3. Increased Na^+ entry ⟶ causing depolarization.

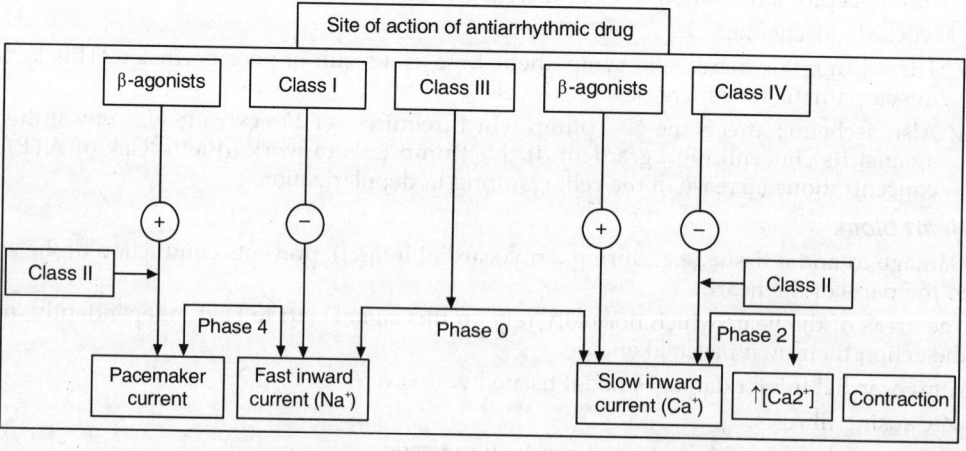

Site of action of antiarrhythmic drug

β-agonists | Class I | Class III | β-agonists | Class IV

Class II

Class II

Phase 4 | Phase 0 | Phase 2

Pacemaker current | Fast inward current (Na⁺) | Slow inward current (Ca⁺) | $\uparrow[Ca^{2+}]$ | Contraction

Table 27.1: Antiarrhythmic drugs work by inhibiting one of these mechanisms

Class	Drugs	Mechanism of action
IA	Quinidine, procainamide, disopyramide	Sodium channel blockade, lengthen refractory period
IB	Lidocaine, phenytoin, tocainide, mexiletine	Sodium channel blockade, shorten duration of action potential
IC	Encainide, flecainide, lorcainide, moricizine, propafenone	Sodium channel blockade, conduction slowed
II	Propranolol, esmolol, acebutolol, *l*-sotalol	Blockade of β-adrenergic receptors, AV conduction time slowed,
III	Amiodarone, bretylium, sotalol (*d*, *l*), dofetilide, ibutilide	Potassium channel blockade, prolonged refractoriness
IV	Verapamil, diltiazem, bepridil	Blockade of slow inward Ca^{2+}
Miscellaneous	Adenosine, digitoxin, digoxin	Miscellaneous

Class IA antiarrhythmic agents

Quinidine   Procainamide   Disopyramide

Class IB antiarrhythmic agents

Lidocaine   Tocainide   Mexiletine   Phenytoin

Class IC antiarrhythmic agents

Encainide   Flecainide   Lorcainide

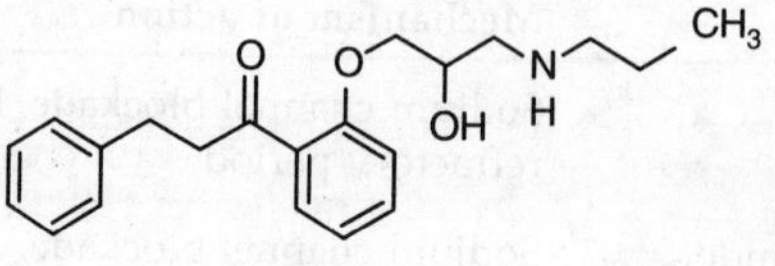

Propafenone

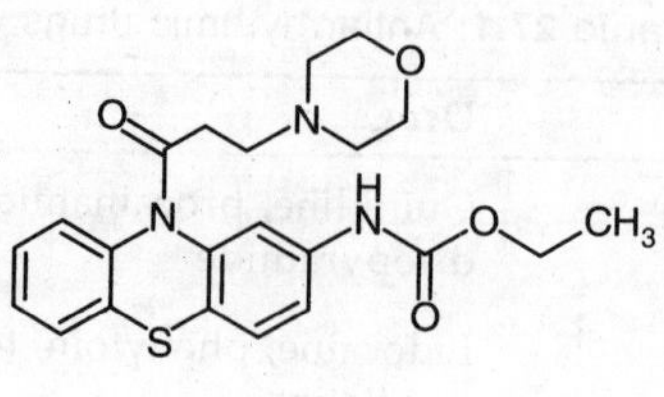

Moricizine

Class II antiarrhythmic agents

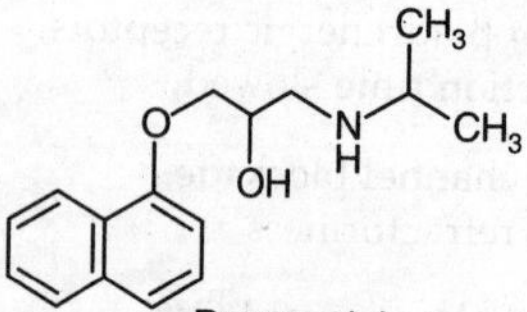

Propranolol

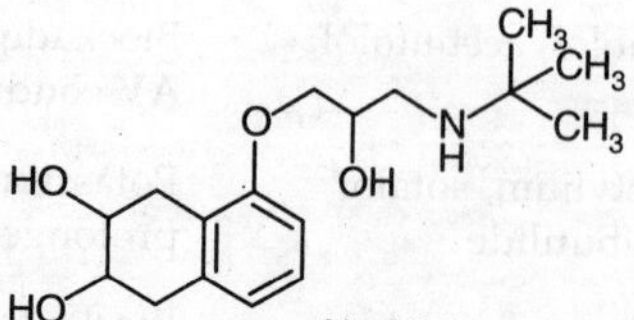

Nadolol

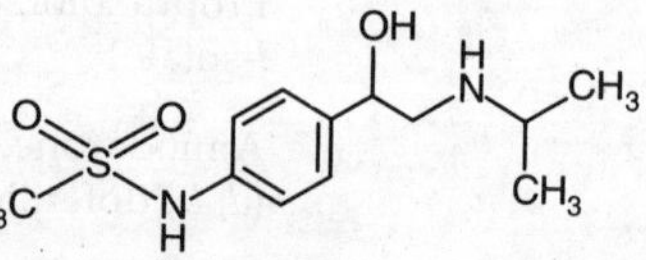

Sotalol

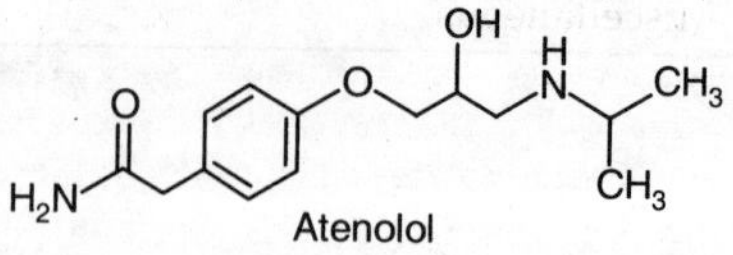

Atenolol

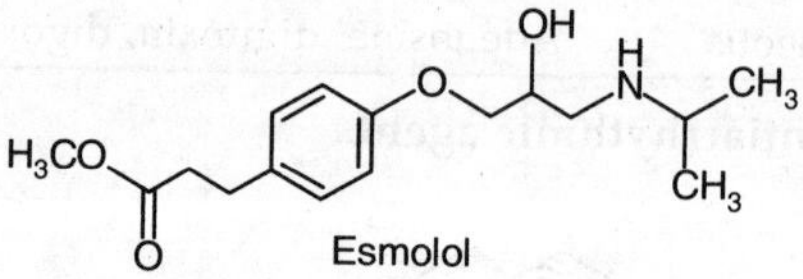

Esmolol

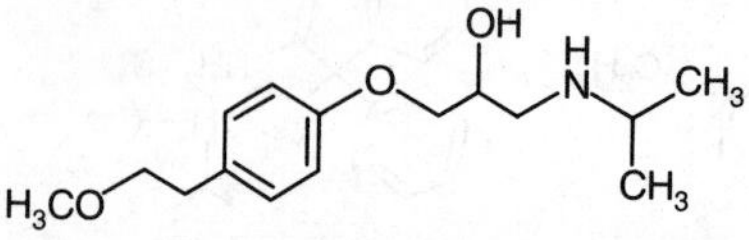

Metoprolol

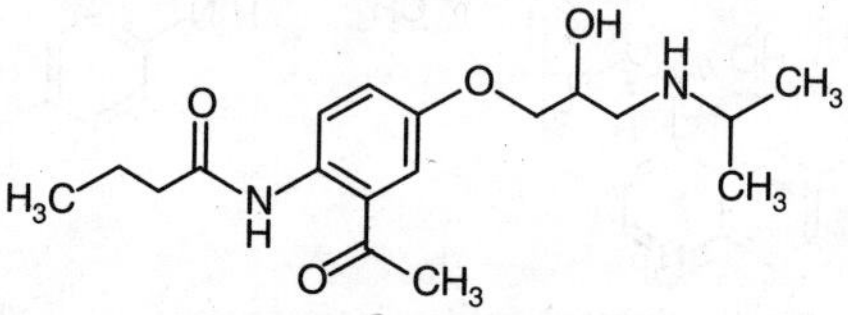

Acebutolol

Class III antiarrhythmic agents

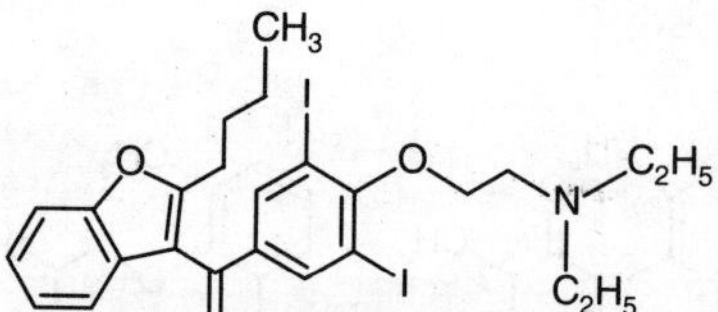

Amiodarone

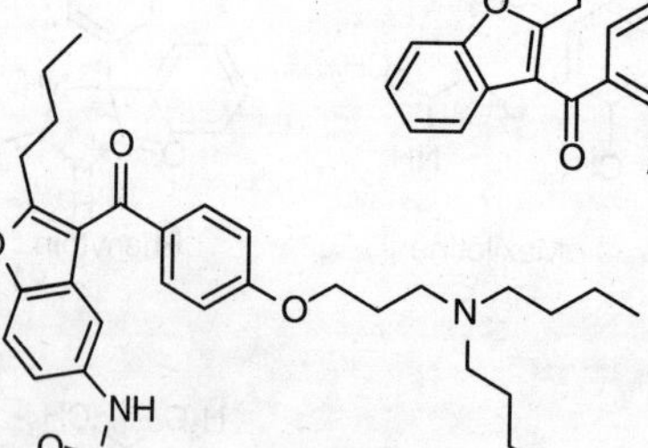

Dronedarone

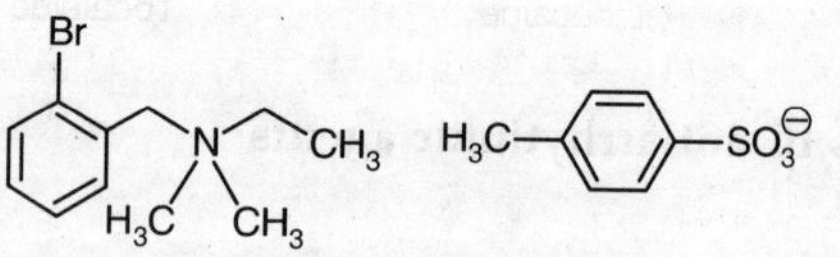

Bretylium tosylate

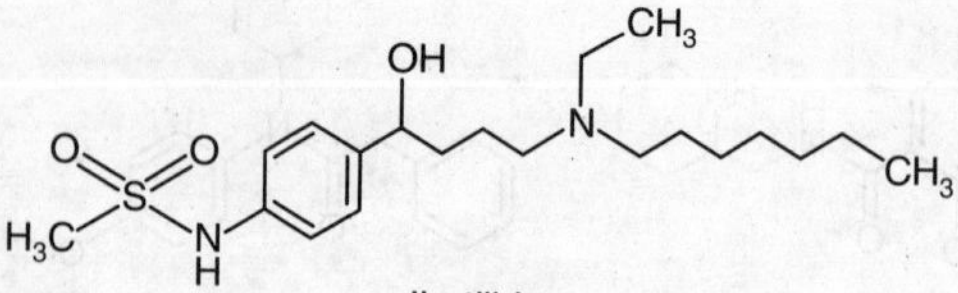

Ibutilide

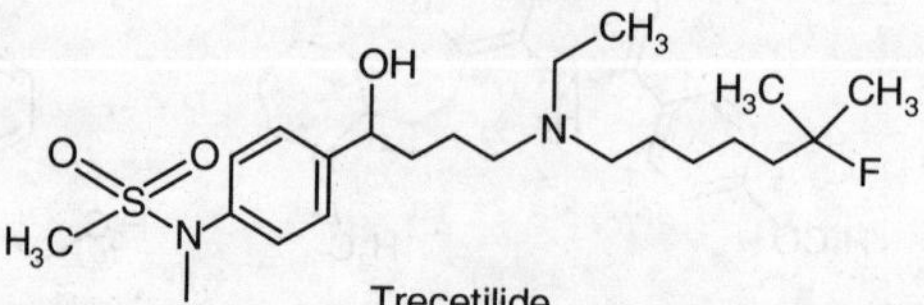

Trecetilide

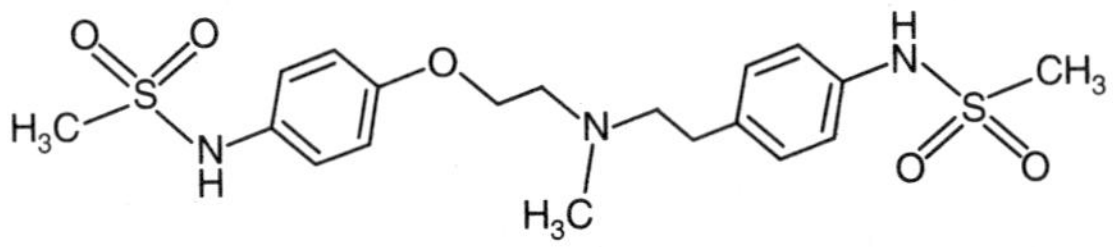

Dofetilide

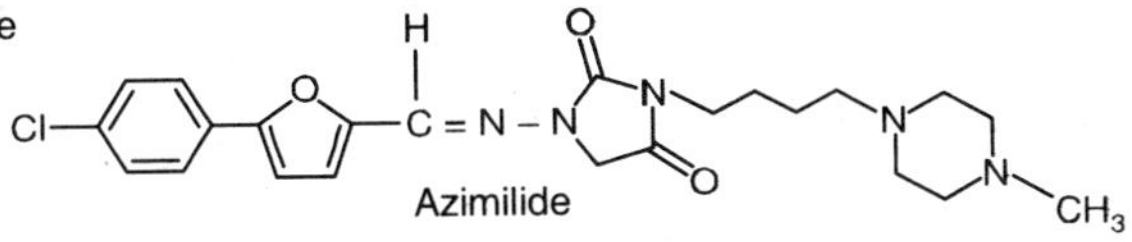

Azimilide

Class IV antiarrhythmic agents

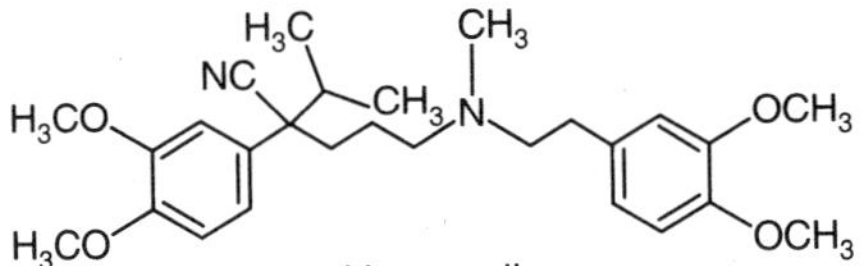

Verapamil

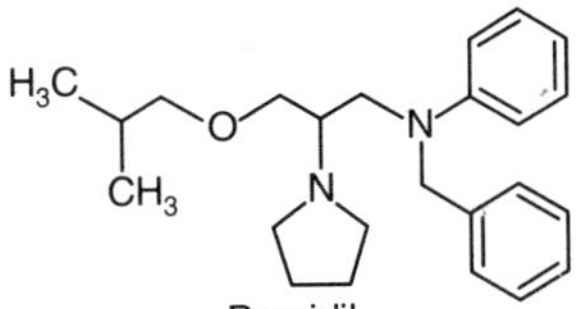

Bepridil

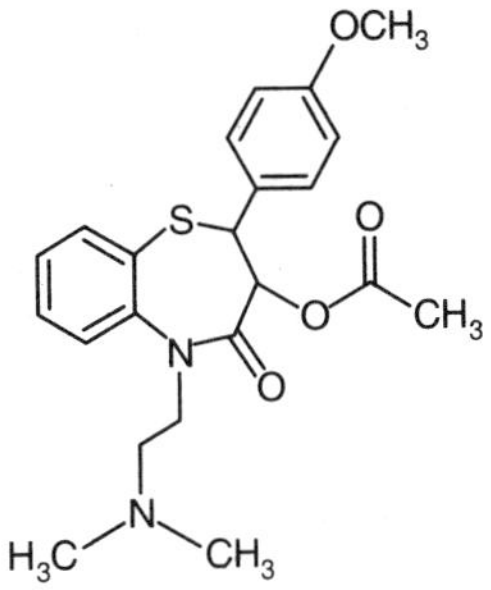

Diltiazem

Class I Drugs

- Block voltage sensitive Na^+ channels.
- Important for the treatment of arrhythmias where Na^+ channels are important (in non-nodal tissues where Na^+ is the predominant ion in the upstroke phase).
- Voltage sensitive Na^+ channels exist in either of 3 forms.
  - o Resting (M gates closed, H gates open).
  - o Open (both M and H gate open).
  - o Refractory (M gates open, H gates closed).
- The refractory state is a state of inactivation, and no further action potentials can be initiated until it returns to the resting phase (i.e. the H gates open and the M gates closed). These drugs bind preferentially to the open or refractory state. In the refractory state, the drugs bind to the closed H gate and prevent it from opening (thus preventing the channel from returning to the resting state).
- The class I drugs are divided into subclasses, according to their rate of dissociation from the channel.

Class IB drugs

- The most used drug is the class IB drug lignocaine. Lignocaine is also used as a local anesthetic.
- Binds preferentially to the refractory channels. Refractory channels occur when the cell is depolarized.

- Lignocaine is useful for ventricular arrhythmias after a myocardial infarct because when ischemia occurs, it causes cells to be partially depolarized, hence the Na^+ channels will be in their refractory state.
- Lignocaine dissociates rapidly. It binds to the channel during phase 0 and dissociates before the arrival of the next action potential (assuming normal rhythm).
- In abnormal rhythms, a premature beat will be prevented from occurring because lignocaine will not have dissociated yet. Administered intravenously.

Adverse effects:

- CNS effects— drowsiness, convulsion.
- CVS effects— reduced cardiac contractility, bradycardia.
- Amino-2', 6'-propionoxylidide; propionamide, 2-amino-N-(2,6-dimethyl-phenyl) Used for prevention and treatment of ventricular arrhythmia.

Class IC drugs

- Not used much any more since it may cause death by increasing ventricular fibrillation after myocardial ischemia.
- Many antiarrhythmics can also be proarrhythmic under particular circumstances. In the case of flecainide, it becomes proarrhythmic under ischemic conditions.
- Slow association and dissociation (10 sec.)
- Reach a steady state level of block which does not vary within the cardiac cycle.
- Cause a general reduction in excitability.
- Used for severe ventricular tachycardia.

Class II Drugs

- These drugs are β-adrenoceptor antagonists.
- They are useful for stress-induced tachycardia or ischemia induced arrhythmias when there is increased sympathetic activity.
- β antagonists are also useful to reduce anxiety associated with increased heart rate.

Class III Drugs

- Mechanism of action unknown.
- They prolong the cardiac action potential, thus increasing the refractory period.
- As a result, they are useful in preventing ventricular and supraventricular arrhythmias.

Toxicity

These drugs have a very long half-life (10 to 100 days). The drug accumulates in tissue causing following adverse effects.

1. **Cornea:** Deposits, causing halos in vision. Reversible if stop taking drug.
2. **Skin:** Photosensitivity, rashes.
3. **Thyroid:** Hypo-or hyperthyroidism (due to high iodine content in the drug).
4. **Lungs:** Fibrosis (may be irreversible).
5. Liver damage.
6. GIT disturbance.

- A class III drug and also α β antagonist. The L isomer is a β blocker. Both the D and the L isomers contribute to its class III activity. Less adverse effects than amiodarone. The adverse effects which do occur are the result of its β blocking effects (e.g. bronchoconstriction, decreased cardiac activity).

Class IV Drugs

- Blocks voltage sensitive Ca^{2+} channels.
- More selective for cardiac tissue than Ca^{2+} channels present elsewhere (e.g. in vascular smooth muscle).
- Shortens phase 2 (plateau phase) of the action potential by reducing the influx of Ca^{2+}. This causes suppression of premature ectopic beats by preventing phase 4 depolarization.
- Reduces cardiac contractility.
- Must not use verapamil in conjunction with β blockers because they both have an additive effect in causing cardiac depression.
- Effective for use in atrial tachycardia (but not ventricular tachycardia).
- Do not use, if there is underlying impairment of cardiac contractility.

Tocainide

2, 6-dimethyl-aniline

2-bromo-propionyl bromide

Tocainide

Flecainide

2, 5-dihydroxy-benzoic acid

2, 2, 2-trifluoro-ethyl trifluoro-methanesulfonate

2, 2, 2-trifluoroethyl 2, 5-bis(2, 2, 2-trifluoro-ethoxy) benzoate

2-aminomethyl-pyridine

(I)

Flecainide

Diisopromine

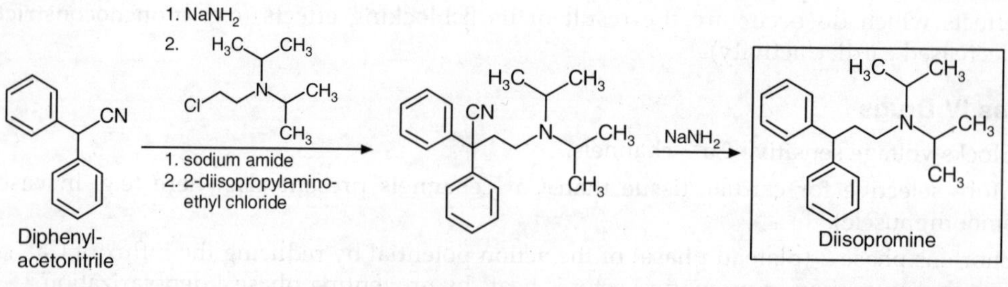

1. NaNH₂
2. H₃C—CH₃ / CH₃ / CH₃ Cl–CH₂CH₂–N

1. sodium amide
2. 2-diisopropylamino-
   ethyl chloride

Diphenyl-
acetonitrile

NaNH₂

Diisopromine

Procainamide

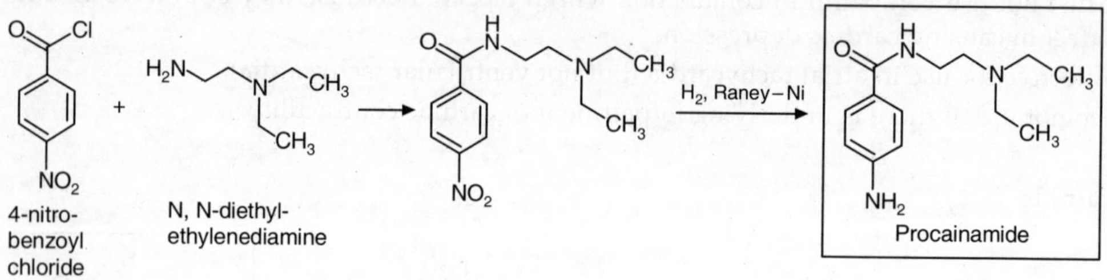

4-nitro-
benzoyl
chloride

N, N-diethyl-
ethylenediamine

H₂, Raney–Ni

Procainamide

Propranolol

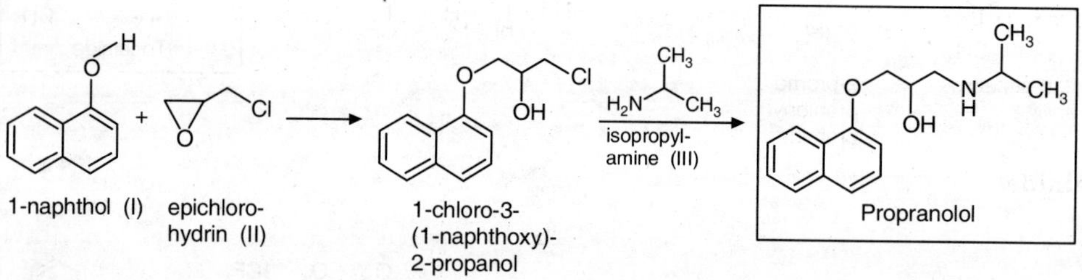

1-naphthol (I)   epichloro-
                  hydrin (II)

1-chloro-3-
(1-naphthoxy)-
2-propanol

isopropyl-
amine (III)

Propranolol

Sotalol

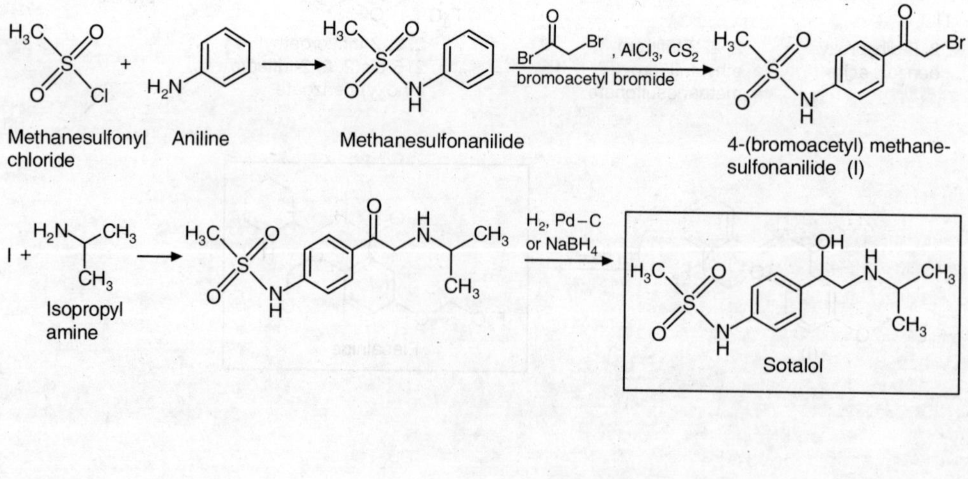

Methanesulfonyl   Aniline
chloride

Methanesulfonanilide

bromoacetyl bromide

4-(bromoacetyl) methane-
sulfonanilide (I)

I +

Isopropyl
amine

H₂, Pd–C
or NaBH₄

Sotalol

Verapamil

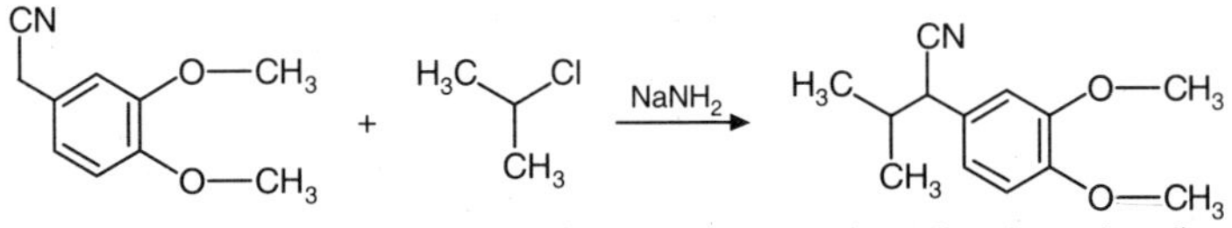

3, 4-dimethoxy-
phenylacetonitrile

Isopropyl
chloride

2-(3, 4-dimethoxyphenyl)-
3-methylbutyronitrile (I)

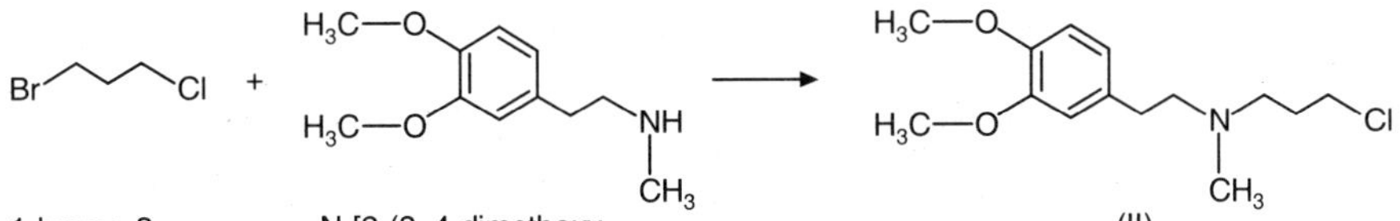

1-bromo-3-
chloropropane

N-[2-(3, 4-dimethoxy-
phenyl)ethyl] methylamine

(II)

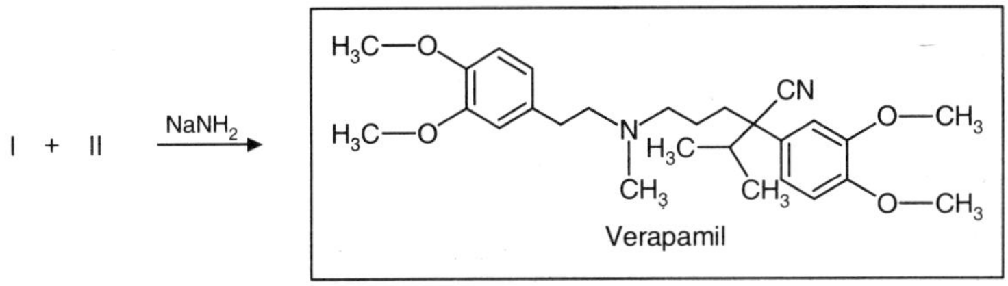

I + II

Verapamil

Amiodarone

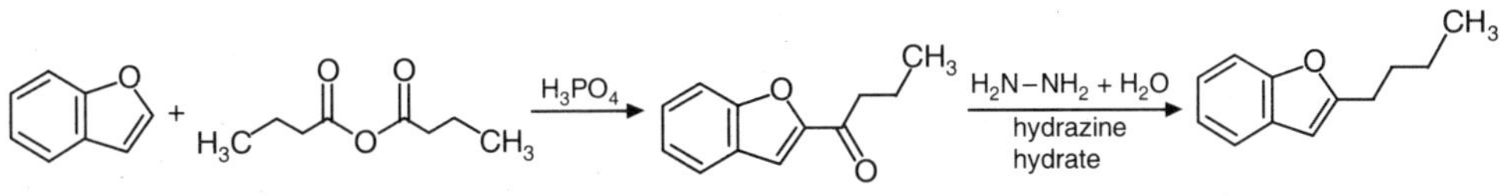

Benzofuran

Butyric anhydride

2-butyrylbenzofuran

2-butyrylbenzofuran (I)

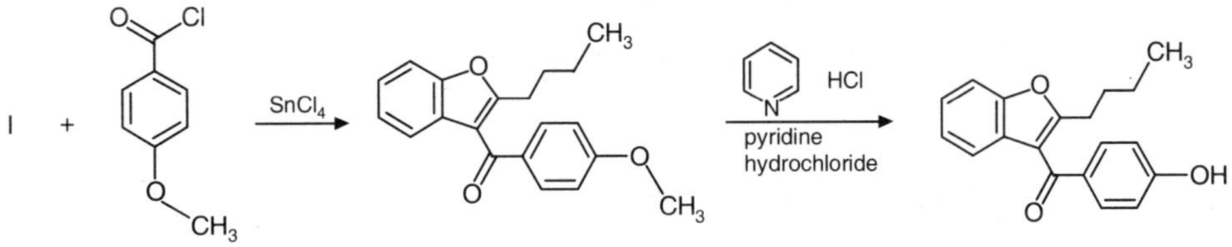

4-methoxy-
benzoyl chloride

2-butyl-3-(4-methoxy-
benzoyl)-benzofuran

2-butyl-3-(4-hydroxy-
benzoyl)-benzofuran (II)

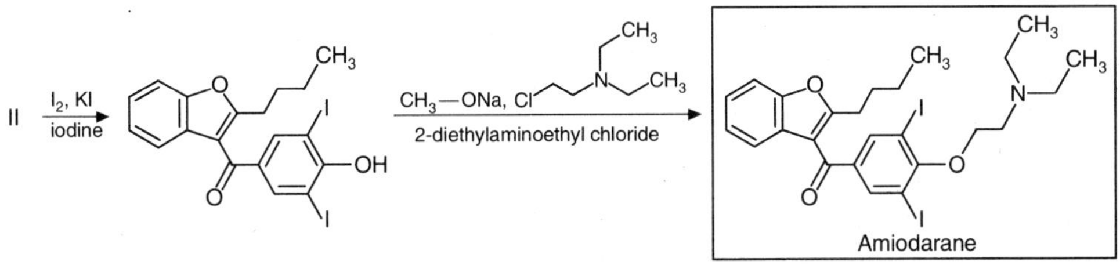

2-diethylaminoethyl chloride

Amiodarane

28

Antihypertensive Agents

Elevation of blood pressure (BP) above the normal level is called hypertension. Normal level of blood pressure is 140 mm Hg (systolic) and 90 mm Hg (diastolic). BP is determined by cardiac output (c.c.) and total peripheral resistance.

▆ TYPES OF HYPERTENSION

Primary Hypertension

- The exact cause of hypertension is not known.

Secondary Hypertension

- This may be because of renal disease, pheochromocytoma, hyperthyroidism and hyperaldosterism leading to a secondary hypertension.

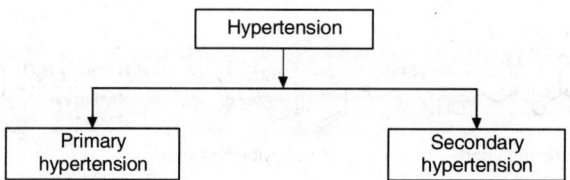

▆ MECHANISM FOR CONTROLLING BLOOD PRESSURE (FIG. 28.1)

Baroreceptor

- Baro reflexes involving sympathetic nervous system are responsible for the rapid moment to moment regulation of blood pressure.
- A fall in blood pressure causes pressure sensitive neurons (baroreceptor in aortic arch and carotid sinus) to send fewer impulses to cardiovascular centers in brain/CNS.
- This prompts a reflex response of increased sympathetic and decreased parasympathetic output to the heart and vasculature resulting in vasoconstriction and increased cardiac output. These changes result in compensatory rise in blood pressure.

Renin–Angiotensin–Aldosterone System

- The kidney provides for the long-term control of blood pressure by altering blood volume. Baroreceptor in kidney responds in reduced arterial blood pressure by releasing the enzyme renin.

- The peptidase converts angiotensinogen to angiotensin-I, which is converted in turn to angiotensin-II in the presence of enzyme angiotensin converting enzyme. Angiotensin-II is the body's most potent circulating vasoconstrictor, causing increase in blood pressure.
- Furthermore angiotensin-II stimulates aldosterone secretion, leading to increased renal sodium reabsorption and increased blood volume, which can contribute to further increase in blood pressure.

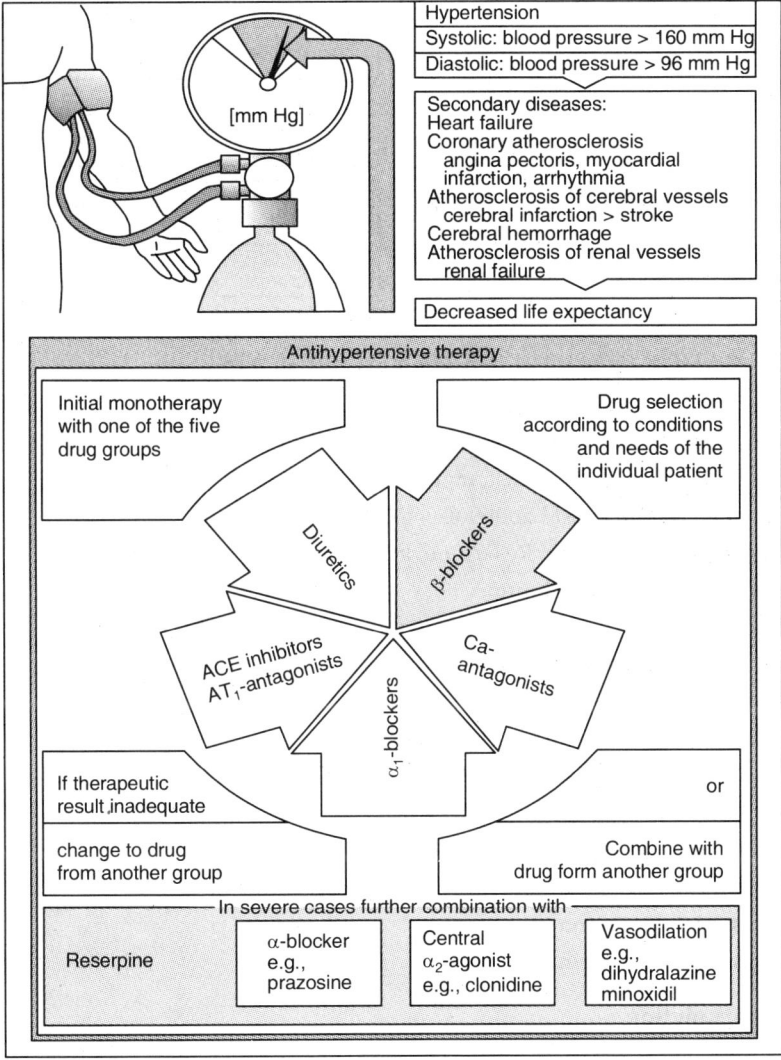

Fig. 28.1: Different approaches to treat hypertension

POSSIBLE APPROACHES FOR TREATMENT OF HYPERTENSION

The approaches for treatment of hypertension are depicted in Flow chart 28.1.

Flow chart 28.1: Treatment of hypertension—possible approaches

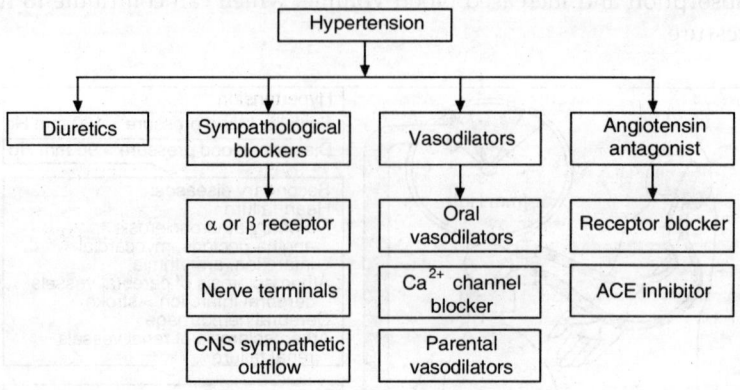

CLASSIFICATION OF ANTIHYPERTENSIVE AGENTS

1. **Central sympatholytics:** Clonidine, methyldopa.
2. **α-adrenergic blocker:** Prazosin, terazosin, phentolamine, phenoxibenzamine.
3. **β-Adrenergic blocker:** Propanolol, metoprolol, atenolol.
4. **α, β-Nonselective blockers:** Labetelol.
5. **Adrenergic neuron blockers:** Reserpine, guanethidine.
6. **Ganglionic blockers:** Pentolinium.
7. **Vasodilators:**
   Calcium channel blocker: Verapamil, diltiazem, nifedipine, amlodipine.
   Directly acting vasodilators:
   Arteriolar: Hydralazine, minoxidil, diazoxide.
   Arteriolar + venous: Sodium nitropruside, pinacidil, and cromakalin.
8. **Diuretics:** Thiazide, furosemide, spironolactone, triamterene.
9. **RAS inhibitors:**
   ACE inhibitors: Captopril, rampril, lisinopril, enalapril
   Angiotesin (AT$_1$) antagonist: Losartan.
10. **5HT antagonist:** Ketanserin.

Central Sympatholytics

Methyldopa

Clonidine

α Adrenergic Blocker

α₁-Selective blocker

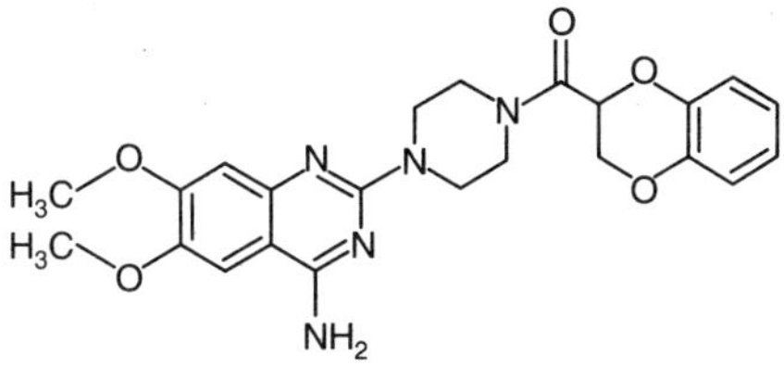

Doxazosin

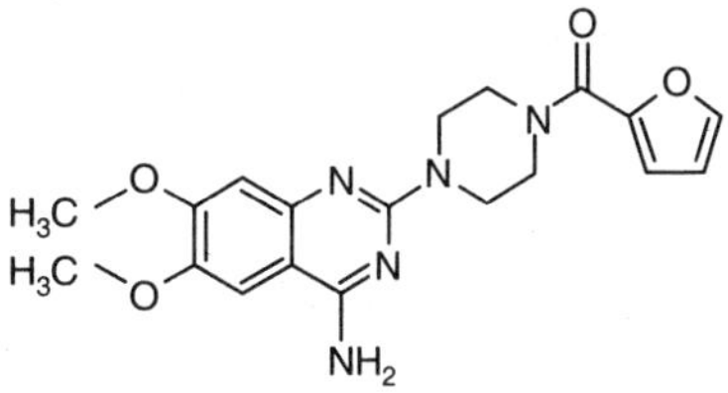

Prazosin

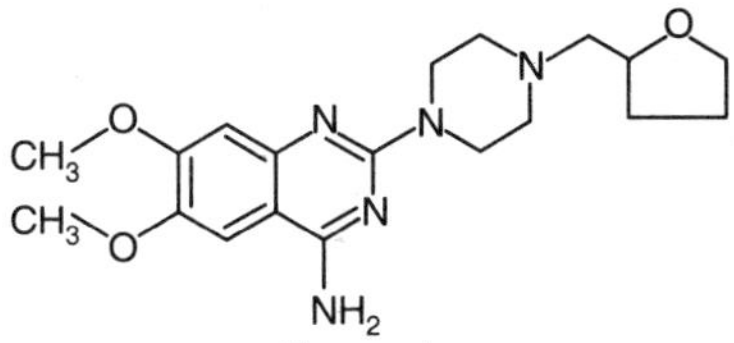

Terazosin

Non-selective α-blocker

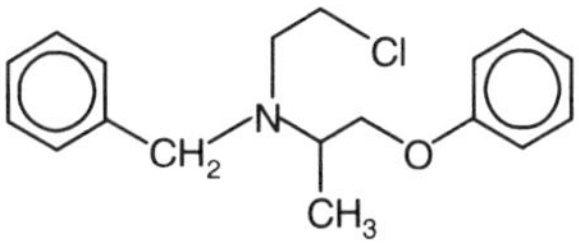

Phenoxybenzamine

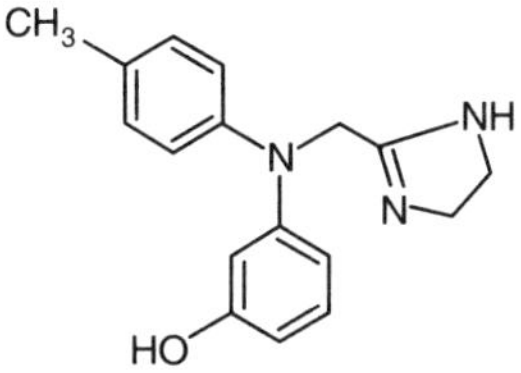

Phentolamine

β-Adrenergic Blocker

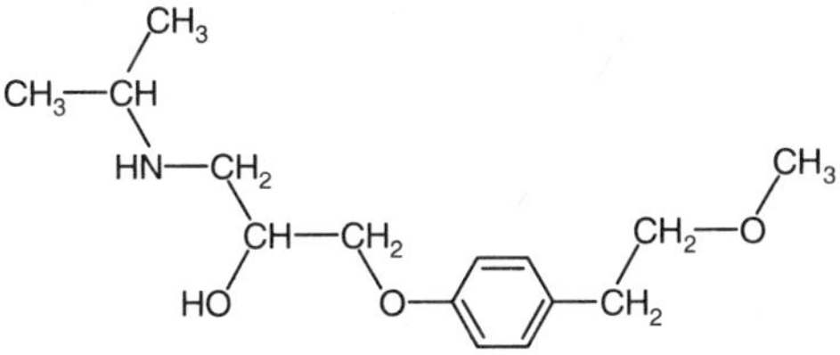

Metoprolol

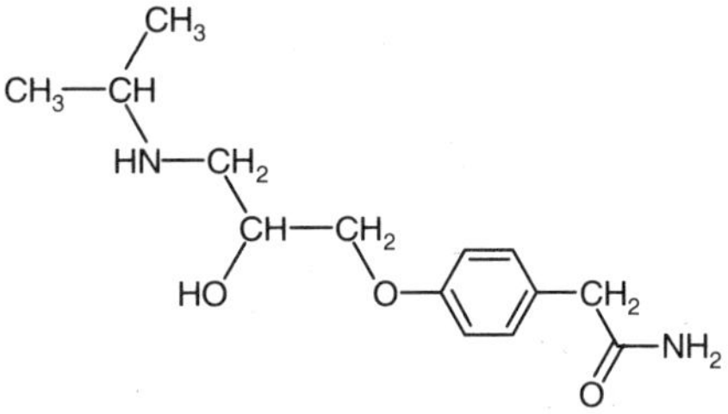

Atenolol

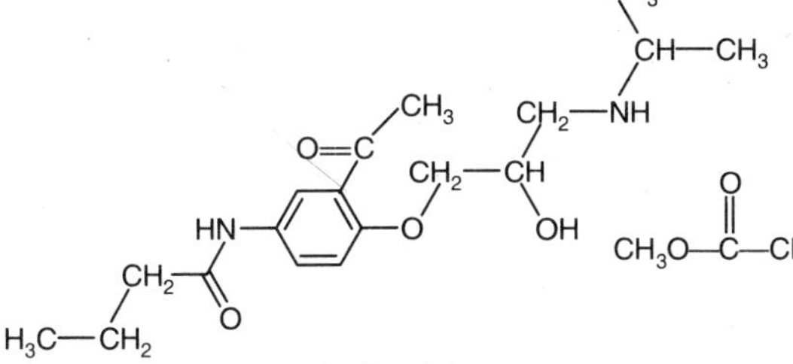

Acebutolol

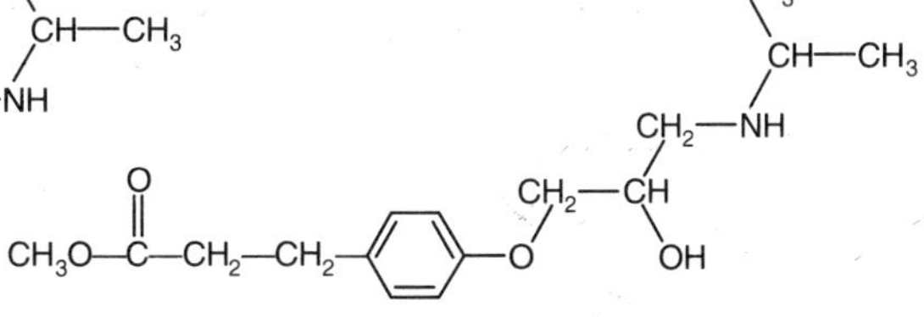

Esmolol

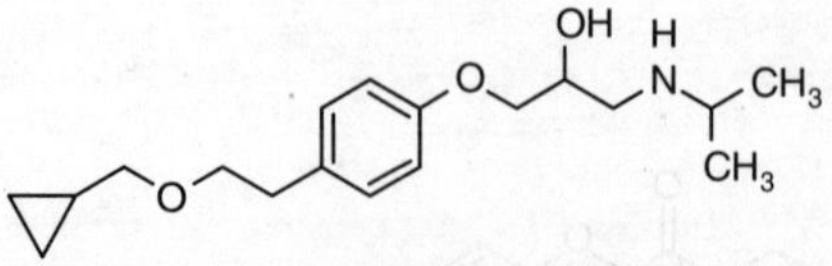

Betaxolol

Adrenergic Neuron Blockers

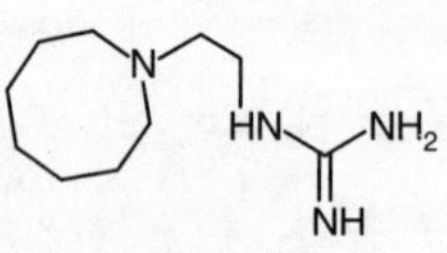

Guanethidine

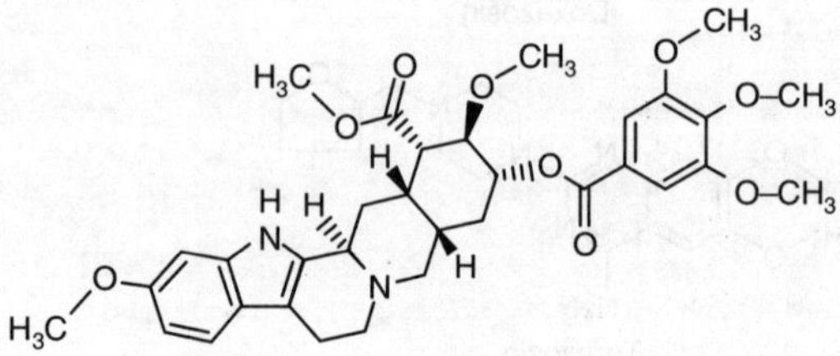

Reserpine

Ganglion Blocker

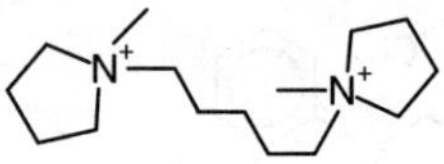

Pentolinium

Vasodilators

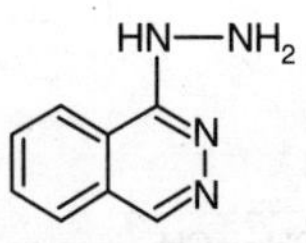

Hydralazine

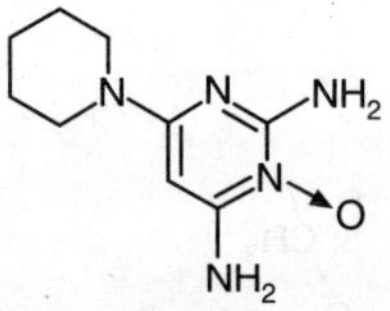

Minoxidil

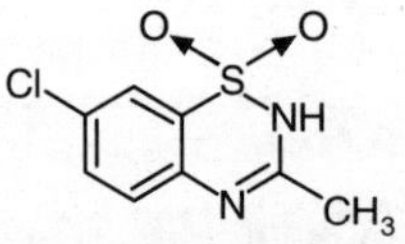

Diazoxide

Calcium Channel Blockers

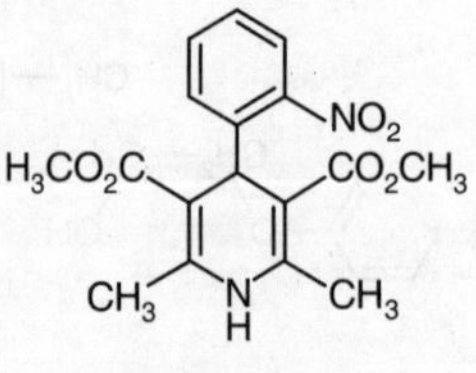

Nifedipine

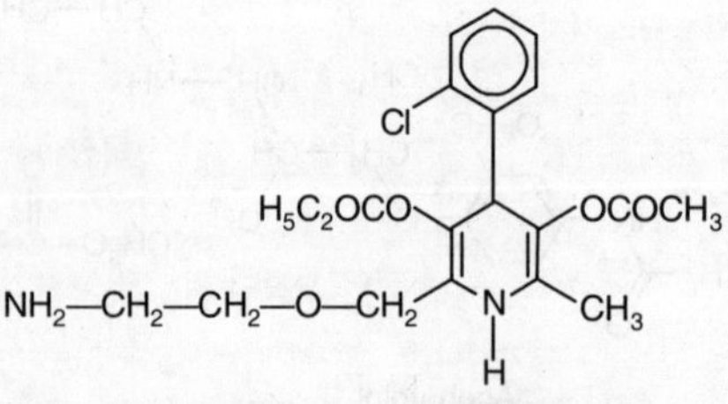

Amlodipine

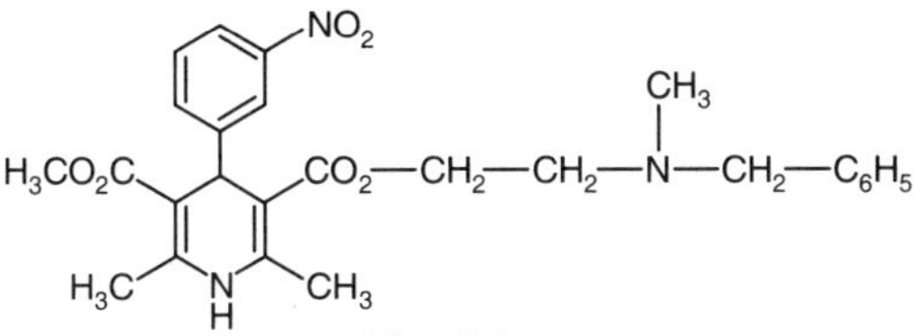

Nicardipine

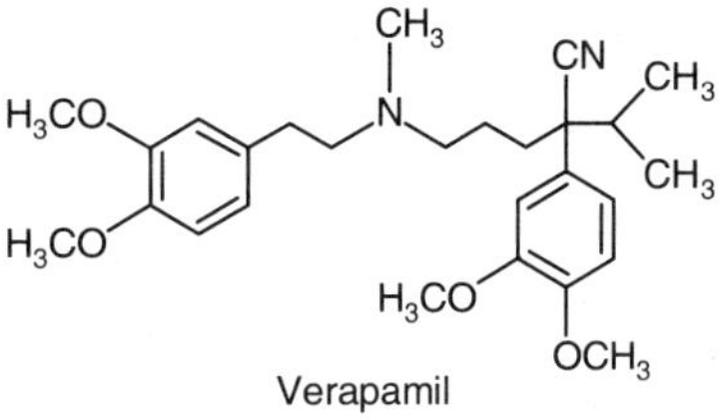

Verapamil

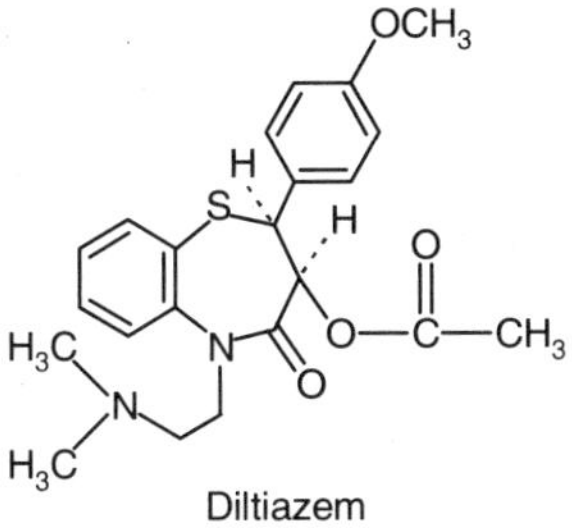

Diltiazem

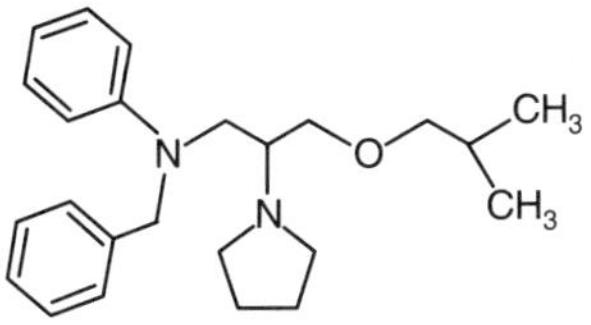

Bepridil

ACE Inhibitors

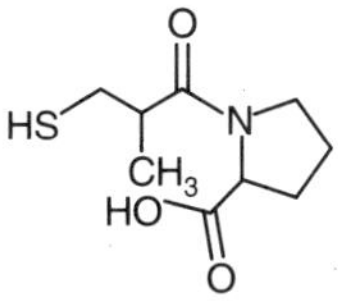

Captopril

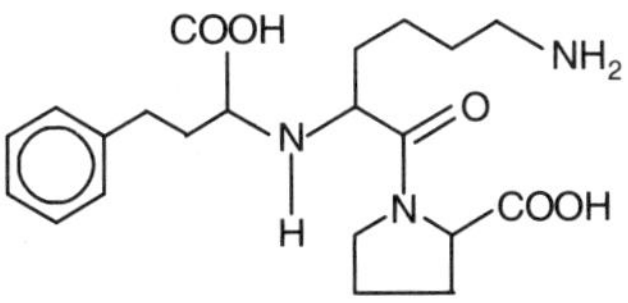

Lisinopril

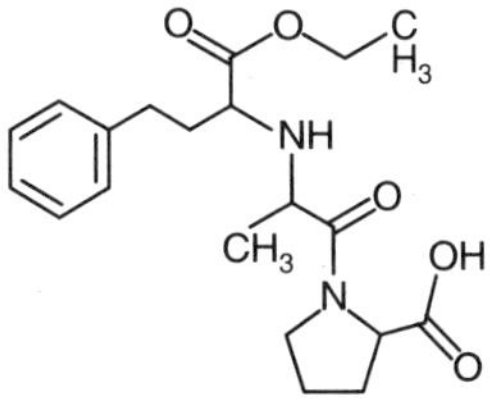

Enalapril

Diuretics

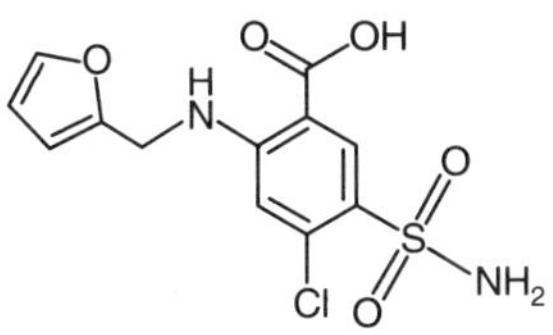

Furosemide

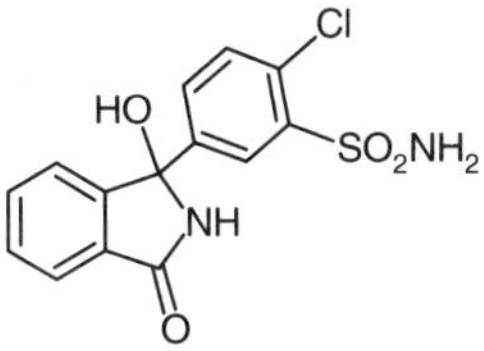

Chlorthalidone

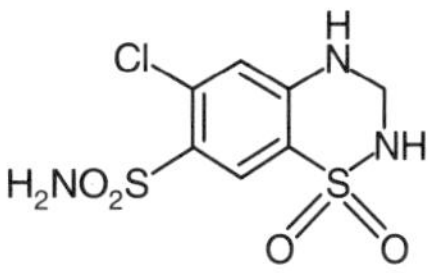

Hydrochlorthiazide

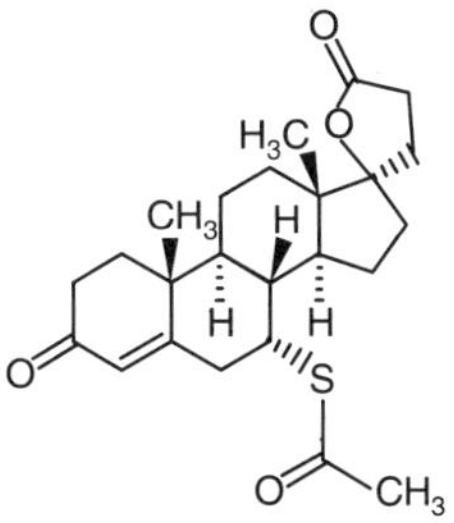

Spiranolactone

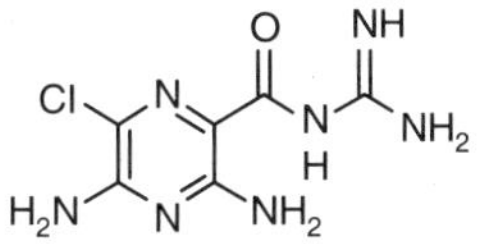

Amiloride

Central Sympatholytics

1. *Methyldopa*

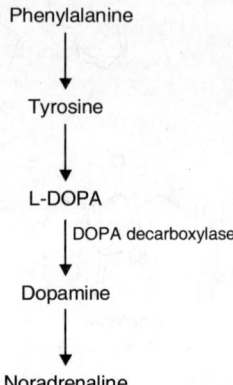

Methyldopa

Mechanism of action

- Earlier it was theorized that methyldopa is an inhibitor of DOPA decarboxylase and thus impairs the conversion of DOPA to dopamine and thereby decrease nor-adrenaline synthesis in the adrenergic neuron. This mode of action latter proved incorrect.

Phenylalanine

↓

Tyrosine

↓

L-DOPA

| DOPA decarboxylase

Dopamine

↓

Noradrenaline

- Later it was postulated that methyldopa itself is a substrate for DOPA decarboxylase and in the neuron is converted to alpha methylnoradrenaline, which acts as a false transmitter and in due course of time leads to noradrenaline depletion.

2. *Clonidine*

Mechanism of action

This thought to stimulate α_2-adrenergic receptor in the vasomotor center of the brain, resulting in the decreased sympathetic outflow to the peripheral vessel.

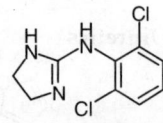

Clonidine

Structure–activity relationship

1. It has been shown that at least one ortho-Cl, Br or CH_3 group is essential but two ortho groups are clearly preferred.
2. The distance between the cationic center to the outer of the aromatic ring be 5.0-5.1 Å and from the cationic center to the plane of the aromatic ring 1.28-1.36 Å.
3. Increase in the size of the imidazolidine ring considerably decreases activity.
4. Replacement of the benzenoid ring by heterocyclic systems gave potent agents. Tiamenidine is one-third potent as clonidine but relatively less sedative.

α Adrenergic Blockers

MOA

They produce their anti-hypertensive effect by blocking post synaptic α1-adrenergic receptors in blood vessels and cause vasodilation of both arteries and veins.

SAR of α₁ Selective Blocker

These are highly selective α_1-receptor antagonist. Structurally, these contain three components:
1. Quinazoline ring.
2. Piperazine ring.
3. Acyl moiety.

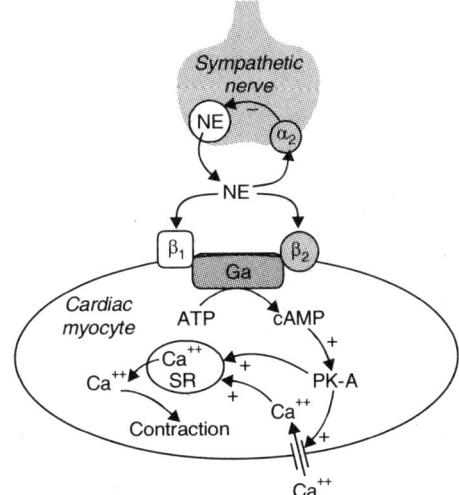

1. 4-amino group on quinazoline is very essential for the activity.
2. Piperazine ring can be replaced by that of other heterocyclic ring without affecting activity.
3. The nature of acyl group has significant role in pharmacokinetic properties.

Uses

- This is used in diagnosis, control and management of malignant and toxemic hypertensive crises, e.g. pheochromocytoma. α1 selective blockers are prazosin, terazosin, doxazosin, etc. while non-selective blockers are phentolamine, phenoxybenzamine, etc.

β-Adrenergic Blockers

MOA (Fig. 28.2)

Blocks β-receptor in heart and thus slows force of contraction and reduces cardiac output, e.g. propanolol, atenolol, metoprolol, etc. They have been used extensively to treat hypertension.

Abbreviations: NE, norepinephrine; Gs, G-stimulatory protein; PK-A, cAMP-dependent protein kinase; SR, sarcoplasmic reticulum

Fig. 28.2: Mode of action of β blockers

Structure–Activity Relationship

$$Ar-O-CH_2-\overset{OH}{\underset{}{CH}}-CH_2-NH-\overset{CH_3}{\underset{CH_3}{\diagdown}}R$$

1. The aryloxypropanolamines are more potent than arylethanolamines.
2. Replacement of the ethereal oxygen in aryloxypropanolamines with S, CH_2 or NCH_3 is determental activity.
3. The most effective amine substituent is isopropyl and tertiary butyl.
4. The beta adrenergic receptor affinity resides chiefly in the D(-) absolute configuration.
5. If we are putting 4-OH group on naphthyl ring of the propanolol, it results into a very potent beta antagonist.

4-hydroxy propanolol

6. The catechol ring (adrenergic drugs) can be replaced by a great variety of other ring system varying from.
   1. Phenylether................Oxprenolol
   2. Sulphonamide..............Sotalol
   3. Amide......................Labetelol
   4. Indoles....................Pindolol
   5. Naphthalene...............Propanolol
7. Substitution of CH_3, Cl or NO_2 groups on the phenyl ring was most favoured at 2 and 3 positions and least favoured at 4-position.
8. Alkenyl and alkenyloxy groups in the ortho position on phenyl ring, provided good activity.

Oxprenolol

Alprenolol

9. Larger alkyl chains are less effective but isopropyl or t-butyl, which gives an optimal basicity or nucleophilicity to the amino group for receptor affinity are most preferred.

10. A major clinical problem with propanolol was its high lipid solubility, which allowed it to penetrate nerve tissue and exert undesirable cardiodepressant effect in addition to its beta blocking action. To solve this problem, methanesulphonamide was considered...and resulting compound practolol is devoid of this side effect.

Practolol

11. Replacement of catechol hydroxyl groups with chlorine to give dichloro-isoproterenol. A classic beta blocker.

Dichloroisoprenaline

12. Replacement of the electron rich hydroxyl groups with an electron rich phenyl at 3, 4 position gives pronethol, which is having good beta blocking activity.

13. Converting the aromatic portion to phenanthrene or anthracene was disadvantageous.

N-Substitution

1. N, N-disubstituted compounds are inactive.
2. Alpha methyl group decreases activity.
3. Methoxyphenyl ethyl groups are added to amine part of the molecule.
4. Cyclic alkyl substituents are better than corresponding open chain substituent at nitrogen atoms of amine.
5. Chain length may extended to a total of four atoms.

Unwanted Effects

The main side effects of b-receptor antagonists result from their receptor-blocking action.

Bronchoconstriction

- This is of little importance in the absence of airway disease, but in asthmatic patients the effect can be dramatic and life-threatening.
- It is also of clinical importance in patients with other forms of obstructive lung disease (e.g. chronic bronchitis, emphysema).

Cardiac depression

Cardiac depression can occur, leading to signs of heart failure, particularly in elderly people. Patients suffering from heart failure who are treated with b-receptor antagonists (see above) often deteriorate in the first few weeks before the beneficial effect develops.

Bradycardia

This side effect can lead to life-threatening heart block and can occur in patients with coronary disease, particularly if they are being treated with antiarrhythmic drugs that impair cardiac conduction.

Hypoglycemia

* Glucose release in response to adrenaline is a safety device that may be important to diabetic patients and to other individuals prone to hypoglycemic attacks.
* The sympathetic response to hypoglycemia produces symptoms (especially tachycardia) that warn patients of the urgent need for carbohydrate (usually in the form of a sugary drink). β-receptor antagonists reduce these symptoms, so incipient hypoglycemia is more likely to go unnoticed by the patient.
* The use of β-receptor antagonists is generally to be avoided in patients with poorly controlled diabetes. There is a theoretical advantage in using β_1-selective agents, because glucose release from the liver is controlled by β_2-receptors.

Fatigue

This is probably due to reduced cardiac output and reduced muscle perfusion in exercise. It is a frequent complaint of patients taking β receptor-blocking drugs.

Cold Extremities

* These are presumably due to a loss of β-receptor-mediated vasodilatation in cutaneous vessels, and are a common side effect.
* Theoretically, β_1-selective drugs are less likely to produce this effect, but it is not clear that this is so in practice.

α + β Nonselective Adrenergic Blockers

For example, labetelol, carvedilol.

Labetelol

Ganglion Blockers

For example, pentolinium.

Pentolinium

Adrenergic Neuron Blockers

MOA

Act on membrane of intraneuronal granules which stores monoamines (NA, 5-HT, DA) and inhibits the active transport of them → depletion of monoamines (neurotransmitters) → slow fall in BP, e.g. reserpine, guanethidine.

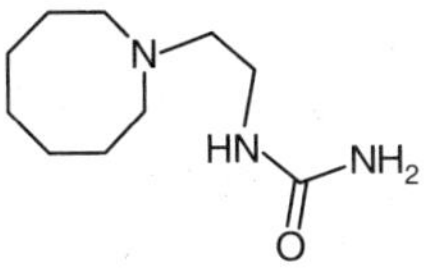

Guanethidine

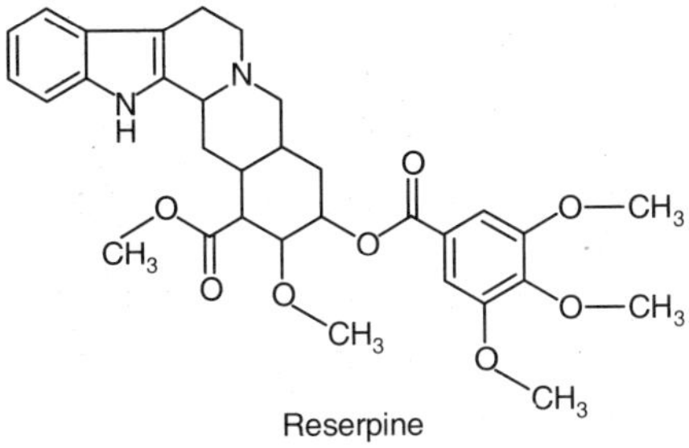

Reserpine

Calcium Channel Blocker

Mode of action (Fig. 28.3)

- It inhibits the cellular influx of calcium, which is responsible for muscle contraction. The calcium channel blockers protect the tissue by inhibiting the entrance of calcium into cardiac and smooth muscle cells of the coronary and systemic arterial beds.
- All calcium channel blockers are therefore vasodilators that ultimately cause dilatation of coronary and peripheral arteries, reduce heart rate.

Uses

1. It reduces oxygen requirement and less likely to aggravate ischemia.
2. In hypertension, in arrhythmia, suppress nocturnal leg cramps.
3. Antihypertension, in angina, in Reynaud's syndrome
4. Amlodipine besylate is used in the treatment of hypertension and chronic stable and vasospastic angina.

Structure–activity relationship (Refer anti-anginal chapter)

Directly Acting Vasodilators

Hydralazine

This is generating NO like nitrates and causes vasodilation (Refer anti-anginal chapters).

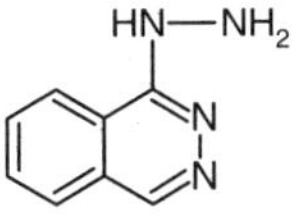

Hydralazine

Minoxidil

This produce active metabolite known as minoxidil sulfate, which is K^+ channel opener and causes direct relaxation of the arteriolar smooth muscle relaxation.

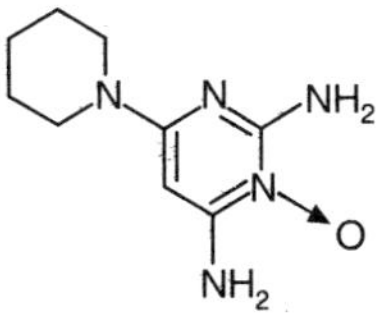

Minoxidil

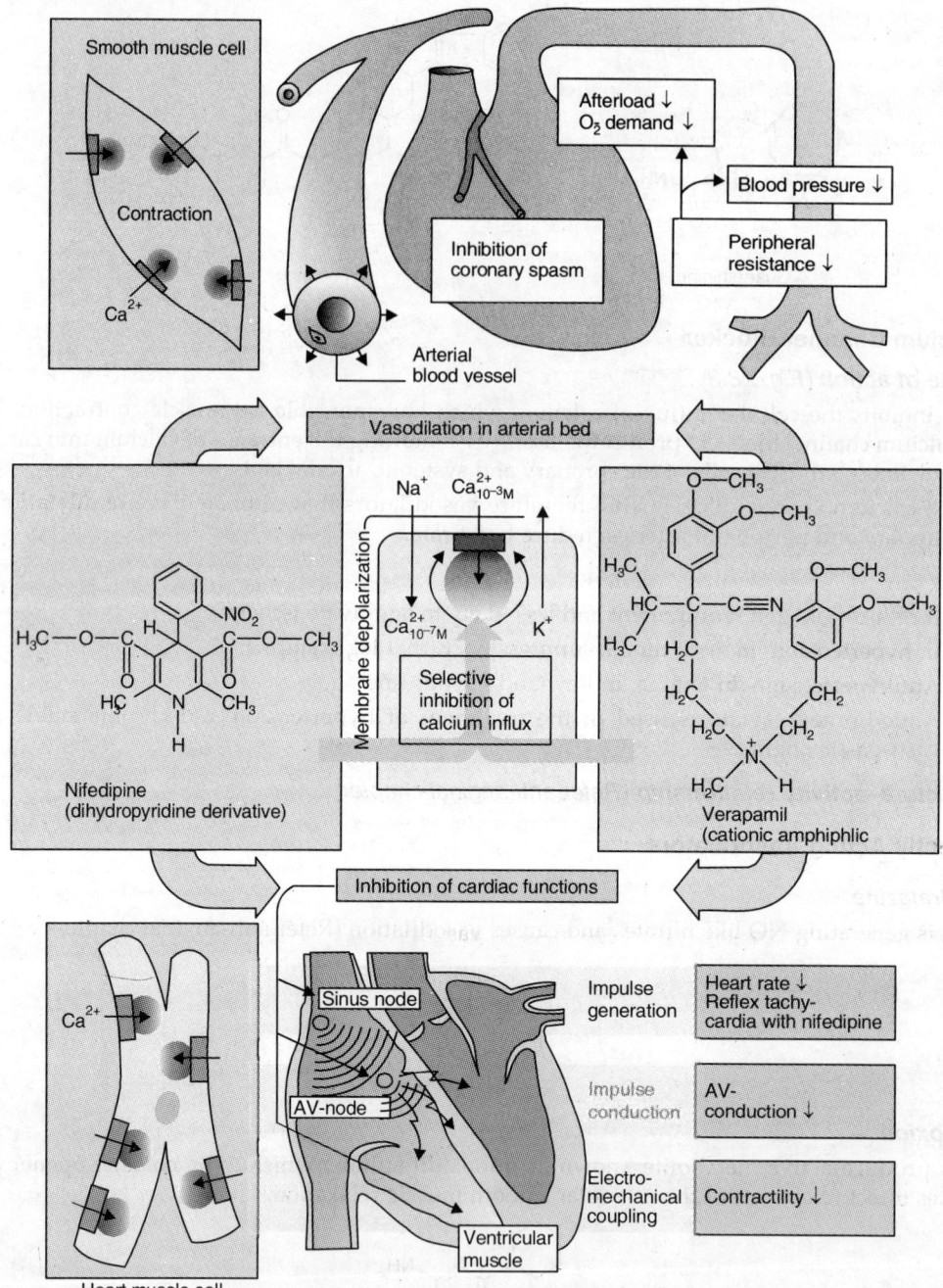

Fig. 28.3: Mode of action of calcium channel blockers

Diazoxide

This is going to open K^+ channel causing arteriolar smooth muscle relaxation.

ACE Inhibitors

Mechanism of Action (Fig. 28.4)

- The principle mechanism of action of ACE inhibitors (angiotensin converting enzyme inhibitors) centers around the renin–angiotensin–aldosterone system.

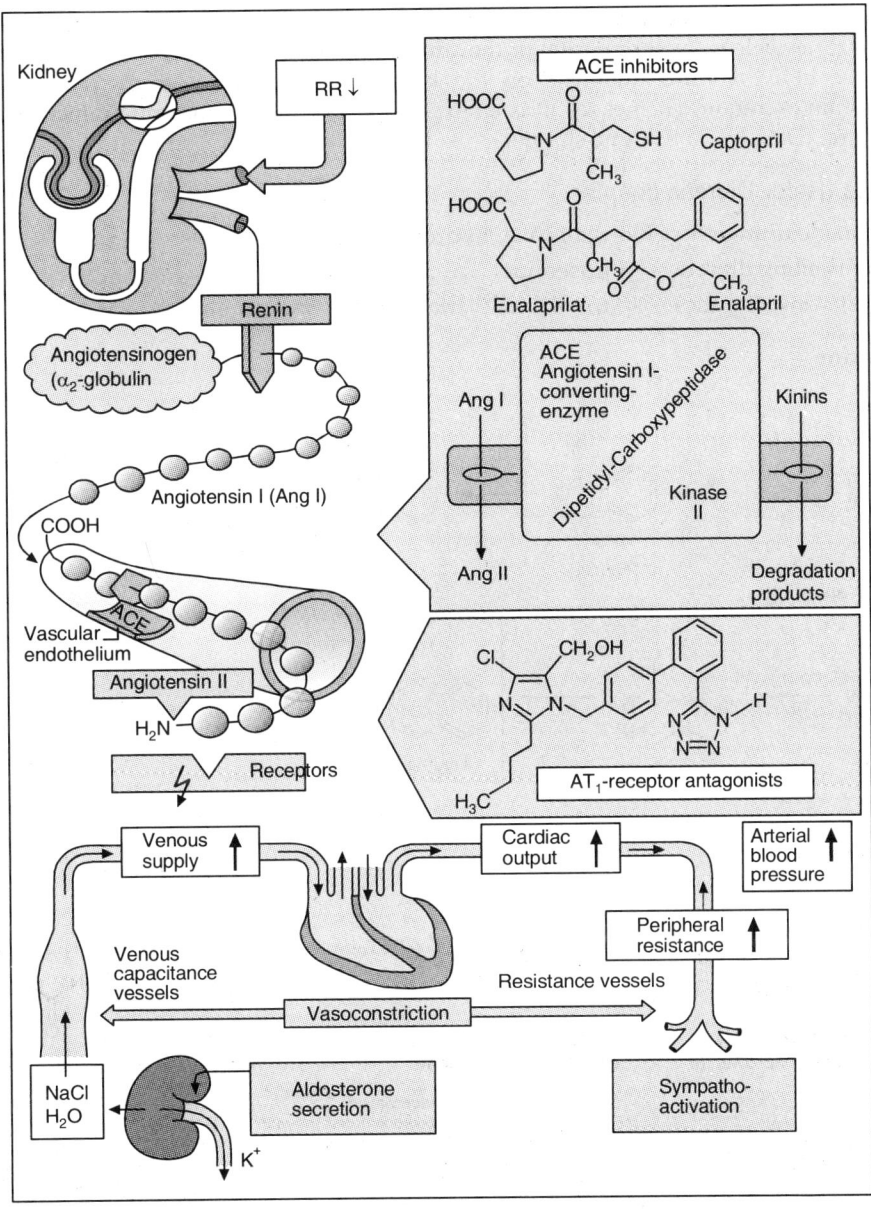

Fig. 28.4: Renin–angiotensin–aldosterone system and inhibitors

- Renin is endogenous enzyme that is produced and secreted in kidney and is released in response to fall in blood pressure. Renin is responsible for the conversion of angiotensinogen to angiotensin-I a relatively weak hormone with little or no pharmacological activity. Following production of angiotensin-I, conversion to the active angiotensin-II occurs in the presence of ACE (angiotensin converting enzyme).

- Angiotensin-II is a potent vasoconstrictor responsible for arterial vasoconstriction and blood pressure, as well as for stimulation of the adrenal gland to produce aldosterone. Aldosterone increase blood volume and acts on the kidney to stimulate sodium reabsorption and potassium excretion. The net result is an expansion of total volume and an increase in blood pressure. (Detailed in diuretic chapter)

Diuretics (Refer Diuretic chapter)

1. Thiazide diuretics— chlorthalidone, hydrochlorothiazide
2. High ceiling diuretics— furosemide
3. K^+ sparing diuretics— spironolactone, triamterene, amiloride

Hydralazine

Phthalic anhydride   Phthalide   phthalazone (II)

Hydralazine

Methyldopa

(3, 4-dimethoxy-phenyl)acetone (I)   Potassium cyanide   Ammonium carbonate   4-methyl-4-(3, 4-di-methoxybenzyl) hydentoin (II)

(±)-3-(3, 4-dimethoxy-phenyl)-2-methylalanine (III)   Methyldopa

Diazoxide

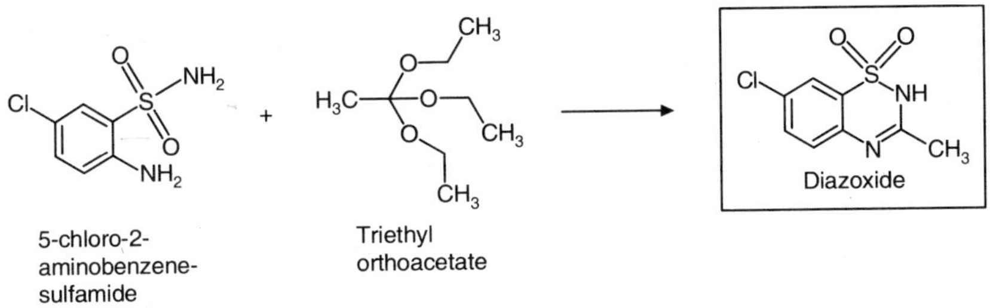

5-chloro-2-
aminobenzene-
sulfamide

Triethyl
orthoacetate

Diazoxide

Clonidine

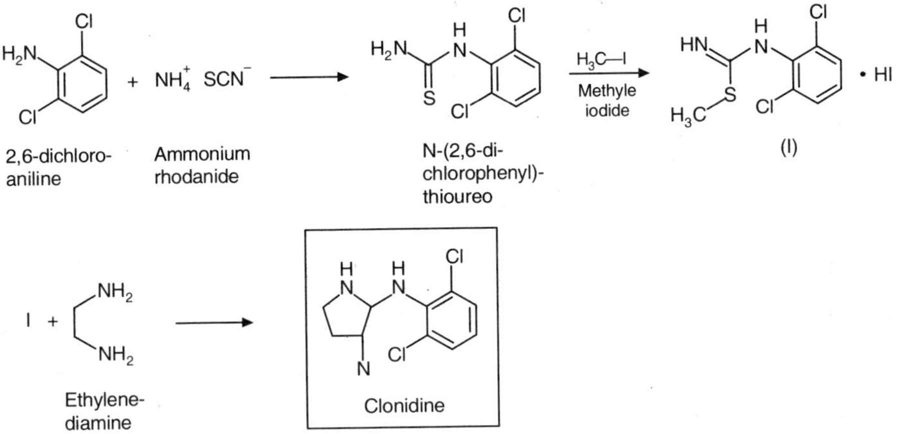

2,6-dichloro-
aniline

Ammonium
rhodanide

N-(2,6-di-
chlorophenyl)-
thioureo

(I)

Ethylene-
diamine

Clonidine

Guanethidine Hydrochloride

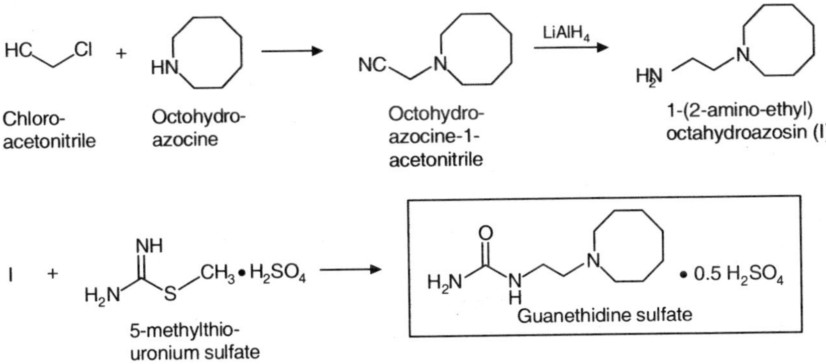

Chloro-
acetonitrile

Octohydro-
azocine

Octohydro-
azocine-1-
acetonitrile

1-(2-amino-ethyl)
octahydroazosin (I)

5-methylthio-
uronium sulfate

Guanethidine sulfate

Minoxidil

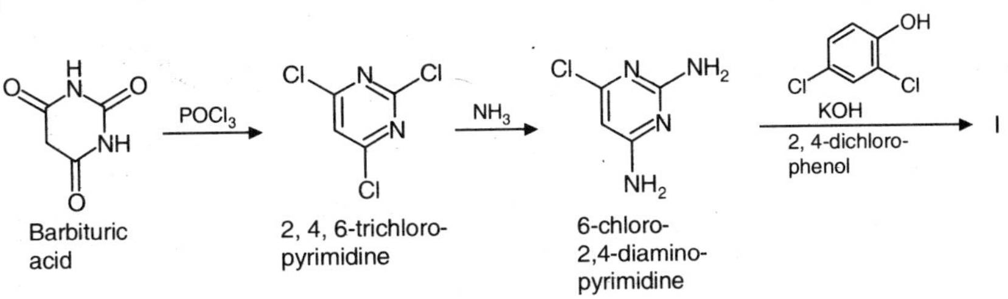

Barbituric
acid

2, 4, 6-trichloro-
pyrimidine

6-chloro-
2,4-diamino-
pyrimidine

2, 4-dichloro-
phenol

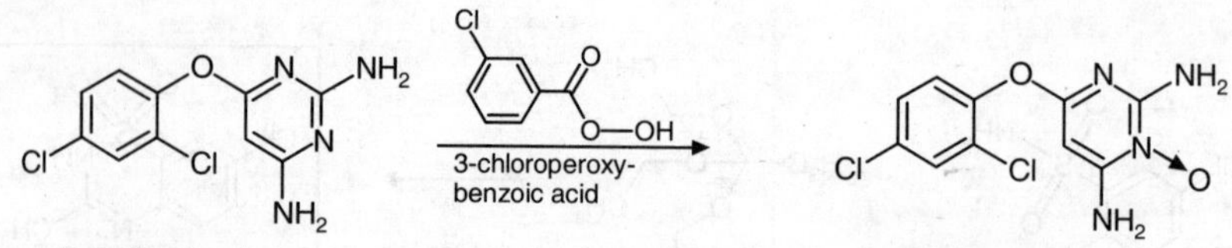

2, 4-diamino-6-
(2, 4-dichlorophenoxy)-
pyrimidine (I)

3-chloroperoxy-
benzoic acid

2, 4-diamino-6-(2, 4-
dichlorophenoxy) pyri-
midine 3-oxide (II)

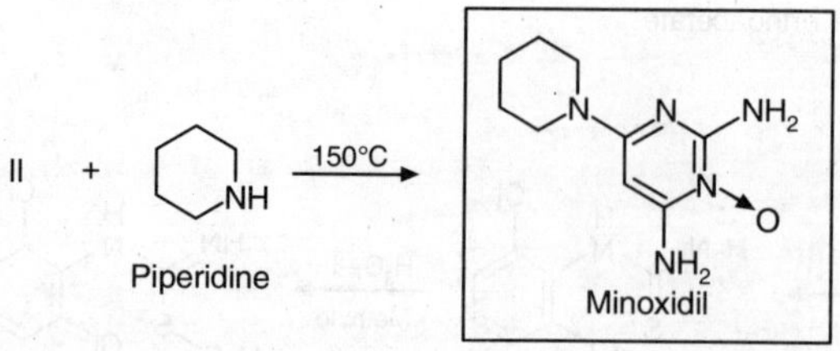

II + Piperidine 150°C

Minoxidil

Captopril

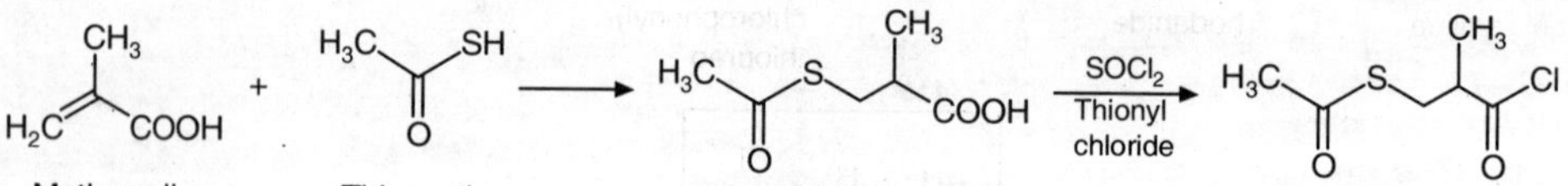

Methacyrlic
acid (I)

Thioacetic
acid

3-acetylthio-2-methyl
propionic acid

SOCl₂
Thionyl
chloride

(II)

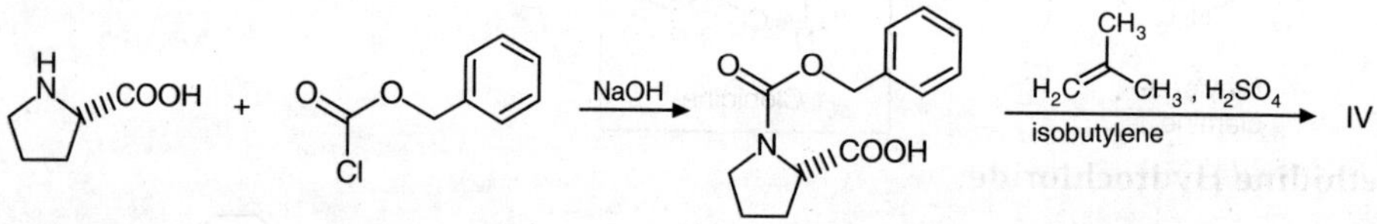

L-proline (III)

Benzyl
chloroformate

NaOH

N-benzyloxycorbony-
L-proline

H₂C=CH₃, H₂SO₄
isobutylene

IV

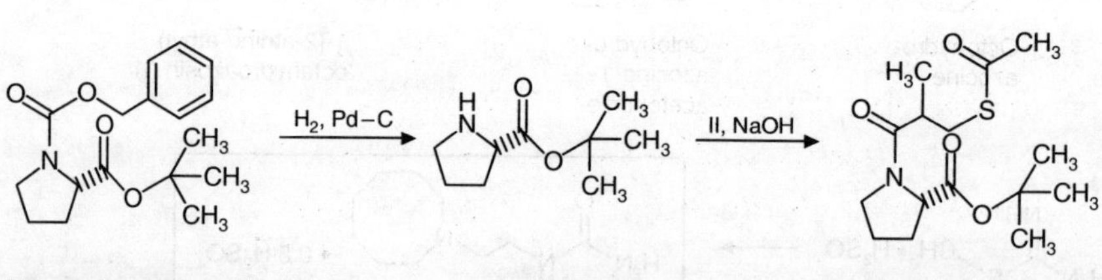

N-benzyloxycarbonyl-L-
proline tert-butyl ester (IV)

H₂, Pd–C

L-proline tert-
butyl ester

II, NaOH

(V)

V   CF₃COOH, Onisole
trifluoroacetic acid

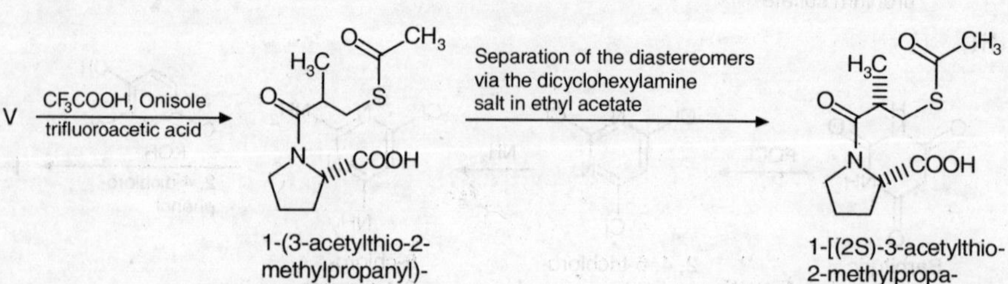

1-(3-acetylthio-2-
methylpropanyl)-
L-proline

Separation of the diastereomers
via the dicyclohexylamine
salt in ethyl acetate

1-[(2S)-3-acetylthio-
2-methylpropa-
nyl]-L-proline (VI)

$$VI \xrightarrow{NH_3, CH_3OH}$$

Captopril

Enalapril

(2-bromoethyl)-benzene

$$\xrightarrow{Mg, THF}$$

$$\xrightarrow[\text{diethyl oxalate}]{THF, -10°C}$$

ethyl 2-oxo-4-phenyl-butyrate (I)

N-tert-butosy-carbonyl-L·alanine

+

L-proline benzyl ester

$$\xrightarrow{DCC, CH_2Cl_2}$$

(II)

$$II \xrightarrow{CF_3COOH}$$

L-alonyl-L-proline benzyl ester (III)

$$\xrightarrow{HBr \text{ or } NaOH}$$

L-alanyl-L-proline (IV)

$$IV + I \xrightarrow[\substack{\text{molecular sieve 0.4 nm} \\ \text{sodium cyanoborohydride}}]{Na[BH3(CN)] \text{ or } H2/Pd - C,}$$

Enalapril

29

Antianginal Drugs

Angina pectoris is a pain syndrome due to induction of adverse oxygen supply or imbalance between demand and need of oxygen in a portion of myocardium.

- It is characterized by sudden, severe pressing chest pain radiating to the neck, jaw and arms. It is caused by coronary blood flow that is insufficient to meet the oxygen demand of myocardium, leading to ischemia.

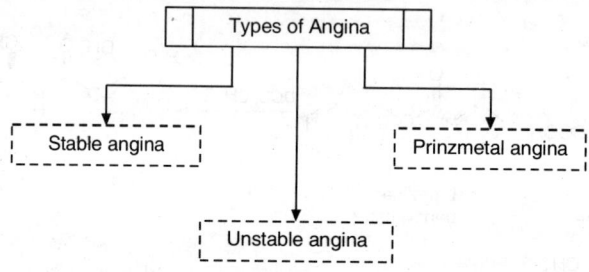

TYPES OF ANGINA

Stable Angina

Attacks are predictably provoked by exercise, emotion, eating and coitus and subside when the increased energy demand is withdrawn. The underlying pathology is severe coronary atherosclerosis, because of which blood flow fails to increase during increased demand.

Unstable Angina

Unstable angina lies between stable angina and myocardial infarction. It is often unrelated to exercise and occurs at rest. The symptoms are not relived by rest or nitroglycerine. Unstable angina may require more aggressive therapy.

Prinzmetal or Variant Angina

This is episodic angina that occurs at rest and is due to coronary artery spasm. The symptoms are caused by decreased blood flow to the heart muscle or by spasm of the coronary artery. Although individual with this form of angina may well have significant coronary atherosclerosis.

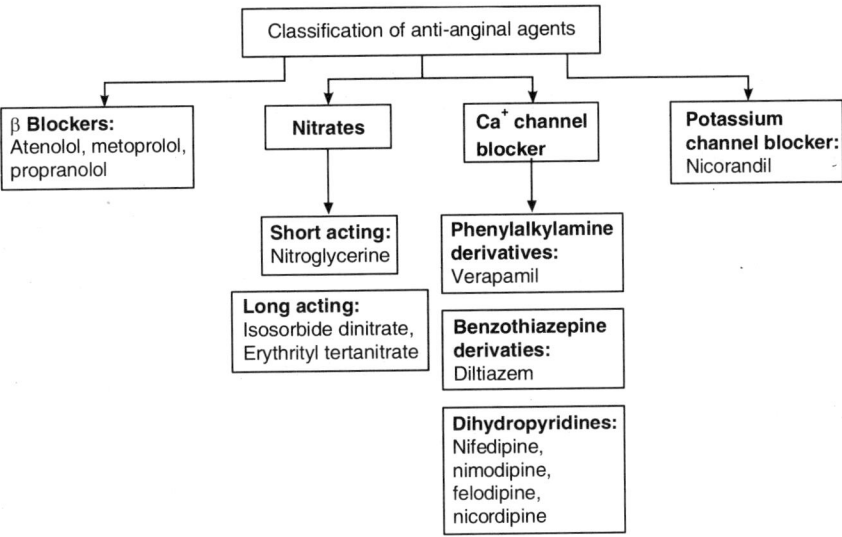

1. Organic Nitrates and Nitrites

Glyceryl trinitrate

Erythrityl tetranitrate

Amyl nitrites

Isosorbide dinartrate

Pentaerythritol tetranitrate

Tenitramine

Propatyl nitrate

2. Beta-blockers

Propranolol

Atenolol

Metaprolol

Esmolol

3. Calcium Channel Blocker

Nicardipine

Verapamil

Diltiazem

▒ ORGANIC NITRATES

Mode of Action (Fig. 29.1)

- Organic nitrates are rapidly denitrated enzymatically in the smooth muscle cell to release the reactive free radical nitric oxide (NO), which activates cytosolic guanylyl cyclase that results in increased cGMP, which causes dephosphorylation of myosin light chain kinase (MLCK) through a cGMP dependant protein kinase.
- Reduced availability of phosphorylated MLCK interferes with activation of myosin. It fails to interact with actin filament to cause contraction. Consequently relaxation occurs. Raised intracellular cGMP also reduces Ca^{2+} entry contributing to relaxation.

Uses

1. Used for unstable angina, coronary vasospasm, in hypertension during surgery.
2. In angina pectoris, in CHF, in myocardial infarction, in biliary colic.
3. In angina pectoris.

Beta Blockers

Mode of Action (Fig. 29.2)

All beta blockers are competitive antagonist they block β_1 and β_2 receptors but has weak activity on β_3 subtype, which reduces contraction by and cause relaxation.

Uses

1. It decreases the frequency and severity of attack and increases exercise tolerance in classical angina.
2. In angina, hypertension and in glaucoma.
3. In hypertension, in myocardial infarction, in pheochromocytoma, thyrotoxicosis, migraine, anxiety.

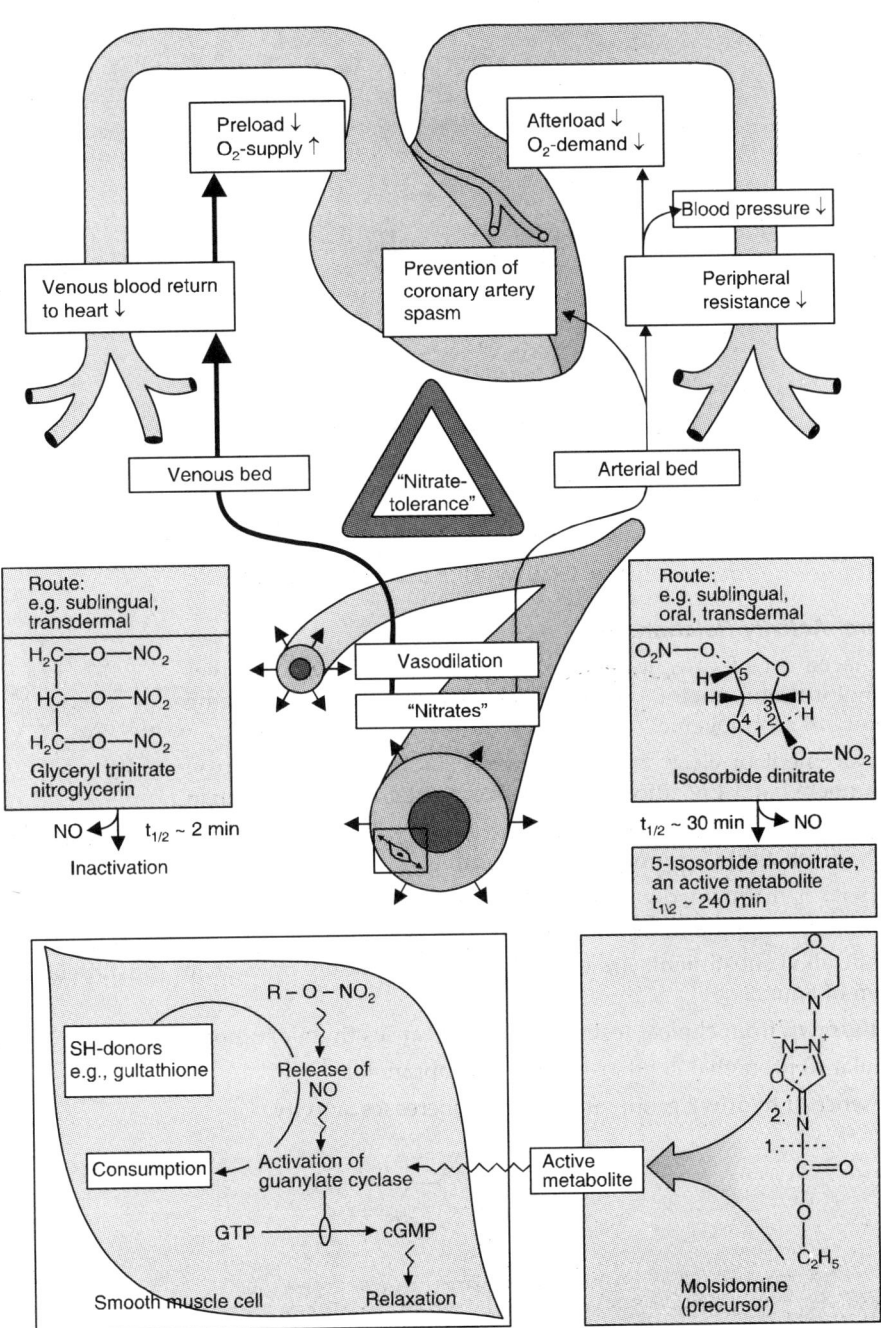

Fig. 29.1: Mode of action of nitrates

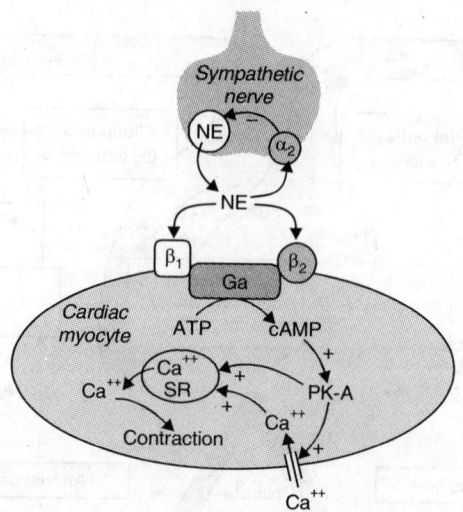

Abbreviations: NE, norepinephrine; Gs, G-stimulatory protein;
PK-A, cAMP-dependent protein kinase; SR, sarcoplasmic reticulum

Fig. 29.2: Mode of action of β blockers

Structure–Activity Relationship

1. Replacement of catechol hydroxyl groups with chlorine gives dicholoroisopropnetol (DCI), which is classical beta blocking agent but carcinogenic.

2. Replacement of electron rich hydroxyl group with an electron rich phenyl at 3,4 positions gives pronethalol, better-blocker than dichloroisoproterenol.

3. N, N-disubstituted compounds are inactive.

4. Activity is maintained when phenyl ethyl, hydroxy phenyl ethyl or methoxy phenyl ethyl groups are added to amine part of the molecule.

5. Cyclic alkyl substituents are better than corresponding open chain substituents at nitrogen atom of amine.

6. Withdrawn from clinical testing because it causes thymic tumors in mice.

7. Similar to pronethalol, other-blocker is propranolol.

8. Presence of hydroxy group at 4-position increases activity.

Dichloroisopropentol

4-hydroxy propranolol

9. N substituents must be bulky to ensure affinity to β-receptor.

10. Substitution of CH_3, Cl, OCH_3 or NO_2 groups on the phenyl ring was most favored at 2 and 3 positions and least favored at 4-position.

11. Alkenyl and alkenyloxy group in the ortho position on phenyl ring increases activity, e.g. oxprenolol.

Oxprenolol

Calcium Channel Blocker

Mode of action (See Fig. 28.3)

- It inhibits the cellular influx of calcium, which is responsible for muscle contraction. The calcium channel blockers protect the tissue by inhibiting the entrance of calcium into cardiac and smooth muscle cells of the coronary and systemic arterial beds.
- All calcium channel blockers are therefore vasodilators that ultimately causes dilatation of coronary and peripheral arteries, reduce heart rate.

Uses

1. It reduces oxygen requirement and less likely to aggravate ischemia.
2. In hypertension, in arrhythmia, suppress nocturnal leg cramps.
3. In antihypertension, in angina, in Reynaud's syndrome.
4. Amlodipine besylate is used in the treatment of hypertension and chronic stable and vasospastic angina.

Structure–Activity Relationship

General structure: A substituted phenyl ring at the C-4 position optimizes activity. Substitution with a non-polar, alkyl or cycloalkyl decreases activity.

1, 4-dihydropyridine

1. If RS is at ortho or meta substituent increases activity.
2. If RS is at para position decreases activity.
3. Electron withdrawing group on phenyl ring at C-4 position have good activity.
4. 1,4-dihydropyridine rings are essential for activity.
5. Substitution at N-1 position decreases activity.

6. Ester group at C-3 or C-5 position optimizes activity.

7. Replacement of C-3 ester of isradipine with NO$_2$ group produces calcium channel activator.

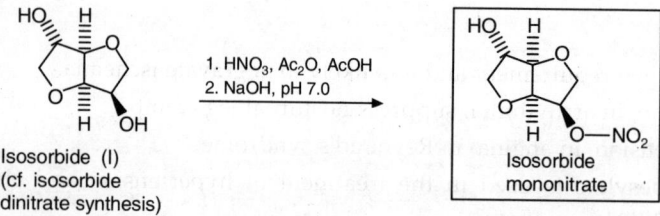

Potassium Channel Opener

Mode of action

K$^+$ channel openers are the smooth muscle relaxant.

Example

1. Minoxidil.
2. Nicorandil.

Isosorbide Mononitrate

HO H

1. HNO$_3$, Ac$_2$O, AcOH
2. NaOH, pH 7.0

HO H

O—NO$_2$

Isosorbide (I)
(cf. isosorbide
dinitrate synthesis)

Isosorbide
mononitrate

Pentaerythrityl Tetranitrate

HO— —OH
HO— —OH

94% HNO$_3$

O$_2$N

NO$_2$

O$_2$N

NO$_2$

Pentaerythritol

Pentaerythrityl tetranitrate

Minoxidil

Barbituric
acid

POCl$_3$

2, 4, 6-trichloro-
pyrimidine

NH$_3$

6-chloro-
2,4-diamino-
pyrimidine

KOH

2, 4-dichloro-
phenol

I

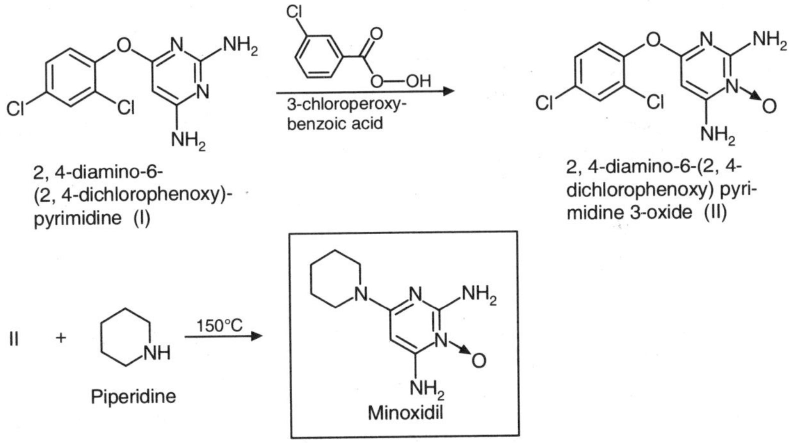

3-chloroperoxy-
benzoic acid

2, 4-diamino-6-
(2, 4-dichlorophenoxy)-
pyrimidine (I)

2, 4-diamino-6-(2, 4-
dichlorophenoxy) pyri-
midine 3-oxide (II)

II + Piperidine →(150°C) Minoxidil

Piperidine

Propranolol

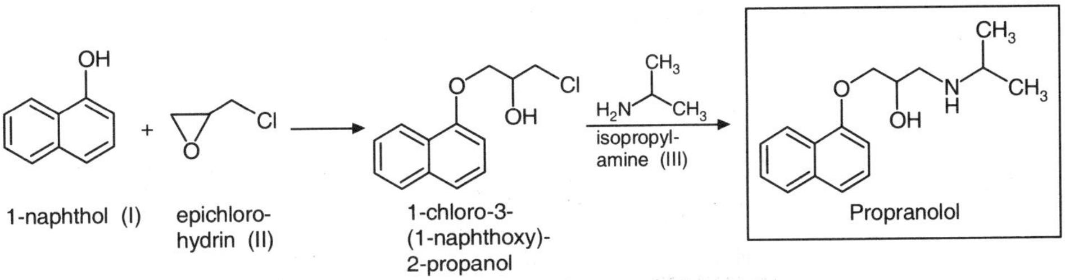

1-naphthol (I) epichloro-hydrin (II) 1-chloro-3-(1-naphthoxy)-2-propanol

isopropyl-amine (III)

Propranolol

Atenolol

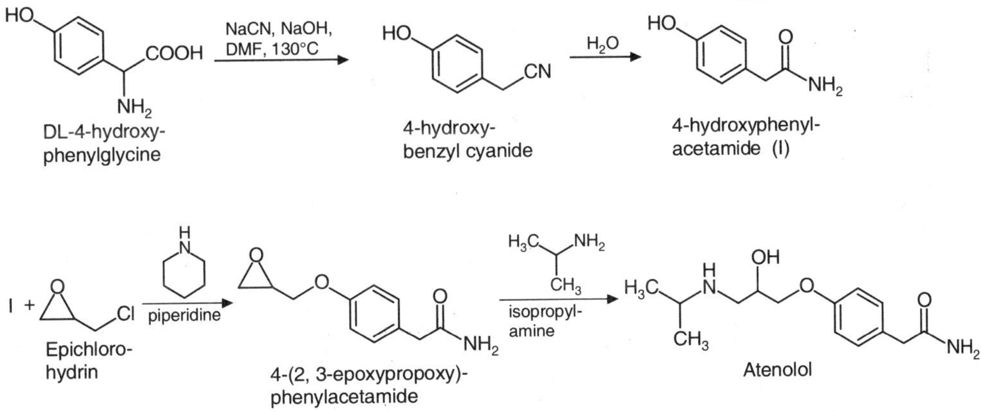

NaCN, NaOH, DMF, 130°C

H_2O

DL-4-hydroxy-phenylglycine 4-hydroxy-benzyl cyanide 4-hydroxyphenyl-acetamide (I)

I + Epichloro-hydrin piperidine 4-(2, 3-epoxypropoxy)-phenylacetamide

isopropyl-amine

Atenolol

Esmolol

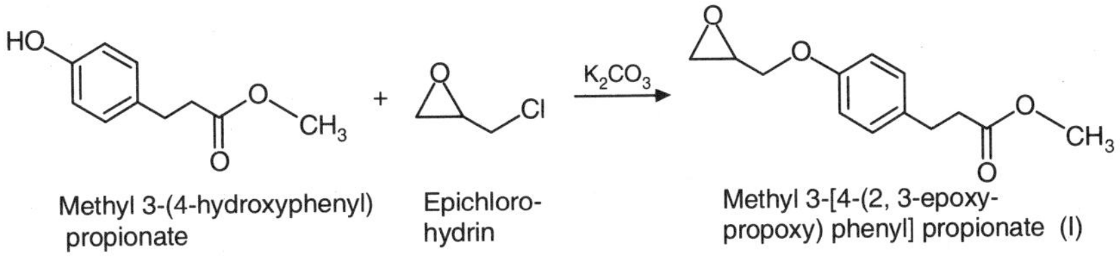

Methyl 3-(4-hydroxyphenyl) propionate + Epichloro-hydrin →(K_2CO_3) Methyl 3-[4-(2, 3-epoxy-propoxy) phenyl] propionate (I)

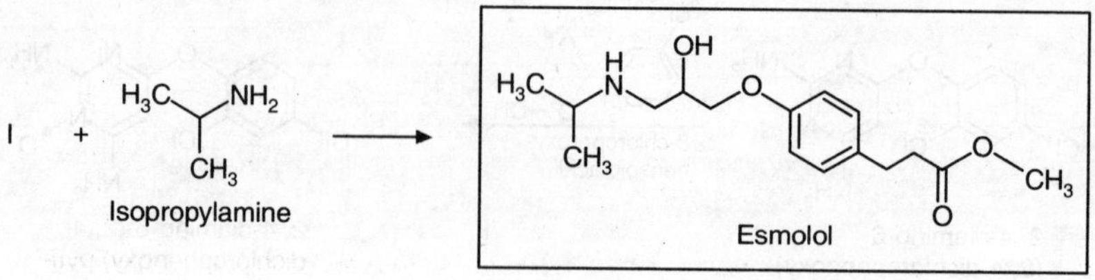

I + [H₃C–CH(CH₃)–NH₂ Isopropylamine] ⟶ Esmolol

Isopropylamine

Nifedipine

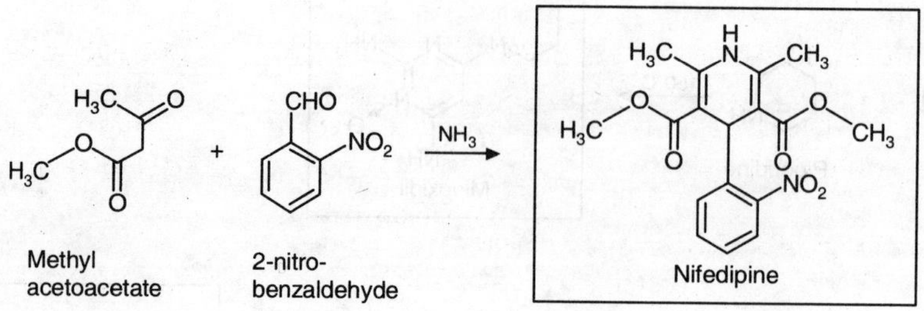

Methyl acetoacetate + 2-nitro-benzaldehyde —NH₃→ Nifedipine

Nicardipine

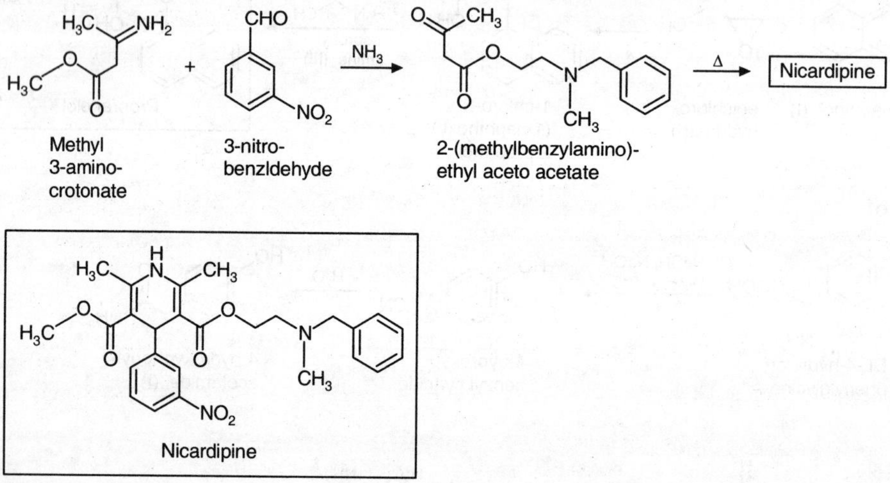

Methyl 3-amino-crotonate + 3-nitro-benzldehyde —NH₃→ 2-(methylbenzylamino)-ethyl aceto acetate —Δ→ Nicardipine

Nicardipine

Nimodipine

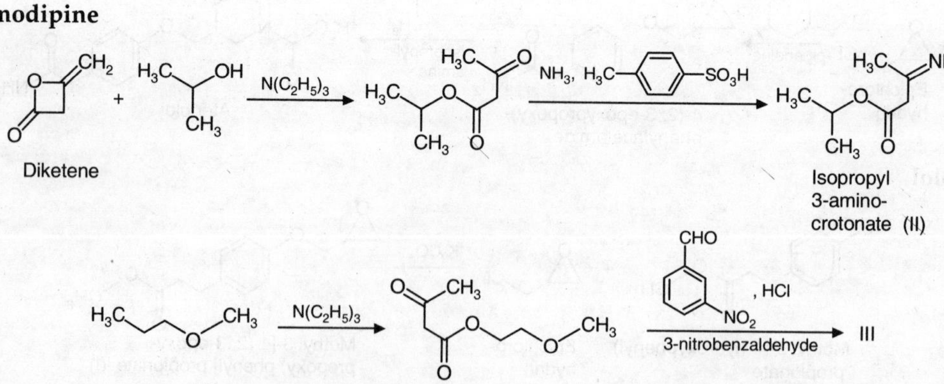

Diketene + H₃C–CH(OH)–CH₃ —N(C₂H₅)₃→ [H₃C...O...CH₃] —NH₃, H₃C–⬡–SO₃H→ Isopropyl 3-amino-crotonate (II)

H₃C–O–CH₃ —N(C₂H₅)₃→ [O...CH₃...O...CH₃] —3-nitrobenzaldehyde, HCl→ III

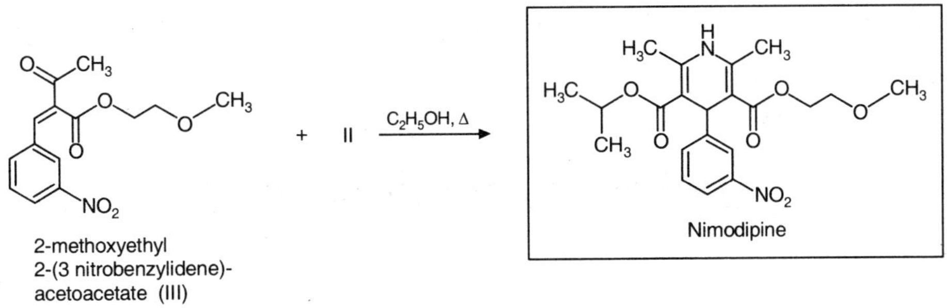

+ II
C_2H_5OH, Δ
Nimodipine
2-methoxyethyl
2-(3 nitrobenzylidene)-
acetoacetate (III)

Verapamil

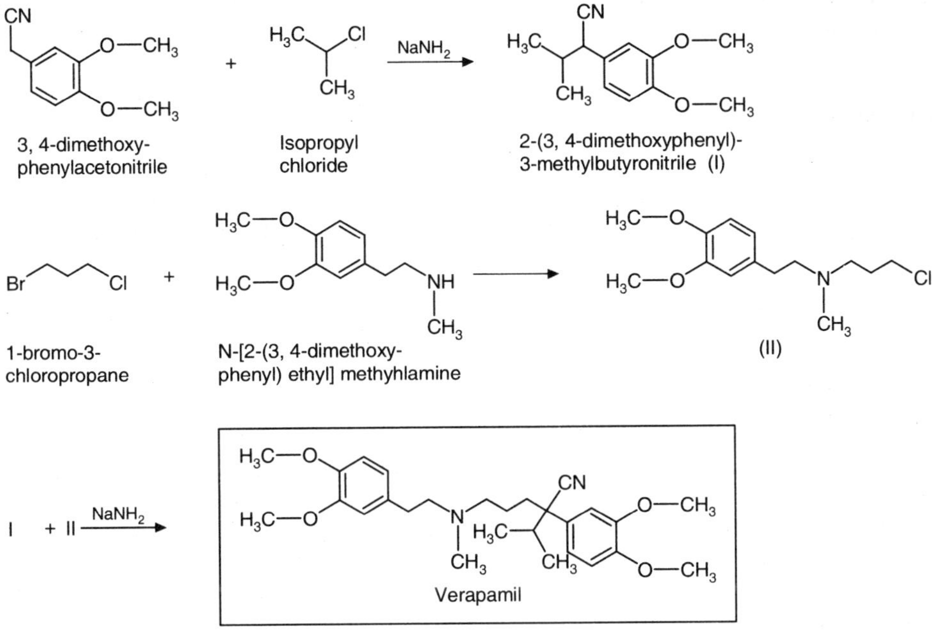

+
$NaNH_2$
3, 4-dimethoxy-
phenylacetonitrile
Isopropyl
chloride
2-(3, 4-dimethoxyphenyl)-
3-methylbutyronitrile (I)
+
1-bromo-3-
chloropropane
N-[2-(3, 4-dimethoxy-
phenyl) ethyl] methyhlamine
(II)
I + II
$NaNH_2$
Verapamil

30

Antihyperlipidemics

An increase in the plasma concentration of lipoprotein is known as hyperlipidemia and the pharmacological agents, which reduce the concentration of plasma lipids are called antihyperlipidemic agents.

PHYSIOLOGY

- Carbohydrates, proteins and fats are the body fuels which provide necessary energy for growth, maintenance and functioning of various organs in human body. Besides acting as the major form of energy storage, fatty acids are also involved in the formation of cell membranes. For example, phospholipids are the essential constituent of a variety of cell membranes.

- Plasma cholesterol can be freely utilized in the synthesis of various endogenous steroids and nerve cell membranes. Except plasma cholesterol, rest of the body lipids is catabolised to give carbondioxide and water as end products. While bile acids are the ultimate end products of cholesterol catabolism.

- Only a small fraction of these bile acids is excreted through faeces while rest is reabsorbed by the enterohepatic circulation. The shedding of epithelial cells from the gut and skin offers the major route of cholesterol excretion. Atherosclerosis, thrombosis, myocardial infarction and pancreatitis are the clinical manifestations of elevated plasma lipid level.

- The term, hyperlipidemia denotes an elevated plasma cholesterol and/or plasma triglyceride level while the term, hyperlipoproteinemias are the conditions in which there is elevated plasma concentration of cholesterol or triglyceride containing lipoproteins. The term lipoprotein was first coined in 1929 by Macheboeuf of Pasteur institute to denote lipoidal macromolecular complexes.

LIPOPROTEIN STRUCTURE (FIG. 30.1)

- Lipids are carried in plasma in the form of lipoprotein after getting associated with several apoproteins; plasma lipid concentration is dependent on the concentration of lipoproteins.

- The core of lipoprotein globules consist of triglycerides, while the outer layer has phospholipids, free cholesterol and apoprotein.

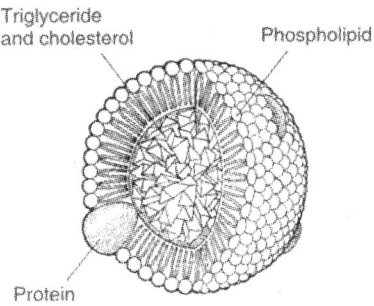

Triglyceride
and cholesterol

Phospholipid

Protein

Fig. 30.1: Structure of lipoprotein

TYPES OF LIPOPROTEINS

- There are separate mechanisms for the transport of lipids from exogenous (i.e. dietary origin) and endogenous (i.e. of hepatic origin) lipids. The dietary triglycerides are hydrolysed to monoglycerides and free fatty acids by pancreatic lipase in the intestinal lumen.

- These dietary triglycerides and cholesterol are trapped by chylomicrons which are large lipoprotein particles having diameter ranging 80-500 nm. Lipoproteins contain a hydrophobic lipid filled core surrounded by a monolayer of ampiphilic lipids and specific proteins, i.e. apoproteins.

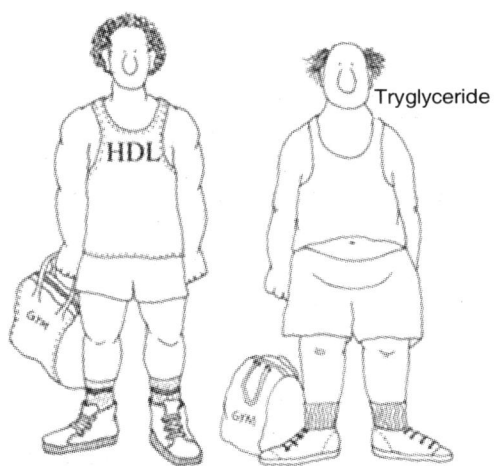

- The hydrophobic core acts as the storage package for triglyceride and cholesteryl esters. Apoproteins are categorised into 5 types, like A, B, C, D and E. Almost 6 classes of lipoproteins are identified in the human body which are involved in the transport of lipids from their sites of absorption and synthesis to the tissues where they are utilised.

- Size, density and the nature of apoprotein in the lipoprotein are the probable points utilized in the classification of lipoproteins. They are categorised as given below.

1. *Chylomicrons*

These are the largest species of triglyceride rich lipoproteins which are involved in the transportation of dietary fat from gut. These are secreted into the lymph and contain apoprotein A and B-48.

2. *Very Low-density lipoprotein (VLDL)*

These are globular particles synthesized in the liver having diameter of 30–80 nm. They contain apoproteins B, C and E. They are involved in the transport of endogenous lipid from liver to the plasma.

3. *Intermediate density lipoprotein (IDL)*

These are the lipoproteins obtained when the triglyceride content of VLDL are partially digested in capillaries by the action of extrahepatic lipoprotein lipase. They have a diameter of 20–35 nm.

4. *Low density lipoprotein (LDL)*

- Due to further action of lipoprotein lipase on IDL in the circulation, most of the remaining triglyceride content of IDL is digested resulting into the loss of apoproteins C and E from their structure.

- The density of particle is increased and diameter is brought down to 18–28 nm. These particles are now termed as LDL which consists of cholesterol, phospholipids and apoprotein B-100. LDL also contains B-74 and B-26. They have longest plasma half-life of about 1.5 days amongst the lipoproteins.

- LDL particles are finally delivered to hepatic and certain extrahepatic tissues for further lysosomal degradation to release the cholesterol, which can be utilised in cell membrane formation.

5. *High density lipoprotein (HDL)*

- This is a group of heterogeneous lipoproteins having low lipid content. A further subclassification in HDL is based upon density value of these particles. HDL apparently enhances the removal of cholesterol from the arterial wall.

- Hence chances of development of atherosclerotic lesions are more when HDL value falls below normal. While the elevated levels of VLDL, IDL and LDL are always correlated with increased risk of atherosclerosis.

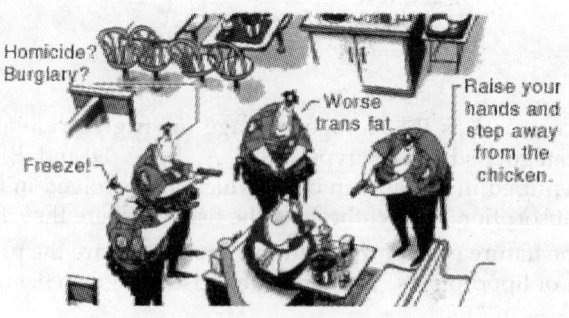

▨ LIPOPROTEIN TRANSPORT MECHANISM (FIG. 30.2)

- Chylomicrons are the lipoproteins that trap the dietary tri-glycerides and cholesterol from the intestinal lumen and cross the intestinal mucosal cells to enter into circulation. In the adipose tissue and muscle, the chylomicrons are partly digested by lipoprotein lipase enzymes present in vascular endothelium resulting into fatty acids (i.e. hydrolysis products of triglycerides).

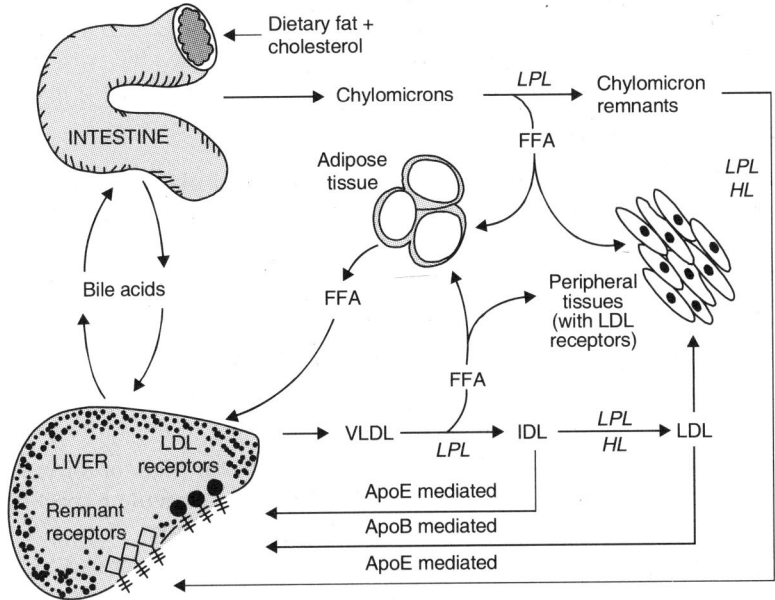

Fig. 30.2: The major pathways involved in the metabolism of chylomicrons synthesized by the intestine and VLDL synthesized by the liver

- These fatty acids then enter into underlying adipocytes or muscle cells where re-esterification to triglycerides occurs.
- The newly formed triglycerides are carried by the lymph and then by the blood to various body tissues for either storage or for utilization as a source of energy.
- The remaining small fraction of triglyceride in the partly digested chylomicrons (now termed as chylomicrons remnant, diameter 30-50 nm) is digested by hepatic lysosomal enzymes to generate free cholesterol. The transporta..on of endogenous, (hepatic origin) lipids is quite similar to the transportation of exogenous (dietary) lipids. Liver releases triglycerides and cholesterol into circulation by packing them into the core of very low density lipoproteins (VLDL).
- Due to the partial digestion of VLDL by lipoprotein lipase-enzymes present in the vascular endothelium, VLDL is then converted into intermediate density lipoprotein (IDL). Some of IDL particles are recycled through liver to get back VLDL while rests of them are further digested to give low density lipoproteins (LDL).
- These particles may be taken up by lysosomes present in the hepatic cells by the activation of LDL-receptors bound to the cell surfaces. The LDL particles thus taken up by receptor-

mediated endocytosis, is digested to liberate free cholesterol for cell use. Hence an elevation in the level of circulating LDL particles may be seen in defective LDL-receptor mechanisms. Some LDL particles are also taken up in certain extrahepatic tissues by receptor-mediated endocytosis process to release free cholesterol. Thus LDL particles in the circulation act as the storage depot for major amount of body cholesterol.

- The cholesterol released during the degeneration of cells in tissue damage is taken up by high-density lipoproteins (HDL) where re-esterification with long-chain fatty acid occur. The resulting cholesteryl esters are then handed over to VLDL or LDL particles by cholesteryl ester transfer protein in plasma. These VLDL or LDL particles loaded with cholesteryl esters, then deliver their content into the liver. Thus cholesterol conservation is maintained.

▓ HYPERLIPOPROTEINEMIA

- Hyperlipoproteinemia is usually characterized by elevated plasma concentration of VLDL (mostly triglycerides) and/or of LDL (mostly cholesterol).
- The condition may arise mainly due to inherent genetic defect in the catabolism of various lipoproteins or due to presence of such diseases which induce generalized metabolic disturbances. Accordingly hyperlipoproteinemia may be categorised as given below.

Primary Hyperlipoproteinemia

- Here the genetic abnormalities in the person are usually responsible. If it arises due to single gene defect, it is known as monogenic hyperlipoproteinemia.
- While if multiple gene defects along with nongenetic factors (i.e. obesity, high fat-riched diet) are involved, then it is known as multifactorial or polygenic hyperlipoproteinemia. Examples of primary hyperlipoproteinemia include the following:
  1. **Abetalipoproteinemia:** It is an inherited genetic disorder characterized by the absence of chylomicrons, VLDL and LDL. The deficiency of all these apobeta lipoproteins leads to deficiency of vitamin E and malabsorption of triglycerides.
  2. **Familial lipoprotein lipase deficiency disorder:** As the name indicates, it is a familial (i.e., genetic) deficiency of lipoprotein lipase enzyme.
  3. **Familial type HI hyperlipoproteinemia (dysbetalipoproteinemia):** The E-3 and E-4 forms of apolipoprotein E are absent resulting into an accumulation of remnant particles in the plasma.
  4. **Familial hypercholesterolaemia:** Due to deficiency of LDL-receptor sites on the cell membrane, hepatic catabolism of LDL-particles decreases. This leads to elevation in the plasma LDL levels.

Secondary Hyperlipoproteinemia

- Elevated levels of VLDL, IDL and LDL particles are seen under certain diseased conditions, e.g., diabetes mellitus, uremia, corticosteroid excess, hypothyroidism, chronic alcoholism, nephrosis, glycogen storage abnormalities, acromegaly, obesity, etc. induce metabolic abnormalities and increase the risk factor for atherosclerosis.
- The elevated levels of VLDL and/or LDL particles hence can be brought to normal range by treating these underlying secondary causes along with the dietary control. Dietary therapy is always the beneficial step for all lipoprotein disorders which minimizes the concentration of lipids in the plasma and it should be strictly observed even if drug therapy has begun.

CLASSIFICATION OF ANTIHYPERLIPIDEMICS

Classification of antihyperlipidemics are given in Flow chart 30.1.

Flow chart 30.1: Classification of antihyperlipidemics

Antihyperlipidaemics

Drugs that lowers
VLDL and LDL level:
Nicotinic acid

Fibric acid derivatives:
Clofibrate, gemfibrozil,
fenofibrate, ciprobibrate

Anti-oxidant:
Probucol

Bile acid binding resin:
Cholestyramine,
colestipole

**HMGCoA reductase
inhibitors:**
Metastatin, lovastatin,
simvastatin

Miscellaneous:
Metformin, neomycin

Drugs that lower VLDL and LDL level

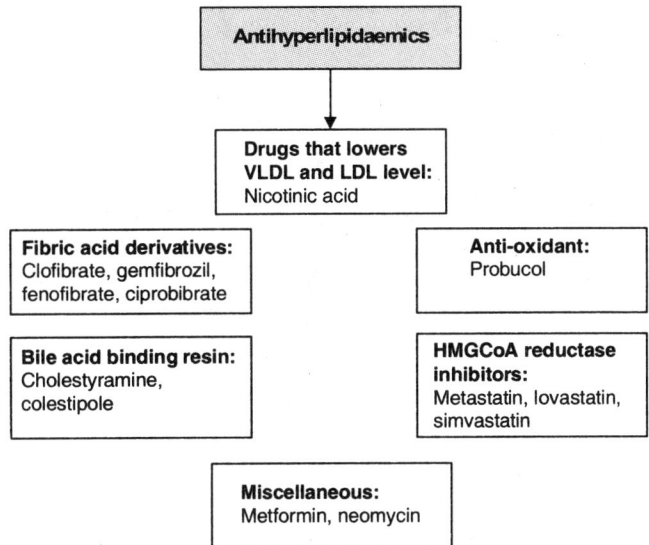

Nicotinic acid

Fibric acid derivatives

Clofibrate

Fenofibrate

Ciprofibrate

Benzafibrate

Gemfibrozil

Antioxidant

Probucol

Bile acid binding resin

Cholestyramine

Colestipole

HMG CoA reductase inhibitors

Pravastatin

Metastatin

Lovastatin

Simvastatin

Atherosclerosis, ischemia and acute pancreatitis are some of the clinical manifestations of hyperlipoproteinemia. During elevated levels of triglycerides (in the range of 300-800 mg/dl) and plasma cholesterol (about 150-200 mg/dl), the risk factor for above diseases is likely to increase.

- It is the elevated level of VLDL and/or LDL particles which is responsible for it. However, the elevated HDL particles (which participates into transport of excess plasma cholesterol into liver) offer safeguard against above conditions and leads to decrease in the risk of coronary atherosclerosis.

- Diet and weight control are the firstline treatment of all patients with high cholesterol or triglyceride blood levels (hyperlipidemia). However, there are patients who do not respond adequately to non-drug management.
- Various drugs used in the treatment of hyperlipoproteinemia may act either by lowering the plasma level of VLDL or LDL particles. Persons with elevations of both VLDL and LDL levels may require combination therapy. These drugs show synergistic effect when used in the combination therapy. On occasions; combination treatment with reduced doses of 2 drugs is more effective than a single agent with fewer adverse effects.

ANTIOXIDANT

Probucol

Mechanism of action (*Fig. 30.3*)

- Oxidised LDL is taken by macrophages to convert it into a foam cell. Group of these foam cells constitute the earliest maker of atherosclerosis.
- The antioxidant inhibits the oxidation of LDL thereby prevent uptake by macrophages.

Pharmacokinetics

It is very poorly soluble in water and only about 1 to 10% of 1 g dose is absorbed from GIT. Since probucol is lipophilic, it associates with lipids in the diet and is absorbed along with them and transported by chylomicrons and VLDL through lymphatics to the systemic circulation.

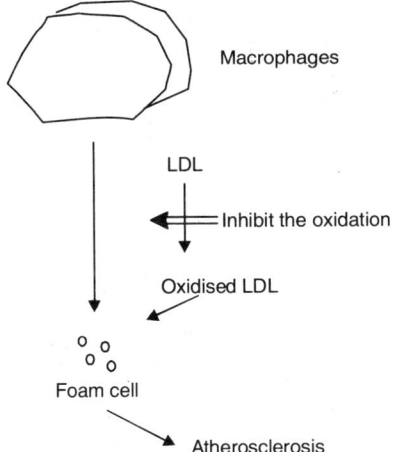

Fig. 30.3: Mechanism of action of probucol

Adverse Effect

- The common adverse effect of probucol is its high lipophilicity due to which it is retained in adipose tissues of the body. Hence its lipid lowering effects are observed for months even after the discontinuation of drug therapy.
- Most of the drug is eliminated in the bile and feces. The common adverse effects of probucol include nausea, flatulence, abdominal pain, diarrhea, eosinophilia and angioneurotic edema. It is contraindicated in pregnancy and in cardiac dysfunction.

■ BILE ACID-BINDING RESINS

Cholestyramine and Colestipole

Mechanism of action (*Fig. 30.4*)

- Bile acids are the metabolic endproducts of cholesterol which are released into the intestine. Major fraction (about 98%) of bile acids released into the gut is reabsorbed through the enterohepatic circulation and suppresses the microsomal hydroxylase enzyme involved in the conversion of cholesterol to the bile acids.

- Thus due to enterohepatic reabsorption of the bile acids, further catabolism of cholesterol is suppressed. Bile acids, through their emulsifying effect, also enhance the absorption of dietary lipids from the gut lumen. If the concentration of gut bile acid is lowered down by promoting their excretion in the faces (and by inhibiting their enterohepatic reabsorption), naturally it will be reflected into;

  1. Increased conversion of cholesterol to bile acids coupled with a compensatory increase the rate of hepatic cholesterol synthesis. The latter needs an increased hepatic uptake and catabolism of circulating LDL particles. The overall result will be lowering of plasma LDL level.

  2. Deficient absorption of dietary lipids into the circulation. This leads to decrease in plasma lipid concentration.

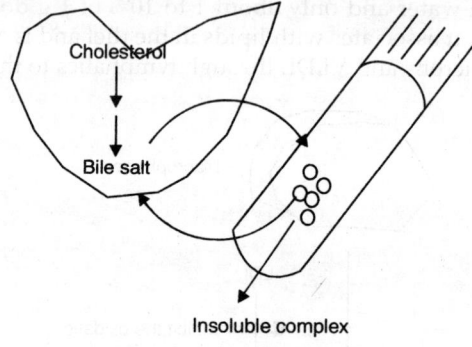

Cholestyramine forms
insoulble complex
with bile acid and salts
preventing their absorption

Fig. 30.4: Mechanism of action of bile acid-binding resin

- Cholestyramine and colestipol are the examples of bile acid-binding resins which form a sort of no absorbable complex with bile acids due to the presence of quaternary nitrogen in their structure. Thus these drugs promote their elimination from the gut and inhibit their reabsorption into the circulation. The fecal excretion of bile acids in fact, has been shown to increase 30 folds by these drugs.

- Both these drugs, cholestyramine and colestipol HCl, are high molecular weight, water insoluble anionic exchange resins. Since these resins carry a positive charge and bile salts carry a negative charge, both bind together to form relatively stable complexes in the intestinal lumen. This drain on the bile acid pool stimulates increased synthesis of bile acids in the liver from cholesterol, thus depleting the hepatic stores of cholesterol. These agents stimulate VLDL production in the liver and hence may increase triglyceride concentrations.

In patients who have both raised plasma cholesterol levels, and raised triglyceride levels it may be necessary to combine the use of resins with nicotinic acid or clofibrate.

Uses

Both these drugs are the examples of anion exchange resins and remain undigested and no absorbable in the GIT. Hence the drugs are considered safest anti-hyperlipidemic agents due to the lack of systemic effects. They are used only in the patients who have elevated LDL levels. They are favored in the treatment of type II hyperlipoproteinemia. In the treatment of familial hypercholesterolemia, usually a combination of cholestyramine and nicotinic acid gives better results. Beside bile acids, these resins also bind with other drugs due to their anionic nature. Thus absorption of thyroxin, vitamin C, digitalis glycosides, iron, and warfarin is reported to be impaired by these resins.

Adverse Effect

The adverse effects include nausea, abdominal pain, flatulence, constipation, acidosis and hypoprothrombinemia. They are contraindicated during the pregnancy.

β-Sitosterol

Mechanism of action

It is a plant sterol. Due to the structural similarity with cholesterol, this agent impedes the absorption of dietary cholesterol and produces a moderate reduction in cholesterol level. Its low efficacy and high cost decrease its popularity as lipid lowering agent.

▓ FIBRIC ACID DERIVATIVES

Clofibrate

Mechanism of action (Fig. 30.5)

- A series of esters of p-chlorophenoxyisobutyric acid has been prepared out of which clofibrate was found to lower the plasma lipid level more efficiently. Several derivatives of clofibrate are also in clinical use. They include bezafibrate, ciprofibrate, fenofibrate and etofibrate. Etofibrate is an ethylene glycol diester of nicotinic acid and clofibric acid.

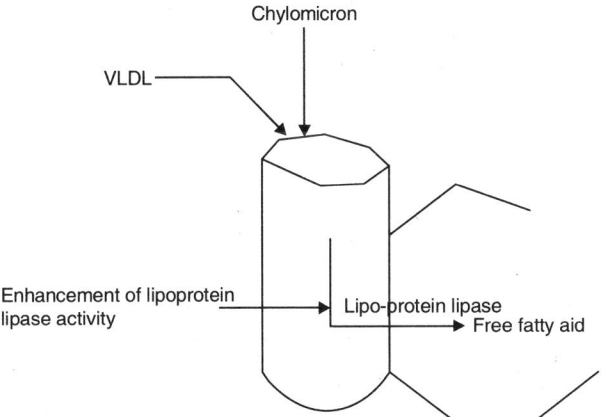

Fig. 30.5: Mechanism of action of clofibrate

- The mechanism of action of clofibrate is not well defined. Various proposed mechanisms include:
  a. Stimulation of lipoprotein lipase enzyme activity.
  b. Increased cholesterol excretion.
  c. Inhibition of hepatic cholesterol synthesis.
  d. Increased intravascular catabolism of VLDL and IDL to LDL.
  e. Inhibition of hepatic VLDL synthesis.
  f. Increase in the plasma thyroxin concentration by clofibrate-induced displacement of thyroxin from albumin.

Drug–drug interaction

Due to displacement ability of clofibrate anion exerted on plasma albumin, potentiation of activities of many drugs (which are bound to albumin) can be seen during clofibrate therapy. Such drugs include sulfonylureas, coumarin and indandione anticoagulants.

Pharmacokinetics

- Clofibrate is well absorbed from GIT. In the circulation, the ester linkage is hydrolysed to release p-chlorophenoxyisobutyric acid which then binds to plasma albumin. The acid metabolite is mainly excreted in the urine along with its glucuronide.
- It hydrolyzes to clofibric acid which is the active form. Following oral administration, maximum plasma concentration is usually attained with 3-6 hours. Clofibric acid is highly protein bound (93–98%) and has half-life of 13–17 hours.

Uses

It is used in the management of a condition in which cholesterol rich VLDL and chylomicrons remnant particles accumulate in the plasma (type III hyperlipidemia).

Adverse effect

Adverse effects include nausea, diarrhea, skin rash, weakness, muscle cramps, impotency and myopathy. The drug is contraindicated during pregnancy and in patients with impaired renal or hepatic functioning.

▓ DRUGS THAT LOWERS VLDL AND LDL

Nicotinic Acid

Mechanism of action

- Its use in the treatment of hyperlipoproteinemia was first made by Altschul in 1955. It brings about hypolipidemic action by decreasing lipolysis and by promoting hepatic storage of lipids.
- It also enhances the activity of lipoprotein lipase resulting into low circulating VLDL level. Since VLDL acts as the precursor for most of the circulating IDL, the low VLDL level results into low level of circulating LDL.
- Nicotinamide, however, lacks hypolipidemic activity. In many cases, nicotinic acid is co-administered along with bile acid-binding resin to get better results.

Pharmacokinetics

- In body, nicotinic acid undergoes extensive metabolism resulting into formation of various metabolites, such as nicotinamide, nicotinuric acid, methyl nicotinamide, N-methyl-2-pyridone-3-carboxamide and N-methyl-2-pyrione-5-carboxamide.
- These metabolites are mainly excreted in the urine along with some unchanged nicotinic acid.

Adverse effect

- Nicotinic acid has a long list of adverse effects. These include vomiting, diarrhoea, peptic ulcer, jaundice, hyperpigmentation, dry skin, postural hypotension, cutaneous vasodilation (flushing) specifically in the upper part of the body.
- Gouty arthritis may develop due to the drug-induced elevation in the plasma uric acid level. It is contraindicated during pregnancy. Due to too many adverse effects of nicotinic acid, it is less frequently used alone in the treatment of hyperlipoproteinemia.

▨ HMG CoA REDUCTASE INHIBITOR

Simvastatin, Lovastatin, Metastatin

Mechanism of action (Fig. 30.6)

- About two-thirds of body cholesterol are synthesized in the liver and intestine and one-third is supplied from diet on a low cholesterol diet, the liver of a healthy adult synthesizes about 800 mg of cholesterol daily, which replaces that lost in the faeces.

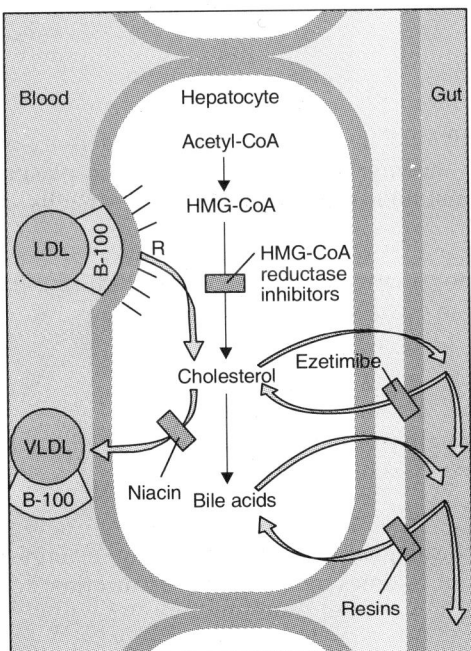

Fig. 30.6: Sites of action of HMG-CoA reductase inhibitors, niacin, ezetimibe, and resins used in treating hyperlipidemia. LDL receptors (R) are increased by treatment with resins and HMG-CoA reductase inhibitors

- The rate limiting step in the synthesis of cholesterol is the enzyme HMG-CoA reductase. The HMG-CoA reductase inhibitors can selectively and competitively inhibit the action of this enzyme, thus reducing body's ability to synthesize cholesterol.

Structuring–activity relationship

1. The activity of HMGRIs is sensitive to the stereochemistry of the lactone ring to be hydrolyzed, and the length of bridge connecting the two ring systems.
2. The bicyclic ring could be replaced with other lipophilic rings and that the size and shape of the other ring system were important to the overall activity of the compounds.
3. The replacement of the bicyclic ring with various substituted, aromatic ring system led to the development of fluvastatin, atorvastatin and cerivastatin.
4. Minor modification of the bicyclic ring and side chain ester of lovastatin produced simvastatin and pravastatin.

Pharmacokinetics

Three statins, lovastatin, simvastatin and pravastatin, have been extensively studied. Simvastatin is a prodrug. The eliminating half-life is relatively short (1-3 hrs), but duration of enzyme inhibition is much longer.

Adverse Effect

Adverse effects are few and of mild nature. Like other hypolipidemic drugs, HMG CoA reductase inhibitors are contraindicated during pregnancy.

▨ MISCELLANEOUS

Neomycin

Mechanism of action

It is an amino glycoside antibiotic. It exerts hypolipidemic activity only in oral administration while if given parenterally, neomycin does not reduce the plasma level of LDL. The poor absorption upon oral administration of neomycin indicates that its site of action is in GIT.

Adverse effect

The adverse effects (like, ototoxicity, nephrotoxicity) seen during parenteral administration of neomycin, are not reported to occur with oral use of the drug.

Acipimox

Mechanism of action

Acipimox is a synthetic derivative of nicotinic acid and like nicotinic acid; it acts by inhibiting adipose tissue lipolysis (hydrolysis of lipid esters).

Adverse effect

It appears to produce less flushing and GI intolerance than nicotinic acid at normal doses (250 mg 2-3 times/day). It is about 20 times more active than nicotinic acid.

Metformin

Chemically it is N, N-dimethyl biguanidine. It has no effect on cholesterol biosynthesis but it affects the lipoprotein composition. It produces about 50% reduction in the serum triglyceride level. It is also a hypoglycemic agent and lowers blood glucose level.

Clofibrate

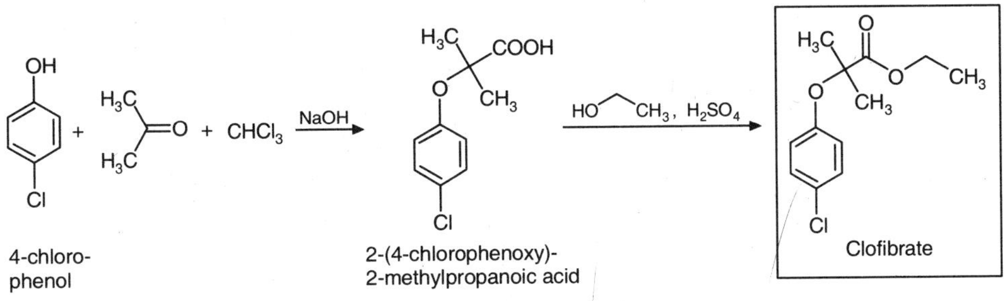
NaOH
HO CH3, H2SO4
4-chloro-phenol
2-(4-chlorophenoxy)-2-methylpropanoic acid
Clofibrate

Ciprofibrate

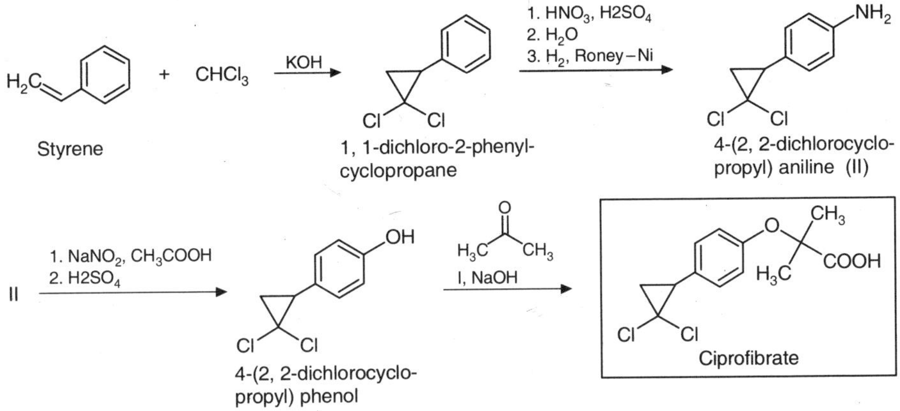
KOH
1. HNO3, H2SO4
2. H2O
3. H2, Roney–Ni
Styrene
1, 1-dichloro-2-phenyl-cyclopropane
4-(2, 2-dichlorocyclo-propyl) aniline (II)
1. NaNO2, CH3COOH
2. H2SO4
I, NaOH
4-(2, 2-dichlorocyclo-propyl) phenol
Ciprofibrate

Fenofibrate

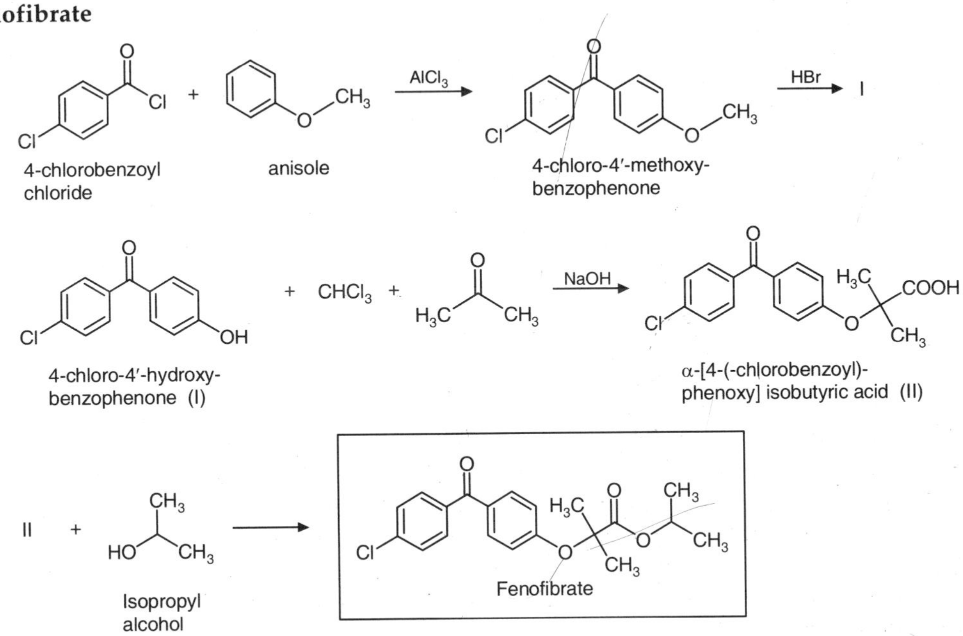
AlCl3
HBr
4-chlorobenzoyl chloride
anisole
4-chloro-4′-methoxy-benzophenone
NaOH
4-chloro-4′-hydroxy-benzophenone (I)
α-[4-(-chlorobenzoyl)-phenoxy] isobutyric acid (II)
Isopropyl alcohol
Fenofibrate

Diuretics

Diuretics are drugs which increase sodium and water excretion by the kidney. The term 'diuresis' means increased urine flow, while the term 'saluresis' means increased urinary sodium excretion. In common usage, however, diuretics have come to mean agents which increase both sodium and water excretion. A diuretic is any drug that elevates the rate of bodily urine excretion (diuresis). There are several categories of diuretics.

- All diuretics increase the excretion of water from the body, although each class of diuretic does so in a distinct way. Chemically, diuretics are a diverse group of compounds that either stimulate or inhibit various hormones that naturally occur in the body to regulate urine production by the kidneys. The primary therapeutic goal of diuretic use is to reduce edema by reducing the ECF volume.
  1. For this to occur, NaCl output must exceed NaCl intake.
  2. Diuretics primarily prevent Na^+ entry into the tubule cell.
- Once a diuretic enters the tubule fluid, the nephron site at which it acts determines its effect. In addition, the site of action also determines which electrolytes, other than Na^+, will be affected. All diuretics except spironolactone exert their effects from the luminal (tubule fluid) side of the nephron.
- Hence, it is necessary for diuretics to get into the tubule fluid in order to be effective. Mannitol does this by filtration at the glomerulus, however, all other diuretics (except spironolactone) are fairly tightly protein bound and undergo little filtration.
- They reach the urine by secretion across the proximal tubule via the organic acid or organic base secretory pathway.

ROLE OF THE NEPHRON (FIG. 31.1)

1. Kidneys control the extracellular fluid (ECF) volume by adjusting NaCl and H_2O excretion.
2. Each day the kidney filters more than 22 moles of Na. To maintain NaCl balance, approximately 3 lbs of NaCl must be reabsorbed by the renal tubules on a daily basis.
3. The body maintains blood pressure at the expense of ECF volume.
4. When NaCl intake > output, i.e. congestive heart failure or renal failure, edema develops.
5. Na^+ reabsorption is driven primarily by Na^+/K^+ adenosine triphosphatase (ATPase) located at the basolateral (blood side) membrane of epithelial cells throughout the nephron.
6. The Na^+/K^+ is an energy-requiring pump which exchanges 1 Na^+ for 2 K^+, thereby keeping a low Na^+ concentration and a high K^+ concentration within the cell.
7. On the luminal side, cell-specific pathways exist for passive movement of Na^+ down its electrochemical gradient from lumen to cell. These cells form the physiologic basis of diuretic action.

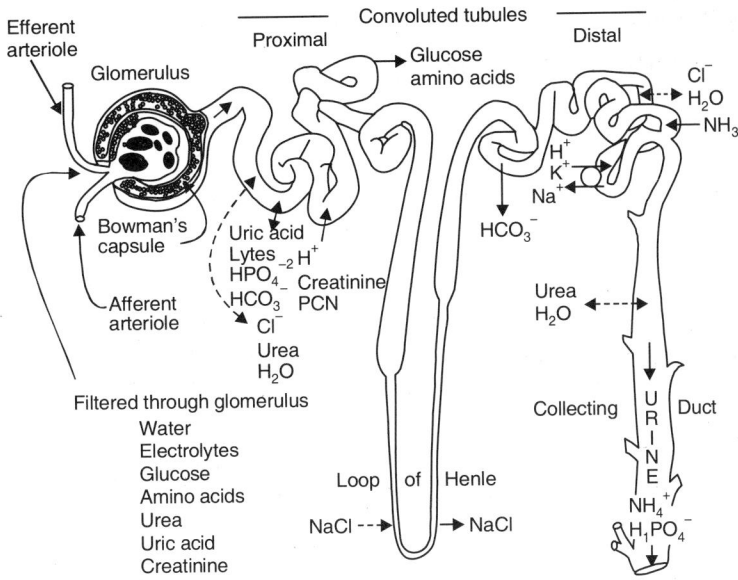

Fig. 31.1: Nephron, the structural and functional unit of kidney

CLASSIFICATION OF DIURETICS

Classification of diuretics is given in Flow chart 31.1.

Flow chart 31.1: Classification of diuretics

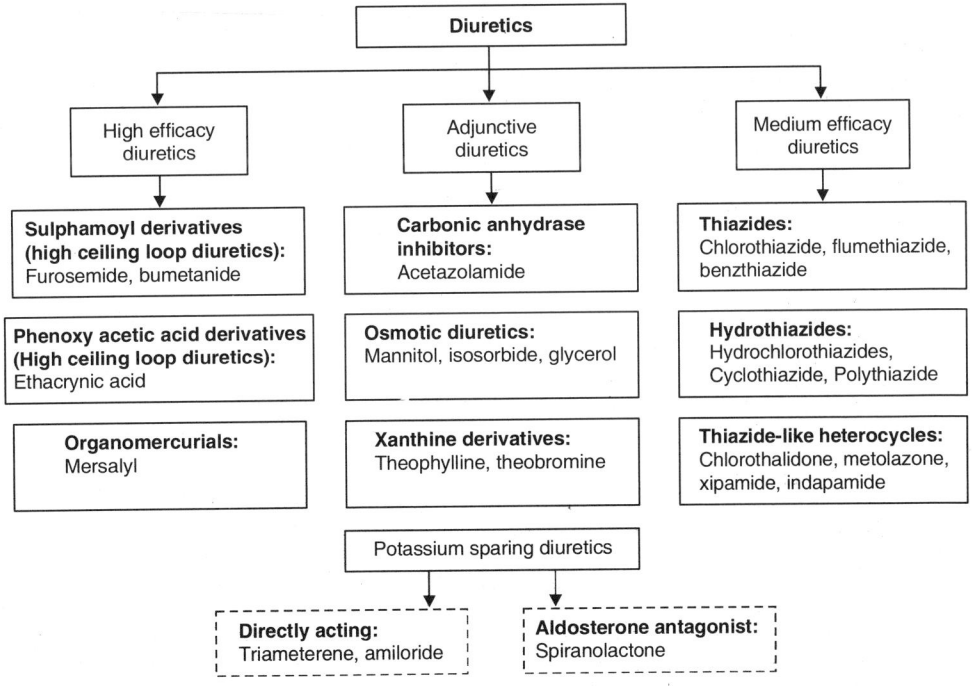

High Efficacy Diuretics

A. Sulphamoyl derivatives (high ceiling loop diuretics)

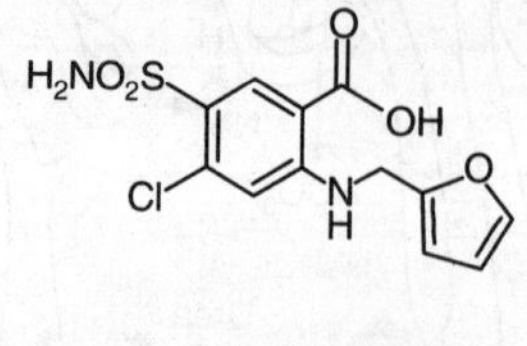

Furosemide

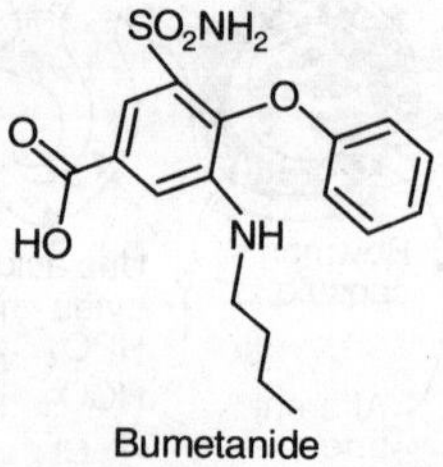

Bumetanide

B. Phenoxy acetic acid derivatives (high ceiling loop diuretics)

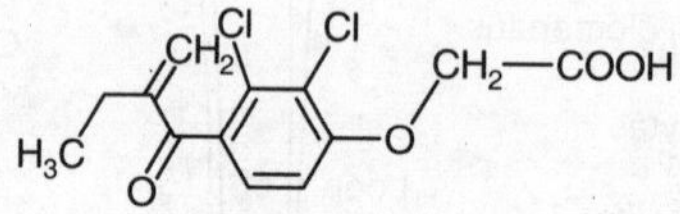

Ethacrynic acid

C. Organomercurials

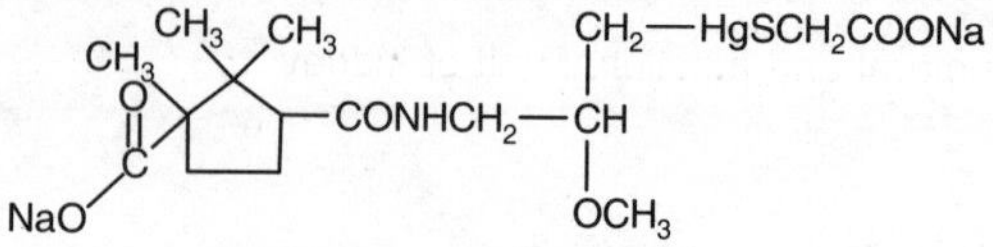

Mercaptomerin sodium

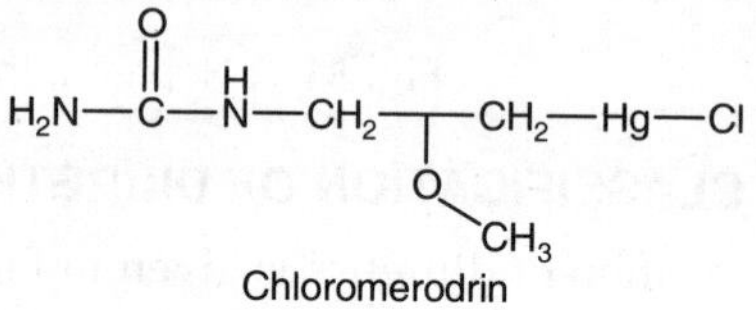

Chloromerodrin

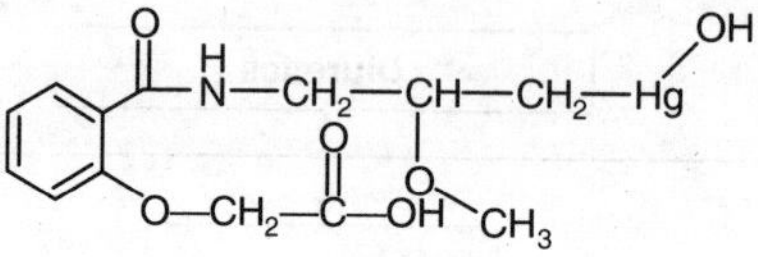

Mersalyl

Medium Efficacy Diuretics

A. Thiazides

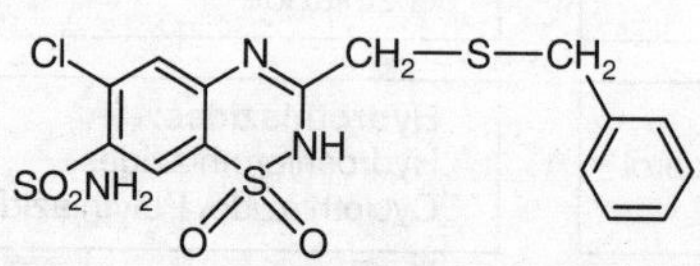

Benzthiazide

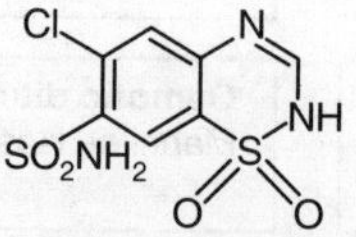

Chlorothiazide

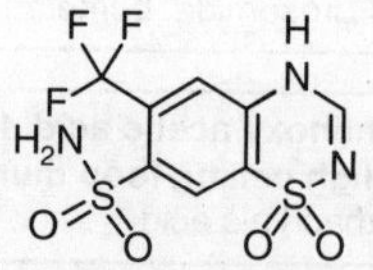

Flumethiazide

B. Hydrothiazides

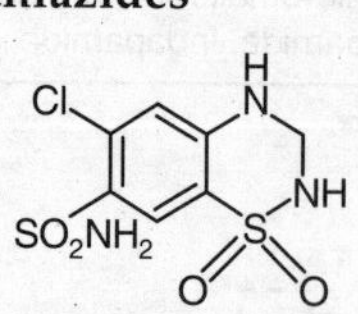

Hydrochlorothiazide

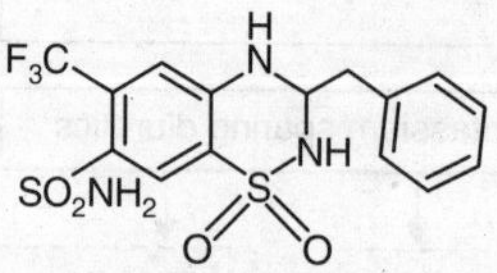

Bendroflumethiazide

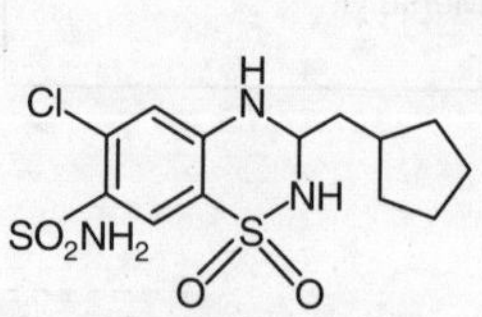

Cyclopenthiazide

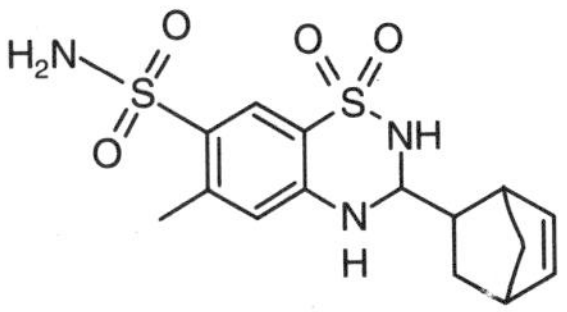

Cyclothiazide

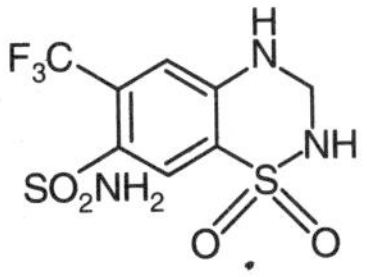

Hydroflumethiazide

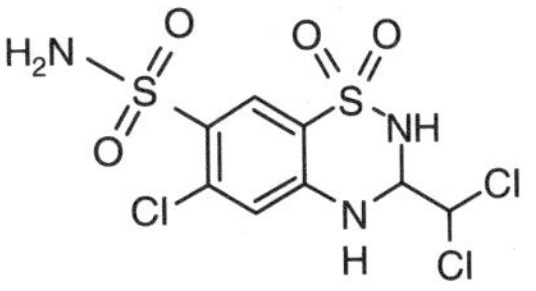

Trichlormethiazide

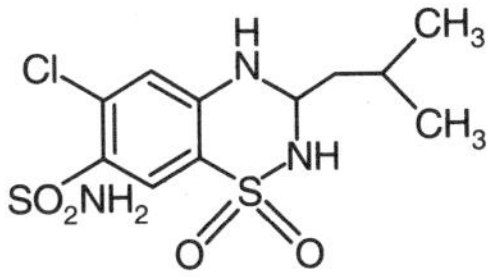

Buthiazide

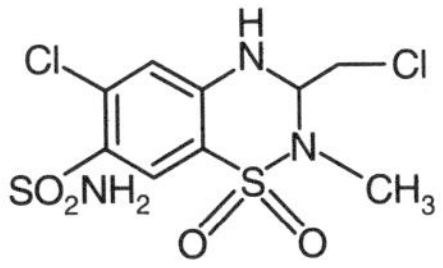

Methyclothiazide

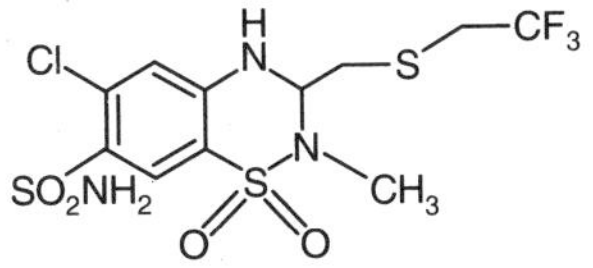

Polythiazide

C. Thiazide like diuretics

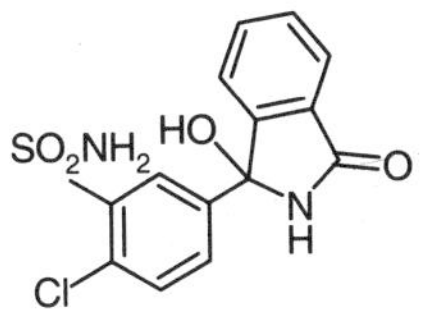

Chlorothalidone

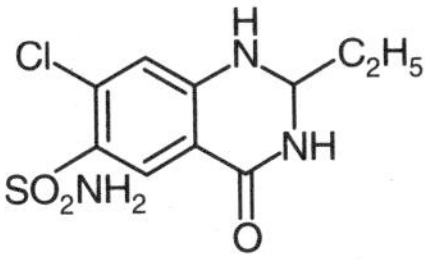

Quinethazone

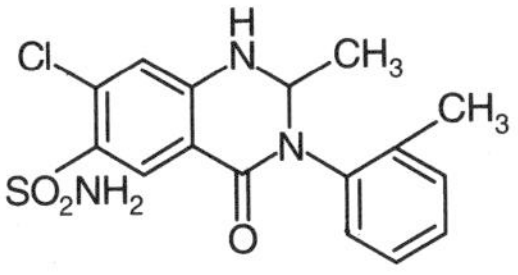

Metolazone

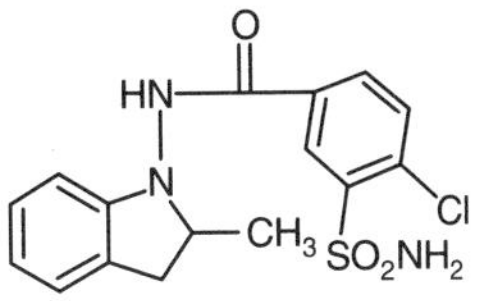

Indapamide

Adjuncitve Diuretics

A. Carbonic anhydrase inhibitors

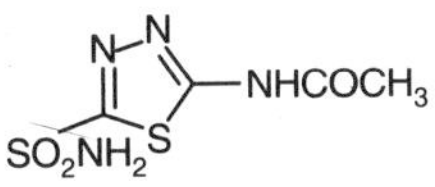

Acetazolamide

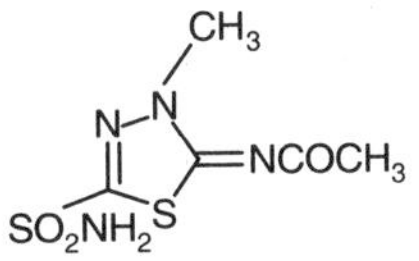

Methazolamide

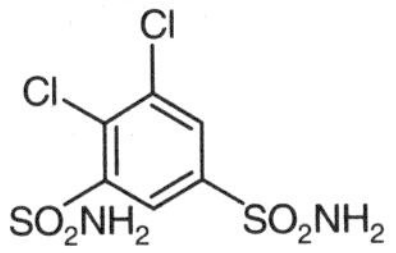

Dichlorophenamide

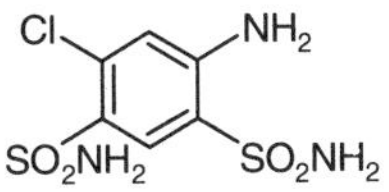

Chloraminophenamide

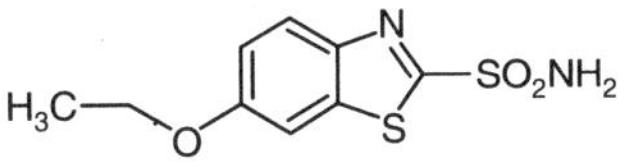

Ethoxzolamide

B. Xanthine derivatives

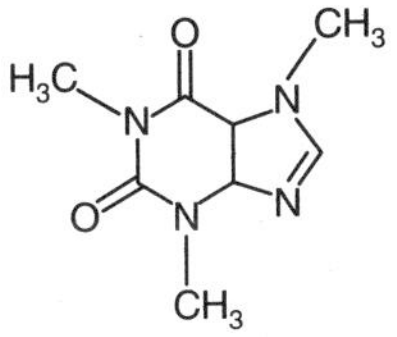

Caffeine

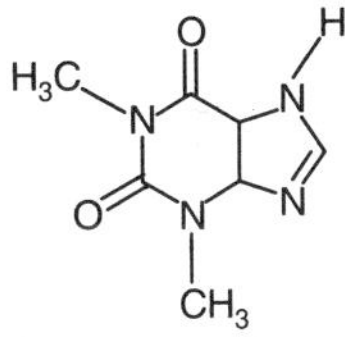

Theophylline

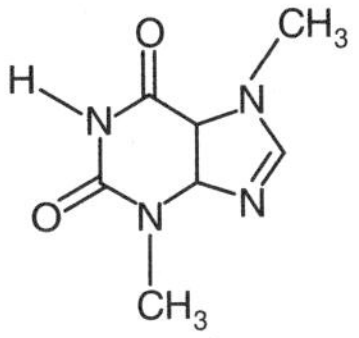

Theobromine

C. Osmotic diuretics

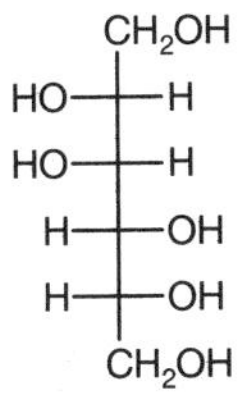

D-mannitol

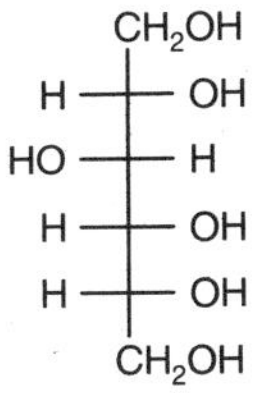

Sorbitol

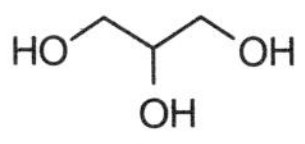

Glycerine

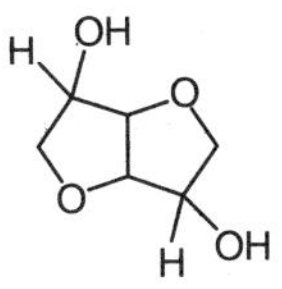

Isosorbide

D. Potassium sparing diuretics

i. Aldosterone antagonist

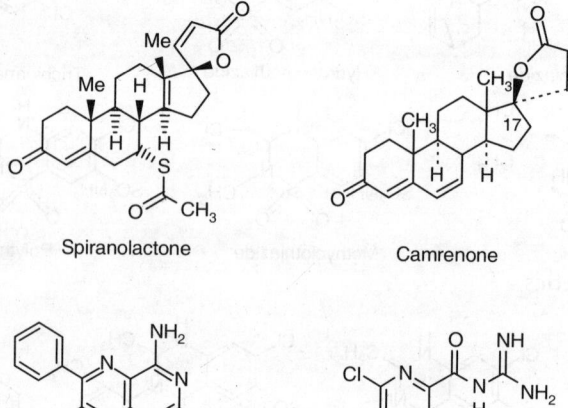

Spiranolactone

Camrenone

ii. Directly acting

Triamterene

Amiloride

HIGH EFFICACY DIURETICS

Furosemide, Bumetanide and Ethacrynic Acid (Loop Diuretics)

- Drugs in this group of diuretics inhibit the activity of the Na^+-K^+-$2Cl^-$ symporter in the thick ascending limb of the loop of Henle; hence these diuretics also are referred to as loop diuretics. Although the proximal tubule reabsorbs approximately 65% of the filtered Na^+, diuretics acting only in the proximal tubule have limited efficacy because the thick ascending limb has a great reabsorptive capacity and reabsorbs most of the rejectate from the proximal tubule.

- Diuretics acting predominantly at sites past the thick ascending limb also have limited efficacy because only a small percentage of the filtered Na^+ load reaches these more distal sites. In contrast, inhibitors of $Na^+ - K^+ - 2Cl^-$ symport in the thick ascending limb are highly efficacious, and for this reason, they sometimes are called high-ceiling diuretics.

- The efficacy of inhibitors of $Na^+ - K^+ - 2Cl^-$ symport in the thick ascending limb of the loop of Henle is due to a combination of two factors:

1. Approximately 25% of the filtered Na^+ load normally is reabsorbed by the thick ascending limb.

2. Nephron segments past the thick ascending limb do not possess the reabsorptive capacity to rescue the flood of rejectate exiting the thick ascending limb.

Mechanism of action (Fig. 31.2)

- Furosemide and others act primarily in the thick ascending limb and inhibit $Na^+ - K^+ - Cl^-$ symport. In the thick ascending limb, flux of $Na^+ - K^+$ and Cl^- from the lumen into the epithelial cell is mediated by $Na^+ - K^+ - 2Cl^-$ symporter.

- This symporter captures the energy in the Na^+ electrochemical gradient established by the basolateral Na^+ pump and provides for uphill transport of K^+ and Cl^- and into the cell. K^+ channels in the luminal membrane provide a conductive pathway for the optical recycling of this cation and basolateral Cl^- channels provide a basolateral exit mechanism for Cl^-.

- Inhibition of $Na^+ - K^+ -2\,Cl^-$ symport binds to the $Na^+ - K^+ - 2Cl^-$ symporter and blocks its function, bringing salt transport in this segment of nephron to virtual standstill. It is suggested that these drugs attach to the binding site of the symporter.
- The $Na^+ - K^+ - 2Cl^-$ symporter has amino acid sequence of 1191 residues containing 12 putative membranes – spanning domains flanked by long N and C termini in the cytoplasm.

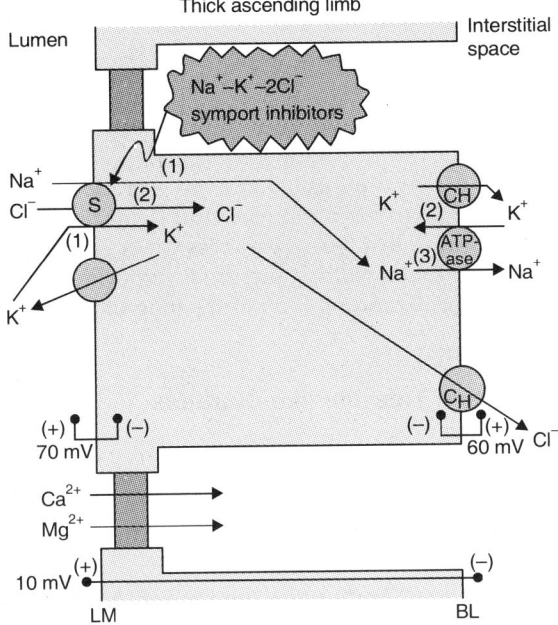

Fig. 31.2: NaCl reabsorption in thick ascending limb and mechanism of diuretic action of $Na^+ - K^+ - 2Cl^-$ symport inhibitors. S = symporter, CH = ion channel

Adverse effect

Over use of these drugs can cause hyponatremia, hypotension and circulatory collapse. They can cause ototoxicity, vertigo. Drug interaction may occur with aminoglycosides, propranolol, probencid and thiazide diuretics.

Uses

1. A major use of loop diuretics is in the treatment of acute pulmonary edema. A rapid increase in venous capacitance in conjunction with a brisk natriuresis reduces left ventricular filling pressures and thereby rapidly relieves pulmonary edema.
2. Loop diuretics are also used widely for the treatment of chronic congestive heart failure when diminution of extracellular fluid volume is desirable to minimize venous and pulmonary congestion. In this regard, a meta-analysis of randomized clinical trials demonstrates that diuretics cause a significant reduction in mortality and the risk of worsening heart failure, as well as an improvement in exercise capacity.

Mercurial Diuretics

Mechanism of action

- Most mercurials have the general structure, in which a chain of at least three carbon atoms, one atom of mercury at one end of the chain. The group R is hydrophilic in nature which determines the distribution and rate of excretion of the compound.

- The nature of X substituent affects the toxicity of the compound, irritation at the site of injection and rate of absorption. In an acidic environment, the mercuric ion dissociates and binds to sulfhydryl enzymes, inactivating them.

$$R—CH_2—\underset{\underset{CH_3}{\overset{|}{O}}}{CH}—CH_2—Hg—X \xrightarrow{\text{Metabolism}} R—CH_2—CH=CH_2 + Hg^{++}$$

$$\underset{\text{Receptor site}}{\overset{SH \quad X}{|\quad\quad|}} + Hg^{++} \longrightarrow \underset{\text{Inactivated receptor}}{\overset{Hg}{\overset{/\quad\backslash}{S\qquad X}}}$$

- As a result, reabsorption of Na^+ is diminished and the excretion of Na^+ and Cl^- is increased. More Cl^- than Na^+ is lost, thus, to maintain electrical neutrality, cations such as hydrogen and to a lesser degree K^+ are also lost. Because excess Cl^- is excreted, bicarbonate remains to maintain balanced anions, and the resulting picture is hypochloremic alkalosis. They inhibit active chloride transport in the ascending limb of the loop of Henle.

■ MEDIUM EFFICACY DIURETICS

Thiazides, Hydrothiazides and Thiazide-like Diuretics

Chemistry

- Inhibitors of Na^+–Cl^- symport are sulfonamides, and many are analogues of 1, 2, 4-benzothiadiazine-1,1-dioxide.
- Because the original inhibitors of Na^+–Cl^- symport were benzothiadiazine derivatives, this class of diuretics became known as thiazide diuretics. Subsequently, drugs that are pharmacologically similar to thiazide diuretics but are not thiazides were developed and are called thiazide-like diuretics. The term thiazide diuretic is used here to refer to all members of the class of inhibitors of Na^+–Cl^- symport.

Mechanism of action (Fig. 31.3)

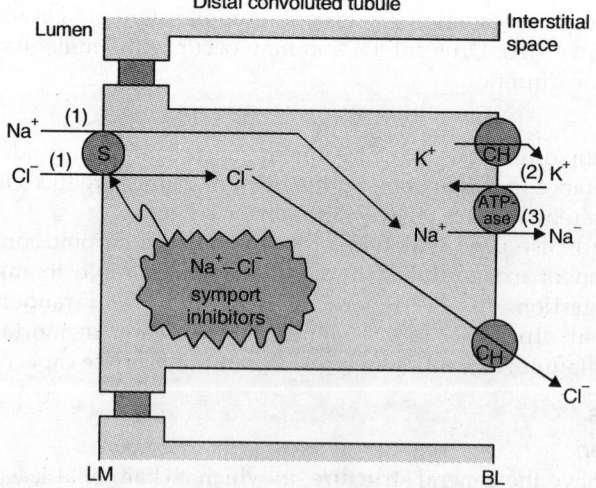

Fig. 31.3: NaCl reabsorption in distal convoluted tubule and mechanism of diuretic action of Na^+–Cl^- symport inhibitors

- The primary site of action of thiazide is the distal convulated tubule,whereas the proximal tubule may represent a secondary site of action. In the distal convulated tubule, transport is powered by an Na^+ pump in the basolateral membrane.
- The energy is the electrochemical gradient for Na is harnessed by an Na^+ –Cl^- into the epithelial cell against its electrochemical gradient. Cl then passively exists the basolateral membrane via a chloride channel. Thiazide diuretics inhibit the Na^+–Cl^-symporter, perhaps by competing for the chloride binding site.
- The Na^+ –Cl^- symporter has a predicted size of 1023 amino acoid residues, has 12 putative membrane spanning domains. These domains exhibit 12 potential membrane-spanning helices and they are flanked by long –NH_2 and COOH terminal nonhydrophobic domains.

Structure–activity relationship

1. The SO_2 group can be replaced with CO with increase in activity.
2. Saturation of 3, 4-double bond increase in activity.
3. Substitution of the ring nitrogen at position 2 with methyl increases activity. However, at position 4 the methyl group reduces activity with the heterocyclic ring more vulnerable to heterocyclic cleavage.
4. Substituent in the position 3, hydrophobic in character, increases 1000 times saluretic activity. Substituents include, –CH_2Cl, –$CHCl_2$, –$CH_2C_6H_5$, CH_2CH_2S-$CH_2C_6H_5$. The increase in activity correlates with the lipid solubility.
5. Substitutions in the 6 position by Cl, Br, or CF_3 increase activity, whereas H, or NH_2 are weakly active.
6. A free sulfamoyl or potentially free sulfamoyl group at 7 position is essential for activity. The loss of sulfamoyl group eliminated the diuretic effect, but not the hypertensive effect.

Adverse effect

The most serious adverse effect is extracellular volume depletion, hypotension, hyponatremia and hypochloremia.

Uses

1. Thiazide diuretics are used for the treatment of the edema associated with heart (congestive heart failure), liver (hepatic cirrhosis), and renal (nephrotic syndrome, chronic renal failure, and acute glomerulonephritis) disease.
2. With the possible exceptions of metolazone and indapamide, most thiazide diuretics are ineffective when the GFR is less than 30 to 40 ml/min.

WEAK OR ADJUNCTIVE DIURETICS

Carbonic Anhydrase Inhibitors

Mechanism of action (31.4)

- Bicarbonate is primarily reabsorbed in the proximal tubule. H^+ ion is secreted into the lumen where it can combine with filtered bicarbonate (HCO_3^-) to form H_2CO_3 that is then converted to CO_2 and H_2O (catalyzed by carbonic anhydrase).
- CO_2 diffuses into the proximal tubule where it combines with H_2O to form H_2CO_3 that then forms H^+ and HCO_3^-. HCO_3^- exits the proximal tubule on the blood side, while H^+ is again secreted into the tubule lumen. This results in HCO_3^- reabsorption.
- If CA activity is inhibited, HCO_3^- reabsorption is reduced and exits the proximal tubule in much larger amounts. Because Na^+ is the most abundant cation present in proximal tubule fluid, it is the major cation which accompanies HCO_3^- out of the proximal tubule.

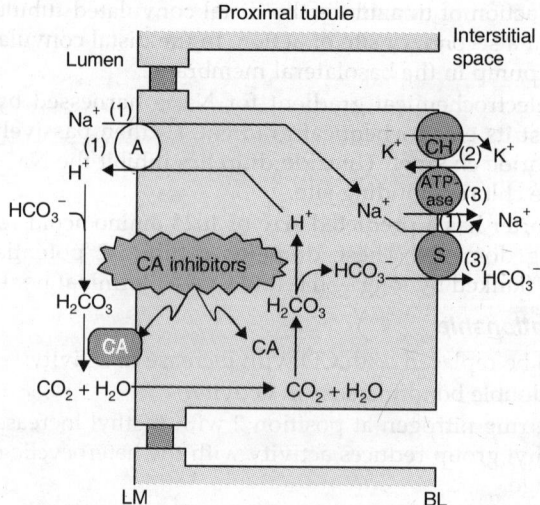

Fig. 31.4: $NaHCO_3$ reabsorption in proximal tubule and mechanism of diuretic action of carbonic anhydrase inhibitors. A, antiporter; S, symporter; CH, ion channel. (The actual reaction catalyzed by carbonic anhydrase is $OH^- + CO_2$ HCO_3^-; however, H_2O $OH^- + H^+$, and $HCO_3^- + H^+$ H_2CO_3, so the net reaction is $H_2O + CO_2$ H_2CO_3.) Numbers in parentheses indicate stoichiometry. BL and LM indicate basolateral and luminal membranes, respectively.

- In the distal nephron, Na^+ is largely reabsorbed (unlike HCO_3^-) and is exchanged for K^+. Therefore, acetazolamide primarily causes an increase in urinary HCO_3^-, K^+, and water excretion. Effectiveness is reduced with continued therapy because plasma $[HCO_3^-]$ fall, reducing the amount of HCO_3^- that appears in the urine.

Structure–activity relationship

Maximal diuretic activity is observed when this position is substituted with: Cl, Br < CF_3 or NO_2

Substitution with an amino ($-NH_2$) group increases saluretic activity, but decreases carbonic anhydrase activity

An substituted sulfamoyl moiety is of paramount importance.

SO_2NH_2 The sulfamoyl moiety can be replaced with a similarly electrophilic group (e.g. carboxyl), carbamoyl, etc.) that may increase diuretic potency while decreasing carbonic anhydrase inhibitory activity.

Dichlorophenamide

Chloraminophenamide

1. Simple heterocyclic sulfonamides yielded the prototypic carbonic anhydrase inhibitor acetazolamide.
2. The sulfamoyl group is essential for the in vitro and in vivo carbonic anhydrase activity.
3. The sulfamoyl nitrogen must remain unsubstituted to retain both in vivo and in vitro activities.
4. Substitution of a methyl group on one of acetazolamide's ring nitrogen yields methazolamide retains carbonic anhydrase inhibitory activity.
5. The moiety to which sulfamoyl group is attached must possess aromatic character.
6. Heterocyclic sulfonamide, the derivative with highest lipid/water partition coefficient and the lowest pKa values has the greatest carbonic anhydrase activity and diuretic activity.

Adverse effect

Serious toxic reactions to carbonic anhydrase inhibitors are infrequent; however, these drugs are sulfonamide derivatives and, like other sulfonamides, may cause bone marrow depression, skin toxicity, sulfonamide like renal lesions, and allergic reactions in patients hypersensitive to sulfonamides. With large doses, many patients exhibit drowsiness and parenthesis. Most adverse effects, contraindications, and drug interactions are secondary to urinary alkalinization or metabolic acidosis, including;

1. Diversion of ammonia of renal origin from urine into the systemic circulation, a process that may induce or worsen hepatic encephalopathy (the drugs are contraindicated in patients with hepatic cirrhosis).
2. Calculus formation and ureteral colic owing to precipitation of calcium phosphate salts in an alkaline urine.
3. Worsening of metabolic or respiratory acidosis (the drugs are contraindicated in patients with hyperchloremic acidosis or severe chronic obstructive pulmonary disease).
4. Reduction of the urinary excretion rate of weak organic bases.

Uses

1. Although *acetazolamide* is used for treatment of edema, the efficacy of carbonic anhydrase inhibitors as single agents is low, and carbonic anhydrase inhibitors are not employed widely in this regard.
2. However, studies indicate that the combination of acetazolamide with diuretics that block Na^+ reabsorption at more distal sites in the nephron causes a marked natriuretic response in patients with low basal fractional excretion of Na^+ (<0.2%) who are resistant to diuretic monotherapy. Even so, the long-term usefulness of carbonic anhydrase inhibitors often is compromised by the development of metabolic acidosis.

Osmotic Diuretics

Mechanism and site of action

- For many years, it was thought that osmotic diuretics act primarily in the proximal tubule. By acting as non-reabsorbable solutes, it was reasoned that osmotic diuretics limit the osmosis of water into the interstitial space and thereby reduce luminal Na^+ concentration to the point that net Na^+ reabsorption ceases.
- Although early micro-puncture studies supported this concept, subsequent studies suggested that this mechanism, while operative, may be of only secondary importance and that the major site of action of osmotic diuretics is the loop of Henle.

- By extracting water from intracellular compartments, osmotic diuretics expand the extracellular fluid volume, decrease blood viscosity, and inhibit renin release. These effects increase RBF, and the increase in renal medullary blood flow removes NaCl and urea from the renal medulla, thus reducing medullary tonicity. Under some circumstances, prostaglandins may contribute to the renal vasodilation and medullary washout induced by osmotic diuretics.

- A reduction in medullary tonicity causes a decrease in the extraction of water from the DTL, which, in turn, limits the concentration of NaCl in the tubular fluid entering the ATL. This latter effect diminishes the passive reabsorption of NaCl in the ATL. In addition, the marked ability of osmotic diuretics to inhibit reabsorption of Mg^{2+}, a cation that is reabsorbed mainly in the thick ascending limb, suggests that osmotic diuretics also interfere with transport processes in the thick ascending limb. The mechanism of this effect is unknown.

- In summary osmotic diuretics act both in the proximal tubule and the loop of Henle, with the latter being the primary site of action. Also, osmotic diuretics probably act by an osmotic effect in the tubules and by reducing medullary tonicity.

Adverse effect

1. Osmotic diuretics are distributed in the extracellular fluid and contribute to the extracellular osmolality. Thus water is extracted from intracellular compartments, and the extracellular fluid volume becomes expanded. In patients with heart failure or pulmonary congestion, this may cause frank pulmonary edema.

2. Extraction of water also causes hyponatremia, which may explain the common adverse effects, including headache, nausea, and vomiting.

3. On the other hand, loss of water in excess of electrolytes can cause hypernatremia and dehydration.

4. Urea may cause thrombosis or pain, if extravasation occurs, and it should not be administered to patients with impaired liver function because of the risk of elevation of blood ammonia levels.

5. Both mannitol and urea are contraindicated in patients with active cranial bleeding. Glycerin is metabolized and can cause hyperglycemia.

Xanthine Diuretics

Mechanism of action

- These are rarely used as diuretic nowaday. Theophylline exerts its diuretic action by inhibiting Na^+ reabsorption in the proximal convulated tubule.

- This drug increases renal plasma flow, promoting a higher glomerular filtration rate. They also increase cardiac output. Adverse effects are CNS stimulation and vomiting.

POTASSIUM SPARING DIURETICS OR ANTI-KALIURETIC AGENTS

- Inhibitors of renal epithelial Na^+ channel. The body as a whole contains more K^+ than Na^+. The saluretic diuretic agents also cause a concomitant increase in K^+ excretion; therefore producing hypokalemia is not desired. Potassium-sparing diuretics produce mild natriuresis and decrease potassium and hydrogen ions secretion.

- Efforts to discover diuretics that would increase Na^+ excretion by inhibiting its exchange with K^+ in the distal convulated tubule produced two classed of potassium sparing agents.

1. Direct acting anti-kaliuretic agents.
2. Aldosterone antagonist

Direct Acting Anti-Kaliuretic

Mechanism of action *(Fig. 31.5)*

- These agents are used in combination with other diuretic agents (thiazide) for the treatment of hypertension, edema associated with chronic congestive heart failure or cirrhosis. These agents inhibit active Na^+ reabsorption.
- The increased excretion of Na^+ and Cl disrupts normal Na^+ transport and produces a net change in the electrogenic force across tubular a membrane, which subsequently reduces the net driving force for K^+ secretion. Their action is independent of aldosterone.

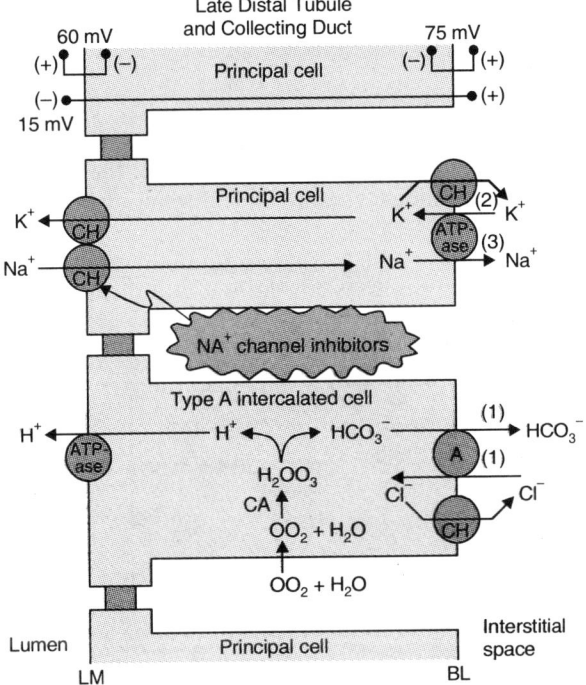

Fig. 31.5: Na^+ reabsorption in late distal tubule, collecting duct and mechanism of diuretic action of epithelial Na^+-channel inhibitors. Cl^- reabsorption (not shown) occurs both paracellularly and transcellularly, and the precise mechanism of Cl^- transport appears to be species-specific. A, antiporter; CH, ion channel; CA, carbonic anhydrase. Numbers in parentheses indicate stoichiometry. Designated voltages are the potential differences across the indicated membrane or cell. BL and LM indicate basolateral and luminal membranes, respectively

Uses

- Because of the mild natriuresis induced by Na^+-channel inhibitors, these drugs seldom are used as sole agents in the treatment of edema or hypertension. Rather, their major utility is in combination with other diuretics. Coadministration of an Na^+-channel inhibitor augments the diuretic and antihypertensive response to thiazide and loop diuretics.
- More important, the ability of Na^+-channel inhibitors to reduce K^+ excretion tends to offset the kaliuretic effects of thiazide and loop diuretics; consequently, the combination of an Na^+-channel inhibitor with a thiazide or loop diuretic tends to result in normal values of plasma K^+.

1. Liddle's syndrome can be treated effectively with Na^+-channel inhibitors. Approximately 5% of people of African origin carry a T594M polymorphism in the β subunit of ENaC, and amiloride is particularly effective in lowering blood pressure in patients with hypertension who carry this polymorphism.

2. Aerosolized amiloride has been shown to improve mucociliary clearance in patients with cystic fibrosis. By inhibiting Na^+ absorption from the surfaces of airway epithelial cells, amiloride augments hydration of respiratory secretions and thereby improves mucociliary clearance.

3. Amiloride is also useful for lithium-induced nephrogenic diabetes insipidus because it blocks Li^+ transport into the cells of the collecting tubules.

Aldosterone Antagonist

Mechanism of action

- Epithelial cells in the late distal tubule and collecting duct contain cytosolic MRs that has a high affinity for aldosterone. This receptor is a member of the superfamily of receptors for steroid hormones, thyroid hormones, vitamin D, and retinoids.

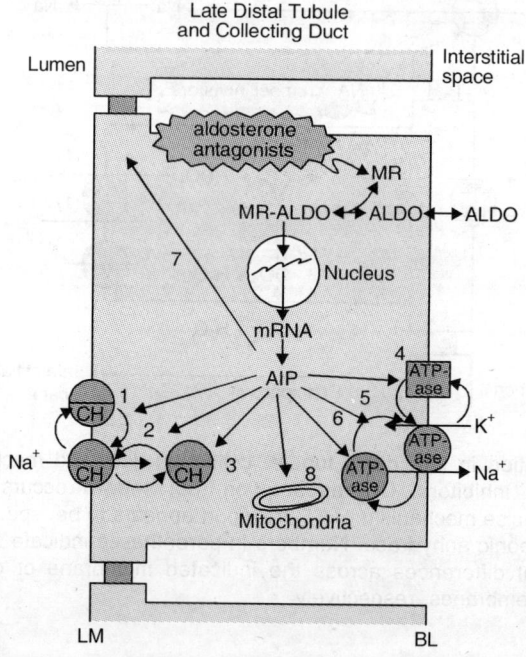

Fig. 31.6: Effects of aldosterone on late distal tubule and collecting duct and diuretic mechanism of aldosterone antagonists. AIP, aldosterone-induced proteins; ALDO, aldosterone; MR, mineralocorticoid receptor; CH, ion channel; 1, activation of membrane-bound Na^+ channels; 2, redistribution of Na^+ channels from cytosol to membrane; 3, de novo synthesis of Na^+ channels; 4, activation of membrane-bound Na^+, K^+-ATPase; 5, redistribution of Na^+,K^+-ATPase from cytosol to membrane; 6, de novo synthesis of Na^+,K^+-ATPase; 7, changes in permeability of tight junctions; 8, increased mitochondrial production of ATP. BL and LM indicate basolateral and luminal membranes, respectively

- Aldosterone enters the epithelial cell from the basolateral membrane and binds to MRs; the MR-aldosterone complex translocates to the nucleus, where it binds to specific sequences of DNA (hormone-responsive elements) and thereby regulates the expression of multiple gene products called aldosterone-induced proteins (AIPs).

- Illustrates some of the proposed effects of AIPs, including activation of 'silent' Na^+ channels and 'silent' Na^+ pumps that pre-exist in the cell membrane, alterations in the cycling of Na^+ channels and Na^+ pumps between the cytosol and cell membrane such that more channels and pumps are located in the membrane, increased expression of Na^+ channels and Na^+ pumps, changes in permeability of the tight junctions, and increased activity of enzymes in the mitochondria that are involved in ATP production.

- The precise mechanisms by which AIPs alter transport are incompletely understood. However, the net effect of AIPs is to increase Na^+ conductance of the luminal membrane and sodium pump activity of the basolateral membrane. Consequently, transepithelial NaCl transport is enhanced, and the lumen-negative transepithelial voltage is increased. The latter effect increases the driving force for secretion of K^+ and H^+ into the tubular lumen.

- Drugs such as spironolactone and eplerenone competitively inhibit the binding of aldosterone to the MR. Unlike the MR-aldosterone complex, the MR-spironolactone complex is not able to induce the synthesis of AIPs. Since spironolactone and eplerenone block the biological effects of aldosterone, these agents also are referred to as aldosterone antagonists. MR antagonists are the only diuretics that do not require access to the tubular lumen to induce diuresis.

Table 31.1: Mechanism of action of diuretics

Classification of common diuretics and their mechanisms of action			
Agent group	Example	Mechanism	Location
	Ethanol, water	Inhibit vasopressin secretion	
Acidifying salts	$CaCl_2$, NH_4Cl		
Carbonic anhyhdrase inhibitors	Acetazolamide, dorzolamide	Inhibit H^+ secretion, resultant promotion of Na^+ and K^+ excretion	Proximal tubule
Loop diuretics	Bumetanide, ethacrynic acid, furosemide, torsemide	Inhibit the Na-K-2Cl symporter	Medullary thick ascending limb
Osmotic diuretics	Glucose (especially in uncontrolled diabetes), mannitol	Promote osmotic diuresis	Proximal tubule, descending G limb
Potassium-sparing diuretics	Amiloride, spironolactone, triamterene	Inhibition of Na^+/K^+ exchange: Spironolactone inhibits aldosterone action, Amiloride inhibits epithelial sodium channels	Cortical collecting ducts
Thiazides	Bendroflumethiazide, hydrochlorothiazide	Inhibit Na^+/Cl^- reabsorption	Distal convoluted tubules
Xanthines	Caffeine,	Inhibit reabsorption of Na^+, increase glomerular filtration rate	Tubules

Uses

1. As with other K^+-sparing diuretics, spironolactone often is coadministered with thiazide or loop diuretics in the treatment of edema and hypertension. Such combinations result in increased mobilization of edema fluid while causing lesser perturbations of K^+ homeostasis.

2. Spironolactone is particularly useful in the treatment of primary hyperaldosteronism (adrenal adenomas or bilateral adrenal hyperplasia) and of refractory edema associated with secondary aldosteronism (cardiac failure, hepatic cirrhosis, nephrotic syndrome, and severe ascites).

3. Spironolactone is considered the diuretic of choice in patients with hepatic cirrhosis. Spironolactone, added to standard therapy, substantially reduces morbidity, mortality and ventricular arrhythmias in patients with heart failure.

Acetazolamide

Ammonium rhodanide   Hydrazine   Hydrazine-1, 2-bis-(thiocarboxamide)   2-amino-5-mercapto-1, 3, 4-thiadiazole (I)

Acetic anhydride   2-acetylamino-1, 3, 4-thiadiazole-5-sulfonyl chloride   2-acetylamino-1, 3, 4-thiadiazole-5-sulfonyl chloride (II)

Acetazolamide

Methazolamide

3-acetylamino-5-benzylthio-1, 3, 4-thiodiazole   Methyl iodide   (I)

Methazolamide

Hydrochlorothiazide

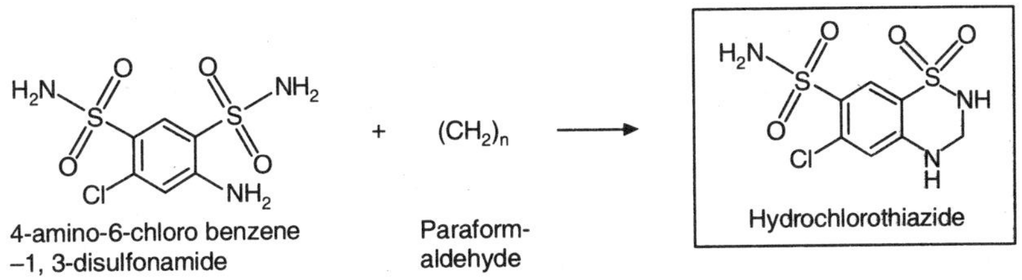
4-amino-6-chloro benzene
–1, 3-disulfonamide
+
$(CH_2)_n$
Paraform-
aldehyde
Hydrochlorothiazide

Cyclothiazide

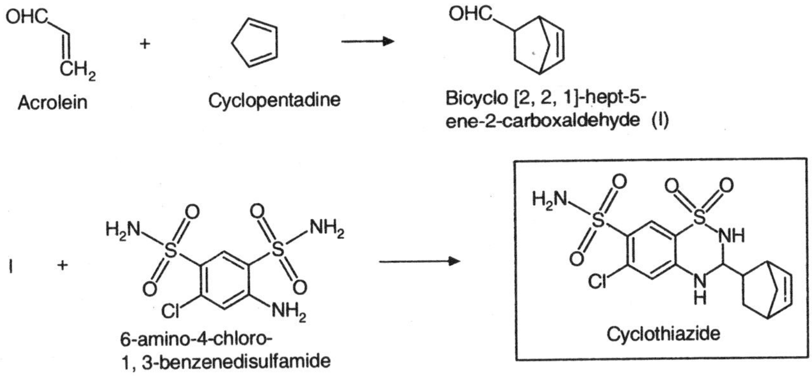
OHC
CH_2
Acrolein
+
Cyclopentadine
OHC
Bicyclo [2, 2, 1]-hept-5-
ene-2-carboxaldehyde (I)
I +
6-amino-4-chloro-
1, 3-benzenedisulfamide
Cyclothiazide

Cyclopenthiazide

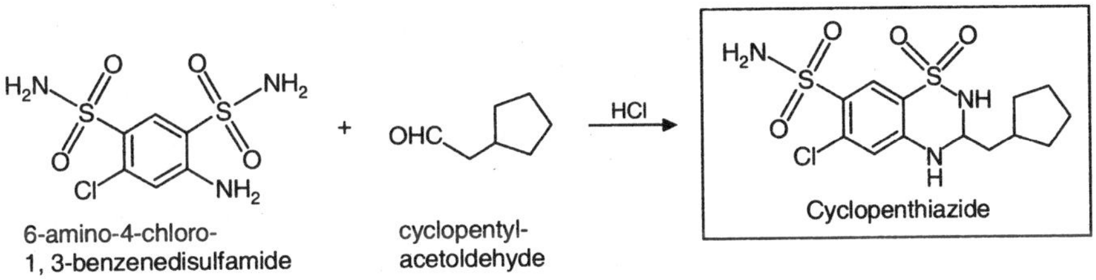
6-amino-4-chloro-
1, 3-benzenedisulfamide
+
OHC
cyclopentyl-
acetoldehyde
HCl
Cyclopenthiazide

Benzothiazide

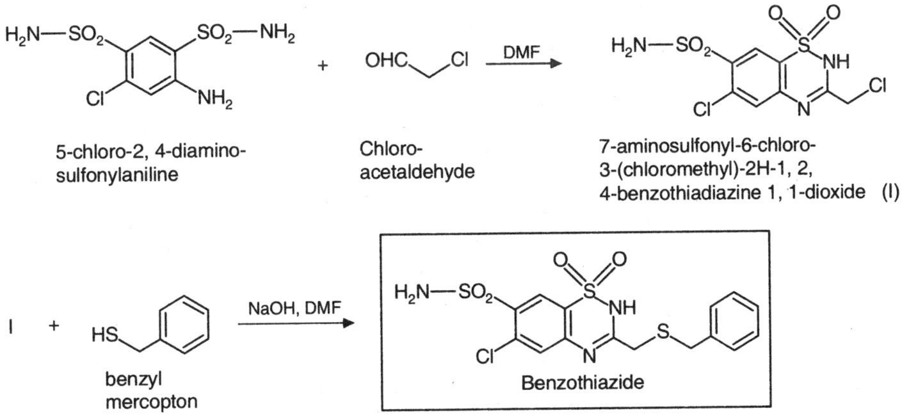
5-chloro-2, 4-diamino-
sulfonylaniline
+
OHC Cl
Chloro-
acetaldehyde
DMF
7-aminosulfonyl-6-chloro-
3-(chloromethyl)-2H-1, 2,
4-benzothiadiazine 1, 1-dioxide (I)
I +
HS
benzyl
mercopton
NaOH, DMF
Benzothiazide

Bendroflumethiazide

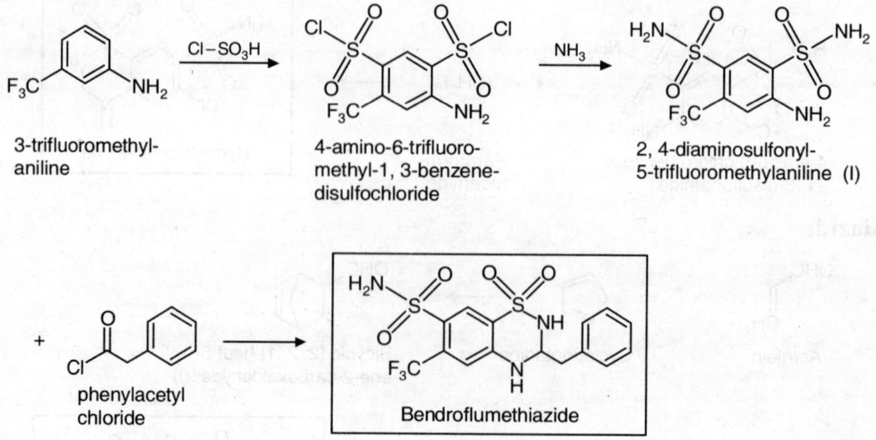

3-trifluoromethyl-
aniline

4-amino-6-trifluoro-
methyl-1, 3-benzene-
disulfochloride

2, 4-diaminosulfonyl-
5-trifluoromethylaniline (I)

phenylacetyl
chloride

Bendroflumethiazide

Indapamide

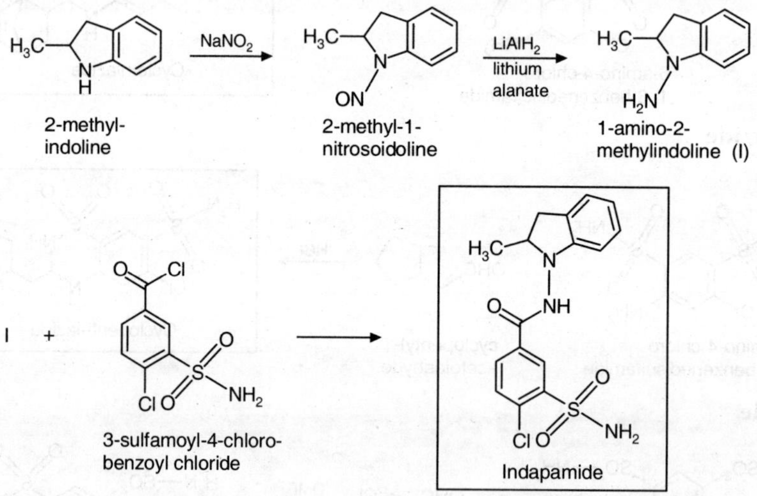

2-methyl-
indoline

2-methyl-1-
nitrosoidoline

1-amino-2-
methylindoline (I)

3-sulfamoyl-4-chloro-
benzoyl chloride

Indapamide

Furosemide

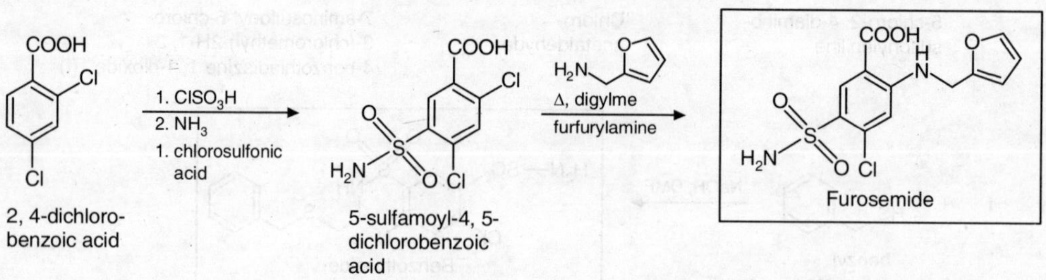

2, 4-dichloro-
benzoic acid

1. ClSO₃H
2. NH₃
1. chlorosulfonic
   acid

5-sulfamoyl-4, 5-
dichlorobenzoic
acid

Δ, digylme
furfurylamine

Furosemide

Bumetanide

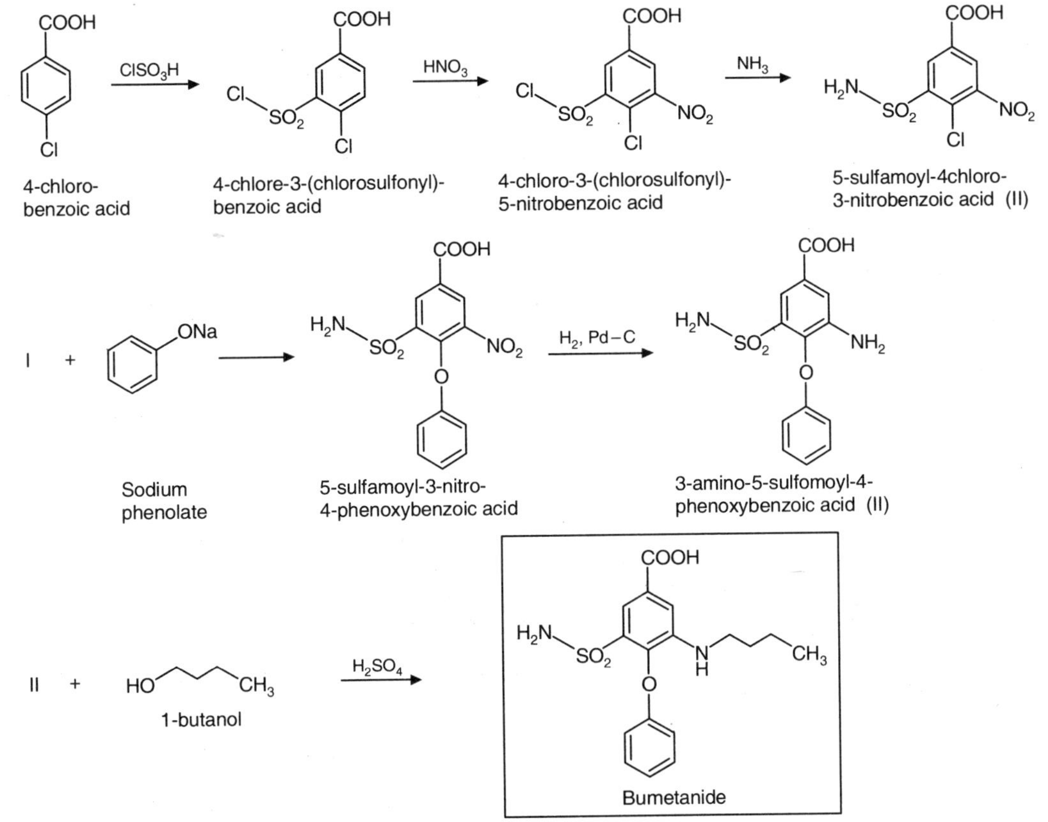
COOH
Cl
ClSO3H
Cl
SO2
HNO3
NO2
NH3
H2N
4-chloro-
benzoic acid
4-chlore-3-(chlorosulfonyl)-
benzoic acid
4-chloro-3-(chlorosulfonyl)-
5-nitrobenzoic acid
5-sulfamoyl-4chloro-
3-nitrobenzoic acid (II)
I +
ONa
H2, Pd–C
NH2
O
Sodium
phenolate
5-sulfamoyl-3-nitro-
4-phenoxybenzoic acid
3-amino-5-sulfomoyl-4-
phenoxybenzoic acid (II)
II +
HO
CH3
1-butanol
H2SO4
N
H
Bumetanide

Amiloride

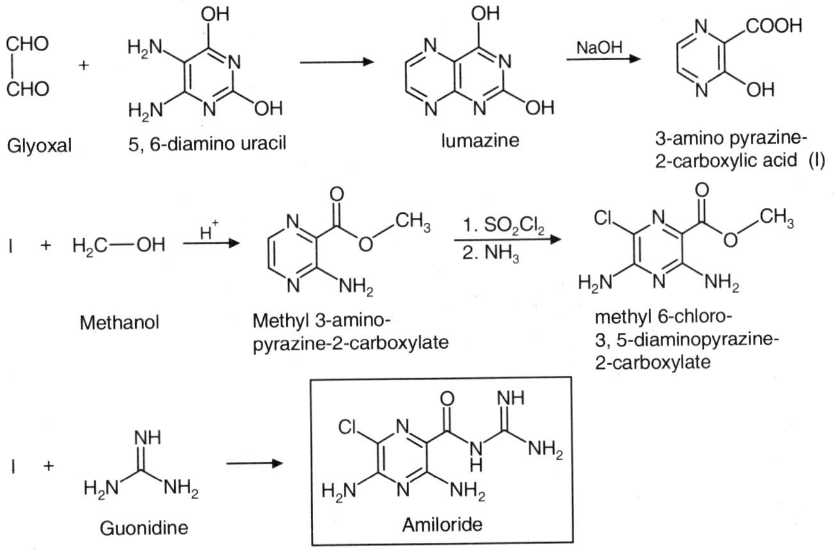
CHO
CHO
+
H2N
OH
N
Glyoxal
5, 6-diamino uracil
lumazine
NaOH
COOH
3-amino pyrazine-
2-carboxylic acid (I)
I + H2C—OH
H+
O
CH3
NH2
1. SO2Cl2
2. NH3
Cl
Methanol
Methyl 3-amino-
pyrazine-2-carboxylate
methyl 6-chloro-
3, 5-diaminopyrazine-
2-carboxylate
I +
NH
Guonidine
H
Amiloride

Triametrene

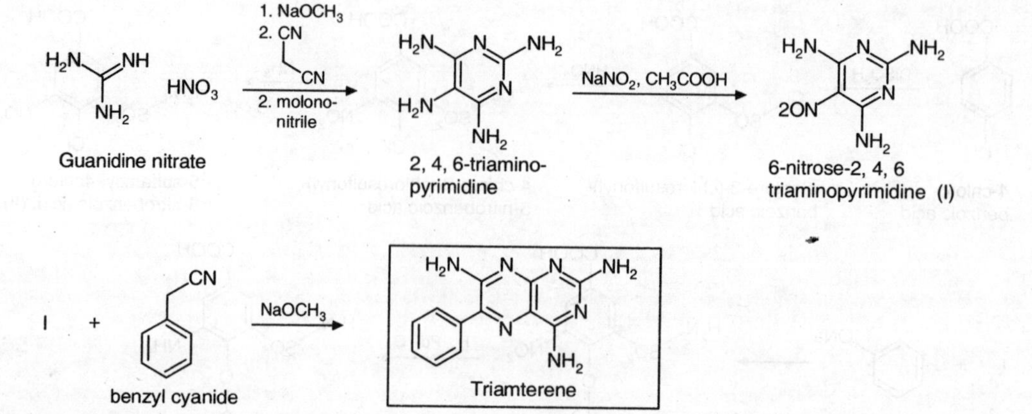

Guanidine nitrate
1. NaOCH3
2. CN CN
2. molono-nitrile
2, 4, 6-triamino-pyrimidine
NaNO2, CH3COOH
6-nitrose-2, 4, 6 triaminopyrimidine (I)
I +
benzyl cyanide
NaOCH3
Triamterene

Spironolactone

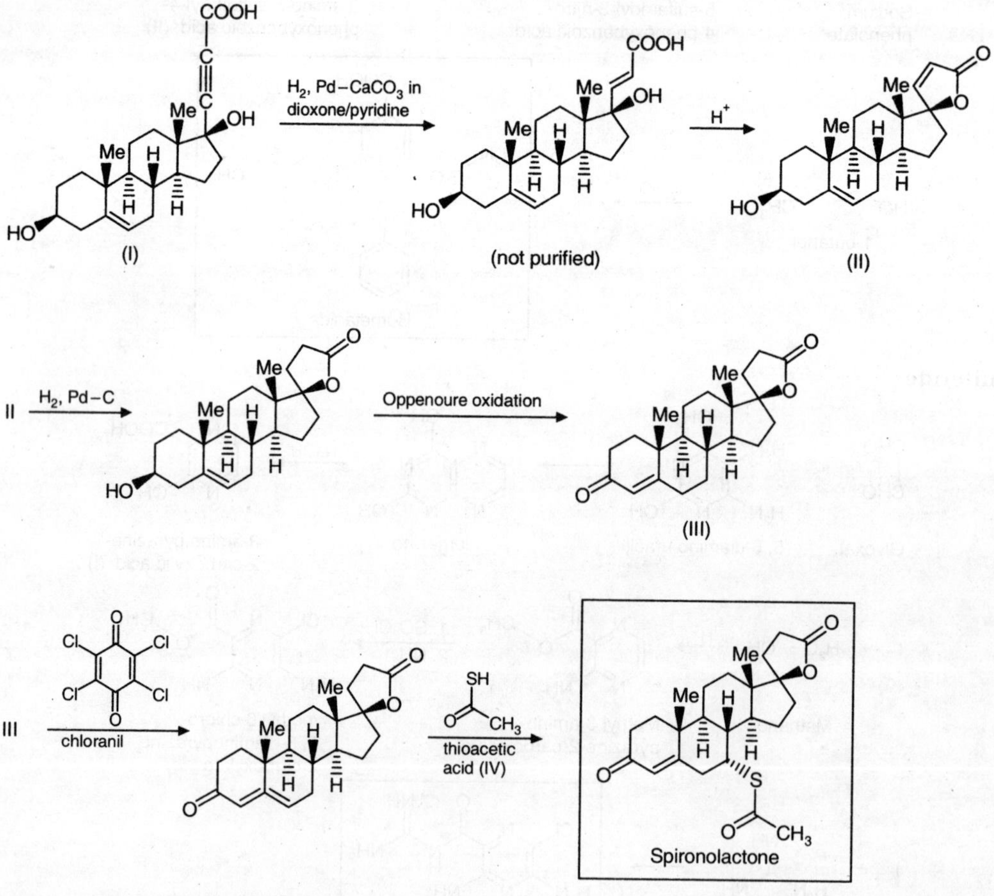

(I)
H2, Pd–CaCO3 in dioxone/pyridine
(not purified)
H+
(II)
II
H2, Pd–C
Oppenoure oxidation
(III)
III
chloranil
thioacetic acid (IV)
Spironolactone

Unit V

Drugs Acting on Blood

32

Coagulants

Blood is a transport agency which carries oxygen from the lungs and dietary elements from the gastrointestinal tract to various body tissues and drains away carbon dioxide and waste metabolic products to their respective sites of excretion, i.e. the lungs and kidneys. It also helps to maintain proper electrolyte balance and pH.

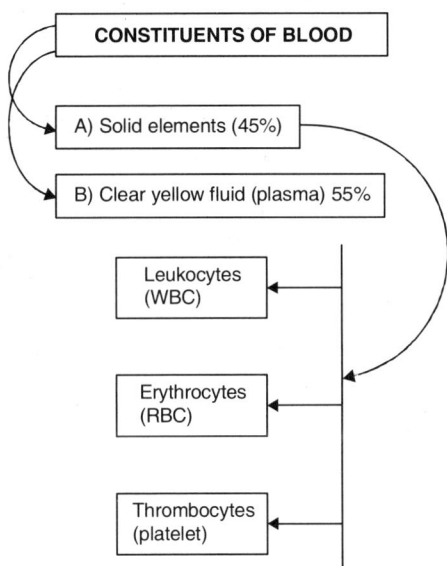

- The leukocytes and the circulating antibodies serve as the defense mechanisms and guard against infection. Red blood cells (Fig. 32.1) survive in the circulation for about 120 days. As on average, a little less than 1% of the circulating red cells are being replaced daily. The circulation is controlled by hemostatic processes mediated by central nervous system and renal mechanisms.

- Besides certain other factors, red cell formation depends upon an adequate supply of iron and certain coenzymes, vitamin B_{12} and tetrahydrofolate.

- Blood is kept fluid in the circulation by hemostatic mechanisms, which can be summarized under following heads.

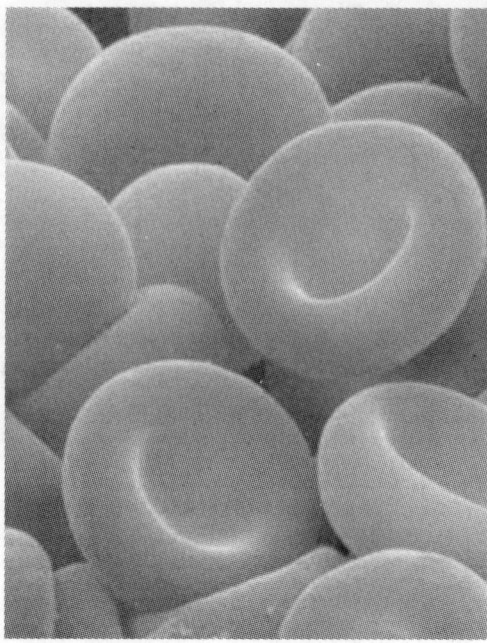

Fig. 32.1: Red blood cells

HAEMOSTATIC MECHANISM

Vascular Mechanisms

- It involves the reactions and surface properties of the blood vessels. After the vascular injury, the precapillary vessels show vasoconstriction.
- Exposure of the subendothelial collagen after injury to thrombocytes or blood platelets results into platelet adhesion. This leads to formation of blood clot through the activation of intrinsic system.

Platelet Factors

- It involves the properties of platelet adhesion. The platelets adhere to the subendothelial collagen of the injured vasculature in the presence of the von Willebrand binding factor.
- Platelets also stick to each other. The structural deformation of the platelets leads to loss of individual cell membranes and the release of the contents of platelet granules. The arrest of bleeding may be achieved through the formation of platelet plug.

Plasma Coagulation Factors

- Platelet adhesion and aggregation are stimulated by the release of ADP, thrombin and epinephrine.
- The platelet adhesion initiates the intrinsic system to cause clotting of blood via activation of Hageman factor XII to XII a.
- The production of thrombin also occurs. Each clotting factor initiates the activation of next clotting factor in the series until ultimately an insoluble fibrin clot is formed.

Fibrinolytic Mechanisms

- This mechanism helps to maintain the blood in fluid state and prevents the spread of effects of clotting elements in the body vasculature.
- During this process, the plasmin formation is initiated which then dissolves thrombi formed into the blood vessel.
- Plasmin causes the lysis of both fibrin clots and fibrin. Fibrinolysis thus can be viewed as a final stage of blood clotting.
- The first three mechanisms promote the blood clotting and prevent the blood loss. These four mechanisms operate with mutual understanding and in mutual benefit of each other with an aim to alter viscosity of blood as per the body need.

▨ PLASMA COAGULATION

- Injury initiates the blood coagulation process. The normal plasma clotting time is 12 seconds. The clot formation involves a series of complicated reactions characterized by vasoconstriction, adhesion and aggregation of platelets and formation of thick gel-like mass.
- The process involves a series of clotting factors (Table 32.1), which interact in the sequential manner that comprises many intermediate reactions.

Table 32.1: Blood clotting factors

Factor	Synonyms	Molecular weight
I	Fibrinogen	3,40,000
II	Prothrombin	68,700
III	Thromboplastin	
IV	Calcium ions	4,00,000
V	Proaccelerin	
VI	Not verified	45,000
VII	Proconvertin	1,00,000
VIII	Antihemophilia A - 1 factor	55,400
IX	Christinas factor	55,000
X	Stuart-Prower factor	1,60,000
XI	Plasma thromboplastin.	74,000
XII	Hageman factor (contact factor)	3,20,000
XIII	Fibrinoligase (fibrin stabilizing factor)	
HMW-K	High molecular weight kininogen	
Ka	Kallikrein	
PL	Platelet phospholipid	

- Except calcium, all these factors are proteins or lipoproteins and remain inactive in proenzymatic form under the resting conditions. They get readily activated by injury to the vascular endothelium.

Mechanism (Fig. 32.2)

- Normally, blood remains in its liquid form as long as it stays within its vessel. If it is drawn from the body, however, it thickenes and forms a gel. Eventually, the gel separates from the liquid. The straw-colored liquid, called serum is simply blood plasma minus the clotting proteins. The gel is called a clot. It consists of a network of insoluble protein fibers called fibrin in which the formed element of blood is trapped.

- The process of gel formation, called clotting or coagulation, is a series of chemical reaction that culminates in formation of fibrin threads. If blood clots too easily, the result can be thrombosis-clotting in an undamaged blood vessel. Clotting involves several substances known as clotting factor. These factors include several inactive enzymes that are synthesized by liver cells and released into the bloodstream, and various molecules associated with platelets or released by damaged tissues. Most clotting factors are identified by Roman numerals that indicate the order of their discovery.

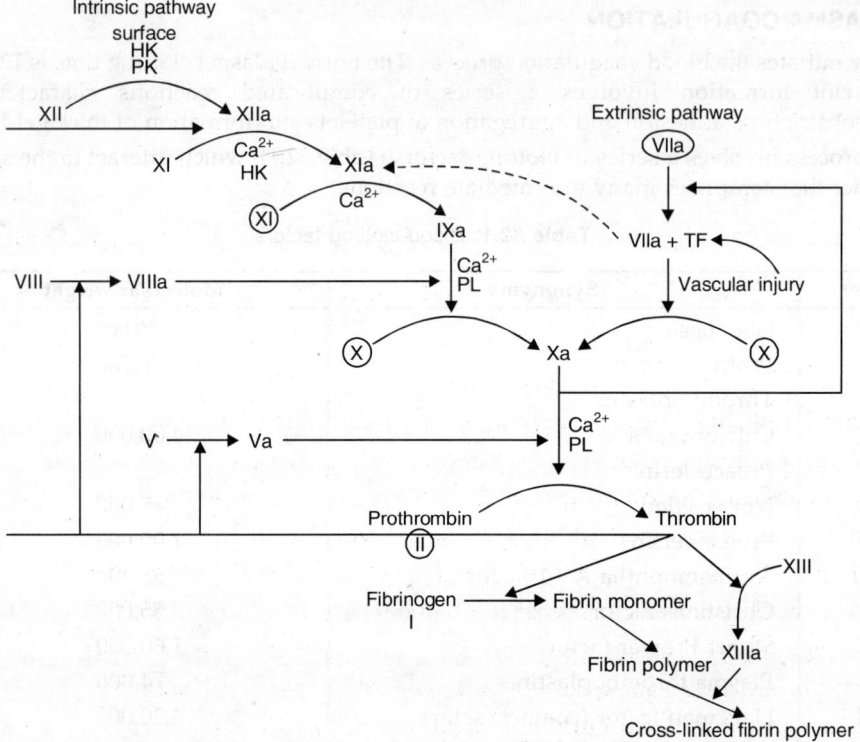

Fig. 32.2: Cascade of clotting factors and clotting mechanism

- Clotting is a complex cascade of enzymatic reaction in which each clotting factor activates many molecules of the next one in a fixed sequence. Finally, a large quantity of product is formed. Clotting can be divided into three stages.
- Two pathways, called the extrinsic pathway and the intrinsic pathway, which will be described shortly, lead to the formation of prothrombinase. Once prothrombinase is formed, the steps involved in the next two stages of clotting are the same for both the extrinsic and intrinsic pathways, and together these two stages are referred to as the common pathway.
- Proyhrombin converts prothrombin into the enzyme thrombin. Thrombin converts soluble fibrinogen into insoluble fibrin. Fibrin forms the thread of clot.

Extrinsic pathway

- The extrinsic pathway of blood clotting has fewer steps than the intrinsic pathway and occurs rapidly – within a matter of second, if trauma is severe.
- It is so named because a tissue protein called tissue factor (TF), also known as thromboplastin, leaks into the blood from cell outside blood vessels and initiates the formation of prothrombinase.
- TF is a complex mixture of lipoproteins and phospholipids released from the surface of damaged cells. In the presence of Ca^{2+}, TF begins a sequence of reaction that ultimately activates clotting factor X. Once factor X is activated, it combines with factor V in the presence of Ca^{2+} to form the active enzyme prothrombinase, completing the extrinsic pathway.

Intrinsic pathway

- The intrinsic pathway of blood clotting is more complex than the extrinsic pathway, and occurs more slowly, usually requiring several minutes. The intrinsic pathway is so named because its activators are either in direct contact with blood or contained within the blood; outside tissue damage is not needed.
- If endothelial cells become roughned or damaged, blood can come in contact with collagen fibers in the connective tissue around the endothelium of the blood vessel. In addition, trauma to endothelial cells causes damage to platelets, resulting in the release of phospholipids by the platelets. Contact with collagen fibers activates clotting factor XII, which begins a sequence of reaction that eventually activates clotting factor X.
- Platelets, phospholipids and Ca^{2+} can also participate in the activation of factor X. Once factor X is activated, it combines with factor V to form the active enzyme prothrombinase like extrinsic pathway, completing the intrinsic pathway.

Common pathway

- The formation of prothrombinase marks the bigning of the common pathway. In the second stage of blood clotting, prothrombinase and Ca^{2+} catalyze the conversion of prothrombin to thrombin. In the third stage, thrombin in the presence of Ca^{2+}, converts fibrinogen, which is soluble, to lose fibrin threads, which are insoluble.
- Thrombin also activates factor XIII, which strengthens and stabilizes the fibrin threads into a sturdy clot. Plasma contains some factor XIII, which is also released by platelets trapped in the clot.
- Thrombin has two positive feedback loops, which involves factor V; it accelerates the formation of prothrombinase. Prothrombinase, in turn, accelerates the production of more thrombi, and so on. In the second positive feedback loop, thrombin activates platelets, which reinforces their aggregation and the release of platelets.

Clot retraction

- Once a clot is formed, it plugs the ruptured area of the blood vessel and thus stops blood loss. Clot retraction is the consolidation or tightening of the fibrin clot.
- The fibrin threads attached to the damaged surface of the blood vessel gradually contract as platelets pull on them. As the clot retracts, it pulls the edges of the damaged vessel closer together, decreasing the risk of further damage.
- During retraction, some serum can escape between the fibrin threads, but the formed elements in blood cannot. Normal retraction depends on an adequate number of platelets in the clot, which release factor XIII and other factors, thereby strengthening and stabilizing the clot.

- Permanent repair of the blood vessels can then take place. In time, fibroblasts form connective tissue in the ruptured area and new endothelial cells repair the vessel lining.

Fibrinolysis

- Fibrinolysis is the last stage of blood clotting process. The process is initiated by conversion of plasminogen (profibrinolysin) into plasmin (fibrinolysin) under the influence of urokinase (fibrinokinase). Kidney is the site of production for plasminogen.

- The formation of plasmin will dissolve the insoluble fibrin clot into soluble inert peptides. These fibrin degradation products also have an ability to inhibit fibrin polymerization.

- Once the blood clotting process at the site of vascular endothelium is initiated, various coagulation factors may spread up into various body organs from the site of injury.

- Antithrombin III (hepann cofactor) is an important part of body's own natural anticoagulation machinery that localizes the fibrin clot at the site of injury and neutralizes the clotting factors at other sites of the body. Though liver is the principal site for its synthesis, antithrombin III is widely distributed in various tissues of the body. Its neutralizing effect is mainly exerted on factors Ha, IXa, Xa, XIa and XIIa.

- Its inhibitory action on blood clotting is due to its binding with thrombin (IIa). Similarly, the heparin–antithrombin III complex also inhibits plasmin and thus may be a factor in regulating fibrinolysis process.

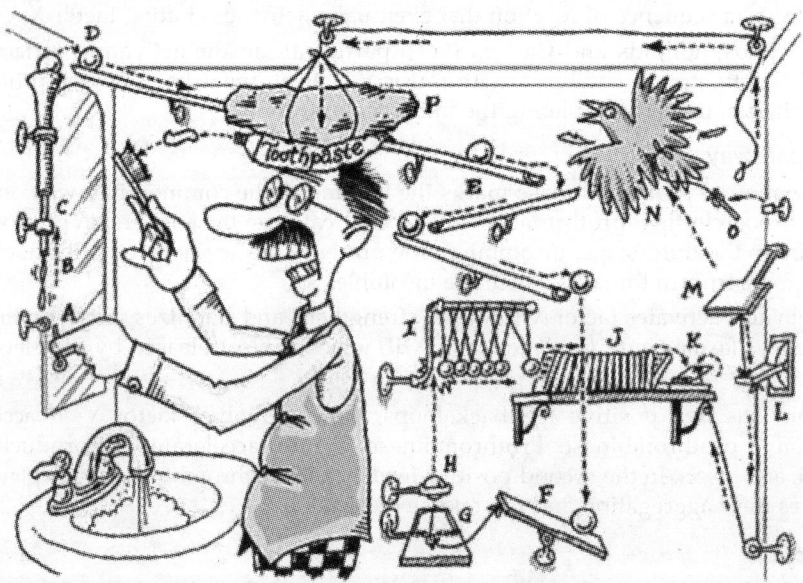

Like this, clotting mechanism might be occurring.......

▓ COAGULANTS

These are the agents which promote coagulation and are indicated in hemorrhagic states. Fresh whole blood or plasma provide all the factors needed for coagulation and are the best therapy for deficiency of any clotting factor; also they act immediately. Other drugs used to restore hemostasis are as given in flow chart 32.1.

Flow chart 32.1: Coagulants

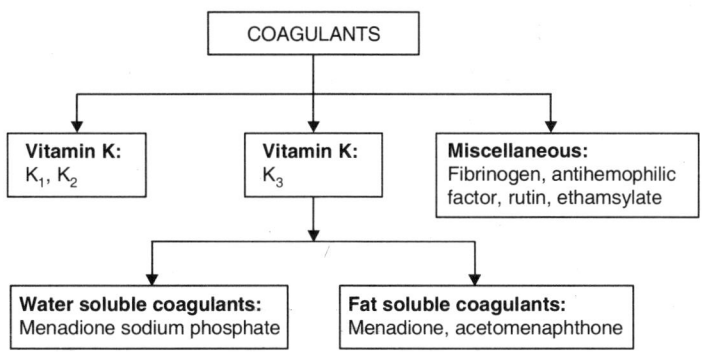

Vitamin K₁, K₂

Vitamin K₁ (Phytomenadione)

Vitamin K₂ (Menaquinones)

Vitamin K₃ (Fat soluble)

Menadione Acetomenaphthone

Vitamin K₃ (Water soluble)

Menadiol sodium diphosphate

VITAMIN K

Chemistry

- Vitamin K has a basic naphthoquinone structure, with or without side chain. The side chain in K_1 is phytyl, in K_2 prenyl, while in K_3 there is no side chain.

Action (Fig. 32.3)

- Liver is the site for the biosynthesis of various blood clotting factors like prothrombin, proconvertin, plasma thromboplastin component and the Stuart factor. These clotting factors are involved in the blood clotting phenomenon.

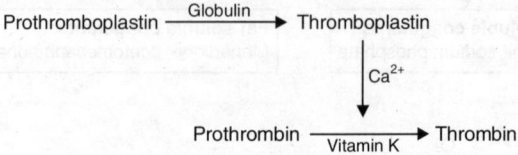

Fig. 32.3: Mode of action of vitamin K

- The above mentioned blood clotting factors remain biologically inactive in the absence of vitamin K. It is clear from the figure that in the clotting phenomenon, Ca^{2+} ions play an important role. γ – caboxyglutamyl residue within the prothrombin structure is necessary to produce strong binding sites for Ca^{2+} ions.
- Vitamin K hydroquinone is a coenzyme in the conversion of glutamyl residue of the prothrombin precursor protein to γ – caboxyglutamyl residue which participate in the complexation of necessary Ca^{2+} ions.

Toxicity

Rapid i.v. injection of emulsified vitamin K produces flushing, breathlessness, a sense of constriction in the chest, fall in BP.

MISCELLANEOUS

Fibrinogen

Mechanism of action

The fibrinogen fraction of human plasma is employed to control bleeding in hemophilia, antihemophilic globulin deficiency and acute afibrinogenemic states.

Antihemophilic Factor

It is concentrated human AHG prepared from pooled human plasma. It is indicated in hemophilia and AHG deficiency. It is highly effective in controlling bleeding episodes, but action is short lasting.

RUTIN

Mechanism of action

- It is plant glycoside claimed to reduce capillary bleeding. It has been used along with vitamin C, which is believed to facillate its action.

Ethamsylate

Mechanism of action

It reduces capillary bleeding when platelets are adequate; probably exerts antihyaluronidase action; improves capillary wall stability. It also claimed to inhibit PGI_2 production and correct abnormal platelet function, but does not stabilize fibrin.

Phytomenadione

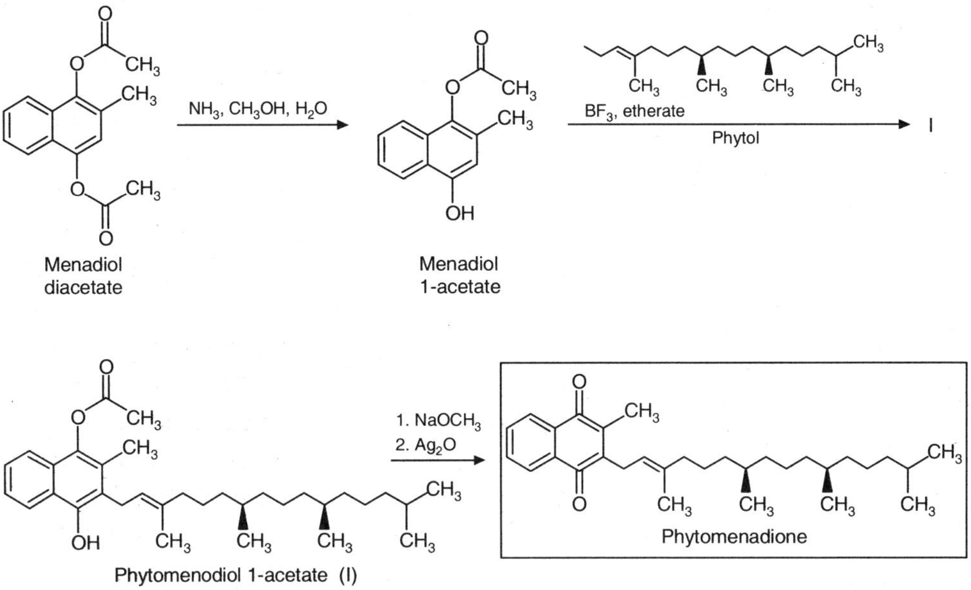

Menadiol diacetate

NH_3, CH_3OH, H_2O

Menadiol 1-acetate

BF_3, etherate

Phytol

I

Phytomenodiol 1-acetate (I)

1. $NaOCH_3$
2. Ag_2O

Phytomenadione

Menadione

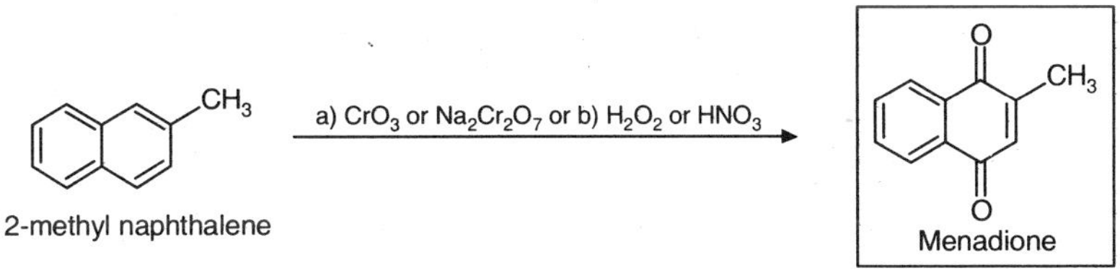

2-methyl naphthalene

a) CrO_3 or $Na_2Cr_2O_7$ or b) H_2O_2 or HNO_3

Menadione

33

Anticoagulants

Anticoagulants are agents that prolong the coagulation time of blood. Anticoagulants are usually administered to patients with cause of myocardial infarction, long-term therapy after acute myocardial infarction, prophylaxis and treatment of pulmonary and venous thrombosis.

PATHOPHYSIOLOGY

- Two distinct pathways contribute to the formation of the blood clot. When the protein factors present in the circulation provide the whole cause and completion of the clotting process, the clot is said to be effected by the intrinsic system. While, when the blood coagulation is activated by the factors which are not originated from the circulating blood (e.g. tissue thromboplastin), the clot is said to be due to the extrinsic system.

- Agents used to modify the stages of clotting process may act by:
  1. Potentiating the natural inhibitory elements of clotting process, e.g. heparin.
  2. Reducing the rate of synthesis of vitamin K dependent clotting factors, e.g. warfarin.
  3. Potentiating fibrinolytic mechanisms, e.g. streptokinase, urokinase, etc.

- Various conditions contribute to bleeding disorders. These include thrombocytopenia (i.e. low platelet count), hemophilias (i.e. genetic defect in the synthesis of clotting factors. In some cases, certain clotting factors are totally missing from the plasma of the patient), etc. These bleeding disorders may lead to the clot formation (i.e. thrombus) in the artery or vein or even in the heart chamber.

- Thromboembolism is the next stage in which reduced blood flow occurs at sites quite distinct to the point of thrombus. Myocardial infarction, peripheral arterial emboli, deep venous thrombosis and pulmonary embolization are some conditions where anticoagulant therapy is generally needed. Many compounds prevent the availability of calcium ions during coagulation process. These include soluble salts of citrate, oxalate, fluoride or EDTA. All these compounds can be used as in vitro anticoagulants.

CLASSIFICATION OF ANTICOAGULANTS

Classification of anticoagulants is given in flow chart 33.1.

Flow chart 33.1: Classification of anticoagulants

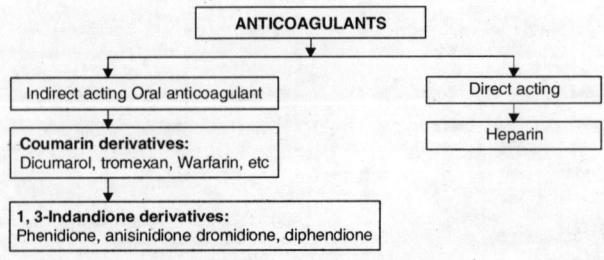

Direct Acting
Heparin

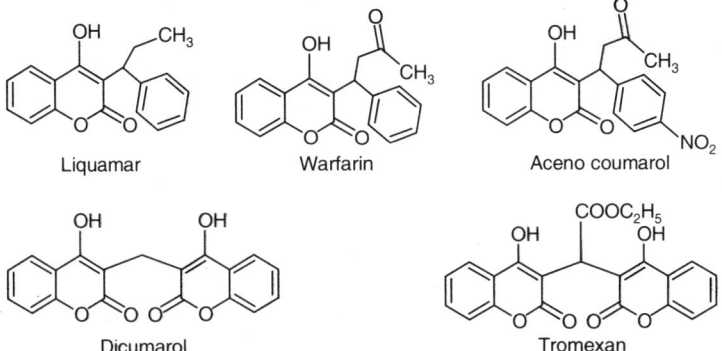

Polymeric nature of heparin

Indirect Acting
Coumarin derivatives

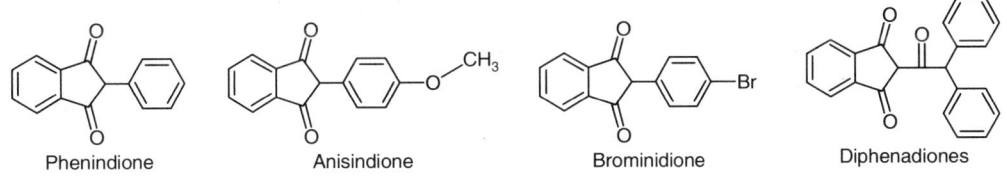

Liquamar	Warfarin	Aceno coumarol

Dicumarol   Tromexan

1,3 Indanedione derivatives

Phenindione   Anisindione   Brominidione   Diphenadiones

DIRECT ACTING

Heparin (Parenteral Anticoagulant)

Chemistry

- Heparin occurs intracellularly, especially concentrated in the basophil cells found in the circulating plasma. Its discovery was reported by Howell in 1922. It was first isolated from liver. Hence it was named as heparin. It is widely distributed in the tissues, particularly in the lungs and liver.

- Jorpes in 1937 established its chemical composition and the first clinical use of heparin was also documented in the same year. Chemically, it is a heterogeneous group of highly electronegative water soluble straight-chain mucopolysaccharides.

Polymeric nature of heparin

- It is a polymer consisting of alternate units of two disaccharides (i.e. D-glucosamine-L-iduronic acid and D-glucosamine-D-glucuronic acid) in addition to sulfuric acid. Besides this, 1 : 1 additional residues of glucuronic acid and fewer residues of N-sulfated glucosamine per heparin molecule are also reported in the structural analysis. Because of its acidic properties, heparin may also be called as heparinic acid.

- Commercially, heparin is mainly obtained from bovine lung or porcine intestinal mucosa. In most of the samples, the number of repeating disaccharide units per molecule ranges from 6 to 15. Hence its molecular weight also ranges from 8,000 to 50,000. The commercial samples of heparin may differ in their degree of polymerization and sulfation but biologically all heparins are almost equivalent. In clinical practice, heparin may be used during and after various types of surgery to reduce or to prevent intravascular clotting and thrombosis.

Mechanism of action (Fig. 33.1)

- As an anticoagulant, heparin is effective both in vivo and in vitro. After its administration, several clotting factors are neutralized by heparin and antithrombin III factor. Heparin neutralizes thromboplastin by forming an inactive complex with it.

- While in the absence of heparin, antithrombin III factor has an ability to neutralize thrombin but at quite slow speed. Heparin induces some sort of conformational changes in the antithrombin III molecule, thus making it highly active.

Thrombin + Antithrombin III $\xrightleftharpoons{\text{slow}}$ Inactive thrombin

Thrombin + Heparin + Antithrombin III $\rightleftharpoons$ Inactive thrombin

Heparin − Antithrombin III complex + Factor Xa $\rightleftharpoons$ Inactivated factor Xa complex

Fig. 33.1: Mechanism of action of heparin

- Hence in the presence of heparin, the molecule of antithrombin III can neutralize thrombin and several other clotting factors (IXa, Xa, XIa, XIIa and kallikrein) at much faster rate by forming inactive complexes with these clotting factors. Thus heparin may act as a catalyst in the neutralization of these clotting factors by antithrombin III factor.

Pharmacokinetics

- Heparin is poorly absorbed (less than 15%) from GIT after oral administration mainly because of its polyanionic character (polarity), large molecular size and its instability in the gastric juice. Since its oral or sublingual administration is not effective, it is given parenterally.

- Because of its acidic properties, it induces local trauma followed by hemotonia formation, if it is administered intramuscularly. Hence when low dose of heparin is required, it is usually administered subcutaneously or at intrafat sites. When large dose of heparin is required (as in pulmonary emboli), the intravenous route is favored.

- Heparin is significantly bound (95%) to plasma proteins. It is partially metabolized in the liver by the enzyme, heparinase. The metabolite, uroheparin has slight antithrombin like activity. The plasma half-life of heparin is estimated to be about one hour at a dose of 100 units/kg.

- However, it is dose-dependent. For example, as the dose of administered heparins increased to 400 units/kg, the plasma half-life also reaches to about 2 hours. In hepatic cirrhosis or renal dysfunctioning, the half-life of heparin becomes significantly longer. Heparin neither crosses the placental barrier nor it appears in the milk of lactating mothers.

Adverse effects

- Heparin itself is of low toxicity and is an excellent anticoagulant for short-term therapy. However, due to its commercial production from animal tissues, it may induce allergic reactions, specifically when given in high doses.

- Heparin also retains an inherent property to induce platelet aggregation. This may lead to thrombocytopenia in some patients.

- The major adverse reaction in heparin therapy is hemorrhage. The specific heparin antagonist, protamine (low molecular weight, positively charged proteins having a high affinity for the negatively charged heparin) may be used to neutralise heparin in the cases of severe hemorrhage.

- Hence heparin therapy is contraindicated in patients having intracranial hemorrhage, thrombocytopenia, severe hypertension, history of allergy or who consume large amounts of ethanol.

- Heparin is an excellent anticoagulant for short-term therapy of 10-15 days. Oral anticoagulants then can be used to extend the anticoagulant effect for desired period.

Heparin antagonists

Protamine:

- Severe hemorrhage may occur in patients receiving high dose of heparin. Protamine sulfate can be used in such cases to antagonise the effect of heparin. Protamines are strongly basic proteins of low molecular weight.

- They were isolated from the sperm or mature testes of the fish belonging to the family Salmonidase. Protamine sulfate is usually administered intravenously to neutralise heparin by forming inactive complex with it. Dyspnea may develop, if the rate of infusion of protamine is rapid. An excess of protamine sulfate has anticoagulant property.

- Heparin may be used as anticoagulant in surgical procedures and in the treatment of myocardial infarction and venous thrombin or thromboembolism.

▨ INDIRECT ACTING (ORAL ANTICOAGULANT)

Coumarin and 1,3 Indanedione Derivatives

History

- The first orally effective anticoagulant was bishydroxy-coumarin. Isolated in 1939 by Link, its structure was established in 1940. In 1941, it was used clinically as the first orally effective anticoagulant (dicoumarol). Thereafter, it has been used clinically for years in patients with a tendency thrombus formation.

- Dicoumarol itself has drawbacks as a therapeutic agent mainly due to its poor and irregular absorption. Many analogs have been prepared. They all are water insoluble and possess either 4-hydroxycoumarin nucleus (coumarin derivatives) or of indan -1, 3-dione nucleus (indandione derivatives). The latter are less preferred due to their greater toxicity.

Chemistry

- Some of these agents (e.g. phenprocoumon, warfarin) contain asymmetric carbon atom in their structure and commercially they are marketed as racemic mixtures. Usually the S (-) - isomers are more potent anticoagulants than are the R (+) isomers All these agents differ from each other in onset and duration of their anticoagulant action. Coumarins do not have in vitro activity.

- They exert in vivo effect after a period of 1–2 days. Their effects last long. Coumarins depress the synthesis of clotting factors (prothrombin, factors VII, VIII and IX) in the liver which result in the gradual decline in the concentration of clotting factors and hence a slow onset of action. Whereas the long duration of action may be due to the time taken by liver to accumulate again the enough concentration of clotting factors.

Mechanism of action (Fig. 33.1)

- Vitamin K appears to be related to the important quinone coenzymes called as ubiquinones. Since the oral anticoagulants have close structural similarity with vitamin K, they exert anticoagulant activity by acting as noncompetitive antagonists of vitamin K.

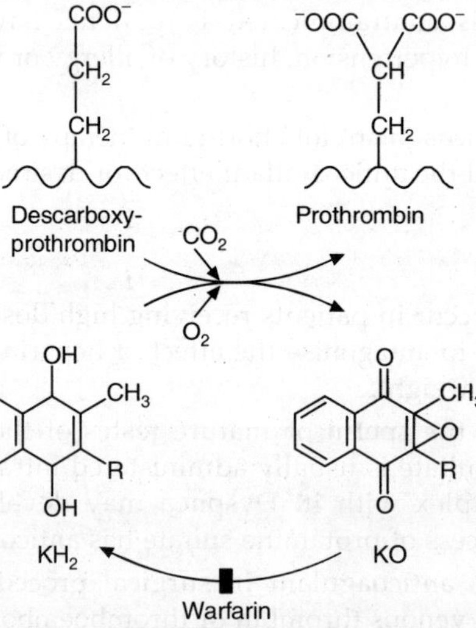

Fig. 33.1: Mechanism of action of oral anticoagulant

- The activation of prothrombin involves formation of γ-carboxyglutamic acid residues which are important for entrapment of calcium ions. Calcium ions are needed at almost every stage to activate the clotting factors. The carboxylation process of prothrombin in hepatic microsomes is catalysed by vitamin K where the vitamin gets converted to its hydroquinone form. In normal circumstances, the inactive hydroquinone form gets back converted to the active vitamin K form by NADH - NAD^+ system.

- The orally active anticoagulants inhibit the conversion of inactive vitamin K hydroquinone to the active vitamin K form. This leads to the accumulation of inactive vitamin hydroquinone and depletion of the active vitamin K form in hepatic tissues. The oral anticoagulant agents thus prevent the hepatic synthesis of the biologically active forms of the vitamin K-dependent clotting factor, mainly prothrombin and factors VII, IX and X.

- The clotting time is prolonged due to the formation of structurally incomplete clotting factors. However, the onset of therapeutic efficacy will be seen only after existing plasma concentration of prothrombin and other vitamin K-dependent clotting factors have been declined.
- The vitamin K-dependent clotting factors have plasma half-life as follows: Factor II (60 hours), VII (6 hours), IX (24 hours) and X (40 hours). Hence all these drugs show a long delay (about 3–5 days) in their onset of action. The rate of onset is independent of the size of the dose. The longer duration of their anticoagulant activity is mainly due to the long time required by the hepatic microsomal enzymes to convert coumarins into inactive hydroxylated metabolites. The mechanism of action and uses of indandione derivatives are similar to coumarins.

Pharmacokinetics

- Warfarin sodium is usually administered in the form of its racemic mixture. It is completely and rapidly absorbed from GIT. In the circulation, it is extensively bound (about 99%) to the plasma proteins. Unlike heparin, warfarin and phenindione do not have dose-dependent plasma half lives. Warfarin has the plasma half-life of about 35 days.
- The more potent levo-isomer of warfarin is metabolised (ring hydroxylation) in the liver to 7-hydroxy warfarin while the dextro-isomer is metabolized by side chain reduction to a secondary alcohol. The formation of a 6-hydroxywarfarin from both isomers is also reported. All these hydroxylated metabolites are inactive and partly undergo glucuronidation.
- They are excreted through urine and stool. Under many pathophysiological conditions, the response of a patient to oral anticoagulant therapy may be altered. For example, deficient bile secretion (decreased absorption of dietary vitamin K from GIT), oral antibiotic treatment (decreased vitamin K synthesis by the intestinal microflora), hepatic diseases (decreased rate of synthesis of clotting factors), all these conditions lead to increased response to oral anticoagulant therapy.
- However during pregnancy, the activity of some clotting factors (i.e., VII, VIII, IX and X) enhances, leading to decrease in the patient's response to oral anticoagulant therapy. Both, warfarin and dicumarol can cross placental barrier and can induce fetal and placental hemorrhage in therapeutic doses.
- Due to their slow onset of action, usually heparin is administered first and the anticoagulant effect is then maintained by oral anticoagulant drugs.

Adverse effects

- The safest and commonly used drugs are warfarin and bishydroxy coumarin. Side effects of coumarin include rash, nausea, vomiting, jaundice, leukopenia and thrombocytopenia. Minor hemorrhage during the therapy may be corrected by discontinuing the therapy.
- While in the cases of overdoses, excessive bleeding and long prothrombin time may be treated by intravenous use of vitamin K or its synthetic derivatives such as menadiol diphosphate. Prothrombin itself may be given in the form of plasma or plasma concentrates, if immediate treatment of overdoses is required.
- Untoward effects with indanedione anticoagulants include leukopenia, hepatitis, agranulocytosis and renal tubular necrosis. These drugs are less preferred than coumarins due to their greater toxicities. Their use is advocated only in patients who cannot tolerate coumarins.
- Oral anticoagulants are contraindicated in bleeding disorders, ulcers, local anesthesia, hepatic or renal diseases.

Warfarin

4-hydroxy-coumarin   benzal acetone   pyridine   Warfarin

Acenocoumarol

methyl salicylate   Acetic anhydride   methyl acetyl salicylate   NaOCH₃   4-hydroxy-coumarin (I)

4-nitro-benzalacetone   Acenocoumarol

Phenprocoumon

2-acetoxybenzoyl chloride   (1-phenylpropyl)malonic acid diethyl ester (sodium salt)   (2-acetoxybenzoyl)(1-phenyl-propyl)malonic acid diethyl ester (I)

NaOCH₃   eq. NaOH   Phenprocoumon

3, 4-dihydro-2, 4-dioxo-3-(1-phenyl-propyl)-2H-1-benzo-pyran-3-carboxylic acid ethyl ester

Diphenadione

dimethyl phthalate   1, 1-diphenyl-acetone   NaOCH₃   Diphenadione

Bromidione

Phthalide   4-bromo-benzaldehyde   NaOC₂H₅   Bromidione

Anisinidione

Phthalide   4-methoxybenzaldehyde   NaOC₂H₅   Anisinidione

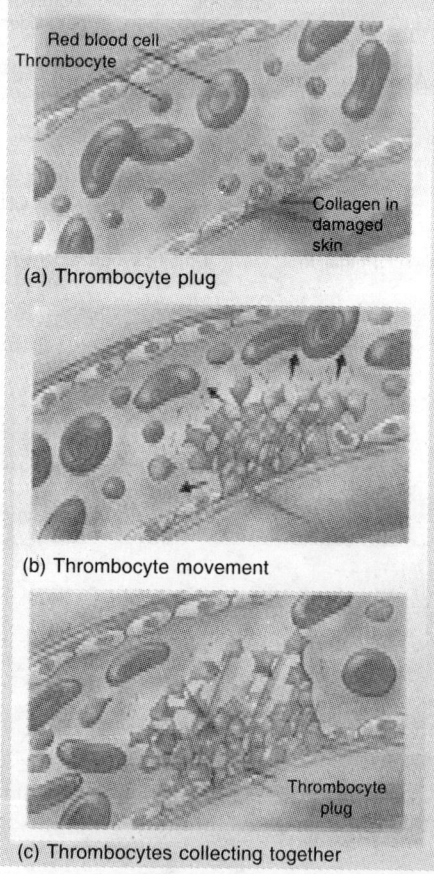

34

Antiplatelet Drugs

Thrombus is a physical occlusion of blood vessel lumen due to the formation of solid mass consisting of platelets, fibrin, red cells and white cells in the arterial or venous circulation. If part of this thrombus in the venous circulation breaks off and enters the right heart, it may be lodged in the pulmonary arterial circulation causing pulmonary embolism. This is reflected in sudden shortness of breath and dull central chest pain.

PATHOPHYSIOLOGY

- Thrombosis may increase the risk of unconsciousness. The peripheral arterial occlusion in the arterial circulation may result either in the lower limbs or in cerebral circulation. In a large deep venous thrombosis which prevents venous return, the leg may become discolored and edematous. The deep vein thrombosis is the common cause of pain, swelling and tenderness of the leg.

- The blood platelets play an important etiological role in the pathogenesis of atherosclerosis, thrombosis, thromboembolism and stroke. The reactivity of platelets, the activity of leukocytes, the coagulation of blood and regulation of blood vessel tone and permeability are in turn governed by the vascular endothelium.

- These functions are mediated by the release of certain bioactive substances by the endothelial cell which include prostacyclin, nitric oxide, platelet activating factor, plasminogen activator, endothelium derived hyperpolarizing factor, and endothelium derived contracting factor and also enzymes that can activate or degrade vasoactive hormones.

- Platelets bind to the collagen in the vessel wall and promote other platelets to adhere. The process is stimulated by ADP released by the already adhered platelets. Arachidonic acid, thrombin and collagen are the other inducers. Collagen is the fibrous protein of connective tissue and the most abundant protein in the human body.

(a) Thrombocyte plug

(b) Thrombocyte movement

(c) Thrombocytes collecting together

Fig. 34.1: Role of platelets in thrombus formation

454

- Collagen is involved in platelet adhesion, activation and homeostasis. It occurs in a variety of forms where type III collagen is more potent stimulant of platelet aggregation than other types. Platelets thus play a critical role in the recognition of vascular injury, formation of effective hemostatic plugs, retraction of clots and wound healing.
- Collagen when binds on the surface of the platelet membrane, induces the changes in the activities of platelet membrane cyclic nucleotides. These changes in turn phosphorylation of certain platelet component proteins which may then trigger the release reaction and culminate in aggregation. The platelet aggregation occurs in following steps.
  1. The initial adhesion of platelets to collagen.
  2. The release of the contents of platelets like ADP, Ca^{2+} serotonin.
  3. The subsequent formation of platelet aggregates under the mediation of released ADP and Ca^{2+}. The release of adenosine diphosphate (ADP) from platelet under release reaction may be mediate.
- It is proposed that the free amino groups of lysine and arginine residues of collagen are critical for the platelet aggregation activity of collagen and the carboxy groups are less important. The platelet activation inhibitory drugs exert their effects by blocking different activation signaling mechanism.
- Inhibitors of platelet activation are also termed as antiplatelet drugs or antithrombotic drugs. The category includes all such compounds that prevent adhesion, aggregation and secretion of platelets.

CLASSIFICATION OF ANTIPLATELET AGENTS

Classification of antiplatelet agents is give in Flow chart 34.1.

Flow chart 34.1: Classification of antiplatelet agents

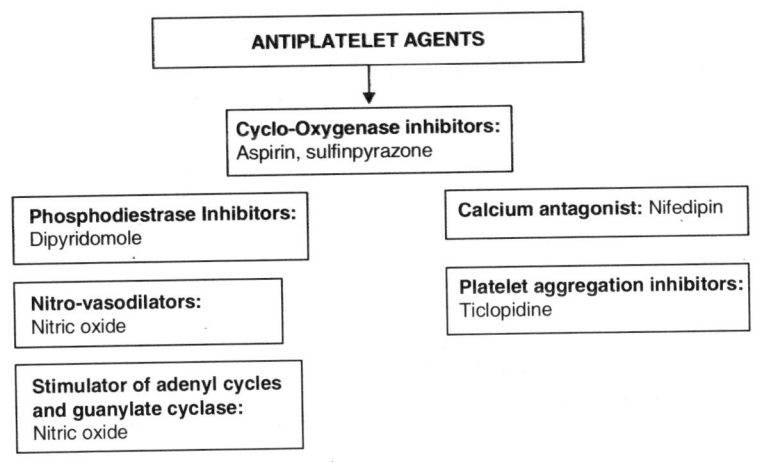

Inhibitors of arachidonic acid metabolism

Aspirin

Platelet aggregation inhibitors

Ticlopidine

Phosphodiestrase inhibitors

Dipyridamole

COX INHIBITORS

Aspirin

Mechanism of action

- Aspirin and other NSAIDs act as antiplatelet drugs by irreversibly inhibiting platelet aggregation by acylating cyclo-oxygenase, a platelet enzyme.
- This in turn, inhibits the synthesis of thromboxane A_2, a powerful vasoconstrictor and inducer of the platelet release reaction and platelet aggregation.

Uses

- Aspirin is the most commonly used antiplatelet drug. It appears to increase survival after myocardial infarction, to prevent reinfarction, to prevent transient cerebral ischemia and to decrease the incidence of stokes.
- It has also proved effective in maintaining potency of bypass grafts.

Sulfinpyrazone

Mechanism of action

It inhibits platelet cyclo-oxygenase in competitive and reversible manner.

Uses

The compound has been reported to reduce the incidence of transient ischemic attacks. Unlike aspirin, sulfinpyrazone neither prolongs bleeding time nor affects platelet aggregation in normal persons and is effective.

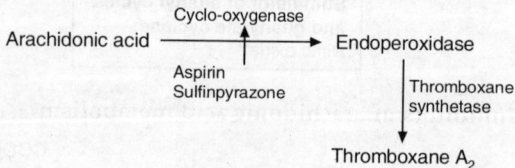

Fig. 34.2: Mechanism of action of sulfinpyrazone and aspirin

PHOSPHODIESTRASE INHIBITORS

Dipyridamole

Mechanism of action

- Dipyridamole effectively inhibits platelet activation. One mechanism is inhibition of platelet phosphodiesterase. Inhibition of this enzyme, coupled with enhancement of adenylcyclase activity by endogenous prostacyclin, increases platelet cyclic AMP and decreases activation.
- Dipyridamole also blocks uptake of adenosine, which acts at A_2 receptors for adenosine to stimulate platelet adenyl cyclase. The drug is effective in combination with aspirin and warfarin.

Uses

It is currently recommended for maintenance of prosthetic heart valves and vascular grafts. It is useful in transient ischemic attacks and secondary prevention of myocardial infarction.

PLATELET AGGREGATION INHIBITORS

Ticlopidine

Mechanism of action (Fig. 34.3)

Ticlopidine acts by inhibition of adenosine diphosphate-induced platelet aggregation, although suppression of PAF and thromboxane A_2 and activation of adenyl cyclase may play a contributing role.

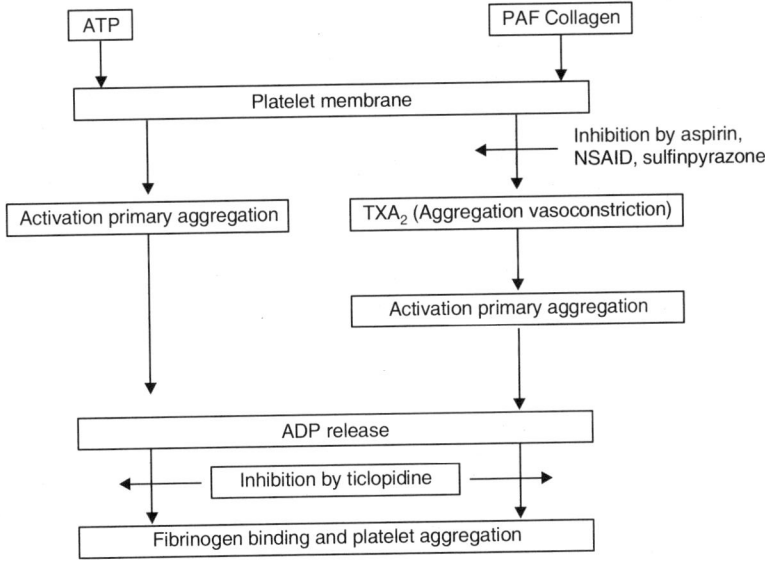

Fig. 34.3: Mechanism of ticlopidine action

Uses

It is indicated in cerebrovascular disease such as transient ischemic attacks, reversible ischemic neurological defects, stroke, coronary disease such as unstable angina, coronary artery bypass-grafts, secondary prevention of myocardial infarction and diabetic neuropathy.

■ NITROVASODILATORS

Nitric Oxide

Mechanism of action (Fig. 34.3)

Nitrovasodilators as a class seem to exert their effect by producing nitric oxide, a potent stimulator of guanylate cyclase. This enzyme is found in soluble form in platelets and is stimulated by carbon monoxide, hydroxyl radicals and nitric oxide. Nitric oxide synthatase is present in a variety of cells including macrophages, neutrophils, endothelial cells and platelets. This enzyme uses L-asparginase as substance and generates nitric oxide and L-citrulin as metabolites.

Aspirin

Salicylic acid   Acetic anhydride   Aspirin

Sulfinpyrazone

Diethyl 2-phenyl-thioethylmalonate   hydrazobenzene   (I)

Sulfinpyrazone

Ticlopidine

4, 5, 6, 7-tetrahydro-thieno-[3, 2-c] pyridine   2-chlorobenzyl chloride (I)   Ticlopidine

Dipyridamole

Urea (I) + Ethyl acetoacetate (II) → 2, 4-dihydroxy-6-methylpyrimidine

HNO₃ → 5-nitroorotic acid (III)

Thiourea + II → 4-hydroxy-2-mercapto-6-methylpyrimidine

HNO₃ → III

SnCl₂ or Na₂S₂O₄ or H₂/Pd–C → IV

5-aminoorotic acid (IV)

I or KOCN potassium cyanate → 2, 4, 6, 8-tetra-hydroxypyrimido-[5, 4-d] pyrimidine

POCl₃, PCl₅ → 2, 4, 6, 8-tetra-chloropyrimido-[5, 5-d] pyrimidine (V)

V + Piperidine → 2, 6-dichloro-4, 8-dipiperidinopyri-mido[5, 4-d] pyrimidine

diethanolamine → Dipyridamole

35

Hematinics

These are the agents required in the formation of the blood and are used for the treatment of anemias.

Anemia occurs when the balance between production and destruction of RBCs is disturbed by:

1. Blood loss (acute chronic).
2. Impaired red cell formation due to deficiency of essential factors, i.e. iron, vitamin B_{12}, folic acid, bone marrow depression, erythropoietin.
3. Increased destruction of RBCs.

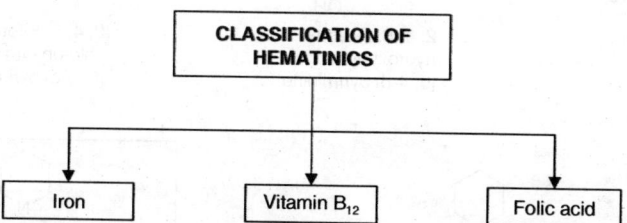

IRON

History

- The first evidence about the presence of iron in the blood was reported in 1713 by Lemery. Nearly 1.1 mg of iron is present per millimeter of the red blood cells. In the food, iron is mainly present in the form of organic ferrous or ferric complexes.

- Due to the digestive action of gastric acid and alkaline environment of small intestine, the dietary iron is then converted to ferrous hydroxide. A carrier intracellular protein known as apoferritin is present in the mucosal cells of small intestine that transports the dietary iron into the portal circulation.

- Certain factors like vitamin C, fats, and meals promote the absorption of iron. In the circulation, iron in the ferrous form gets converted to ferric form which is important for attachment with transferin, a glycoprotein plasma carrier for iron. Laurell in 1947 identified and named it as transferrin.

- It has a molecular weight of about 76,000. The serum iron is present only in the form of transferrin–iron complex which is then taken up to various intracellular sites by receptor-mediated endocytosis. The iron then mobilizes into the cell while transferrin returns back to pick up other ferric ions.

Physiology

- The oxygen carrying capacity of the blood is due to the presence of erythrocytes or red blood cells that contain hemoglobin. Each erythrocyte, on an average, contains 280 million molecules of hemoglobin, thus normal human blood contains about 15 g of hemoglobin per 100 ml of blood. It is synthesized in the erythrocyte precursor cells of bone marrow.

- Structurally, it is a conjugated protein consisting of the globin (protein fraction) and four nonprotein iron-containing fragments known as heme.

- In the lungs, oxygen reacts with these pigments to give oxyhemoglobin that exchanges free oxygen for carbon dioxide at the tissue level and get converted to carbaminohemoglobin. It is the form in which, carbon dioxide is transported to the lungs for excretion resulting into regeneration of hemoglobin.

- Red bone marrow of cranium, ribs, sternum, and proximal epiphyses of humerus and femur are the sites for production of RBCs. Red blood cells survive in the circulation for about 120 days after which they are catabolized by the reticuloendothelium.

- On an average, a little less than 1% of the circulating red cells are replaced daily as the part of hemostatic processes mediated through central nervous system and renal mechanisms.

- The metabolic products of worn out RBCs include iron (which later associates with a protein to form hemosiderin), bilirubin pigment and globin. In bone marrow, the iron from hemosiderin is reutilised to produce new RBCs. Bilirubin is passed into the bile while globin is defragmented by the liver to yield amino acids which are then utilized into biochemical reactions.

- One molecule of hemoglobin contains four atoms of iron. The total body content of iron is about 50 mg/kg for male and 37 mg/kg for female. Out of this, about 60% is utilized for hemoglobin formation. 20% is present in the iron stores (mainly in the form of ferritin, hemosiderin and transferrin.

- Ferritin is a complex of ferric ions with a protein, apoferritin found mostly in the liver, spleen and bone marrow and remaining 20% is present in myoglobin, cytochrome, catalyase and other iron containing enzymes (i.e. hemenzymes). Hence iron deficiency may lead to;

  1. Hypochromic (iron deficient) anemia.
  2. Disturbances in muscle metabolism.
  3. Slow-down of the activities of hemenzymes.
  4. Abnormalities in catecholamine metabolism and heat production.

Pharmacokinetics

- The recommended daily intake of iron is estimated to be 12 mg. However, only 1–15 mg of iron is usually absorbed from dietary elements in humans. The major fraction of the absorbed iron is made available for the formation of hemoglobin in the marrow or extramedullary hemopoietic tissues.

- In normal man, iron is usually excreted out in the form of extravasated red cells, exfoliated iron-containing mucosal cells of the skin and GIT, bile, loss of hair and nails in the urine. Women are more susceptible to iron deficiency than men due to extra iron loss during menstruation, pregnancy and lactation.

- Approximately 20 – 40 mg of iron is lost during each menstrual cycle in addition to other normal losses. In pregnancy and lactation, nearly 15 mg per day of iron may be needed.

Role of Iron

- Iron is an important constituent of hemoglobin and thus it is required for erythropoiesis (poiesis = to make). Iron deficiency or iron loss may therefore result into a decrease in hemoglobin synthesis. Various conditions may give rise to iron deficient erythropoiesis.

- These include nutritional iron deficiency, blood loss, inadequate absorption or its improper utilization. Beside this, nutritional deficiencies of copper, cobalt, folic acid, vitamin C and vitamin B_{12} also contribute for inferior erythropoiesis.

- This leads to the development of anemic conditions. Anemia occurs when the hemoglobin concentration of the blood is decreased below normal levels. Various forms of anemia are recognized. For example, cell hypo-proliferation leads to aplastic anemia; excessive destruction of red blood cells leads to hemolytic anemia while iron-deficient anemia and megaloblastic anemia may result due to abnormalities in the maturation process of red blood cells.

- Increased demands for hemoglobin are registered during growth, menstruation and pregnancy. If they are not fulfilled, anemia is likely to result.

Iron Deficient Anemia

- In iron-deficient anemia, symptoms include, fatigue, weakness, loss of appetite, breathlessness, difficulty in swallowing and inflammation of mouth. The only important use of iron in modern medicine today is in the treatment of iron-deficient anemia.

- Beside anemia, the deficiency of iron may also lead to decrease in the activity of iron-containing enzymes, abnormalities in the biochemical processes (where iron serves as the cofactor) and disturbed nucleic acid synthesis.

Preparation and Doses

Various iron salts are used in the treatment of anemia. The most commonly used are, ferrous sulfate, ferrous fumarate, ferrous succinate, ferrous gluconate, ferrous lactate and ferric ammonium citrate.

Oral preparation

Ferrous salts: Ferrous salts are more rapidly absorbed than ferric salts, if given orally. Ferrous sulfate is the most favoured iron salt due to its low cost. These iron salts are usually administered in the fasting state in order to enhance absorption. However, these preparations when given orally usually induce gastrointestinal disturbances.

Adverse effect: The common adverse effects of oral therapy include nausea, vomiting, abdominal pain, diarrhoea and heart-burn. Staining of teeth in young children and Hack stools may be observed.

Parenteral preparation

- If patient does not tolerate oral administration of iron, it may be given intramuscularly or intravenously. The intramuscular iron preparations include, iron-sorbitex injection, ferric ammonium citrate, ferrous gluconate, iron adenylate, iron polyisomaltose, etc. The oral iron preparations take their own time in saturation of body's iron store. Beside this maximally 40–60 mg of iron per day can be supplied to erythroid marrow by the oral therapy. These drawbacks are overcome by the parenteral administration of iron.

- Several forms of iron-dextran complexes are in use for intravenous administration. This route has an advantage over intramuscular route in that, it neither allows deposition of iron in muscle nor it induces local discoloration of the skin at the site of injection. Iron–dextran injection (imferon) contains ferric hydroxide complexed with partially hydrolyzed dextran of low molecular weight ranging from 5000 to 7000 daltons in a colloidal solution form. Each ml contains the equivalent of 50 mg element iron and may be given either by intramuscular or intravenous route. In circulation, iron gets dissociated, from the sugar part of the dextran and is made available to the body tissues.
- Yet another iron-sorbitex injection (jectofer) is available for intramuscular iron therapy. It is a solution of complex of iron, sorbitol and citric acid stabilized with dextrin and excess of sorbitol. It contains an equivalent of 50 mg iron per ml.

Adverse effect:
- The usual adverse effects of parenteral iron therapy include headache, fever, urticaria and rheumatoid arthritis.
- The systemic toxicities due to overdose include anaphylactic reaction, dizziness and tachycardia. In severe cases, cyanosis and circulatory collapse may occur which is followed by death.

Iron Poisoning

- The toxicities due to iron overdoses may be treated by gastric levage with sodium bicarbonate or phosphate solution.
- Milk and egg neutralise excess of iron by forming protein complexes with iron. Deferoxamine may be given, if plasma iron concentration is quite high.

▒ HEMOPOIETIC VITAMINS

Folic Acid and Cobalamin

- Folic acid and cyanocobalamin (vitamin B_{12}) collectively are called as hemopoietic vitamins because these vitamins are involved in the formation of red blood cells. Their deficiency may cut short the lifespan of these cells and may lead to ineffective erythropoiesis. Other signs include constipation, anorexia, weight loss, atrophic glossitis and elevation of serum bilirubin.

Cobalamin

- Before folic acid can function, it must be reduced to 5, 6, 7, 8-tetrahydrofolate. The reducing agent is NADPH and the enzyme dihydrofolate reductase catalyses this conversion. Vitamin B_{12} cofactors participate in the regeneration of tetrahydrofolate from methyl tetrahydrofolate. The folates are also involved in gluconeogenesis.

Pernicious Anemia

- Well-marked neurological symptoms (i.e. peripheral neuritis, atrophy of optic nerves, mental deterioration and degeneration of spinal cord) are often associated with pernicious anemia. Both these vitamins are used to cure pernicious anemia.

- Although vitamin B_{12} does not cure the anemia caused by folic acid deficiency, folic acid does relieve some of the symptoms of anemia caused by vitamin B_{12} deficiency. However, folic acid does not prevent the development of neurological changes seen in pernicious anemia.

- A possible explanation may be that folic acid is the essential factor (required for the proper development of erythrocytes) and cobalamin is a cofactor, which is needed to maintain normal nervous functioning.

Megaloblastic Anemia

- Megaloblastic or macrocytic anemia may result due to the dietary deficiency of cobalamins or folates. This results due to the abnormality in the erythrocyte maturation process.

- They are decreased in number but increased in the size resulting in overall deficiency of hemoglobin. Beside this polymorphonuclear leukocytes and giant platelets are also formed due to altered synthesis of genetic material.

- Morphological changes are also reported to occur in mucosal layer of mouth, stomach, intestine and vagina. Cobalamins are also necessary for proper functioning of the central nervous system.

Unit VI

Drugs Affecting the Endocrine System

36

Insulin

The ancient Greek and Roman physicians used the term 'Diabetes' to mean large urine volume. The adjective 'mellitus', a Latin word (meaning honey), was added in 1674 by Thomas Willis. The large urine volume is due to the large amounts of glucose and urea in the urine (osmotic diuresis).

- Early references in Ayurveda to this disease had also been reported. Charaka referred to diabetes as a 'diseased flow of urine' and mentioned that ants are attracted by urine of a person affected with this disease.

- Von Mering and Minkowski were first to link the functioning of pancreas with the onset of this disease. In 1889, they induced similar diabetic symptoms in dogs by pancreatectomized them implicating the lack of a pancreatic hormone in the etiology of the disease.

- It is now agreed that diabetes is characterized by a deficiency of effective insulin which is a pancreatic hormone. Banting and Best through a simple experiment on pancreatic duct ligated dog demonstrated the role of insulin in diabetes. It was on the midnight of July 30, 1921 that they injected a pancreatic extract to a depancreatised diabetic dog on the verge of coma. Urine sugar abolished and blood sugar came down to normal after one hour. Insulin was thus born.

DIABETES

The normal blood glucose level in humans ranges between 70–90 mg per 100 ml. Hyperglycemia is characterized by more than normal concentration of the blood sugar and hypoglycemia develops when the blood sugar level falls below the normal range. Diabetes mellitus is the condition arising due to abnormal metabolism of carbohydrates, fats and proteins. It is characterised mainly by an unusually high sugar level in the blood (hyperglycemia) and the presence of sugar in the urine (glucosuria).

Symptoms (Fig. 36.1)

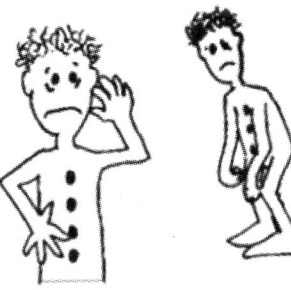 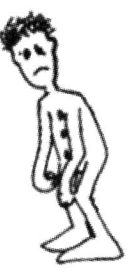 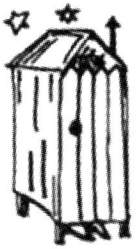 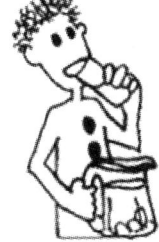

Feeling unwell   Feeling tired   Passing more urine   Thirst

Fig. 36.1: Symptoms of diabetes

1. These include, hyperglycemia, hyperlipemia, glucosuria, polyuria (loss of water and salts), polydipsia (increase in thirst), polyphagia (excessive hunger), ketonemia (ketone bodies and fatty acids in the blood), ketonuria (ketone bodies in the urine), azoturia (increased production and excretion of urea and ammonia), poor wound healing and infection.

2. Sometimes the disease eventually causes serious complications like, kidney damage, retina degeneration, premature atherosclerosis, cataract, heart disease, neurological dysfunction and a predisposition to gangrene (Figs. 36.2 and 36.6).

Etiology

- The etiology of the disease involves a complex interplay of endocrinal, immunological, infectious and genetic factors.

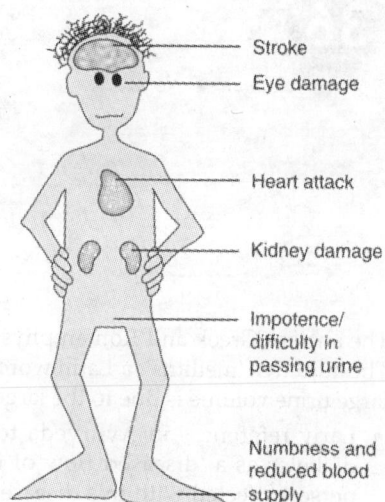

Fig. 36.2: Possible complication associated with diabetes

- Functioning of the pancreas with the onset of diabetes was linked first by Von Mering and Minkowski in 1889. They induced similar diabetic symptoms in pancreatectomized dogs thus implicating the lack of a pancreatic hormone in the etiology of the disease.

- Deficiency of effective insulin, a pancreatic hormone, is well characterized in diabetes. Through a simple but intellectual experiment on pancreatic duct ligated dog, Banting and Best demonstrated the role of insulin in diabetes. They injected a pancreatic extract to a depancreatised diabetic dog on the verge of coma; urine sugar abolished and blood sugar came down to normal after one hour. Insulin was thus born.

- Not only the deficiency of insulin but also the disturbances in the level of certain other substances like adrenaline, pituitary hormones, corticosteroids, aldosterone, oestrogen, thyroid hormones and glucagon can cause diabetes. All these bioactive substances exert their own influence on the blood-sugar level. Determination of glucose tolerance curve is the most useful pathological test for diabetes.

- Diabetes could be caused not only by a deficiency of insulin but also by disturbances in the level of certain other substances like, adrenaline, pituitary hormones, corticosteroids, aldosterone, estrogen, thyroid hormones and glucagon. All these bioactive substances exert their

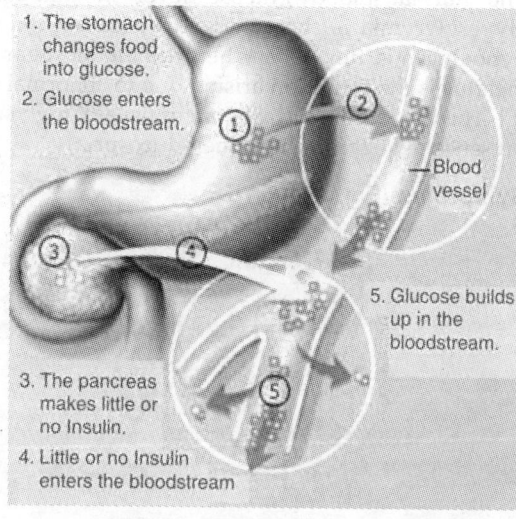

Fig. 36.3: Role of insulin in glucose transport

own influence on blood sugar level. Determination of glucose tolerance curve is the most useful pathological test for diabetes.

PANCREAS (FIG. 36.4)

- In human, pancreas (the organ lying behind the upper intestine) contains about a million islets of Langerhans, which constitute, about 1–2% of the pancreatic tissue. The cells from these islets can be categorised as:

  1. α cells which are mainly present in the outer cortex and represent about 25% of the islet cells. They secrete glucagon.
  2. α cells which are concentrated mainly in the medulla and constitute about 60% of the islet population. Insulin is secreted by these cells.
  3. D cells or δ cells are involved in the secretion of somatostatin which inhibits the release of both, glucagon and insulin.
  4. PP or F cells are responsible for the release of pancreatic polypeptide. Thus glucagon (a - cells), insulin (P cells) and somatostatin along with gastrin (D cells) are the principal hormones secreted and released by the islets.

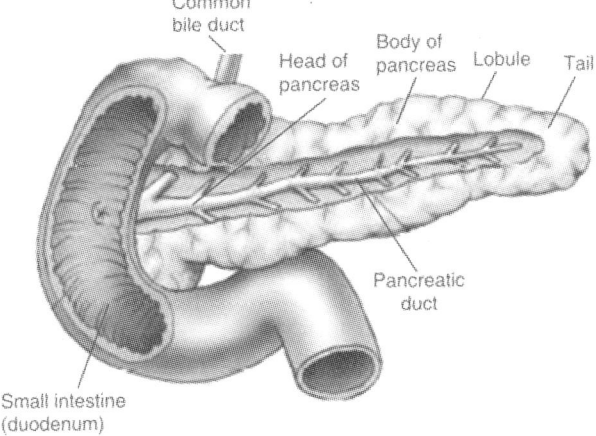

Fig. 36.4: Pancreatic gland

- Proteolytic destruction of insulin by the digestive enzymes of pancreas during the course of extraction has been reported. Insulin may be regarded principally as a hormone of anabolism while glucagon as a hormone of catabolism.
- That is to say, insulin will pull out the excess of blood sugar under the glucostatic function of the liver where excess glucose is converted to glycogen.
- Similarly when glucagon secretion is more (as in the fasting state), the body's energy needs are fulfilled by promoting conversion of glycogen to glucose in the liver and thus increasing the blood sugar concentration.
- Pancreatic somatostatin can inhibit the secretion of both insulin and glucagon. It may be having its role in maintaining the proper ratio of insulin to glucagon.
- Thus, it is not the absolute blood level of insulin but, the insulin-glucagon molar ratio (I/G) in the blood that determines the blood sugar level. It means in diabetes, the I/G molar ratio

is disturbed instead of insulin secretion alone. Nowadays glucometers are available to check the blood glucose level (Fig. 36.5).

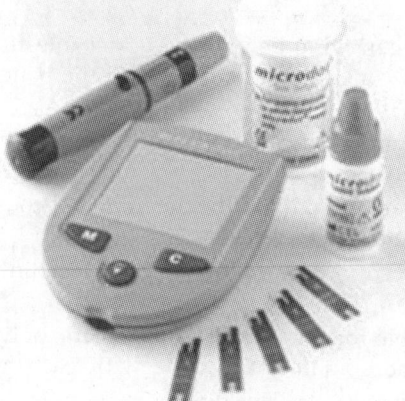

Fig. 36.5: Glucometer

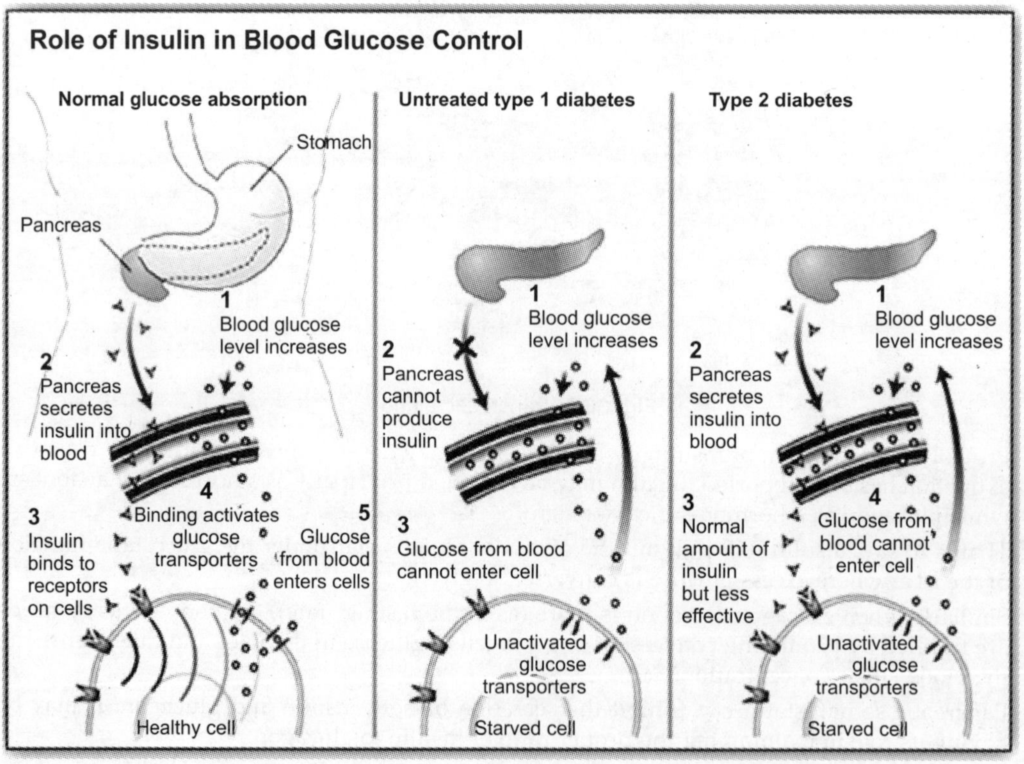

Role of Insulin in Blood Glucose Control

Normal glucose absorption

Stomach

Pancreas

1 Blood glucose level increases

2 Pancreas secretes insulin into blood

3 Insulin binds to receptors on cells

4 Binding activates glucose transporters

5 Glucose from blood enters cells

Healthy cell

Untreated type 1 diabetes

1 Blood glucose level increases

2 Pancreas cannot produce insulin

3 Glucose from blood cannot enter cell

Unactivated glucose transporters

Starved cell

Type 2 diabetes

1 Blood glucose level increases

2 Pancreas secretes insulin into blood

3 Normal amount of insulin but less effective

4 Glucose from blood cannot enter cell

Unactivated glucose transporters

Starved cell

Fig. 36.6: Role of insulin and diabetes

EFFECTS OF DIABETES ON METABOLISM

Effect on Glucose Metabolism

- As a result, the blood sugar concentration increases which leads to higher rate of excretion of glucose through the urine along with large amounts of water (osmosis diuresis).
- Due to the disturbed I/G ratio, the insulin dependent entry of glucose into the muscles and other peripheral tissues get paralyzed. Hence to meet the energy demands for their normal metabolic activities, these tissues utilize the deposited fat as a source of energy.

Effect on Lipid Metabolism

- The increased mobilization of fat (lipolysis) from the peripheral fat depots leads to increased formation of ketone bodies (ketosis). Proteineous material also undergoes metabolism, releasing nitrogenous waste products.
- Since some of the ketone bodies are organic acids, acidosis (ketoacidosis) develops due partly to the loss of Na^+ and K^+ ions with ketone bodies in the form of their salts in the urine. If the condition does not receive attention, the chronic loss of water and electrolytes coupled with accumulation of HT^1 ions can lead to diabetic acidosis and coma.

Effect on Protein Metabolism

Insulin stimulates the transport of certain amino acids into tissue and favour the protein synthesis. In absence of insulin, this process is get affected.

In short:

1. Conversion of liver glycogen to glucose.
2. Conversion of fatty substances to glucose.
3. Conversion of proteins to glucose.

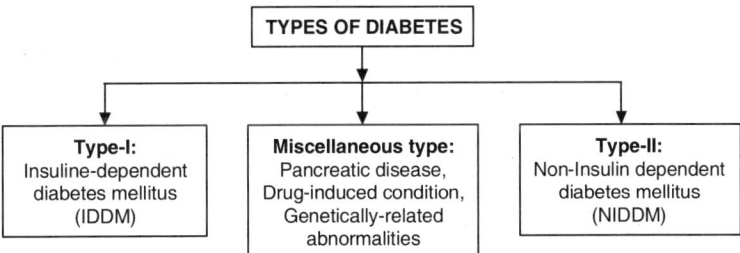

Under current clinical terms, diabetes mellitus can be categorised as under:

1. Insulin-dependent or type I (IDDM or juvenile or brittle or unstable diabetes).
2. Non-insulin-dependent or type II (NIDDM or adult onset or maturity onset diabetes).
3. Other types:
   a. Insulin receptor abnormalities.
   b. Hormonal etiology, e.g acromegaly.
   c. Pancreatic disease.
   d. Genetically related abnormalities.
   e. Drug-induced conditions.

- Another term 'diabetes insipidus' is sometimes used in which the urine of the patient remains tasteless. Nowadays the term 'diabetes insipidus' is reserved for the conditions produced by the disorders of the pituitary gland and the term, diabetes mellitus is used to describe the actual diabetes.

▩ INSULIN-DEPENDENT DIABETES MELLITUS (IDDM)

Etiology

This condition results when there is under production of insulin in childhood or adolescence. The principal derangement is the failure of β-cells to produce insulin in full capacity.

Pathophysiology

- The insignificant amounts of insulin fail to properly utilise and metabolise carbohydrate as the available source of energy. To overcome the shortage in energy production, body attempts to find out other alternative pathways.
- To meet the demand of energy, fat and protein metabolism gets accelerated. These metabolic alterations are symptomized by the presence of increased amounts of ketone bodies and nitrogenous waste material both, in the blood and in the urine.
- In severe ketosis, coma follows in less severe cases, poor wound healing, infection, nausea, vomiting, restlessness and drowsiness constitute as main symptoms. Evidences are gathering to suggest that juvenile diabetes may have a viral origin.

Table 36.1: Insulin-dependent versus non-insulin-dependent forms of diabetes mellitus

IDDM	NIDDM
1. Lacks the ability to synthesize and release insulin due to destruction of some p cells.	1. Can synthesize and release insulin but not enough to meet the requirement
2. Occurs at an early age.	2. Occurs in the people usually over the age of forty.
3. Obesity is not the common factor.	3. Obesity is generally a contributing factor.
4. May be of viral origin.	4. May be of hereditary origin.
5. Equally affects male and female.	5. Females are more attacked than males.
6. The mass of a, D and PP cells remain unchanged.	6. The mass of p, D and PP cells remain unchanged.
7. Characterized by decreased secretion of insulin.	7. Characterized by increased secretion of glucagon.
8. Insulin therapy is the only answer.	8. Oral hypoglycemic agents can serve the purpose.

- The communicable nature of this type of diabetes adds to the evidence. The persons, having genetic susceptibility to get affected by virus easily get diabetic. Recently 'encephalomyocarditis' virus was reported to produce diabetes when injected into mice.
- It is proposed that a viral attack may trigger an autoimmune reaction which destroys some of the pancreatic p cells and thus cuts off partially the source of insulin. Though there is marked reduction in the number of p cells, the number of a, D and PP cells appears to be unaffected.
- The number of P cells may get decreased due to the patients' exposure to certain chemicals. These chemicals selectively destroy pancreatic p cells and reduce the secretion of insulin. Such agents include alloxan, uric acid, dehydroascorbic acid, quinolones and streptozocin.
- If viral etiology proves its correctness in near future, alone a suitable vaccine treatment would assure an easy and effective solution to this problem.

NON-INSULIN-DEPENDENT DIABETES MELLITUS (NIDDM)

- This type has more definite genetic and hereditary characteristics. This disease type announces its presence quite late. More often this is a disease of affluent and old aged people and is more common in women than in men. The patient retains a considerable number of functioning p cells making insulin deficiency less severe. However, the population of a-cells is increased without major changes in D or PP cells. Ketosis does not occur and wasting is not a common feature. This indicates that this type may not need any treatment except a strict dietary restriction.

- Other types include latent diabetes where the symptoms arise only under the conditions of strain and stress. In some patients, biochemical tests confirm the presence of the disease but the persons enjoy the life like any normal person (i.e. mild non-obese diabetes). Similarly due to complex hormonal and metabolic changes that occur during infection or pregnancy, gestational diabetes may develop.

Symptoms and Complications

Gangrene

Diabetes, if not treated with insulin or with any other oral hypoglycemic agent, may result into thickening of capillary basement membrane. Gangrene of the extremities and degenerative diseases of retina, nerve tissues and arterioles which accompany the disease can be explained on this basis.

Retinopathy (Fig. 36.7)

Cataracts and nerve lesions may be seen due to covalent interaction of glucose with tissue proteins in the lens and the nerve. Swelling occurs due to the accumulation of sugar in these lesions.

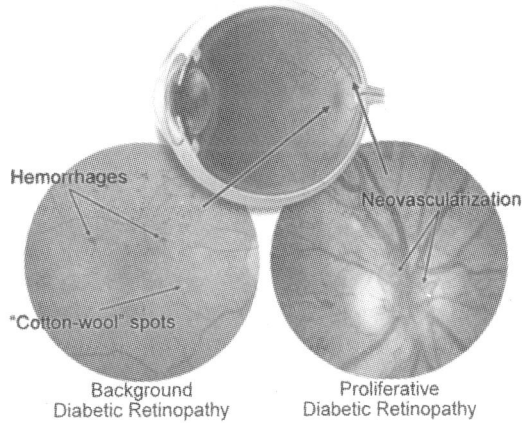

Fig. 36.7: Retinopathy one of the complications of diabetes

Ketoacidosis (Fig. 36.8)

- Mobilization of fat (lipolysis) is the process governed by insulin, glucagon and anterior pituitary hormone. Insulin has antilipolytic action. Hence in insulin deficiency, lipolysis is facilitated. The resulting fatty acid flow is directed to the liver where they are oxidised to acetyl CoA. The latter is converted into various ketone bodies.

- These include acetoacetic acid, P-hydroxy butyric acid and acetone. In ketosis, overproductions of ketone bodies occur. They enter the bloodstream for distribution and oxidation in the kidneys, muscle, heart, brain and testes. Acetone is exhaled in the breath and the person has a characteristic acetone breath.

- It occurs in starvation, in severe diabetes, in the acidosis of childhood and during anesthesia, where it serves as an important sign of the attack of coma.

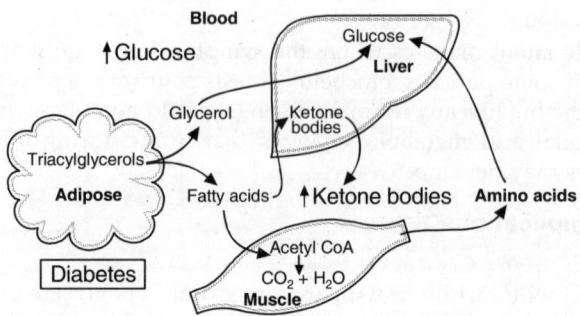

Fig. 36.8: Formation of ketone bodies

Hyperglycemia

- Insulin acts primarily by controlling and rectifying the disturbances in carbohydrate, fat and protein metabolism. It suppresses lipogenesis and prevents hyperlipemia and ketogenesis. The free fatty acids are again re-esterified to triglycerides in adipose tissues. Some of them are routinely utilized as a source of energy in tissues except brain, erythrocytes and adrenal medulla.

- During insulin deficient state, glucose continues to get synthesized from amino acids and triglyceride, despite the high levels of circulating blood glucose. Insulin prevents this undesired protein and fat metabolism and promotes protein synthesis. Its anabolic effect is exerted through the catalysis of various enzymatic steps in glucogenolysis. During hyperglycemia, insulin promotes lipogenesis by:
  a. Increasing the glucose transport in adipose tissues.
  b. Exerting antilipolytic effects.

Limitation

Though all this is true, the clinical evaluation of insulin does not certify it as an ideal antidiabetic agent. Regardless of its ability to control certain symptoms and to prevent ketoacidosis and impending coma in diabetic patient. It is having certain limitations:

1. Insulin must be injected, because given orally it is destroyed by pepsin and trypsin. (It is not orally effective due to its proteinous nature. It gets easily destroyed in the gastric environment of stomach.)

2. Allergic reactions, local or generalized, in sensitive individuals.

3. Antibody formation against insulin, requiring increasing doses or occasionally inducing insulin resistance. Available insulin are prepared chemical structure, differ in one terminal amino acid where alanine is replaced by threonine; a preparation identical to human insulin is still sought. Desalanino pork insulin recently synthesized and tested in animals, may have the same hypoglycemic properties and be less likely to induce antibody.

4. The proteinous nature of the hormone triggers allergic reactions at the site of injection when given parenterally.

5. Insulin fails to give expected result— if the restriction of the diet and exercise is not strictly observed.

6. Insulin does not abolish or prevent development of diabetic complications such as vascular changes, neuropathy and cataract formation. In diabetic patients, the disturbances in basic biochemical reactions lead to the alterations in the thickening of the basement membranes of many tissues, especially that of kidney and arterioles. Though insulin therapy rectifies the cause of the disease, already occurred consequences as mentioned above are left untouched. This gets reflected in long-term complications in cardiovascular, renal, neural and visual systems. Only when diabetic patient begins to develop cardiac and renal problems at a rate greater than the normal person, one realises that insulin therapy alone could not be the only answer to the treatment of diabetes. Disturbed carbohydrate metabolism alone does not constitute the etiology of the disease but remains only one of the segments of this complex disease. As time went by, the etiology of this disease was found to be many folded; ranging from purely endocrine nature to immunological, infectious and genetic origin.

7. Diabetes may also accompany diseases of other organ like that of liver, kidney, adrenal cortex, thyroid and pituitary gland. Glucocorticoidal therapy is reported to aggreviate the disease conditions. Many drugs (e.g. thiazide diuretics) may also precipitate it in certain cases.

BIOSYNTHESIS OF INSULIN

- In to the polyribosome of the rough endoplasmic reticulum of the β-cells. Preproinsulin is converted to the proinsulin, which contains 86 amino acids. This proinsulin is then transferred toward the golgi apparatus and enteres the storage granules, where proinsulin is converted to the insulin (Fig. 36.9).

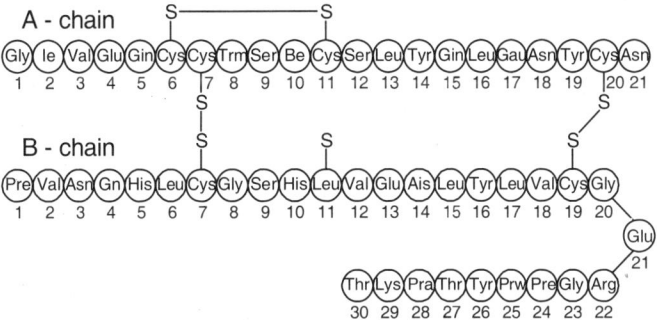

Fig. 36.9: Structure of insulin

- Actually proinsulin consists of the 86 amino acids. These amino acids are broken-down at specific amino acid by specific enzyme and that result into the formation of insulin.
- Endopeptidase enzyme causes the removal of the Arg-Arg residue at 31 and 32 positions and Arg-Lys residue at positions 64 and 65 that result in the formation of insulin and C-peptide.
- The resulting insulin molecule consists of chain A and B containing 21and 30 amino acids, respectively. The chains are connected by two disulfide linkage, with an additional disulfide linkage within chain A.

- Insulin, with a molecular weight of about 6,000 is made up of two chains A (acidic) and B (basic), containing 21 and 30 amino acids, respectively. Thus total 51 ammo acids are present in insulin molecule.

SECRETION OF INSULIN

- The capacity of pancreas to secrete insulin ranges from 1–2 mg per day. However, under fasting conditions, the insulin secretion may be increased to 20 ug per hour. The glucose concentration in the blood serves as a stimulus to the biochemical reactions needed to initiate insulin release. Other hypotheses stress the importance of glucose metabolites (e.g. ATP, glucose-6-phosphate, phosphoenolpyruvate, etc.) and try to link the increase in the concentration of these metabolites with insulin release. Beside this, several hormones from GIT (e.g. secretin, gastrin, pancreozytnin- cholecystokinin, vasoactive intestinal polypeptide, etc.) also enhance the rate of insulin release.

- The islets are richly innervated by adrenergic and cholinergic nerves. Within the pancreatic cells, glucagon and vagal nerve stimulate the secretion of insulin and Somatostatin. somatostatin inhibits the secretion of both, insulin and glucagon while insulin prevents the release of glucagon. This explains the interhormonal autoregulation of the insulin release. Under the conditions of strain and stress (i.e. increased catecholamine release), the insulin secretion is suppressed through the activation of α-adrenoceptors. Thus depending upon quality and quantity of the food ingested, hypothalamus regulates the insulin secretion from p-cells through autonomic nervous system.

- The breaking of storage granules of insulin requires the presence of intracellular calcium in an energy consuming process. The secretory granules contain about 10% of insulin of their total storage capacity. The secreted insulin is taken in the pancreatic vein that ultimately transports it to the portal vein. During its passage through the liver, a large fraction of released insulin (about 40 – 60%) from the portal blood is removed and metabolized by the action of metabolizing enzymes like,

  1. Glutathione–insulin–transhydrogenase which breaks the disulfide linkages through reductive cleavage.

  2. Insulinase enzymes that further dearrange the chains A and B to smaller peptides and amino acids.

  3. Some peptide bonds present in the insulin may be hydrolyzed by pepsin and chymotrypsin.

- The remaining amount is made available to the systemic circulation. The insulin concentration in the plasma ranges from 6–26 nU/ml. It is mainly present in the free form while slight amount of the circulating insulin may be bound to α and β globulins. The half-life of insulin in plasma ranges from 6.5 to 9.0 minutes.

PHYSIOLOGICAL FUNCTION OF INSULIN (FIG. 36.10)

- Insulin is an anabolic hormone. It catalyses the synthesis of various macromolecules and prevents undue breakdown of proteins, carbohydrates and fat. Thus it promotes cell growth by deposition of carbohydrates, lipids and proteins.

- It regulates the redox-potential gradient at the cell surface and by increasing the total number of hexose transporters; it facilitates the entry of glucose molecules to adipose tissues, cardiac tissues and skeletal muscles with minimum expenditure of energy. In the muscles and adipose tissues, glucose metabolises to acetyl CoA which is then utilised in the synthesis of fatty acids.

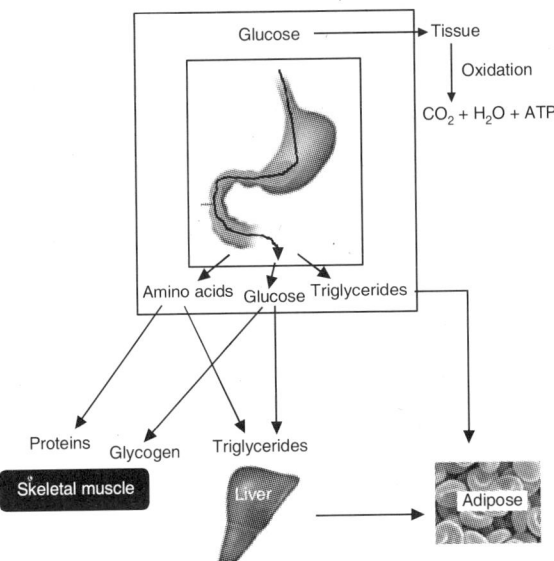

Fig. 36.10: Physiological function of insulin

- While in the liver, various enzymes (glucokinase, phosphofructokinase and pyruvate kinase) involved in the glucose metabolism are directed in such a way to favour glycogenesis while decreasing glycogenolysis. This explains the role of insulin in lowering down the blood glucose levels.

CHEMISTRY OF INSULIN

- In 1926, Abel isolated insulin in a crystalline form by using X-ray crystallography techniques, Dorothy Hodgkin and her associates reported three-dimensional arrangement of atoms in insulin molecule. For such excellent work, she had been awarded Nobel Prize. In the early 1960s, Sanger et al established the exact sequence of amino acids in this polypeptide hormone. Utilizing the data of Sanger, the complete chemical synthesis of insulin was reported in 1963–64 by Meienhofer et al and Kotsoyannis et al but independently. To date, structural elucidations of insulins from at least 25 species are documented in the literature. The first total chemical synthesis of human insulin was claimed by Rittel et al. In human insulin, B-strand possesses a helical pattern in which A strand appears to get entrapped.

- Insulin is composed of 51 amino acids arranged in two polypeptide chains, designated A and B, which are linked together by two disulfide bridge between amino acids residues 6 and 11 of the A chain.

- In the rhombohedral crystal, the unit cell consists of six insulin molecules arranged as three equivalent dimmers in three-fold symmetry. The compact packing of the hexamer produces an oblate spheroid, with polar amino acid side chains covering its surface. The two zinc ions are situated, $17A°$ apart, on the three-fold crystal axis and co-ordinated to three equivalent β_{10} histidine.

▨ SAR STUDIES

- The natural sources of insulin are mainly porcine and bovine pancreatic tissues. In comparison to synthetic insulin, natural is cheaper and is readily obtained in large amounts. SAR studies carried out on insulin revealed the following points:

  1. There exist a definite relationship between the conformation of insulin molecule and its activity. Any attempt to change this conformation leads to decrease in activity.
  2. Disturbance in the sequence of amino acids in chain A reduces the activity while amino acids from one to six and 28 to 30 can be removed from chain B, without significantly affecting the activity.
  3. Reduction of either chain abolishes the activity.
  4. Any modification of the side chain carboxyl groups or the tyrosine residues tend to decrease the activity.
  5. It may be concluded that chemical modifications in the insulin structure fail to potentiate the hormone activity. Some analogs have been prepared but are of limited use to study insulin receptors.
  6. The therapeutic importance of zinc and chromium in the treatment of diabetes is recently reviewed. Zinc, being an integral part of the insulin structure, is also found to affect carbohydrate metabolism while chromium activates insulin at its receptor sites and is found to increase both, the affinity and intrinsic activity of insulin.

B-chain

1. Several residues of the β-chain are not required for full bioactivity. The first four to six and the last three residues are dispensible.
2. As further residues from COOH terminus (B 28–30) are dispensible. As further residues from the COOH terminus (B 27–26, etc.) are omitted one by one, the biological activity decreases gradually desheptapeptide (B 26–30) insulin, which is totally inactive. Residues 24–26 occupy important parts of the receptor binding area of the insulin.

A-chain

1. The A chain cannot be shortened. Omission of A1 glycine reduces the hormonal potency to less than 1% and omission of A 21 asparagine abolishes the activity. However, replacement of A21 Aspn by alanine preserves full activity.
2. The A1 guanidinated insulin is the most active derivative. A positive charge increases (for A1 Lys and Arg-insulin) and a negative charge decreases activities (for the A1 Glu derivative).

Fast-acting analouges

1. Human insulin analogs Lys B28, Pro B29 have desirable pharmacokinetic and pharmacodynamic properties.
2. Asp B10 insulin (wherein the naturally occurring at the 10 position of the B-chain is replaced by aspartic acid) is 3–4 times more active than that of human insulin.

Slow-acting analogs

Human diarginyl insulins Arg B3, Arg B32 are more slowly absorbed from the subcutaneous tissues. Two extra arginines shift the isoelectric point from 5.4 to 7.0, thereby, giving insoluble insulin. Glycin was substituted for asparagine at A21. This modification gives extended duration of action of the diarginyl insulin.

MECHANISM OF ACTION (FIG. 36.11)

Insulin Receptor

The insulin receptor is synthesized as a single polypeptide that is glycosylated and cleaved into α and β subunits, which are then assembled into a tetramer linked by disulfide bonds. A hydrophobic domain in each β-subunit spans the plasma membrane. The extracellular α-subunit contains the insulin binding site. The cytosolic domains of the β-subunit is a tyrosine kinase, which is activated by insulin.

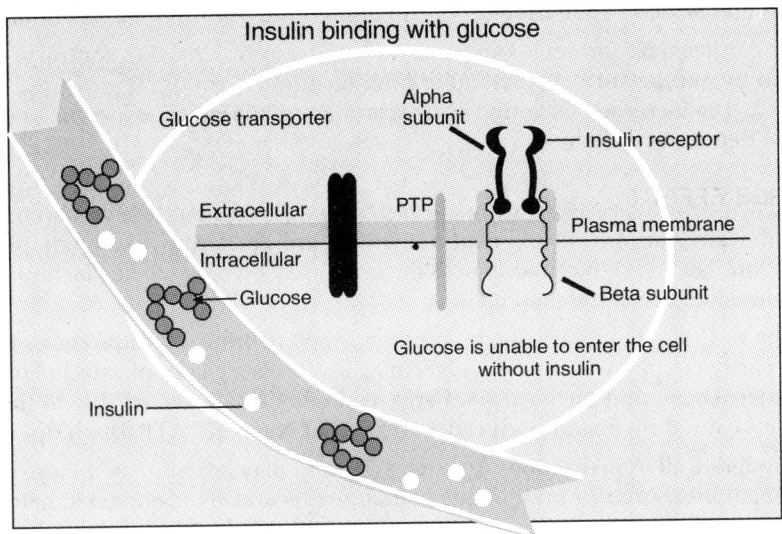

Fig. 36.11: Mechanism of action of insulin

Signal Transduction

- The binding of insulin to the α-subunits of the insulin receptor induces conformational changes that are transduced to the β-subunits (it possesses tyrosine kinase activity).
- Due to the attachment of insulin to the receptor, the β-subunit or tyrosine kinase get autophosphorylated that results in increased activity of tyrosine kinase towards the intracellular signaling protein.
- The activated tyrosine kinases further phosphorylation of the intracellular protein, which stimulate the different enzymes such as glycogen synthetase, pyruvate dehydrogenase. This enzyme is further responsible for transformation of glucose to glycogen, amino acid to protein as well as formation of lipids.

Insulin Deficiency

- The most prominent effects of insulin are exerted mainly on the liver, adipose tissues and skeletal muscle. These effects are anabolic in nature. Hence the deficiency of insulin is mainly characterized by hyperglycemia, hyperlipemia, ketonemia, acidosis and azoturia.
- During insulin deficiency, various routes of glucose utilization are suppressed. The rate of glucose transport across the cell membrane is also reduced (except brain, erythrocytes, leukocytes).

- However, the rates of hepatic conversion of glycogen, fatty acids and proteins to glucose are accelerated. The overall result of such underutilization and overproduction of glucose is hyperglycemia and elimination of excess glucose in the urine of the patient.

- Insulin exerts antilipolytic action. In its deficiency, mobilization of fat (lipolysis) proceeds uninhibited resulting into high plasma levels of free fatty acids. This leads to hyperlipemia. Lipogenesis from pyruvate-acetyl CoA system is also suppressed. Hence acetyl CoA is utilized only in the production of ketone bodies, some of which are relatively strong acids. Ketonemia and acidosis thus develop due to higher rate of formation of ketone bodies.

- In insulin deficiency, protein synthesis is suppressed. On the contrary, proteins are catabolised to glucose at relatively higher rate. As a result, production of urea and ammonia is enhanced. The increased excretion of urea and ammonia in urine (azoturia) is thus seen in the insulin deficient patients.

ADVERSE EFFECT

- Most of the adverse effects of insulin therapy are seen due to higher plasma insulin concentration. The hypoglycemic state in the brain may give rise to headache, blurred vision, mental confusion, coma and convulsions.

- Some of the early symptoms are due to secretion of epinephrine which promotes glycogenolysis and thus partly counteracts the hypoglycemia. The reflex release of catecholamines leads to sweating, weakness, and tachycardia. Peripheral edema also occurs due to the retention of sodium ions caused by insulin-induced activation of $Na^+ - K^+$ ATPase pump.

- Mild to moderate allergic reactions (itching, swelling) may accompany the use of commercial insulin preparations due to proteinious contaminants and their antigenic nature. In certain cases, the use of antihistaminic agents can be advised. In more severe forms, however, insulin therapy has to be replaced by oral hypoglycemic agents.

INSULIN-RESISTANT DIABETES (FIG. 36.12)

- Patient is said to be insulin-resistant when he does not respond to insulin therapy. In such cases, the insulin requirement may exceed 200 units per day. This may occur due to involvement of certain genetic or autoimmune factors.

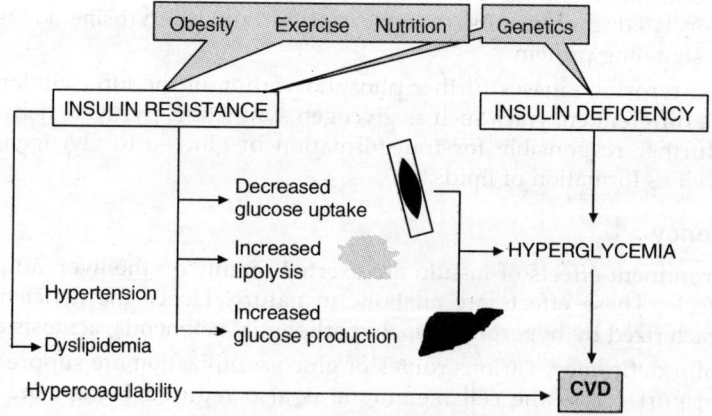

Fig. 36.12: Insulin-resistant diabetes

- For example, proinsulin may not be efficiently converted to insulin at the expected rate due to genetic defaults. Since proinsulin is weak hypoglycemic agent (only about 5% as active as insulin), diabetic condition may develop.
- Even though insulin secretion is normal, the low intensity of biological effects of insulin may be due to decrease in both, the receptor sites and binding sites in the tissues.
- Due to some autoimmune mechanisms, the anti-insulin antibodies may be generated and insulin-receptor interaction may be inhibited by these antibodies.
- Over secretion of physiological antagonists for insulin (e.g. glucagon, epinephrine) may be one of the reasons in insulin resistant diabetic patients.

INSULIN PREPARATION

Short-acting Insulin Preparations

- As the plasma half-life of intravenously injected insulin is not enough to meet the requirements, one has to search for such insulin preparations, having quick onset and prolong duration of action. Presently available insulin preparations differ only with respect to onset and duration of action. First clinically used form was amorphous insulin which was highly soluble in body fluids.
- This leads to its rapid excretion and hence it was to be replaced by other insulin preparations. In early 1940s came 'regular insulin' which is a buffered solution of crystalline zinc insulin. Duration of action of this preparation still needs improvement. Chemically, pure zinc insulin has physiologic action essentially identical to that of regular noncrystalline insulin as far as onset, duration and rate of blood sugar reduction are concerned.

Intermediate and Long-acting Insulin Preparations

1. Protamine–insulin preparations: The longer duration of action is due to protamine, a basic protein that leaves the site of injection more slowly.

2. Protamine–zinc–insulin preparations: Prolonged duration of action of insulin, a long time objective, was finally achieved by Hagedorn in 1935 with protamine zinc insulin. Developed in 1936, these suspensions were proved to be better than 'protamine insuline' duration of action. This is prepared by complexing insulin with zinc and protamine. The products are available with 40–80 units/ml.

3. Globin–zinc–insulin preparation: Developed in 1939, its duration of action (12–18 hours) is less than protamine zinc insulin preparations (24–36 hours).

4. Isophane–insulin suspensions: Developed in 1946, these suspensions contain protamine, zinc and insulin. It differs from 'protamine–zinc–insulin' in the method of preparation and contains less protamine than 'protamine–zinc–insulin'.

- This preparation has 'time activity best adapted to the requirements of majority of diabetic patients. This has a blood-sugar lowering effect usually lasting over 24 hours.

5. Lante insulins:

- The solubility pattern of insulin (and hence its absorption) is mainly governed by its physical state. For example, large crystals of insulin with high zinc content will be less soluble in body fluids and naturally produce long duration of action due to slow absorption. Such preparations are known as ultralante insulin.
- This concept was utilized to develop such preparations which do not need a protein modifier (e.g. protamine or globin) to prolong their action. Stretching the same concept ahead, amorphous insulin exhibits rapid absorption and hence rapid onset of action. Such insulin zinc suspension is known as semilante insulin.

- A proper combination of ultralante insulin (7 parts) and semilante insulin (3 parts) will naturally constitute a preparation having a rapid onset and intermediate duration of action; both the properties desirable for well-clinical acceptance of the preparation.

Very Long-acting Insulin Preparations

- Attempts to formulate insulin preparations with very long duration of action are made. The solubility of insulin at physiological pH 7.4 is mainly controlled by the amount of $ZnCl_2$, which is increased to 5–10 times than normally required to prepare 'soluble zinc insulin'.
- The increased concentration of zinc ions form low solubility complexes with insulin molecules, if the buffer is changed from phosphate to acetate. Such suspensions are reported in USP.

■ LIMITATION OF INSULIN THERAPY

Present evidences regarding insulin therapy uncovered the limitations of insulin and do not agree to recognize insulin as an ideal hypoglycemic agent. Various problems encountered in insulin therapy are listed below.

1. In the long-term therapy, there is a risk of development of tumors at the site of injection.
2. Due to its proteinous nature, insulin triggers local allergic reactions in sensitive patients. Anaphylactic shock may occur in extreme cases.
3. Fluctuations in blood glucose levels may lead to visual disturbances which may extend to blindness. This is mainly due to disturbed osmotic equilibrium in the eyes.
4. If the dose schedule is not properly corrected according to the requirement, insulin therapy leads to hypoglycemic shock.
5. Thickening of basement membrane of several tissues (due to poor control of blood glucose level), particularly of kidney and vasculature leads to renal and cardiovascular impairments.
6. Every exogenous protein is associated with antigenic properties to less or more extent. Naturally insulin administration in almost every patient leads to the production of insulin antibodies, which bind insulin and decrease its effectiveness. This is known as insulin resistance. This is the most severe problem of insulin therapy where the daily insulin requirement exceeds 200 units in comparison to the normal requirement of 50 units a day. This resistance thus, has an immunological basis and can be solved by shifting:

   a. From conventional to purified insulin therapy, or

   b. From one insulin type (e.g. bovine insulin) to another insulin type (e.g. porcine insulin).

   Here the insulin from another origin will be new to the body and resistance to this insulin would not occur at least for couple of months. This is due to the failure of the body mechanistic to recognize immediately the new insulin type (and therefore to generate antibodies for it).

37

Oral Hypoglycemic Agents

Insulin, due to its proteineous nature, is destroyed in the gastric environment of the stomach. Some peptide bonds present in insulin structure are hydrolyzed by pepsin and chymotrypsin in GIT. Hence it is orally ineffective. Therefore, it is usually given by subcutaneous injection.

The most attractive and direct approach to treat diabetes, however, will be administration of orally active hypoglycemic agents. Various limitations of insulin therapy along with its inactivation in GIT encouraged medicinal chemists to find out potent and orally active hypoglycemic candidates which may stand firmly as alternative or substitute to insulin therapy in maturity onset type of diabetes. In juvenile type, strict dietary control along with exogenously administered insulin constitutes the only treatment.

CLASSIFICATION OF ORAL HYPOGLYCEMIC AGENTS

Flow chart 37.1 depicts the classification of oral hypoglycemic agents.

Flow chart 37.1: Oral hyproglycemic agents–classification

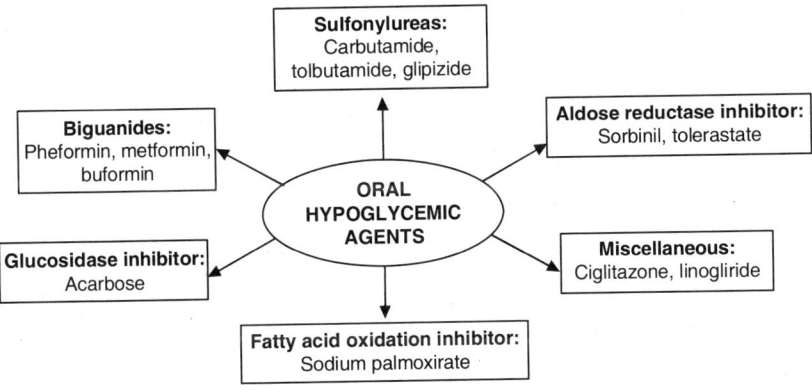

Sulfonylureas

1. First generation

Carbutamide

Tolbutamide

Tolazamide

483

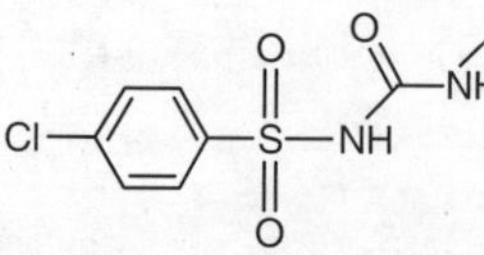

Chlorpropramide

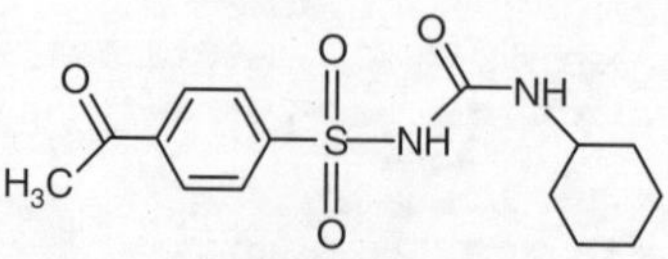

Acetohexamide

2. Second generation

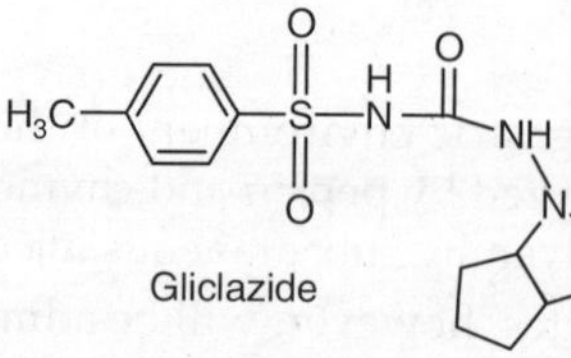

Gliclazide

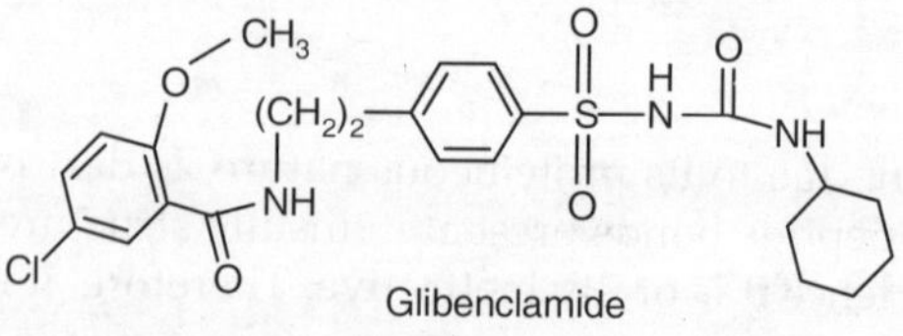

Glibenclamide

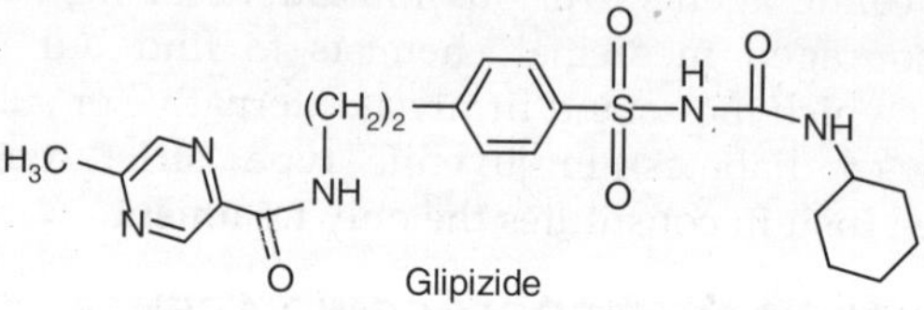

Glipizide

Biguanides

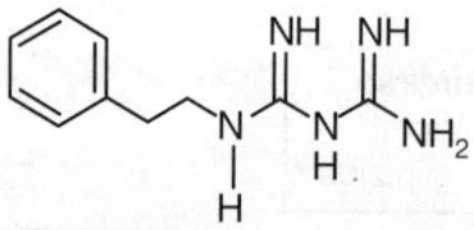

Phenformin

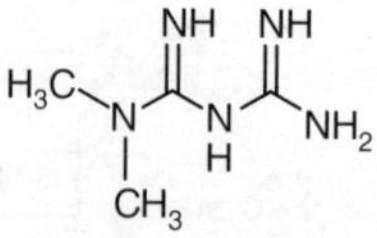

Metformin

Aldose Reductase Inhibitor

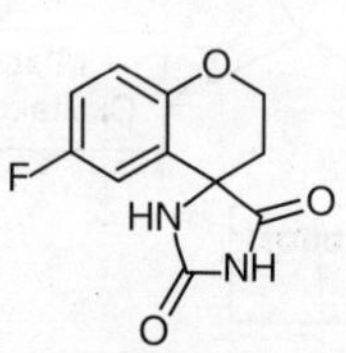

Sorbinil

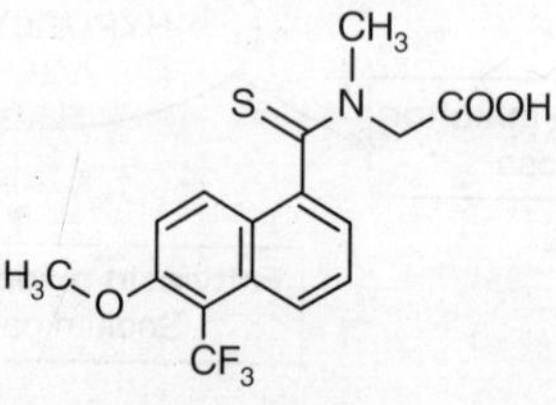

Tolrestat

Glucosidase Inhibitor

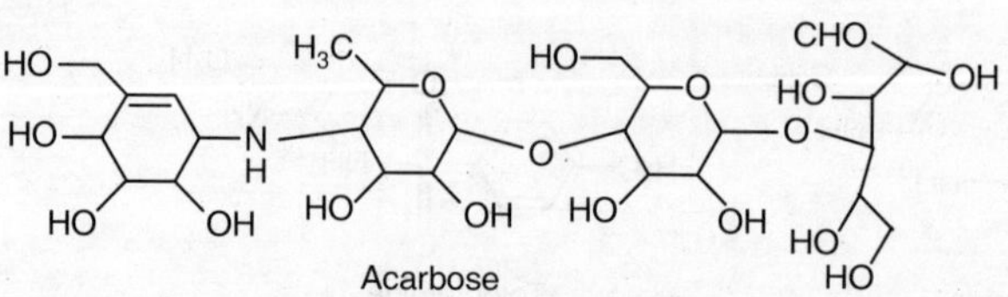

Acarbose

Fatty Acid Oxidation Inhibitors

$$H_3C-(CH_2)_{13}$$

Sodium palmoxirate

Miscellaneous

Pirogliride

Linogliride

SULFONYLUREAS

Mechanism of Action (Fig. 37.1)

- Sulfonylureas stimulate insulin secretion from pancreatic β-cell without entering the cell. This occurs in the absence of glucose. Intact pancreatic β-cells are essential for the hypoglycemic action of sulfonylureas. β-cells contain sulfonylurea receptors that appear to be linked to an ATPase K^+ channel and the inhibition of K^+ efflux leads to depolarization of the β-cell membrane and opens voltage dependent Ca^{2+} channels.

- Increased entry of Ca^{2+} and intracellular binding to calmodulin could activate kinases involved in exocytosis of secretory granules. Thus more insulin is released for a given increment of blood glucose.

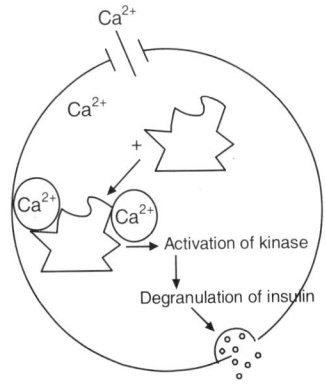

Fig. 37.1: Mode of action of sulfonylureas

The order of potency of sulfonylurea in binding to β-cells approximates its potency in stimulating the release of insulin and inhibiting the effect of K^+. In addition, sulfonylureas appear to act synergistically with insulin possibly by increasing insulin sensitivity at post-receptor level.

SAR Studies

It can be summarized into following points:

1. Certain substituents when placed at paraposition in benzene ring tend to potentiate the activity, e.g. halogens, amino, acetyl, methyl, methylthio and trifluoromethyl groups.

2. The size of terminal nitrogen along with its aliphatic substituent R, determines lipophilic properties of the molecule. Optimum activity results when R consists of 3 to 6 carbon atoms.

Sulfonylureas

3. The nature of para-substituent in benzene ring (-X-) appears to govern the duration of action of the compound.

4. Aliphatic substituent (R) at the terminal nitrogen may also be replaced by an alicyclic or heterocyclic ring.

5. Hypoglycemic activity can be related to the nature of sulfonyl grouping.

6. Replacement of a metabolically easily oxidised group, like a CH_3 group by less readily oxidised chlorine was used to transform the short-acting tolbutamide into long-acting chlorpropramide, with a half-life six-fold greater than its parent.

Pharmacokinetics

1. These drugs are extensively bound to plasma proteins and mainly metabolized in liver. Except tolbutamide whose chief metabolite (i.e. butyl-carboxyphenyl sulfonylurea is in the form of carboxylic acid due to carboxylation of its methyl group, other sulfonylureas undergo metabolism rather slowly into more active and longer lasting metabolites.

2. Acetohexamide undergoes reduction to give hydroxyhexamide. Much of its hypoglycemic activity can be assigned to this metabolite.

3. Tolazamide metabolizes to number of weakly active metabolites. Glipizide and glyburide undergo slow metabolism to inactive hydroxylated derivatives which appear in the conjugate forms in the urine. Chlorpropamide appears in urine in unchanged form together with its metabolites.

Adverse Effect

If overdoses of sulfonylureas are continued for prolonged period, it leads to degranulation of pancreatic β-cells. The common adverse reactions of this class can be categorized as:

1. Cutaneous reactions, e.g. skin rashes and photosensitivity.

2. Gastrointestinal reactions: Nausea, vomiting, anorexia, mild toxic hepatitis with jaundice.

3. Cardiovascular reactions: Increased risk of cardiac dysfunctioning, transient leucopenia, agranulocytosis, thrombocytopenia and fetal aplastic anemia.

4. These reactions, except the cardiovascular effects are usually not severe and the incidence of these effects is also low. However, under the conditions of strain, stress, infection and dysfunctioning of renal, hepatic or cardiac origin, these drugs should not be used.

5. Sulfonylureas should be reserved only in the treatment of either non-insulin dependent diabetic patient or such patient where insulin therapy alone is inadequate or inconvenient. In certain cases, sulfonylurea therapy may be used to lower down the insulin-dose in insulin resistant patients.

■■ GUANIDINE DERIVATIVES

Phenformin and Metformin

History

- The parent lead compound of this series, guanidine was reported to lower blood glucose levels in animals in 1918. High toxicities associated with its use necessitated the search for better drug in this series.

- Subsequently phenformin was reported which is comparatively safer, non-toxic biguanide. It was soon followed by metformin, another biguanide.

Mechanism of action

- Biguanide derivatives lower the blood sugar in the absence of pancreatic islet cells; they act in pancreatectomized animals and man but do not appreciably lower the blood sugar level in normal subjects. Peripheral utilization of glucose is increased.

- Biguanides may inhibit oxidative phosphorylation by inhibiting such oxidative enzymes is succinic dehydrogenase. Respiratory enzyme inhibition results in cellular hypoxia; subsequently, glucose uptake by the peripheral muscles increases and anaerobic glycolysis follows.
- Owing to decrease in oxidation of adipose tissue, lipogenesis is also decreased. Because of these differences in action, applications and usefulness, these preparations differ from those of the sulfonylurea compounds. They often lower the blood sugar content in patients resistant to sulfonylurea compounds.
- The possible mechanisms of action of these hypoglycemic biguanides include :
  1. Inhibition of intestinal transport and absorption of sugars.
  2. Potentiation of the action of insulin on glucose transfer processes into the cell.
  3. Inhibition of hepatic gluconeogenesis.
  4. Enhancement of glucose utilization processes and/or inhibition of oxidative phosphorylation in the peripheral tissues.

Adverse effect

- Phenformin and metformin are similar in their actions. The normal therapeutic dose for both these biguanides ranges from 25–150 mg/day.
- They do not stimulate insulin release but remain ineffective in the absence of insulin. Because of lactic acidosis associated with the use of phenformin, it was withdrawn from the market.

ALDOSE REDUCTASE INHIBITORS

Sorbinil and Tolrestat

Mechanism of action

- Chronic diabetes mellitus causes development of microvascular and neurologic complications like retinopathy and neuropathy. The tissues involved are the lens, retina, nerves, kidney and blood vessels which do not require insulin for glucose uptake. Aldose reductase has been implicated in cataract formation, retinopathy and diabetic neuropathy.

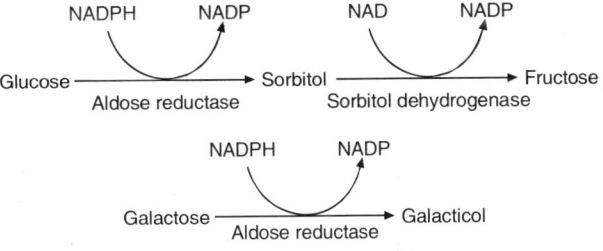

Fig. 37.2: The polyol pathway

- The accumulation of sorbitol is implicated in this disease. In diabetic complication, the high concentration of glucose is converted to sorbitol by aldose reductase by the polyol pathway (Fig. 37.2). Sorbitol is subsequently converted to fructose and these products accumulate in such tissues.
- Galactose is converted to galacticol which is not further metabolized. Because sorbitol and other polyols do not readily pass through cell membranes, they cause osmotic swelling and eventual cell disruption.

- Aldose reductase inhibitors interfere in the polyol pathway of sorbitol and fructose and thereby cause hypoglycemic effects.

α-D-GLUCOSIDASE INHIBITORS

Acarbose

Mechanism of action

- Alpha glucosidases are found in the brush border of the small intestinal mucosa. This enzyme is responsible for breaking down complex polysaccharides and sucrose to monosaccharides, which are then absorbed α-glucosidase inhibitors, decreases the rate of breakdown of glucose. They are also called starch blockers. These inhibitors are useful adjunct to insulin in the treatment of both type I and type II diabetes mellitus. These agents might be of value in obese diabetic patients.

Adverse effect

A limited side effect is flatulence, production of intestinal gas.

FATTY ACID OXIDATION INHIBITORS

Sodium Palmoxirate

Mechanism of action

Glucose and lipid level in the blood affect each others metabolism. In diabetes, the metabolism of sugar is disturbed, due to this, fatty acid oxidation is an alternate pathway for food. Inhibitor of fatty acid oxidation could reverse the cycle in favor of glucose utilization. Based on this hypothesis sodium palmoxirate, has proved a potential oral antidiabetic.

MISCELLANEOUS

Ciglitazone and Pirogliride

Mechanism of action

It suppose to enhance the action in the harmone target tissue, e.g. liver, muscle. They are known as insulin sensitizers.

DIETARY MEASURES

- Diabetes is a disease, which cannot be cured but can be controlled, i.e. controlled by means of proper drug treatment and proper diet measures.
- A report published in 1970 by an American group (University Group Diabetes Program, UGDP) revealed that diabetic patients receiving oral hypoglycemic treatment, more easily develop cardiovascular diseases than, those who are merely on placebo treatment.
- This report inclined people's, mind for not to use drugs unless there appears no other way of controlling diabetes. If proper dietary measures are followed which will supply the bulk of calories, exactly needed, the dependence on drug therapy can greatly be reduced.

Carbutamide

4-acetamido-benzenesulfonamide   Phosgene

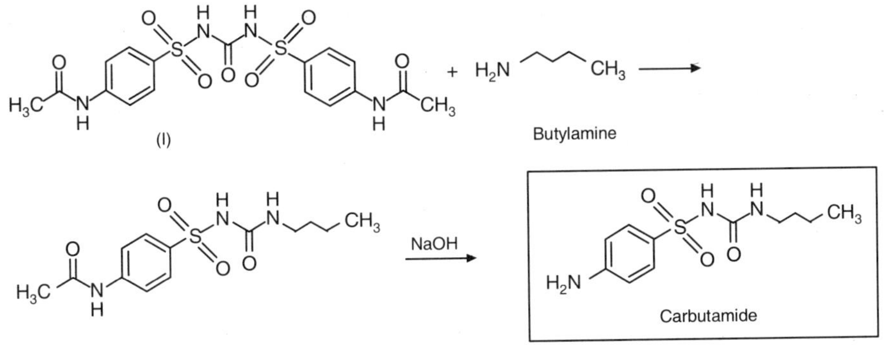

(I) + H₂N⌒⌒CH₃ Butylamine

NaOH → Carbutamide

Tolbutamide

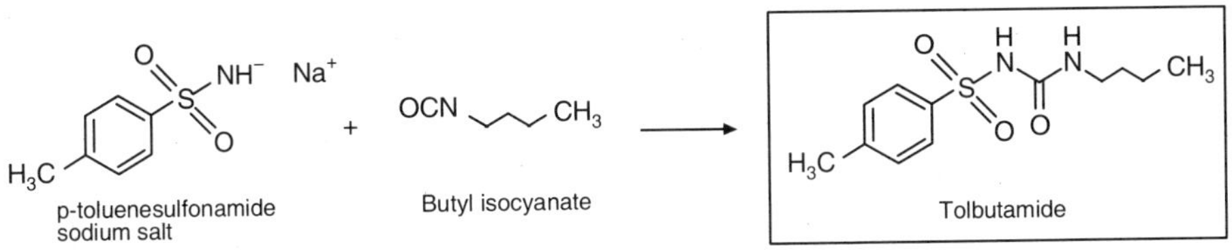

p-toluenesulfonamide sodium salt + Butyl isocyanate → Tolbutamide

Chlorpropamide

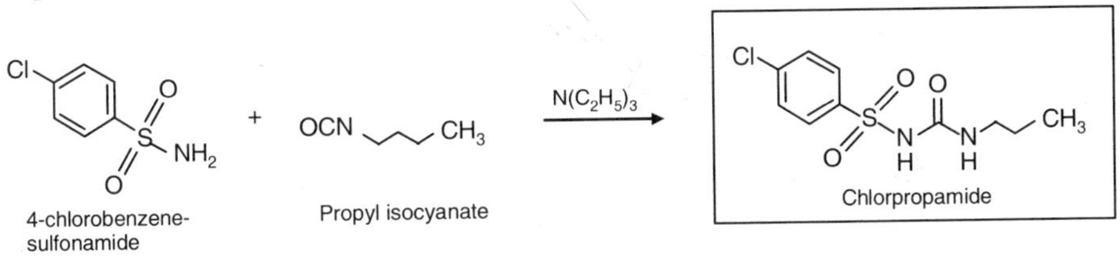

4-chlorobenzene-sulfonamide + Propyl isocyanate → N(C₂H₅)₃ → Chlorpropamide

Tolazamide

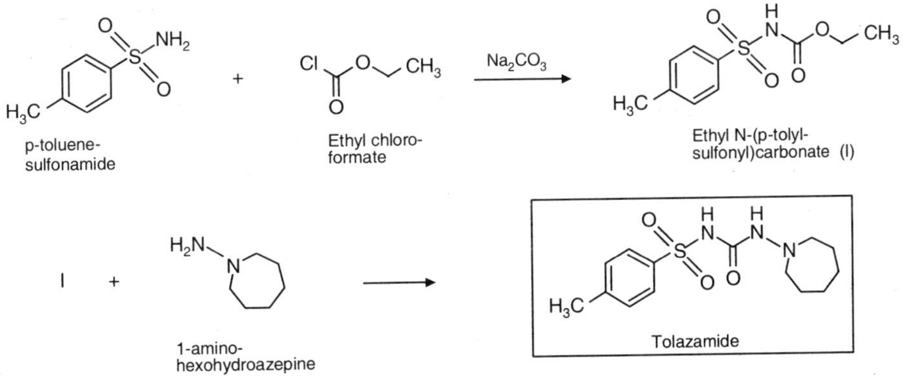

p-toluene-sulfonamide + Ethyl chloro-formate → Na₂CO₃ → Ethyl N-(p-tolyl-sulfonyl)carbonate (I)

I + 1-amino-hexohydroazepine → Tolazamide

Glibenclamide

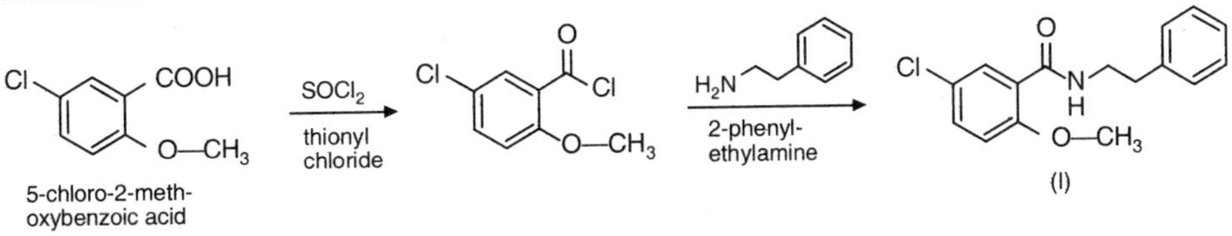

5-chloro-2-meth-oxybenzoic acid → SOCl₂ thionyl chloride → H₂N 2-phenyl-ethylamine → (I)

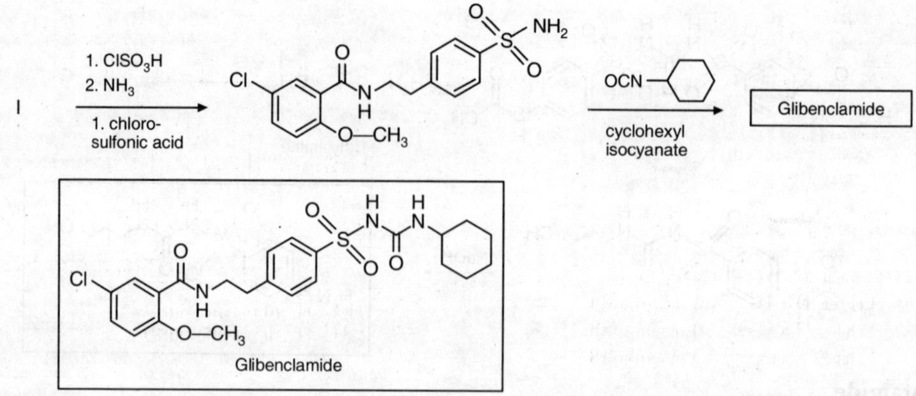
I
1. ClSO3H
2. NH3
1. chloro-
sulfonic acid
Cl
O
N
H
O—CH3
S
O
O
NH2
OCN
cyclohexyl
isocyanate
Glibenclamide
Glibenclamide

Glipizide

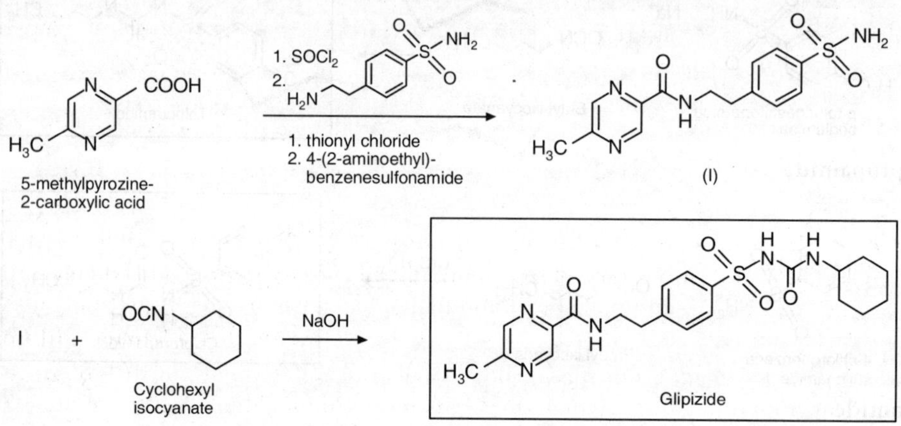
N
COOH
H3C
N
5-methylpyrozine-
2-carboxylic acid
1. SOCl2
2.
H2N
S
O
O
NH2
1. thionyl chloride
2. 4-(2-aminoethyl)-
benzenesulfonamide
(I)
I
+
OCN
Cyclohexyl
isocyanate
NaOH
Glipizide

Gliclazide

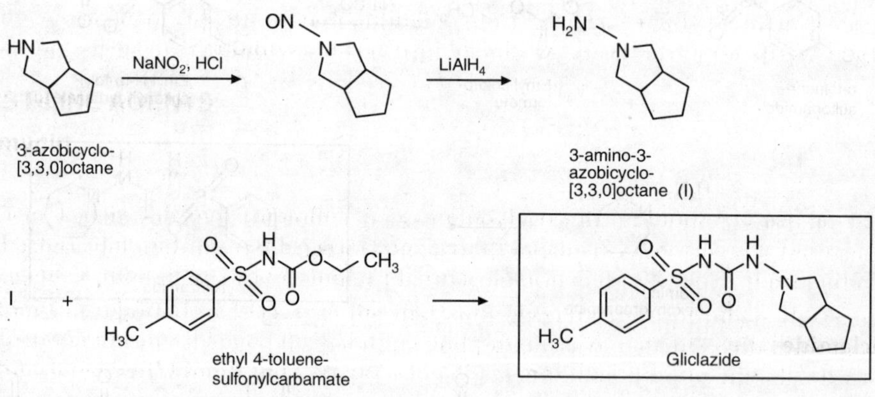
HN
3-azobicyclo-
[3,3,0]octane
NaNO2, HCl
ON
N
LiAlH4
H2N
N
3-amino-3-
azobicyclo-
[3,3,0]octane (I)
I
+
H3C
CH3
ethyl 4-toluene-
sulfonylcarbamate
Gliclazide

38

Thyroid Hormones and Antithyroid Drugs

All vertebrates have thyroid glands. It is not essential to life but it is necessary for growth and mental well-being. In a healthy adult, it weighs about 25 g and is composed of two lobes which lie one on either side of the larynx. It is larger in women than in men.

▦ THYROID GLAND (Fig. 38.1)

- At the posterior surface of each thyroid gland, can be seen the parathyroid gland. Thyroid gland consists of cells arranged in a close spherical fashion to create hollow spheres (follicles), which are the functional units of thyroid gland.

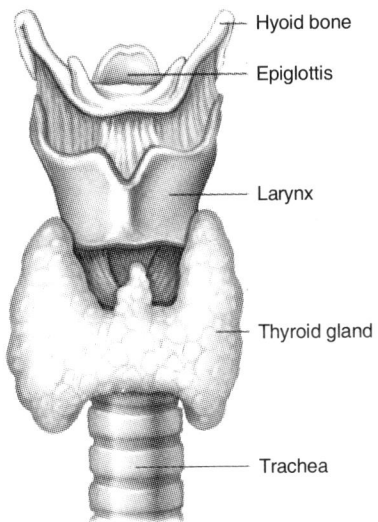

Fig. 38.1: Thyroid gland

- The follicles are filled with structureless, gelatinous, amber-colored protein material, the 'colloid'. It contains the thyroid hormone 'thyroglobulin'. The hormone has molecular weight of about 6, 80,000 and it contains organically bound iodine.
- A large quantity of iodine (0.06 %) which is present in thyroid gland, almost all of which is firmly bound to protein largely in the form of the thyroid hormones. On hydrolysis, thyroglobulin is converted to several iodinated tyrosine derivatives. Thyroid hormones are part of thyroglobulin molecule which is formed in the microsomes of the follicular cells.

491

- Thyroxine (T4) and tri-iodotyrosine(T3) are the principal thyroid hormones. Chemically, they are amino acids containing iodinated diphenyl ethers. Tri-iodotyrosine is more active than thyroxine.

Role of Thyroid Hormones

1. Oxygen consumption, heat production and metabolism of carbohydrates, fats and proteins.
2. Proper functioning of the gastrointestinal, cardiovascular, reproductive, skeletal and neuromuscular systems.
3. Optimal functioning of catecholamines, antidiuretic hormone and glucocorticoids.
4. Normal growth and differentiation.

Biosynthesis, Storage and Metabolism of Thyroid Hormones (Fig. 38.2)

- The biosynthesis of thyroid hormones is regulated by variations in the plasma levels of thyroid-stimulating hormone (TSH) from the anterior pituitary gland. The conversion of inorganic iodide to thyroid hormone involves following steps:
  1. Iodine uptake by the gland.
  2. Oxidation of iodine and iodination of tyrosyl groups.
  3. Formation of thyroxine and tri-iodothyromone from iodotyrosines.
  4. Release of thyroxine and tri-iodothyrone.
- The inorganic iodide is taken up from the blood and is accumulated in the acinar cells of thyroid. The process is accelerated by TSH and is inhibited by perchlorate, thiocyanate or cardiac glycosides.
- Iodine is oxidised by cytochrome system and in this form iodine is incorporated into tyrosine part of the thyroglobulin to form monoiodo-and di-iodotyrosines. Thyroxine and tri-iodothyronine are formed after oxidative coupling.

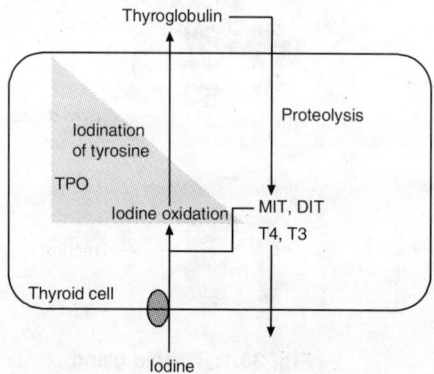

Fig. 38.2: Synthesis of thyroid hormone

- The enzyme, iodotyrosine deiodinase brings about the conversion of thyroxine to tri-iodothyrone by removal of one atom of iodine.
- Both these hormones are stored in the colloid in peptide linkage within the thyroglobulin molecule. Under stimulation by TSH (thyrotropin) and thyrotropine-releasing hormone (from hypothalamus), the thyroglobulin fuses with lysosomes and is hydrolyzed by a proteolytic enzyme to release thyroxine and di-iodothyronine into the circulation.

- The mono-and di-iodotyrosines formed are retained in the glands and are metabolised to release iodide which is reused.
- In circulation, thyroid hormones speed up the consumption of oxygen, affect oxidative phosphorylation and cause swelling of mitochondria. Most of the hormone is deiodinated. A small fraction undergoes deamination, decarboxylation or remains even unchanged. During their metabolism, the diphenyl ether skeleton remains unaffected. They are excreted as glucoronides and as sulfates through the bile.
- The production and release of thyroid hormones is regulated by the thyrotropin (TSH) hormone of the anterior pituitary gland through a feedback inhibition mechanism. It thus helps to maintain a constant amount of thyroid hormones in the circulation and in the tissues.

SAR Studies of Thyroid Hormones

1. The two phenyl rings must be connected by an ether, thioether or methylene linkage in order to maintain the activity.

$$HO - \underset{3'}{\overset{5'}{\boxed{B}}} - X - \boxed{A} - \text{Side chain}$$

2. A carboxyl group must be present in the aliphatic side chain.
3. Halogen or methyl substituents may be placed at 3' and 5' positions.
4. The 3'-monosubstituted analogs are more active than the 3', 5'-disubstituted compounds.
5. For maximal activity, position 4' should be occupied by a hydroxyl group.
6. The bulky and lipophilic groups at 3' position enhance the activity.
7. The 3'-substituent should be distal (away from) and the 5'-substituent should be proximal (above) to the side chain bearing ring in order to maintain the hormone molecule in the active conformation.

▨ DISEASE OF THYROID GLAND

Simple Goiter (Fig. 38.3)

- Normal secretion by the thyroid requires an adequate intake of iodine. If it does not meet the requirement, thyrotrophin is released in higher concentration which results in enlargement of thyroid gland.

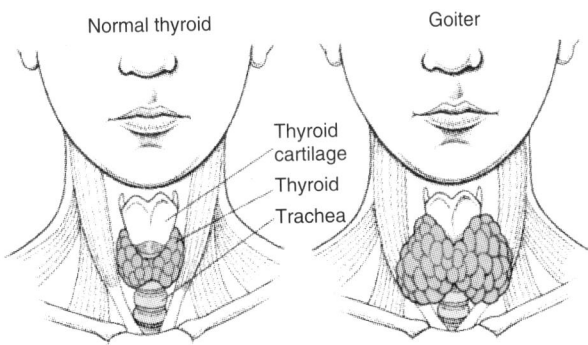

Fig. 38.3: Enlarged thyroid gland in goiter

- This enlargement of thyroid gland is known as a goitre (French word goitre, meaning a neck). Depending upon situations, goitre may be associated with over-secretion, under secretion or with no alteration in the hormone secretions.

- Simple or non-toxic goitre results when an essentially normal thyroid gland secretes the hormones which do not meet the increased body's demand during puberty, menstruation and pregnancy. This is usually treated with adding iodine to the diet, often in combination with salt.

Myxedema

- Thyroid hormone deficiency may result due to spontaneous degeneration of glandular tissues, biosynthetic defects or impaired secretions of the hormones synthesized. Myxedema is a case of severe hypothyroidism which causes the infiltration of the intercellular spaces of skin and muscle with mucopolysaccharide.
- The skin remains dry, the hairs loose, the body becomes cold, the pulse is slow and the mental functions are impaired. The clinical manifestations of hypothyroidism attack virtually every organ system.
- The metabolic rate falls and cholesterol starts accumulating in the blood. To face this situation though higher amount of hormone are secreted, they are immediately inactivated by autoimmune reaction. Causes of myxedema include, atrophy of thyroid gland, pituitary deficiency, overdosage with antithyroidal drugs, etc.

Cretinism (Fig. 38.4)

- It is a case of severe hypothyroidism in infant unassociated with a goiter. It involves similar symptoms to that of myxedema and results in neurological, sexual, mental and physical retardations.
- The basal metabolic rate is depressed. It usually occurs in infants having congenital defects in thyroid development.

Treatment

- Myxedema and cretinism, both deficiencies are treated with thyroxine or tri-iodothyronine. The thyroid hormone replacement therapy is reliable and nonallergic.

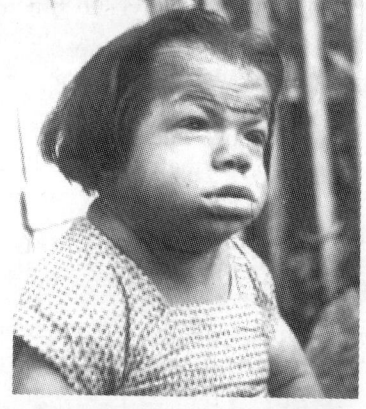

Fig. 38.4: Child with cretinism

- In the treatment of simple goitre, iodides (e.g. potassium iodide) are preferred, while in the treatment of large multinodular goitre, thyroid hormone (L-thyroxine or levothyroxine) preparations may be beneficial.
- Some preparations contain a mixture of both thyroxine and tri-iodothyronine, e.g. Liotrix is a 4:1 mixture of levothyroxine sodium and liothyronine sodium. In therapeutic doses, no adverse reactions are reported.

Hyperthyroidism

Graves' disease (Fig. 38.5), toxic adenoma, toxic multinodular goitre, thyroiditis are some of the diseases of thyroid gland where the gland secretes excessive quantities of hormone. A long acting thyroid stimulator has been isolated from the blood of some patients suffering from hyperactivity of thyroid gland.

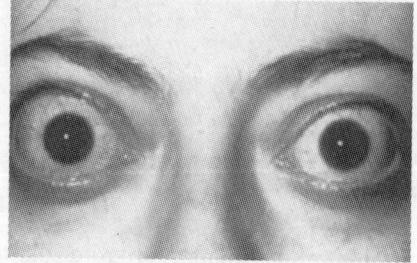

Fig. 38.5: Exophthalamous in Graves disease

Etiology

- This stimulator is a component of the immunoglobulin G fraction of the plasma protein and much behaves like autoantibodies to cause hyperthyroidism.

Symptoms

- The most striking features of hyperthyroidism include, protrusion of the eyeballs with retraction of the upper lids, rise in metabolic rate but the body temperature is not usually raised (extra heat is lost by vasodilation and sweating).
- Metabolism of carbohydrates, fats and proteins increases, leading to an increase in the nitrogen excretion in urine. This results in the general loss of body weight. Skeletal muscle weakness occurs along with tremours. Changes in the cardiovascular system (tachycardia, increase in the pulse rate, arrhythmias) have also been reported.

Treatment

Hyperthyroidism may be treated by reducing the hyperactivity of the thyroid gland. This is achieved by partial thyroidectomy (removal of part of the thyroid gland) or by radioactive iodine or by antithyroid drugs.

▓ DRUGS USED IN HYPERTHYROIDISM

Classification of antithyroid drugs is given in Flow chart 38.1.

Flow chart 38.1: Classification of antithyroid drugs

```
                    ┌─────────────────────┐
                    │  ANTITHYROID DRUGS  │
                    └─────────────────────┘
                              │
                              ▼
┌────────────────┐  ┌──────────────────────────┐  ┌──────────────────────┐
│ Radioactive    │  │ Thioamide derivatives:   │  │ Ionic inhibitors:    │
│ iodine         │  │ Thiourea, thiouracil,    │  │ Potassium perchlorate,│
│                │  │ polythiouracil, methimazole,│ │ thiocyanate          │
│                │  │ cabimazole               │  │                      │
└────────────────┘  └──────────────────────────┘  └──────────────────────┘

┌────────────────────────┐  ┌──────────────────────┐  ┌──────────────────────┐
│ Adrenergic blockers:   │  │ Lithium carbonate:   │  │ Polyhydric phenols:  │
│ Reserpine, Propranolol │  │                      │  │ Resorcinol           │
└────────────────────────┘  └──────────────────────┘  └──────────────────────┘

                    ┌──────────────────────────┐
                    │ Aniline derivatives:     │
                    │ Sulfanilamide, carbutamide,│
                    │ sulphaguanidine          │
                    └──────────────────────────┘
```

Thioamides

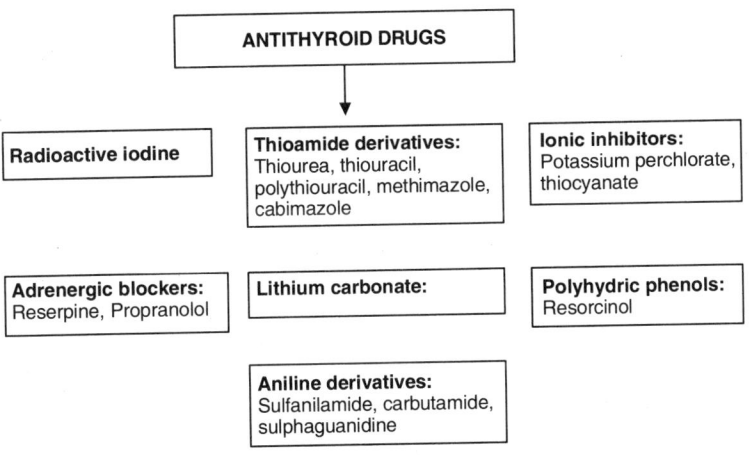

Thiourea   Thiouracil derivatives   Polythiouracil   Carbimazole   Methimazole

Aniline Derivatives

| Sulfanilamide | Sulfaguanidine | P-amino salicylic acid | Carbutamide |

Polyhydric Phenols

Resorcinol

■ RADIOACTIVE IODINE

Mechanism of action

- The radioactive isotope (^{131}I) causes selective depression of thyroid activity by emitting p - rays which effectively destroy some of the secretory parts of the gland.
- Since thyroid gland absorbs most of the iodide supplied to the body other organs remains unaffected. Sodium iodide (^{131}I) is a safe and effective compound which impairs thyroid function by radiation damage.

■ ANTITHYROID DRUGS

- These drugs act by inhibition of the synthesis of thyroid hormone. They exert immediate effect since they act at the first stage of iodine incorporation by the gland.
- They are categorised as under (i) Thioamides, (ii) Aniline derivatives, (iii) Polyhydric phenols, (iv) Ionic inhibitors' that block the uptake of iodine by the gland and (v) Miscellaneous agents.

Thioamides

Mechanism of action

- Thiourea and thiouracil derivatives are among the primary drugs to treat thyroid hyperactivity. The methyl and propylthiouracil are effective drugs.
- They prevent iodine incorporation into the organic form perhaps by antagonizing the iodide oxidation, by peroxidase.
- They are also found to prevent coupling of iodotyrosines to form iodothyronines. They do not influence the breakdown or release of thyroid hormones. Skin rashes and agranulocytosis are the most common side effects of these drugs.

Aniline Derivatives

Mechanism of action

- These agents interfere some of the processes catalyzed by thyroid peroxidase like, iodide oxidation, organisation and coupling of iodo-tyrosines.

- The carbutamide (an oral hypoglycemic agent) interferes in the uptake of iodine. It also interferes with the thyroid peroxidase activity.

Polyhydric Phenols

Mechanism of action

The only clinical agent from this category is resorcinol. It possesses same mechanism of action to that of thioamides.

Ionic Inhibitors

Mechanism of action

- These anions resemble iodide ions and affect the power of thyroid gland to accumulate iodine. Examples include potassium perchlorate and thiocyanate.
- They are inhibitors of the iodide transport into the thyroid gland. Potassium perchlorate sometimes may lead to fatal aplastic anemia. This severely limits its therapeutic value.

Adrenergic Blockers

Mechanism of action

- Because hyperthyroidism has some of the symptoms common with adrenergic overstimulation, the adrenergic blockers are sometimes used in alleviating many of the signs and symptoms of hyperthyroidism, usually in short-term treatment.
- Examples include reserpine, guanethidine and propranolol. They may reduce hyperthyroid-induced tachycardia, tremor, anxiety, sweating and heat intolerance.

Lithium Carbonate

Mechanism of action

Lithium appears to prevent the release of both hormonal and nonhormonal iodines from the thyroid gland. It is less preferred agent due to its adverse effects which include tremors with high risk of cardiac failure.

▨ PARATHYROID HORMONES

Parathyroid Gland (Fig. 38.6)

- The four small parathyroid glands are attached to the surface of thyroid glands. They weigh from 0.05 to 0.3 gm. The normal function of parathyroid glands is to keep the blood calcium level constant. Removal of glands results in the decrease in the plasma calcium level. The parathyroid hormone exerts calcium mobilizing activity and phosphaturic activity (increased excretion of phosphate into urine).
- The homeostatic regulation of extracellular calcium and inorganic phosphate is principally governed by parathyroid hormone (PTH), calcitonin (CT) and various metabolites of vitamin D. Human PTH is a protein composed of 84 amino acids, devoid of disulfide bonds and having a molecular weight of about 9,500.
- Calcitonins are single-chain polypeptides present in parathyroid glands. They all are composed of 32 amino acids with a molecular weight of about 3,600. Various bioactive forms of vitamin D are produced during the metabolic biconversions of vitamin D in liver and skin.

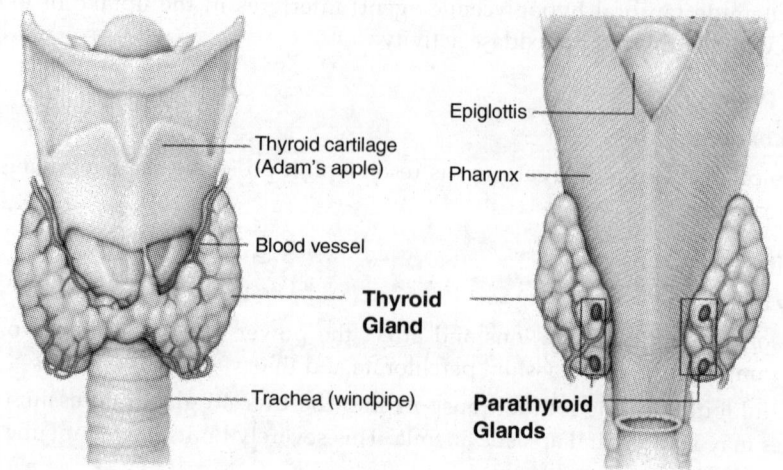

Fig. 38.6: Parathyroid gland

Mechanism of action

The parathyroid hormone acts mainly on kidney, bone and gastrointestinal tract and regulates the plasma calcium level by following ways:

1. Promoting absorption of calcium from gastrointestinal tract.
2. Mobilizing the calcium in the bones.
3. Decreasing calcium excretion in urine, faeces, sweat and milk.

Deficiency

- Deficiency of this hormone leads to fall in the plasma, a calcium ion, which causes tetany. Parathyroid hormone is used therapeutically only for the early control of this tetany.
- Thyrocalcitonin is yet another hormone having opposite action to that of parathyroid hormone. It reduces the circulating calcium levels the plasma calcium exists mainly as: (i) ionized form (50%), (ii) protein bound (45%) and (iii) organic bound form (5%). It is maintained by the proper ratio of parathyroid hormone and thyrocalcitonin.

Methylthiouracil

Ethyl acetoacetate + Thiourea → Methylthiouracil

Carbimazole

Bromoacet-aldehyde ethylene acetal + Methylamine + Potassium thiocyanate → 3-methyl-Δ⁴-imidazol-2-thione → (ethyl chloroformate, pyridine) → Carbimazole

39

Oxytocin and Vasopressin Hormones

Hormones of posterior pituitary lobe, vasopressin and oxytocin are synthesized in the hypothalamous, transported to the posterior pituitary and released in response to specific physiological signal such as high plasma osmolarity or parturition, respectively.

OXYTOCIN

Structure (Figs. 39.1 and 39.3)

- The backbone conformation of the 20-membered cyclic moiety of oxytocin in dimethyl sulfoxide is characterized by 11 β type turn involving the sequence— Tyr-Ile-Gln-Asn. Thus the chain is folded sheet conformation with the disulfide bridge closing the ring and stabilizing the structure. The backbone –NH of the Asn5 residue is hydrogen bonded to the C=O of the Tyr2 residue and provides additional intermolecular stabilization.

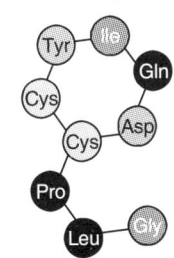

Fig. 39.1: Structure of oxytocin

- The $CONH_2$ terminal tail moiety form a second β-turn (type-I) comprizing residues—Cys-Pro-Leu-Gly, which folds the tail over one side of the ring and is stabilized by another hydroxyl bond between the NH of Leu and the side chain C=O of the Asn5 residue. All peptides bonds are trans configuration.
- During its interaction with receptors, oxytocin is proposed to assume a conformation in which the tyrosine side chain is folded over the 20-membered ring of oxytocin. In this model, the tyrosine hydroxyl group, appears as the predominant active element initiating the oxytoxic response.

Synthesis (Fig. 39.2)

- Du, Vignaeud et al, first synthesized the hormone. The sequence of reactions is shown. A tripeptide (sequence 3-5) was coupled with a tetrapeptide (sequence 6-9) and the ensuring heptapeptide was joined with a disulfide.
- The protecting group was removed by sodium in liquid ammonia. Disulfide bond formation was carried out at high dilution.

Structure–Activity Relationship

1. A 20-membered ring of the neurohypophyseal hormone is essential for bioactivity. Enlargement or loss of activity. Noncyclic structures are inactive.
2. Analogs in which the sulfur atoms for the disulfide bridges are replaced by CH_2 (carbon analogs)exhibit high activity.

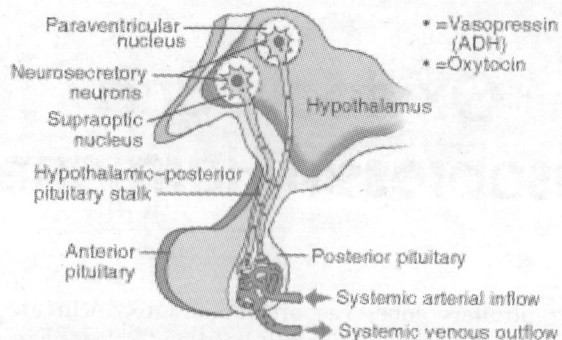

Fig. 39.2: Synthesis and action of oxytocin hormone

3. The hydroxyl group of the tyrosine side chain–folded over the 20-membered ring of the oxytocin acting co-operatively with the aspargine carboxamide group is considered to be the active element.

4. Introduction of 4-L-threonine, 7-glycine increases the oxytocin activity several-thousand fold.

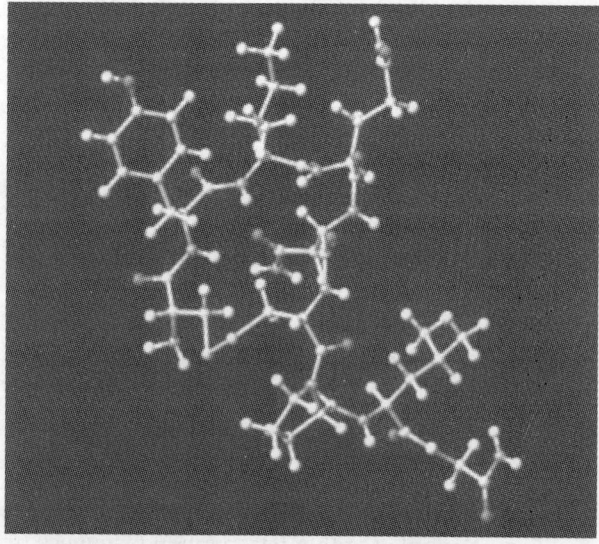

Fig. 39.3: Ball and stick model of oxytocin hormone

Mechanism of Action

- Oxytocin has dual effects in the uterus. It regulates the contractile properties of myometrial cells and elicite prostaglandin production by endometrial decidual cells. These effects are mediated by two distinct receptor subtypes.

- Receptor occupancy has been coupled to activation of phospholipase C and release of intracellular Ca^{++} by inositol-1, 4, 5-trisphosphate as well as direct or depolarization-induced activation of voltage sensitive Ca^{++} channels.

Pharmacokinetics

Oxytocin is effective after administration by any parental route. It can also be given by intranasal spray. The half-life is 5–12 minutes.

Adverse Effect

Due to its weak antidiuretic property, large doses can cause water intoxication with convulsion and coma. Pelvic hematomas and allergic reactions may occur in the mouth.

Uses

Uterus

- Oxytocin stimulates both the frequency and force of contractile activity in uterine smooth muscle.
- Oxytocin is used antepartum when an early vaginal delivery is desired. It is the drug of choice for the maintenance of labor once the pregnancy is at term. It may be used to assist an ongoing abortion.

Mammary Gland

Oxytocin induces contraction of the myoepithelial cells around the breast alveoli, thus squeezing milk into the larger ducts and increasing flow through the nipple and it is occasionally used in the treatment of breast engorgement or to increase milk flow to the sucking infant.

Cardiovascular System

Oxytocin causes a marked but transient relaxation of vascular smooth muscle when large amounts are administered to human beings. It can cause an antidiuretic effect as well. Oxytocin also can suppress the action of ACTH.

▨ VASOPRESSIN (ANTIDIURETIC HORMONE, ADH) (Fig. 39.4)

- Vasopressin is structurally related to oxytocin. With the emergence of life on land, Vasopressin became the mediator of remarkable regulatory system for the conservation of water. Vasopressin is a potent vasopressor and its name was originally chosen in recognition of its vasoconstrictor action. A number of vasopressin-like peptides occurs naturally.

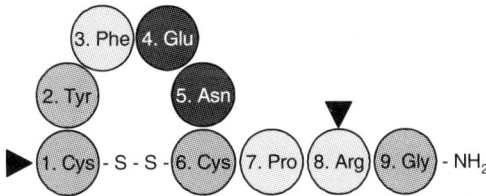

Fig. 39.4: Amino acid of vasopressin

- All are nonapeptides, contain cysteine residues in position 1 and 6; have an intermolecular disulfide-bridge between the two cysteine residues (essential for agonist activity); have additional conserved amino acid in position 5, 7 and 9 (aspargine, proline, and glycine, respectively); contain a basic amino acid in position 8; and are amidated on the carboxyl terminus.

- In all mammals except swine, the neurohypophyseal peptide is 8-arginine vasopressin, and the terms vasopressin, arginine-vasopressin, and antidiuretic hormone are used interchangeably.

Structure–Activity Relationship (Fig. 39.5)

1. New vasopressin analogs have been synthesized with the goals of increasing duration of action and selectivity for vasopressin receptor subtypes.

2. Replacement with various basic amino acids diaminobutyric acid enhances vasopressin activity.

3. Whereas the D-enetiomers of these basic amino acids increase the selectivity for antidiuretic action.

4. Deamination at position 1 increases duration of action and increases antidiuretic activity without increasing vasopressor activity. Desmopressin, 1-diamino-8-D-arginine vasopressin is approximately 3000-fold greater than that for vasopressin. Desmopressin is the preferred drug for the treatment of central diabetes insipidus.

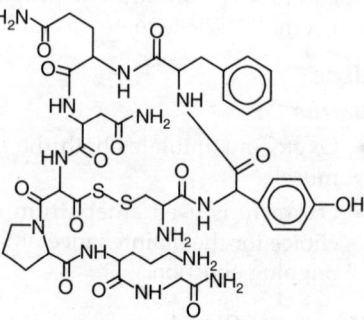

Fig. 39.5: Structure of vasopressin

5. Substitution of valine for glutamine in position for further increases the anti-diuretic selectivity. Deamino (Val4)D-Arg8) AVP has approximately 11,000 fold greater antidiuretic to pressor ratio than that for vasopressin.

6. 1-Deamino, 7-(3, 4-dehydroproline) arginine-vasopressin and [1-deamino, 2-phenylalanine, 7-(-3, 4-dehydroproline), arginine-vasopressin exhibit high anti-diuretic activity.

Mechanism of Action

- There is evidence that two distinct types of receptor (V1 and V2) are responsible for the effects of vasopressin. The renal effect, mediated through V2 receptors, occurs at very low concentration of vasopressin and involves activation of adenylate cyclase and an increase in intracellular cAMP concentration.

- The other effects (e.g. on smooth muscle) mediated through V1 receptors, require much higher concentration and involve intracellular calcium mobilization via the phosphatidylinositol mechanism.

Unit VII

Steroids

Introduction to Steroids

Steroids consist of the 1, 2 – cyclopentanophenanthrene skeleton in which four rings are fused. Rings A, B and C are completely saturated derivative of phenanthrene while D is a five-membered cyclopentane ring.

1, 2-Cyclopentanophenanthrene

NOMENCLATURE, NUMBERING AND STEREOCHEMISTRY

1. Nearly all steroids are named as derivatives of any one of the following basic steroidal rings.

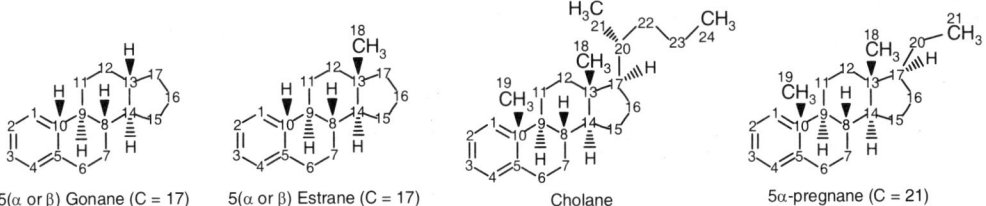

5(α or β) Gonane (C = 17)   5(α or β) Estrane (C = 17)   Cholane   5α-pregnane (C = 21)

2. The ring juncture of backbone carbons are shown in the structure of 5α-cholestane with a dotted line.

3. Solid lines denote group above the plane of the nucleous (β-configuration) and dotted or broken lines denote groups below the plane (α). If the configuration of substituent is unknown, its bond to the nucleus is drawn as wavy line.

5α- cholestane (C=27)

4. The configuration of the H at C-5 is always indicated in the name.

5. Circles were sometimes used to indicate α-hydrogens and dark dots to indicate β-hydrogens.

6. Compounds with 5α-cholestane, belong to allo-series while compounds derived from 5β-cholestane, belong to the normal series.

7. If the double bond is not between sequentially numbered carbons, in such cases both carbons are indicated in the name.

8. When a methyl group is missing from the side chain, this is indicated by the prefix 'nor' with the number of the C-atom, which has disappeared.

505

9. The symbol Δ is often used to designate a C=C bond in a steroid. If C=C is in between carbons 5 and 4, the compound is referred to as Δ^4 – steroid; and if the C=C bond is between position 5 and 10 the compound is designated as $\Delta^{5(10)}$ steroid.

Since 17β-estradiol contains 18 carbon atoms. It is considered as derivatives of estrane, a basic nucleus.

17β-estradiol

Stereochemistry

1. The absolute stereochemistry of the molecule and any substituent is shown with solid (β) and dashed (α) bonds; a (axial) bond is perpendicular to the plane of molecule while (equatorial bond) is horizontal to the plane of the molecule.

2. The aliphatic side chain at position 17 is always assumed to be of β configuration.

5 α-androstane

3. The terms cis and trans are occasionally used to indicate the backbone stereochemistry between rings. For example, 5α-steroids are A/B trans: and 5β-steroids are A/B cis. The terms syn and anti are used analogously to trans and cis.

Conformation

1. Cholestane, androstane and pregnane can exist into two conformations, i.e. chair form and boat form.

5 α– cholestane (in chair form)

2. Chair conformation is more stable than boat conformation due to less angle strain and hence all cyclohexane rings in the steroid nucleus exist in the chair conformation.

Estrogens

The mammalian ovary is a source of steroid hormones that maintain reproductive function. Though ovary is the main site of estrogen secretion in the female, placenta, testes, adrenal cortex, liver, fat, skeletal muscle and hair follicles can form significant quantities of estrogen from the steroid precursors. They are largely responsible for the development of secondary sex characteristics in women at puberty.

OCCURRENCE, BIOSYNTHESIS AND METABOLISM

• Estrogen is produced in the female by the ovary, placenta and adrenal cortex and in the male by the testis and adrenal cortex. Some other tissue, such as liver muscle, fat and hair follicles, can also convert steroid precursor into estrogen.

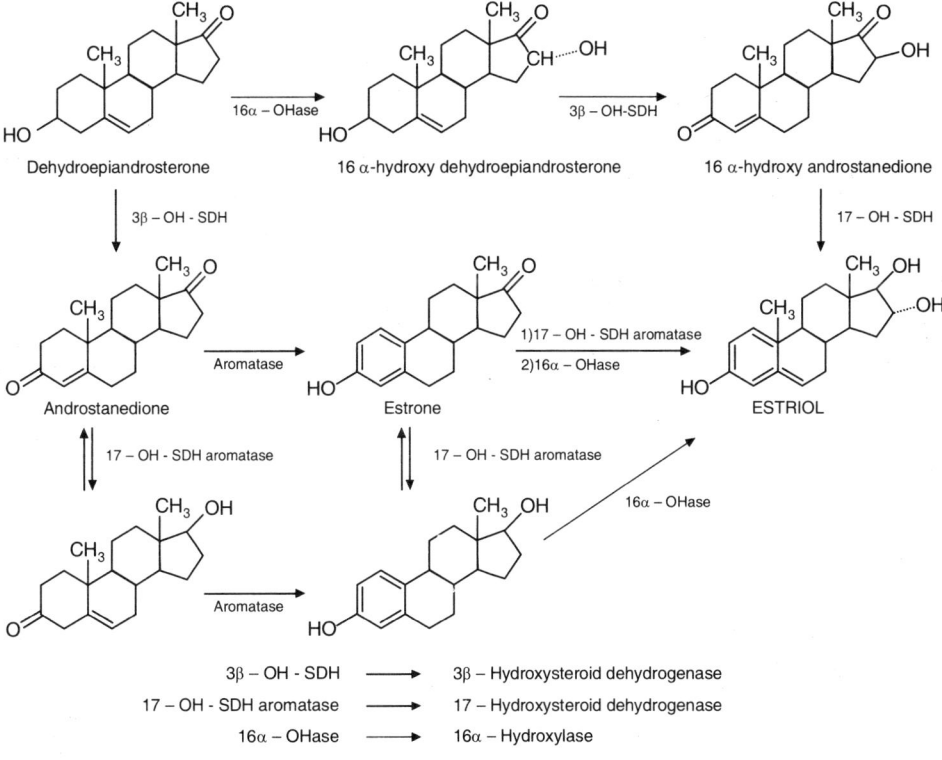

- The starting substance for estrogen biosynthesis is cholesterol. The immediate precursor to the estrogen is androgenic substances androstanedione or testosterone. The most significant reaction is aromatization of ring A of the steroid molecule.
- This reaction is catalysed in three steps by a mono-oxygenase enzyme complex that uses NADPH and molecular oxygen as co-substrates. In the first step of this reaction, C19 the angular methyl group on C10 of the androgen precursor is hydroxylated. A second hydroxylation results in the elimination of the newly formed C19 hydroxymethyl group, and a final hydroxylation of C-2 results in the formation of unstable intermediate that rearranges to form phenolic A ring. The entire reaction consumes three molecules of oxygen and three molecules of NADPH.
- Aromatase activity resides within a transmembrane glycoprotein CP450 family of mono-oxygenase; a ubiquitous flavoprotein, NADPH-cytochrome P450 reductase, also is essential. Both proteins are localized in the endoplasmic reticulum of ovarian granulse cells, testicular Sertoli and Leyding cells, stromal cells of adipose tissue, placental and various brain regions.
- Secreted estradiol is oxidized reversibily to estrone by 17-hydroxyl steroid dehydrogenase and both of these estrogens can be converted to estriol. Another significant alteration of estrones is its conversion to 2-hydroxyestrone, which is further metabolized to 2-methoxy 1 estrone.

▒ PHARMACOKINETIC ASPECT

- Both the natural and synthetic oestrogen used in the therapy are well absorbed in the gastrointestinal tract, but after absorption the natural estrogens are rapidly metabolized in the liver, whereas the synthetic estrogens and non-steroidal estrogens like compounds are less rapidly degraded.
- Most estrogens are readily absorbed from skin and mucous membranes and can be given topically in the vagina as creams. In the plasma, natural estrogen is bound to albumin and to sex steroid binding globulin. Natural oestrogens are excreted in the urine as glucuronides and sulfate.

▒ PHARMACOLOGICAL ACTION

- Estrogens stimulate the development of the secondary sexual characteristics and the phase of accelerated growth. Their main use in adult women is for oral contraception. They may also be used to reduce menopausal symptoms associated with the decline in estrogen production, hot flush, palpitation and atrophic virginities. They decrease postmenopausal osteoporosis.
- Estrogen causes some degree of retention of salts and water. They have mild anabolic action. Estrogens increase the coagulability of the blood.

▒ CLINICAL USES

Estrogen may be used for:

1. Replacement therapy, to treat menopausal symptom, or for post-menopausal replacement therapy.
2. Contraception.
3. Therapy of prostatic cancer and for some cases of breast cancer in postmenopausal patients.
4. Menstrual diseases such as dysmenorrhea.
5. Suppression of lactation.
6. Acne.
7. Vaginitis (topical oestrogen is used).
8. Osteoporosis.

ADVERSE EFFECT

- In general, the unwanted effects of estrogen are tenderness in the breast, nausea, vomiting, anorexia, alteration of carbohydrate metabolism and retention of salt and water with resultant edema.
- Long-term use in postmenopausal also increases the risk of gallbladder disease and endometrial carcinoma. When administered to male, estrogens result in feminization.

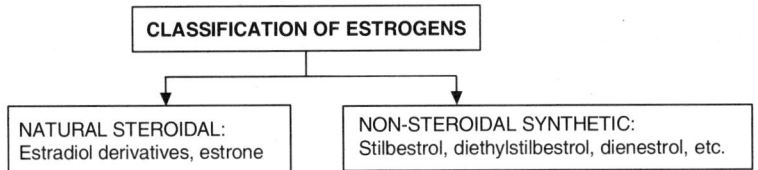

Natural Steroidal Estrogens

Estradiol

Estradiol valerate

Estradiol cypionate

Estradiol dipropionate

Estradiol benzoate

Ethinyl estradiol

Mestranol

Quinestrol

Estrone

Estriol

Synthetic or Non-steroidal Esterogens

Diethylstilbestrol

Chlorotrianisene

Dienestrol

Benzestrol   Trans-stilbene   Hexestrol   Methallenestrill

Structure–Activity Relationship

1. 17β-estradiol is potent estrogenic agent. Many structural modification of 17β-estradiol were carried out since it rapidly gets oxidized to estrone, in liver and hence ineffective orally. Adding a 17β-alkyl group (particularly 17β-ethinyl derivative) to estradiol blocks this oxidation and makes the compound orally active. Another estrogen, synthesized by this similar route is mestranol which is used in oral contraceptives.

2. The esterification of 17β-hydroxy and 3-hydroxy function also prolongs the duration where slow rate of absorption is due to low water solubility. 3-benzoate; 3,17-dipropionate, 17-valerate and 17-cyclopentylpropionate are the most commonly used ester forms. Slow hydrolysis of these esters releases the free estrogen over a prolonged period of time, hence ester forms are termed as prodrug.

3. Steroidal nucleus is not an essential feature of estrogenic activity, e.g. plant estrogen like genistein and coumestrol.

Genistein   Zearalenone   Allenolic acid   Coumestrol

4. The intensity of activity changes if route of administration is changed, e.g. for oral route:
   Estriol>Estradiol>Estrone
   For subcutaneous route: Estradiol> Estrone> Estriol

5. Substitution on estrone nucleus significantly modifies the estrogenic activity.

6. Insertion of hydroxyl groups at 6, 7 and 11 positions reduces the activity.

7. Removal of oxygen function at 3 and 17 position or epimerization to α configuration results in less active compounds.

8. Introduction of unsaturation in ring β reduces the activity.

9. Expansion of ring D in both, estradiol and estrone greatly reduces the estrogenic activity.

10. If ring D is removed in estrone or estradiol, activity remains the same, e.g. estradiol on treatment with strong base gives doisynolic acid which has same activity as that of estradiol. Hence ring D is not necessary for the activity.

11. According to Schueler, hypothesis to have optimal estrogenic activity, a molecule should have a distance of about 8.55 Å between the groups that can form H-bonds (e.g. ketones, phenolic and alcoholic hydroxyl groups). The activity of non-

D - homoestradiol

Doisynolic acid

steroidal synthetic estrogens can be explained on this hypothesis, this critical distance is 12.1Å and in estradiol it is 10.9Å.

12. Many other potent steroidal and non-steroidal estrogens confirm this hypothesis.

13. A number of heterocyclic analogues of the estrogens (steroidal) are being prepared and evaluated biologically. Among the most common are the aza analogs. The –NH- group is isosteric to a methylene group.

METABOLISM

1. The three primary estrogens in women are 17β-estradiol, estrone and estriol. These hormones are metabolized mainly in liver and are largely excreted as water soluble glucuronide conjugates.

Sodium glucuronide of estriol

2. Other tissues such as kidney and intestine may also act as sites of metabolism. 17β-estradiol first gets oxidized to estrone, which upon further oxidation, gives estriol, the major estrogen found in human urine.

3. 2 Hydroxy and 2-methoxy metabolites are also found in considerable amounts. Bile also serves as the route of excretion but estrogens and their various metabolites, excreted through bile may be reabsorbed so that several days are required for complete excretion of a given dose.

MODE OF ACTION

• Cellular components of uterus are responsible for the binding of estrogens. At the subcellular level, estradiol binds with both the cytoplasmic portion and nucleus of the cell. The uptake and transportation of estrogens is governed by extranuclear receptors while estrogen retention and growth initiation is controlled by nuclear receptors.

• Estrogen increases the synthesis of RNA in the target cells. This RNA is thought to be responsible for several uterine effects that are seen with normal estrogen stimulation. The increased RNA synthesis eventually leads to an increase in the synthesis of specific proteins which affect the activity of various enzyme systems.

Diethylstilbestrol

Anethole

HBr, toluene
Hydrogen bromide

1. NaNH$_2$, NH$_3$, – 80°C
2. KOH, glycol, 224°C

1. Sodium amide

Diethylstibestrol

Dienestrol

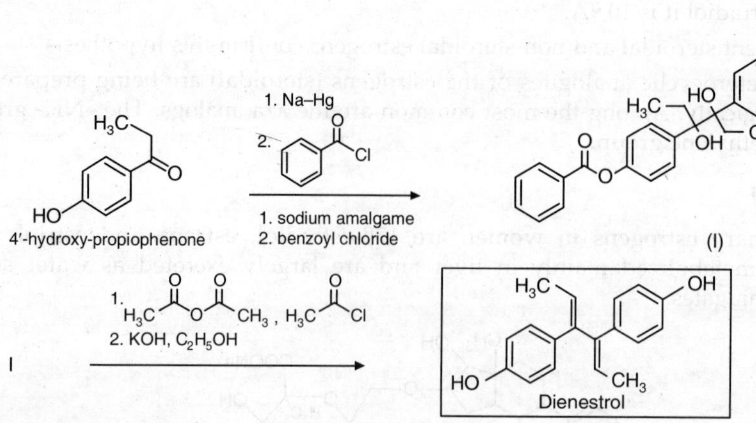

4′-hydroxy-propiophenone

1. Na–Hg

2. benzoyl chloride

1. sodium amalgame
2. benzoyl chloride

(I)

I

1. H_3C—CO—O—CO—CH_3 , H_3C—CO—Cl
2. KOH, C_2H_5OH

Dienestrol

Chlorotrianisene

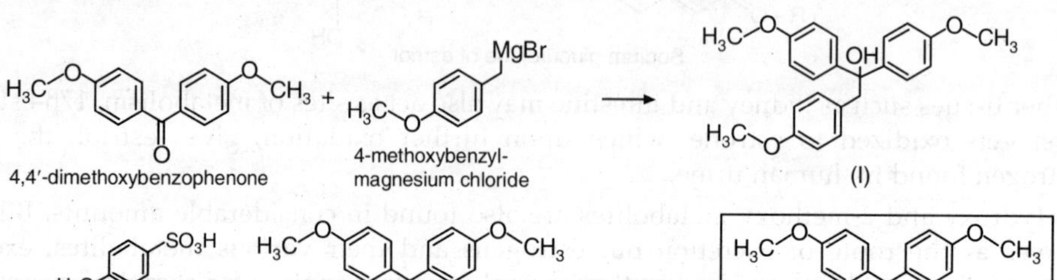

4,4′-dimethoxybenzophenone + 4-methoxybenzyl-magnesium chloride

(I)

I

SO_3H / H_3C

Cl_2, CCl_4

Chlorotrianisene

Quinestrol

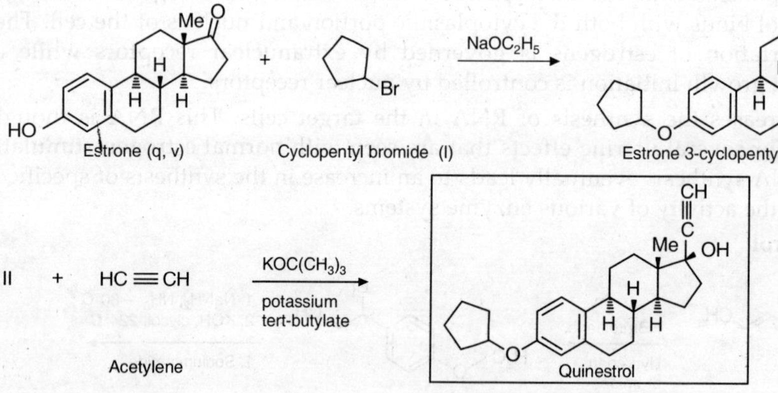

Estrone (q, v) + Cyclopentyl bromide (I)

$NaOC_2H_5$

Estrone 3-cyclopentyl ether (II)

II + HC≡CH

$KOC(CH_3)_3$

potassium tert-butylate

Acetylene

Quinestrol

Estrone

Androstenolone

H_2, Pd–C

CrO_3

Chromium (VI) oxide

Br_2, CH_3COOH

bromine

I

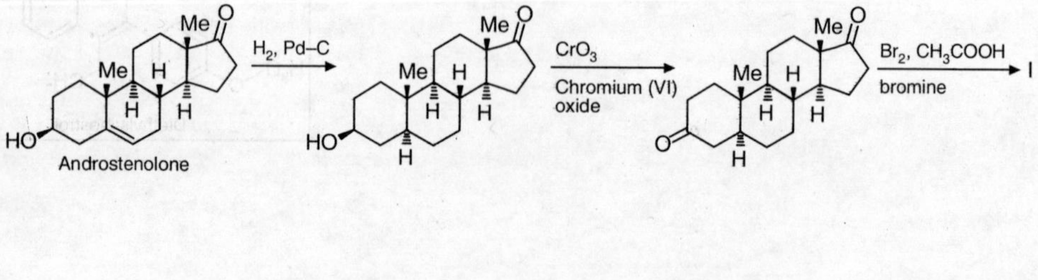

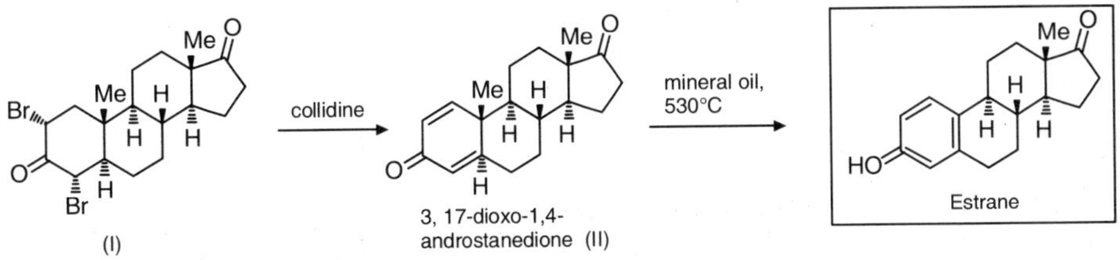
(I)
collidine
3, 17-dioxo-1,4-androstanedione (II)
mineral oil, 530°C
Estrane

Mestranol

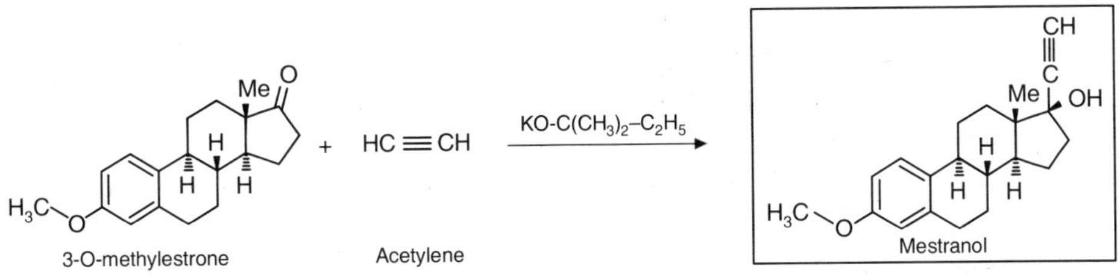
3-O-methylestrone
Acetylene
KO-C(CH3)2–C2H5
Mestranol

Estradiol

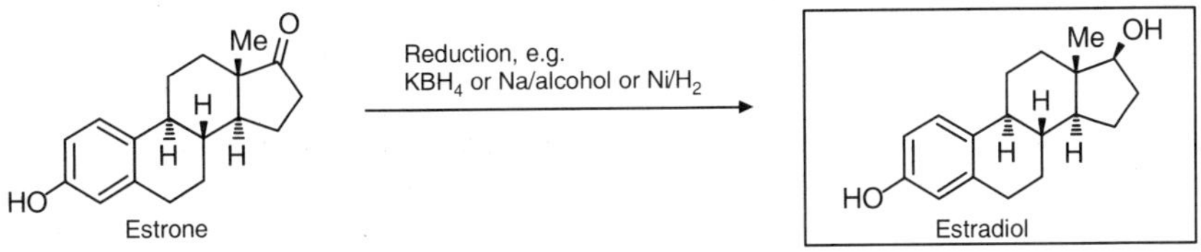
Estrone
Reduction, e.g.
KBH4 or Na/alcohol or Ni/H2
Estradiol

Estradiol Benzoate

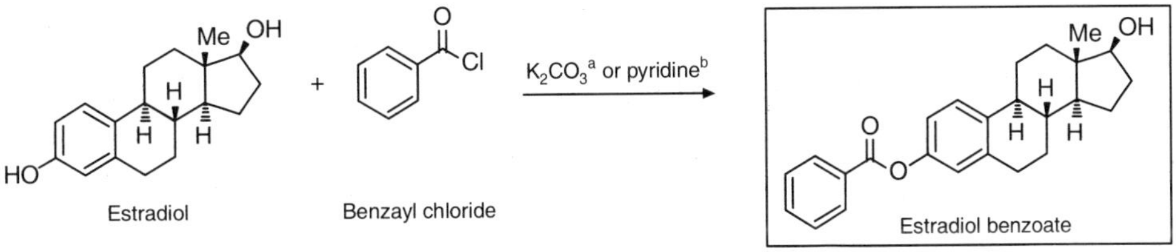
Estradiol
Benzayl chloride
K2CO3a or pyridineb
Estradiol benzoate

Estradiol Cypionate

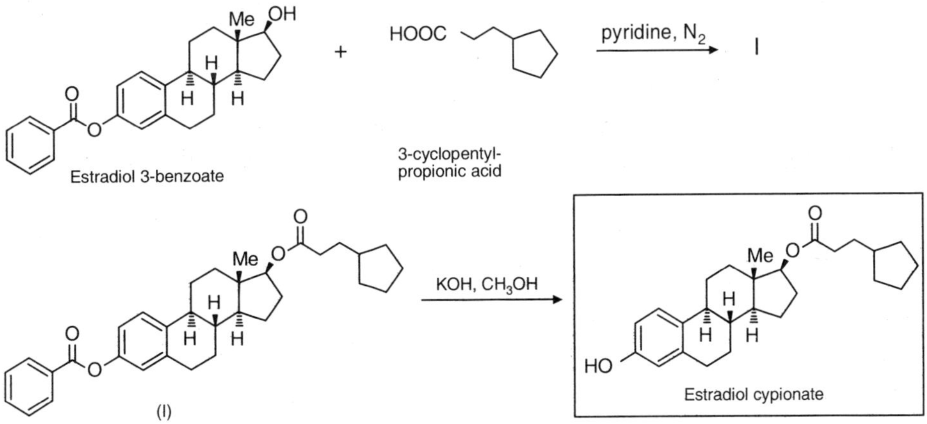
Estradiol 3-benzoate
3-cyclopentyl-propionic acid
pyridine, N2
I
(I)
KOH, CH3OH
Estradiol cypionate

Progesterones

The natural progestational hormone or progestagen is progesterone, which is secreted mainly by the corpus luteum in the second part of menstrual cycle. Small amounts are also secreted by the testis in the male and the adrenal cortex in both the sexes, and large amounts are secreted by the placenta. Corner and Allen (1933) originally isolated a hormone from the corpora lutea of cows, named it "progestin".

BIOSYNTHESIS

- The corpus luteum, which is formed from the ruptured follicle after ovulation, starts the secretion of progesterone, which is responsible for the maintenance of vascularity of uterine endometrium.

- The corpus luteum continues the secretion of progesterone to suppress the secretion of the FSH and LH by feedback inhibitory mechanism and thus prevent ovulation during pregnancy. It also inhibits the release of oxytocin which causes uterine contraction, thus avoiding dislodgement of the fertilized egg or embryo.

Progesterone

19-nortestosterone

- Progesterone is naturally secreted by corpus luteum and placenta. It is also synthesized by the adrenal glands and testes, where it acts as a precursor of various steroidal hormones. The placental progesterone besides having its physiological effects on maternal organs also acts as an important precursor for fetal corticosteroids and androgens.

- Progesterone is rapidly metabolized to 5β-pregnenediol glucuronide. The measurement of urinary excretion of this metabolite can be used as an index of corpus luteum and placenta activity and a premature drop in its urine level of a pregnant woman may be warning for possible abortion.

5 β-pregnanediol glucuronide

514

- The 19-nortestosterone derivatives have marked ovulation-inhibiting activity and thus can be used as oral contraceptive along with progestins. The weak androgenic property can be reduced by the structural modification.

PHARMACOLOGICAL ACTION

Reproductive Tracts

- Progesterone released during the luteal phase of the cycle decreases estrogen driven endometrial proliferation and leads to the development of a secondary endometrium. The abrupt decline in the release of progesterone from the corpus luteum at the end of the cycle is the main determinant of the onset of menstruation.
- The estrogen-induced maturation of the human vaginal epithelium is modified toward condition of pregnancy by the action of progesterone. It is very important for the maintenance of pregnancy. Major action of the hormone as to suppress menstruation and uterine contractility.

Mammary Gland

- Progestins have the ability to stimulate development of the glandular portion of the mammae. During pregnancy and to a minor degree during the luteal phase of the cycle, progesterone acting with estrogen brings about a proliferation of the acini fill with secretion and the vasculature of the gland is notably increased.
- During the normal menstrual cycle, mitotic activity in the breast epithelium is very low in the follicular phase and then peaks in the luteal phase. This pattern is due to progesterone, which triggers a single round of mitotic activity in the mammary epithelium.

Metabolic effects

Progesterone increases basal insulin levels. It also stimulated lipoprotein lipase activity and seems to enhance fat depositions.

CNS effects

Throughout menstrual cycle, an increase of temperature about 1° F may be noted at midcycle, this correlate with ovulation. This increase in temperature is clearly due to progesterone. It may also have depressant and hypnotic actions in the CNS.

THERAPEUTIC APPLICATION

1. It prevents habitual abortion.
2. For treatment of functional uterine bleeding resulting due to the lack of estrogen and progesterone.
3. For treatment of dysmenorrhea or painful menstruation. In order to produce more closely condition, which are seen in normal menstrual cycle. Estrogen used in the treatment of dysmenorrhea may be supplemented with progestins during the last four days of each period.
4. Pregnancy diagnosis.
5. Oral contraceptive.
6. For treatment of advanced carcinoma of breast.
7. To treat premature discomfort in the breasts.

▨ CLASSIFICATION OF PROGESTERONE

Flow chart 40.1 depicts the classification of progesterone.

Flow chart 40.1: Classification of progesterone

```
                        ┌─────────────────┐
                        │ CLASSIFICATION  │
                        └─────────────────┘
```

TESTOSTERONE DERIVATIVES	PROGESTERONE DERIVATIVES	19-NORTESTOSTERONE DERIVATIVES

| Ethisterone | Esteres of 17α-hydroxy- progesterone derivatives: 17α-Acetoxyprogesterone, 17α Hydroxyprogesterone - 17 caproate, Retroprogesterone, Dydrogesterone | 19-Nortestosterone, Norethynodrel, Norgestrel, Norgestimate |

C_6–Substituted 17α-hydroxy-progesterone derivatives: Medroxy progesterone acetate, Megestrol acetate

Dehydrogesterons:- Chlormadinone acetate, Dehydrogesterone

Progesterone Derivatives

A. Esteres of 17 α-Hydroxyprogesterone derivatives

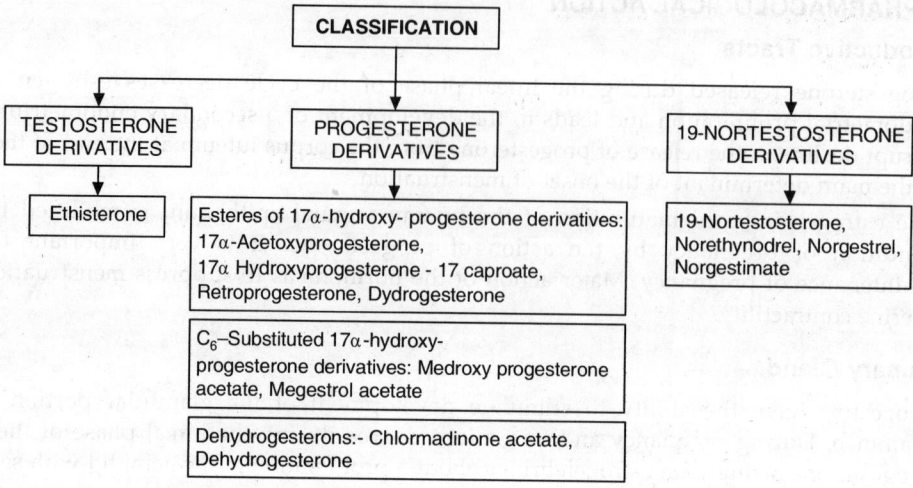

17α - Acetoxyprogesterone

17α - Acetoxyprogesterone - 17 caproate

Retroprogesterone

Dydrogesterone

16α, 17-dihydroxyprogesterone acetophenide

B. C_6 – Substituted 17 α-Hydroxyprogesterone Derivatives

Medroxy progesterone acetate

Megestrol acetate

C. Dehydrogestrones

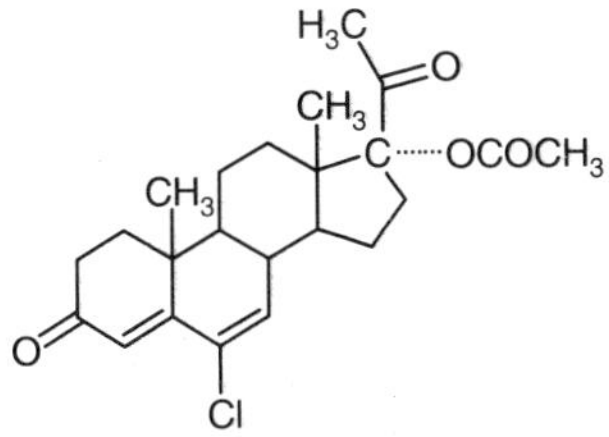

Chlomadinone acetate

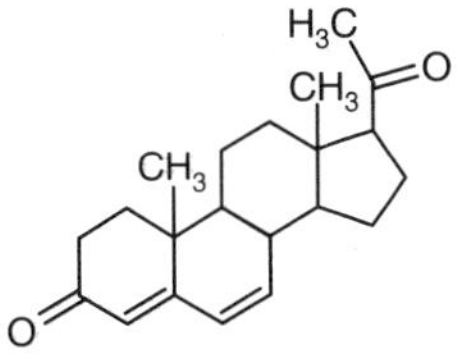

Dehydroprogesterone

Testosterone Derivatives

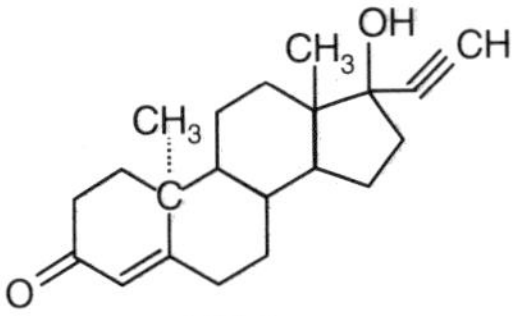

Ethisterone

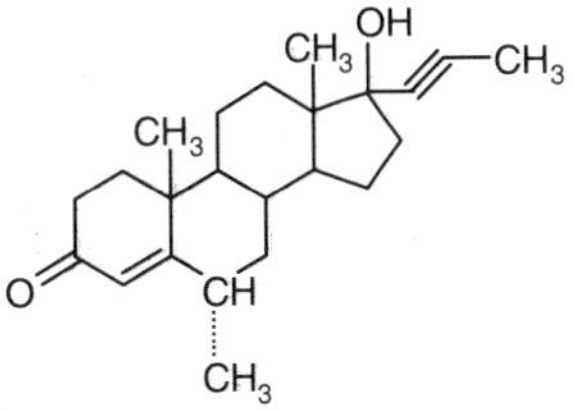

Dimethisterone

19-Nortestosterone Derivatives

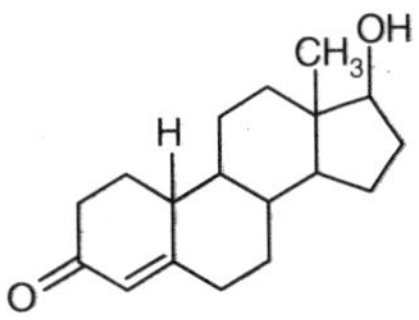

19-Nortestosterone

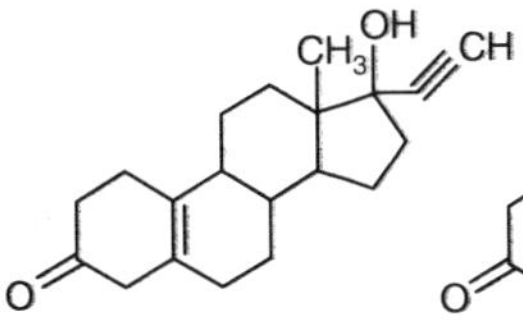

Norethynodrel

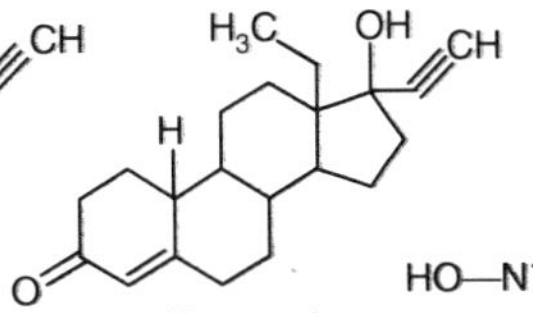

Norgestrel

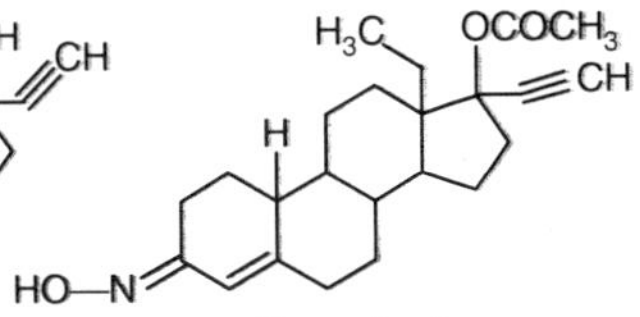

Norgestimate

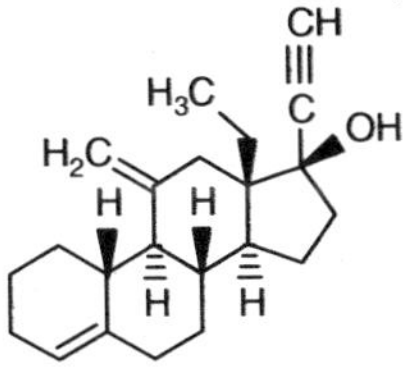

Desogestrel

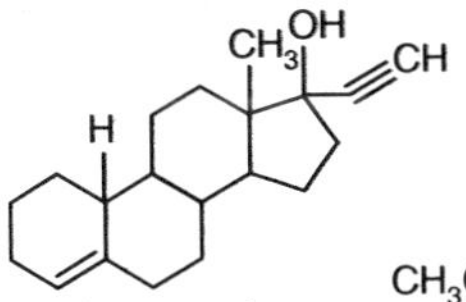

Lynesternol

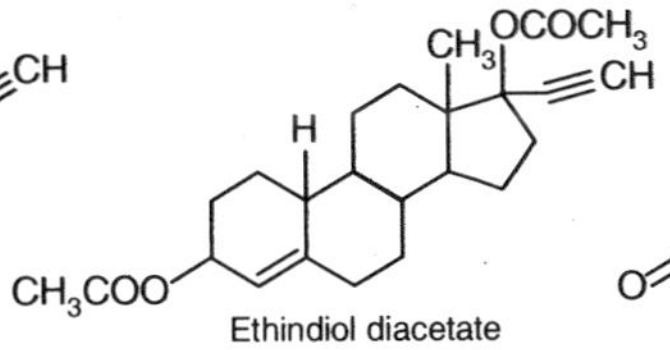

Ethindiol diacetate

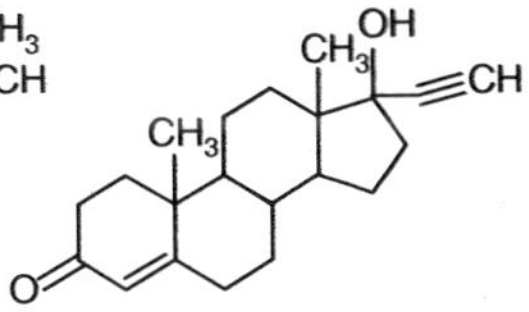

Ethisterone

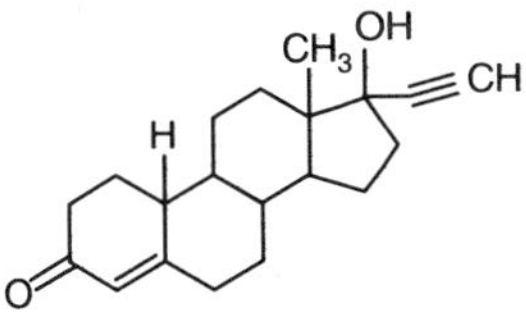

Norethisterone

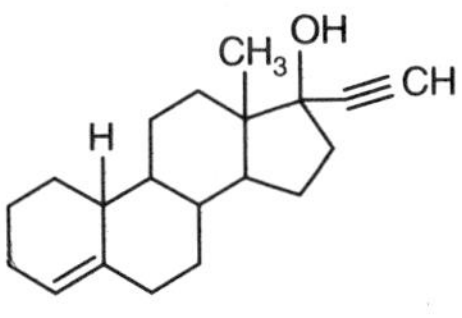

Lynesternol

▓ STRUCTURE–ACTIVITY RELATIONSHIP

SAR or Progesterone Derivatives

Esteres of 17 α-Hydroxyprogesterone

1. Since the natural hormone progesterone, has a very low potency when administered orally, its ester derivatives were prepared which have good oral activity.

17α–Acetoxyprogesterone

17α–Acetoxyprogesterone -17 caproate

Activity of 17α-hydroxyprogesteron can be increased by;

17α–Hydroxyprogesterone

2. Unsaturation at positions 6 and 7.

3. Substitution of a methyl group or a halogen atom at 6th carbon.

4. Introducing a methyl group at position 11. The above modification probably prevents metabolic reduction of two carbonyl groups and metabolic oxidation at position 6.

5. Substitution of a fluro group at position 21 prevents hydroxylation at this point and enhances the oral effectiveness.

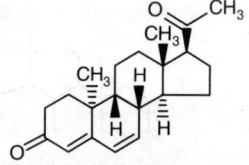

6. Inversion of the configuration at positions 10 and 19 in progesterone leads to retroprogesterone, which is more active parenterally and orally than progesterone.

Retroprogestron

7. Further unsaturation at positions 6 and 7 gives dehydrogesterone which is orally active.

Dehydrogesterone

8. A progestin with a prolonged duration of action is 16α, 17-dihydroprogesterone acetophenide, which is devoid of androgenic and estrogenic activities when given parenterally.

16α, 17-dihydroprogesterone acetophenide

C6 –Substituted 17α-Hydroxyprogesterone derivatives

Further structural modification of 17a-hydroxyprogesterone at sixth carbon, hinders the catabolism of the compounds and increase their lipid solubility, resulting in enhanced biological effect, e.g. medroxyprogesterone acetate and megestrol acetate.

Medroxyprogesterone acetate   Megestrol acetate

Dehydrogesterones

Progestational activity is further enhanced by introducing a double bond between carbon 6 and 7 in substituted 17α-hydroxyprogesterone derivatives.

Chlomadinone acetate   Dehydroprogesterone

SAR of Testosterone Derivatives

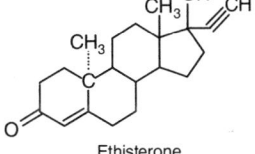

Ethisterone

1. The first synthetic progestin, ethisterone, was prepared by Inhoffen et al in 1937 in an attempt to find an orally active androgen but later proved to be effective an oral progestin.

2. Ethisterone became the first orally effective progestogen. However, its oral activity is still low.

3. In dimethisterone which is a modified structure of ethisterone, introduction of CH_3 groups in the C-6α and C-21 positions, enhance progestational activity.

Dimethisterone

SAR of 19-Nortestosterone Derivatives

1. Ethrenstein in 1944 found that the C-19 methyl group is not essential for progestational activity, which leads to this new series of progestins, e.g. 19-nortestosterone, norethynodrel, norgestrel, etc.

19-Nortestosterone Norethynodrel Norgestrel Norgestimate

Desogestrel Lynesternol Ethindiol diacetate

2. Introduction of an alkyl group at C-17 of 19-nortestosterone blocks its oxidation to inactivate compounds and increases its progestational activity.

19 - Nortestosterone

3. As in 17α-ethinyl analog, increasing its electron density at C-17, one can simultaneously decrease its anabolic activity and promote good progestational activity, e.g. ethisterone. Ethisterone is an orally effective progestin, with slight androgenic activity.

Ethisterone

4. Removal of 19 –CH₃ group (19-nor analog) further decreases its androgenic activity, e.g. norethisterone.

Norethisterone

5. Following modification of 19-nortestosterone leads to even more effective progestins.

   1. Substituting a chlorine atom at C-21.

   2. Adding methyl group at C-18, e.g. norgestrel.

   3. Unsaturation of the ring B or C.

   4. Introduction of halogen or methyl at 6α or 7α position.

Norgestrel

5. Acetylation of the 17β- OH results in longer duration of action.
6. Removal of the keto function at C-3

Lynesternol

SAR of 11-Substituted Analogues

1. Bulky 11β-substituents induce through 1,3-diaxial interaction with 18-methyl group, a change in the shape of the steroid skeleton leading to better binding to the progesterone receptor and decreased binding to serum proteins. This enhances the potency of the compound.
2. By contrast, long substituent interferes with the receptor binding and so decreases the potency. The potent 11-substituted analogues were studied for their selectivity of action and this led to the selection of desogestrel for further development.

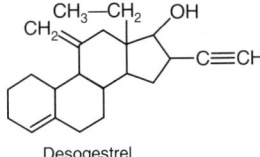

Desogestrel

MODE OF ACTION

1. Progesterone has a biphasic feedback effect on ovulation, i.e. first it stimulates ovulation process and effects of estrogens. Following this initial phase, however, ovulation and estrogenic effects are inhibited.
2. It has blocking effect on the rhythmic contractions of myometrium.
3. It potentiates the synthesis of only one specific oviduct protein, avidin.
4. To induce above effects, progesterone may require gene activation and transcription of chromosomal information through the stimulated m-RNA synthesis.

Pharmacological Actions

• It acts on both, the endometrium (inner mucous lining of uterus) and the myometrium (muscle mass of uterus). It induces the secretory phase in endometrium during which the endometrial glands grow and secrete large amount of carbohydrate that will possibly be utilized by the fertilized ovum as a source of energy.
• On myometrium, progesterone stops the spontaneous rhythmic contraction of the uterus to prevent abortion.

SIDE EFFECTS

• The commonly associated side effects with progestin therapy are—nausea, vomiting, drowsiness, edema, irregular bleeding.

Progesterone

Pregnenolone

cyclo-hexanone   aluminum triisopropylate

Progesterone

Hydroxyprogesterone Caproate

17-hydroxyprogesterone + Caproic anhydride → Hydroxyprogesterone caproate (Tos–OH)

Medroxyprogesterone Acetate

5α, 17α-dihydroxy-3,20-dioxo-6β-methyl-pregnane → 17-hydroxy-6α-methylprogesterone (I) (HCl, CHCl₃)

I + acetic anhydride → Medroxyprogesterone acetate (CH₃COOH, Tos–OH)

Megestrol Acetate

Medroxyprogesterone → Megestrol (I)

I + acetic anhydride → Megestrol acetate (Tos–OH)

Norethisterone

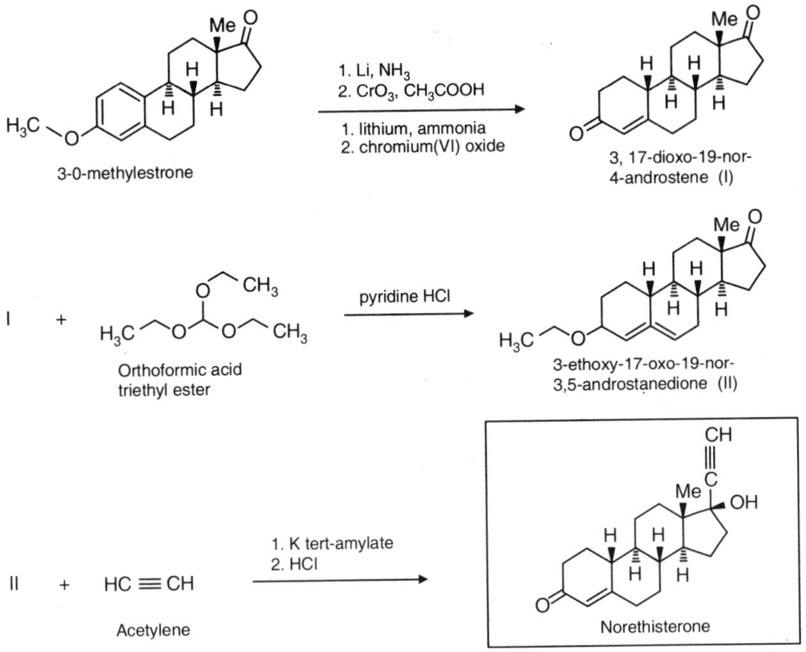

3-0-methylestrone

1. Li, NH₃
2. CrO₃, CH₃COOH

1. lithium, ammonia
2. chromium(VI) oxide

3, 17-dioxo-19-nor-
4-androstene (I)

I +

Orthoformic acid
triethyl ester

pyridine HCl

3-ethoxy-17-oxo-19-nor-
3,5-androstanedione (II)

II + HC≡CH

Acetylene

1. K tert-amylate
2. HCl

Norethisterone

Desogestrel

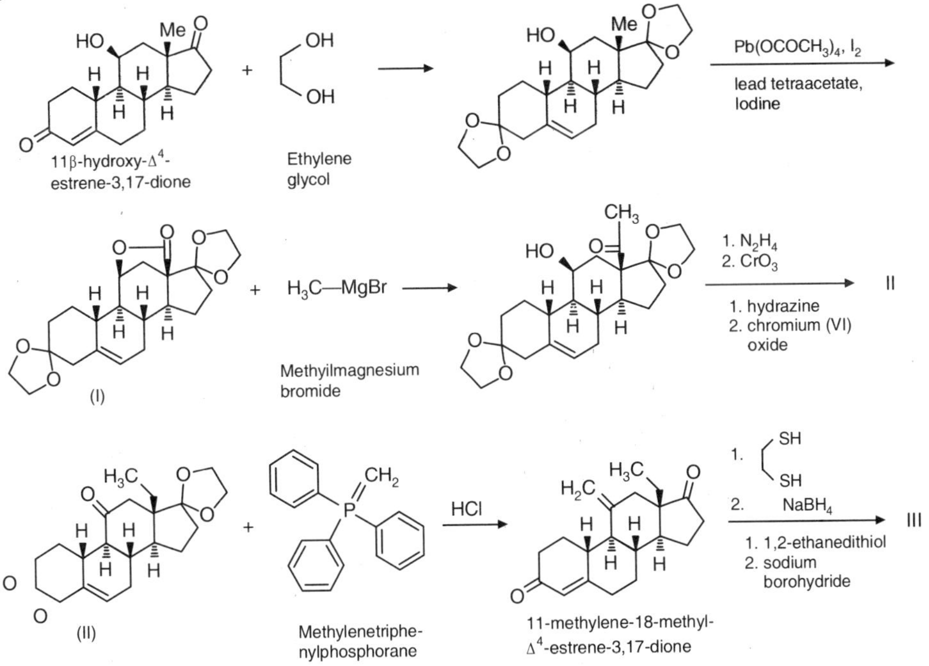

11β-hydroxy-Δ⁴-
estrene-3,17-dione

Ethylene
glycol

Pb(OCOCH₃)₄, I₂

lead tetraacetate,
Iodine

(I) + H₃C—MgBr

Methyilmagnesium
bromide

1. N₂H₄
2. CrO₃

1. hydrazine
2. chromium (VI)
oxide

II

(II) +

Methylenetriphe-
nylphosphorane

HCl

11-methylene-18-methyl-
Δ⁴-estrene-3,17-dione

1.

2. NaBH₄

1. 1,2-ethanedithiol
2. sodium
borohydride

III

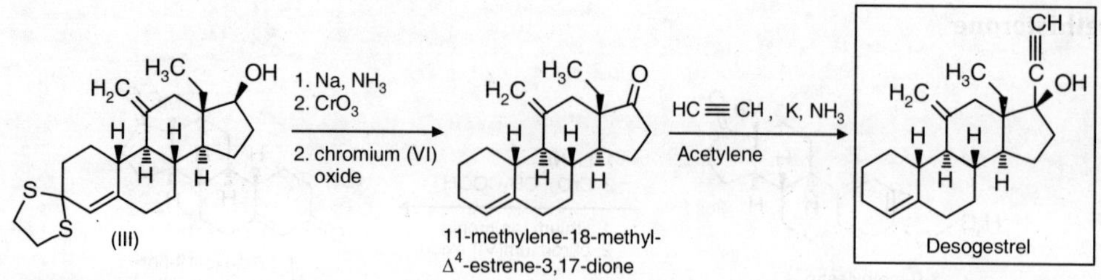
1. Na, NH_3
2. CrO_3
2. chromium (VI) oxide
(III)
11-methylene-18-methyl-Δ^4-estrene-3,17-dione
$HC \equiv CH$, K, NH_3
Acetylene
Desogestrel

Norgestrel

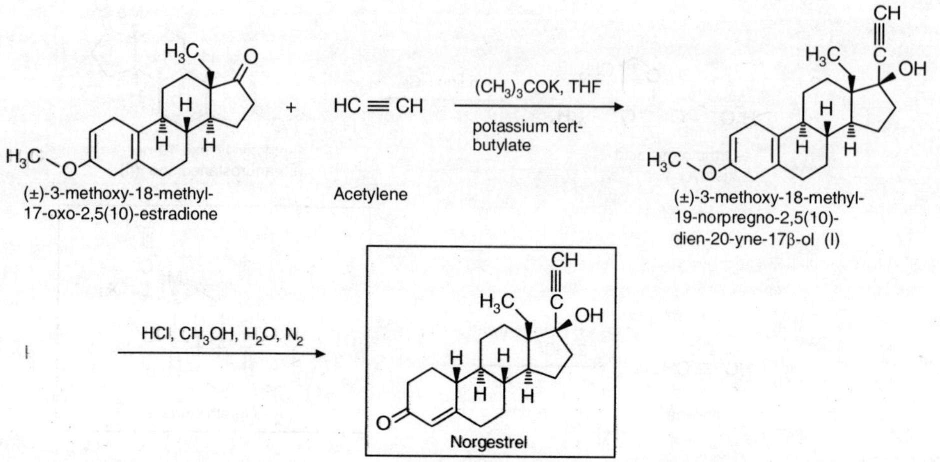
(±)-3-methoxy-18-methyl-17-oxo-2,5(10)-estradione
+
$HC \equiv CH$
Acetylene
$(CH_3)_3COK$, THF
potassium tert-butylate
(±)-3-methoxy-18-methyl-19-norpregno-2,5(10)-dien-20-yne-17β-ol (I)
I
HCl, CH_3OH, H_2O, N_2
Norgestrel

43

Androgen and Anabolic Agents

Androgen or male sex hormones are synthesized from cholesterol in the testes and adrenal cortex. In the liver, androgens are formed from C-21 steroids.

BIOSYNTHESIS (Fig. 43.1)

- Testosterone is secreted by the testis and is the main androgen in the plasma of men. In women, testosterone is synthesized in small amount by both ovary and adrenal gland.

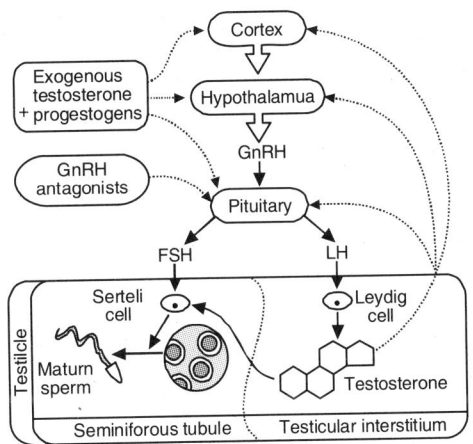

Fig. 43.1: Biosynthesis of testosterone

- In man, the gonadotropin releasing hormone (GnRH) controls the secretion of gonadotropin by the anterior pituitary.
- Follicular stimulating hormone (FSH) is responsible for the integrity of the seminiferous tubules and after puberty is important in gametogenesis through action on the sertoli cell, which nourishes and supports the developing spermatozoa. LH, which in the male is also called "interstial cell stimulating hormone (ICSH)", stimulates the interstitial cells, to secrete 'Testosterone' a male gonadotropic hormone, responsible for anabolic effect, fertility, bone growth.

PHARMACOKINETIC ASPECTS

- Virtually all testosterone in the circulation is bound to plasma protein mainly to the sex steroid-binding globulin. The half-life of free testosterone is 10–20 minutes. It is inactivated in liver by conversion to androstanedione which is having weak androgenic activity and 90% of its metabolite is excreted in urine.

- Testosterone is reduced at the 5α-position to dihydrotestosterone, which serve as intracellular mediator of most action of the hormone. Dihydrotestosterone binds to the intracellular androgen receptor protein more tightly than does testosterone, and the dihydrotestosterone-receptor complex is more stable than the testosterone-receptor complex; its greater androgenic potency is thereby explained. Testosterone also can be aromatized to estradiol in a variety of extraglandular tissue, a pathway that accounts for most estrogen system in men and postmenopausal women. Other interactive metabolites include androsterone and etiocholanone.

THERAPEUTIC USES

1. Introduction of puberty and maintenance of sex characteristics an adult with testicular failure, accidental castration, or hypogonadism.
2. Stimulation of erythropoietin secretion in some types of refractory anemia.
3. Introduction of anabolic effects (weight gain) in under nourished patient or in the terminally ill (drug abuse professional athletes).
4. Replacement therapy in women with hypopituitarism; androgens are given in conjuction with other hormones (i.e. thyroid, growth, adrenal corticosteroid, estrogen hormones).
5. Breast cancer therapy because of its antiestrogenic effects.
6. Treatment of short stature not due to pituitary insufficiency.
7. Treatment of hereditary anginoneurotic edema.

ADVERSE EFFECT

1. During long-term treatment, musculization in women occurs.
2. Facial hair in women, depending of voice, menstrual irregularities.
3. Edema in both the sex.
4. 17α-alkyl androgens may cause accumulation of bile in the biliary capillaries of the hepatic lobules; if possible their use should be avoided in patient with hepatic dysfunction.

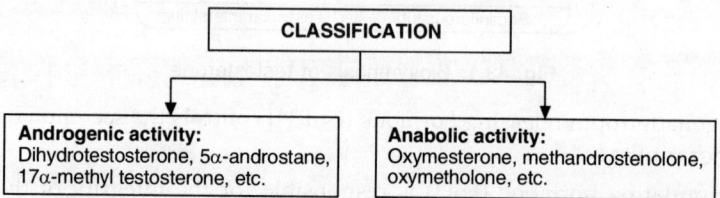

5. On long-term treatment, anabolic steroids can suppress endogenous production of testosterone and may lead to impotence after their withdrawal.
6. They are incompatible with many drugs.

- The active androgenic principle of testes is testosterone. It has two main activities:

1. Androgenic or male sex characteristic promoting activity: It includes normal development, functioning and maintenance of the male sex organs and sexual characteristics.

2. Anabolic or muscle building activity: It causes nitrogen retention by increasing the rate of protein synthesis, decreasing the rate of protein catabolism and thus promotes laying down of new tissue.

- It also stimulates the thickness rise and linear growth of the bones to some extent. Hence it helps in the development of skeletal musculature and emotional gate up of male type.
- The distinction of anabolic therapy of such wasting condition as cancer, trauma, osteoporosis and effects of immobilizations. The condition necessitates nitrogen and mineral retention.

Steroids with Androgenic Activity

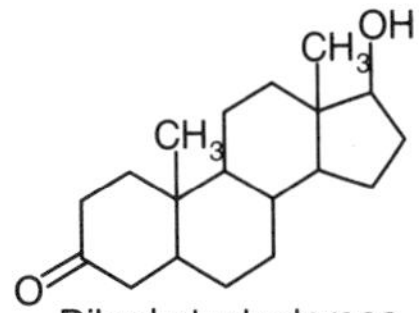

Dihydrotestosterone

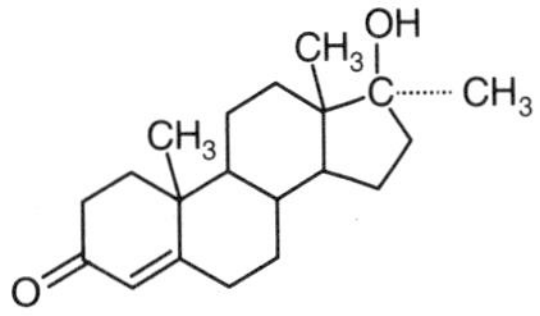

17 α-methyl testosterone

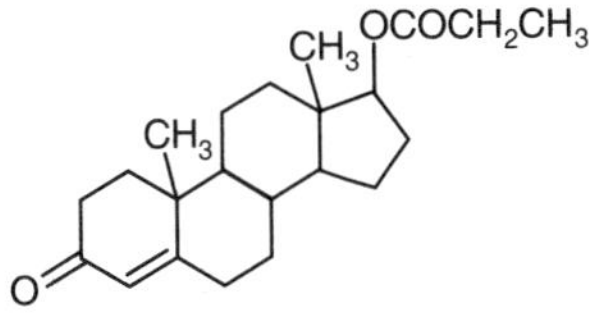

Testosterone propionate

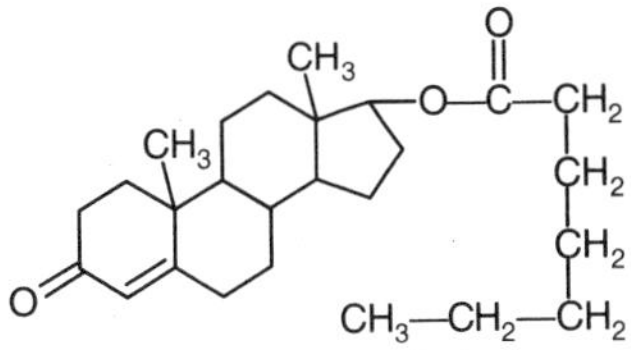

Testosterone enathate

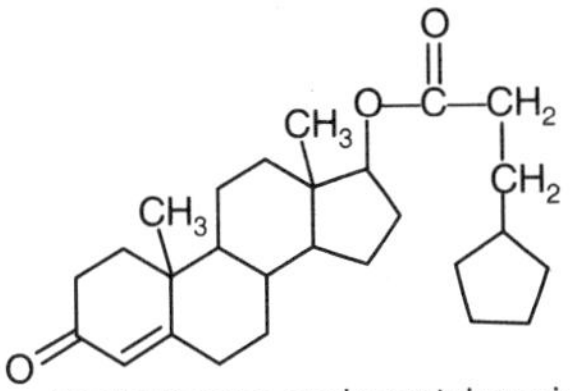

Testosterone cyclopentylpropionate

Steroids with Anabolic Activity

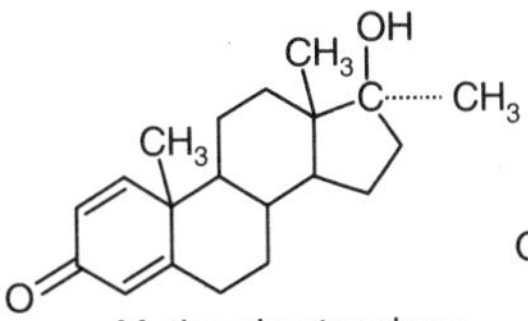

Methandrostenolone

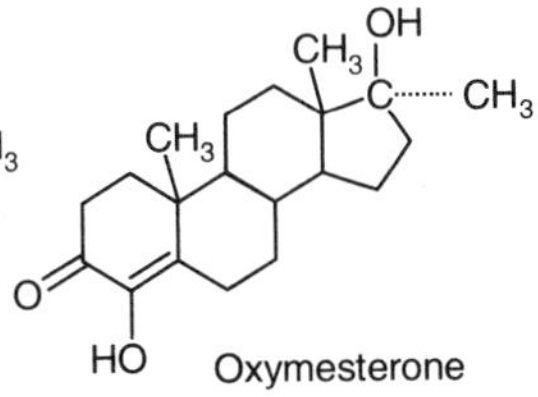

Oxymesterone

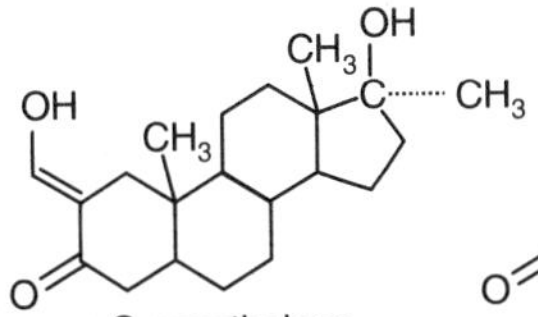

Oxymetholone

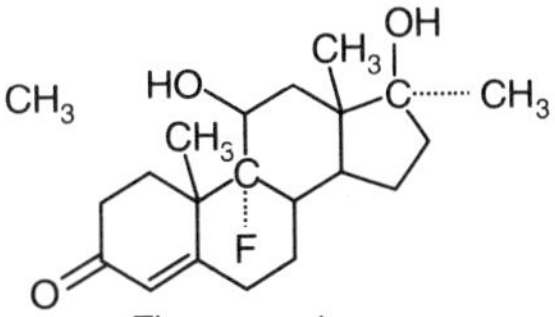

Fluoxymesterone

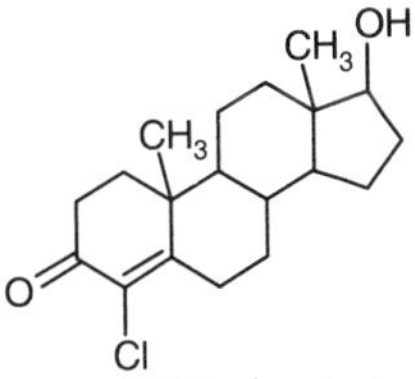

4-Chlorotestosterone

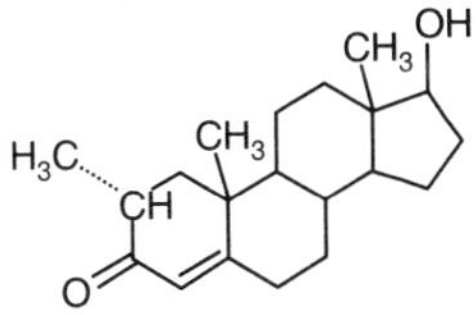

Dromostanolone

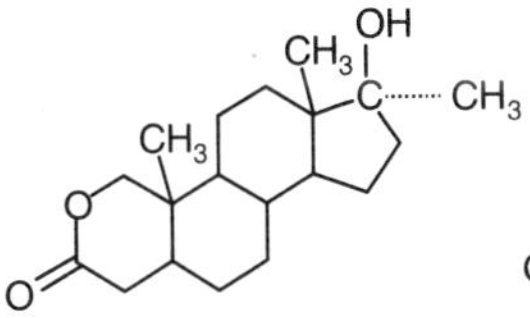

Oxandrolone

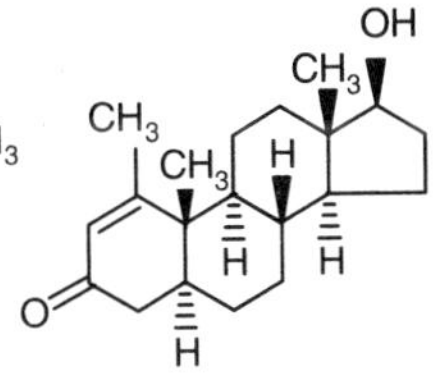

methenolone

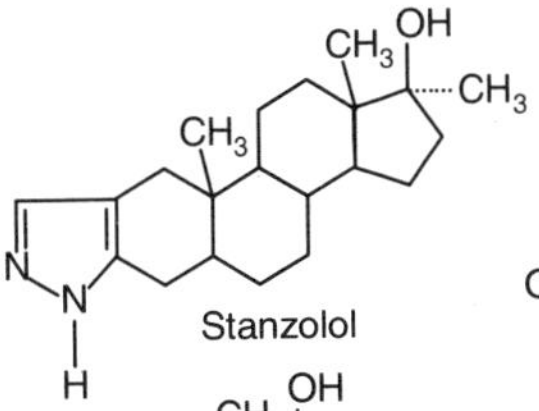

Stanzolol

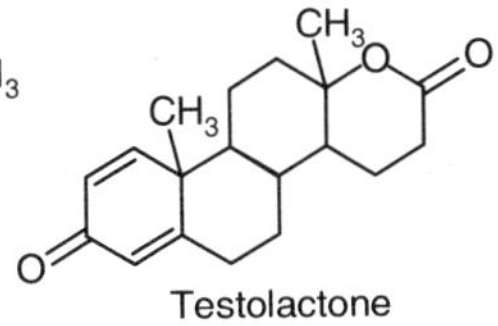

Testolactone

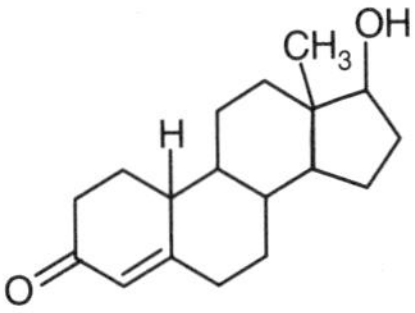

19-nortestosterone

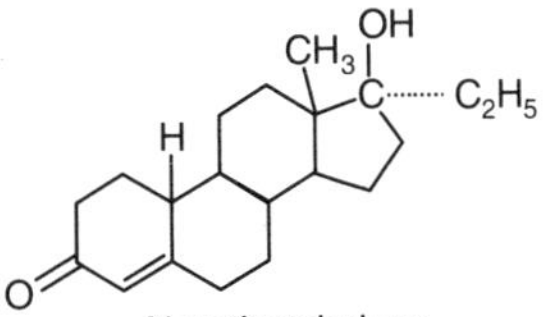

Norethandrolone

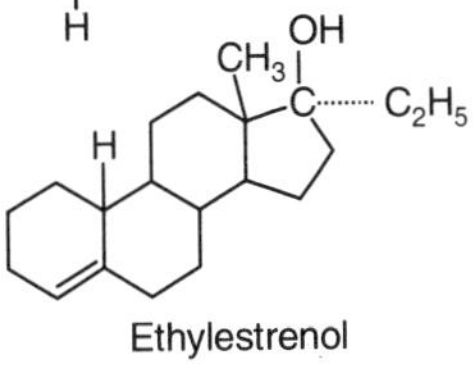

Ethylestrenol

STRUCTURE–ACTIVITY RELATIONSHIP

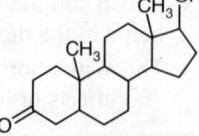

1. Androgens are regarded as derivatives of androstane. Testosterone exerts its physiological activity after its conversion to the dihydrotestosterone.

Dihydrotestosterone

2. A steroidal skeleton is minimum structural requirement to have androgenic activity.

3. The basic nucleus 5α-androstane has androgenic activity.

5α androstane

4. Ring expansion, ring contraction and change in configuration at C-5, significantly reduce or destroy the androgenic activity.

5. Testosterone is not effective, because metabolic changes occur at 17-β oxygen, which is important for the attachment to the receptor site. Hence 17α-alkyl groups are incorporated to prevent these metabolic changes and to render the compound orally active.

17α-methyl testosterone

6. Increasing the length of the alkyl side chain at 17α-position results in reduced activity.

7. Esterification of testosterone at C-17 with a number of acid results into a long duration of action when used parenterally.

Testosterone enanthate   Testosterone cyclopentylpropionate   Testosterone propionate

8. A hydroxyl group at 17α-position does not increase or decrease androgenic or anabolic activity.

9. Several modification of 17α-methyltestosterone lead to potent, orally active anabolic agents.

Methandrostenolone   Oxymesterone

10. Introduction of SP² hybridized carbon atom into the ring A renders the ring more planer resulting in greater anabolic activity.

Oxymetholone

11. Generally, halogen derivatives of testosterone produce compounds with decreased activity except when inserted in to position 4 or 9.

4-Chlorotestosterone

Fluoxymesterone

12. Introducing an α-methyl group at C-2 or replacement of C-2 atom by oxygen results n potent anabolic agents.

Oxandrolone

Dromostanolone

13. Certain substituent at 1, 2, 4, 7 and 17 results in good anabolic agent.

14. Heterocyclic rings are also incorporated to yield good anabolic agents.

Stanazolol

15. Using Birch reduction, 19-norandrogens were synthesized some of which were found to be effective anabolic agents.

19-nortestosterone

Norethandrolone

Ethylestrenol

16. The only compound with purely anabolic but minimum androgenic activity is testolactone. It is used in the treatment of breast cancer.

Testolactone

Testosterone Propionate

Methyl Testosterone

Oxandrolone

Stanozolol

Danazol

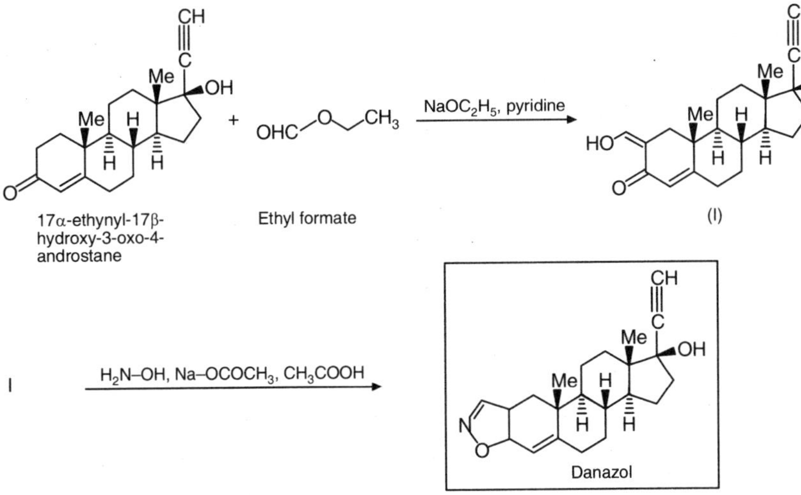

17α-ethynyl-17β-
hydroxy-3-oxo-4-
androstane

Ethyl formate

NaOC$_2$H$_5$, pyridine

(I)

I $\xrightarrow{\text{H}_2\text{N–OH, Na–OCOCH}_3,\ \text{CH}_3\text{COOH}}$

Danazol

Nandrolone

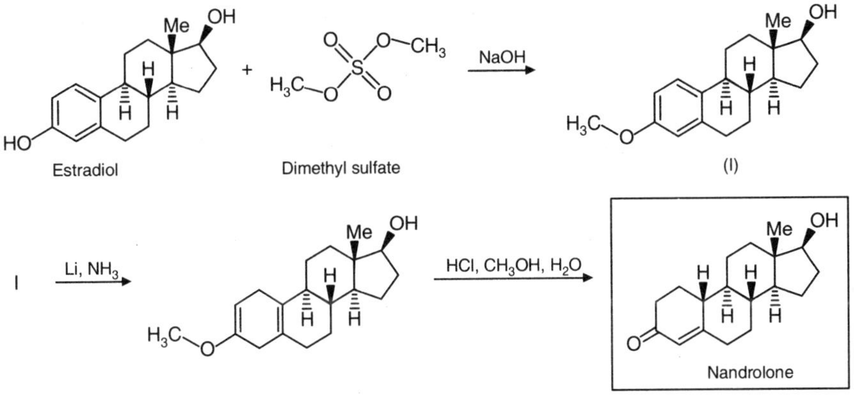

Estradiol

Dimethyl sulfate

NaOH

(I)

I $\xrightarrow{\text{Li, NH}_3}$

$\xrightarrow{\text{HCl, CH}_3\text{OH, H}_2\text{O}}$

Nandrolone

Adrenocorticoids

Adrenal gland is a cap-like organ sitting on top of kidney. Histologically, the gland consists of the inner medulla, the site of catecholamines synthesis, and the outer cortex where steroids synthesis takes place. The adrenal cortex is regulated by the hypothalamous–pituitary peptides.

- The hypothalamus secretes corticotropic releasing factor (CRF) which controls the release of adrenocorticotropic (ACTH), a 39-amino acid peptide. A corticotropin secretion is under the control of higher CNS centers, stress or adrenaline can increase corticosteroid production.
- On the basis of biochemical effects, three groups of corticosteroids can be distinguished as given in Flow chart 44.1.

Flow chart 44.1: Classification of adrenocorticoids

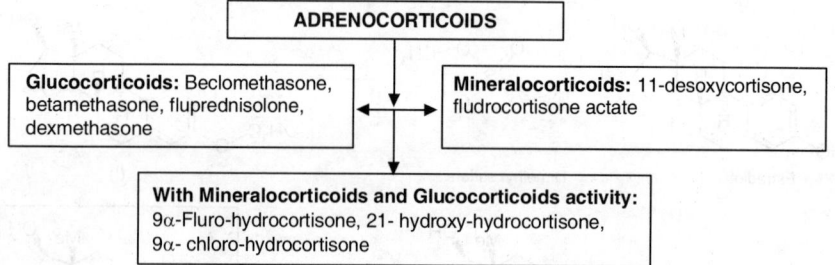

Glucocorticoids

Triamcinolone

Methylprednisolone

Prednisone

Prednisolone

Dexmethasone

Betamethasone

Paramethasone acetate

Fluprednisolone

532

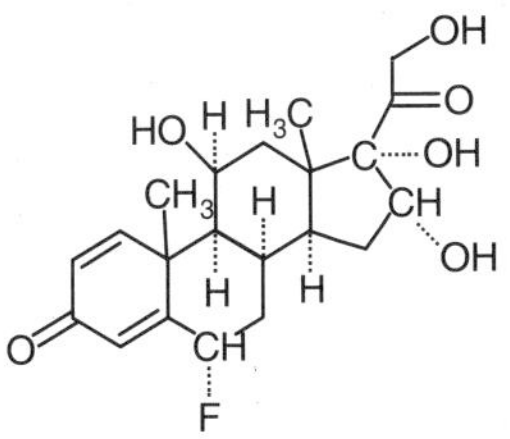

Fluandrenolone

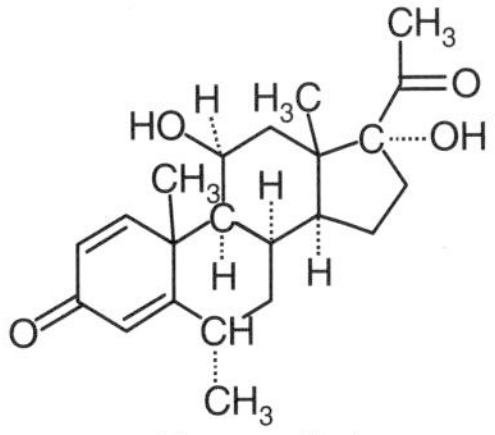

Fluromethalone

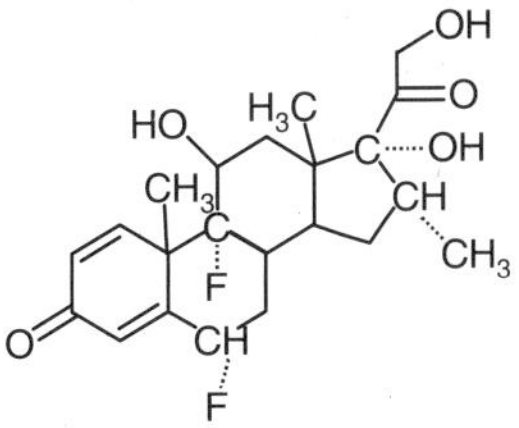

Flumethasone

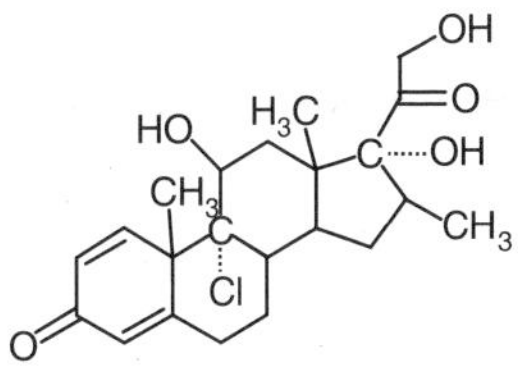

Beclomethasone

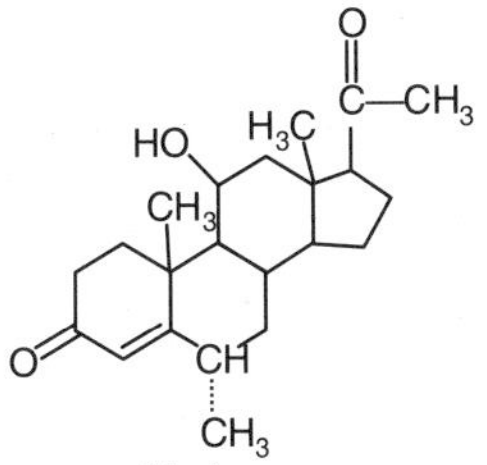

Medrysone

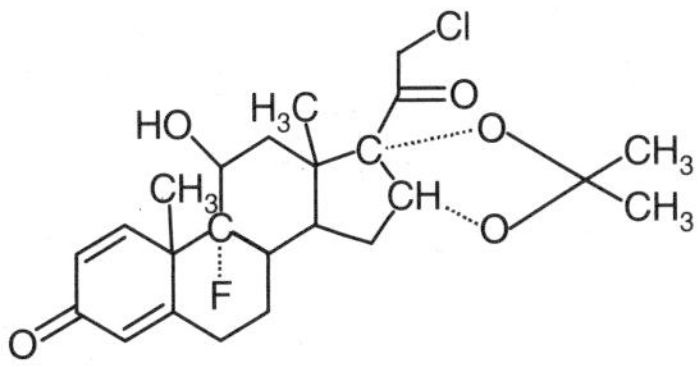

Halcinonide

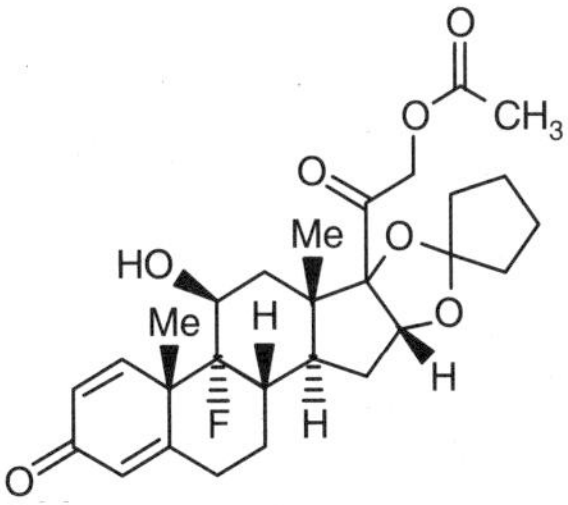

Amcinonide

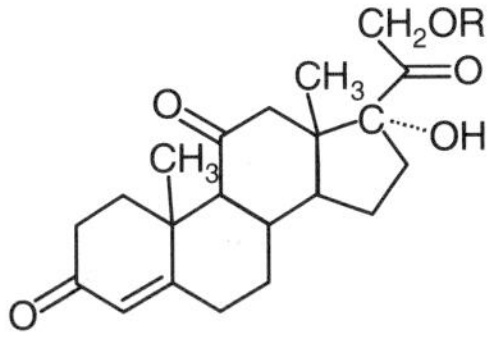

Cortisone R = H
Cortisone acetate R = OCOCH$_3$

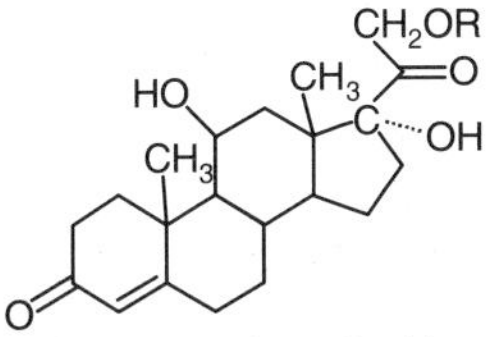

Hydrocortisone R = H
Hydrocortisone acetate R = OCOCH$_3$

With Mineralocorticoid and Glucocorticoid Activity

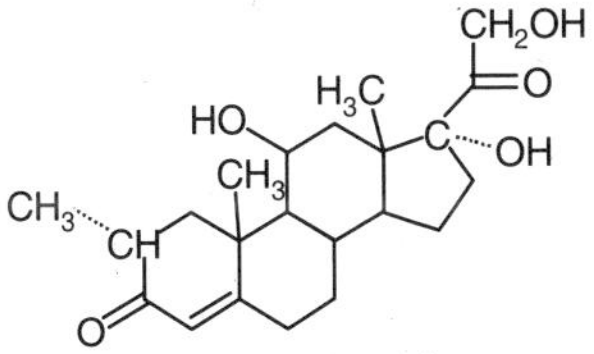

2α methyl hydrocortisone

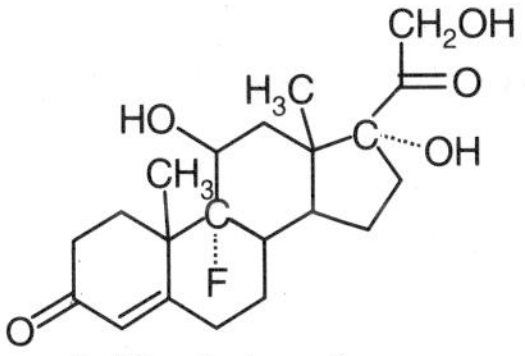

9α Fluro hydrocortisone

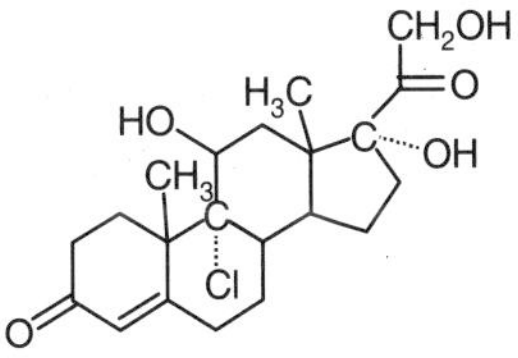

9α Chloro hydrocortisone

Mineralocorticoids

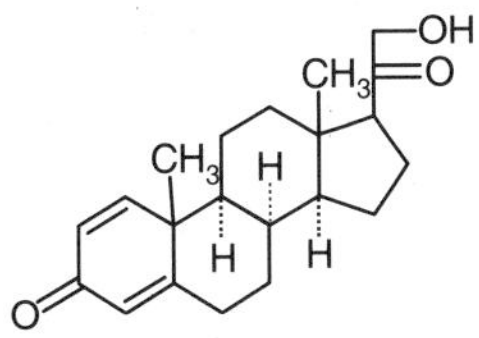

11 - Desoxycorticosterone

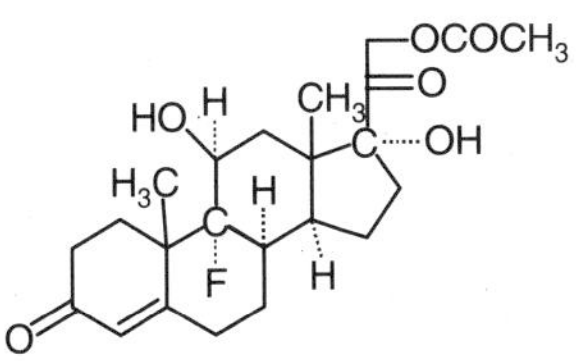

Fludrocortisone acetate

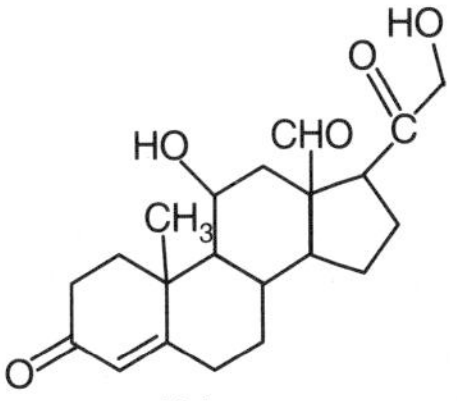

Aldosterone

Glucocorticoids

Which are involved primarily in carbohydrate metabolism but also have anti-inflammatory and immunosuppressive, corticotrophin suppressing and anabolic activities; in general, they enhance glucose availability and stimulate protein catabolism and lipolysis, e.g. cortisone and hydrocortisone.

Mineralocorticoids

Which act primarily as regulation of electrolyte and water balance, they promote reabsorption of small but significant amount filtered sodium in the distal tubule, e.g. aldosterone and deoxycorticosterone.

Biosynthesis and Release, Glucocorticoids

- Adrenal steroids are not stored performed; they are synthesized and released as needed and released as needed and the main physiological stimulus for the synthesis and release of the glucocorticoids is corticotropin (adrenocorticotropic hormone or ACTH) secreted from the anterior pituitary gland. Corticotropin secretion is regulated partly by corticotropin-releasing factor (CRF) derived from the hypothalamus and partly by the level of glucocorticoids in the blood.

- Emotional changes may affect the release of CRF, as many stimuli such as excessive heat or cold, injury or infection; this is the mechanism in fact, by which the pituitary adrenal system is activated in response to a threading environment.

- The starting substance for synthesis of glucocorticoids is cholesterol, which is obtained mostly from the plasma and is present in the lipid granules of the cells of the fascicular zone the middle layer of cells in the adrenal cortex.

- The first step in the conversion of cholesterol to pregnolone is the rate-limiting step and is regulated by ACTH and catalysed by the cholesterol side chain cleavage enzyme, designated P-450.

- The ACTH stimulates the translocation of cholesterol to the inner mitochondrial matrix by a 30-KDa phosphoprotein in all primary steroidogenesis in tissue. This phosphoprotein, steroidogenic, acute regulatory protein plays a key role to the steroid biosynthetic pathways.

▨ BIOLOGICAL ACTION OF ADRENOCORTICOIDS

Carbohydrate, Protein and Fat Metabolism

1. Corticosteroid therapy leads to an increase in liver glycogen deposition, resulting due to:
   a. Increase in glucose formation.
   b. Reduction in glucose peripheral utilization.
   c. Conversion of glucose to glycogen.
2. Proteins are also broken down to amino acids which, in liver, serve as substrate for enzymes involved in production of glucose and glycogen.
3. Corticosteroids stimulate the mobilization of fat from the peripheral fat depots. There is a gain of fat in the back of the neck (buffalo hump), super-clavicular area and face (moon face).

Electrolyte and Water Balance

1. Mineralocorticoids enhance the reabsorption of sodium ions from the distal tubule of kidney into the plasma; and increase the urinary excretation of both potassium and hydrogen ions.
2. They act on the distal tubules of the kidney to enhance the reabsorption of sodium ions from the tubular fluid into the plasma; they increase the urinary excretion of both potassium and H ions.

3. In mineralocorticoid deficiency, proportionately more sodium than water is excreted through the kidney with resultant decrease in extracellular sodium concentration; extracellular fluid becomes hypo-osmotic, and water shifts from the extracellular into the the intracellular compartments. The shift results in a marked reduction in the volume of the extracellular fluid; cells are hydrated and erythrocytes also swell.

4. The shrinkage of extracellular fluid volume, the cellular hydration and the hypodynamic state of the cardiovascular system combine to cause circulatory collapse, renal failure and death, e.g. Addison's disease. Hyperkalemia, acidosis and muscular weakness are the manifestation of aldosterone deficiency.

5. Aldosterone exerts similar effects on kidney, salivary glands, the sweat glands, pancreas and the mucosa of GIT.

6. Glucocorticoids antagonize the action of vitamin D on the gut and reduce the absorption of calcium. The long-term treatment may cause improper development of cartilage and linear growth in children may be inhibited. Thus reduced Ca^{2+} absorption and proteins catabolism inhibit the formation of new bony tissue.

Cardiovascular system: Overdose of corticosteroids may cause hypertension due to high Na^+ concentration, which is retained in plasma. In absence of the corticosteroids there is increased permeability of capillaries and reduction in cardiac size and output.

Skeletal muscle: Adequate concentration of corticoids maintains the normal function of skeletalmuscle. Overdose may result in muscle weakness due to the hypokalemia.

Nervous system: Corticosteroids may affect the mood, behavior, the EEG and brain excitability. Long-term treatment may result in the production of euphoric state.

Anti-inflammatory properties: They inhibit the inflammatory response of any origin but the underlying cause of the disease still remains. The inflammatory manifestations are merely suppressed. In addition, they stimulate erythropoiesis.

Anti-allergic and immunosupressive action: Glucocorticoids inhibit phagocytosis of antigens and their subsequent intracellular digestion by the macrophages. They modify the clinical course of a variety of disease in which hypersensitivity is important. It has been proposed that the initial increase in blood glucose and glycogen deposition is the biological expression of the hormones function.

MOA of Glucocorticoids

- Glucocorticoids appear to exert their anti-inflammatory action in the microcirculation of inflamed tissue by inhibiting the production or activity of prostaglandins, kinins, histamine.
- These glucocorticoids are seemed to be responsible for production of 'Macrocortin' a protein that inhibits the phospholipase A2 activity by binding with Glucocorticoids receptor.
- Bradykinin is considered as a potent inflammatory agent because of its effect on smooth muscle and vascular systeme. It causes vasodilation, increased vascular permeability and hypertension. Glucocorticoids decrease PG-synthesis and hence it is not surprising that they inhibit a bradykinin-induced inflammation that depends upon on arachidonic acid production and metabolism.
- These drugs reduce the increased permeability of capillaries.
- They inhibit the leakage of inflammation producing lysosomal enzymes into the surrounding tissue by stabilizing the lysosomal membrane.
- Theses damaging lysosomal enzymes are released when antigen–antibody complexes are engulfed by white blood cells and cortisone inhibits such an engulfing process.

- The reduced permeability of capillaries inhibits the migration of white cells out of the bloodstream, which inturn decreases the number of such cells to permit leakage of their lysosomal enzymes into the surrounding tissue.
- These drugs maintain the integrity of the cell membrane even in the presence of toxins and thus inhibit the cellular swelling.
- They interfere with prostaglandins and collagenase synthesis and the circulatory distribution of leucocytes in inflamed tissue.

MOA of Mineralocorticoids

- Like other steroids, aldosterone probably acts to initiate transcription of RNA that serves as template for the synthesis of carrier protein or proteins that subsequently facillate the crossing of Na^+ ion through the rate limiting permeability barrier of the mucosal surface.
- Progesterone, the diuretic agent spironolactone, actinomycin and puromycin block the aldosterone stimulated transport of Na^+. Such inhibitors have no effects on non-hormonal basal transport systeme of Na^+.

Structure–activity Relationship

- Hydrocortisone is the natural glucocorticoid with mineralocorticoid activity. The aim of the medicinal chemist has been to modify this structure in increasing glucocorticoid potency and decreasing sodium retention. From the modification in cortisole molecule, following SAR has emerged.

Modification in ring A

1. The introduction of a double bond at C-1 leads to enhanced anti-inflammatory activity, e.g. betamethasone.
2. The introduction of a 2α-methyl group into cortisol increases activity; a 2-bromosubtituent is virtually without systemic effect.
3. Almost all inactive steroids have a carboxyl group at C-3. The carbonyl group could be fused with a heterocyclic moiety to yield "soft drug: A 3-spirofused thiazolidine derivative (A) was found active and this derivative considerably reduced the thinning of the skin, generally found in corticosteroids. This is due to the fact, that such analogs bind to skin tissue through formation of disulfide bonds between prodrug and –SH containing amino acids residue in skin proteins.

Betamethasone

A

B

4. The Δ^4 double bond is important but not essential for anti-inflammatory activity.
5. Ring A can fused with pyrazole ring. Compound (B) a has 2000 times the potency of cortisol, but also lacks mineralocorticoid activity.

Modification in ring B

1. Substitution at 6α-position by hydrophobic group, such as alkyl or halogens tends to increase activity. 6α-methyl, chloro and fluro group enhances activity markedly.
2. Substitutions at 9 positions have drastically influenced the anti-inflammatory potency of corticosteroids. The group introduced were F, Cl, Br, I,-OH and CH_3. The activity of the compound rises with increasing hydrophobic bonding of the 9α substituents. The function of the electron withdrawing group at C-9 was to increase the acidity of the neighboring 11β-hydroxy group and that the corticoid activity of an 11β-hydroxysteroid increases with increasing the acidity of the11β-hydroxy group.
3. Removal of the 19-angular methyl group reduces anti-inflammatory activity.

Modification in ring C

1. The C-11 oxygen group is not essential for anti-inflammatory activity. But it can be replaced by such group, e.g. Cl, which can be converted to the hydroxyl group *in vivo*.
2. Ester substituents at C-12 have shown anti-inflammatory activity. Potency follows the order: propionyl>butyl>isovaleryl.

Modification in ring D

1. Presence of 16α-hydroxy and 17α-hydroxy groups resulted in potent compounds. These two groups could also form acetonide derivatives which are more potent than the corresponding 16, 17-dihydroxy derivatives.
2. At C-16, a carbonyl group increases topical activity and various esters have been prepared with increased local anti-inflammatory activity.
3. At C-16, introduction of chloro, methyl groups increase activity.
4. The 17α-hydroxy group is not essential for activity. However, it can form ketals and esters to give compounds with increased activity.

Modification in the sidechain at C-17

1. The classical hydroxylethanone corticosteroid side chain attached at C-17 is not a requirement for activity. Tipredane, a 17-thioketal is a potent topical anti-inflammatory drug.

Tipredane

Fluticasone

2. Ketalization of the C-20 carbonyl group of corticosteroids with ethylene glycols gives ketals that retain anti-inflammatory activity.
3. Replacement of the hydroxyl group at C-21 by a chloro, fluro enhances activity.
4. Replacement of the 21-carbons by sulfur fluticasone provided 21 thioesteres, which have found clinical activity.
5. Replacement of hydroxymethyl group with an aldehyde (C) was active with some systemic absorption.
6. Acetonide formation across the 17, 20-diol arrangement led to more potent analogs compared to free diols.

(C)

7. The C-21 hydroxyl group is converted to various esters to give lipophilic compounds for respiratory use.

8. Introduction of activating groups at C-21; conversion of hydroxymethyl group to a CH_3 group, such as medrysone (D) gives clinically useful ophthalmic anti-inflammatory with relatively little effect on intraocular pressure.

(D)

9. Fried and Borman were among the first to recognize that certain modification of the steroid skeleton had predictable effects on corticoid activity and assigned 'enhancement factors' to various modification found to increase glucocorticoid and anti-inflammatory activities. Later, an ever increasing number of findings revealed the invalidity of applying animal test results to man. So based on the observation that a measure of anti-inflammatory potency of steroid manifests itself in eosinopenic responses in man, which can be easily measured. Ringler and his associatetes showed that eosinopenic and hyperglycemic clinical assay correlated closely with the anti-inflammatory efficacy of clinically used gluco-corticoids in man. In comparison with Fried and Borman enhancement factors, these new values are in general slightly lower.

Table 44.1: Enhancement factors for various functional groups

Functional Group	Anti-inflammatory activity
9α Fluro	7 - 10
9α Chloro	3
9α Bromo	-
12α Fluro	-
1-Dehydro	3 - 4
6-Dehydro	-
2α-Methyl	1 - 4
6α-Methyl	1 - 2
21-Hydroxy	25

Cortisone

Dihydrocortisone 21-acetate
(from deoxycholic acid)

(I)

21-O-acetylcortisone (II)

$$\text{II} \xrightarrow{\text{KHCO}_3,\ \text{CH}_3\text{OH}}$$

Cortisone

Hydrocortisone Acetate

Hydrocortisone + Acetic anhydride $\xrightarrow{\text{pyridine}}$ Hydrocortisone acetate

Hydrocortisone

16-dehydropregnenolone $\xrightarrow{\text{H}_2\text{O}_2,\ \text{NaOH}}$ $\xrightarrow{\text{HBr}}$ (I)

I $\xrightarrow[\substack{\text{2. HCOOH,}\\ \text{TosOH}}]{\text{1. H}_2,\ \text{Pd–C}}$ $\xrightarrow{\text{Br}_2}$ $\xrightarrow{\text{NaI}}$ II

(II) $\xrightarrow{\substack{1.\ \text{H}_3\text{C–CO–OK} \\ 2.\ \text{(CH}_3\text{CO)}_2\text{O},\ \text{Tos-OH}}}$ (III)

III $\xrightarrow[\substack{\text{Al[OCH(CH}_3)_2]_3 \\ \text{2. KOH}}]{\text{1.}\ \text{cyclohexanone}}$ Reichstein's substance S $\xrightarrow[\text{[Curvularia lunata]}]{\text{Microbiological hydroxylation}}$ Hydrocortisone

Prednisolone

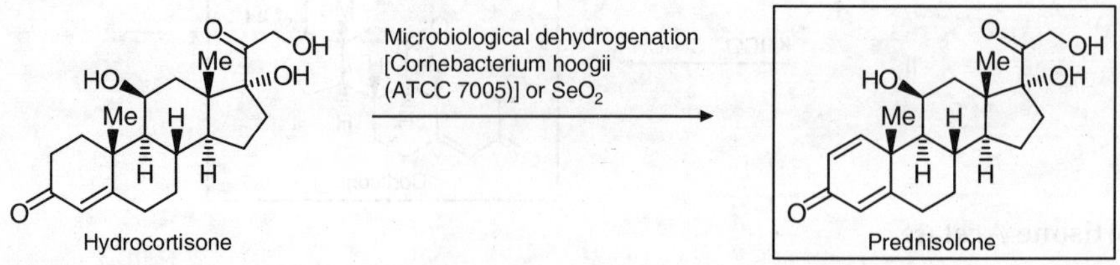

Microbiological dehydrogenation
[Cornebacterium hoogii
(ATCC 7005)] or SeO$_2$

Hydrocortisone

Prednisolone

Prednisolone Acetate

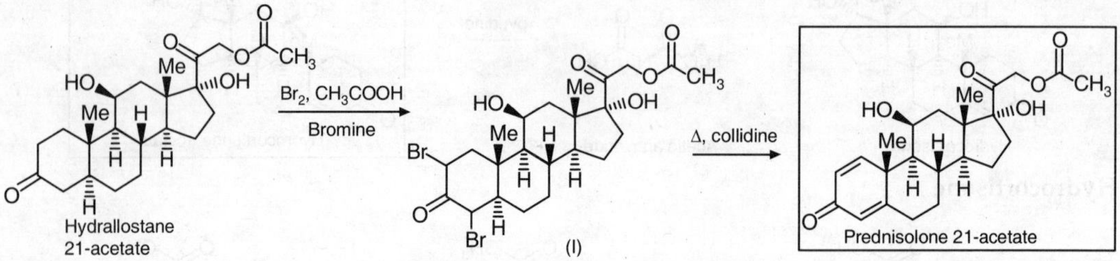

Br$_2$, CH$_3$COOH

Bromine

Hydrallostane
21-acetate

(I)

Δ, collidine

Prednisolone 21-acetate

Fludrocortisone

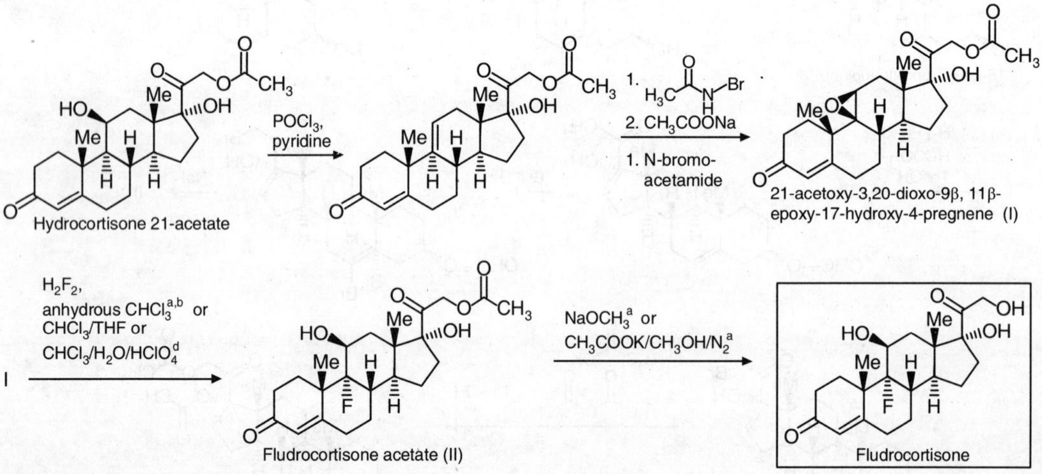

POCl$_3$,
pyridine

Hydrocortisone 21-acetate

1. H$_3$C—C(O)—N(H)—Br
2. CH$_3$COONa

1. N-bromo-
acetamide

21-acetoxy-3,20-dioxo-9β, 11β-
epoxy-17-hydroxy-4-pregnene (I)

H$_2$F$_2$,
anhydrous CHCl$_3^{a,b}$ or
CHCl$_3$/THF or
CHCl$_3$/H$_2$O/HClO$_4^d$

I

Fludrocortisone acetate (II)

NaOCH$_3^a$ or
CH$_3$COOK/CH$_3$OH/N$_2^a$

Fludrocortisone

Dexamethasone

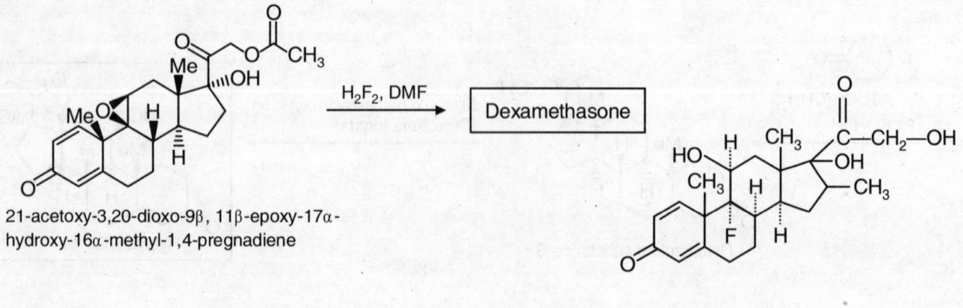

H$_2$F$_2$, DMF

Dexamethasone

21-acetoxy-3,20-dioxo-9β, 11β-epoxy-17α-
hydroxy-16α-methyl-1,4-pregnadiene

Betamethasone Acetate

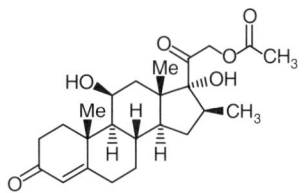

16β-methylprednisolone
21-acetate (from
meprednisone acetate)

1. CH₃–SO₂–Cl, pyridine
2. CH₃–CO–NH–Br, dioxane
3. KO–COCH₃, CH₃OH
4. H₂F₂, CHCl₃

1. methanesulfanyl chloride
2. N-bromoacetamide
3. potassium acetate
4. hydrogen fluoride

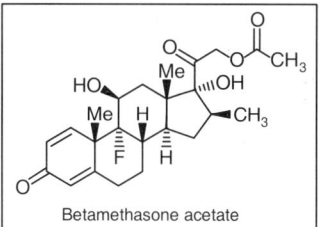

Betamethasone acetate

Betamethasone Valerate

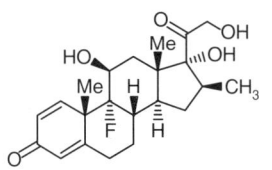

Betamethasone   +   Trimethyl orthovalerate

1. H₃C—⬡—SO₃H
2. H₂SO₄, CH₃OH, H₂O

1. p-toluene-
   sulfonic acid
2. sulfuric acid

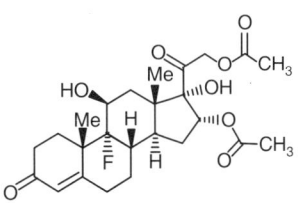

Betamethasone valerate

Triamcinolone Diacetate

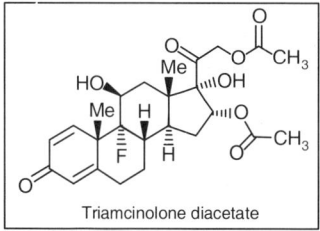

16α,21-diacetoxy-11β,17-dihydroxy-3,
20-dioxo-9-fluoro-4-pregnene

1. SeO₂, (CH₃)₃COH
   or
2. Corynebacterium simplex

1. selenium dioxide,
   tert-butanol

Triamcinolone diacetate

Beclomethasone

21-acetoxy-17-hydroxy-16β-
methylpregna-1,4,9(11)-triene-3,20-dione

N-chloro-succinimide , HClO₄, H₃C–CO–CH₃

Beclomethasone 21-acetate (I)

I —→ H₂O, HClO₄

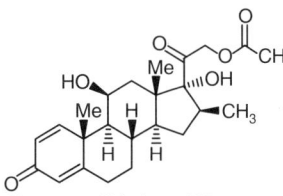

Beclomethasone

Unit VIII

Drugs Affecting the Gastrointestinal System

45

Antiulcer and Antispasmodics

Peptic ulcer disease [PUD] is a group of upper GIT disorder that results from the erosive action of acid of pepsin. Duodenal ulcer and gastric ulcer are the most common forms, although PUD may occur in the esophagus or small intestine. Factors involves in pathogenesis and recurrence of PUD include hypersecretion of acid pepsin and GI infection by *H.pyroli*, cigarette smoking, chronic use of ulcerogenic drugs.

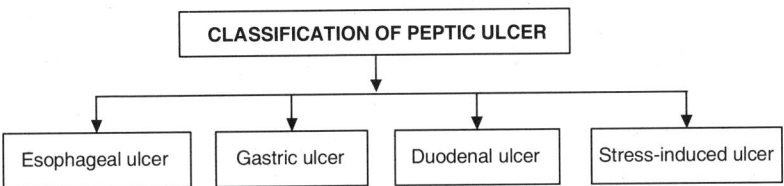

Peptic ulcer consists of a group of ulcerative disorders affecting the upper gastrointestinal tract. It is thought to occur from an imbalance between the effects of destructive factors (acid, pepsin, bile salts) and protective factors (mucus, bicarbonate, blood flow, epithelial cell regeneration and prostaglandin synthesis). Depending upon the location, ulcers can be classified as follows:

1. **Esophageal ulcers**: They affect esophagus.
2. **Gastric ulcers:** They affect gastric mucosa.
3. **Duodenal ulcers:** They affect duodenum.
4. **Stress-induced or drug-induced ulcers.**

MECHANISM OF ULCER

- In digestion of food, the important constituents of gastric juice are pepsin (a proteolytic enzyme) and hydrochloric acid. Pepsin is produced from pepsinogens which are located in mucous neck cells of oxyntic gland area, mucous neck cells of pyloric gland and in Brunner's gland. It has molecular weight of 35,000 and it is maximum active at pH 2.0. Hydrochloric acid is secreted by the oxyntic (or parietal) cells of the stomach.

- This secretion is under the control of acetylcholine, histamine and gastrin. Gastrin, a heptadecapeptide was first reported in 1905 by Edkins. It contains 17 amino acids out of which, only four at the acid end are concerned with its role in the stimulation of acid secretion.

- It is released from antrum of stomach while secretin and pancreozymin are released from duodenal wall in response to a fall in pH and stimulate the secretion of pancreatic juices. Pentagastrin, one of the gastrin analogs, is a powerful stimulant of acid secretion. All the three bases, i.e. histamine, acetylcholine and gastrin, through an interlinked mechanism, control the turnover of gastric acid. Gastric acid has important role in:

1. Formation of proteolytic enzyme, pepsin form an inactive precursor, pepsinogens. Gastric acid also provides lower pH to make the pepsin activated.

2. Inducing the release of secretin.

- Gastric acid secretion is governed by histamine receptors, muscarinic receptors and gastrin receptors. Histamine, acetylcholine and gastrin promote the secretion of gastric acid by activating these respective receptor sites. Histamine is released by mast cells located in the lamina propria, acetylcholine is released by postganglionic vagal neurons and gastrin is released from the G cells located in the gastric mucosal antrum.

- $H^+ – K^+ – $ATPase pump is involved in the secretion of gastric acid. It is located in the apical membrane of the parietal cell. The release of gastric acid (i.e. intracellular hydrogen ions) occurs through this pump by one to one exchange with luminal potassium ions. It is an energy-dependent process. Cyclic-AMP and calcium ions stimulate this proton pump resulting into the secretion of gastric acid. While prostaglandins, somatostatin, calcitonin, glucagon, dopamine and vasoactive intestinal peptide inhibit gastric acid secretion. Usually, the basal acid secretion is high in the night hours with the low levels of acid secretion occurring during the daytime hours.

- Mucus is the thick, viscous, physiological barrier which protects the gastric mucosa from the attack of pepsin and gastric acid. It is secreted from the surface epithelium columnar cells and the mucous neck cells of the cardiac, oxyntic and pyloric gland areas. It is secreted along with an alkaline fluid. It increases the life-span of gastric epithelial cells by providing a tenacious, slimy and alkaline coat over the inner surface of gastric mucosa (Fig. 45.1).

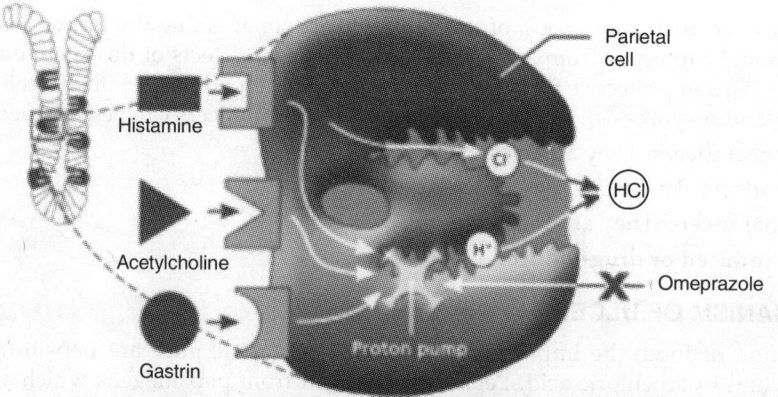

Fig. 45.1: Mechanism of acid formation in stomach

- One of the serious complications of hyperacidity is peptic ulcer which results due to the digestive action of pepsin and hydrochloric acid on the inner wall of stomach and duodenum. This results due to the failure of protective mechanisms of mucosa to prevent the autodigestion process. The feeling of gastric irritation is further potentiated due to increased spasms of GIT. The goals in peptic ulcer treatment are to reduce pain, accelerate healing rate, prevent complications and prevent ulcer recurrence.

- When an ulcer is formed, the gastric acid present in the stomach causes pain and spasm. This in turn, inhibits healing process. The severity of hyperacidity ranges from gastritis (mucosal inflammation) to peptic ulcer. Most peptic ulcers are chronic in nature and visit the patient in the periodic fashion. Recurrence is associated with the development of complications, such as bleeding, perforation, penetration and obstruction. Depending upon the severity and location of an ulcer, one can start the treatment.

1. Relaxation of the GIT smooth muscles (i.e. spasmolytic action). It is brought about by anticholinergic agents. However, they are now replaced by more potent and specific antisecretory agents which have fewer side effects.

2. Reduction in the gastric acid secretion rate (i.e. antacids and H_2-blockers).

- If drug treatment fails to achieve satisfactory results, bed rest and surgery may be needed to manage this chronic, relapsing condition.

- People with hyperacidity should avoid taking alcohol, coffee and cigarette smoking (stimulants of acid secretion) and mucosa irritating diet.

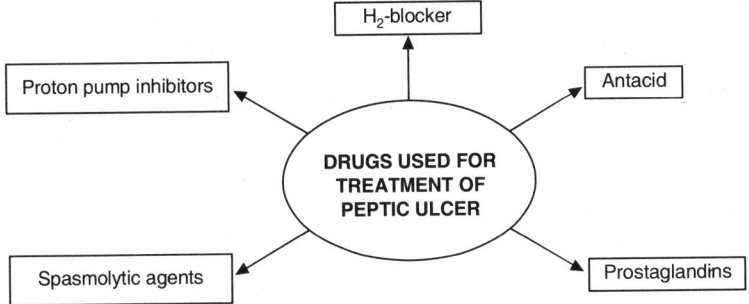

Spasmolytic Agents (Anticholinergic Drugs)

Dicyclomine   Hyoscine butyl bromide   Propantheline bromide   Telenzepine   Pirenzepine

H_2-Receptor Antagonist

Ranitidine   Nizatidine   Roxatidine acetate

Metiamide   Tiotidine   Oxmetidine

Lupitidine

Zolantidine

Proton Pump Inhibitor

Omeprazole (Astra AB)

Pantoprazole (Byk Gulden)

Rabeprazole (Eisai Co. Ltd.)

Lansoprazole (Takeda Industries Ltd.)

Esomeprazole (Astra AB)

▨ GASTRIC ANTACID

- The stomach pH ranges from pH 1 when empty to 7 when food is present. In normal adult, about 22 mEq of acid is secreted per hour by about 1 billion parietal cells present in the gastric mucosa. In duodenal and gastric ulcers, the amount of acid secreted per hour reaches to 42 mEq, and 18 mEq respectively.
- Emotional status of the person, smoking, alcohol and spicy food are known to be predisposing factors in peptic ulcer disease. To avoid this, mixture of antacids are often used. Antacids are weak bases and they raise the gastric pH above 4 (certain antacids like sodium bicarbonate may even elevate the pH to 7).
- It results into reduction in the proteolytic action of pepsin. Antacids also help to reduce spasms and cause symptomatic relief to pain.
- Absorption of antacids may disturb the acid-base balance of the body and cause alkalosis and local effects like, constipation or diarrhea.
- Because the actual mechanism for relieving pain is not known, the evaluation of antacids is done quantitatively in terms of their acid-neutralising capacity (ANC value).

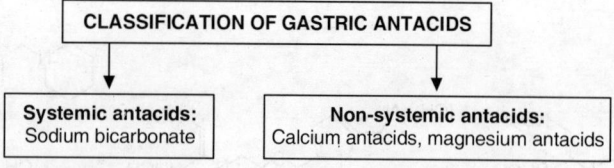

Systemic Antacids (Alkalotic Agents)

Mechanism

They get easily absorbed into systemic circulation and therefore are capable of changing pH of the blood. They may cause systemic alkalosis. Such alkalosis is enhanced by chloride loss (vomiting, gastric suction or diarrhea) and by Na^+ ion absorption. Examples of antacids belonging to the category include sodium bicarbonate and sodium citrate.

Adverse effect

Side effects of these agents include nausea, vomiting, diarrhea, abdominal pain, irritability, headache, insomnia, myalgia and tetany.

Sodium Bicarbonate (Baking Soda)

Mechanism

- It is a popular and widely used antacid. Due to its high water solubility, it neutralises gastric acid very quickly. Thus it has a rapid onset but relatively very short duration of action. The pH may be significantly increased up to 7.
- It is given orally. Major fraction appears in the urine while small amounts are decomposed to release carbon dioxide which is exhaled through the lungs.

$$NaHCO_3 + HCl \rightarrow NaCl + CO_2$$

- The carbon dioxide evolved during the reaction can cause bleaching and flatulence along with carminative action. In many antacid preparations, sodium bicarbonate is one of the ingredients. It is used in the dose of 1 - 5 g to give rapid relief from heart burn and dyspepsia. In general, the carbonate and bicarbonate antacids are preferably used when short-term antacid treatment is required.

Adverse effect

- Adverse effects include nausea, vomiting, anorexia, stomach cramps, headache, frequent urination, weakness, nervousness, muscle cramps and irregular heart beats.
- It is mainly used to treat metabolic acidosis (i.e. excessively high concentration of the acid in the urine like, cysteine in cystinuria or uric acid in hyperuricemia) due to a variety of conditions, including renal disease, diabetes, shock, dehydration or cardiac arrest.
- A 0.05 N solution may be used for continuous nasogastric irritation. Similarly a 5% solution is recommended for the repair of dehydration.

Non-systemic Antacids

Mechanism

- They are insoluble in water and are poorly absorbed due to their cationic nature. Since they do not have direct effect upon the acid-base equilibrium of the blood, systemic alkalosis does not result. Examples include aluminium hydroxide gel, magnesium trisilicate, etc.
- Systemic antacids are used to combat acidosis while local antacids are used in the treatment of peptic ulcer and hyperacidity.
- Most of the marketed antacid preparations contain aluminium and magnesium hydroxides. However due to the toxicity reactions of sodium and calcium ions, their salts are not used for this purpose.

1. Compounds of Aluminium

Mechanism

- These include aluminium hydroxide, aluminium oxide hydrate, aluminium carbonate, dihydroxy-aluminium aminoacetate, dihydroxyaluminium sodium carbonate and aluminium phosphate. All these aluminium compounds are used as antacids.
- These preparations possess both, the neutralizing activity and protective activity on the tender mucosal surface of the stomach and duodenum. They are used in the form of colloidal, viscous suspension and are found to possess a steady and prolonged action. The antacid activity is due to the liberation of aluminium cations.

- They also possess adsorbent activity for various gases and toxins. Independent to their buffering effect on gastric pH, they may also inhibit pepsin activity.

Adverse effect

- These preparations impede peristalsis and tend to induce constipation. But this drawback can be overcome by their combination with magnesium salts. For example, aluminium hydroxide is marketed mostly in combination with magnesium hydroxide. In prolonged use, aluminium salts produce phosphate deficiency.
- This is due to the reaction of aluminium chloride and dietary phosphate in the stomach to form insoluble aluminium phosphate. Due to the increased fecal phosphate excretion, additional dietary supplements of phosphate are to be given.

Preparation

- The commercially available aluminium hydroxide gel is generally a mixture of the hydroxide, the hydrated oxide and a small amount of the basic carbonate. Various other preparations include aluminium phosphate gel, aluminium carbonate, aluminium glycinate (i.e. dihydroxyaluminium aminoacetate) and dihydroxy aluminium sodium carbonate.
- In pharmacopoiea, aluminium hydroxide gel is described under suspension and dried forms. In both dosage forms, aluminium hydroxide gel is popularly used. A loss of antacid property of the gels during the aging process is reported. Hence the gel preparations are needed to be stabilized.

2. Magnesium Containing Antacids

Mechanism

- A large number of official antacid preparations contains magnesium in the form of magnesium oxide (MgO) light magnesium carbonate ($3 MgCO_3$; $Mg (OH)_2$; $3H_2O$), heavy magnesium carbonate, magnesium hydroxide, magnesium phosphate and magnesium trisilicate.
- Due to their insoluble nature, these compounds do not cause systemic alkalosis. Their antacid mechanism does not involve the liberation of CO_2 gas.
- The anion portion of magnesium salts seems to be important for their antacid property. They all function in the same manner, with magnesium trisilicate remains the only exception.

$$MgO + 2 HCl \rightarrow MgCl_2 + H_2O$$

- The newly formed magnesium chloride undergoes second reaction with the bicarbonate, (of the pancreatic juice) in the intestinal juice to form magnesium carbonate. The antacid action of magnesium trisilicate is slow, prolonged and powerful.

$$2 MgO . 3 SiO_2. XH_2O + 4 HCl \rightarrow MgCl_2 + 3 SiO_2 + (X + 2)$$

- The neutralizing reaction yields hydrated silicon oxide which serves as an adsorbent and provides the protective coating over the mucosal layer and thus protects it from further attack of acid and pepsin. It may also absorb the pepsin.
- Thus the activity of trisilicate may be considered as a protective and as an adsorbent. This group of antacids is found to possess purgative action due to magnesium chloride and magnesium carbonate (formed in the GIT). For this reason, they are generally used with such antacids (e.g. aluminium or calcium salts), which cause constipation. For example, gelusil is a preparation containing aluminium hydroxide gel and magnesium trisilicate combination. Similarly, magaldrate is a chemical combination of aluminium hydroxide and magnesium hydroxide.

Adverse effect

In patients with impaired renal function, magnesium ion retention may lead to magnesium poisoning. Hence magnesium salts are contraindicated in such patients.

3. Calcium Antacids

Mechanism

- This category includes calcium carbonate and calcium hydroxide. They have quick onset of action. They raise gastric pH to nearly 7.
- They do not cause systemic alkalosis. Chalk is a natural calcium carbonate. It interacts with gastric acid in the stomach as per the following equation:

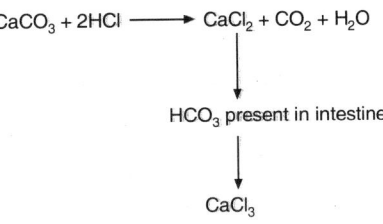

$$CaCO_3 + 2HCl \longrightarrow CaCl_2 + CO_2 + H_2O$$

HCO_3 present in intestine

$$CaCl_3$$

- The carbonate present in the intestine leads to constipation just similar to aluminium antacids. But unlike aluminium salts, their action is dependent upon their basic properties rather than on any amphoteric effect.

Adverse effect

- To counteract calcium constipating effect, most of the calcium carbonate preparations are given in combination with magnesium antacids. Calcium antacids are contraindicated in patients having impaired renal function because they may increase the serum calcium level during prolonged use.
- The release of carbon dioxide in acid neutralization reaction adds to discomfort in some patients. Combination preparations of aluminium hydroxide gel, magnesium antacid and calcium carbonate are also available.

4. Bismuth Containing Compounds

Mechanism

- These agents are commonly used for the treatment of mild diarrhea. Bismuth carbonate and subnitrate also possess antacid property. This property is due to their ability to cover the gastrointestinal mucosa with a dry, inert and protective coating.
- Tripotassium dicitratobismuthate is one of the agents from this category which is used in the treatment of ulcer. Along with the protective activity, this compound has antipepsin and spasmolytic activities. It actually promotes the healing of ulcers and also prevents their reoccurrence.

5. Milk

Mechanism

It is regarded as a weak antacid having an additional protective action. Recently antacid formulations have come up with dried milk plus calcium carbonate and magnesium salts.

Adverse effect

The prolonged administration of such antacid formulations leads to the milk-alkali syndrome. This syndrome is characterized by hypercalcemia, hypoparathyroidism, acute alkalosis and renal damage. Usually, the syndrome disappears as one discontinues the treatment.

■ H₂-RECEPTOR ANTAGONIST

History

- Histamine is a powerful stimulant of hydrochloric acid secretion in gastric mucosa. In larger doses, histamine also augments the secretion of pepsin. These actions of histamine are mediated via H_2-receptors.

- Hence H_2-receptor antagonists are also termed as antisecretory drugs. In 1972, Black et al first described selective H_2-receptor blockade for acid secretion.

- With the successful introduction of cimetidine in 1977, other analogs like ranitidine, famotidine and nizatidine are now available for the treatment of peptic ulcer.

- Histamine is a powerful stimulant of hydrochloric acid secretion in gastric mucosa. Hence this is also termed as antisecretory drug. All agents of this class act as a reversible dose dependent competitive antagonists at H_2-receptor resulting in inhibition of gastric acid secretion.

SAR of H₂ Receptor Antagonists

1. In cimetidine methylation at 5th position, imidazole heterocycle of histamine produces a selective agonist at atrial histamine receptor.

2. The guanidino analog of histamine possesses weak antagonistic activity to the acid-secretory actions of histamine.

3. Increasing the length of side chain from two to four carbons coupled with replacement of the strongly basic Guanidino group by neutral methylthiourea function leads to burimamide, the first antagonist to be developed lacking detectable agonist activity in laboratory assays.

4. Low potency of burimamide is postulated to be related to its nonbasic electron releasing side chain, which favors the nonpharmacophoric imidazole tautomer over the basic electron withdrawing side chain in histamine which predominantly presents the higher affinity imidazole tautomer to the receptor.

5. Insertion of an electronegative thioether function in side chain in place of methylene group favours the tautomer.

6. Toxicity associated with the thiourea structural feature is eliminated by replacing the thiourea sulfur with a cyano-imino function to produce cimetidine.

7. Separation of the ring and the nitrogen group with the equivalent of c-chain appears to be necessary for optimal antagonistic activity.

Therapeutic Application of H₂ Receptor Blockers

- Duodenal ulcers.
- Gastric ulcers.
- Pathological hypersensitivity.
- Upper GI bleeding.
- Gastroesophageal reflux disease (GERD).

Mechanism of action

- All these agents act as reversible, dose-dependent competitive antagonists at H_2-receptor site resulting in inhibition of gastric acid secretion.

- They do not reduce gastric secretion of pepsin or pancreatic secretion of bicarbonate or enzymes.

Cimetidine

Mechanism of action

- Cimetidine has been shown to inhibit competitively the action of histamine at the H_2-receptor.
- Duodenal ulcers using cimetidine to inhibit most of the night time basal and food-stimulated secretion of gastric acid in duodenal ulcer patients permits healing of the ulcer.

Ranitidine

Chemistry

- Isosteric modification of the imidazole nucleus resulted in the development of a furan derivative. Ranitidine in which basic properties are retained by substitution of a dimethyl amino methyl group on the heterocyclic ring.
- The substituted guanidine group has also been isosterically modified by utilizing a nitromethenyl moiety to reduce basicity.

Mechanism of action

Cimetidine has been shown to inhibit competitively the action of histamine at the H_2-receptor.

Famotidine and Nizatidine

- Famotidine and nizatidine consist of a thiazole ring. In addition; nizatidine has the same ring side chain of ranitidine.
- Famotidine has potency 50–80 times more than that of cimetidine and 9–15 times than that of ranitidine, while nizatidine is 6–10 times more potent than cimetidine.

Uses

- Famotidine currently is indicated for the treatment of active duodenal ulcer and active benign gastric ulcer and for the treatment of pathological hypersecretory conditions (e.g. Zollinger-Ellison syndrome, multiple endocrine adenomas, etc.)
- Nizatidine is indicated for the treatment of active duodenal ulcer and maintenance therapy for duodenal ulcer patients. Both, famotidine and nizatidine may also be used in the treatment of gastroesophageal reflux disease, systemic mastocytosis and in the prophylaxis of stress ulceration.

ANTIMUSCARINIC AGENTS

Pirenzepine

Mechanism of action

- It is an antimuscarinic agent having structural similarity with tricyclic antidepressant agents. However, it lacks antidepressant activity because of its poor penetration ability in the CNS.
- It selectively inhibits cholinergic receptors present in the gastrointestinal tract due to its greater affinity for the muscarinic receptors located in the gastric mucosa.

Adverse effect

Adverse effects are few and include dry mouth, blurred vision, constipation and urinary retention. It is used orally to heal gastric and duodenal ulcers in the dose of 100–150 mg per day.

▨ TRICYCLIC ANTIDEPRESSANTS

MOA

These agents possess anticholinergic activity. The reduction in the gastric acid secretion is also brought about by their antagonistic action on both, H_1 and H_2 -receptors. Doxepin and trimipramine are undergoing clinical investigation, for their utility in the treatment of gastric and duodenal ulcers.

Adverse Effect

Adverse effects include drowsiness and anticholinergic features. These agents may be used in patients unresponsive to conventional drug regimens.

▨ H⁺-K⁺-ATPASE INHIBITORS

Mechanism of Action

Proton pump inhibitors are both more potent and of longer duration than H_2-receptor antagonists and therefore are frequently the drug of choice for the treatment of diseases associated with the secretion of gastric acid. PPIs inhibit gastric acid secretion by inhibiting the enzyme H^+/K^+ -ATPase, which is located on the luminal surface of gastric parietal cells.

SAR of Proton Pump Inhibitors (PPIs)

1. If the introduction of fl009uromethyl group instead methoxy group leads to increase the metabolism that leads to decrease in pharmacologic action.
2. If the introduction of difluroaldehyde group at 6th position of omeprazole to increase in pharmacological action because it can be oxidize.
3. If the trimethyl group introduced instead of methoxy group leads to decreasing metabolite in increasing activity.

Clinical Uses

- PPIs are currently the most rapid, potent, and long-lasting treatment for hyperacidity disorders. Omeprazole was first marketed in 1988 and still remains the drug of choice for many patients. Like omeprazole, the majority of subsequently marketed PPIs, pantoprazole, lansoprazole, and esomperazole, bind irreversibly to the proton pump.
- Acid secretion can be restored only through endogenous synthesis of new H^+/K^+-ATPase, which has a half-life of production of approximately 50 h.
- Rabeprazole, however, H^+/K^+-ATPase is converted more rapidly into its activated forms and dissociates more readily from the, resulting in a faster rate of inhibition and a shorter duration of action. This property of rabeprazole is most likely linked to its activation.

Omeprazole

MOA

- It is an orally effective benzimidazole derivative. It reversibly inhibits H^+-K^+-ATPase pump system in the parietal cell membranes resulting into decrease in the gastric acid secretion.
- It blocks the terminal phase of acid production by binding to an enzyme, hydrogen/potassium adenosine triphosphatase that is needed for extrusion of hydrogen ions into the gastric lumen. Suppression of gastric acid with omeprazole is long-lasting and may persist for three days or longer.

Adverse effect

- Adverse effects include nausea, diarrhea and insomnia. It promotes rapid healing of peptic ulcers.
- It is used in the treatment of peptic and duodenal ulcers. In large oral dose, it is effective to control severe gastric acid hypersecretion seen in Zollinger-Ellison syndrome. Adult oral dose is 30-80 mg per day prior to breakfast.

PROSTAGLANDINS

MOA

- These are naturally occurring substances that mediate almost every biological function in the body. Chemically they are 20-carbon oxygenated fatty acid derivatives of prostanoic acid. Prostaglandins inhibit gastric acid secretion stimulated by feeding, histamine or gastrin. Reduction in gastric acid secretion results in reductions in the gastric volume of secretions, acidity and pepsin content.
- Prostaglandins, especially of the E class (e.g. 15, 15-dimethyl PGE_2 and 16, 16 - dimethyl PGE_2), possess antisecretory and cytoprotective (i.e. mucosal protective action) effects in the gastrointestinal tract. They appear to protect the mucosal layers by stimulating gastric mucus secretion and gastric and duodenal bicarbonate production. They also reduce acid back diffusion. They also allow substantial movement of water and electrolytes in the intestinal lumen.

Example

Misoprostol, a synthetic prostaglandin has been clinically used for the prevention of gastric ulcers caused by prolonged use of nonsteroidal anti-inflammatory agents. Other synthetic prostaglandins which are under clinical trials include abraprostil, enprostil, riboprostil and trimoprostil.

MISCELLANEOUS AGENTS

Carbenoxolone

Chemistry

It is orally well-absorbed oleandane derivative of glycyrrhizinic acid, which is a constituent of liquorice. Due to its ability to stimulate the production of 11-hydroxy corticosteroids, it possesses anti-inflammatory activity.

Pharmacokinetic

- It is orally absorbed rapidly when pH is 2 or less. More than 99.9% of absorbed dose is bound to the plasma-proteins.
- Small amount undergoes metabolism to yield inactive glucuronide and sulfuric acid conjugates which are excreted in the bile. Minor amounts also appear in the urine.

Uses

- It is used as an antiulcer agent to promote healing of gastric ulcers and duodenal ulcers. Its activity is due to its protective antipepsin and mucus secretion promoting properties.
- It also increases the volume of mucus secreted and increases its effectiveness. It reduces acid backs diffusion and possibly augments secretin release.

Adverse effect

- Adverse effects include alkalosis, edema and hypokalemia; all are due to the mineralocorticoidal nature of the drug.
- It is contraindicated in cardiac failure and hypertensive patients. Adult oral dose is 100 mg two to three times a day for 4–8 weeks.

Deglycyrrhizinated Liquorice

MOA

It contains about 1–3% glycyrrhizinic acid. It possesses weak antispasmodic activity. It minimally depresses gastric acid secretion. It does not affect mucous secretion.

Metoclopramide

MOA

- Basically, this drug is a good antiemetic because of its dopaminergic blocking action. It does not affect the secretion of either gastric acid or pepsin.
- It promotes gastric emptying and relieves flatulence, dyspepsia and heart burn. Due to its indirect actions on peristalsis and ability to abolish the enterogastric reflux of bile, it is of value in the treatment of gastric ulcer.

Adverse effect

Adverse effects include nausea, bowel disturbances, headache, facial grimacing, fatigue, drowsiness, lassitude, insomnia, restlessness, involuntary movement, dizziness and extrapyramidal effects.

Uses

- It is used in the treatment of gastric and peptic ulcer. It is also employed in the management of reflux esphagitis and the control of gastroparesis in diabetes.
- Adult oral dose is 10 mg which is given about 30 minutes before each meal and at the bedtime.

Sucralfate

MOA

- It is a complex of sulfated sucrose and polyaluminium hydroxide. It acts as a gastric mucosa protectant by adhering strongly with epithelial cells.
- It forms a protective barrier on the ulcer and prevents gastric acid, pepsin and bile salts from aggravating the ulceratic lesions.
- It also adsorbs pepsin, trypsin and bile acids. However, it does not have acid neutralizing capacity.

Pharmacokinetics

- About 3–5% dose is orally absorbed. Rest fraction appears unchanged in the feces. Systemically absorbed drug appears in the urine in the form of sulfate disaccharide.

Adverse effect

- Adverse effects include dry mouth, stomach discomfort, constipation, nausea, vomiting, xerostomia, dizziness and elevated plasma aluminium concentration.

Uses

- It is used to promote healing rate in duodenal and gastric ulcers. It is more effective in duodenal than in gastric ulcers.
- Antacids should not be taken for 30 minutes prior and after the dose of sucralfate. Adult oral dose is 1 g which is given about one hour before meal and at the bedtime.

Gefarmate

MOA

It is a synthetic terpene that contains a number of isoprene units. Originally, it was extracted from the white-headed cabbage. It has antipepsin activity.

Uses

It is used in the treatment of gastric ulcer in the dose of 200–400 mg every 8 hours, however, it is not effective in the treatment of duodenal ulcer.

Maintenance Therapy

- Maintenance therapy is indicated in patients having a history of frequent relapses of hyperacidity. It reduces the rate of ulcer recurrences as long as the therapy is continued.
- It consists of continuous low-dose treatment with one of the H_2-receptor antagonists cimetidine-400 mg at bedtime; famotidine-20 mg at bedtime or nizatidine-150 mg at bed-time.
- Other miscellaneous drugs include urogastrone and sulglycotide. Urogastrone is a 52 amino acid polypeptide isolated from human urine.
- It is found to depress gastric acid secretion after parenteral administration. While sulglycotide is isolated from porcine duodenal mucosa. It was found to reduce peptic activity.

ANTISPASMODICS (SPASMOLYTIC AGENTS)

Classification

These are the agents that have an ability to relax smooth muscles of gastrointestinal tract. On the chemical basis, antispasmodic agents can be classified as.

1. Atropine and its synthetic analogs.
2. Synthetic aminoalcohol esters.
3. Aminoalcohol ethers.
4. Aminoalcohols.
5. Aminoamides, and
6. Papaverine and its synthetic analogs.

Mechanism of Action

- Out of these, from class 1 to 5 acts by anticholinergic mechanism while class 6 does not act by interfering with cholinergic nerve transmission.
- Anticholinergic compounds have some structural similarity with acetylcholine and contain some additional substituents that enhance their binding with cholinergic receptors. The acetylcholine molecule does not cover all the area of receptor.
- The area of a receptor which is not covered by acetylcholine molecule appears to be chiefly hydrophobic in nature.

- Hence hydrophobic substituents increase the affinity of the antagonist for the receptor surface. The large hydrophobic group may not only increase the affinity of the blocking agent but through an 'umbrella effect' may also block the access of acetylcholine to the receptor site.

Papaverine

MOA

- Papaverine and its analogs do not produce antispasmodic effect by interfering with cholinergic nerve transmission. It is believed to inhibit phosphodiesterase activity and adenosine uptake into the muscle cells.
- Since cholinergic nerve stimulation increases peristaltic movements of GIT (spasmodic), adrenergic nerve stimulation will produce antispasmodic effect through the stimulation of P-adrenergic receptor.
- Cyclic-AMP is the active factor which is a product of the response of adrenergic receptors. Papaverine and its analogs are inhibitors of phosphodiesterase, an enzyme that degrades cyclic-AMP.

Pirenzepine

Cimetidine

Ranitidine

Omeprazole

Lansoprazole

Emetics

EMESIS

Nausea and vomiting are the most usual side effects of many drugs. When a toxic or irritant substance is ingested, the body will try to expel it out and vomiting results. In sick condition, vomiting or nausea may often occur as a symptom of the disease.

Mechanism of Emesis

- Nausea, an unpleasant sensation is generally associated with vomiting. Severe nausea may sometimes occur in the absence of vomiting and severe vomiting can occur without the nauseating feeling. Vomiting (emesis) is a complex physiological event.

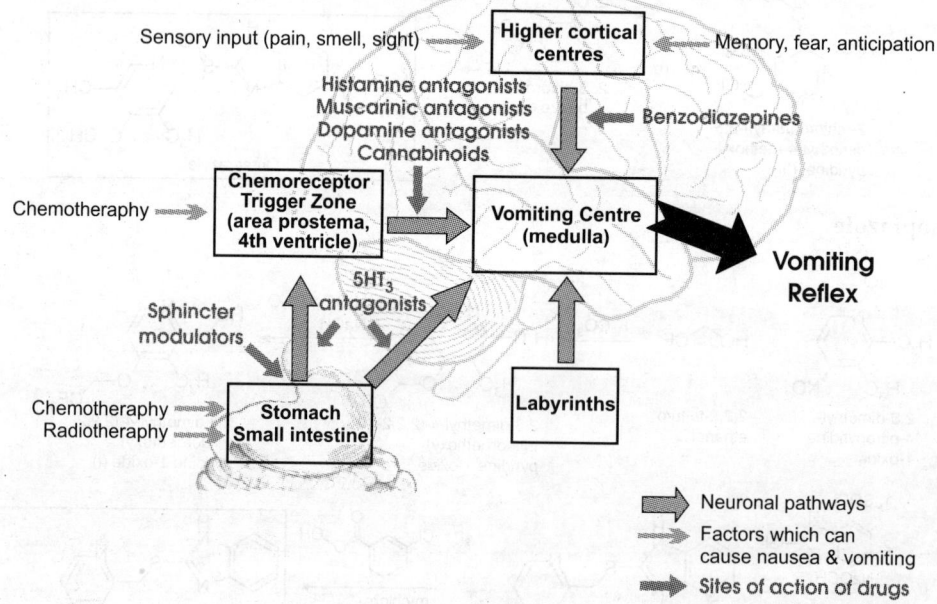

Fig. 46.1: Mechanism of emesis and different drugs which blocks it

- Emetic centers present in the lateral reticular formation of medulla oblongata, regulate the process. These centers may get stimulated due to mechanical, chemical or peripheral stimuli. Sometimes, certain drugs may also activate these centers and vomiting results.

- The chemoreceptor trigger zone (CTZ) plays an important role in stimulating the emetic process. It contains dopaminergic receptors. Since it lies outside the blood-brain barrier, it can be easily activated by the attack of drugs. Certain drugs (e.g. apomorphine) activates CTZ and lead to vomiting.
- While some drugs depress the CTZ activity (e.g. chlorpromazine) and lead to antiemetic activity. In the medulla other important controlling centers of autonomic, cardiovascular and respiratory systems are also located in vicinity of emetic centers.
- Hence vomiting is usually proceeded by the signs of autonomic stimulation, sweating, salivation, pallor, bradycardia and other cardiovascular effects. Psychological factors play an important role in both, the emesis and antiemetic processes.

EMETICS

- These drugs constitute a valuable part of treatment in poisoning cases. They are sometimes also used in low doses in cough preparations to simulate flow of respiratory tract secretions. These drugs act either by local irritation (reflux) mechanisms or directly on the chemoreceptor trigger zone (i.e. central mechanism).

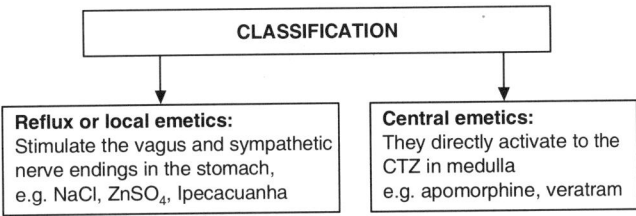

Reflux or Local Emetics

Mechanism

- These drugs cause vomiting by stimulating both, the vagus and the sympathetic nerve endings in the stomach and refluxly stimulate the emetic centers present in the medulla. The commonly used examples of this class include **sodium chloride, mustard, copper sulfate, zinc sulfate, ammonium bicarbonate** and ipecacuanha. In case, if vomiting is not induced by copper sulfate, its absorption into the circulation may lead to serious toxic effect.
- Ipecacuanha tincture, in larger doses, has a strong emetic action and is very safe in use. It is prepared from the dried roots of Cephaelis ipecacuanha. It contains emetine, an alkaloid as an active constituent. It acts directly on CTZ as well as indirectly by irritating stomach. Action is enhanced, if 200–300 ml water is ingested immediately after the administration of the syrup.

Adverse effects

Adverse effects include stomach cramps, headache, itching, muscle stiffness, weakness, faintness, mild drowsiness, sweating and hypotension.

Uses

- It should not be given to semiconscious or unconscious patients because of the risk of passing the vomited material into the lungs.
- Syrup of ipecacuanha is used to induce vomiting in the cases of drug overdoses or poisoning due to other chemicals. Adult oral dose is 15–30 ml of syrup of ipecac.

Central Emetics

Mechanism

- These drugs activate the chemoreceptor trigger zone (CTZ) in medulla which then sends impulses to the vomiting centre itself. Examples include **apomorphine, cardiac glycosides, morphine, veratrum alkaloids, nicotine, lobeline, etc.** Apomorphine is morphine analog.
- It is a very short-acting central and peripheral dopaminergic agonist obtained by exposure of morphine to strong mineral acids. It is devoid of analgesic activity and exerts emetic effect by stimulating chemoreceptor zone in the brainstem which is connected with the vomiting center.

Adverse effect

Opioids may cause respiratory depression along with circulatory collapse, if it is given in higher doses. Other adverse effects include depression, euphoria, restlessness and tremors.

Uses

- It is used in the management of poisoning due to oral ingestion of poisons or drug overdoses. When given subcutaneously or by intramuscular— in dosage up to 8 mg, it leads to vomiting within few minutes.
- Due to its short duration of action and adverse effects, it is not preferred in the treatment of Parkinson's disease.

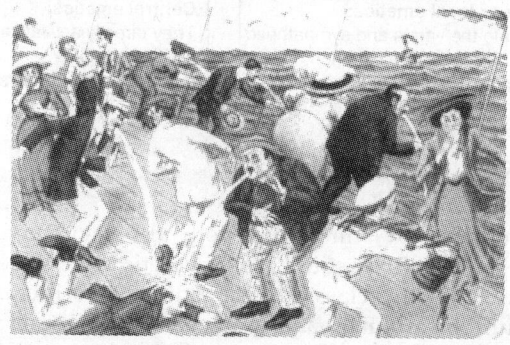

47

Antiemetics

These drugs are used to reduce or to prevent vomiting in conditions where it is common or may be expected. Most of the antiemetic agents possess at least some degree of central depressant action.

- Many anticholinergics and antihistaminergic agents possess antiemetic property. The vomiting of pregnancy does not need the drug treatment, at least for first trimester Thereafter, apparently safer drugs are to be used to avoid the possibility of teratogenic effects of the drugs.
- The commonly used drugs in such cases are phenothiazines (e.g., chlorpromazine, prochlorperazine and promazine). Pyridoxine, one of B-complex vitamins, is also used in various combinations. Drowsiness, dry mouth and related side effects are due to the anticholinergic and antihistaminic nature of these drugs.

CLASSIFICATION OF ANTIEMETICS

Classification of antiemetics is given in Flow chart 47.1

Flow chart 47.1: Classification of antiemetics

```
                    CLASSIFICATION

    ► Anticholinergics: Hyoscine, dicycloamine

    ► H₁ anti-histaminics: Promethazine, cyclizine

    ► Neuroleptics: Chlorpromazine, haloperidol

    ► Prokinetic drugs: Metaclopramide, cisapride,
      Domperidone

    ► 5-HT₃ antagonist: Ondansterone, granisteron

    ► Adjuvant antiemetics: Dexmethasone,
      canabinoids benzodiazepines
```

Anticholinergics

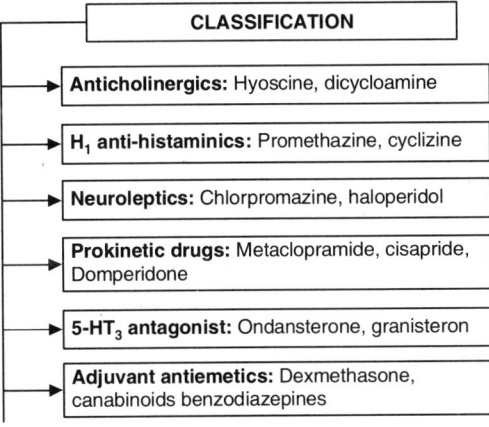

Dicycloamine

563

H₁-Antihistaminics

Diphenhydramine   Cyclizine   Promethazine   Meclozine

Neuroleptics

Chlorpromazine   Prochlorperazine   Haloperidol

Prokinetic Agents

Domperidone

5-HT₃ Antagonist

Ondansterone

Neuroleptics

MOA

These are potent antiemetic; act by blocking D_2 receptors in the CTZ; antagonize apomorphine induced vomiting.

Adverse effect

- Most of these drugs produce significant degree of sedation. Acute muscle dystonia may occur after a single dose, especially in children and girls.
- They are not effective in motion sickness—the vestibular pathway probably does not involve dopaminergic link.

Uses

- Drug-induced vomiting and post-anesthetic nausea.
- Disease induced vomiting and cancer chemotherapy.
- Radiation sickness vomiting.

Anticholinergic Agents

Hyoscine

MOA: It acts probably by blocking conduction of nerve impulses across a cholinergic link in the pathway leading from the vestibular apparatus to the vomiting center.

Adverse effect: It produces sedation and anticholinergic side effects.

Uses: It is most effective drug for motion sickness.

Dicycloamine

Uses: It is used for prophylaxis of motion sickness and for morning sickness.

Antihistaminic Agents

MOA

- Histamine causes the contractions of smooth muscles of GIT. It also acts as a central neurotransmitter.
- Thus antihistaminics act by both, relaxing the smooth muscles and also act centrally to depress vomiting centers.
- Examples include dimenhydrinate, buclizine, cyclizine, meclozine and promethazine. The selective activity of these drugs contributes further to their antiemetic activity.
- Some of these agents also possess anticholinergic action. All agents from this class are H_1-receptor blockers.

Promethazine and Diphenhydramine

- They afford protection of motion sickness for 4–6 hours, but produce sedation and dryness of mouth.
- By their central anticholinergic action, they block the extrapyramidal side effects of metaclopramide while supplementing its antiemetic action.

Cyclizine and Meclozine

- These are less sedative and less anticholinergic. Meclozine is long acting protecting against sea sickness for nearly 24 hours.

Prokinetic Agent

These are drugs which promote gastrointestinal transit and speed gastric emptying.

1. Metaclopramide

MOA

D_2 Antagonism:

- Dopamine is an inhibitory transmitter in GIT normally acts to delay gastric emptying when food is present in stomach.

- It also appears to cause gastric dilation and LES relaxation attending nausea and vomiting. Metaclopramide blocks D_2 receptors and has an opposite effect hastening gastric emptying and enhancing LES tone.

5-HT$_4$ Agonism:

- It acts in the GIT to enhance ACh release from myenteric neurons. This results from 5-HT$_4$ receptor activation on interneurons which promote ACh release from the primary motor neurons innervating the smooth muscles.
- The gastric hurrying effect is mainly due to this action which is synergized by bethanecol and attenuated by atropine.

5-HT$_3$ Antagonism:

- At high concentration, metaclopramide can block 5-HT$_3$ receptors present on inhibitory myenteric interneurons and in NTS/CTZ.
- The central action appears to be significant only when large doses are used to control chemotherapy induced vomiting.

Pharmacokinetics: Metaclopramide is rapidly absorbed orally, enters brain, crosses placenta and is secreted in milk. It is partly conjugated in liver and excreted in urine within 24 hours.

Adverse effect: Sedation, dizziness, diarrhea, muscle dystonias are the main side effects. Long-term use can cause Parkinsonism, galactorrhea and gynecomastia.

2. Domperidone

MOA: It is D_2 receptor antagonist in upper GIT. Unlike metaclopramide its prokinetic action is not blocked by atropine.

Pharmacokinetics: It is absorbed orally, but bio-availability is only 15% due to first pass metabolism. It is completely biotransformed and metabolites are excreted in urine.

Adverse Effect: Dry mouth, loose stools, headache, rashes, galactorrhoea, cardiac arrhythmias have developed on rapid i.v. injection.

5-HT$_3$ Antagonist

Ondansteron

MOA: It blocks the depolarizing action of 5-HT through 5-HT$_3$ receptors on vagal afferents in the GIT as well as in NTS and CTZ.

Adverse Effect: Ondansteron is generally well-tolerated. The common side effect is headache. Mild constipation or diarrhea and abdominal discomfort occur in few patients. Rashes and allergic reaction occur, especially after i.v. injection.

Adjuvant Antiemetics

Tetrahydrocannabinol

MOA: It is a psychoactive substance isolated from the flowering heads of hemp plant, Cannabis sativa. It possesses antiemetic activity against moderately emetogenic chemotherapy. It probably acts at higher centers or at vomiting center itself.

Pharmacokinetics: Though it is orally absorbed, it undergoes an extensive first pass metabolism. It has a biphasic plasma half-life. Initial half-life is 10–20 minutes while terminal half-life is 30 hours. Principal metabolites include 11-hydroxy -A -TEC (active) and 11 - nor - A -THC - 9-carboxylic acid (inactive). They are excreted in urine as well as in faeces.

Adverse effect: Adverse effects include dry mouth, dizziness, somnolence, confusion, hallucination, dysphoria, euphoria, depersonalization, conjunctivitis, hypotension, tachycardia, tolerance and addiction.

Uses: It is used as an antiemetic agent to control nausea and vomiting induced by cancer chemotherapeutic agents. It may be given orally or by smoke.

Dicycloamine

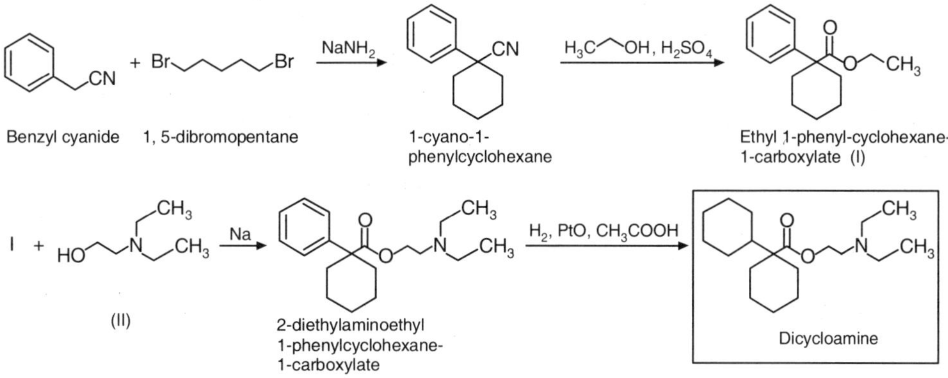
Benzyl cyanide
1, 5-dibromopentane
NaNH2
1-cyano-1-phenylcyclohexane
H3C OH, H2SO4
Ethyl 1-phenyl-cyclohexane-1-carboxylate (I)
I +
(II)
Na
2-diethylaminoethyl 1-phenylcyclohexane-1-carboxylate
H2, PtO, CH3COOH
Dicycloamine

Cyclizine

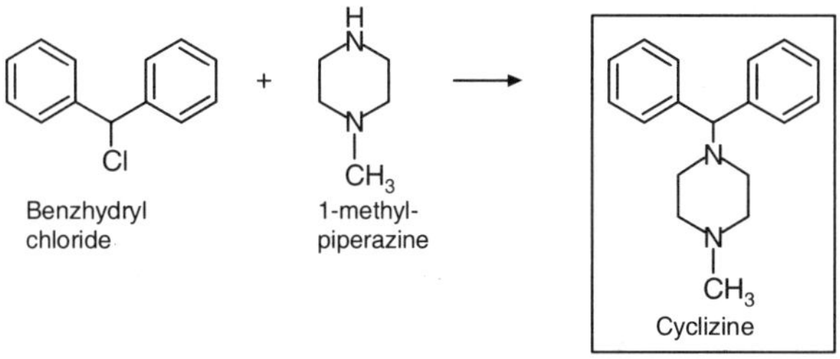
Benzhydryl chloride
1-methyl-piperazine
Cyclizine

Meclozine

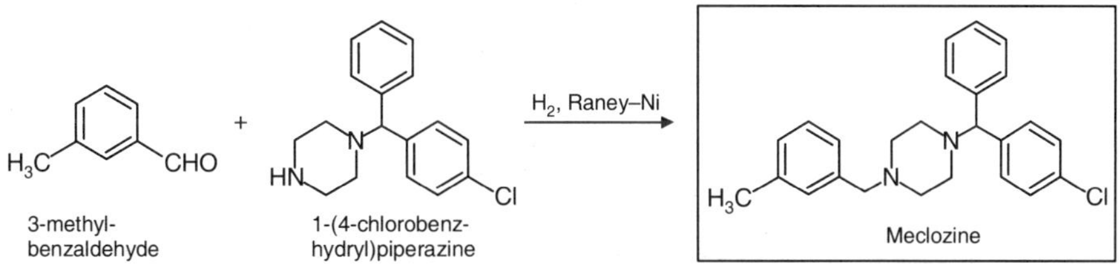
3-methyl-benzaldehyde
1-(4-chlorobenz-hydryl)piperazine
H2, Raney–Ni
Meclozine

Diphenhydramine

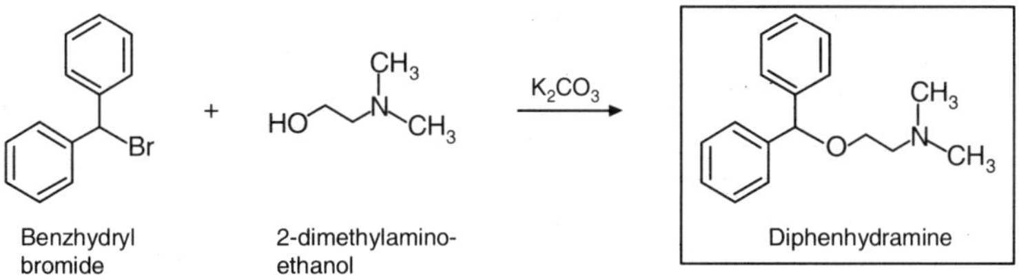
Benzhydryl bromide
2-dimethylamino-ethanol
K2CO3
Diphenhydramine

48

Laxatives and Purgatives

These are drugs that promote evacuation of bowel. A distinction is sometimes made according to the intensity of action.

- **Laxatives:** These are milder acting, eliminate soft but formed tools.
- **Purgatives or cathartics:** These are stronger action resulting in more fluid evacuation. Many drugs in low doses act as laxative and in larger doses as purgatives.

MECHANISM OF ACTION

- Constipation and illness have historically been associated with each other. Constipation is the infrequent or delayed evacuation of the feces. It is a battle between the bowl and bowel. Regularity of the bowel movement is necessary to avoid a vague feeling of discomfort. Constipation is different from dysphasia (i.e., difficulty in defecation).

- In a normal adult, approximately 9 litres of fluid and partly undigested food reach the cecum per day. Fecal fluid content of 200–300 ml usually results in some softening of stool. Large amounts of fluids can be retained in large intestine due to the hydrophilic properties of laxative. This increased pressure then facilitates the process of defecation. Fecal fluid values greater than 300 ml usually result in diarrhea.

- Cathartic (Greek term, katharsis = purification) is the general term used to describe all such agents which promote the passage of feces. This category includes aperient, laxative, purgative and drastic, all of which have intensity of cathartic action in increasing order. Drastic agents include colocynth, croton oil, jalap and podophyllum. Since they have potent cathartic action, they may induce severe mucosal irritation and gastroenteritis. Laxatives are the drugs which stimulate peristalsis, promote evacuation through the powerful contractions of the bowel. Defecation results due to powerful peristalsis.

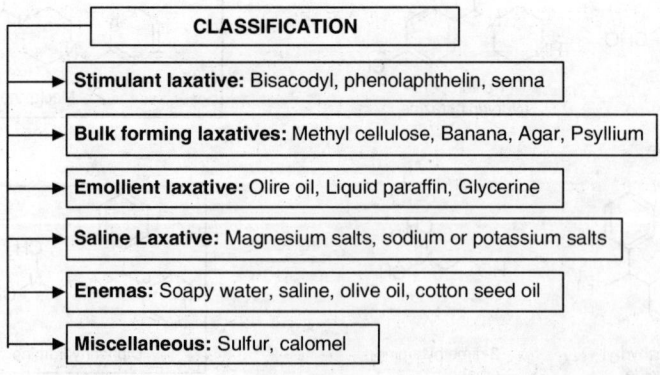

CLASSIFICATION

Stimulant laxative: Bisacodyl, phenolaphthelin, senna

Bulk forming laxatives: Methyl cellulose, Banana, Agar, Psyllium

Emollient laxative: Olire oil, Liquid paraffin, Glycerine

Saline Laxative: Magnesium salts, sodium or potassium salts

Enemas: Soapy water, saline, olive oil, cotton seed oil

Miscellaneous: Sulfur, calomel

Phenolphthalein

Bisacodyl

Danthrone

▓ STIMULANT OR IRRITANT LAXATIVES

Anthraquinone, Castor Oil, Bisacodyl and Phenolphthalein

- These agents irritate the intestinal mucosa. This results into quick response to the distention. They also lead to the accumulation of fluids in the colon resulting into an increased pressure and stool softening effects.
- Examples include anthraquinone derivatives; castor oil, diphenylmethane derivatives (phenolphthalein and bisacodyl) and bile acids. All above agents produce laxative effect by stimulating peristalsis by irritation. They induce reflux increase in the gut motility. They are inactive, given parenterally.

Castor Oil
MOA

It contains the triglyceride of ricinoleic acid which undergoes enzyme; hydrolysis in body to give glycerol and cinoleate. The laxative action of castor oil is mainly due to ricinoleate. In addition, it has an emollient activity. It is obtained from the plant, Ricinus communis. Adult oral dose is 15–30 ml per day.

Anthraquinone Glycosides
MOA

- Senna, rhubarb, aloe and cascara are the main sources of anthraquinone glycosides. These plants contain various oxymethyl quinines present, partly in free form and partly as inactive glycosides.
- These glycosides are released in the intestinal lumen under the influence of microbial flora. Emodin (trioxymethyl anthraquinone) and chrysophanic acid (dioxymethyl anthraquinone) are the active laxative constituents of anthraquinone glycosides.
- Emodin increases the retention of water and sodium ions in the lumen by inhibiting $Na^+ - K^+ - ATPase$ pump present in the lumen mucosa. Danthron is a synthetic derivative of anthraquinone glycoside.

Sources
Anthraquinone glycoside is obtained from:
1. Dried leaves of *Cassia acutifolia* and *Cassia angustifolia* (Senna leaves)
2. Dried roots and rhizomes of *Rheum officinale* Rhubarb.
3. Bark of *Rhamnus purshiana* (*Cascara sagrada*), and
4. Juice *of Aloe perryi* (Aloe)

Adverse effect

Adverse effects of stimulant laxatives include excessive purgative action. Sometimes larger doses of these agents may produce nephritis. They should not be used in pregnancy.

▓ BULK FORMING LAXATIVES

Methylcellulose, Isapghula, Agar, Banana and Psyllium Seeds and Bran

- If the diet contains a bulk of non-absorbable residue, this part, by filling the intestine, exerts the pressure on the bowel wall. This pressure serves as a stimulus for normal defecation. Since part of their activity can be attributed to their ability to absorb water (i.e. a hydrogel), patients should drink adequate amount of water to avoid dehydration.
- They act as the mechanical laxatives and are used when the faeces are dry and hard. Most of them are marketed in the form of granules which absorb water and swell up into the thick mucilage that is not digested but excreted unchanged. They indirectly stimulate peristalsis by their water content and their content of undigestible matter. The hydrogel which is formed facilitates defecation by lubrication of fecal mass because of its emollient property.

Bran

- This is yet another example of bulk-forming laxatives. It comprises all undigestible fiber material derived from both fruits and vegetables or from cereals.
- It mainly contains carbohydrates in the form of cellulose, lignin and pectin. It is usually used in the treatment of diverticulitis.

▓ EMOLLIENT LAXATIVES (LUBRICANTS)

These agents are also called as stool softners. They act simply by lubricating intestinal mucosa. Softening of stool is assisted by reducing intestinal electrolyte and fluid transport. Examples include olive oil, glycerin, liquid paraffin, etc.

Liquid Paraffin

MOA

- Liquid paraffin is a mixture of liquid hydrocarbons, used as an emollient to lubricate and soften the fecal matter in constipation. It is available as oil or as a white emulsion, when given orally, it is not absorbed. Its continued use is contraindicated.
- It is a thick, clear mineral oil which passes into the intestine in undigested form, softens the bowel contents, lubricates the intestinal channel resulting into the smooth, painless movements. It is usually prescribed in the form of emulsion to which agar or phenolphthalein is sometimes added. Dose ranges from 8 to 30 ml.

Docusate Sodium

MOA

- Docusate sodium (dioctyl sodium sulphosuccinate) is yet another example of this category. It is an anionic type of surfactant having a wide variety of emulsifying, wetting and dispersing applications. It is used as a fecal softener due to its emulsifying action. It increases the secretion of water and electrolytes into intestinal lumen.
- It apparently hydrates and softens the stool. It is incorporated into retention enemas. Because of detergent nature, it allows water to penetrate and soften the hard fecal matter. It is available in the form of docusate sodium, docusate calcium and docusate potassium. Adult oral dose is 50–300 mg per day— while adult rectal dose is 50–100 mg as 0.10% solution.

SALINE LAXATIVES (OSMOTIC LAXATIVE)

- They are salts of poorly absorbable anions and sometimes cations. Here the word, "saline" indicates certain compounds of sodium and magnesium; this class includes water soluble inorganic salts that contain multivalent cations or anions.
- Because of their ionic nature, these ions are slowly or incompletely absorbed from intestine. Consequently water is retained in the intestinal lumen through osmotic effect exerted by these nonabsorbed ions.
- Osmotic pressure depends upon molecular weight of the drug and concentration of such unabsorbed ions. The resulting semifluid fecal matter exerts a pressure on the luminal wall. Peristalsis is induced by the activation of stretch receptor present in the GIT mucosa resulting into a laxative effect. Magnesium salts, in addition stimulate the secretion of cholecystokinin-pancreozymin, a hormone that stimulates the fluid secretion and motility and reduces absorption of sodium chloride.
- More commonly used saline purgatives include:
  1. Magnesium salts, e.g. magnesium sulfate and milk of magnesia (magnesium hydroxide).
  2. Sodium or potassium salts, e.g. tartrate, sulfate, phosphate and biphosphate.
  3. Potassium sodium tartrate (Rochelle salt) and
  4. Lactulose.

Magnesium sulfate

- Magnesium sulfate (epsom salt) is the most powerful saline laxative since both ions are least absorbed. It is used as a cathartic to provide complete evacuation of small and large intestine in patients with chronic liver disease. Adult oral dose is 5–20 g per day in divided doses.

Adverse effect

In patients with renal dysfunctioning, higher blood concentration of magnesium is reported to occur due to inadequate removal of magnesium ions from blood. This may lead to CNS depression or coma. Hence its use is contraindicated in patients with renal dysfunctioning.

Lactulose

MOA

- Lactulose is a semisynthetic disaccharide sugar. About 2–3% dose is orally absorbed. The unabsorbed dose is metabolized by intestinal bacterial (lactobacilli, bactericides species, *E. coli* and clostridia species) to lactic, acetic and formic acids and carbon dioxide. These low molecular weight acids initiate an osmotic drive.
- Systemically absorbed portion appears in urine in unchanged form. Each 15 ml contains 10 g of lactulose and minor amounts of other sugars like galactose and lactose, it is used orally (7–10 g) along with sufficient water to treat constipation.

Adverse effect

- Adverse effects of saline laxatives include; anorexia, headache, hypogastric pain, bloating, flatulence, dehydration, weakness, myalgias, (depression, and disturbance in water–electrolyte balance).
- Chronic treatment with saline laxatives may cause damage to colonic mucosa resulting into proctocolitis. In certain cases, systemic toxicity is reported to occur. Adequate fluid intake should be maintained to avoid dehydration due to hypertonic solution of the saline laxatives.

ENEMAS

- These are the detergent containing preparations which are introduced through the rectum. Soapy water, saline, olive oil, cotton seed oil, glycerin, sodium phosphate or sodium diphosphate are the common ingredients of enema preparations.
- Hypertonic saline solution offers certain advantages over the detergent substances. They soften feces and produce laxation either by fragmentation, liquefaction or lubrication. They increase the muscle tone of colon and rectum. Phosphate enemas lower the serum calcium level by inducing considerable loss of calcium.

MISCELLANEOUS

Sulfur

MOA

- Chemically sulfur is very active element. It is therapeutically employed both internally as well as topically. Topically, it acts as fungicide and keratolytic agent.
- If used internally, it exhibits a mild cathartic action, which is due to its reduction to the sulphide anion in the intestine.
- This sulphide anion (S~) neutralises excess gastric acid to give hydrogen sulphide which is a mild intestinal irritant.

Calomel

MOA

- Chemically, it is mercurous chloride. Its cathartic action is due to the strong intestinal irritant property of mercuric cation (i.e. mercury albuminate) formed in the small intestine. The possibility of mercury poisoning has posed limitations on its use.

49

Antidiarrheals

Diarrhea means loose bowel movements resulting into the frequent passage of watery, uniformed stools with or without mucous and blood.

Etiology

- This condition may arise due to the change in the nature of diet and routine or sometimes due to bacterial infection. The former type of diarrhea is the mild form while the infective diarrhea is more powerful and persistent.
- Organism escapes from gastric acid and other digestive processes and reaches the bowel. Its metabolic products irritate the nerve ending of intestinal wall leading to severe diarrhea.
- In this condition, to compensate the loss of body fluids, a mixture of salt (sodium chloride or sodium bicarbonate) and water is to be given frequently.
- The simple type of diarrhea may be controlled just by using intestinal adsorbents while infected diarrhea needs the use of intestinal antiseptics.

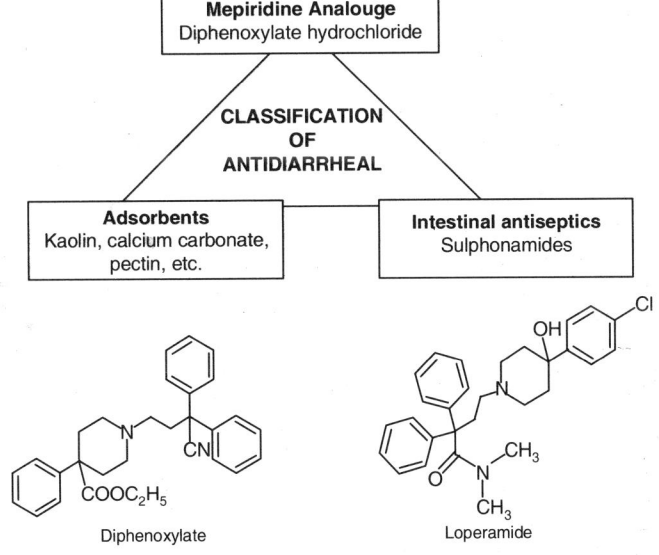

ADSORBENTS

- These substances have the power of adsorbing gases, bacteria or toxins without undergoing any chemical reaction.

- In addition to adsorbent action, they also possess the protective property. They form a coating over the intestinal mucosa to reduce its irritation.

1. Kaolin
MOA
- It is a hydrated aluminium silicate used internally and externally in the form of very finely powder for its adsorbent properties. It adsorbs irritant toxins and bacterial toxins, reduces mucous secretion and binds water.
- It also provides a sort of protective coating over the inflamed mucosal walls. It is often used alone with pectin (kaopectate is a mixture of 20% kaolin, pectin and hydrated aluminium silicate) for the symptomatic treatment of chronic diarrhea.

Uses
Adult oral dose is 45–90 ml after each loose bowel movement. Kaolin and morphine mixture is useful in the treatment of mild diarrhea. Because of its constipatory effect, morphine increases effectiveness of this preparation.

2. Calcium Carbonate (Chalk)

Its properties are quite similar to those of kaolin. Chalk and opium mixture is also available. It also helps to release flatulence and distension.

3. Magnesium Trisilicate and Aluminium Hydroxide

They have adsorbent property which is beneficial in the treatment of acidity and diarrhea. They are also used in the treatment of flatulence and distension.

4. Pectin
Chemistry
- It is a purified carbohydrate product obtained from an acid extraction of the rind of citrus fruits or from apple pomace.
- It is mainly made up of polygalacturonic acid with some of the methylated hydroxyl functional groups.

Uses
- It is used along with kaolin as an adsorbent and demulcent in the treatment of diarrhea. Each 30 ml of this preparation contains 5.85 g of kaolin and 130 mg of pectin. Activated charcoal and bentonite are also used in the treatment of mild diarrhea.

5. Bismuth Subsalicylate
MOA
- Because of adsorbent property, it binds with intestinal toxins and provides protective coating to mucosal surfaces. Its administration leads to formation of gray-black discoloration of stools.

6. Polycarbophil and Various Psyllium Seed Derivatives
MOA
- It binds water and bile salts. It is used to control diarrhea that is associated with passing of excessively watery stools.

MEPERIDINE DERIVATIVES

1. Diphenoxylate Hydrochloride

MOA

Because of its constipating effect, it is used for the symptomatic relief of diarrhea in patients with mild chronic inflammatory bowel disease and for infectious gastroenteritis. Atropine is added in subtherapeutic dose because of its spasmolytic activity. In lomotil, a mixture of diphenoxylate and atropine is present. Adult parenteral dose is 20 mg per day.

Pharmacokinetics

It is a weak meperidine congener lacking analgesic activity. It has the plasma half-life of 2.5 hours. Upon metabolism, diphenoxylic acid (active metabolite) and hydroxydiphenoxylic acid are excreted in the feces.

Adverse effect

- Adverse effects include nausea, vomiting, abdominal discomfort, miosis, blurred vision, dry mouth, flushing, sedation and tachycardia.
- It is contraindicated in children under 2 years and in patients with obstructive jaundice.

2. Loperamide

MOA

Loperamide exerts spasmolytic effect on GIT muscles by depressing slow cholinergic phase and rapid prostaglandin-mediated phase of smooth muscle contraction. It may act on intestinal nerve endings or ganglia.

Pharmacokinetics

- It is a synthetic meperidine congener devoid of sedative or respiratory depressant actions. It is orally used as an antidiarrheal agent.
- About 97% administered dose is bound to the plasma proteins. It has a plasma half-life of 7–14 hours. Major portion of administered dose appears unchanged in the feces. Inactive metabolites are excreted in the urine along with 10% dose in unchanged form.

Adverse effect

- Adverse effects include nausea, vomiting, anorexia, skin rashes, crampy abdominal pain, dry mouth and drowsiness.
- It is used in the symptomatic treatment of both acute nonspecific diarrhea and chronic diarrhea. Adult oral dose is 4 – 8 mg per day.

INTESTINAL ANTISEPTICS

MOA

These agents are used to treat severe diarrheal forms which are due to microbial infection. They mainly comprise of certain members of the sulphonamides and antibiotics that are poorly absorbable in GIT and thus reach in high concentration to the small and large bowel. Examples include sulphasalazine, sulphaguanidine, phthalyl sulfathiazole, succinyl sulfathiazole, etc.

Combination

- Various combinations of sulphonamides and antibiotics along with kaolin are available either in the form of cream or suspension. Streptomycin, neomycin, chloramphenicol, tetracyclines, nystatin are the examples of such antibiotics used for this purpose.
- A reduction in fecal volume contributes to the effectiveness of any antidiarrhoeal preparation. This is achieved by inclusion of a strong water-absorbing agent (e.g. methyl cellulose) in the formulation.

Loperamide

Ethylene oxide

Ethyl diphenyl-acetate

3,3-diphenyl-2-oxo-tetrahydrofuran

4-bromo-2,2-diphenyl-butyric acid (I)

4-bromo-2,2-diphenylbutyryl chloride

Dimethyl-amine

Dimethyl-(3,3-diphenyltetra-hydro-2-furylidene)-ammonium bromide (II)

4-(4-chlorophenyl)-4-hydroxypiperidine

Loperamide

Diphenoxylate

4-bromo-2,2-diphenylbutyronitrile

Ethyl 4-phenyl-piperidine-4-carboxylate

Diphenoxylate

Unit IX

Drugs Affecting the Respiratory System

50

Expectorants

Expectorants are the drugs that increases the volume of sputum and promote the expulsion of secretion or exudates from the respiratory tract. They also reduce the viscosity of tenacious sputum. The increase in volume of fluids from the respiratory tract by coughing is a measure of the effectiveness of an expectorant.

```
                    CLASSIFICATION OF EXPECTORANT

   Directly acting: Guaiphenesin,                 Mucolytics: Bromohexine,
   Potassium iodide, potassium citrate,           ambroxo 1, carbocisteine,
   potassium acetate, vasaka, terpinhydrate       acetylcysteine

                    Reflexly acting: Ammonium
                    chloride, potassium iodide,
                    ammonium carbonate
```

These drugs increase the bronchial secretion or reduce its viscosity, facilitating its removal by coughing. They are believed to loosen cough, which becomes less tiring and more productive.

Direct Acting

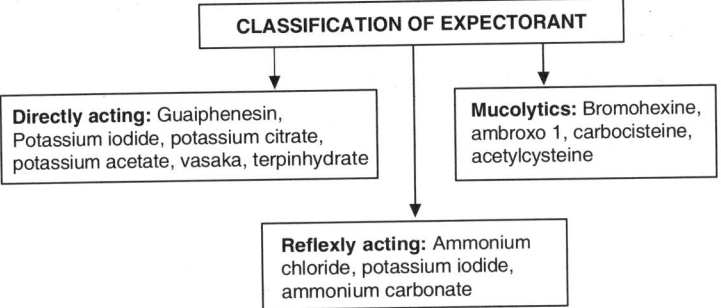

Terpinhydrate   Vasicine   Guaiphenesin

Mucolytics

Carbocisteine   Ambroxol   Bromohexine   Acetylcysteine

■ DIRECTLY ACTING

Sodium and Potassium Citrate or Acetate

These are believed to increase bronchial secretion by salt action.

Potassium Iodide

MOA: It is secreted by bronchial glands and in this process irritates them, increasing the volume of secretion. This irritant action is not desirable if bronchial mucosa is actually inflamed. It is also a gastric irritant, acts refluxly as well.

Adverse effect: It is dangerous in patient sensitive to iodine and interferes with thyroid function test. Prolonged use can induce goiter and hypothyroidism. Given to pregnant or nursing mother, fetal or infantile goiter and hypothyroidism has occurred.

Guaiphenesin

It is believed to act directly increase the bronchial secretion and mucosal ciliary action, when after absorption from gut they are secreted by tracheobronchial glands. Gastric upset and rash can occur.

Tolu Balsum, Vasaka Syrup, Terpin Hydrate

These act in the same manner as that of Guaiphenesin.

■ REFLEXLY ACTING

Ammonium Salts

MOA: These are gastric irritants; reflxly enhances bronchial secretion and sweating. Expectorant doses are subemetic but often nauseating because of unpleasant taste.

■ MUCOLYTICS

Bromohexine
MOA

- A derivative of the alkaloid vasicine obtained from *Adhatoda vasica*, is a potent mucolytic and mucokinetic, capable of inducing thin copious bronchial secretion.
- It depolymerises mucopolysaccharides directly as well as liberating lysosomal enzymes, network of fiberes in tenacious sputum is broken. It is particularly useful if mucus plugs are present.

Adverse effect: These are rhinorrhea and lacrymation, gastric irritation and hypersensitivity.

Ambroxol

A metabolite of bromohexine having similar effects.

Acetylcysteine

MOA: It opens disulfide bonds in mucoproteins present in sputum, makes it less viscous, but have to be administered directly into the respiratory tract.

Carbocisteine

MOA: It liquefies viscid sputum in the same as acetylcysteine and is administered orally. Side effects are GI irritation and rashes.

Guainphenesin

Guaiacol (I) + 3-chloropropane-1,2-diol → (NaOH) → Guaiphenesin

Acetylcysteine

L-cysteine hydrochloride monohydrate + Acetic anhydride → (CH₃COONa) → Acetylcysteine

Ambroxol

Paracetamol → (H₂, Rh) → trans-4-acet-amidocyclohexanol → (NaOH) → trans-4-acet-amidocyclohexanol (I)

2-amino-3,5-dibromobenzaldehyde → trans-4-(2-amino-3,5-dibromobenzylidenamino)-cyclohexanol → (NaBH₄ or HCOOH) → Ambroxol

Antiasthmatic Drugs

Bronchial asthma is characterized by hyper-responsiveness of tracheobronchial smooth muscle to a variety of stimuli, resulting in narrowing of air tube, often accompanied by increased secretion, mucosal edema and mucus plugging.

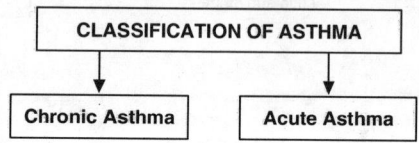

1. Chronic Asthma

- In chronic asthma, the individual has intermittent attacks of dyspnea (disorder of breathing), wheezing, and cough, the dyspnea consisting of difficulty in breathing out.
- Note that the term reversible as applied to chronic asthma needs to be qualified since it is only the acute attack of dyspnea that is reversible—the underlying pathological change may not be reversible and indeed can progress.

2. Acute Asthma

- Acute severe asthma (also known as *status asthmaticus*) is not easily reversed. It can be fatal and requires prompt and energetic treatment. Hospitalization may be necessary.
- It is currently recognised that the characteristic features of most cases of asthma are:
  1. Inflammatory changes in the airways
  2. Bronchial hyper-reactivity.

ETIOLOGY

- The term bronchial hyper-reactivity (or hyper-responsiveness) refers to abnormal sensitivity to a wide range of stimuli such as irritant chemicals, cold air, stimulant drugs, etc., all of which can result in bronchoconstriction. Stimuli that cause the actual asthma attacks are many and varied and include allergens (in sensitized individuals), exercise (in which the stimulus may be cold air), respiratory infections and atmospheric pollutants such as sulfur dioxide.
- The non-steroidal anti-inflammatory drugs (NSAIDs), especially aspirin, can precipitate asthma in sensitive individuals.

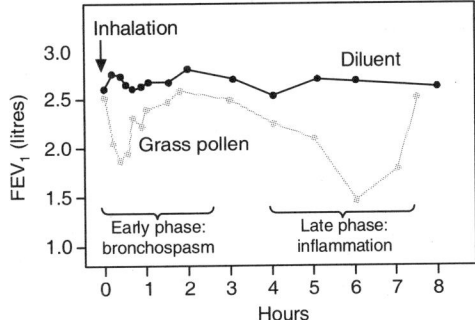

Fig. 51.1: The two phases of asthma as demonstrated by the changes in the forced expiratory volume in 1 second (FEV$_1$) after inhalation of grass pollen in an allergic subject.

- The development of allergic asthma probably involves both genetic and environmental factors, and the asthmatic attack itself consists, in many subjects, of two main phases—the immediate phase and the late (or delayed) phase. These phases can be demonstrated by tests of FEV$_1$ after allergen challenge (Fig. 51.1).
- This division into two phases is fairly arbitrary—indeed, in some subjects, only one of the phases may be obvious—but it provides a useful basis for discussing the physiopathological changes in the bronchi as well as the locus of action and the effects of drugs used in treatment.
- Numerous cells and mediators play a part in the pathogenesis of asthma and the full details of the complex events involved are still a matter of debate. The following account is, therefore, necessarily simplified. Nevertheless, it should provide a useful basis for understanding the rational use of current (and future) drugs in the treatment of asthma.

▨ THE DEVELOPMENT OF ALLERGIC ASTHMA

- In allergic asthma, there is predominant activation of the T helper (Th) type 2 cell wing of the immune response. Sensitization involves exposure of genetically predisposed individuals to allergens such as pollen or proteins of the house dust mite; environmental factors (e.g. atmospheric pollutants) may contribute (Fig. 51.2).
- The allergens interact with dendritic cells and the helper lymphocytes giving rise to a clone of Th2 lymphocytes, which then:
  1. Generate a cytokine environment that switches B cells/plasma cells to the production and release of IgE.
  2. Generate cytokines such as interleukin-5 (IL-5), which promotes differentiation and activation of eosinophils generate various cytokines (e.g. IL-4 and IL-13) that induce expression of IgE receptors, mainly on mast cells but also on eosinophils; IL-4 also induces endothelium to express receptors that specifically attract eosinophils.
- The system thus becomes primed so that subsequent re-exposure to the relevant allergen will cause an asthmatic attack.

The Immediate Phase of Asthmatic Attack

- In allergic asthma, the immediate phase (i.e. the initial response to allergen provocation) occurs abruptly and is mainly caused by spasm of the bronchial smooth muscle. Allergen interaction with mast cell-fixed IgE causes release of several spasmogens—histamine, the cysteinyl-leukotrienes (LTC_4 and LTD_4) and prostaglandin D_2 (PGD_2).

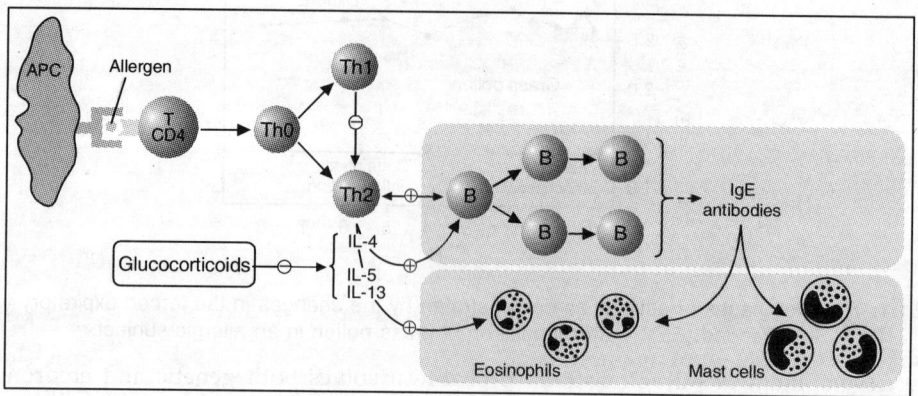

Fig. 51.2: The part played by T lymphocytes in asthma.

- In genetically susceptible individuals, allergen (green circle) interacts with dendritic cells and $CD4^+$ T cells, leading to the development of Th0 helper lymphocytes, which give rise to a clone of helper Th2 lymphocytes.

- These then (i) generate a cytokine environment that switches B cells/plasma cells to the production and release of IgE; (ii) generate cytokines such as interleukin (IL)-5, which promote differentiation and activation of eosinophils; and (iii) generate various cytokines (e.g. IL-4 and IL-13) that induce expression of IgE receptors, mainly on mast cells but also on eosinophils.

- The role of these cells and cytokines in asthma is depicted in Fig. 51.2. It is believed that a decrease in activation of the Th1 wing of the response (shown greyed) allows for the allergen-induced priming of the immune response for asthma. Glucocorticoids inhibit the action of the cytokines specified. (APC, antigen-presenting dendritic cell; B, B cell; Th, T helper cell; P, plasma cell.)

- Important mediators and cells are emphasised. (CysLTs, cysteinyl-leukotrienes (leukotrienes C_4 and D_4); H, histamine; EMBP, eosinophil major basic protein; ECP, eosinophil cationic protein; iNO, induced nitric oxide. For more detail of the Th2-derived cytokines and chemokines, Note that not all asthmatic subjects respond to cromoglicate or nedocromil, and that theophylline and the cysteinyl-leukotriene receptor antagonists are only second-line drugs.

- Other mediators released include IL-4, IL-5, IL-13, macrophage inflammatory protein-1α and tumour necrosis factor-α (TNF-α).

- Various chemotaxins and chemokines attract leucocytes, particularly eosinophils and mononuclear cells, into the area, setting the stage for the delayed phase.

- Once IgE binds to mast cells (or activated eosinophils), an amplification system operates since the cells not only release the spasmogens and other mediators specified but also can stimulate B cells to produce more IgE. Furthermore, the production of IL-4, IL-5 and IL-13 amplifies the Th2-mediated events described in Fig. 51.3.

- Most exercise-induced asthma appears to involve mainly the phenomena of this first phase.

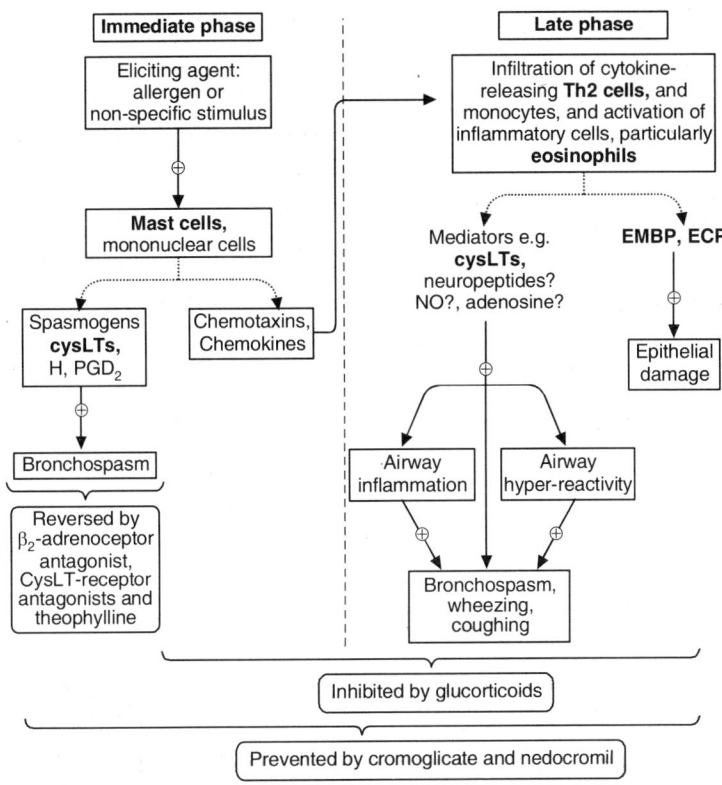

Fig. 51.3: Outline of the reactions thought to occur in asthma, with the actions of the main drugs.

The Late Phase (Fig. 51.4)

- The second, late phase or delayed response occurs at a variable time after exposure to the eliciting stimulus and may be nocturnal. This phase is in essence a progressing inflammatory reaction, initiation of which occurred during the first phase, the influx of Th2 lymphocytes being of particular importance.
- The inflammation is different from that seen, e.g. in bronchitis. It has special characteristics in that there is infiltration not only by the usual inflammatory cells but also, and more specifically, by activated cytokine-releasing Th2 cells and by activated eosinophils. The physiological importance of these later cells is in the defence against invading organisms, particularly helminths.
- But in the context of asthma, they are inappropriately activated and release cysteinyl-leukotrienes, cytokines IL-3 and IL-5, chemokine IL-8 and the toxic proteins, eosinophil cationic protein, major basic protein and eosinophil-derived neurotoxin. These substances play an important part in the events of the late phase, the toxic proteins causing damage and loss of epithelium.
- Growth factors released from inflammatory cells act on smooth muscle cells, causing hypertrophy and hyperplasia, and the smooth muscle can itself release pro-inflammatory mediators and autocrine growth factors shows schematically the changes that take place in the bronchioles.

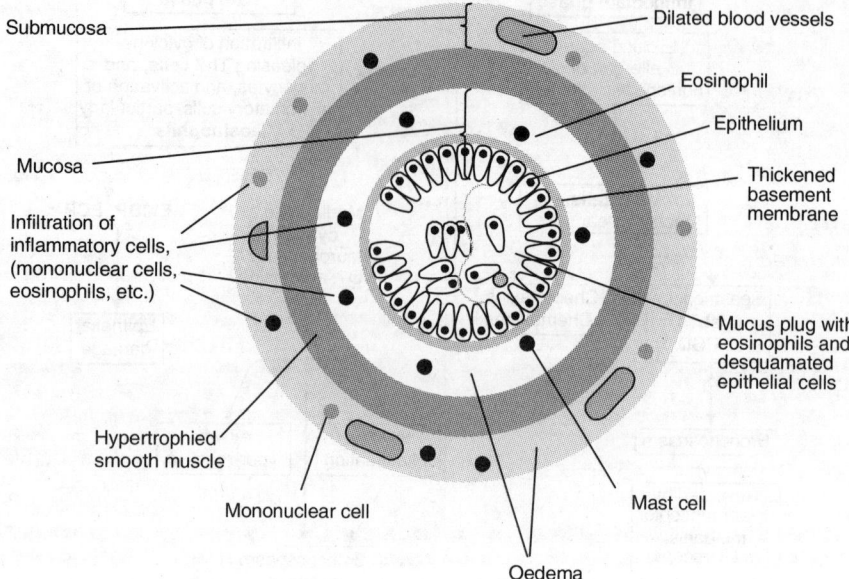

Fig. 51.4: Schematic diagram of a cross-section of a bronchiole showing the changes that can occur with severe chronic asthma.

- The epithelial loss means that irritant receptors and C fibres are more accessible to irritant stimuli; this is thought to be the main basis of the hyperreactivity.

CLASSIFICATION OF ANTIASTHMATIC AGENTS

Classification of antiasthmatic agents is depicted in Flow chart 51.1.

Flow chart 51.1: Classification of antiasthmatic agents

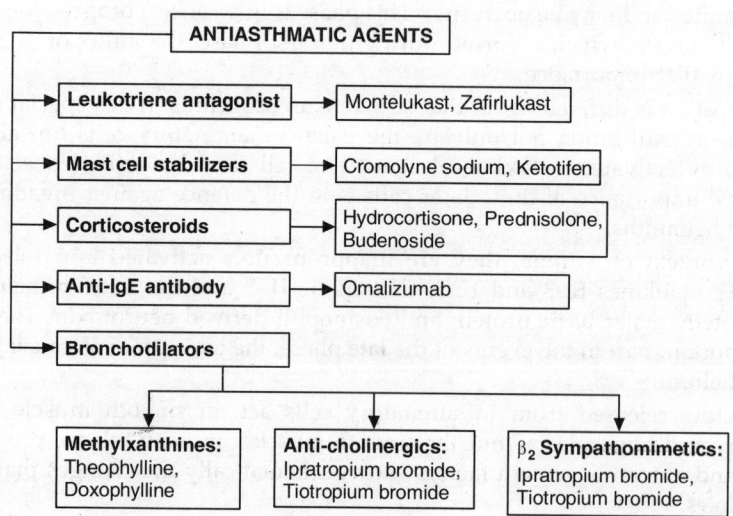

Bronchodilators

A. β₂ Sympathomimetics

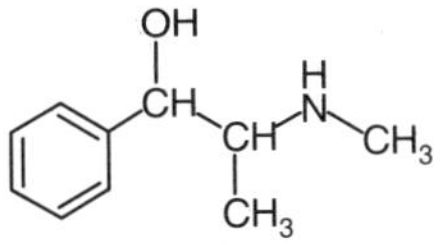

Ephedrine

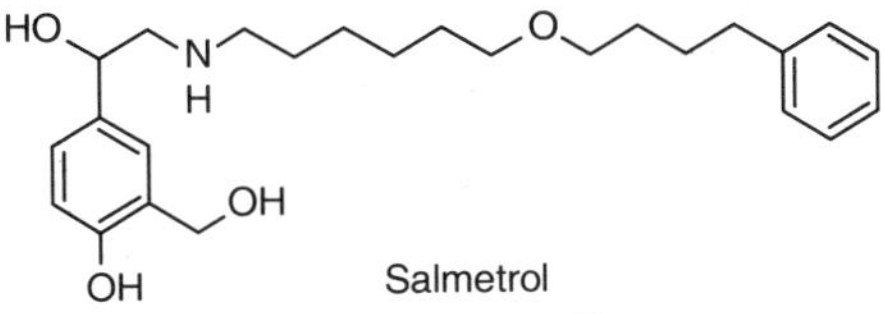

Salmetrol

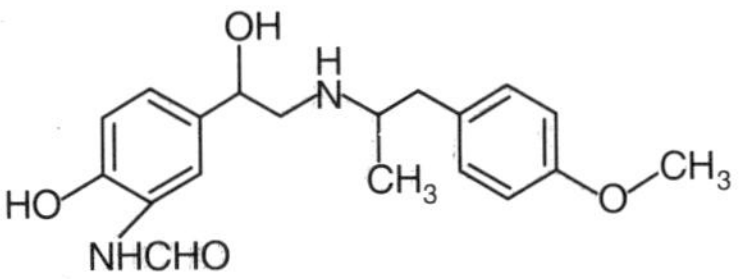

Formoterol

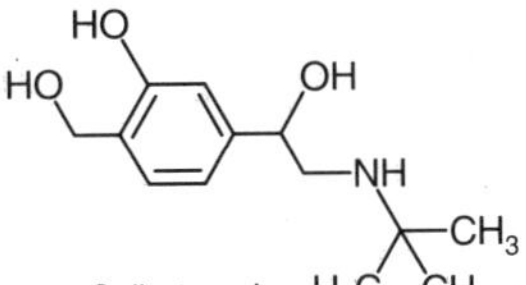

Salbutamol

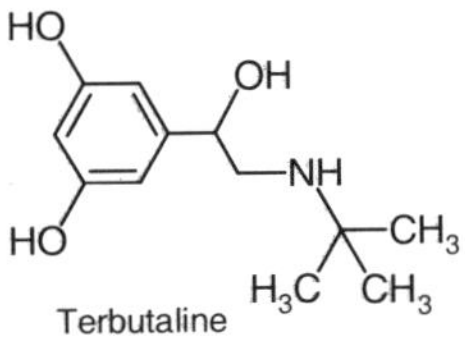

Terbutaline

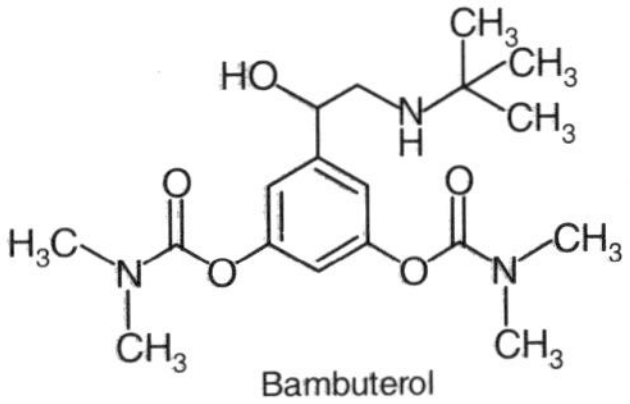

Bambuterol

B. Methylxanthines

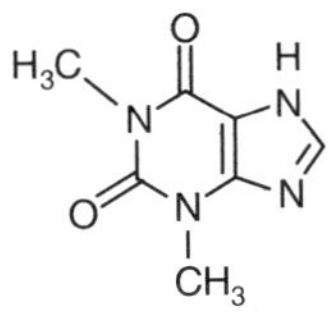

Theophylline

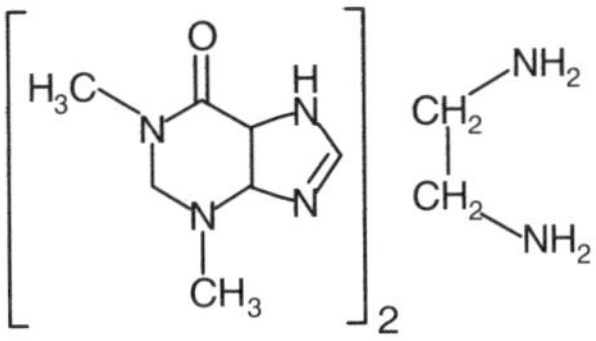

Aminophylline

C. Anticholinergics

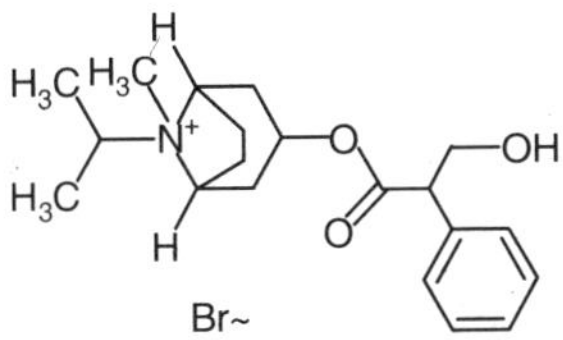

Br~
Ipratropium

Leukotriene Antagonist

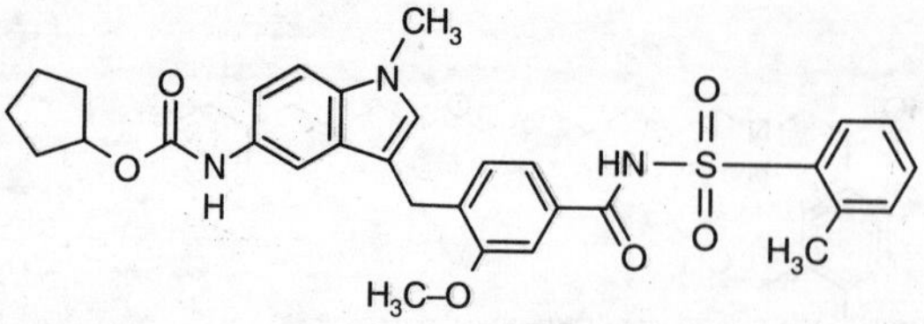

Zafirlukast

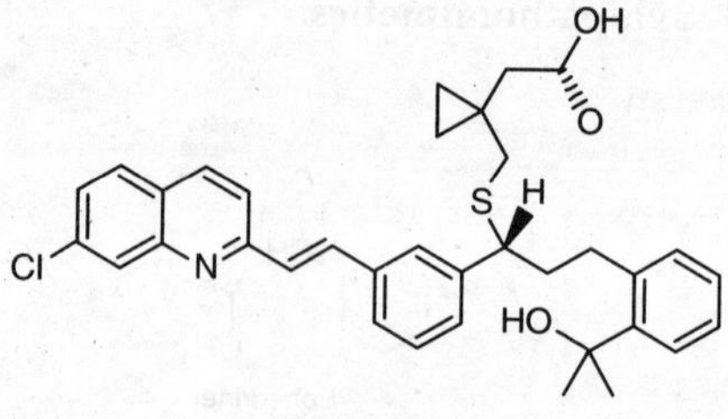

Montelukast

Mast Cell Stabilizers

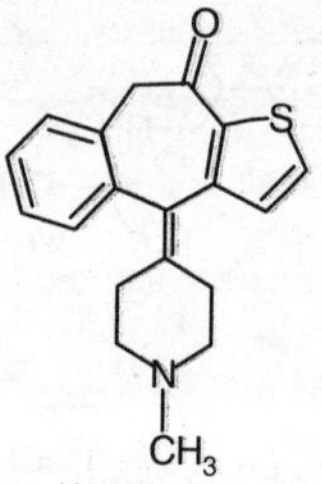

Ketotifen

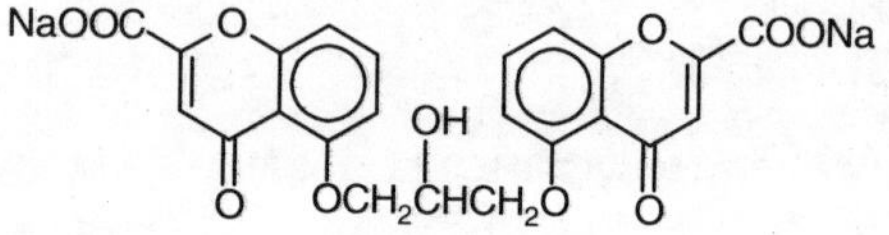

Cromolyn sodium

Glucocorticoids

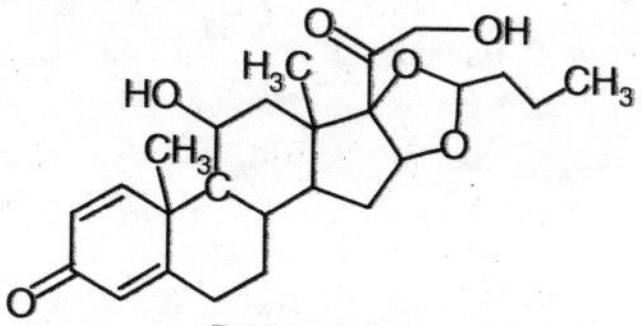

Budenoside

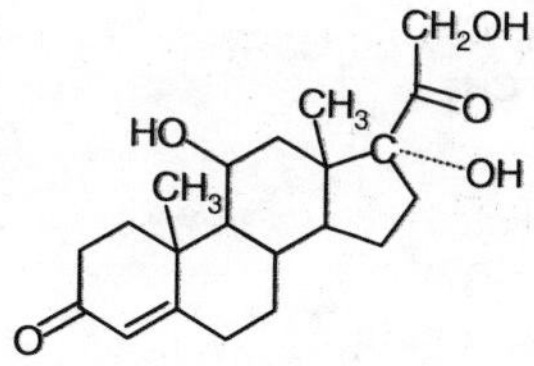

Hydrocortisone

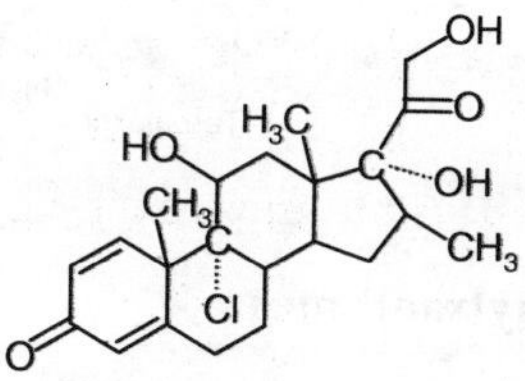

Beclomethasone

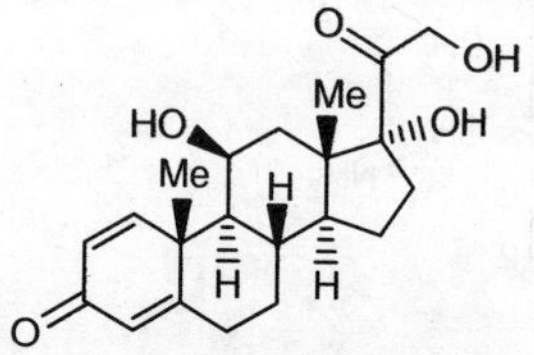

Prednisolone

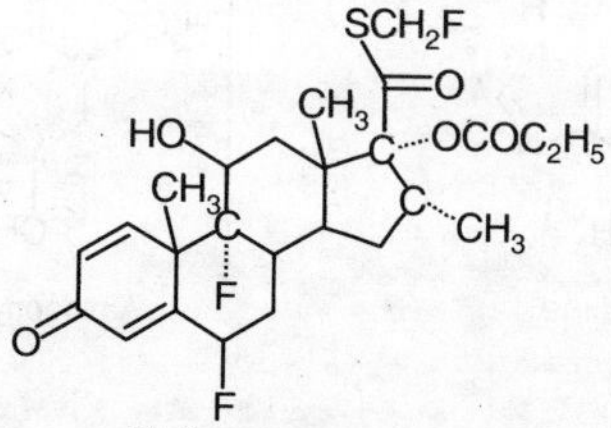

Fluticasone

▨ BRONCHODILATORS

▨ 1. β_2 SYMPATHOMIMETICS

Salbutamol, Terbutaline, Bambuter, Salmetrol and Formetrol

Mechanism of action

- The mechanism of antiasthmatic action of β adrenergic receptor agonists is undoubtedly linked to the direct relaxation of airway smooth muscle and consequent bronchodilation.

Although human bronchial smooth muscle receives little or no sympathetic innervation, it nevertheless contains large numbers of β_2 adrenergic receptors.

- Stimulation of these receptors activates the G_s adenylyl cyclase-cyclic AMP pathway with a consequent reduction in smooth muscle tone. β_2 adrenergic receptor agonists also increase the conductance of large Ca^{2+}-sensitive K^+ channels in airway smooth muscle, leading to membrane hyperpolarization and relaxation.

- This occurs at least partly by mechanisms independent of adenylyl cyclase activity and cyclic AMP production and may involve the regulation of capacitative Ca^{2+} entry by small G proteins.

- There are β_2 adrenergic receptors on cell types in the airways other than bronchial smooth muscle. Of particular interest, stimulation of β_2 adrenergic receptors inhibits the function of numerous inflammatory cells, including mast cells, basophils, eosinophils, neutrophils, and lymphocytes. In general, stimulating β_2 adrenergic receptors in these cell types increases intracellular cyclic AMP, activating a signaling cascade that inhibits the release of inflammatory mediators and cytokines.

Adverse reaction

- Owing to their β_2-receptor selectivity and topical delivery, inhaled β adrenergic receptor agonists at recommended doses have relatively few side effects. A portion of inhaled drug is inevitably absorbed into the systemic circulation.

- At higher doses, therefore, these drugs may lead to increased heart rate, cardiac arrhythmias, and central nervous system (CNS) effects associated with β adrenergic receptor activation. This is of particular concern in patients with poorly controlled asthma, in whom there may be excessive and inappropriate reliance on symptomatic treatment with short-acting β receptor agonists.

2. METHYLXANTHINES

Theophylline, Aminophylline, Cholline, Theophyllinate and Doxophylline

Mechanism of action

- Theophylline inhibits cyclic nucleotide phosphodiestrase (PDEs), thereby preventing breakdown of cyclic AMP and cyclic GMP to 5c-AMP and 5c-GMP, respectively. Inhibition of PDEs will lead to an accumulation of cyclic AMP and cyclic GMP, thereby increasing signal transduction through these pathways. The cyclic nucleotide PDEs are members of a superfamily of genetically distinct enzymes. Theophylline and related methylxanthines are relatively nonselective in the PDE subtypes they inhibit.

- Cyclic nucleotide production is regulated by endogenous receptor-ligand interactions leading to activation of adenylyl cyclase and guanylyl cyclase. Inhibitors of PDEs therefore can be thought of as drugs that enhance the activity of endogenous autacoids, hormones, and neurotransmitters that signal via cyclic nucleotide messengers. This may explain why the *in vivo* potency often exceeds that observed *in vitro*.

- Theophylline is a competitive antagonist at adenosine receptors. Adenosine can act as an autacoid and transmitter with myriad biological actions. Of particular relevance to asthma are the observations that adenosine can cause bronchoconstriction in asthmatics and potentiate immunologically induced mediator release from human lung mast cells. Inhibition of the actions of adenosine therefore also must be considered when attempting to explain the mechanism of action of theophylline.

- Theophylline also may owe part of its anti-inflammatory action to its ability to activate histone deacetylases in the nucleus. In theory, the deacetylation of histones could decrease the transcription of several proinflammatory genes and potentiate the effect of corticosteroids.

ANTI-CHOLINERGICS

Ipratropium Bromide and Tiotropium Bromide

Mechanism of action

- The cholinergic receptor subtype responsible for bronchial smooth muscle contraction is the muscarinic M_3 receptor. Although iprotropium and related compounds block all five muscarinic receptor subtypes with similar affinity, it is likely that M_3-receptor antagonism alone accounts for the bronchodilating effect.
- The bronchodilation produced by ipratropium in asthmatic subjects develops more slowly and usually is less intense than that produced by adrenergic agonists. Some asthmatic patients may experience a useful response lasting up to 6 hours.
- The variability in the response of asthmatic subjects to ipratropium presumably reflects differences in the strength of parasympathetic tone and in the degree to which reflex activation of cholinergic pathways participates in generating symptoms in individual patients. Hence the utility of ipratropium must be assessed on an individual basis by a therapeutic trial.

CORTICOSTEROIDS

Hydrocortisone, Prednisolone, Beclomethasone, Budenoside and Fluticasone

Mechanism of action

- Asthma is associated with airway inflammation, airway hyper-reactivity, and acute bronchoconstriction. Glucocorticoids do not directly relax airway smooth muscle and thus have little effect on acute bronchoconstriction.
- By contrast, these agents are singularly effective in inhibiting airway inflammation. Very few mechanisms of inflammation escape the inhibitory effects of these drugs.
- The anti-inflammatory effects of glucocorticoids in asthma include modulation of cytokine and chemokine production; inhibition of eicosanoid synthesis; marked inhibition of accumulation of basophils, eosinophils, and other leukocytes in lung tissue; and decreased vascular permeability.
- The profound and generalized anti-inflammatory action of this class of drugs explains why they are currently the most effective drugs used in the treatment of asthma.

LEUKOTRIENE ANTAGONIST

Montelukast and Zafirlukast

Mechanism of action

Leukotriene-modifying drugs act either as competitive antagonist of leukotriene receptors or by inhibiting the synthesis of leukotrienes. The pharmacological properties of leukotrienes are discussed in detail.

Leukotriene-receptor antagonists

- Cysteinyl leukotrienes (cys-LTs) include leukotriene C4 (LTC4), leukotriene D4 (LTD4), and leukotriene E4 (LTE4). All the cys-LTs are potent constrictors of bronchial smooth muscle.

On a molar basis, LTD4 is approximately 1000 times more potent than is histamine as a bronchoconstrictor.

- The receptor responsible for the bronchoconstrictor effect of leukotrienes is the cys-LT1 receptor. Although each of the cys-LTs is an agonist at the cys-LT1 receptor, LTE4 is less potent than either LTC4 or LTD4.

- Zafirlukast and montelukast are selective high-affinity competitive antagonists for the cys-LT1 receptor. *Pranlukast* is another cys-LT1-receptor antagonist used in some countries in the treatment of asthma, but it is not approved for use in the United States.

- Inhibition of cys-LT-induced bronchial smooth muscle contraction likely is involved in the therapeutic effects of these agents to relieve the symptoms of asthma. The effects of cys-LTs that are potentially relevant to bronchial asthma are not limited to bronchial smooth muscle contraction.

- Cys-LTs can increase microvascular leakage, increase mucous production, and enhance eosinophil and basophil influx into the airways. The extent to which inhibiting these non-smooth muscle effects of leukotrienes contributes to the therapeutic effects of the drugs is not known. It may be noteworthy; however, that zafirlukast significantly inhibits the influx of basophils and lymphocytes entering the airways following experimental allergen challenge in asthmatic subject.

Leukotriene–synthesis Inhibitors

- The formation of leukotrienes depends on lipooxygenation of arachidonic acid by 5-lipooxygenase. Zileuton is a potent and selective inhibitor of 5-lipooxygenase activity and thus inhibits the formation of all 5-lipooxygenase products.

- Thus, in addition to inhibiting the formation of the cys-LTs, zileuton also inhibits the formation of leukotriene B4 (LTB4), a potent chemotactic autacoid, and other eicosanoids that depend on leukotriene A4 (LTA4) synthesis.

- In theory, the therapeutic effects of a 5-lipooxygenase inhibitor would include all those observed with the cys-LT1-receptor antagonists, as well as other effects that may result from inhibiting the formation of LTB4 and other 5-lipooxygenase products. The pharmacological actions of cys-LTs are not fully accounted for by activation of the cys-LT1 receptor.

Adverse reaction

- There are few adverse effects directly associated with inhibition of leukotriene synthesis or function. This likely is due to the fact that leukotriene production is limited predominantly to sites of inflammation.

▨ ANTI-IgE ANTIBODY

Mechanism of Action

- The Fc region of IgE binds with high affinity to the Fc epsilon receptor I (FceRI). FceRI is expressed on the surfaces of mast cells and basophils, as well as several other cell types. When an allergen interacts with the antigen-binding domains of IgE bound to FceRI on mast cells and basophils, it cross-links the receptors and activates the cell.

- This, in turn, triggers the release of preformed granule-associated mediators such as histamine and tryptase. In addition, it results in the immediate production of eicosanoids, most notably LTC4 and prostaglandin D2 (PGD2) and, on a time scale of hours instead of minutes, the synthesis of various cytokines. Omalizumab is an IgG antibody for which the antigen is the Fc region of the IgE antibody. Omalizumab binds tightly to free IgE in the circulation to form omalizumab-IgE complexes that have no affinity for FceRI.

- At the recommended doses, omalizumab reduces free IgE by more than 95%, thereby limiting the amount of IgE bound to FceRI-bearing cells. Omalizumab treatment also decreases the amount of FceRI expressed on basophils and mast cells.

- Thus the effectiveness of omalizumab in reducing the amount of allergen-specific IgE bound to mast cells and basophils depends on the reduction of both free IgE and available FceRIs on cell surfaces.

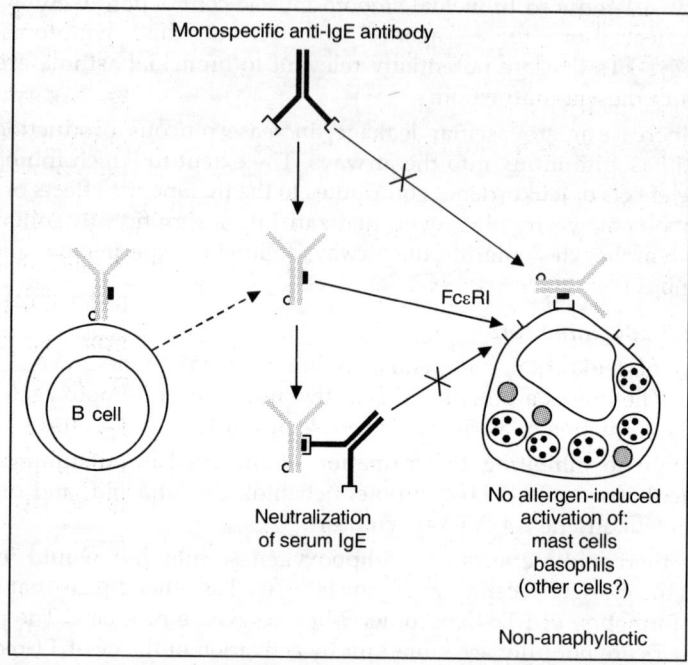

Fig. 51.5: Omalizumab is a monospecific anti-IgE antibody. Specific Blymphocytes produce IgE antibodies. The Fc region of IgE heavy chains binds with high affinity to receptors (FceRI) in the plasma membranes of mast cells and basophils (and other cells). Allergen interacts with the antigen-binding site of cell-bound IgE, causing FceRI cross-linking and cell activation. Omalizumab neutralizes the free IgE in the serum by binding to the Fc regions of the heavy chains to form high-affinity IgE-anti-IgE complexes. This prevents the IgE from binding to FceRI, thereby blocking allergen-induced cell activation.

- Normally, IgE-mediated basophil activation is extremely efficacious, requiring antigen to interact with only a small fraction of the bound IgE to evoke a half-maximal response.

■ MAST CELL STABILIZERS

Cromolyn Sodium and Ketotifen

Mechanism of action

- Cromolyn and nedocromil have a variety of activities that may relate to their therapeutic efficacy in asthma. These include inhibiting mediator release from bronchial mast cells; reversing increased functional activation in leukocytes obtained from the blood of asthmatic patients; suppressing the activating effects of chemotactic peptides on human neutrophils, eosinophils, and monocytes; inhibiting parasympathetic and cough reflexes; and inhibiting leukocyte trafficking in asthmatic airways. Suffice it to say that the mechanism of action of cromolyn and nedocromil in asthma is not known.

Adverse Effect

- Cromolyn and nedocromil generally are well tolerated by patients. Adverse reactions are infrequent and minor and include bronchospasm, cough or wheezing, laryngeal edema, joint swelling and pain, angioedema, headache, rash, and nausea.
- Such reactions have been reported at a frequency of less than 1 in 10,000 patients. Very rare instances of anaphylaxis also have been documented. Nedocromil and cromolyn can cause a bad taste.

Budenoside

16a-hydroxyprednisolone   Butyraldehyde   Budesonide

Bambuterol

3,5-dihydroxy-
acetophenone

Dimethyl-
carbamayl
chloride

3,5-bis(dimethylcarbamayloxy)
acetophenone (I)

1. Br₂
2. H₃C N H
   H₃C CH₃
2. N-benzyl-tert-
butylamine

3,5-bis(dimethylcarbamayloxy)
acetophenone (I)

Bambuterol

52

Chronic Obstructive Pulmonary Disease (COPD)

Chronic obstructive pulmonary disease (COPD) is a progressive disease with emphysema (alveolar destruction) and bronchiolar fibrosis in variable proportion (Fig. 52.1). The expiratory air flow limitation does not fluctuate markedly over long periods of time but there are exacerbations precipitated by respiratory infections, pollutants, etc. It is clearly related to smoking and characterstically starts after the age 40. Quiting of smoking reduces rate of decline in lung function.

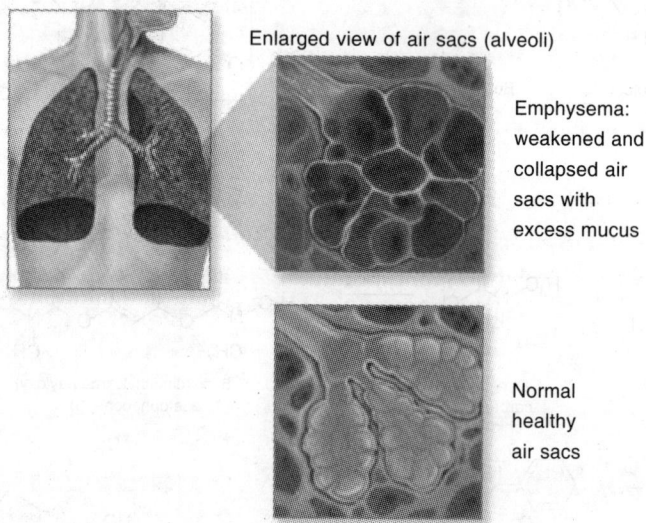

Enlarged view of air sacs (alveoli)

Emphysema: weakened and collapsed air sacs with excess mucus

Normal healthy air sacs

Fig. 52.1: COPD emphysema

- COPD (chronic obstructive pulmonary disease) is a disease of the airways and lungs that results in people having difficulty breathing air out (expiration); other symptoms include chronic coughing, difficulty walking due to shortness of breath, and frequent chest infections.

- In healthy people, the airways are elastic and springy so that when a person breathes in air, the airways fill up like small balloons, and when a person breathes out, the balloons deflate. However, in a person suffering from COPD, the airways lose their shape, resembling floppy balloons, and less air is able to pass in and out.

- In COPD, air flow is reduced during expiration because of inflammation (swelling and mucus buildup) in the lining of the air passages, or damage to some of the air passages, or a combination. In order for people to breath easily, the airways and lungs need to be wide open. However, in patients with COPD, the airways and lungs are partially or completely blocked.

- Medications such as salbutamol, a bronchodilator, can open up these airways allowing air to flow more easily. These medications are used by people with asthma, however, there is a very important difference between COPD and asthma. In asthma, medications can help a blocked airway become fully unblocked, and this is called reversible airway obstruction, whereas in COPD, these medications can only partially unblock the airways. This is called airway obstruction that is not fully reversible. Even with medical testing, it is sometimes difficult to tell if someone has COPD or asthma. Furthermore, it is possible for someone to have both COPD and asthma.

- To summarize, there are four problems affecting the airways in COPD, leading to airway obstruction that is not fully reversible where by a person with this disease experiences shortness of breath and a limited ability to exercise. These problems include:

1. The elastic fibers that allow the airways to expand and contract become less elastic, like old rubber bands.
2. The walls of many of the air passages are destroyed.
3. The walls of the airways swell and thicken.
4. Mucus builds up in the airways.

SYMPTOMS

1. Cough.
2. Sputum (mucus) production or a change in color of sputum can indicate a chest infection.
3. Shortness of breath, especially with exercise.
4. Wheezing (a whistling or squeaky sound when you breathe).
5. Chest tightness.
6. When a person with COPD is given the right treatment, she or he will experience none or fewer symptoms on a day -to-day basis. However, if a 'flare up' occurs, not only may his or her symptoms become more severe, but they may experience new symptoms as well. A symptom 'flare up,' also called an exacerbation, is commonly triggered by chest infections or environmental factors like temperature changes and air pollutants. A flare up requires medical treatment to avoid significant deterioration in the ability to breathe.

ETIOLOGY

1. In the United States, the leading cause of COPD is cigarette smoking by either smokers or former smokers; inhaled pipe and cigar smoke can also contribute to COPD.
2. In the United States, at least 400,000 people die each year as a result of diseases related to cigarette smoking. In COPD, most of the damage to the airways and lungs caused by cigarette smoking is not reversible. However, stopping smoking can definitely reduce further damage and reduce many symptoms of COPD such as chronic coughing and shortness of breath.
3. Other factors and conditions that contribute to the development of COPD are not fully understood, but they include asthma, exposure to air pollutants at home and in the workplace, and genetic factors.
4. Some evidence suggests that there is a genetic role in the development of COPD. In rare cases, COPD is caused by a gene-related disorder called alpha-1-antitrypsin (an-te-TRIP-sin) deficiency.

Alpha-1-antitrypsin deficiency accounts for 2 to 3% of COPD cases in the United States. Alpha-1-antitrypsin is a protein in the blood that helps counteract destructive proteins, but when levels of alpha-1-antitrypsin are low, destructive proteins in the body thrive.

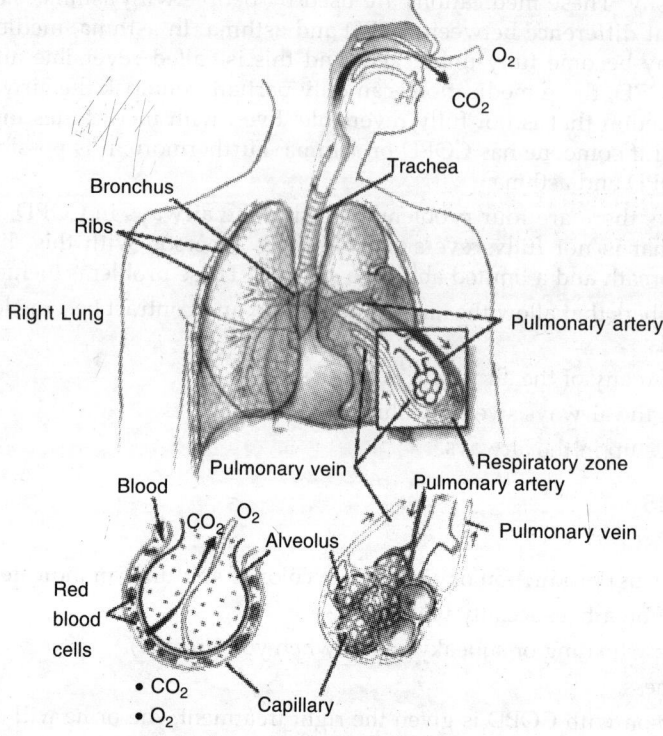

Fig. 52.2: Mechanism of respiration

TYPES OF COPD

- With asthma, airway obstruction is reversible; however, with COPD, airway obstruction is not fully reversible or is irreversible.
- The leading characteristic of COPD is reversible airway obstruction, thus any condition or disease that causes this problem may be referred to as COPD.
- Several common conditions can cause irreversible airway obstruction and therefore be considered a form of COPD. Although sometimes in COPD sufferers, these conditions occur together, rather than as a single condition.

Chronic Bronchitis

Chronic bronchitis is a condition characterized by a chronic wet cough persisting for 3 months a year for 2 successive years. The cough is not caused by an infection, asthma, or medication, and there is no medical explanation for its cause.

Emphysema

Emphysema is a disease in which there is permanent damage to airways, which become floppy and enlarged. Emphysema is common in people who have severe forms of COPD.

Asthma

- Asthma is a chronic condition of the airways caused by inflammation (swelling and mucus build-up) that blocks or obstructs the airways. Symptoms similar to COPD include trouble breathing, particularly when breathing out, except that in asthma the airway blockage or obstruction is reversible when treated.
- Sometimes people who are thought to have asthma fail to reverse their airway blockage after using medications (e.g. bronchodilators), and are subsequently diagnosed as having COPD. Furthermore, long-term, poorly controlled asthma can eventually worsen leading to irreversible airway obstruction.
- It is important to know which of the above conditions in the individual is causing COPD, because each can cause slightly different symptoms requiring different treatments. Most importantly in diagnosing COPD is determining an irreversible airway obstruction or blockage exists and its severity.

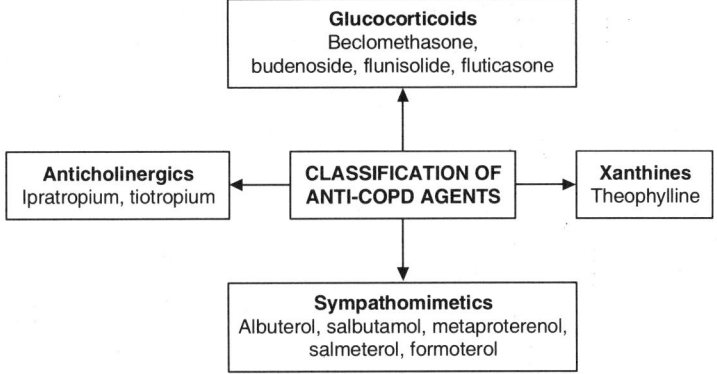

Anti-COPD Agents

1. Bronchodilators

- — Beta agonists short- and long-acting.
- — Anticholinergics short- and long-acting.
- — Theophylline.
- Bronchodilators relax the muscles around the airways to allow air to flow in and out of the lungs more easily.

2. Anti-inflammatories (Glucocorticoids)

- — Inhaled corticosteroids or "inhaled steroids"
- Anti-inflammatory drugs reduce the swelling and mucus in the airways causing them to open up and become wider again. Inhaled steroids can take 4 to 6 weeks to have an effect, while oral steroids act more rapidly.

3. Treatments for exacerbation (antibiotics): Exacerbations are often caused by a chest infection, which is suspected if there is a change in sputum color and/or volume. Antibiotics are required to clear up bacterial infections.

4. Oxygen therapy (at home or in a hospital): People with severe cases of COPD get inadequate oxygen in their bloodstream to sustain life, and consequently require supplemental oxygen at home and/or in a hospital.

For classification and synthesis refer Anti-asthma chapter.

▓ PREVENTION

1. One of the most important goals in the management of COPD is to prevent deterioration of the lungs—in other words, to maintain the best level of lung health possible. Preventive treatment in COPD also involves preventing exacerbations or "flare-ups."

2. The most important way to prevent deteriorations of the lungs in COPD is by quitting smoking and avoiding exposure to second-hand smoke. Avoiding smoking will also reduce the chances of developing COPD in the first place. Your healthcare provider can suggest to you ways to quit smoking, including nicotine replacement and other medications.

3. Annual influenza vaccination as well as vaccination against pneumococcal infection (a type of pneumonia) for COPD patients, independent of their age, will prevent these lung infections and reduce the risk of COPD exacerbations. For pneumococcal protection, after the initial vaccination, a further booster is required after 5 years.

4. Many who suffer from COPD are undernourished and generally less able to defend themselves against infection or cope with their underlying disease. Consulting a dietitian who can recommend food supplements and sample meal plans is helpful for many patients.

53

Antiallergic Rhinitis Agents

Allergic rhinitis is an allergic disease which affects many people worldwide. Rhinitis means 'inflammation of the nose', whilst the term allergic describes a normal but exaggerated response to a substance.

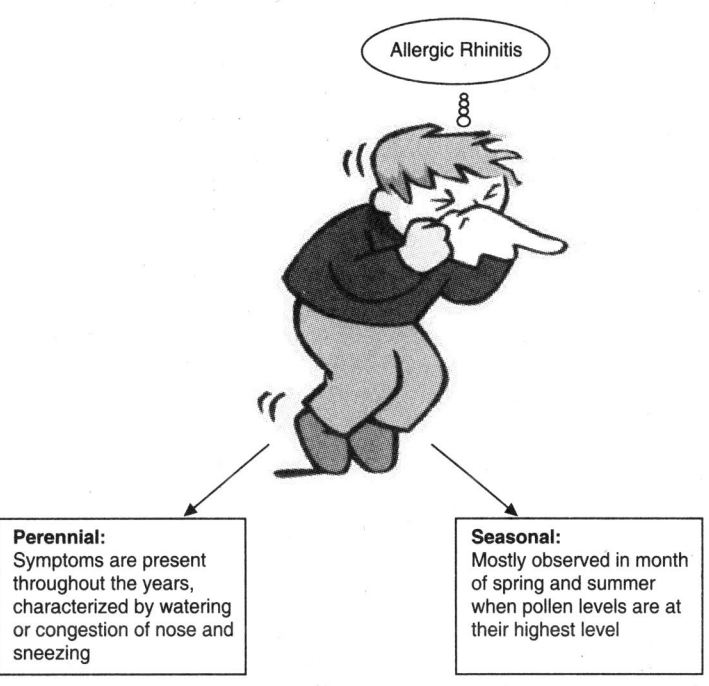

Allergic Rhinitis

Perennial:
Symptoms are present throughout the years, characterized by watering or congestion of nose and sneezing

Seasonal:
Mostly observed in month of spring and summer when pollen levels are at their highest level

- It may be perennial, which means symptoms are present throughout the year, or seasonal, with symptoms peaking during the months of spring and summer when pollen levels are at their highest. Perennial rhinitis is characterized primarily by nasal symptoms including watering or congestion of the nose and sneezing.

- It occurs due to an exaggerated response to an environmental trigger which results in inflammation of the lining of the nose. It is similar to hay fever; however, the substances which cause the allergic reaction are present all year round. Common causes include the faecal matter of the house dust-mite, animal proteins from domestic pets, and industrial dusts and fumes.

■ ETIOLOGY

- You develop an allergy when your immune system becomes hypersensitive to a normally harmless substance, such as inhaled pollen or dust mite particles or feces. Once sensitized, the immune system overreacts every time it's exposed, even to very tiny amounts.

- Not everyone has allergies. Some people are genetically predisposed (one or both parents have allergies), and others may develop allergies in response to the environment.

- One theory, called the 'hygiene hypothesis,' holds that allergies are the price we pay for protecting our children from germs with modern sanitation and antibiotics. The idea is that lack of exposure to dirt, dust, and certain childhood infections early in life makes the immune system hypersensitive later on.

- For example, studies in Europe have found that children growing up in regular contact with farm animals and barns have less hay fever than children in urban environments, who do not live on farms. On the other hand, repeated exposure to certain allergens, such as dust mites, may further predispose the offspring of allergic parents to develop allergies.

Common Offending Allergens (Fig. 53.1)

- A substance that provokes allergic rhinitis in one person may have no effect in another. Some substances are more allergenic than others.

Pollens

- These tiny male reproductive cells of flowering plants are ideally suited to travel on wayward breezes — right into your nose, throat, and eyes. Pollen season starts as early as January in southern states; further north, it may begin in March or April and run through October.

- The major culprits are not the big, showy bloomers; their pollen is generally too heavy to become air borne. The real trouble makers are plants whose blossoms are so inconspicuous that you may be hardly aware that they flower.

- The most common pollen allergens come from trees (alder, ash, birch, box elder, cypress, elm, hickory, maple, mulberry, oak, poplar, sycamore, walnut, and western red cedar); grasses (Bermuda, blue grasses, orchard, meadow fescue, rye, sour dock, sweet vernal, and timothy); and weeds (burning bush, cockleweed, ragweed, pigweed, Russian thistle, sagebrush, and tumbleweed).

Molds

- Though less notorious than pollen, mold spores are an equivalent source of misery. Among the most ubiquitous and allergenic are Alternaria, Cladosporium, Aspergillus, and Penicillium. You can encounter them both indoors and outdoors.

- Indoor molds grow in basements, bathrooms, humidifiers, garbage cans — wherever there's moisture.

- Outdoor molds, which are active from spring until the first frost, also thrive in damp conditions; they love rotting wood, leaf piles, and compost bins. (Mold spore allergens are not the same as the mold-produced toxins that can make you sick, if you eat them.)

Dust mites

These microscopic relatives of spiders and ticks live in fabric — bedding, carpets, and upholstery — and feed off the skin cells we shed. Decayed dust mite carcasses and droppings contain a highly allergenic protein.

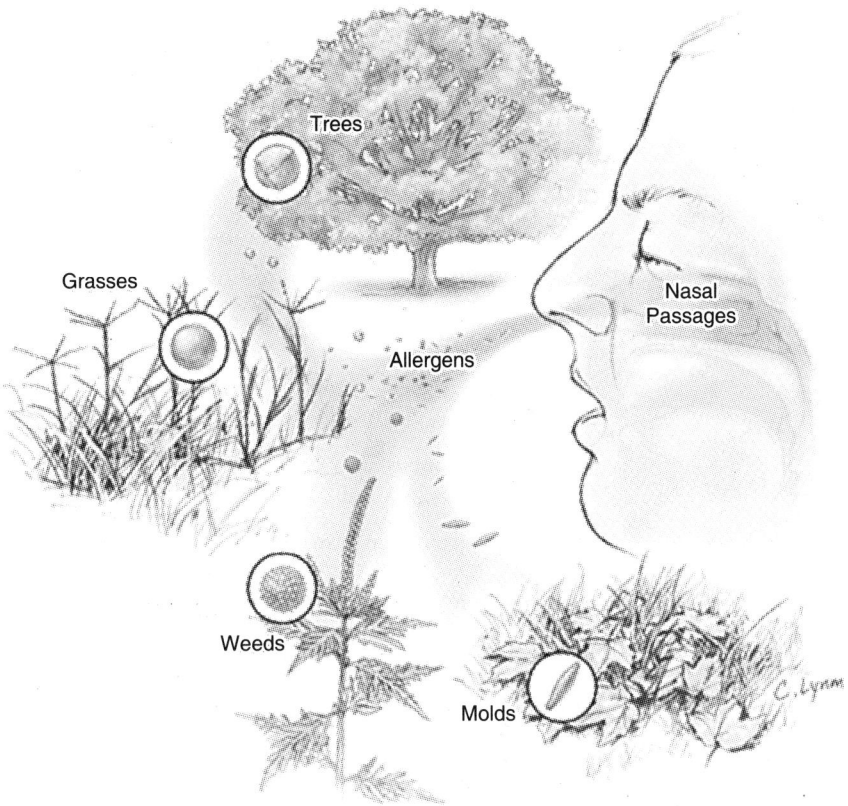

Fig. 53.1: Different sources of allergens

Perts and pests

- A salivary protein that animals, especially cats, collect on their skin and fur when they groom themselves is a potent allergen.
- So is the dander, or skin flakes, that pets shed. Rat urine and cockroach droppings also contain allergenic proteins.

PATHOPHYSIOLOGY (FIG. 53.2)

- In allergic rhinitis, an allergen — pollen, for example — dissolves in the mucosal lining of the nose, throat, or airways, where it comes into contact with sensitized immune cells called mast cells.
- These cells carry immunoglobulin E (IgE) antibodies, the result of the body's earlier encounter with the allergen. IgE-activated mast cells trigger the release of histamines, setting off a process that involves other inflammatory substances, such as leukotrienes and prostaglandins.
- The resulting dilated blood vessels, inflamed tissues, narrowed nasal passages, and congested sinuses cause sneezing, coughing, wheezing, runny nose, weepy eyes, and itchiness. The reaction may worsen and can damage tissue if it is not stopped.

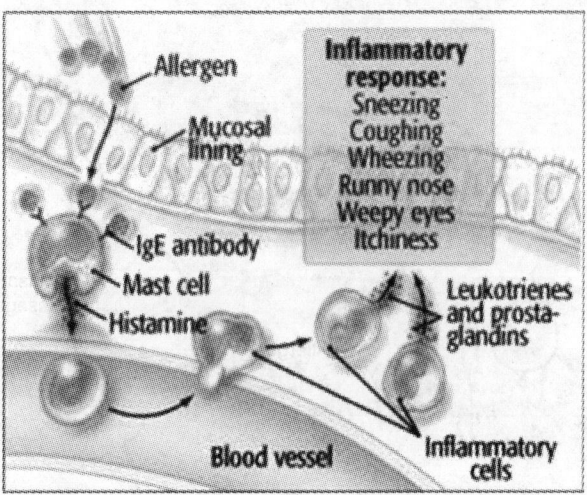

Fig. 53.2: Mechanism of rhinitis

CLASSIFICATION OF ANTIALLERGIC RHINITIS

Classification of antiallergic rhinitis is given in Flow chart 53.1.

Flow chart 53.1: Classification of antiallergic rhinitis

ANTIALLERGIC RHINITIS	
Antihistaminics:	Acrivastine, cetrizine, foxyfenadine, loratadine, azelastine
Mast cell stabilizers:	Cromolyn sodium, nedocromil
Glucocorticoids:	Beclomethasone, budenoside, flunisolide, fluticasone, momentasone
Leukotriene antagonist:	Montelukast
Nasal decongestant:	Phenylpherine, xylometazoline, naphazoline, oxymetazoline, tetrahydrozoline, phenylpropanolamine

Antihistaminics

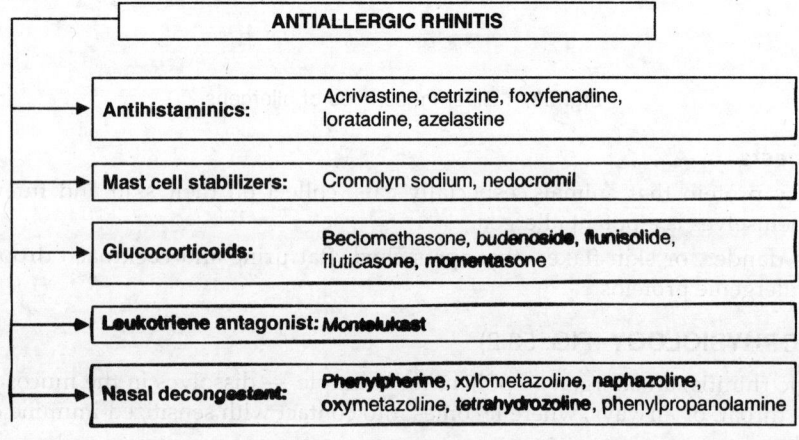

Acrivastine   Cetrizine

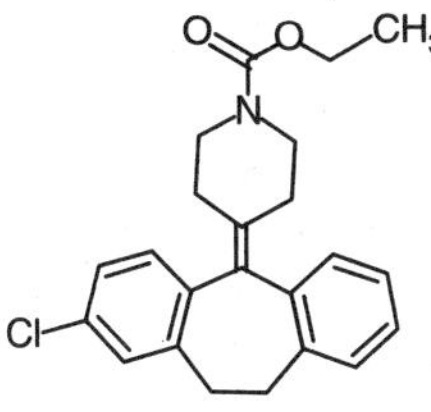

Loratadine

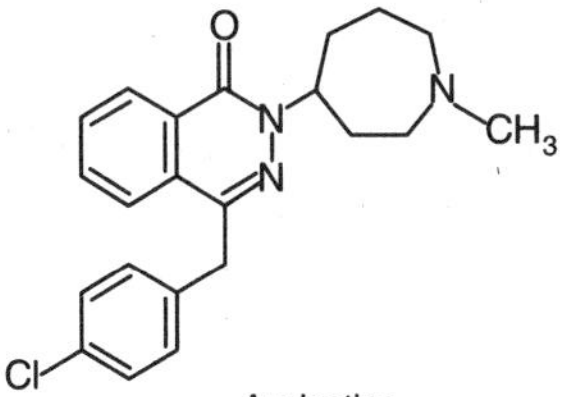

Azelastine

Mast cell stabilizers

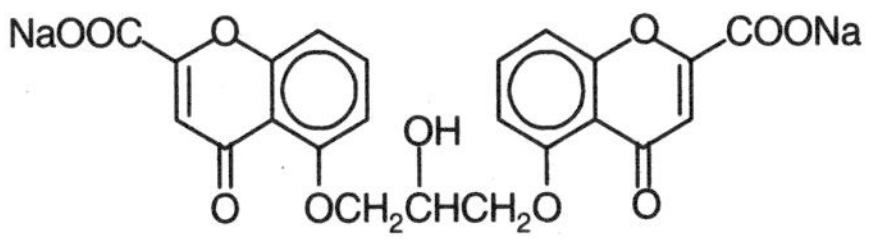

Cromolyn sodium

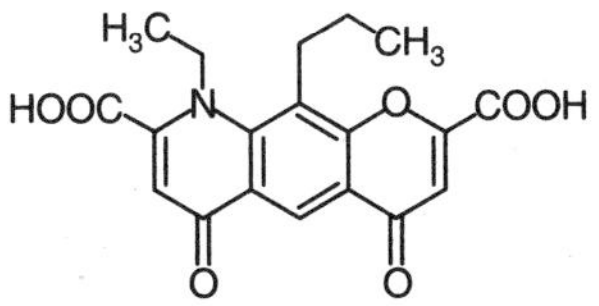

Nedocromil

Glucocorticoids

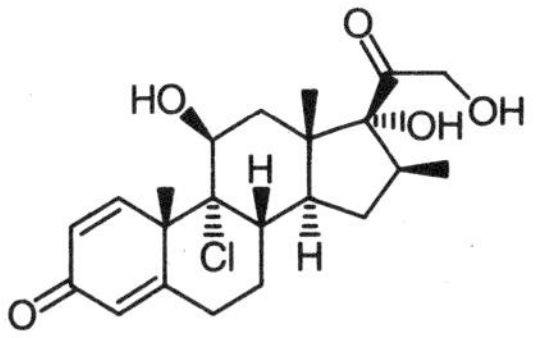

Beclomethasone

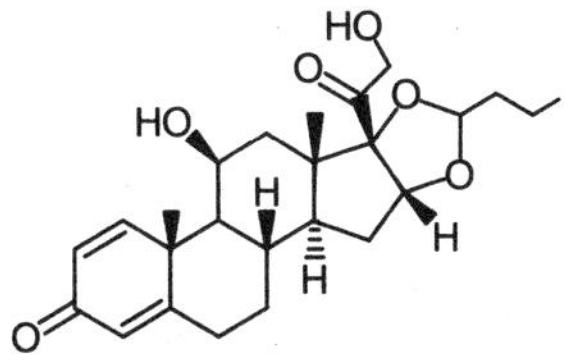

Budenoside

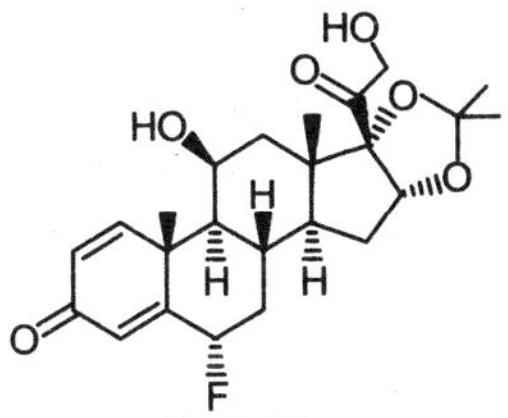

Flunisolide

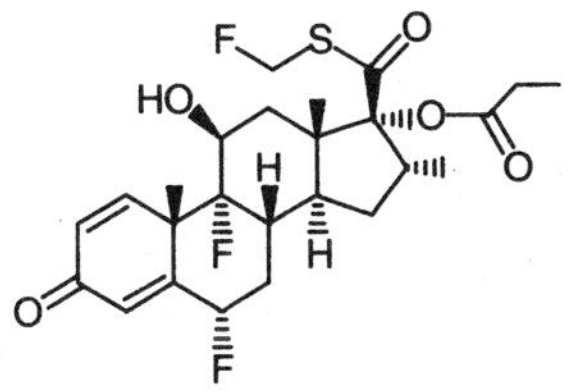

Flucatisone

Leukotriene antagonist

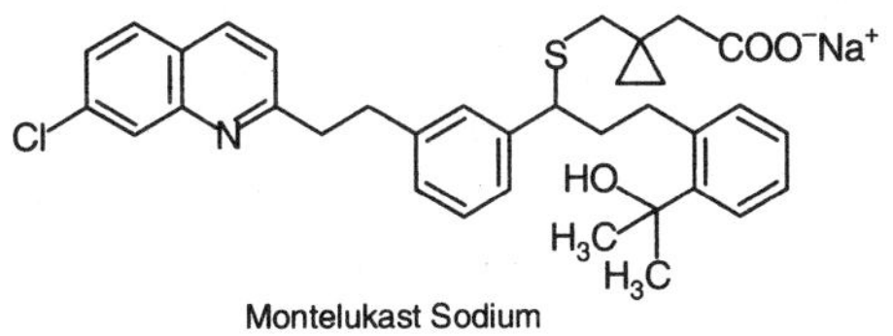

Montelukast Sodium

Decongestant

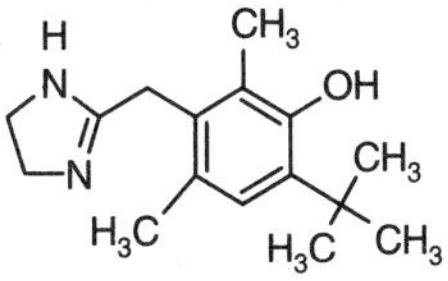

Oxymetazoline

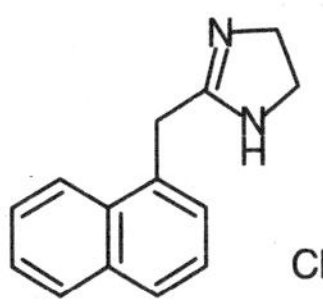

Naphazoline

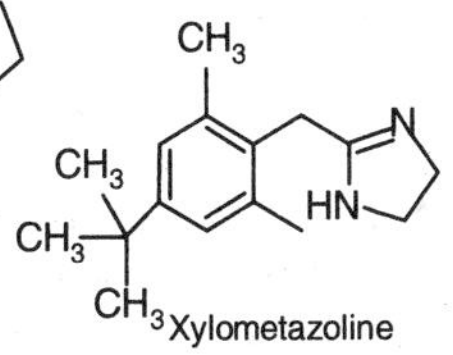

Xylometazoline

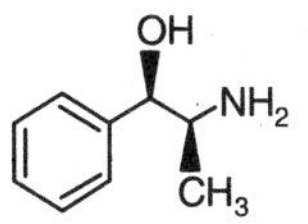

Phenylpropanolamine

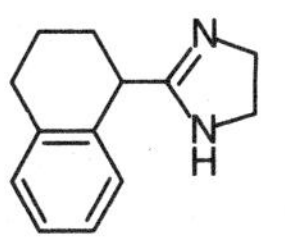

Tetrahydrozoline

Decongestant

Mechanism of action

- These are the agents used to cause a relief or reduction of accumulated fluid because of excessive nasal secretions in the glands of nasal and paranasal area. Beside inflammatory and allergic response, nasal obstruction is also caused by excessive nasal secretions.
- Vasoconstriction of nasal capillary bed is brought about by activation of local α-adrenergic receptors.
- Vasoconstriction of engorged nasal mucosa would allow the inhibition of vascular leakage, drainage of sinuses and clearing of airways. This results into reduction in nasal secretory rate. Hence α-adrenergic agonists may be used locally or systemically to exert decongestant action.
- Locally used decongesants include ephedrine (1% aqueous solution), phenylephrine (solutions of 0.125-1.0%) oxymetazoline (as a 0.05% solution), naphazoline (0.05% solution), tetrahydrozoline (0.05-0.1% solution) and xylometazoline (0.05-1% solution). All these are sympathomimetic agents that produce α-adrenergic stimulation at low concentration when applied locally. However, their duration of action is shorter than that of systemic decongestants. Phenylephrine is most favoured local decongestant because of high potency, minimal systemic effects and lack of CNS-depressant action. It is also used as a systemic decongestant.

Adverse effect

- However when used orally, these drugs may cause urinary retention (by stimulating urinary sphincter) and hypertension. Similarly anticholinergic agents may be used as decongestant because of their antisecretory effect on the glands of nasal and paranasal area.
- The clinically used examples of systemic decongestant include phenylephrine, phenylepropanolamine, ephedrine and pseudoephedrine. However, these drugs have a stimulant effect on CNS and heart because of their activity on α-adrenergic receptors. Main adverse effects include hallucinations, restlessness, tachycardia, nausea, vomiting, anorexia and hypertension. Phenylephrine is usually given in combination with chlorpheniramine (antihistaminic agent) or with phenylpropanolamine. While 1-ephedrine is an orally effective, longer acting bronchodilator having pronounced CNS effects.

Uses

- It is used in bronchospasm, in Strokes-Adams syndrome, as a nasal decongestant, as a sympathomimetic mydriatic and in certain allergic disorders.
- It may also be used to relieve the paroxysms of whooping cough. Adult oral dose is 25 mg per day in divided doses. Pseudoephedrine has poor bronchodilatory effect and better decongestant action. It is widely used decongestant in adult oral dose of 30–60 mg per day.

Antihistaminics

Mechanism of Action

- These medications, also called H1 antagonists, block the action of histamine, a major cause of allergic rhinitis symptoms. Antihistamines are often recommended first because many of them are available over the counter.
- Older drugs may make you drowsy that's less likely with the newer generation of less-sedating or non-sedating antihistamines. These drugs can also be taken once a day, instead of every four to six hours. Antihistamines work well for sneezing, runny nose, and itchy, watery eyes, but not as well as nasal corticosteroids for congestion.

Nasal Corticoids

MOA

- Anti-inflammatory nasal sprays are the most effective medical treatment for allergic rhinitis. They help turn off the immune reaction in the nasal passages and provide sustained relief.
- Nasal corticosteroids can irritate the nasal membranes, but they do not have the troubling side effects associated with oral, injected, or inhaled steroids, such as bone loss and weight gain.

Anti-leukotrienes

MOA: These oral drugs block the effects of leukotrienes, chemicals that cause inflammation. They are an alternative to antihistamines.

Mast Cell Stabilizers

MOA: These drugs reduce swelling and secretions by interfering with the release of certain chemicals from mast cells. They are very safe but not as effective as nasal corticosteroids.

Immunotherapy

MOA

- Better known as allergy shots, immunotherapy involves injecting an allergen under the skin in small and increasing doses every week for several months, then monthly for 3 to 5 years. The object is to accustom the immune system to the substance so that it does not provoke an allergic attack.
- Immunotherapy can markedly reduce the need for medication, and it also cuts the risk that allergic rhinitis will progress to asthma. The drug omalizumab represents a different approach to immunotherapy, dubbed anti-IgE. It is FDA-approved only for asthma but has shown promise in preventing allergic rhinitis.

Anti-inflammatory Drugs and Autacoids

Non-steroidal
Anti-inflammatory Agents

Inflammation can be defined as a defensive but exaggerated local tissue reaction in response to exogenous or endogenous injury. It is a complex phenomenon, comprising of biochemical as well as immunological factors. It is recognized by following symptoms:

1. Calor (heat).
2. Rubor (redness).
3. Tumour (swelling).
4. Dolor (pain).

- Tissue damage initiates or activates the local release of various chemotactic factors that provoke directly or indirectly the appearance of the mediators of pain and inflammation. These factors include:

1. Amines – histamine, serotonin.
2. Proteases – kallikrein, plasmin mast cells, polymorphonuclear leucocytes and platelets.
3. Prostaglandins.
4. Hageman factor.

- Other factor – leucotoxin, lymph node permeability factor. The non-steroidal anti-inflammatory drugs (NSAIDs) are among the most frequently used drugs to treat the disorder caused due to inflammation.
- Inflammation is an attempt to dispose of microbes, toxins, or foreign material at the site to injury, to prevent their spread to other tissues, and to prepare the site for repair in an attempt to restore tissue homeostasis.

Because inflammation is one of body's non-specific resistance mechanism, the response of a tissue to a cut is similar to the response to damaged caused by burns, radiation or bacterial or viral invasion. In each, the inflammatory response has three basic stages:

1. Vasodilation and increased permeability.
2. Emigration of phagocyte from the blood into intestinal fluid.
3. Tissue repair.

STAGES IN INFLAMMATION

Vasodilation and Increased Permeability of Blood (Fig. 54.1)

- Two immediate changes occur in the blood vessels in a region of tissue injury— vasodilation (increase in diameter of blood arterioles) and increased permeability of the capillaries. Increased permeability means the substances normally retained in blood are permitted to pass through blood vessels.
- Vasodilation allows more blood to flow through the damaged area and increased permeability permits defensive proteins such as antibodies and clotting factor to enter the

injured area from the blood. Among the substances that contribute to vasodilation and increased permeability are given below.

Histamine

In response to injury, mast cell in connective tissue, basophils and platelets in blood release histamine. Neutrophils and macrophages attracted to the site of injury also stimulate the release of the histamine, which causes vasodilation and increased permeability of blood vessels.

Kinins

These polypeptides, formed in blood from inactive precursors, induce vasodilation and increased permeability and serve as chemotactic agents for phagocytes. An example of kinin is bradykinin.

Prostaglandins

These lipids, especially those of the E series, are released by damaged cells and intensify the effects of histamine and kinins. PGs also may stimulate the emigration of phagocyte through capillary walls.

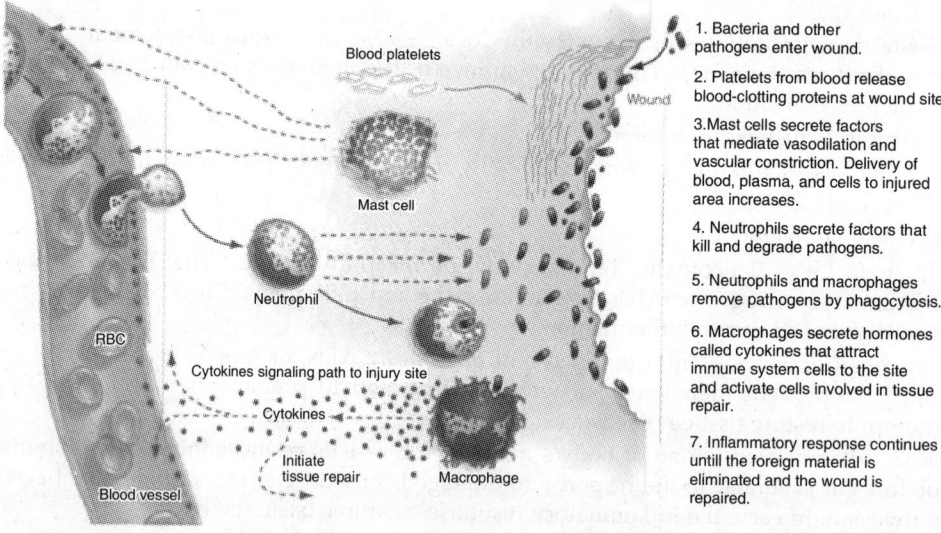

Fig. 54.1: Mechanism of inflammation

Leukotrines

Produced by basophils and mast cells, LTs cause increased permeability; they also function in adherence of phagocytes to pathogens and as chemotactic agents that attract phagocytes.

Complement

- Different components of the complement system stimulate histamine release, attract neutrophils by chemotaxis and promote phagocytosis; some components can also destroy bacteria.
- Dilation of arterioles and increased permeability of capillaries produce three of the symptoms of inflammation— heat, redness and swelling. Heat and redness result from the large amount of blood that accumulates in the damaged area.

- As the local temperature rise slightly, metabolic reaction proceeds more rapidly and release additional heat, which permits more fluid to move from blood plasma into tissue space. Pain is a prime symptom of inflammation. It results from injury to neurons and from toxic chemicals released by microbes.
- Kinins affect some nerve endings, causing much of the pain associated with inflammation. Prostaglandins intensify and prolong the pain associated with inflammation. Pain may also be due to increased pressure from edema.
- The increased permeability of capillaries allows leakage of blood-clotting factors into tissue. The clotting sequence is set into motion and fibrinogen is ultimately converted to an insoluble, thick mesh fibrin threads that localizes and traps invading microbes and blocks their spread.

Emigration of Phagocytosis

- Generally, within an hour after the inflammatory process starts, phagocyte appears on the screen. As large amount of blood accumulates; neutrophils begin to stick to the inner surface of endothelium in blood vessels. Then the neutrophils begin to squeeze through the wall of the blood vessel to reach the damaged area.
- This process, called emigration, depends on chemotaxis. Neutrophils attempt to destroy the invading microbes by phagocytosis. A steady stream of neutrophils is ensured by the production and release of additional cells from red bone marrow. Such an increase in white blood cells in the blood is termed as leukocytosis.
- Although neutrophils predominate in the early stage of infection, they die off rapidly. As the inflammatory response continues, monocytes follow the neutrophils into the infected area. Once in the tissue, monocytes transform into wandering macrophages that add to the phagocytic activity of the fixed macrophages already present. True to their name, macrophages are much more potent phagocytes than neutrophils. They are large enough to engulf damaged tissue, worn-out neutrophils and invanding microbes.

Tissue Repair

- Eventually, macrophages also die. Within a few days, a pocket of dead phagocytes and damaged tissue forms; this collection of dead cells and fluid is called as pus.
- Pus formation occurs in most inflammatory responses and usually continues until the infection subsides. At time, pus reaches the surface of the body or drains into an internal cavity and is dispersed; on other occasion, the pus remains even after the infection is terminated. In this case, the pus is gradually destroyed over a period of days and is absorbed (Fig. 54.2).

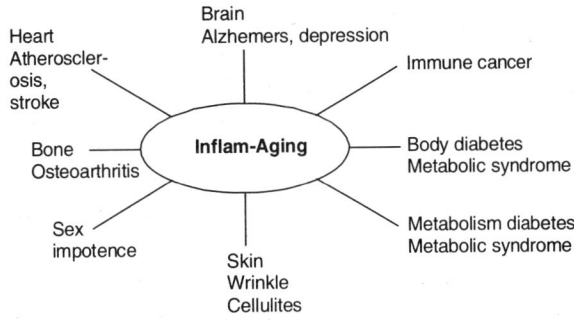

Fig. 54.2: Causes of Inflammation

▨ MODE OF ACTION (FIG. 54.3)

The hypothesis concerning MOA of anti-inflammatory drugs studied as:

    A. Biochemical mechanism.

    B. Cellular or immunologic mechanism.

Biochemical Mechanism

It was recognized that process of inflammation required considerable amount of energy. According to this concept, some NSAIDs modify the oxidative phosphorylation which is the main source of generation of energy but no clear link made between clinical anti-inflammatory activity and the particular biochemical parameter as follows.

1. Inhibition of hydrolytic enzymes: This concept is related with the lysosomes which contain hydrolytic enzymes and participates in the process of inflammation are inhibited to release hydrolytic enzyme by NSAIDs.

2. Inhibition of arachidonic acid (prostaglandins) metabolism

- Prostaglandin play an important role in erythema, oedema, pain, and fever associated with inflammation by direct action.

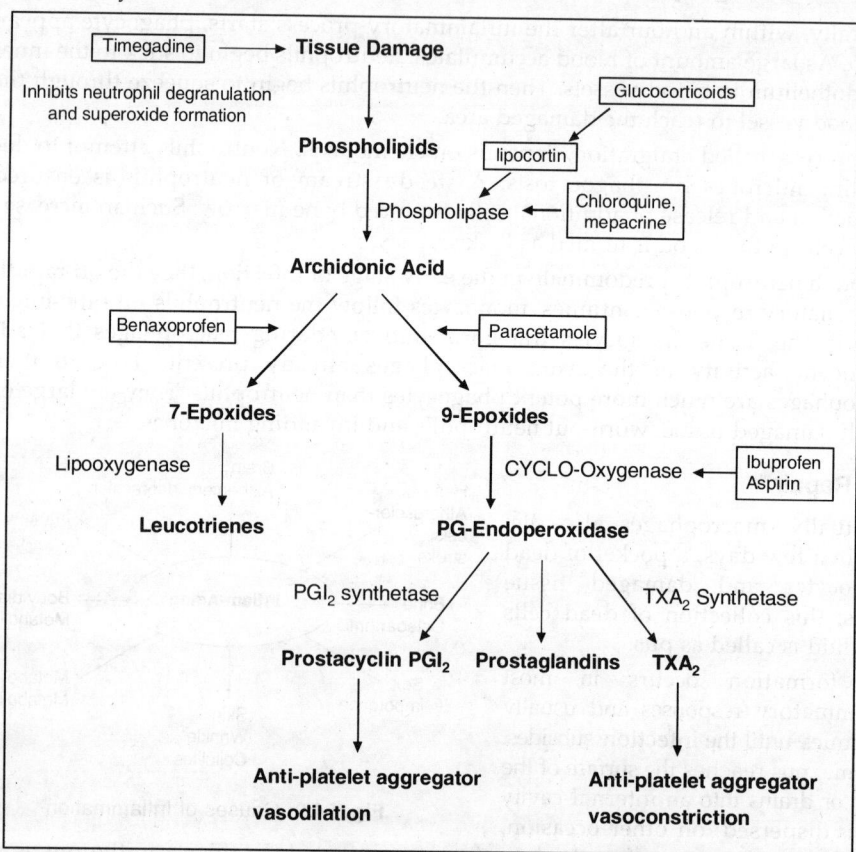

Fig. 54.3: Possible mode of action of NSAIDs

- Most of the NSAIDs inhibit the formation of prostaglandins and leukotrienes which are metabolic product of arachidonic acid and are responsible for inflammation. This occurs by two important pathways known as :

  i. Inhibition of prostaglandin synthatase (fatty acid cyclooxygenase): In this pathway, NSAIDs attach to or interact with cyclooxygenase enzyme and inhibit the formation of prostacyclin (PGI_2). Thromboxane A_2 or the classic prostanoids PGE_2, PGF_2.

ii. **Inhibition of lipooxygenase pathway:** The lipoxygenase pathway produces other arachidonic acid metabolites. The important are LTB4 and 12 HETE detected in inflammation. Both have a chemo-attractant action of leukocytes which may in turn lower the firing of pain fibres. The cyclooxygenase inhibitors have relatively little inhibitory action on lipooxygenase pathway. However, both *diclofenac and indomethain* decrease the production of leucotrienes by leukocytes.

3. Inhibition of free radical generation: Biochemical studies of arachidonic acid generate a no. of free radical species which may participate in process of inflammation. A no. of NSAIDs interferes with the process *in vitro* studies data are less convincing.

Cellular or Immunologic Mechanism

a. **Inhibition of polymorphonuclear leukocytes (PMN):** PMN is recognized as the first cell to arrival at the sites of inflammation and anti-inflammatory drugs suppose to restrict their arrival at the site of inflammation.

b. **Monocyte modification:** It has been proposed that monocytes are the central cell in the inflammatory response. NSAIDs modify the movement and\or function of these cells in the process of inflammation.

c. **Action through lymphocytes:** The 2nd line drugs such as penicilamine, gold salts, chloramines and dapsone are studied in the treatment of inflammation disorder and found that lymphocytes may influence chronic inflammation.

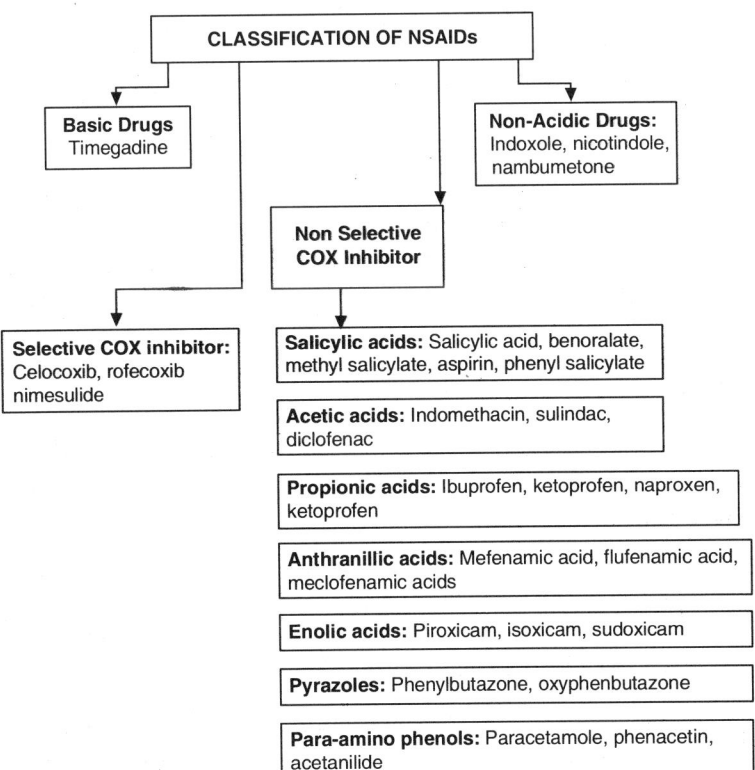

Non-Selective COX Inhibitor
Salicylic Acid Derivatives

Salicylic acid Methyl salicylate Sodium salicylate Phenyl salicylate Acetyl salicylic acid

Salicylamide Flufenisol Diflunisal Benorylate

Acetic Acid Derivatives

Sulindac Indomethacin Tolmetin sodium

Zomepirac sodium Diclofenac sodium Nabumetone

Propionic Acid Derivatives

Ibuprofen Flurbiprofen Ketoprofen

Fenoprofen Naproxan

Anthranillic Acid Derivatives (Fenmate)

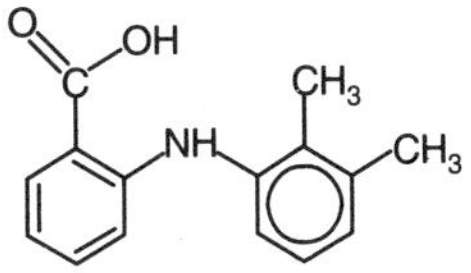

Mefenamic acid

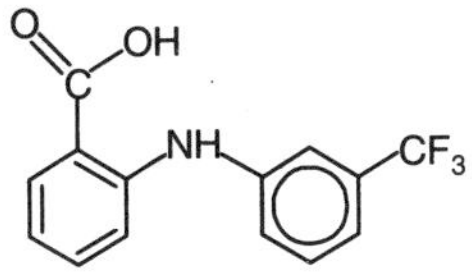

Flufenamic acid

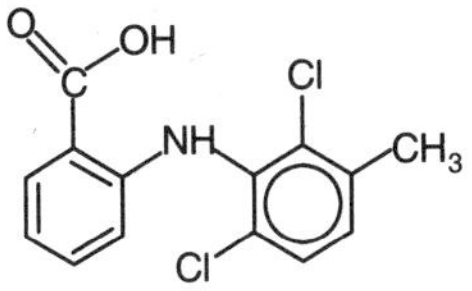

Meclofenamic acid

Oxicams

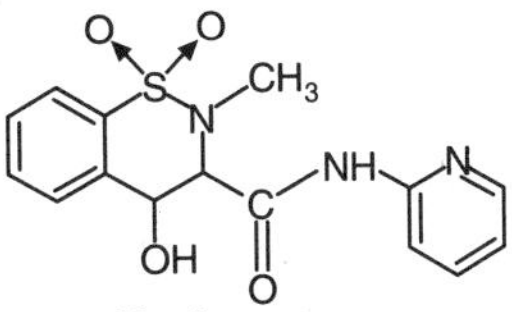

Piroxicam

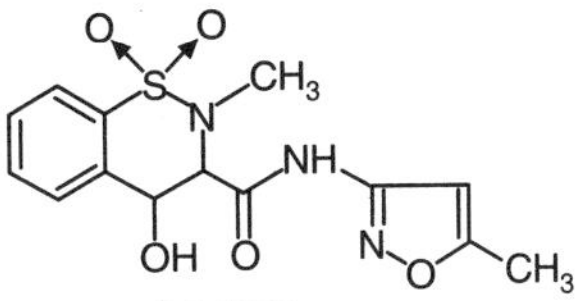

Isoxicam

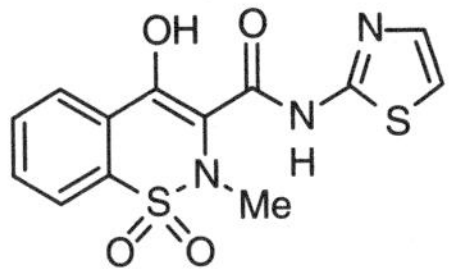

Sudoxicam

Pyrazoles

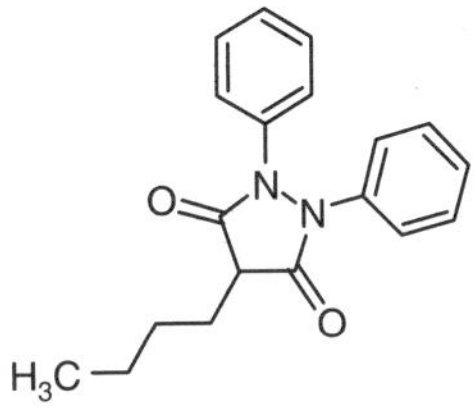

Phenylbutazone

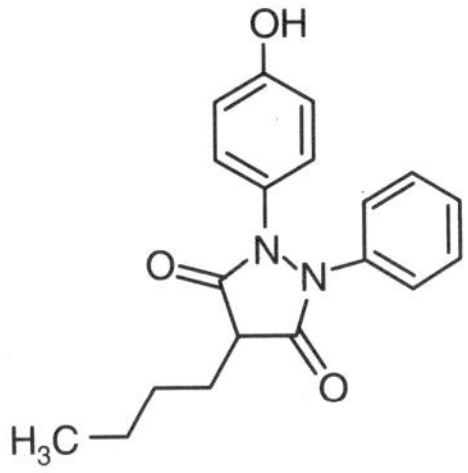

Oxyphenbutazone

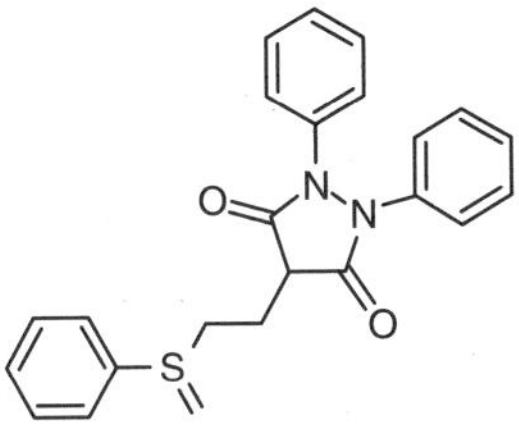

Sulfinpyrazone

Para-amino phenol derivatives

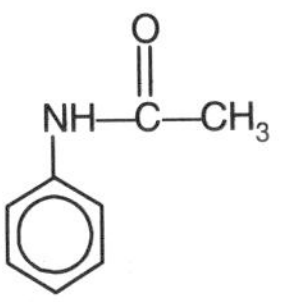

Acetanilide

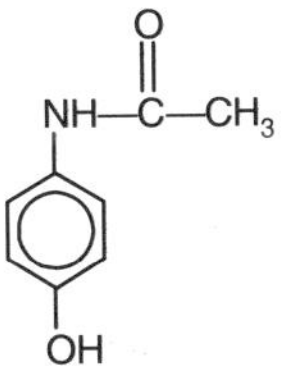

Paracetamol

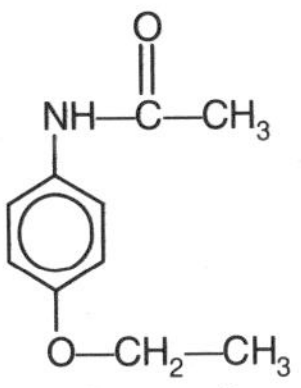

Phenacetin

Selective COX Inhibitor

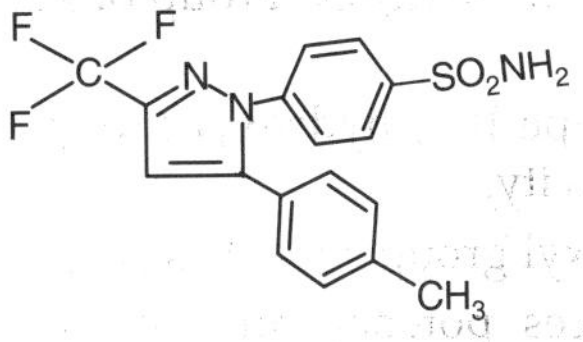

Celocoxib

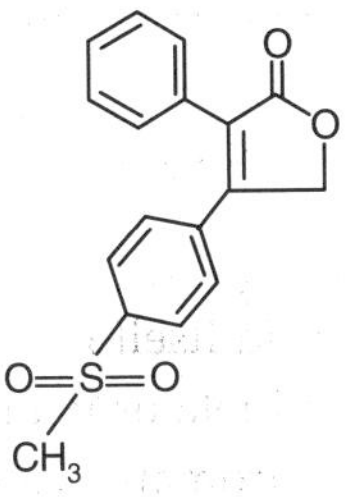

Refecoxib

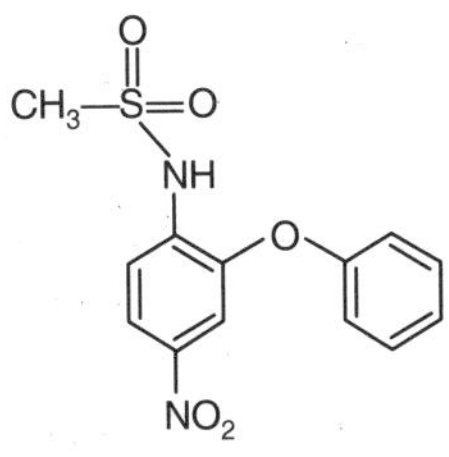

Nimusulide

Drugs Used in Gout

Allopurinol   Probencid   Gold thioglucose

Hydroxychloroquine   Azathiopurine   Colchicine

NON-SELECTIVE COX INHIBITOR

Salicylic Acid Derivatives

Structuring-activity relationship

1. The drug most widely used to treat arthritis is salicylic acid. The simplest active anti-inflammatory compound is salicylic acid. The active moiety appears to be the salicylates anion. The carboxyl group is necessary for activity and the carboxyl group must be adjacent to it. Side effects of salicylates, particularly the GI effects, appear to be associated with the carboxylic acid functional group.

2. Reducing activity of this group (carboxylic acid group) by converting to an amide – salicylamide maintains the analgesic action of salicylic acid derivative but eliminates the anti-inflammatory properties.

3. The derivative of salicylic acid are of two types – type I and type II (a and b)

Type I   Type II (a)   Type II (b)

Type I – represents those that are formed by modifying the carboxyl groups, e.g. salts, ester or amide.

Type II (a and b) – those that are derived by substitution on the hydroxyl group of salicylic acid.

4. Substitution on either the carboxyl (type I) or phenolic (type II a) hydroxyl groups may affect potency and toxicity. Benzoic acid itself has weak activity.

5. Placing the phenolic hydroxyl group Meta or Para to carboxyl group abolishes activity.

6. Substitution of halogen atoms on aromatic ring enhances potency and toxicity, e.g 5-chlorosalicylic acid.

7. 4-aminosalicylic acid is at active substitution of amino group at position 4 abolishes activity.
8. Introduction of a methyl group (adjacent to the phenolic OH group) in aspirin and in salicylic acid produces 3-methyl aspirin and 3-salicylic acid have slower metabolic excretion.
9. Substitution of aromatic ring at position 5 of salicylic acid increases anti-inflammatory activity, e.g. diflunisal.
10. Aspirin acetyl salicylic acid potent agent but has more adverse effect due to presence of ortho-acetyl group, e.g. blood loss due to GIT hemorrhage. Diflunisal has fewer side effects than aspirin.
11. The acute gastric irritancy of salicylates associated with its carboxylic acid group. It can be reduced by modification of the acidic characteristic of the carboxylic group of compound, e.g. by esterification of carboxylic group.

Type II (b) derivative of salicylic acid

Mechanism of action

Aspirin modifies COX by acetylating Ser-530 of COX – 1 and Ser-516 of COX – 2. It is 10 – 100 times more potent against COX – 1 and COX – 2. Its action on COX – 1 prevents both endoperoxide and 15-peroxidation of arachidonic acid but its action on COX – 2 does not prevent formation of arachidonic acid.

Salol Principle

Ester of two toxic substances is called salol principles. This concept was introduced by Necki in 1886.

True salol

Here two toxic substances (phenol and salicylic acid) were combined into an ester that taken, internally slowly hydrolyzes in the intestine to give antiseptic action of its components, e.g. β- naphthol benzoate, guanicol benzoate.

Partial salol

The esters in which only one component, like alcohol or the acids, is toxic, called as partial salol, e.g. methyl salicylate, ethyl salicylate.

Acetic Acid Derivatives or Phenyl Acetic Acid Derivatives

Structure-activity relationship

1. Substitution R1 useful for increasing anti-inflammatory activity as ranked as $C_6H_4CH_2$>Alkyl>H
2. R2 substituent for improved activity is ranked as CH_3>H.
3. X substituent is ranked as 5-OCH_3 > $(CH_3)_2$N>CH_3>H.

4. The carboxyl group at C-3 is essential for activity.
5. A chloro group in indomethacin can be replaced by that of CF_3 or SCH_3, such compounds are having better anti-inflammatory activity.

6. At position 2 in indomethacin, a methyl group is better than an aryl group.
7. At position 5 of the ring, methoxy, alkoxy, dimethylamino, acetyl methyl and fluro function are superior to hydrogen or chlorine.
8. At position 3, acetic acid side chain is free to rotate to assume different conformation.

Propionic Acid Derivatives

Ibuprofen

SAR:

1. R1 should be isobutyl substituent, if we increase or decrease the chain, activity will reduce.
2. The maximal activity is seen when $R_2 = CH_3$, if we increase or decrease the chain activity will diminish.
3. The 'COOH' functional group is essential for activity, if we are replacing it by ester, alcohol or amide, such compounds do exhibit it by ester a little anti-inflammatory activity.
4. This compound is active only in S (+) isomer form.

MOA: This is a rapid and reversible competitive inhibitor of COX enzyme.

Naproxan

SAR:

1. Activity is reduced when – OCH_3 (SCH_3) is larger.
2. The carboxyl group may be replaced by alcohol and aldehyde.
3. Dextro-rotatory is 11 times more active.

Fenmates (Anthranilic Acid Derivatives)

SAR

1. Anthranilic acid is o-substituted benzoic acid

2. Derivative of anthranilic acid (e.g. mefenamic acid, meclofenamic acid and flufenamic acid) are nitrogen analogues of salicylic acid. They are potent analgesic and anti-inflammatory agents.

   • Mefenamic acid:
     $R_1 = R_2 = CH_3; R_3 = H.$
   • Meclofenamic acid:
     $R_1 = R_3 = Cl; R_2 = CH_3$
   • Flufenamic acid:
     $R_1 = R_3 = H; R_2 = CF_3$

3. So the most active anthranilic acid derivative have substituents at position 2, 3 and 6 of the ring attached to the anthranilic acid nitrogen atom.
4. Substitution on the anthranilic acid ring generally reduces activity whereas substitution of N–aryl ring can lead to enhance activity.

5. For monosubstitution order of activity is 3>2>>4, e.g. 3-CF3 derivatives, (flufenamic acid) is more potent.

6. In substituted derivative, where the nature of the two substituents is same, 2, 3-disubstitution appears to be the most active. Substituents on the N-aryl ring for *o*- this ring to be on co-planar with the anthranilic acid ring should enhance binding at active site and thus enhance activity. In other words the most active disubstituted compounds are 2, 3-derivative. This indicates that most activity reside in compound I which is the N-aryl moiety is kept out of coplanirity with the anthranilic acid by ortho substituents, e.g. methyl and chloro function in the mefenamic acid and meclofenamic acid.

7. The resulting non-planar structures are of fitting the hypothetical anti- inflammatory receptor site. This may account for the enhanced anti-inflammatory activity of meclofenamic acid (which has two ortho substituents forcing the ring out of the plane of anthranilic acid ring) over flufenamic acid (one ortho substituents). Meclofenamic acid possesses 25 times greater anti-inflammatory activity than mefenamic acid.

8. The NH moiety of anthranilic acid appears too essential for activity since replacement of the NH function with O, CH_2, S SO_2, $N-CH_3$ or $N-COCH_3$ functionalities significantly reduces the activity.

9. The position, rather than the nature, of the acidic function is critical for activity. Anthranilic acid derivatives are active whereas the meta and para amino benzoic acid derivatives are not.

Oxicams or Enolic Acid Derivatives

SAR

1. The most active analogue have the substituent CH_3 on the nitrogen and electron withdrawing substituent on the anilide phenyl group such as chloro and trifluromethyl.

2. The introduction of heterocyclic ring in the amide oxide chain significantly increases the anti-inflammatory activity.

3. 2-thazolyl derivative, sudoxicam is more potent than, indomethacin.

4. Metabolic studies in animal suggests that chlorine substituted at position -4 of the phenyl ring have extended half-life and duration of action.

5. The tautomeric structure imparts further stability to the enolate anion. Such stabilization of the enolate anion would thereby contribute to a further increase in the acidity of conjugated acids.

6. The enhanced acid properties of these cyclic β-diketones were responsible in part for their biological activities.

MOA

This is a rapid and reversible competitive inhibitor of COX enzyme. Hydrophobic forces are important in this interaction.

Pyrazoles

SAR

1. Propyl or allyl group may replace the butyl group of carbon.

2. The presence of keto group in gama position of the butyl side chain produces the active compound.

3. Meta substitution of the aryl ring of phenylbutazone gives inactive compound. Para – substitution such as methyl, chloro, nitro or OH of one or both rings retain activity.

4. Replacement of one nitrogen atoms in the pyrazolidine with oxygen atoms yields isooxazole analogs, which is active as pyrazolidine derivative.

5. A parabolic relationship was derived between lipophilicity and anti-inflammatory activity.

6. Decreasing pKa values of phenyl butazone analogs correlate with short half-life.

7. Enolizable β-dicarboxyl system is essential because substitution at carbon 4 of pheylbutazone by a methyl group destroy anti-inflammatory activity.

MOA

1. Reactive oxygen radicals produced by neutrophils and macrophages are thought to be implicated not only in eicosanoid production but in tissue damage. NSAIDs that have strong O_2 radical scavenging effects as well as cyclo-oxygenase inhibitory activity may decrease tissue damage.

2. Other proposed mode of action is that Pyrazoles may interfere with binding of mediators such as the chemotactic peptides, peptides derived from bacteria to their receptors on inflammatory cells.

GOUT ARTHRITIS

Gout is purine metabolism disorder resulting from an excess of uric acid in the blood (hyperuricemia), due to either its overproduction or faulty elimination.

Pathophysiology

- Crystals of monosodium urate begin to preciptates and get deposited in joints, skin, kidney and other tissue. Classically, the great toe is involved, characterized by pain, swelling, tenderness and other signs of inflammation.

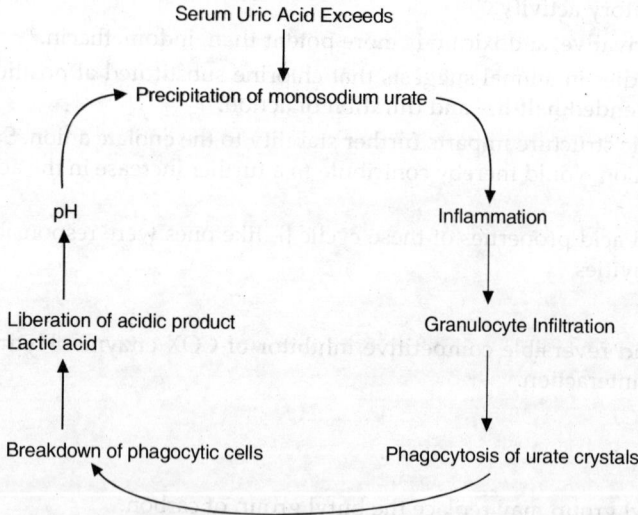

- At the site, there is infiltration of granulocyte that phagocyte the urate crystals. The granulocytes ultimately breakdown and liberate lactic acid and other acidic products, which lower the regional pH and favour further precipitation of urate crystals.

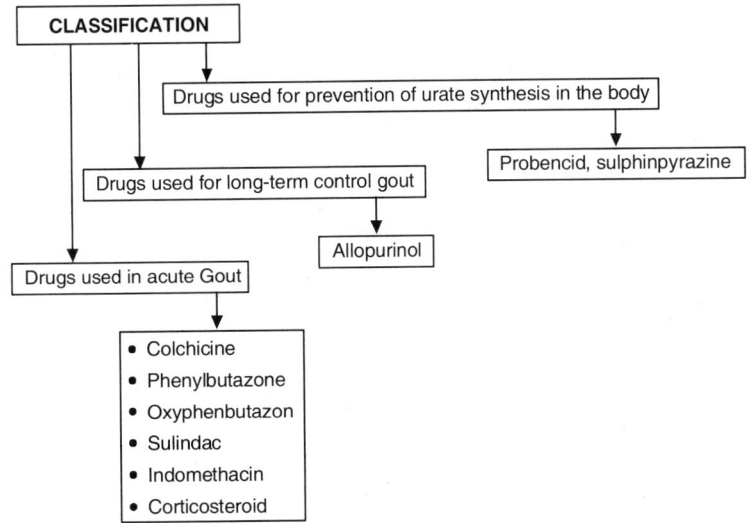

- The nucleic acid from the cells is first converted to the purine bases—hypoxanthine and xanthine. The enzyme xanthine oxidase then catalyzes the metabolic breakdown of these purines to uric acid. Thus, uric acid is the end product in the metabolism of the purines.
- Uric acid is filtered by the glomerulus, but 98% is actively reabsorbed in the proximal tubule. It is also excreted into the distal tubule via an active transport system.
- It is more soluble in alkaline urine and a factor in the development of uric acid stones is an impaired ability to excrete alkaline urine. And the remainder is excreted into gut and is broken down by the intestinal bacteria.

Allopurinol

MOA: Allopurinol inhibits the xanthine oxidase enzyme, which converts hypoxanthine to the uric acid and thus inhibits the conversion and reduce the concentration of uric acid in blood.

Colchicine

MOA: It inhibits the migration of granulocyte to inflamed joints and phagocytosis is inhibited. It inhibits leukocytes, which get into the joint from releasing lactic acid and lysosomal enzymes.

Uricosuric Agents

Probencid and sulfinpyrazone

MOA: Probenecid acts by inhibiting renal tubular reabsorption of uric acid, thereby greater amounts of uric acid are eliminated in the urine. The concentration of urates in the plasma falls gradually towards the normal.

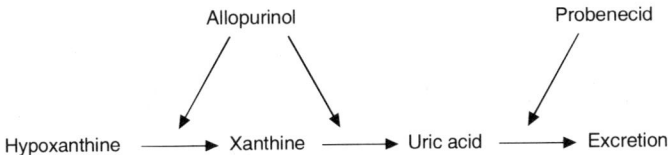

Side Effects of NSAIDs

1. GIT side effects. The most common effects are dyspepsia, nausea, and vomiting, diarrhoea also occurs and ulcer crater disease.
2. Renal disease, chronic consumption of phenacetin or paracetamol could cause chronic nephritis and renal papillary necrosis.
3. Skin reaction, mefenamic acid and sulindac could produce mild skin rashes, urticaria.
4. Other effects include bone marrow disturbance and liver disorders.

Aspirin

Salicylic Acid

Benorylate

Diclofenac

Indomethacin

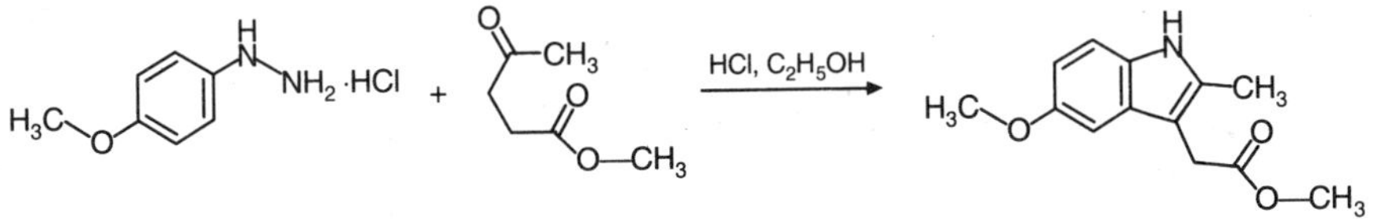

(4-methoxyphenyl)-
hydrazine hydrochloride (I)

methyl
levulinate (II)

methyl 5-methoxy-2-methylindole-
3-acetate (III)

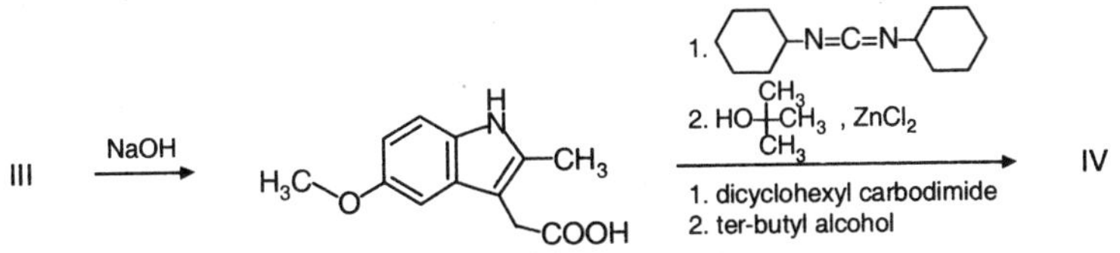

III → NaOH →

5-methoxy-2-methylindole-
3-acetic acid

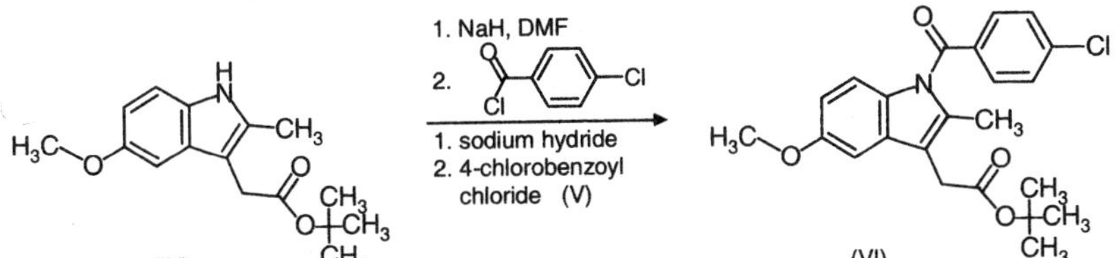

1. ⟨cyclohexyl⟩—N=C=N—⟨cyclohexyl⟩
2. HO—CH₃ , ZnCl₂

1. dicyclohexyl carbodimide
2. ter-butyl alcohol

→ IV

(IV)

1. NaH, DMF
2. 4-chlorobenzoyl chloride (V)

1. sodium hydride
2. 4-chlorobenzoyl
   chloride (V)

(VI)

VI → 210°C →

Indomethacin

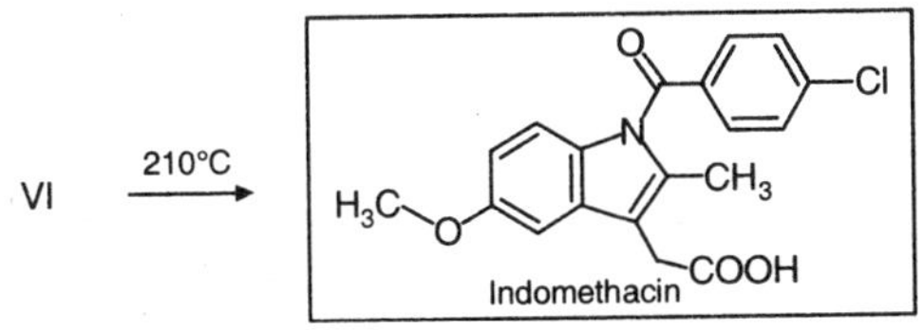

Fenoprofen

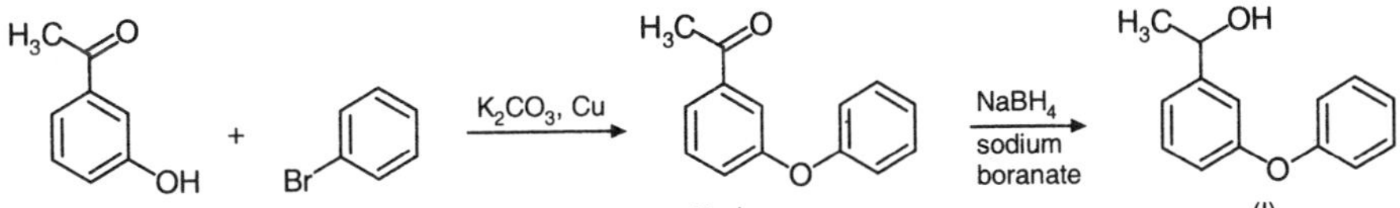

3'-hydroxy-
acetophenone

+ bromobenzene

K₂CO₃, Cu →

3'-phenoxy-
acetophenone

NaBH₄
sodium
boranate

(I)

I → PBr₃
phosphorus (II)
bromide →

NaCN →

aq. NaOH →

Fenoprofen

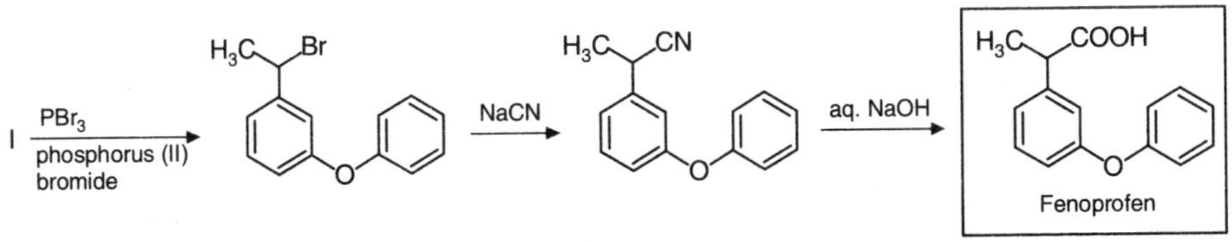

Flufenamic Acid

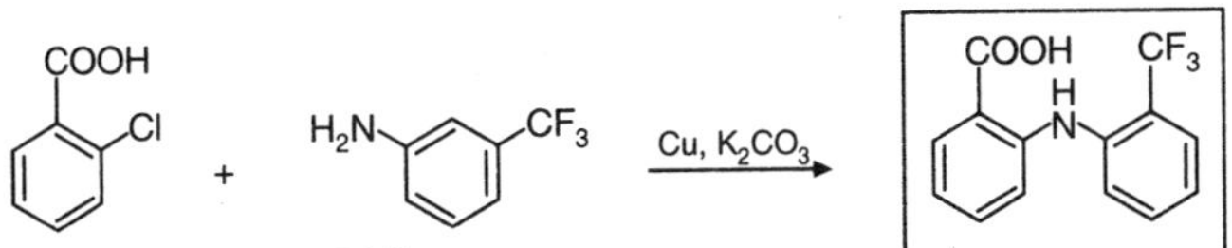

2-chloro-
benzoic acid

+ 3-trifluoro-
methylaniline

Cu, K₂CO₃ →

Flufenamic aciu

Phenylbutazone

Oxyphenbutazone

Sulfinpyrazone

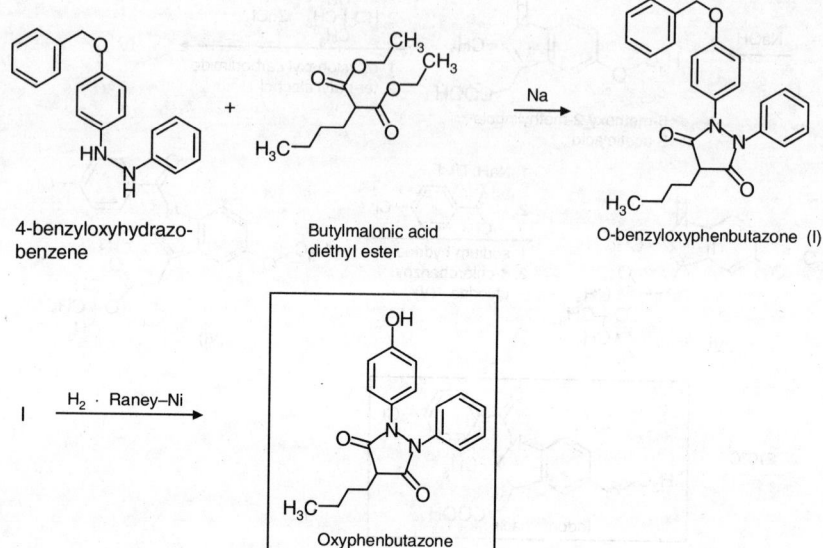

Piroxicam

Saccharin sodium (I) + Methyl chloroacetate (II) → (reaction) → NaOCH₃, OMSO → 3-methoxycarbonyl-4-oxo-3, 4-dihydro-2H-1,2-benzothiazine 1,1-dioxide (III)

III + H₃C—I → NaOH → (V) → H₂N-pyridine, 2-amino-pyridine (VI) → Piroxicam

(IV)

Probenecid

Dipropylamine + 4-carboxybenzene-sulfonyl chloride → Probenecid

Paracetamol

Phenol → HNO₃ nitric acid → 4-nitrophenol → H₂, Roney–Ni → 4-aminophenol → acetic anhydride (II) → Paracetamol

Sulindac

4-fluorobenz-aldehyde + Prapionic anhydride → H₃C–CH₂–COONa → 4-fluoro-α-methyl-cinnamic acid → H₂, Pd–C → I

4-fluoro-α-methyl-dihydrocinnamic acid (I) → polyphosphoric acid 95°C → 5-fluoro-2-methyl-3-indanone →
1. NC–CH₂COOH, CH3COONH₄ —COOH
2. KOH
3. HCl
1. cyanoacetic acid → II

5-fluoro-2-methyl-indane-3-acetic acid (II) + 4-methylthio-benzaldehyde → (NaOCH₃) → 5-fluoro-2-methyl-1-(4-methylthiobenzylidene)-indene-3-acetic acid (III)

III → NaOCH₃, sodium periodate → Sulindac

Ketoprofen

3-methylbenzophenone → (Br₂, Br⌢Br) → 3-bromomethylbenzophenone → (NaCN) → I

(3-benzoylphenyl)-acetonitrite (I) + Diethyl carbonate → (NaOC₂H₅) → (II)

II + H₃C—I → (Methyl iodide) → → (H₂SO₄) → Ketoprofen

Tolmetin

1-methyl-pyrrole + H₂C=O + Dimethylamine (Form-aldehyde) → 2-dimethylamino-methyl-1-methyl-pyrrole → (I—CH₃) → (I)

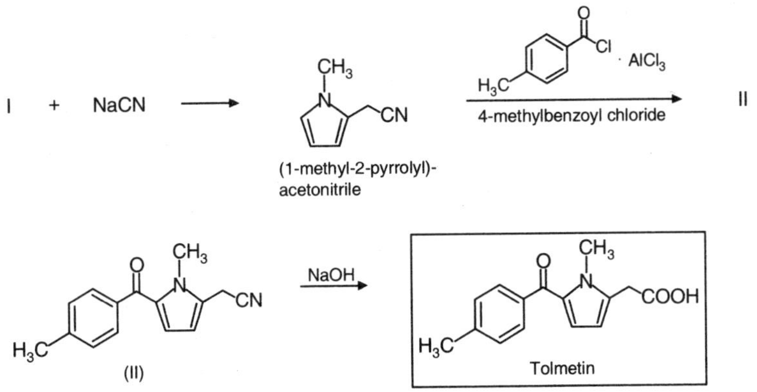

I + NaCN → (1-methyl-2-pyrrolyl)-acetonitrile

4-methylbenzoyl chloride · AlCl₃ → II

(II) NaOH → Tolmetin

Ibuprofen

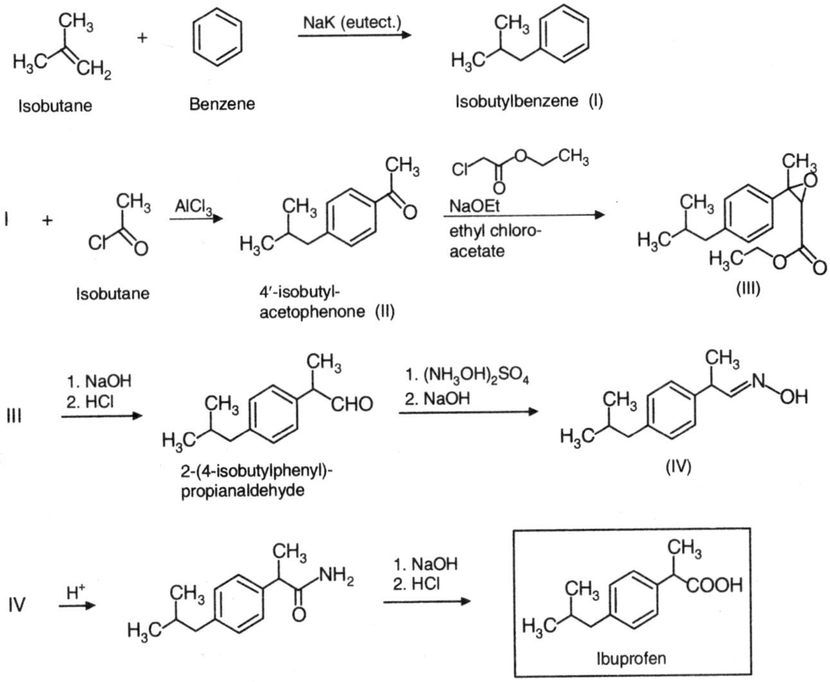

Isobutane + Benzene → NaK (eutect.) → Isobutylbenzene (I)

I + Isobutane → AlCl₃ → 4'-isobutyl-acetophenone (II)

ethyl chloro-acetate / NaOEt → (III)

III → 1. NaOH 2. HCl → 2-(4-isobutylphenyl)-propianaldehyde → 1. (NH₃OH)₂SO₄ 2. NaOH → (IV)

IV → H⁺ → 1. NaOH 2. HCl → Ibuprofen

Naproxen

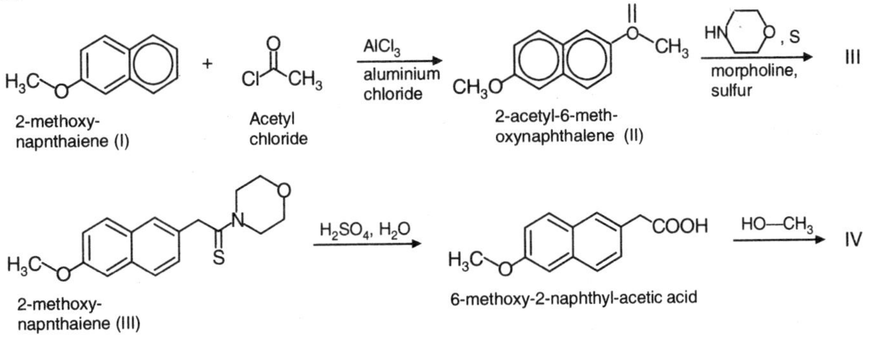

2-methoxy-napnthaiene (I) + Acetyl chloride → AlCl₃ aluminium chloride → 2-acetyl-6-methoxynaphthalene (II)

morpholine, sulfur → III

2-methoxy-napnthaiene (III) → H₂SO₄, H₂O → 6-methoxy-2-naphthyl-acetic acid → HO—CH₃ → IV methyl 6-methoxy-2-naphthylacetate (IV) + methyl isodide → (NaH, Sodium hydride) → methyl DL-2-(6-methoxy-1-naphthyl)propionate (V)

V → (NaOH) → methyl DL-2-(6-methoxy-2-naphthyl)propionic acid (VI)

VI → racemate resolution with cinchonidine → Naproxen

Mefenamic Acid

Potassium 2-bromo-benzoate + 2,3-dimethyl-aniline → (copper (II) acetate) → Mofenamic acid

Isoxicam

3-ethoxycarbonyl-4-hydroxy-2-methyl-2H-1,2-benzothiazine1,1-dioxide + 3-amino-5-methyl-isoxazole → Isoxicam

Phenacetin

4-nitrophenol + Chloro-ethane → (NaOH) → 4-nitrophenetole → (H₂/Pd–C or Raney–Ni) → I

p-phenetidine (I) + chloro-ethane → Phenacetin

55

Antihistaminics

An antihistamine is a drug which serves to reduce or eliminate effects mediated by histamine, an endogenous chemical mediator released during allergic reactions, through action at the histamine receptor. Only agents where the main therapeutic effect is mediated by negative modulation of histamine receptors are termed antihistamines—other agents may have antihistaminergic action but are not true antihistamines.

SYNTHESIS OF HISTAMINE

- Histamine is β-imidazolyl ethylamine. It is synthesized locally from amino acid histidine and degraded rapidly by oxidation and methylation into the methyl histamine and methyl imidazole acetic acid. In mast cell, histamine is stored along with acidic protein and heparin within intracellular process. Structurally, histamine is 4-(2-aminoethyl) imidazole. It exists in two tautomeric forms.

- At physiological pH, the amino nitrogen atom of the side chain is protonated. Histamine occurs, therefore, as a monovalent cation, which forms as an intramolecular hydrogen bond between the amino group of the lateral chain and a nitrogen of the imidazole ring.

- Histamine is widely distributed in plants and animal tissue due to wide occurrence in body tissue, it was named histamine which means tissue amine.

STORAGE

- Most histamine in body tissue is found in granules in mast cells (Fig. 55.1) or basophils. Mast cells are especially numerous at sites of potential injury—the nose, mouth, and feet; internal

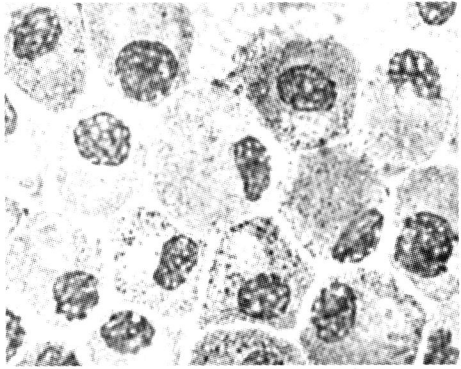

Fig. 55.1: Mast cell

629

body surfaces; and blood vessels. Non-mast cell histamine is found in several tissues, including the brain, where it functions as a neurotransmitter.

- Another important site of histamine storage and release is the enterochromaffin-like (ECL) cell of the stomach. The most important pathophysiology mechanism of mast cell and basophile histamine release is immunologic.

- These cells, if sensitized by IgE antibodies attached to their membranes, degranulate when exposed to the appropriate antigen. Certain amines, including such drugs as morphine and tubocurarine, can displace histamine in granules and cause its release.

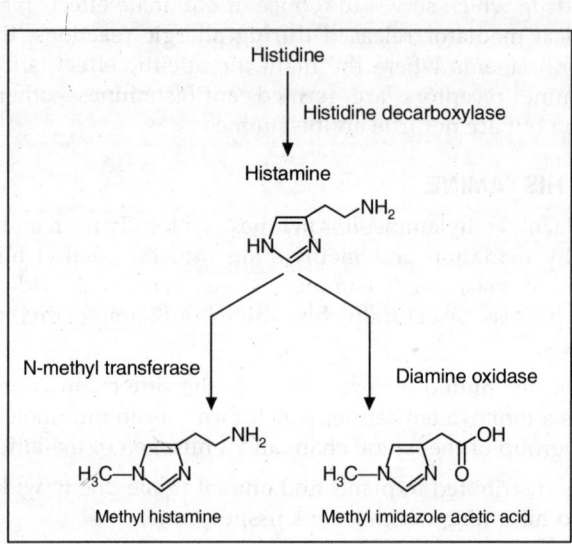

RELEASE

- It is released in body, usually, in response to tissue injury inflammation and allergic or hypersensitivity reactions. In allergic reactions, an allergen (a type of antigen) interacts with and cross-links surface IgE antibodies on mast cells and basophils.

- Once the mast cell–antibody–antigen complex is formed, a complex series of events occurs that eventually leads to cell degranulation and the release of histamine (and other chemical mediators) from the mast cell or basophil.

- Once released, histamine can react with local or widespread tissues through histamine receptors. Histamine, acting on H1-receptors, produces pruritus, vasodilatation, hypotension, flushing, headache, tachycardia, bronchoconstriction, increases vascular permeability, potentiates pain, and more while H1-antihistamines help against these effects, they only work if taken before contact with the allergen.

- In severe allergies, such as anaphylaxis or angioedema, these effects may be so severe as to be life-threatening. Epinephrine, often in the form of an auto-injector, is required by people with such hypersensitivities.

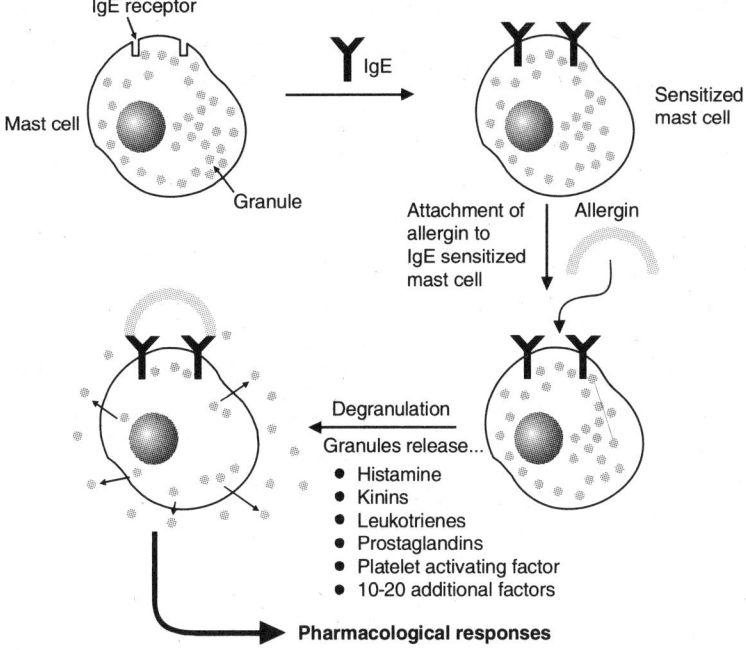

Fig. 55.2: Mechanism of allergic response

MECHANISM OF ACTION (FIG. 55.2)

* Histamine exerts its actions by combining with specific cellular receptors located on cells. The four histamine receptors that have been discovered are designated H1 through H4.

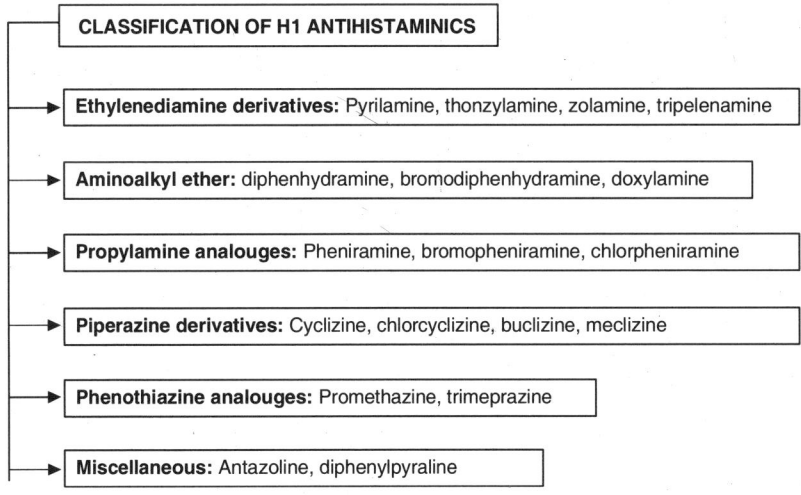

Table 55.1: Histaminic receptors–location and functions

Type	Location	Function
H1 histamine receptor	Found on smooth muscle, endothelium, and central nervous system tissue	Causes vasodilation, bronchoconstriction, smooth muscle activation, separation of endothelial cells (responsible for hives), and pain and itching due to insect stings; the primary receptors involved in allergic rhinitis symptoms and motion sickness.
H2 histamine receptor	Located on parietal cells	Primarily regulate gastric acid secretion
H3 histamine receptor	-	Decreased neurotransmitter release: histamine, acetylcholine, norepinephrine, serotonin
H4 histamine receptor	Found primarily in the thymus, small intestine, spleen, and colon. It is also found on basophils and in the bone marrow.	Unknown physiological role.

First Generation Agents

Ethylenediamine Derivatives

Pyrilamine

Thonzylamine

Tripelenamine

Zolamine

Aminoalkyl Ether

Diphenhydramine

Doxylamine

Bromodiphenhydramine

Methyldiphenhydramine

Medrylamine

Piperazine Derivatives

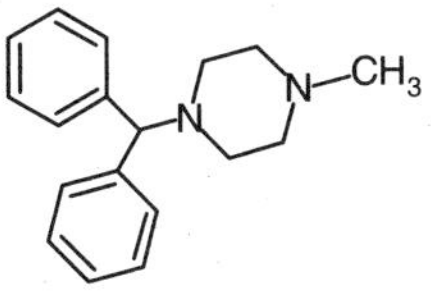

Cyclizine

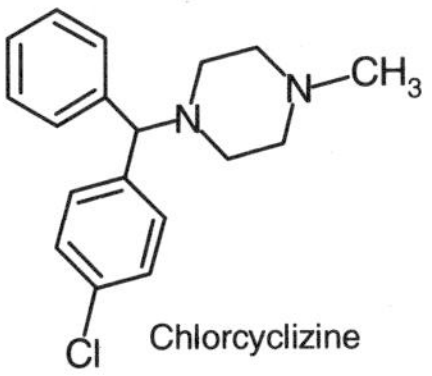

Chlorcyclizine

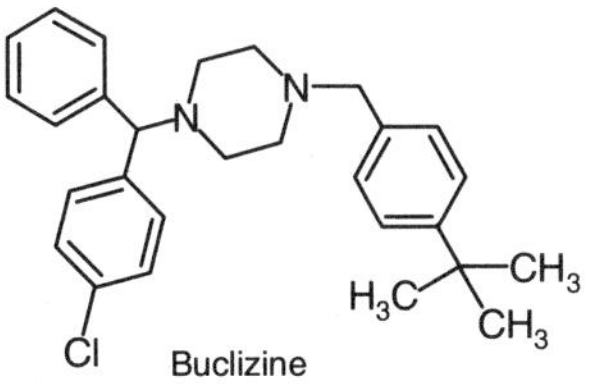

Buclizine

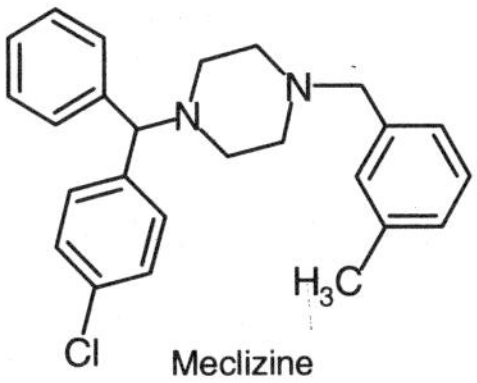

Meclizine

Propylamine Derivatives

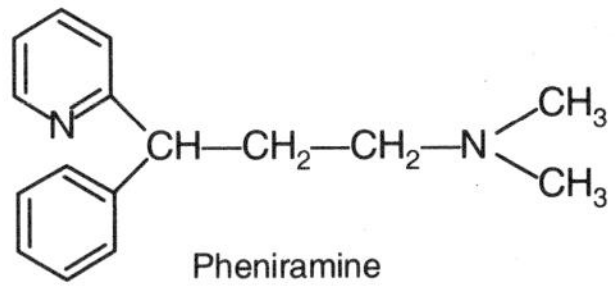

Pheniramine

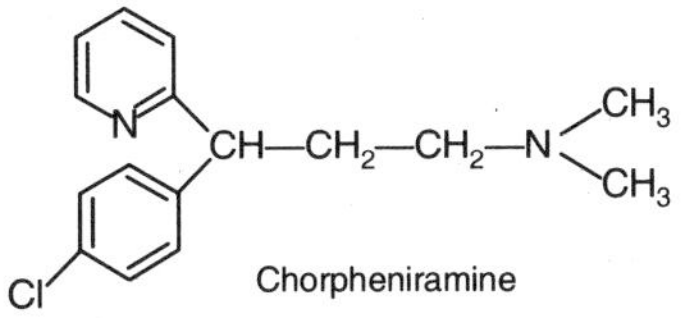

Chorpheniramine

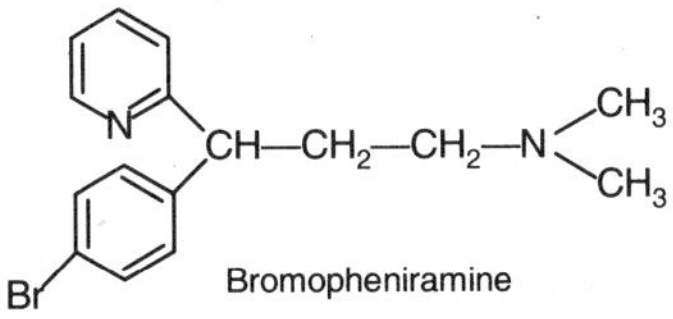

Bromopheniramine

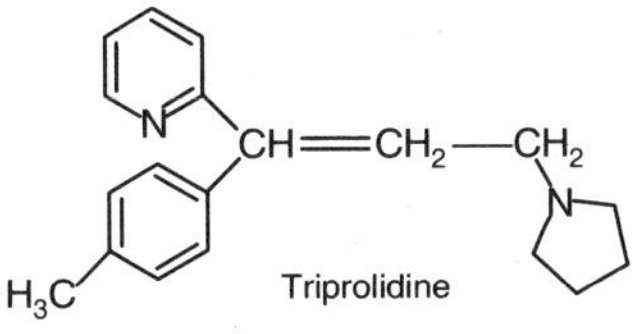

Triprolidine

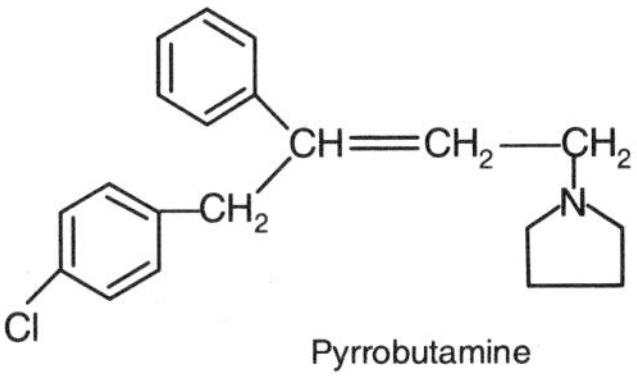

Pyrrobutamine

Phenothiazine Derivatives

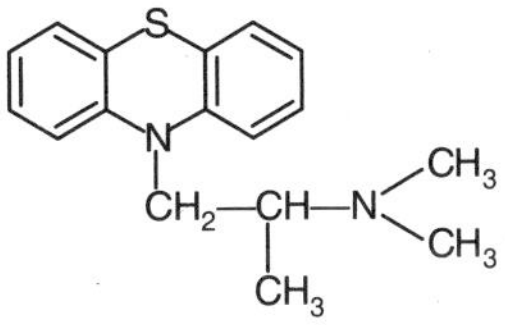

Promethazine

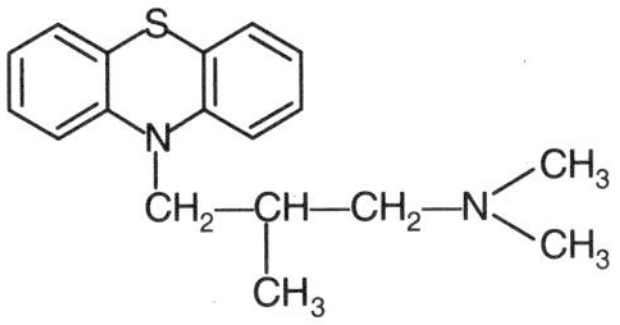

Trimeprazine

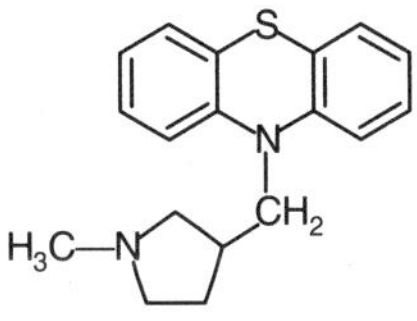

Methdiazine

Miscellaneous Agents

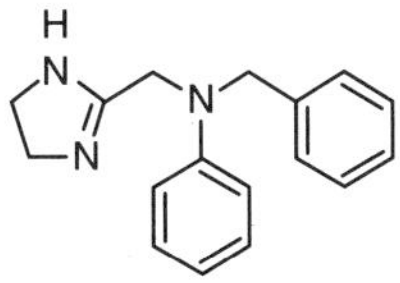

Antazoline

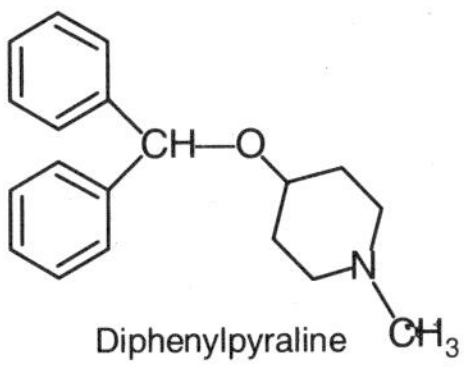

Diphenylpyraline

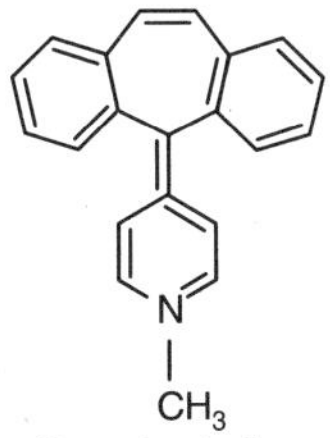

Cyproheptadine

Second Generation Agents

Acrivastine

Cetirizine

■ SECOND GENERATION H1 RECEPTOR ANTAGONIST

- These are newer drugs that are much more selective for peripheral H1 receptors in preference to the central nervous system histaminergic and cholinergic receptors.
- This selectivity significantly reduces the occurrence of adverse drug reactions compared with first-generation agents, while still providing effective relief of allergic conditions. Structure of these drugs varies from case to case. There is no common structural feature for the second generation H1-receptor antagonists.

■ THIRD GENERATION H1 RECEPTOR ANTAGONIST

- These are the active enantiomer (levocetirizine) or metabolite (desloratadine and fexofenadine) derivatives of second-generation drugs intended to have increased efficacy with fewer adverse drug reactions.
- Indeed, fexofenadine is associated with a decreased risk of cardiac arrhythmia compared to terfenadine. However, there is little evidence for any advantage of levocetirizine or desloratadine, compared to cetirizine or loratadine, respectively.

Mechanism of Action

- All antihistamines are reversible, competitive antagonists at histaminic (H1) receptors. They act by inhibiting binding of circulating histamine to its receptor site, but do not prevent histamine release. Administration of an antihistamine results in inhibition of respiratory, vascular, and gastrointestinal smooth muscle constriction, a decrease in histamine-activated secretions from salivary and lacrimal glands, and anti-inflammatory effects. Antihistamines also decrease capillary permeability, which reduces the wheal and flare response to an allergen, as well as diminishes itching.
- The second generation antihistamines are selective for peripheral H1 receptors. These agents are associated with less sedation and anticholinergic effects than the non-selective first generation antihistamines. The current agents also lack the cardiotoxic effects of the first peripherally-selective agents, terfenadine and astemizole.

Structure–Activity Relationship

Structural Requirement

1. Two aromatic rings, connected to a central carbon, nitrogen or CO.
2. Spacer between the central X and the amine, usually 2–3 carbons in length, linear, ring, branched, saturated or unsaturated.

3. Amine is substituted with small alkyl groups, e.g. CH_3.
4. Chirality at X can increase both the potency and selectivity for H1-receptors.
5. For maximum potency, the two aromatic rings should be orientated in different planes.

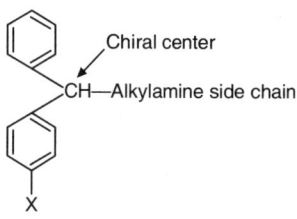

For example, tricyclic ring system is slightly puckered and the two aromatic rings lie in different geometrical planes, giving the drug a very high potency.

Aryl group

In the above structure, one Ar is aryl (including phenyl and heteroaryl group like 2-pyridyl) and second Ar is aryl or arylmethyl group.

Nature of X

It provides the basis of chemical classification of classic anti-histamines, e.g.

When X = Oxygen (aminoalkyl ether analogue).

When X = Nitrogen (ethylene-diamine derivative).

When X = Carbon (monoaminopropyl analogue).

Sometimes, the two aromatic rings are bridge, which constitutes tricyclic ring derivatives.

The alkyl chain

1. Most of the structure of classic antihistamines contains an ethylene chain. Extension or branching of this chain results in less active compounds (promethazine is possibly an exception).
2. Homologation has played an important role in the development of neuroleptic and tricyclic antidepressant from antihistaminic. All contain in general, the chain -C-C-NR2 although some of them have a neuroleptic component, antipsychotic activity is not unveiled in most cases until the carbon chain is lengthened to C3-NR2.

Terminal nitrogen atom

1. In general, the terminal N atom should be a tertiary amine for maximum activity. Unlike many anticholinergic and local anesthetic, here the dimethylamine derivatives are found to possess better antagonistic activity.
2. The terminal nitrogen may be part of heterocyclic ring as in antazoline and in chlocyclizine and retains high antihistaminic activity. However, substitution on the aromatic group with small basic heterocyclic rings increased branching on ethylene chain and substitution between X and N, all modify the potency, metabolism, ability to reach the site of action, toxicity and side reaction in vivo.
3. Since the structure of antihistaminic have a close resemblance with structure of cholinergic blocking agents, most of the classic antihistaminic do exhibit anticholinergics activity. The reverse is also true.

Physical Properties

1. **Lipophilicity:** They are generally lipophilic molecule. Studies show that its activity correlates with the lipophilicity of only one aromatic ring, i.e. the cis ring. It appears that only one aromatic group interacts with the receptor via hydrophobic bonding.
2. **Molecular size:** The two aromatic rings of antihistamines have different size of space available at the receptor for interaction. In a series of emedastine derivative, the length of

the substituent and the size of the nitrogen containing alicyclic ring determine the antihistaminic property.

3. **Side chain basicity:** The majority of the potent antihistamines have basic tertiary amines which are protonated at physiological pH. A quadratic relationship has been found between the basicity of the side chain and antihistaminic activity of the drug. The optimal pKa value was calculated to be 8.6. However, other compound, e.g. cicletamide which do not have basic amine centers in their molecule, yet they exhibits antihistaminic property.

Stereochemistry

- Steric structure in antihistaminic antagonist has profound effects on antihistaminic activity. Many antihistaminic H1-receptor antagonist shares the silent feature of diaryl fuction, e.g. benhydral, structural modification in this molecule often result in chiral molecule. Since diaryl function plays an important role in the interaction with H1-receptor, enantiomers resulted from such a chiral center possess different antihistaminic activity. Carbinoxamine which having the non-identical 2-pyridyl and 4-chlorophenyl group at its benzylic carbon exist in a pair of enantiomers possessing different antihistaminic activity.

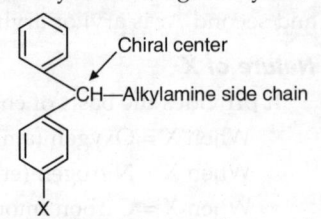

- Its levo form is 64 times more potent than the dextro form. The dextro form of chlorpheniramine is 200 times more potent than levo form. The dextro form of cetirizine is 10 times more potent than the levo form. When chiral center in many compounds away from the benzhydryl carbon, the enantiomers are equally potent.

- Cyroheptidine, rigid analogues give two conformational isomers. The levo isomer of 3-methoxy. Cyproheptidine is 8 fold more active than the dextro isomer.

- From the above fact that the configuration of a chiral center close to the diaryl unit is very important for the steroselectivity. The dispositions of the two aryl group about a double bond, e.g. triprolidine are exemplified. Even if double bond reduced, the relative orientation of the two aromatic rings remains the same due to hybridization changes of the amino alkyl chain. The binding site accommodating two aromatic groups, one so called trans ring, an unsubstituted phenyl and the other cis ring, a para substituted phenyl.

Gepometric isomerism and antihistaminic activity

- E-triprolidine, for example, is 1000-fold more potent than Z-triprolidine. This difference relates to the positioning and fit of the molecules in the histamine H1-receptor binding site.

- Alkylamines are considered to have relatively fewer sedative and gastrointestinal adverse effects, but relatively greater incidence of paradoxical CNS stimulation. The aryl cis to the pyrrolidinomethyl group may be involved in a pi-pi interaction with the receptor because the aromatic nature of this ring seems to be indispensible for H1 reactivity. When aryl trans to the pyrrolidinomethyl may involved in interaction whereas a potential H-bonding group is beneficial.

- Doxepine, a potent tricyclic antihistaminic, its Z-isomer is 3 and 1/2 times more potent than the its E-isomer.

Uses

H1-antihistamines are clinically used in the treatment of histamine-mediated allergic conditions. Specifically, these indications may include:

1. Allergic rhinitis.
2. Allergic conjunctivitis.

3. Allergic dermatological conditions (contact dermatitis).
4. Urticaria.
5. Angioedema.
6. Pruritus (atopic dermatitis, insect bites).
7. Anaphylactic or anaphylactoid reactions—adjunct only.
8. Nausea and vomiting (first-generation H1-antihistamines).
9. Sedation (first-generation H1-antihistamines).

Buclizine

| 4-chlorobenz-hydryl chloride | Ethyl piperazine-N-carboxylate | | Ethyl 4-(4-chlorobenzhydryl) piperazine-1-carboxylate (I) |

1-(4-chlorobenz-hydryl)piperazine   4-tert-butyl-benzyl chloride   Buclizine

Diphenhydramine

| Benzhydryl bromide | 2-dimethylamino-ethanol | Diphenhydramine |

Chlorpheniramine

| 4-chlorobenzyl chloride | Pyridine | 2-(4-chlorobenzyl)-pyridine | Chlorpheniramino |

Buclizine

Diphenhydramine

Chlorphenamine

Unit XI

Chemotherapeutic Agents

56

Antibiotics

The term chemotherapy can be defined as the treatment of diseases caused due to infective parasites or organisms without causing destruction of their host. Modern chemotherapy began with the work of Paul Ehlrich (1854–1915) (Fig. 56.1). Due to his pioneer discoveries in this field, he is regarded as "Father of Chemotherapy".

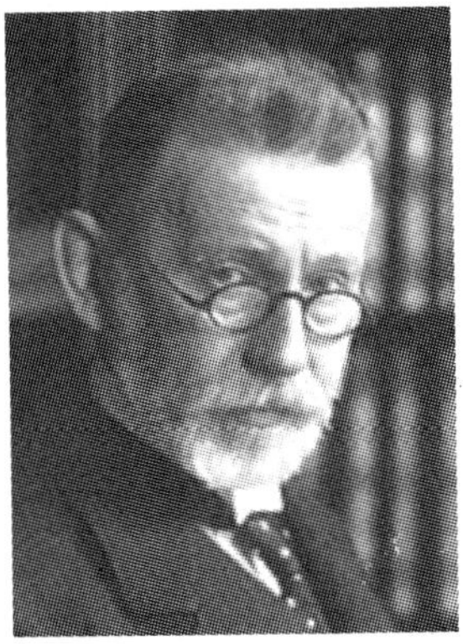

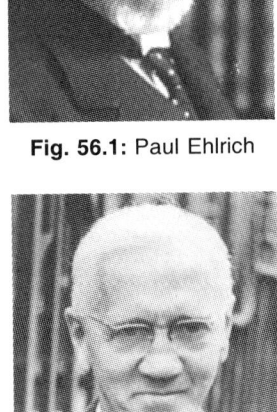

Fig. 56.1: Paul Ehlrich

- The second phase of revolution emerged in the1930s (following the discovery of the British bacteriologist Alexander Fleming (Fig. 56.2) when he tested the filtrate of a broth culture of a penicilium mold for its antibacterial activity.

- The term antibiotic has its origin in the word antibiosis (i.e. against the life); the latter being first time used by Vuillemin in 1889 in an attempt to describe the concept of survival of the fittest.

- Although the discovery of penicillin is named after Sir Fleming in 1928, it was not until 1940 at Oxford that Florey and Chain and their associates isolated it and described its properties in detail, and thus turning Fleming's discovery of practical significance.

- Among the many attempts to define the term antibiotic, the most appropriate one may be stated as,

  "An antibiotic is a chemical compound derived from or metabolically produced by microorganism and that in high dilution antagonizes the growth and/or the survival of one or more species of microorganism".

- The probable points of differences amongst the antibiotics may be physical, chemical and pharmacological properties, antibacterial spectra and mechanism of action.

Fig. 56.2: Alexander Fleming

- With advances made by the medical chemists to modify naturally occurring antibiotics and to prepare synthetic analogues, it has become necessary to permit the inclusion of semisynthetic and synthetic derivatives in the definition. Therefore, a substance is classified as an antibiotics, if the following conditions are met.

  1. It is the product of metabolism.
  2. It is a synthetic product, produced as a structurally similar with naturally occurring antibiotics.

3. It antagonizes the growth or survival of one or more species of micro-organisms.
4. It is effective in low concentration.

CLASSIFICATION OF ANTIBIOTICS

Classification of antibiotics is given in Flow chart 56.1.

Flow chart 56.1: Classification of antibiotics

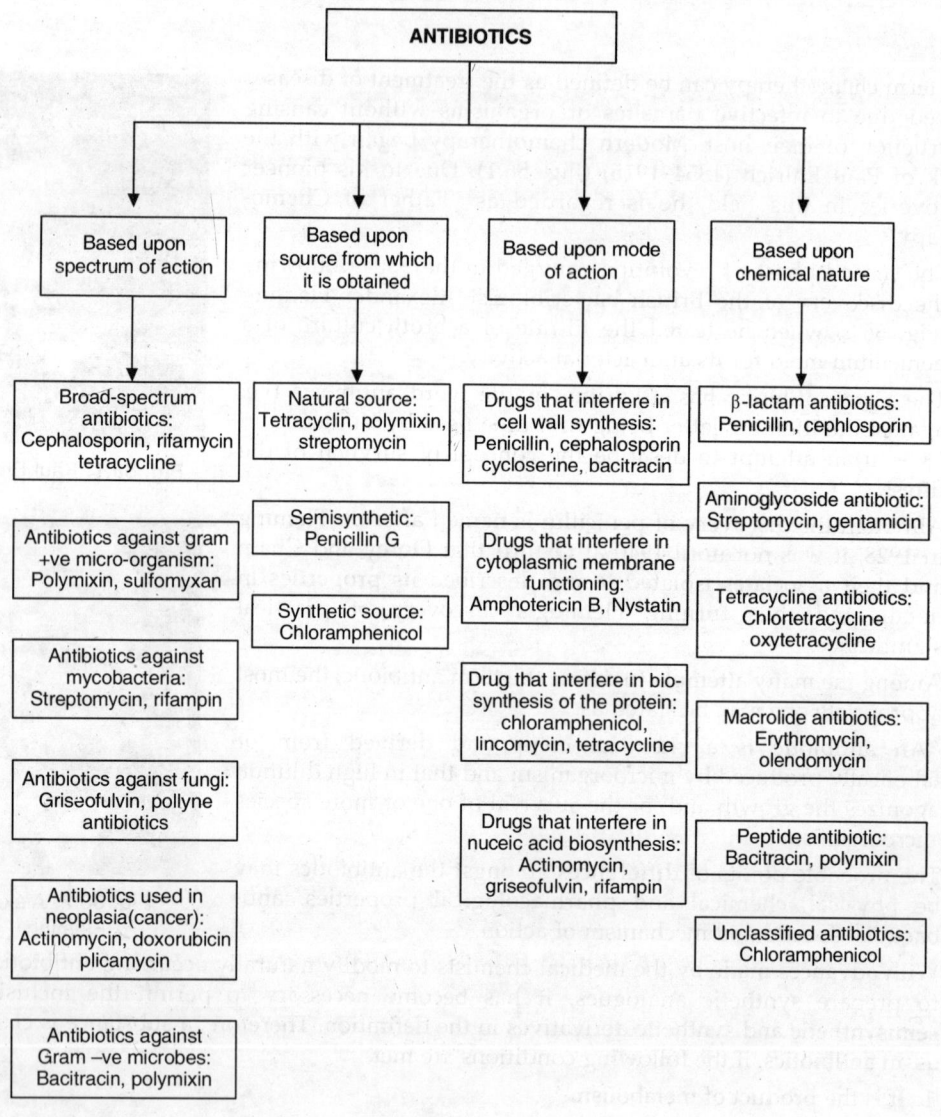

Based Upon Spectrum of Action

Broad-spectrum antibiotics

Cephalosporin derivatives

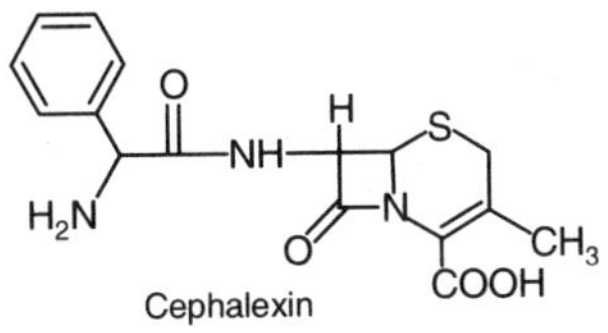

Cephalexin

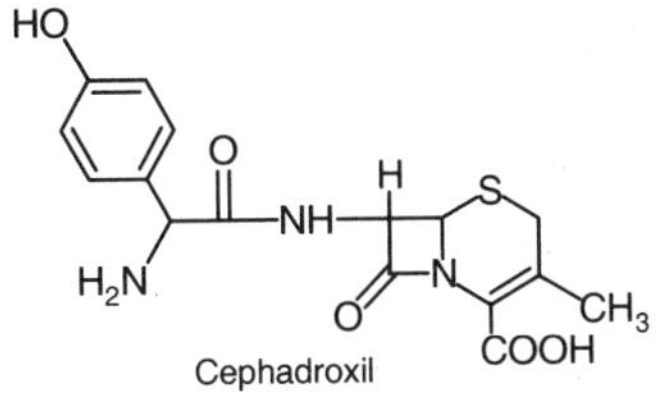

Cephadroxil

Tetracycline derivatives

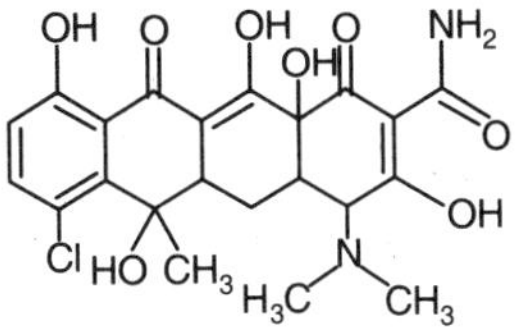

7-chlorotetracycline

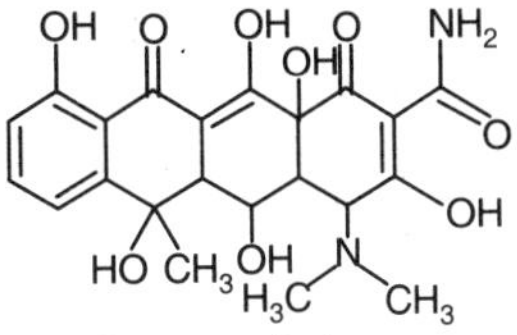

Oxytetracycline

Antibiotics against gram+ve microorganism

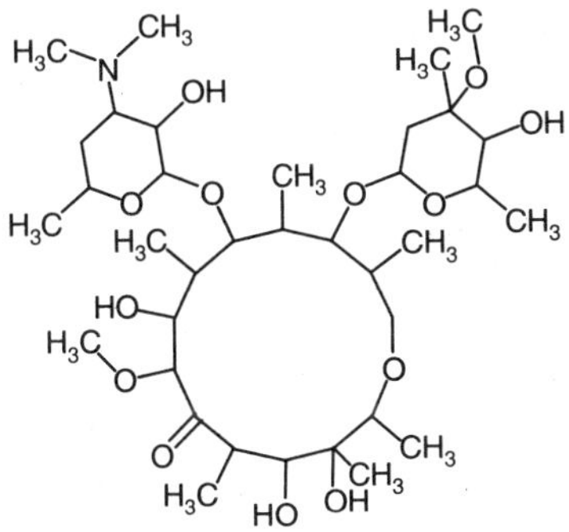

Olendomycin

Antibiotics against gram-ve microorganism

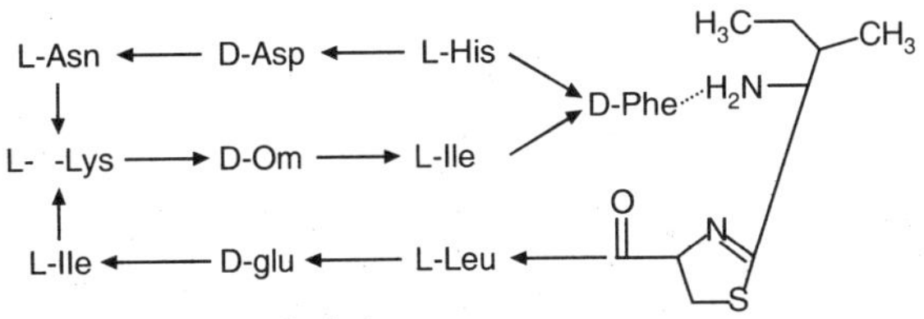

Bacitrcin

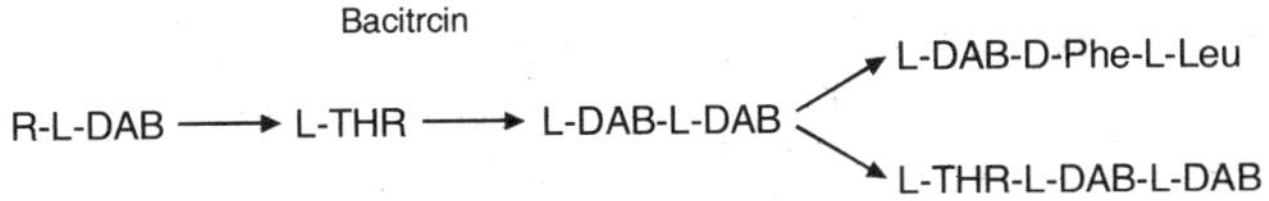

Polymixin

Antibiotics against mycobacteria

Rifampicin

Streptomycin

$3.H_2SO_4$

Antibiotics against fungi

Amphotericin B

Nystatin A_1

Griseofulvin

Anticancer antibiotic

	R_1	R_2
Daunorubicin	$COCH_3$	OH
Doxorubicin	$COCH_2OH$	OH
Esorubicin	$COCH_2OH$	H

Based Upon Source from which Antibiotics are Obtained

Natural source

Polymixin

Streptomycin

$3.H_2SO_4$

Semisynthetic

Ampicillin

Penicillin G

Synthetic source

Chloramphenicol

Based Upon Mode of Action

Drugs that interfere in cell wall synthesis

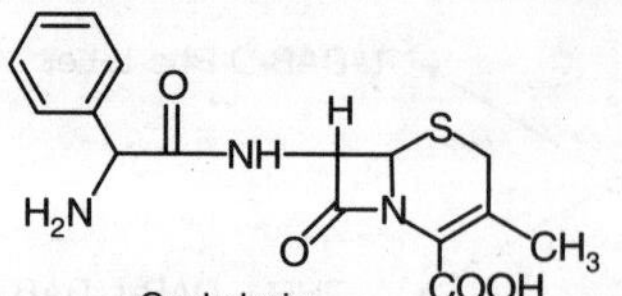

Cephalexin

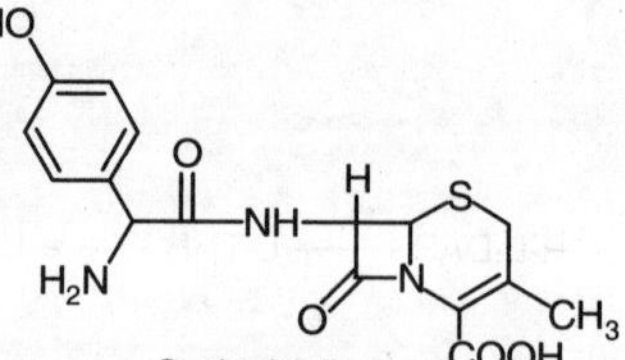

Cephadroxil

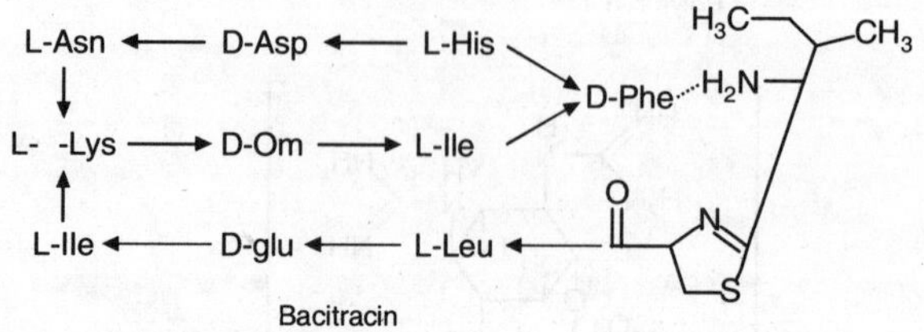

L-Asn ← D-Asp ← L-His

D-Phe····H₂N

L-·-Lys → D-Orn → L-Ile

L-Ile ← D-glu ← L-Leu ←

Bacitracin

Cephalosporin derivatives; Penicillin derivatives
(Refer above structure)

Drugs that interfere in cytoplasmic functioning

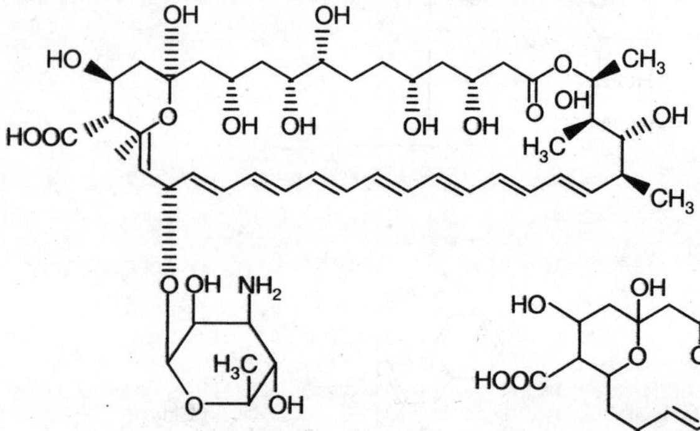

Amphotericin B

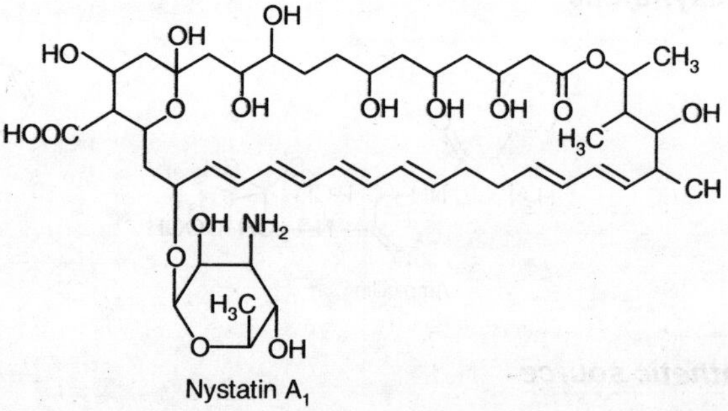

Nystatin A₁

Drugs that interfere in protein synthesis

    Erythromycin

    Lincomycin

    Tetracycline

    Chloramphenicol……….. structure mentioned above

Drugs that interfere in nucleic acid synthesis

    Rifampin

    Griseofulvin……….for structure refer above pages

Based Upon Chemical Nature

β-*Lactam antibiotics*

Cephalosporins

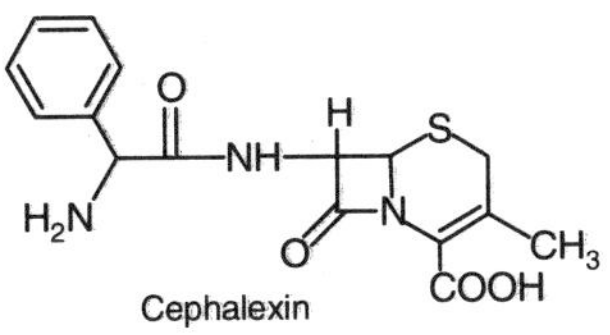

Cephalexin

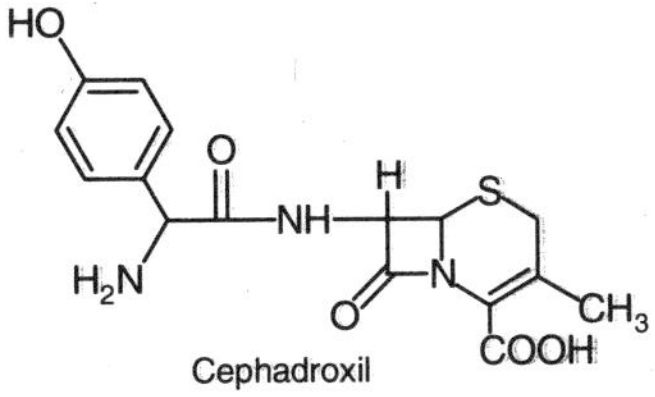

Cephadroxil

Penicillins

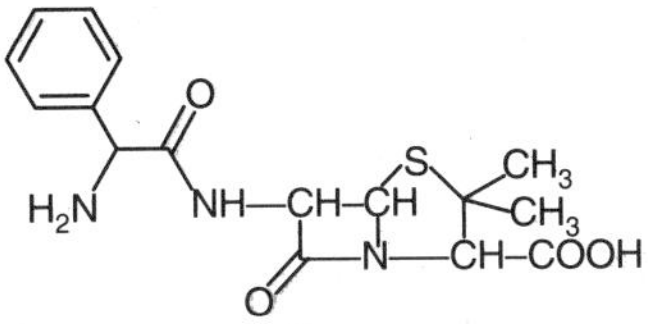

Ampicillin

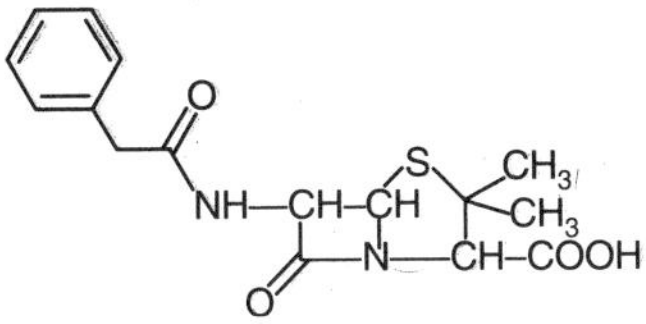

Penicillin G

Aminoglycosides

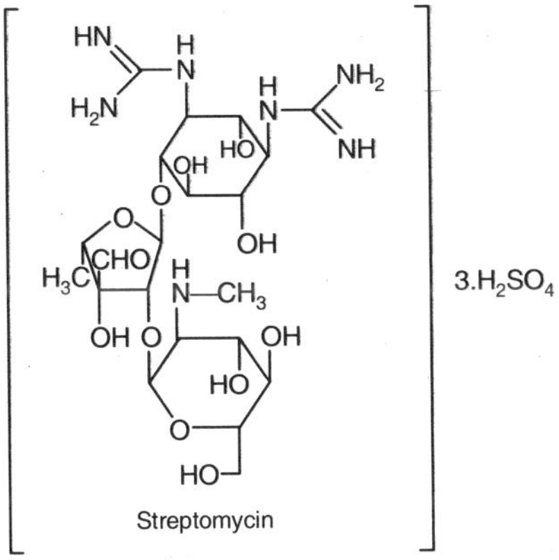

$3.H_2SO_4$

Streptomycin

Tetracyclines

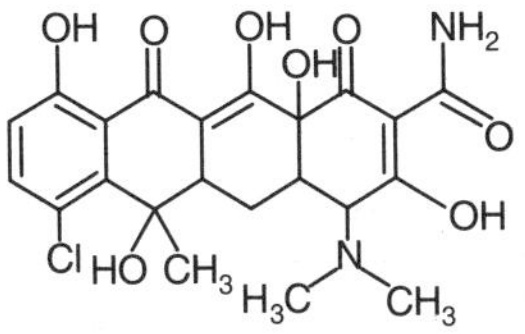

7-chlorotetracycline

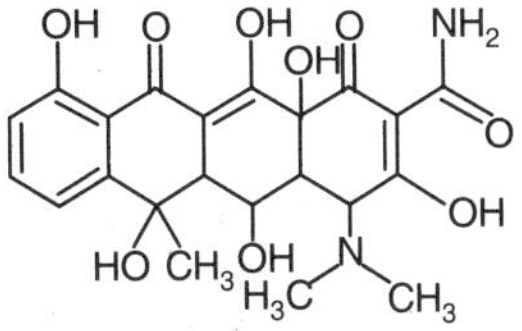

Oxytetracycline

Peptide antibiotics

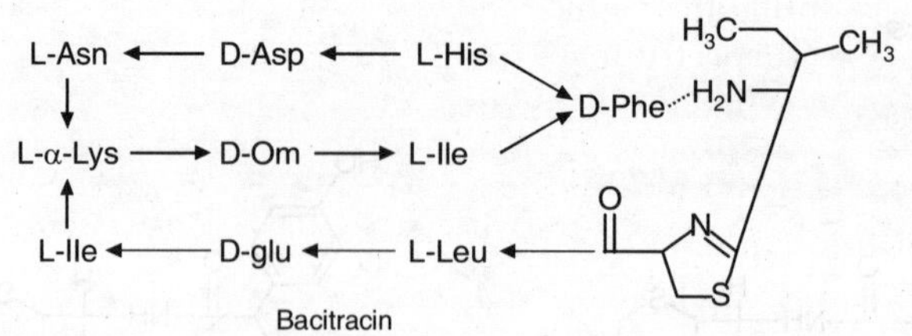

Bacitracin

Macrolide antibiotics

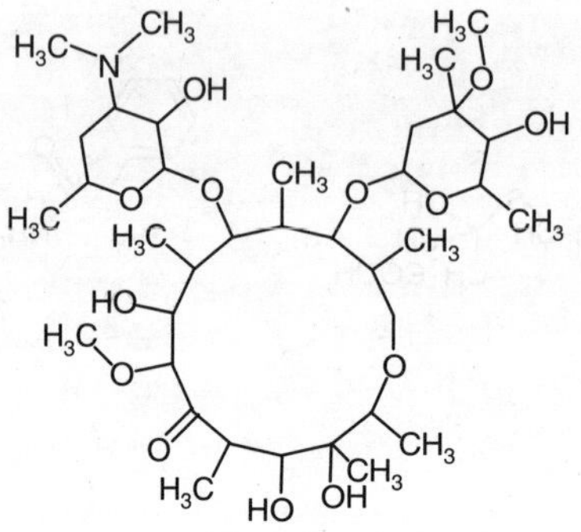

Olendomycin

Unclassifieds

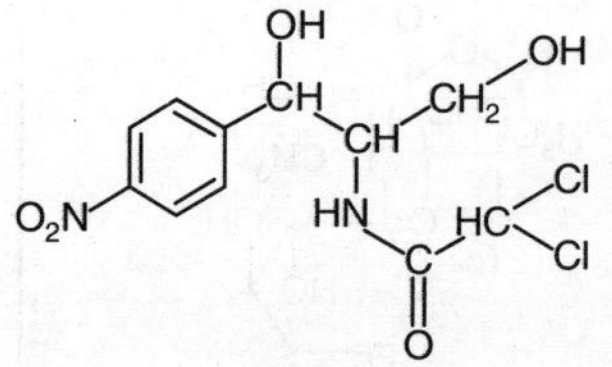

Chloramphenicol

Depending Upon the Sources from which Antibiotics is Obtained

Natural

These antibiotics are obtained from the large-scale fermentation of microorganisms, e.g. bacitracin, and polymixin are obtained from some bacilli while streptomycin, tetracyclines, etc, from *Streptomyces* species.

Semisynthetic

The observation that 6-aminopenicillanic acid can be obtained from cultures of *P. chrysogenum* that were depleted of side chain precursors led to the development of this class. For example, during the commercial production of benzyl penicillin (penicillin G), phenylacetic acid is added to the medium in order to achieve predominance of the product.

Synthetic

This class includes antibiotics which are having purely synthetic origin. For example, chloramphenicol, a broad-spectrum antibiotic initially isolated from a fermented media in 1947 and later was produced synthetically on a commercial basis.

Classification Based Upon Mode of Action

1. **Drugs that interfere in the biosynthesis of bacterial cell wall,** e.g. penicillins, cephalosporins, cycloserine, bacitracin and vancomycin.
2. **Drugs that interfere in the functioning of cytoplasmic membrane,** e.g. polymixins, amphotericin B and nystatin.
3. **Drugs that interfere in the protein biosynthesis,** e.g. erythromycin, lincomycins, tetracyclines, and chloramphenicol.
4. **Drugs that interfere in the nucleic acid biosynthesis,** e.g. actinomycin, griseofulvin and rifampin.

Based on chemical nature

- β-lactam antibiotics.
- Aminoglycoside antibiotics.
- Tetracycline antibiotics.
- Peptide antibiotics.
- Macrolide antibiotic.
- Unclassified antibiotics.

56.1

β-Lactam Antibiotics (Penicillins)

Even though penicillin had been discovered in 1928, and is a member of β-lactam antibiotic, the term β-lactam antibiotic has to wait till 1942 to get registered in the dictionary of medicinal chemists. Thanks to Prof. Howard W. Florey and Dr. Ernst B. Chain, working at that time at the William Dunn School of Pathology, Oxford with their sincere efforts, isolated and characterised the basic structure of the penicillins. This work was supplimented by the efforts of the chemists Dr. Abraham and Dr. Heatley. The clinical effectiveness of penicillin was first tested on 12 February, 1941 in the form of a sodium salt.

- Thus long after the antibiotic projected its appearance on the screen of research, the structure of penicillin was determined.
- Thus penicillins can be considered as the amido derivatives of the 6-aminopenicillanic acid.

Basic skeleton of penicillins

- In the basic skeleton, a thiazolidine ring (A) is fused with a beta-lactam ring (B) which is a 4-membered cyclic amide.

- The penicillins differ from each other in antibacterial and pharmacological characteristics due to variation in the structure of acid moiety of the amide side chain at C-6. After about 45 years of clinical use, remain an extremely effective and the only natural penicillin used clinically.

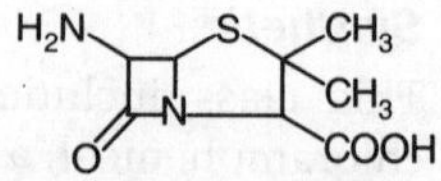

6-aminopenicillanic acid

- Acylation of 6-APA with appropriate carboxylic acids resulted in new penicillins, some of which are broad-spectrum antibiotics.

STEREOCHEMISTRY

1. Penicillin molecule contains 3 assymetric carbon atoms such as C-3, C-5, C-6.
2. All naturally occurring and active synthetic and semisynthetic penicillins have the same absolute configuration at three asymmetric centers.

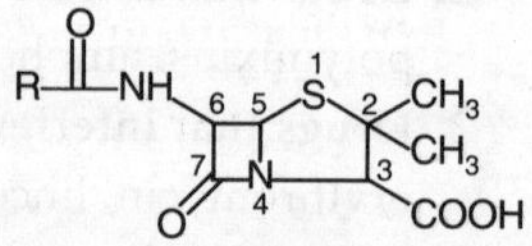

Penicillins

3. The carbon atom bearing the acylamino group C-6 has the L-configuration, whereas the carbon to which COOH group attached has the D-configuration. Thus the acylamino and carboxyl group are trans to each other.
4. The atom comprising the 6-aminopenicillanic acid portion structure is derived biosynthetically.
5. The absolute stereochemistry of penicillin is designated as 3S:5R:6R.

CHEMISTRY

1. The penicillins can be considered as derivatives of the 6-aminopenicillanic acid.

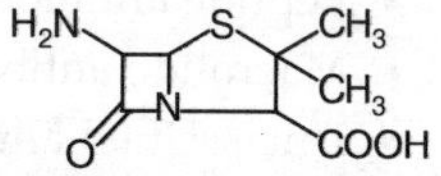

6-aminopenicillanic acid

2. The basic skeleton of penicillins consists of the thiazolidine ring which is fused with the β-lactam ring.

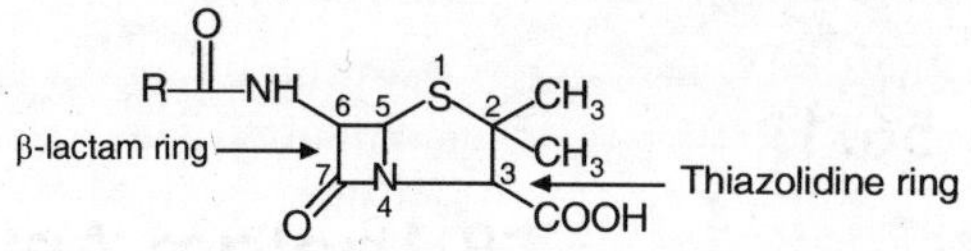

Penicillins

3. The early commercial penicillin was a yellow-brown or red amorphous powder that was so unstable that refrigeration was required to maintain potency, even for short period of time (Fig. 56.1.1).

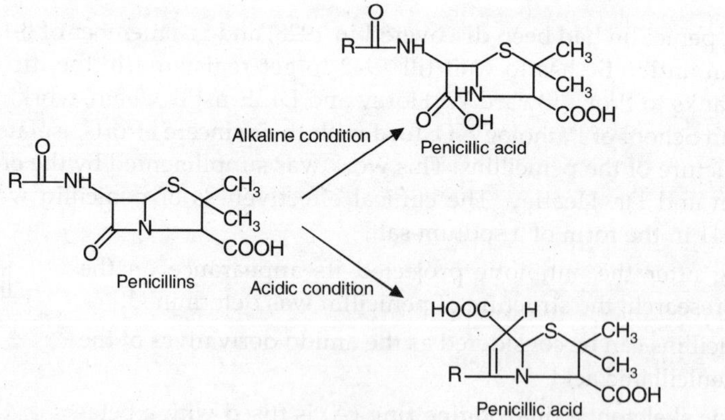

Fig. 56.1.1: Degradation of penicillin in alkaline and acidic condition

4. For stability purpose, penicillin is converted into salt form, which is crystalline white in nature and we can store such penicillin for years without refrigeration, only required thing is that it should be protected from moisture.

5. The sodium and potassium salts of most of the penicillins are water soluble and readily absorbed when given by injection or orally, but the less stable, free acid is not suitable for incorporation into the dosage form.

6. Treatment of penicillins with strong mineral acid or mercuric chloride causes breakdown of the molecule to penicillamine and a penaldic acid, which are unstable.

7. Alkalies and the specific enzyme penicillinase are more selective in their action, attacking only the β-lactam ring to yield penicilloic acid causing inactivation.

8. Similar reaction is also shown by alcohols and amines.

9. The strong gastric acid leads to hydrolysis of the amide side chain and opening of the β-lactam ring, with resultant loss of activity.

▨ DEGRADATION PRODUCTS OF PENICILLINS

Natural penicillins are acid and base unstable. Instability in acid media logically precludes their oral administration due to the highly acidic pH in stomach. At acidic pH, a sort of molecular rearrangement results. The structure is known as a penillic acid and loses its activity. Similarly at basic pH, penicillin molecule gets converted to penicilloic acid which is again an inactive form. The mechanism of degradation is described below.

Degradation of Penicillin (Fig. 56.1.2)

The first step involve the protonation of the β-lactam nitrogen, followed by the nucleophilic attack of the acyl oxygen atom on the β-lactam carbonyl carbon that results in opening of both the rings, which leads to the formation of penicillenic acid. Penicillenic acid is unstable and experiences the two major degradation pathways.

- **Path-I:** Here the oxazolone ring of penicillenic acid undergoes to the hydrolysis to form unstable penamaldic acid. Penamaldic acid further yields penicillamine and penaldic acid on hydrolysis. Next step involves the formation of penicilloaldehyde by decarboxylation of penaldic acid.

- **Path-II:** The second pathway involves a complex rearrangement of penicillenic acid to a penillic acid through a series of intramolecular processes. Penillic acid upon decarboxylation and hydrolytic cleavage under acidic condition gives rise to penilloic acid.

- **Path-III:** Under weakly acidic or alkaline as well as enzymatic hydrolysis condition, penicilloic acid is formed, which is not observed as intermediate under strongly acidic condition. However, it is known to exist in equilibrium with penamaldic acid and undergoes decarboxylation in acid to form penilloic acid.

Certain strains of microorganisms can destroy beta-lactam antibiotics enzymatically. The enzymes more popularly known as penicillinases or β-lactamases can open the β-lactam bond. The difference in the susceptibility to the β-lactamase enzymes depends upon the nature of the amide side-chain at C-6. It also depends upon the bacterial strain involved.

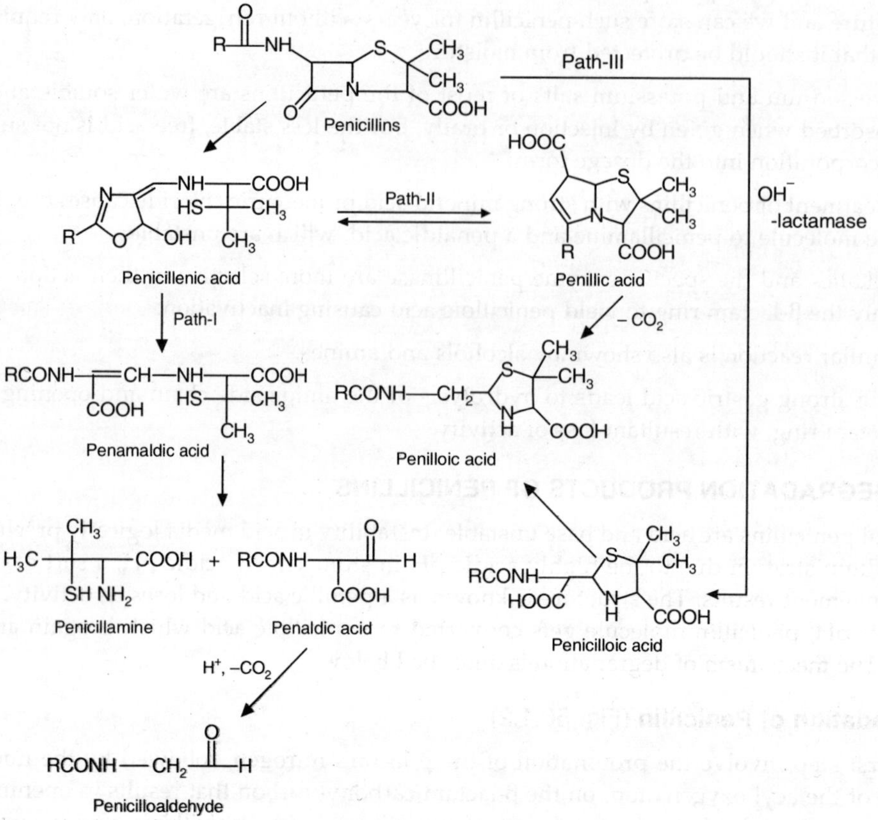

Fig. 56.1.2: Degradation of penicillin

SAR OF β-LACTAM ANTIBIOTICS

1. Introduction of α-aryloxy alkyl penicillins in the side chain gives increased acid stability and oral absorption.

2. Substitution of α-carbon atom of the side chain with amino, chloro, etc. displays good resistance to inactivation by acids.

3. Substitution of α-carbon atom of the side chain with bulky group increases the activity against β-lactamase.

4. Introduction of an ionised or polar group into the α-position of the side chain increases the activity against gram-negative bacilli.

5. D-isomer is 2 to 8 times more effective than L-isomer.

6. The acyl side chain replaced by hydroxymethyl groups increases the activity against gram-negative bacteria.

7. N-acylated ampicillin has increased activity against *Pseudomonas*.

8. Many esters of carboxyl group attached to C-3 prepared as prodrug to increase the lipophilicity and acid stability.

9. Introduction of C-6α-methoxy confers greater stability against β-lactamase without significant loss of activity.
10. The sulfur of the thiazolidine ring can be replaced with O, CH_2...etc. with increase in broad-spectrum activity.

MECHANISM OF ACTION

• Generally it is assume that penicillins act on microorganism by interfering with the development of cell wall.
• Specifically, they inhibit the biosynthesis of dipeptidoglycan that is needed to provide strength and rigidity to cell wall.
• Penicillins acylate the enzyme transpeptidase by opening the lactam ring, there by inactivating it because of which it cannot form cross-link of two linear peptidoglycan strands by transpeptidation and elimination of D-alanine (Fig. 56.1.3).

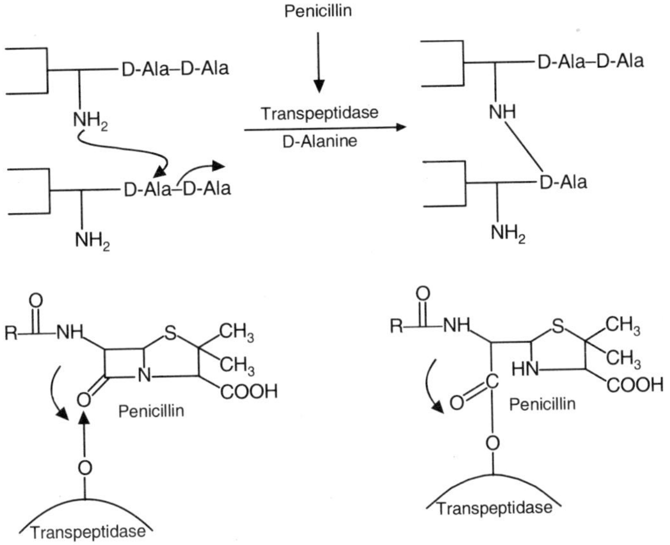

Fig. 56.1.3: Mechanism showing acylation of transpeptidase

SEMISYNTHETIC PENICILLIN (FIG. 56.1.4)

Semisynthetic penicillin is the need of time since penicillin is completely degraded in the presence of acid that results in a poor oral absorption of penicillin. The semisynthetic penicillin should possess following criteria.

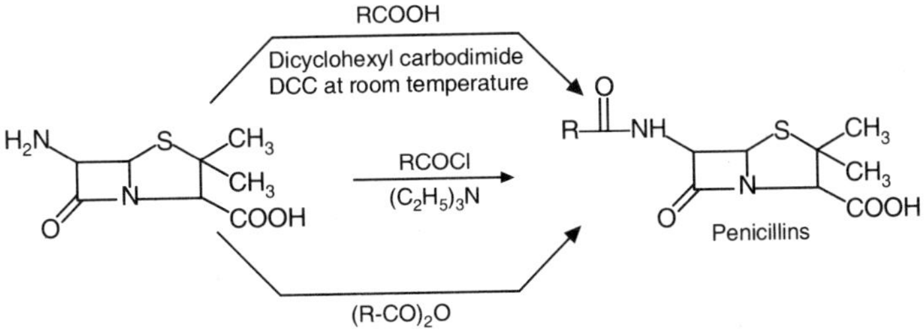

Fig. 56.1.4: Methods to synthesize semisynthetic penicillin

1. Improvement of acidic and metabolic stability.
2. Broadening of the spectrum of antibacterial activity.
3. Improvement of pharmacokinetic parameters.
4. Decreased side effects.

CLASSIFICATION OF PENICILLINS

Classification of penicillin is given in Flow chart 56.1.

Flow chart 56.1.1: Classification of penicillin

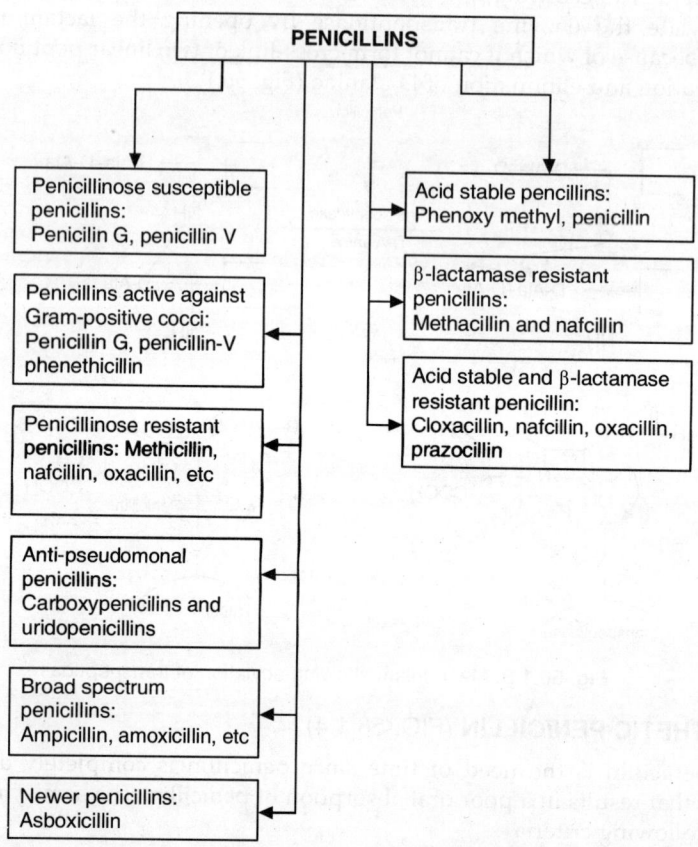

PENICILLINS

Penicillinose susceptible penicillins:
Penicilin G, penicillin V

Penicillins active against Gram-positive cocci:
Penicillin G, penicillin-V phenethicillin

Penicillinose resistant penicillins: Methicillin, nafcillin, oxacillin, etc

Anti-pseudomonal penicillins:
Carboxypenicilins and uridopenicillins

Broad spectrum penicillins:
Ampicillin, amoxicillin, etc

Newer penicillins:
Asboxicillin

Acid stable pencillins:
Phenoxy methyl, penicillin

β-lactamase resistant penicillins:
Methacillin and nafcillin

Acid stable and β-lactamase resistant penicillin:
Cloxacillin, nafcillin, oxacillin, prazocillin

Penicillinase Susceptible Penicillins

Penicillin G

Penicillin V

Penicillinase Resistant Penicillins

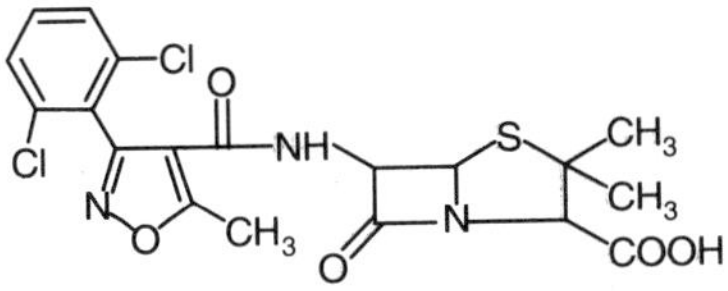

Dicloxacillin

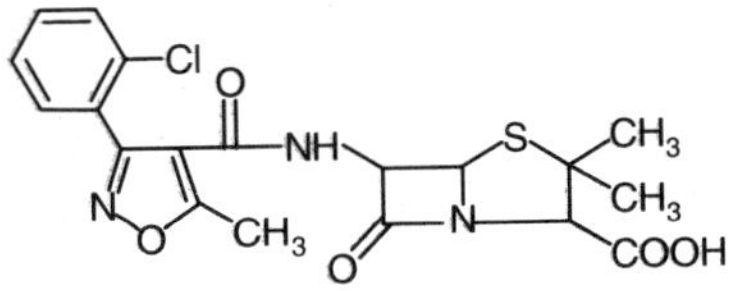

Cloxacillin

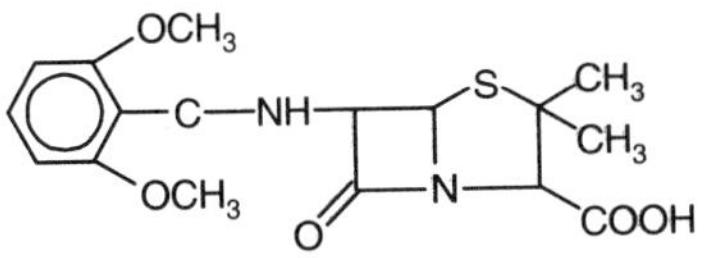

Methicillin

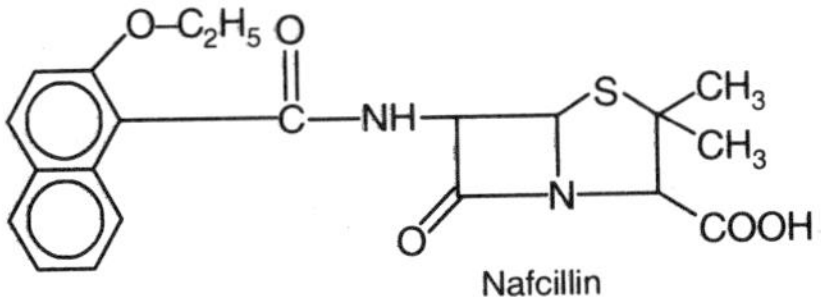

Nafcillin

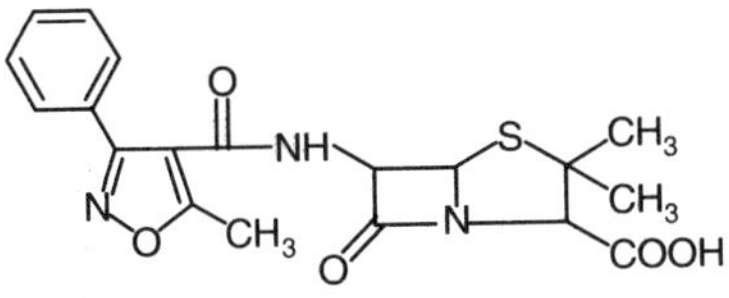

Oxacillin

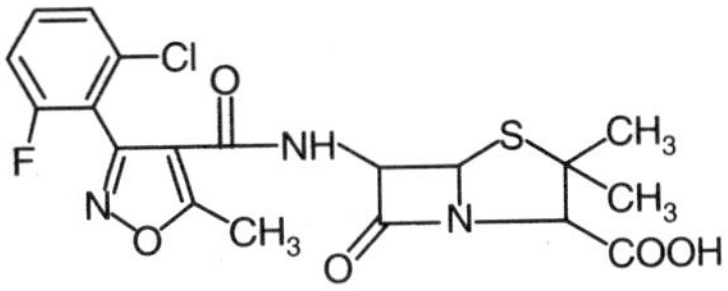

Floxacillin

Broad Spectrum Antibiotics

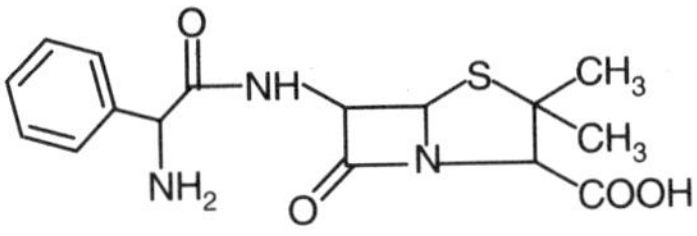

Ampicillin

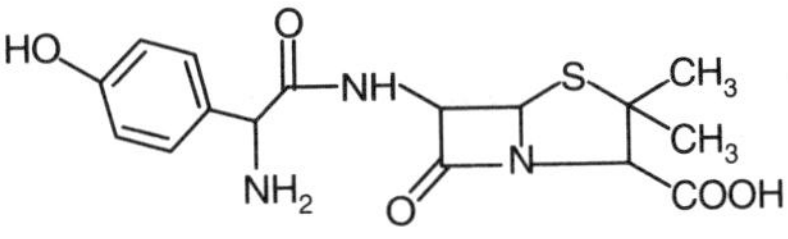

Amoxicillin

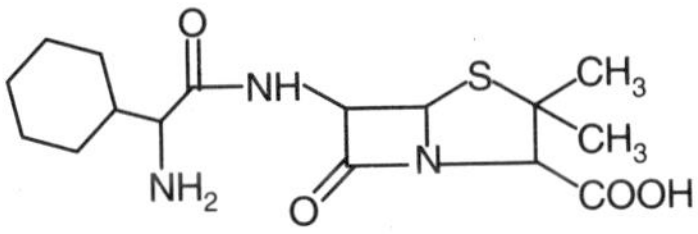

Cyclocillin

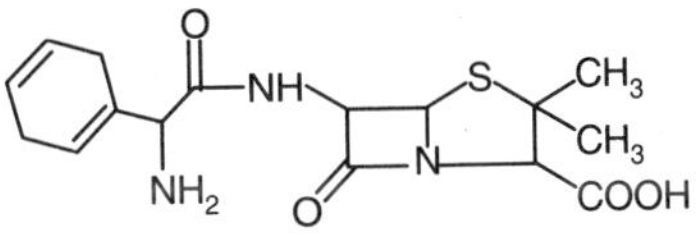

Epicillin

Anti-pseudomonal penicillins

[A] *Carboxypenicillin*

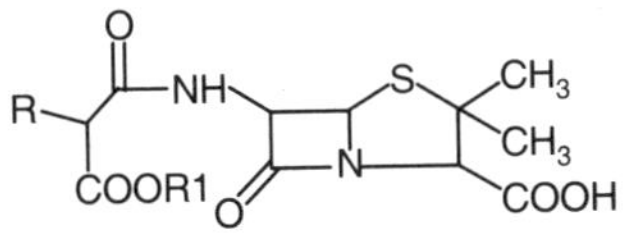

Drug	R	R1
Carbenicillin	C_6H_5	H
Carfecillin	C_6H_5	C_6H_5
Ticarcillin	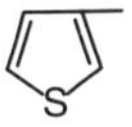	H

[B] *Urido penicillins*

Sr. No.	Penicillins	R
1.	Aziocillin	
2.	Mezlocillin	
3.	Piperacillin	

* Penicillins active against Gram-positive microbes:

Sr. No.	Penicillins	R
1.	Penicillin G	$-CH_2-$
2.	Penicillin V	$-CH_2-O-$
3.	Phenethicillin	

* Acid stable penicillins:

Phenoxy methyl penicillin

* **β-lactamase penicillins:**

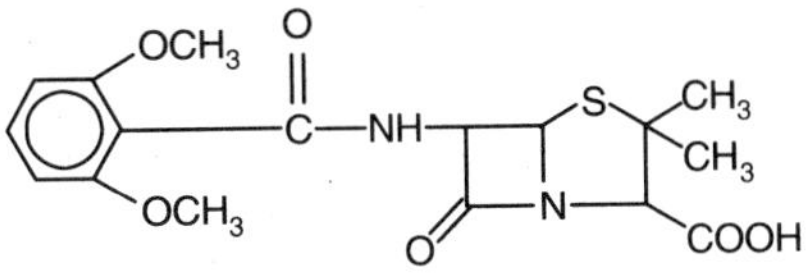

Methicillin

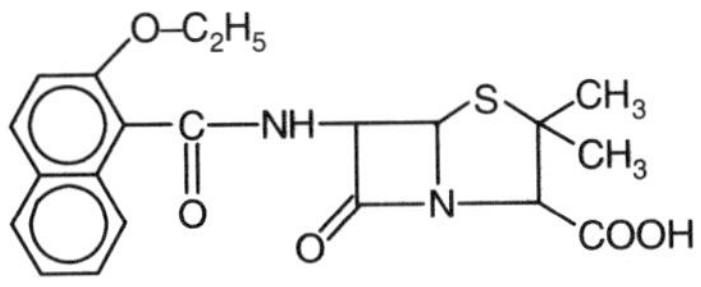

Nafcillin

* **Acid stable and β-lactamase resistant penicillin:**

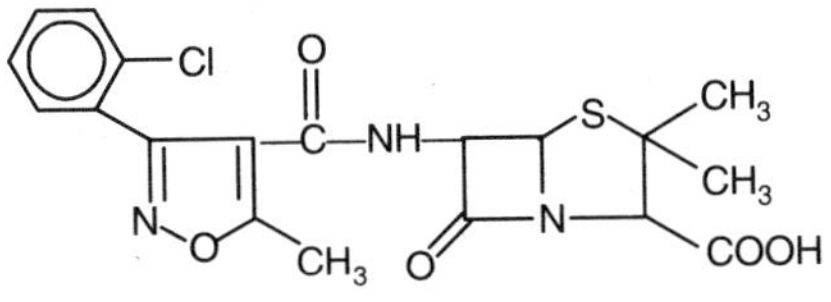

Cloxacillin

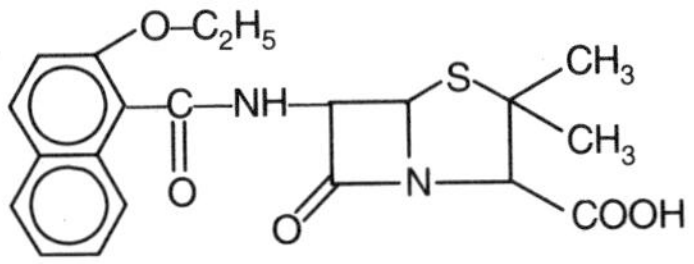

Nafcillin

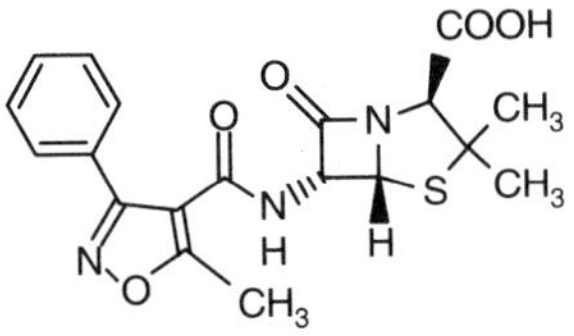

Oxacillin

* **Newer penicillins**

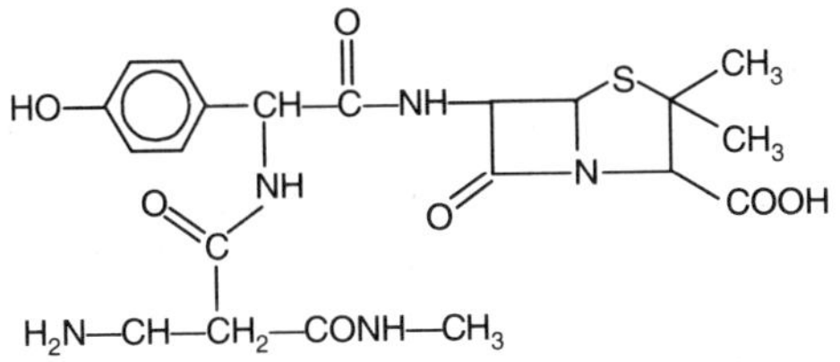

Absoxicillin

EVOLUTION OF THE SERIES OF β-LACTAM ANTIBIOTICS

- The β-lactam antibiotics are cell-wall inhibitors towards susceptible bacteria. It just means that they cannot kill or inhibit all bacteria, e.g. penicillin G (benzyl penicillin) has a fairly narrow antibacterial spectrum. In particular, fungi and many gram-negative bacteria are relatively insensitive to this agent. It is readily hydrolysed by the enzyme penicillinase. The pronounced hydrolytic susceptibility of the β-lactam bond to penicillinase, hindered early progress in working with penicillins.

- Following the realization that the presence of phenyl acetic acid in the fermentation leads to predominance of the product, benzylpenicillin, wide variety of other acids were added to the growing culture. Thus the second generation known as semi-synthetic penicillins born. The proper design of the side chains thus accessible has served not only to overcome many of the drawbacks of the early penicillins (like enzyme susceptibility, acid liability and lack of oral activity) but also helped to develop broad-spectrum antibiotics.

- The involvement of acyl carbon of the side chain in the hydrolytic cleavage of β-lactam bond was recognised. Improvement in clinical qualities was then achieved by creating steric hindrances to this acyl carbon, thus making it less reactive. The fact was attested by attachment of an aromatic or heterocyclic ring directly to the amide carbonyl affords antibiotics with increased penicillinase resistance, e.g. methicillin, oxacillin family and nafacillin.

- One of the most successful penicillin candidates is ampicillin which is prototype of third generation β-lactam antibiotics. It is characterized by increased oral activity than its precursor. The early observation that drugs acylated by amino acids had somewhat greater oral activity turned to be an inspiration behind its development. Thus addition of an amino group to benzylpenicillin also leads to broadening of spectrum of activity along with increased oral activity. The next congener is amoxicillin. The aminopenicillins still suffer from the major drawback, i.e. susceptible to beta lactamase enzymes and thus are ineffective for most staphylococcal infections. In an attempt to improve further, the pharmacodynamic characteristics, prodrug development program of ampicillin was undertaken. As a result, bacampicillin, hetacillin and talampicillin appeared on the screen.

- The fourth generation of β-lactam adds to the list of chemotherapeutic agents in the form of carboxypenicillins. Carboxylic acid group if introduced into the primary amine moiety of ampicillin and other allied skeleton may significantly affects the biological spectrum of the lead, was noted seriously and served as an impulse in the generation of this class. The examples can be glanced at, are carbenicillin family and ticarcillin.

- A parallel observation is also registered stating that acylation of the amino group of ampicillin broadens the antimicrobial spectrum of the prototype drug. Azlocillin is a front-line drug in this series which was named under ureidopenicillins. Recently new impetus has been added to the chemotherapy by the discovery of new ring systems in fermentation liquors.

- Despite the enormous efforts expanded during the past three decades, the β-lactam antibiotic field remains still a field of severe competition within itself. The new drugs coming up differ from benzyl penicillin (natural penicillin) in one or more of four ways–acid sensitivity, susceptibility to inactivation by penicillinase, antibiotic potency and spectrum of antibacterial activity.

- When the acid stability of penicillin is increased, the drug would not be destroyed by gastric acid and thus can be orally administered. The penicillinase resistant penicillins are not hydrolysed by the enzymes produced by *Staphylococcus aureus* and hence they are effectively used to treat the infections caused by resistant strains of microorganisms.

■ BIOCHEMICAL MECHANISMS OF BACTERIAL RESISTANCE TO β-LACTAM ANTIBIOTICS

- It should be noted that penicillin resistance may not always be due to penicillinase production, even among the staphylococci, certain other mechanisms of resistance may be operative, like a change in antibiotic target site, which may not be vital for microbial survival, thus resulting into drug resistance.

1. Inability of the agent to penetrate to its site of action.
2. A reduction in cellular permeability to the antibiotic.

3. The antibiotic agent, instead of attacking the microorganisms, may be utilised to antagonise a biochemical intermediate released by microbes.

4. A sensitive strain may undergo mutational change and thereafter acquires resistant to antibiotic agent.

• Thus penicillin resistance develops into sensitive strains of microbes due to a single or sometimes due to overlapping of one or more mechanisms mentioned above.

Hypersensitivity or allergic reaction

Hypersensitivity reactions may occur with any dosage form of penicillin. In some cases, the reaction is mild and disappears even while the use of drug is continued. While in others, reactions may persist for 1 or 2 weeks or longer after therapy has been stopped. These reactions include immediate or delayed type skin allergies, fever, bronchospasm, serum sickness and anaphylactic reactions.

These manifestations may be due to the following reasons:

1. A breakdown product, penicilloyl moiety results due to opening of β-lactam ring. This fraction is considered to be the most important antigenic intermediate of penicillins.

2. Certain other contaminants (mycelial residues) of high molecular weight originating from fermentation process may serve as a cause of manifestations.

3. A non-protein polymer of unknown origin may also be present in penicillin and may be antigenic.

4. The degradation products, penicillenic acid and/or penicilloate may interact with sulfhydryl/amino groups present in vital tissue proteins. The resulting complexes may serve themselves as penicillin antigens. Thus above mentioned reactions are responsible for releasing foreign proteins in the body which ultimately leads to the generation of allergic reactions to penicillins.

Ampicillin

D(–)-Cbo-phenylglycine   Ethyl chloro-formate (I)   D-Cbo-phenylglycine anhydride with monoethyl carbonate (II)

6-amino-penicillanic acid (III)

Cbo-ampicillin sodium salt (IV)

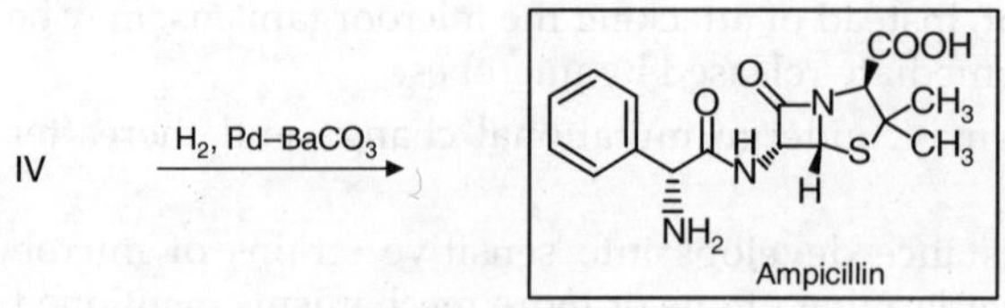

IV $\xrightarrow{\text{H}_2, \text{Pd–BaCO}_3}$ Ampicillin

Amoxicillin

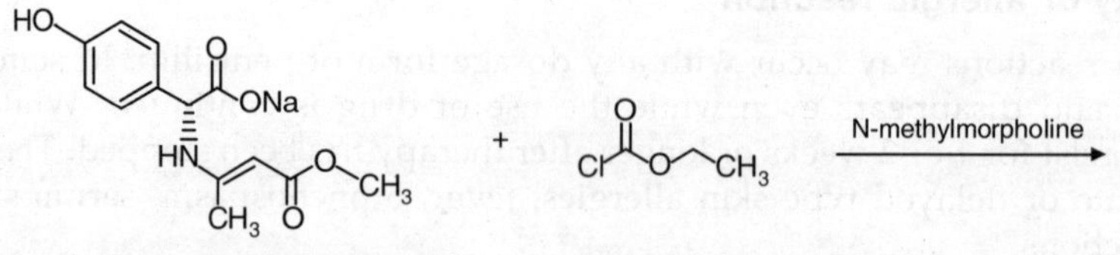

sodium D(−)-α-(4-hydroxy-phenyl)-
α-(2-methoxy-carbony-1-methylethenyl-
amino)acetate (DANE salt)

ethyl chloroformate

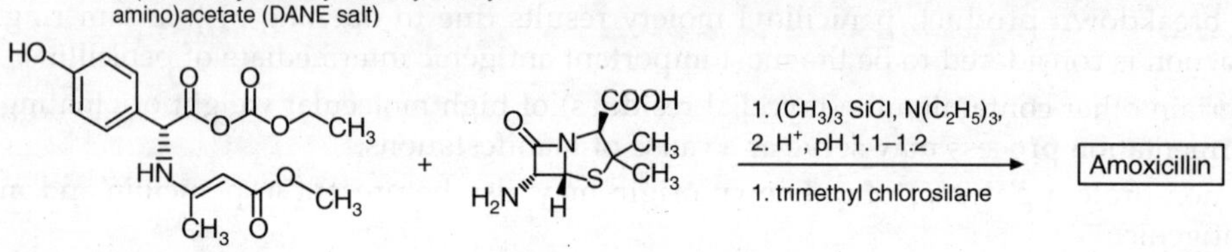

$\xrightarrow{\text{N-methylmorpholine}}$ I

D-α-(4-hydroxyphenyl)-α-(2-
methoxycarbonyl-1-methyl-
ethenylamino)acetic acid
anhydride with monoethyl
carbonate (I)

6-amino-
penicillanic acid (II)

1. $(CH_3)_3$ SiCl, $N(C_2H_5)_3$,
2. H^+, pH 1.1–1.2

1. trimethyl chlorosilane

Amoxicillin

Amoxicillin

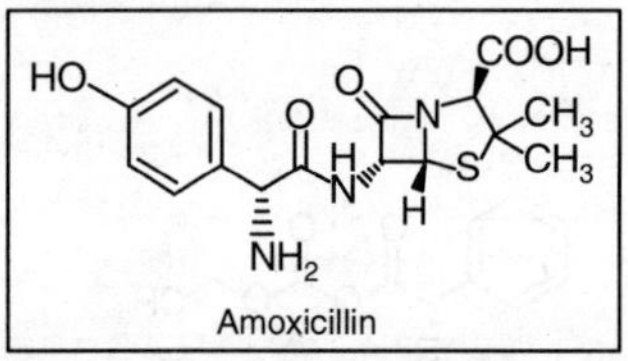

Carbenicillin

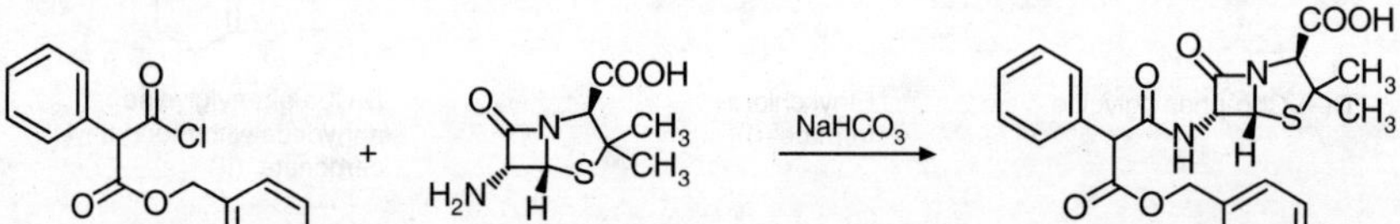

Phenylmalonic acid
benzyl ester chloride

6-amino-
penicillanic acid (II)

$\xrightarrow{\text{NaHCO}_3}$

Carbenicillin benzyl ester (I)

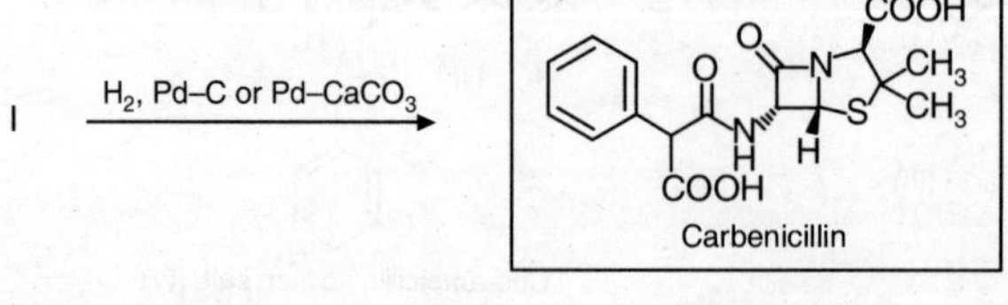

I $\xrightarrow{\text{H}_2, \text{Pd–C or Pd–CaCO}_3}$

Carbenicillin

Ticarcillin

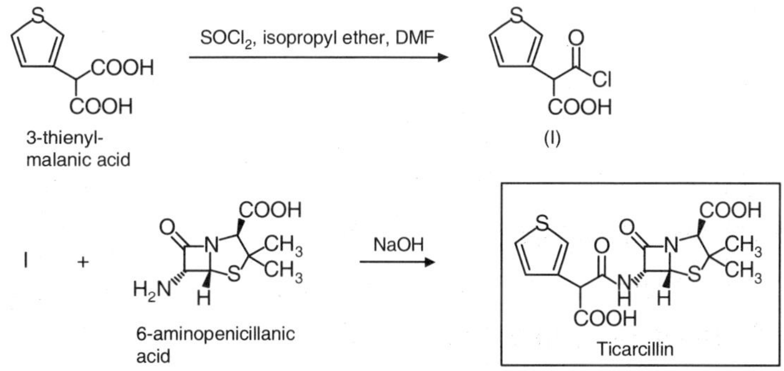

3-thienyl-
malanic acid

SOCl₂, isopropyl ether, DMF

(I)

6-aminopenicillanic
acid

NaOH

Ticarcillin

Oxacillin

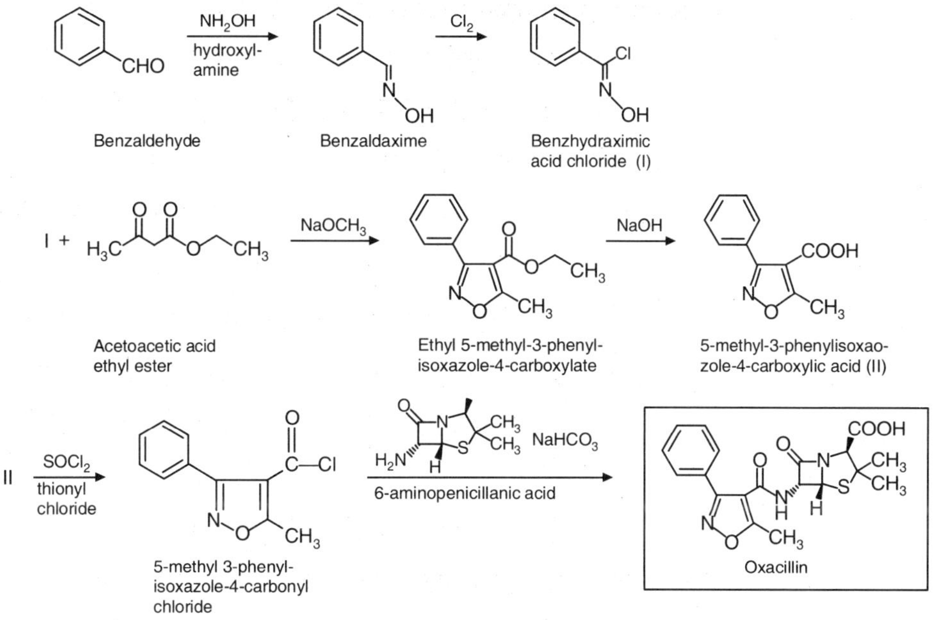

Benzaldehyde

NH₂OH
hydroxyl-
amine

Benzaldaxime

Cl₂

Benzhydraximic
acid chloride (I)

I + Acetoacetic acid
ethyl ester

NaOCH₃

Ethyl 5-methyl-3-phenyl-
isoxazole-4-carboxylate

NaOH

5-methyl-3-phenylisoxao-
zole-4-carboxylic acid (II)

II SOCl₂
thionyl
chloride

5-methyl 3-phenyl-
isoxazole-4-carbonyl
chloride

6-aminopenicillanic acid

NaHCO₃

Oxacillin

56.2

β-Lactam Antibiotics (Cephalosporins)

The concept that certain antibiotics producing fungi may occur in soils and further environments rich in bacteria led to a worldwide examination of soils, sewage, sludges and related material for new antibiotic. The concept crystallized out with some signal successes. A species of Cephalosporium, isolated near a sewage outfall of the Sardinian coast by Brotzu in 1948 was studied at Oxford. The mould produced three antibiotics which were named as, cephalosporin N, cephalosporin P and cephalosporin C.

▨ CEPHALOSPORIN N

It is penicillin like structure being a derivative of 6-aminopenicillanic acid.

▨ CEPHALOSPORIN P

An acidic antibiotic, which is steroidal in nature. A compound similar to cephalosporin P is fusidic acid, an antibiotic produced by the mould *fusidium coccineum*. Both, cephalosporin P and fusidic acid are steroidal in nature.

▨ CEPHALOSPORIN C

- It is a true cephalosporin and is a derivative of 7-amino-cephalosporanic acid. The latter served as a lead nucleus for the development of totally new series of compounds, cephalosporins.
- Widespread clinical acceptance continues to be accorded to the cephalosporins and the field is extremely active in searching out new drugs adding better oral activity and broader antimicrobial activity.
- Cephalosporin C contains a side chain derived from D-aminoadipic acid, which is attached with 7-aminocephalosporanic acid. Regardless of the structure of the side chains, cephalosporins are relatively more acid-stable and penicillinase resistant than penicillin family.

Classification of Cephalosporins

Flow chart 56.1 describes classification of cephalosporins.

Flow chart 56.2.1: Classification of cephalosporin

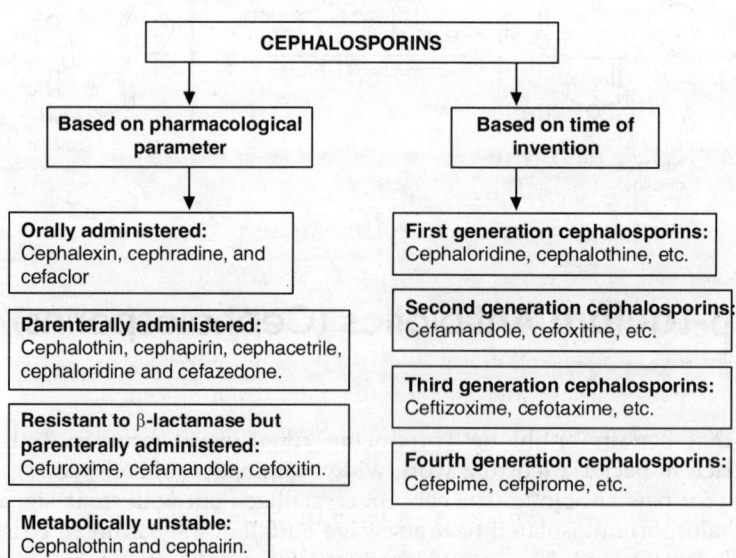

Classification Based on Pharmacological Parameter

Oral Cephalosporins

Cephalexin   Cephaclor   Cephaglycine

Parentral Cephalosporins

Cephapirin   Cephaloridine

Cephalothin

Resistance to β-lactamase

Cefoxitin

Classification based on generation

First Generation

Cephaloridine   Cephalothine

Cephapirin   Cephalexin

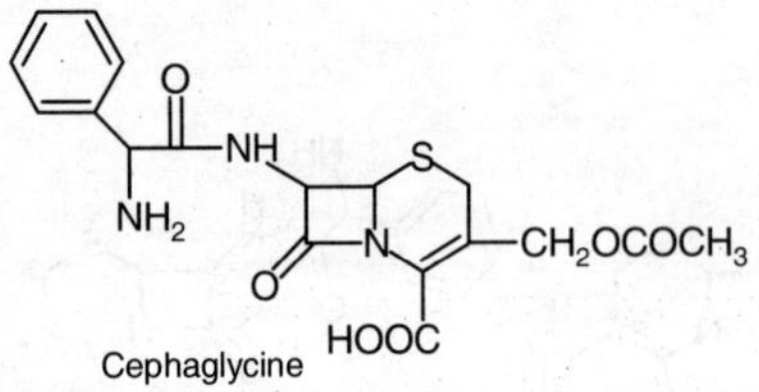

Cephaglycine

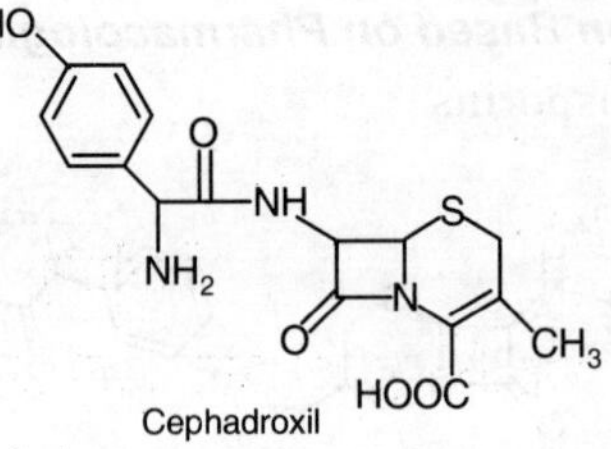

Cephadroxil

Second Generation

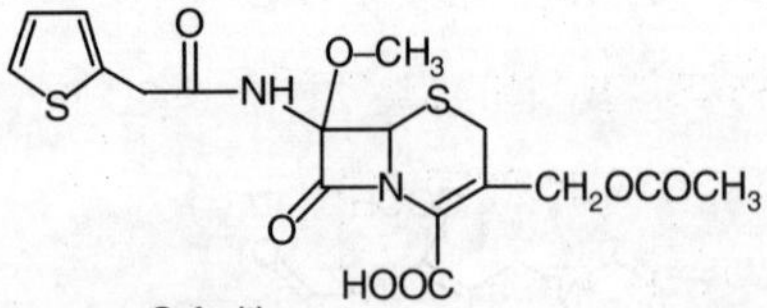

Cefoxitin

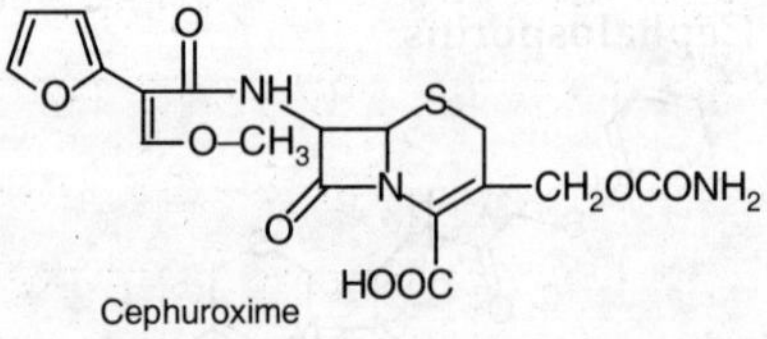

Cephuroxime

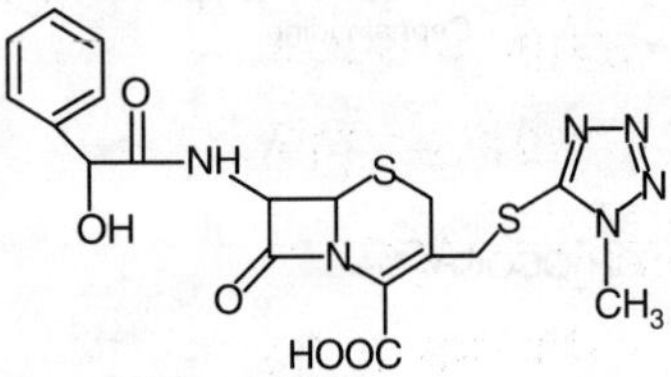

Cefamandole

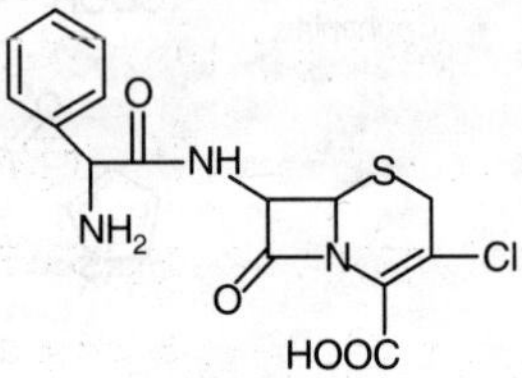

Cafaclore

Third Generation

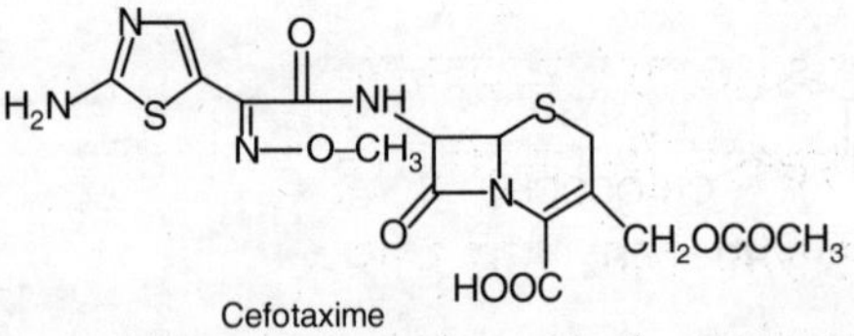

Cefotaxime

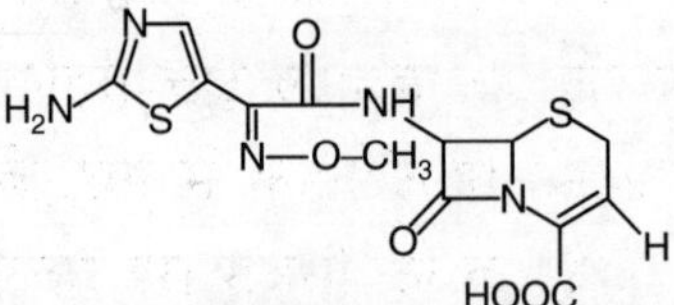

Ceftizoxime

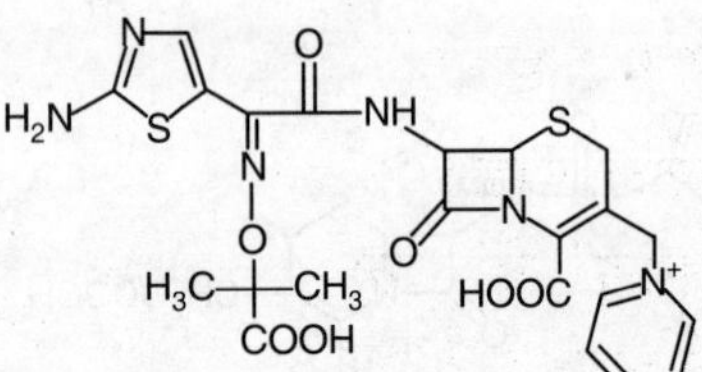

Cefatazidime

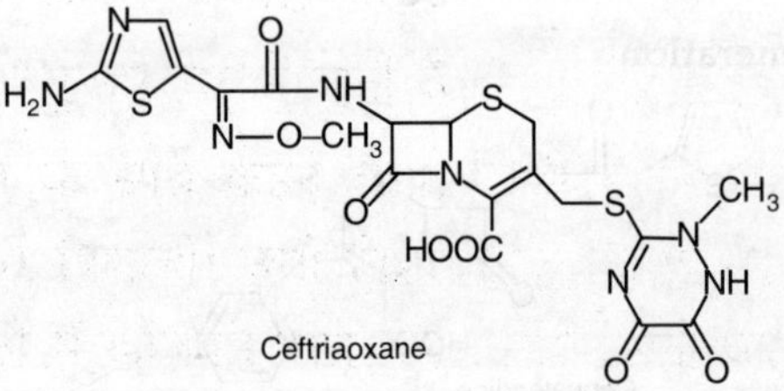

Ceftriaoxane

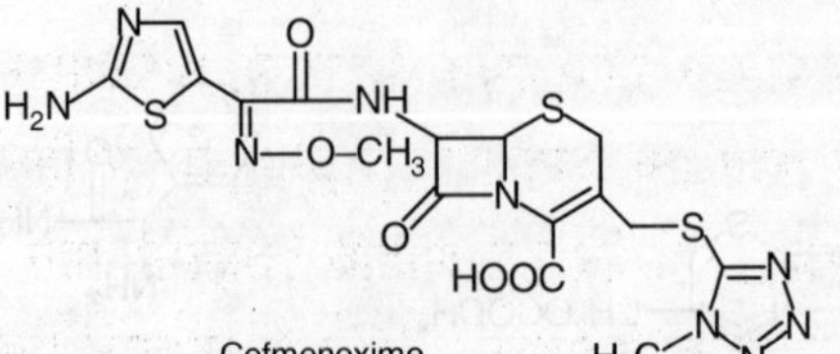

Cefmenoxime

Fourth Generation

Cefepime

Cefpirome

SAR of Cephalosporins

7-Acylamino Modification

1. Acylation of amino group generally results in an increase in gram-positive activity, but it is accompanied by decrease in gram-negative potency.

2. Replacement or attachment of any other heterocycle in side chain increases the gram-positive activity.

3. Presence of catechol group in side chain enhances activity, particularly against *Pseudomonas aeruginosa*, which not only exhibit antipseudomonas activity, but also retain some gram-positive activity which is unused for a catechol cephalosporin.

4. There is reduction of gram-negative activity when the lipophilicity of this side chain is increased and the enhancing effects of polar α-substitution (OH, NH_2, SO_3H, COOH).

5. The aminothiazole group improves gram-negative activity and in combination with the synoximino grouping confers resistance to β-lactamases.

Modification at C-3 substituent

1. The nature of C-3 substituent more noticibaly influences pharmacokinetic and pharmacological properties as well as antibacterial activity. The 3-acetoxymethyl group of cephalosporins is the most reactive site, which readily undergoes solvolysis in strongly acidic solution to form the desacetylcephalosporin. The latter lactonizes to give inactive derivative. Modifications at C-3 position have been made to reduce this degradation of cephalosporins.

2. The derivatives such as ester, amide, nitrogen nucleophile, sulphur nucleophile at C-3 result in improvement of pharmacokinetic properties.

3. The displacement of 3-acetoxy group by aromatic thiols results in enhancement of intrinsic activity specially against gram negative bacteria.

4. Replacement of the acetoxymethyl group at 3 position by chloro has resulted in some compounds showing oral absorption, e.g. cephaclor.

Modification at C-7 substituent

(C-7)-a-formamidino derivatives showed advantage over the cephamycins in conferring high β-lactamase stability.

Modification of ring

- Initially, it was reported that oxidation of the ring sulfur in penicillins or cephalosporins to a sulfoxide or sulphone greatly diminishes or destroy antibacterial activity. But now it has been proved that sulphoxide is very potent antibiotic especially against lactamase forming gram-negative strains.
- Replacement of sulfur by oxygen in ring inceases antibacterial activity and the rate of hydrolysis, because it enhances the acylating power.

Modification at 4-COOH group

Conversion of carboxy group of position C-4 to ester results in the prodrug characteristic that results into the increase in bioavailability of cephalosporins, e.g. cefpodoxime.

C3–C4 linkage is essential for antibacterial activity. Isomerization of the double bond to 2–3 position leads to great loss of antibiotic activity.

MOA: It is similar to penicillin.

▓ OTHER β-LACTAM ANTIBIOTICS

- The story of β-lactam antibiotics began in 1929, had propogated through two distinct phases, one marked by penicillin analogs and second phase dominated by cephalosporin family. The day to day research is still adding new entities to antibiotic field and exposing the one or more clinical deficiencies perceived in existing drugs.
- The new basic skeletons encountered whether will reach the market place or add to the volumes of dead stock in the literature is yet uncertain. Recently three new classes of beta lactam antibiotics have come up. They are: (1) Thienamycins, (2) Nocardicins and (3) Clavulanic acid.

Thienamycins

- The research groups at Merck were the first, to isolate and characterized this antibiotic from *Streptomyces cattleya*. Like penicillins and cephalosporins, it contains a fused bicyclic ring system containing β-lactam and a 3-carboxylic group but instead of β-acylamido side chain, it is a -1-hydroxyethyl group.

Thienamycin

- Two distinct features of thienamycin and cephalosporins are its broad-spectrum of activity and its beta-lactamase resistant property which make it effective against many strains resistant to penicillins and cephalosporins.

Nocardicins

- It is a group of about seven antibiotics isolated from various *Nocardia* species. Here we do not observe a fused bicyclic ring-system.
- This is characteristic of beta-lactam antibiotics. Nocardicin A is a narrow spectrum antibiotic and their status in future clinic still remains to be established.

Nocardicins

Clavulanic Acids

These are produced from streptomyces clavuligerus

β-LACTAMASE INHIBITORS

- The emergence of antibiotic-resistance strains of microorganisms proved to be a major limitation to the clinical utility of antibiotics, beta-lactamases can hydrolyze the beta-lactam ring of different beta-lactam antibiotics including penicillins, cephalosporins, carbapenems and monolactams. Various measures were then undertaken to develop such inhibitors that will bind or inactivate beta-lactamases present in the microorganisms.

- In microorganism, beta-lactamases may be present at extracellular as well as intracellular sites. These enzymes when released into external environment will prevent the access of antibiotic towards the microorganisms by rapidly inactivating the drug. While the membrane bound intracellular beta-lactamase will protect the organism from the residual antibiotic escaped from the attack of extracellular enzyme.

- Inactivation of beta-lactam antibiotics is brought about by these enzymes through the cleavage of CON bond present in the beta-lactam ring. Enzymes form a sort of irreversible complex with the carbonyl group. Studies with several different beta-lactamases have implicated a serine residue as acylation site. Regeneration of the active enzyme from this complex then occurs through hydrolysis of the acyl linkage.

- By providing false substrates having very high affinity for beta-lactamase enzyme with long-term occupying capacity (i.e. very low rate of deacylation), we can effectively increase potency of beta-lactamase sensitive antibiotics. Such substrates are known as beta-lactamase inhibitors. However, such agents must be able to inhibit not only extracellular beta-lactamases but also should penetrate the bacterial cell-wall at adequate concentration to inhibit intracellular beta-lactamases. They should also have the broad-spectrum of activity covering beta-lactamases present in both, gram-positive and gram-negative bacteria.

Table 56.2.1: Non-classical beta-lactam antibiotics

Examples	Year of Introduction
1. 7 α-methoxy cephalosporins (cephamycins)	1971
2. Amidinopenicillins	1972
3. Nocardicins	1976
4. Clavulanic acid	1976
5. Carapenems	
a. Olivanic acids	1976
b. Thienamycins	1978
c. Epithienamycins	1977
d. Asperenomycins	1982
e. Pluracidomycins	1982
f. Carpetimycins	1981
6. Oxacephems	1978
7. Caracephems	1984
8. Monobactams	1981

- Examples of clinically used beta-lactamase inhibitors include clavulanic acid, sulbactam, olivanic acids and halogenated sulfone derivatives. These inhibitors in general possess weak antibacterial activity of their own.

- These agents exhibit weak broad-spectrum antibacterial activity and therefore are not entitled to be used as effective antibiotics. However, they have an affinity for beta-lactamases and served as potent irreversible inhibitors of many beta-lactamases produced by gram-positive and gram-negative bacteria. Due to these pharmacological features, they are not used as primarily, but are combined usually with the conventional beta-lactam antibiotics that are substrates for these enzymes. This usually results into potentiation of activity of beta-lactam antibiotics. Examples from this category are given below:

1. Clavulanic acid: These are produced by Streptomyces clavuligerus.

2. Salbactam: Similar in structure to clavulanic acid.

3. Imipenam: It is the N-formimidoyl derivative of thienamycin. It is having a beta-lactam structure which is resistant to most of the beta lactamases.

Calvulanic acid

Salbactam

Imipenam

Bipenam

Meropenam

5. Oxacephems: In these compounds, at one hand as the oxygen atom unstablizes the molecule, the introduction 7 α-methoxy group works as a compensation. Moxalactam an example from this class is a broad-spectrum antibiotic, having beta-lactam resistant property.

6. 1-Carbapenems: They are structural analoges of penicillins where sulfur atom is replaced by carbon. Olivanic acids stand as example of this class. They are broad-spectrum antibiotics isolated from *Streptomyces olivaceus*.

Oxacephems

1-Carbapenams

7. Monobactams:

These are monocyclic beta-lactam antibiotics isolated from *Cliromobacterium violaceum*. The basic nucleus is 3-amino mono bactamic acid (3-AMA).

Azactam is an example of this class which is active against most of gram-negative bacteria and resistant to most of beta-lactamase enzymes.

Cefalexin

Azabactem

Cefologlycine (I)

H₂, Pd–BaSO₄

Cefalexin

Cefaloridine

Cefalotin + Pyridine → (pH 6,5) → Cefaloridine

Cefuroxime

2-acetylfuran → (NaNO$_2$, conc. HCl) → 2-furyl-glyoxyllic acid → (H$_2$N–O–CH$_3$ HCl, O-methylhydroxyl-amine hydrochloride) → syn-2-methoxy-imino-2-(2-furyl)-acetic acid (I)

I → 1. oxalyl chloride 2. diphenylmethyl 7-amino-cephalosporanate → (II)

II → 1. H$_2$O, OH– or esterases 2. ClSO$_2$–NCO, acetonitrile 3. H$_2$O 4. F$_3$CCOOH, anisole 2. chlorosulfonyl isocyanate → Cefuroxime

Cefoxitin

Cephamycin C (I) + Trichloroethoxy-carbonyl chloride → 1. pH 9.1 2. 2. diphenyl-diazamethane (II) → III

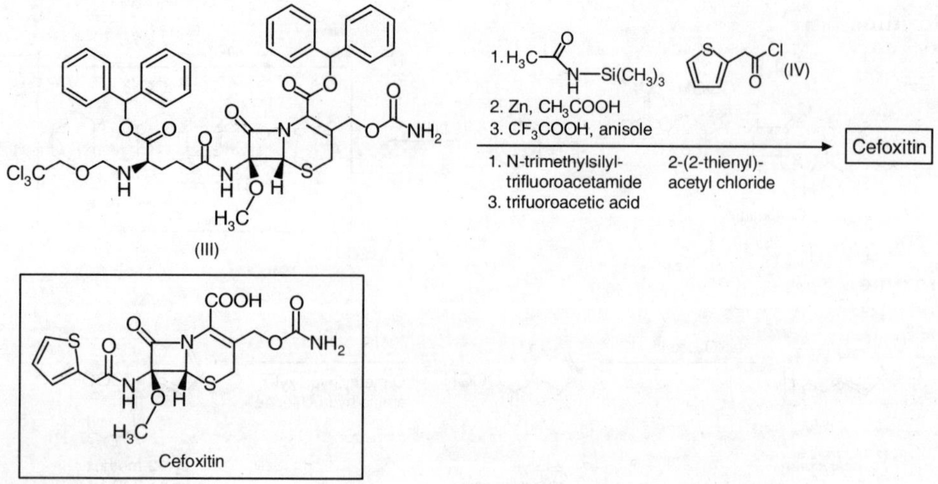

(III)

1. H₃C—C(=O)—N(H)—Si(CH₃)₃
2. Zn, CH₃COOH
3. CF₃COOH, anisole

1. N-trimethylsilyl-trifluoroacetamide
2. 2-(2-thienyl)-acetyl chloride
3. trifuoroacetic acid

(IV)

→ Cefoxitin

Cefoxitin

Cefamandole

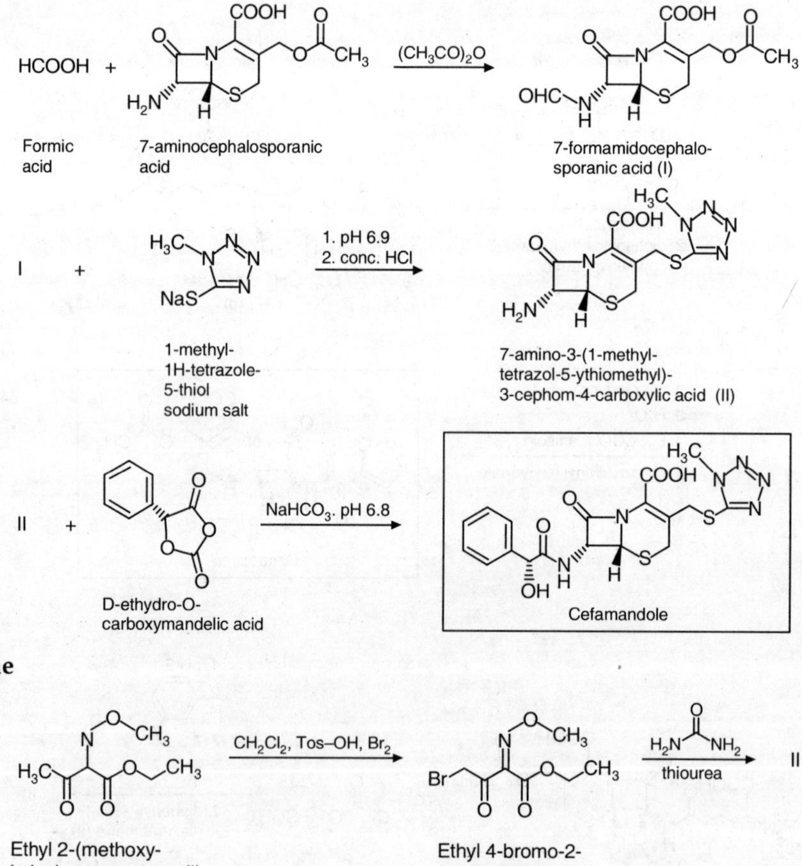

HCOOH +

Formic acid

7-aminocephalosporanic acid

(CH₃CO)₂O →

7-formamidocephalo-sporanic acid (I)

I +

H₃C—tetrazole—NaS

1. pH 6.9
2. conc. HCl →

1-methyl-1H-tetrazole-5-thiol sodium salt

7-amino-3-(1-methyl-tetrazol-5-ythiomethyl)-3-cephom-4-carboxylic acid (II)

II +

D-ethydro-O-carboxymandelic acid

NaHCO₃. pH 6.8 →

Cefamandole

Cefotaxime

Ethyl 2-(methoxy-imino)acetoacetate (I)

CH₂Cl₂, Tos–OH, Br₂ →

Ethyl 4-bromo-2-(methoxyimino)-acetoacetate

H₂N—C(=O)—NH₂
thiourea →

II

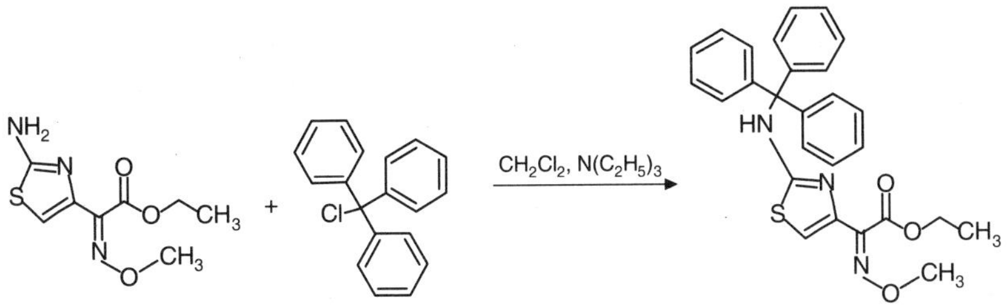

ethyl 2-(2-amino-
4-thiazolyl)-2-(meth-
oxyimino)acetate (II)

trityl
chloride

CH_2Cl_2, $N(C_2H_5)_3$

ethyl 2-(methoxy-
imino)-2-[2-(trityl-
amino)-4-thiazolyl]-
acetate (III)

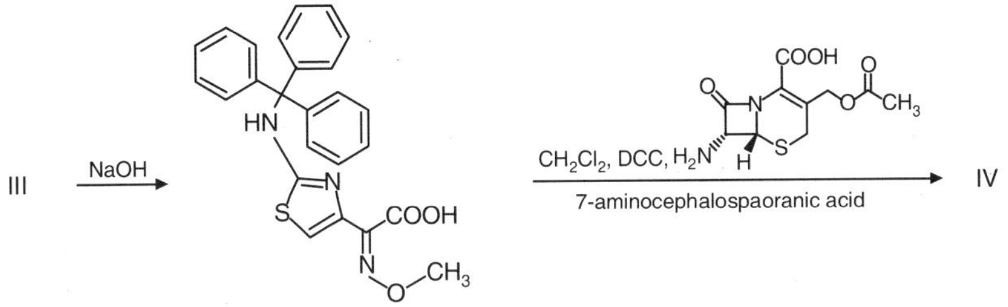

III → NaOH

CH_2Cl_2, DCC, H_2N

7-aminocephalospaoranic acid

IV

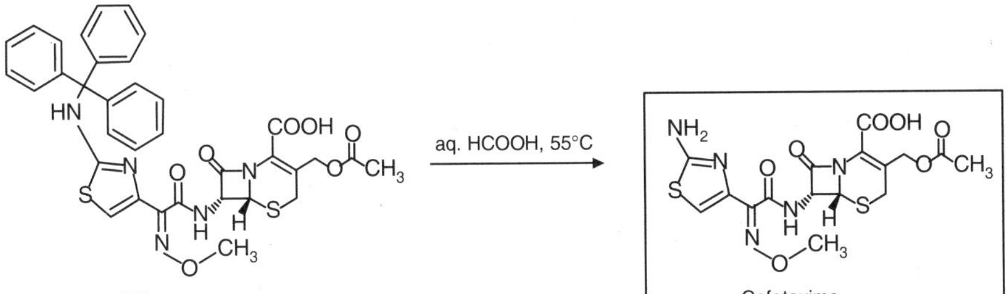

aq. HCOOH, 55°C

(IV)

Cefotaxime

56.3

Tetracyclines

A clear cut division of work is observed amongst previous two classes of antibiotics; penicillins being active against gram-positive organisms while Streptomycin family being in charge of gram-negative affairs. Generation of the tetracyclines was the result of a need to develop such antibiotics which can effectively cover both microbial faculties.

- 7-chlortetracycline discovered in 1948 by Duggar. They are obtained either as metabolic by products from various species of Streptomyces or as semisynthetic derivatives of the natural products.

- Tetracyclines are all yellow amphoteric compounds, forming salts with either acids or bases. They exist as zwitter ions at pH 7.
- Although they are not completely absorbed from GIT, tetracyclines are known for their oral use. Exception is rolitetracycline which is given parenterally. Epimerization at C-4 is witnessed with tetracyclines in the solutions of intermediate pH range. Epitetracyclines, as these isomers are known by, exhibit much less activity than the neutral isomers.
- Resistance to the tetracyclines develops relatively slowly, cross-resistance (i.e. an organism resistant to one drug shows resistance to all other members of the series) is also reported.
- Most of the members safely escape the metabolic degradation after absorption but chlortetracycline and doxycycline do not adopt this tendency.

CHEMISTRY

Chemistry and Stereochemistry

- Tetracyclines are the most important and broad-spectrum antibiotics as they are active against gram+ve, gram-ve bacteria, ricketsia, protozoa, etc.

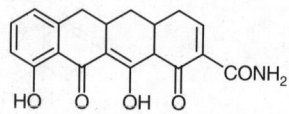

Basic nucleus naphthacenecarboxamide

- This is mainly given when a person is suffering from cholera and acne. These are considered as derivatives of the octahydronaphthacene and basic nucleus is naphthacenecarboxamide.

1. Tetracycline possesses 4, 4a, 5a, 6 and 12a potentially asymmetric carbon atoms. Oxytetracycline and doxycycline have 6 asymmetric centers, whereas other contains only 5 asymmetric centers.

2. Determination of absolute stereochemistry of tetracyclines was a difficult job. Detailed X-ray differaction study eshtablished the stereochemical formula .These studies also confirm that conjugate system exists in the structure from C-10 through C-12 and from C-1 through C-3.

3. Tetracyclines are amphoteric in nature, forming salts either with acids or bases. In neutral solutions, these substances exist mainly as Zwitterions.

4. All the tetracyclines undergo epimerization at carbon-4 in solution between pH 2 and 6 reducing the antibacterial activity of tetracyclines.

Epitetracycline   Tetracycline

5. Strong acid attacks the tetracyclines at hydroxyl group C-6 atom, causing the loss of activity through modification of the C-ring that results in the formation of inactive tetracyclines like anhydrotetracyclines.

Tetracycline   5, 6-anhydrotetrcycline

6. On the other hand bases promote reaction between 6-hydroxyl group and the ketone group at the 11-position that causes the formation of the lactone ring which is inactive and named as isotetracyclines.

7. Stable chelate complexes are formed by the tetracyclines with metals such as calcium, magnesium and iron. Such chelates are usually insoluble in water so that absorption of tetracyclines through GIT is prohibited.

8. Tetracyclines have affinity for calcium, causes their deposition in newly formed bones and teeth as tetracycline-calcium orthophosphate complex. Deposition of these antibiotics causes a yellow discoloration of teeth that darkenes teeth overtime that is why it is prohibited in small children below age of 8-10 years.

9. Tetracycline crosses the placental barrier and enter into the fetus, so it should not be given to pregnant women.

Structure of Activity Relationship

Tetracycline

Name	R_1	R_2	R_3	R_4	R_5	Source
7-chlortetracycline	Cl	CH_3	OH	H	H	S.aureofaciens
Oxytetracycline	H	CH_3	OH	OH	H	S. rimosus
Tetracyclin	H	CH_3	OH	H	H	Semi-synthetically from chlortetracycline
Demeclocycline	Cl	H	OH	H	H	Mutant strain of S.aureofaciens
Methacycline	H		$=CH_2$	OH	H	Semi-syntheticall from oxytetracycline
Doxycycline	H	CH_3	H	OH	H	Semi-synthetically from oxytetracycline
Minocycline	$N(CH_3)_2$	H	H	H	H	Semi-synthetically from oxytetracycline
Rolitetracycline	H	CH_3	OH	H	X	Semi-synthetically from tetracycline
Lymecycline	H	CH_3	OH	H	Y	Mannich base of Tetracycline
Clomocycline	Cl	CH_3	OH	H	CH_2OH	Semi-synthetically from chlortetracycline

$$X = -CH_2-N\square$$

$$Y = -CH_2-NH-CH-(CH_2)_4-NH_2$$
$$\underset{COOH}{|}$$

1. The carbon system present at carbons 1 to 3 must be intact for good activity.
2. The amide function at C-2 is essential for the activity.
3. Epitetracyclines are very much less active than the neutral isomers.
4. Substitution at C-6 decreases chemical stability, e.g. oxytetracycline is chemically less stable than doxycycline.
5. In general, C-6 methylated analogs achieve higher blood levels.
6. 7 substitution results in increased potency and the drug may sometimes be active against resistant microbial strains.
7. Strong acid dehydrates tetracyclines utilising a 6-hydroxyl group and the 5α-hydrogen. This route led to development of 6-deoxytetracycline.
8. A cis type fusion between A/B with hydroxyl group at 12α is necessary for retention of activity.
9. Electron withdrawing groups and electron donating groups both are equally respected at C-7, e.g. chlortetracycline contains an electron withdrawing group at C-7 and minocycline possesses an electron releasing (dimethyl anilino) group at C-7.
10. The SAR of 8-substituted analogs is yet not augmented.
11. The SAR of positions 5, 6, 7 and 9 in brief can summarized by stating that these sites can be modified by various substituents resulting into retention and in some cases, improvement of antibiotic activity.
12. Thiatetracyclines in a preliminary report are showing excellent superior pattern of activity. They contain a sulfur atom at C-6. A recent derivative thiacycline is found to be more active than minocycline against tetracycline-resistant bacteria.
13. Tetracyclines have low solubility in water which may be overcomed by aminoalkylation at carboxamido group. The clinically effective mannich bases are rolitetracycline (pyrrolidino-methyl-tetracycline), lymecycline (tetracyc-line-L-methylenelysine) and clomocycline (N-methylol-7-chlortetracycline).
14. Semisynthetic analogs have also been obtained in an attempt to achieve advances in chemotherapy. Methacycline, doxycycline and minocycline are some results of such deliveries. For example, chlortetracycline through a catalytic de-halogenation can be converted to tetracycline. Methacycline is obtained from oxytetracycline while hydrogenation of methacycline offers doxycycline.

Mechanism of Action (Fig. 56.3.1)

- The main target of tetracycline is to inhibit the protein synthesis. We know very well that tetracycline is having affinity for the metal.
- The tetracycline binds to the 30S ribosomal subunit and forms chelate with that of Mg^+. When t-RNA comes by taking one amino acid to its end to bind with m-RNA but it does not get attached with m-RNA due to the lack of magnesium. Further process of protein synthesis automatically stops.

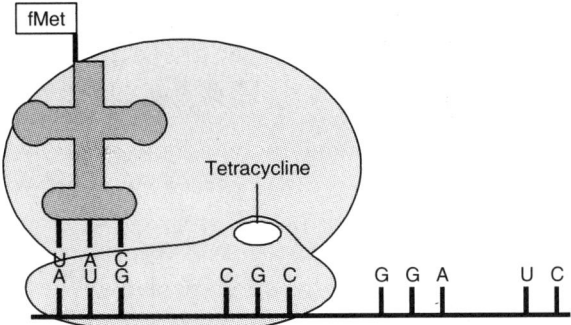

Fig. 56.3.1: Mode of action of tetracycline

▓ TETRACYCLINES IN PREGNANCY

1. Tetracyclines chelate easily with many metals like calcium, magnesium, aluminium and iron. The chelates formed are insoluble in water thus render the drug absorption.

2. The deposition of tetracyclines in newly forming teeth and bones is favoured by chelation process. The tetracycline calcium orthophosphate complex formed is characterized initially by a yellow fluorescence on teeth which may develop into brown discoloration over a period of time.

3. Their untoward effects on calcium present in newly forming teeth and bone blacklisted their use in pregnancy or in children under 8 years of age.

4. The tetracyclines are truely broad-spectrum antibiotics with the broadest spectrum than any of the presently viable antibiotics.

5. The basic nucleus common to all tetracyclines is a polycyclic napthacenecarboxamide which is comprised of four fused, six-membered rings A, B, C and D.

6. The group name tetracycline thus describes the pattern of backbone skeleton-k. A tetracyclic backbone skeleton is essential for activity.

Doxycycline

Oxytetracycline (I) H_2, Rh–C   →   Doxycycline

Minocycline

6-demethyltetracycline H_2, Rh–C   → KNO_3, liq. HF   →   I

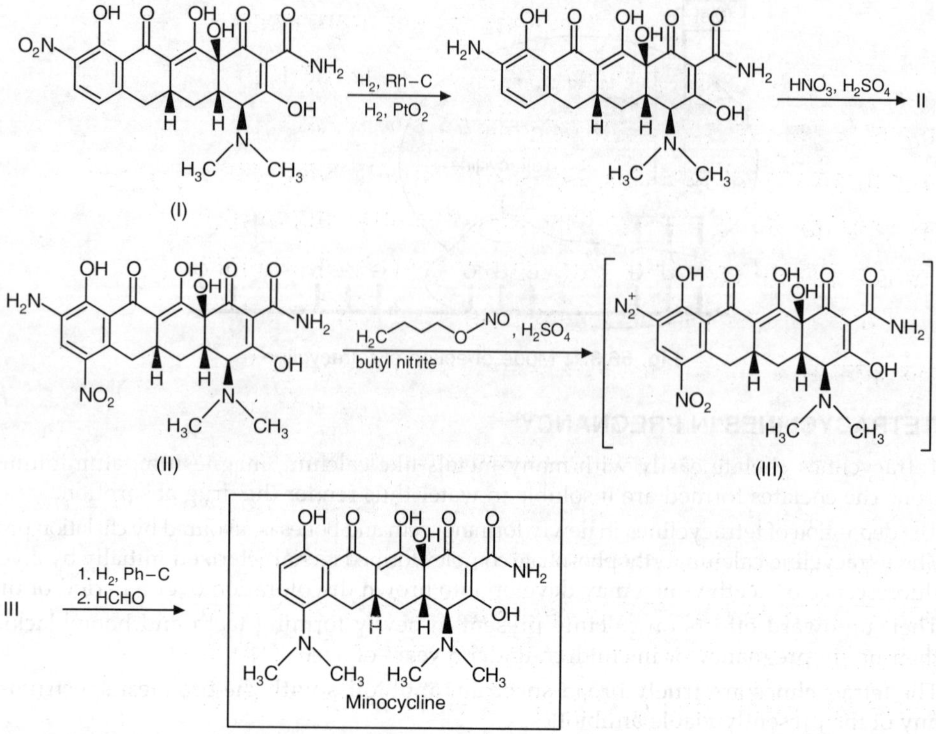

(I) → H₂, Rh–C / H₂, PtO₂ → (converts NO₂ to NH₂) → HNO₃, H₂SO₄ → II

(II) → H₂C—O—NO, H₂SO₄ / butyl nitrite → (III)

III → 1. H₂, Ph–C / 2. HCHO → Minocycline

56.4

Aminoglycosides

The aminoglycosides consist of two or more amino sugars joined in glycoside linkage to a highly substituted 1.3-diaminocyclohexane centrally placed ring. This ring is 2-deoxy streptamine in all aminoglycosides except streptomycin where it is streptidine.

Thus:

1. In kanamycin and gentamicin families, two amino sugars are attached to 2-deoxy-streptamine.

2. In streptomycin, two amino sugars are attached to streptidine.

3. In neomycin family, there are three amino sugars attached to 2-deoxystreptamine

Streptidine

L-streptose

N-methyl-L-glucosamine

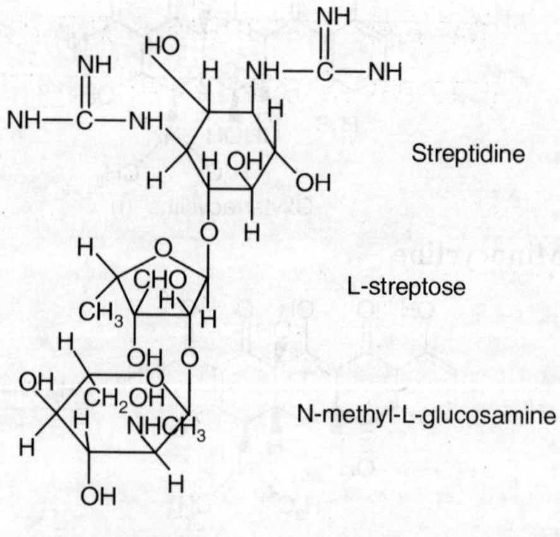

Streptomycin

In summary, the aminoglycoside antibiotics contain two important structural features:
1. Amino sugar portion.
2. Centrally placed hexose ring either 2-deoxystreptamine or streptidine.
- This series includes streptomycin, gentamiycin, neomycin, kanamycin, tobramycin, amikacin, netilmicin, spectinomycin and framycetin.
- These consist of amino sugars linked glycosidically. They are all mixture of water soluble, basic carbohydrates that are closely related chemically.
- They inhibit the growth of gram-positive, gram-negative and mycobacteria. Except for the gentamicins, all are the products of species of streptomyces.
- They are characterized by the presence of at least one aminohexose but some prefer pentose lacking an amino group (e.g. streptomycin).

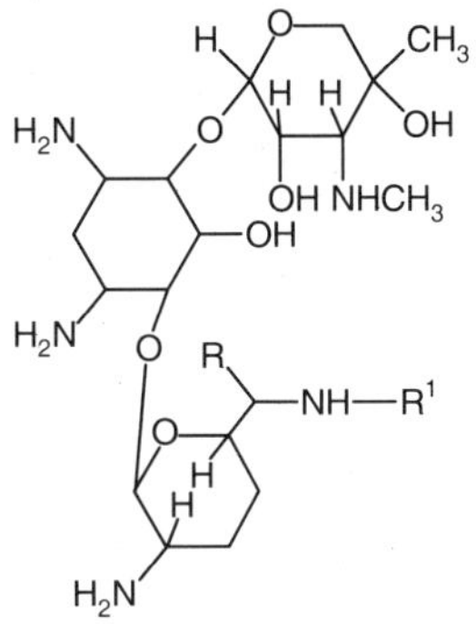

Gentamicins

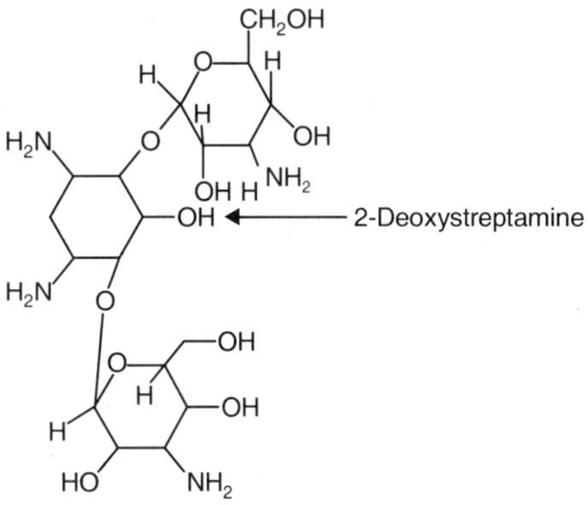

Kanamycins

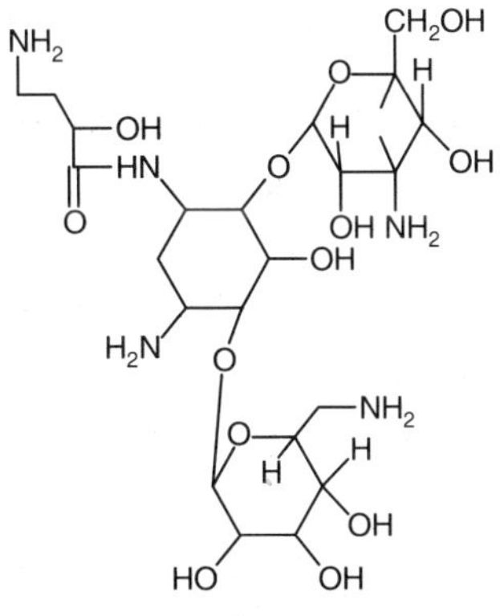

Amikacins

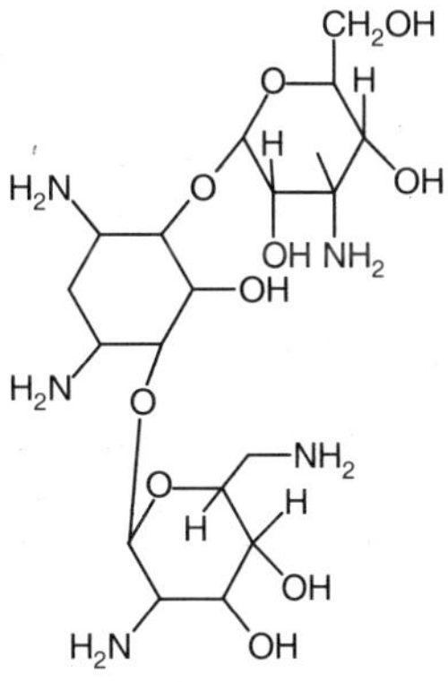

Tobramycins

Table 56.4.1: Different aminoglycoside antibiotics and their source

S. No	Antibiotic	Source	Year of Introduction
1	Streptomycin	*Streptomyces griseus*	1944; Waksman.
2	Neomycin	*S. fradiae*	1949; Waksman
3	Kanamycin	*S. kanamyceticus*	1957; Limezawa
4	Gentamicin	Micromonospora species	1963; Wemstem

5	Netilmicin	*S. tenebrarius*	1967; Higgms
6	Tobramycin	*S. decaris*	1959
7	Nebramycin	*S. rimosus* from paromomycinus	1972; Kawaguchi
8	Framycetin,	Semisynthetic product from kanamycin	
9	Soframycin	Semisynthetic product from sisomicin	

■ SAR OF AMINOGLYCOSIDE ANTIBIOTICS

1. The aminoglycosides consist of two or more amino sugars joined in glycoside linkage to a highly substituted 1, 3-diaminocyclohexane (aminocyclitol) centrally placed ring. This ring is 2-deoxystreptamine in all aminoglycosides except streptomycin and dihydro-streptomycin where it is streptidine.

   Thus:

   a. In kanamycin and gentamicin families, two amino sugars are attached to 2-deoxystreptamine.

   b. In streptomycin, two amino sugars are attached to streptidine.

   c. In neomycin family, there are three amino sugars attached to 2-deoxystreptamine.

2. The aminoglycoside antibiotics contain two important structural features:

   1. Amino sugar portion

   2. Centrally placed hexose ring either 2-deoxystreptamine or streptidine.

SAR of First Amino Sugar Portion

a. The amino functions at C-6 and C-2 serve as a major target sites for bacterial inactivating enzymes.

b. Methylation at C-6 positions does not decrease the activity; instead increases enzyme resistance.

c. Cleavage of 3-hydroxyl or the 4-hydroxyl or both groups does not affect the activity.

d. This ring is an essential for characteristic broad-spectrum antibacterial activity. This ring is mainly responsible for inactivating the bacterial enzyme.

Common structure of aminoglycoside

SAR of Centrally Placed Hexose Ring

a. Various modifications at C-1 amino group have been tested. The acylation (e.g. amikacin) and ethylation (e.g. 1- N-ethylsisomicin) though not increases the activity helps to retain the antibacterial potency.

b. In sisomicin series, 2-hydroxylation and 5-deoxygenation results in increased inhibition of bacterial inactivating enzyme systems.

c. Thus very few modifications of the central ring are possible which do not violate the activity spectrum of aminoglycosides.

SAR of Second Amino Sugar Portion

a. Here functional changes are less sensitive as compared to that of first amino sugar.

b. Only replacement of 2-OH by amino may increase the activity.

c. Similarly replacement at C-3 by secondary and tertiary amine for primary amine increases the antibacterial activity.

Mode of Action (Fig. 56.4.1)

We know very well about protein synthesis. On that basis, three modes of action are possible.

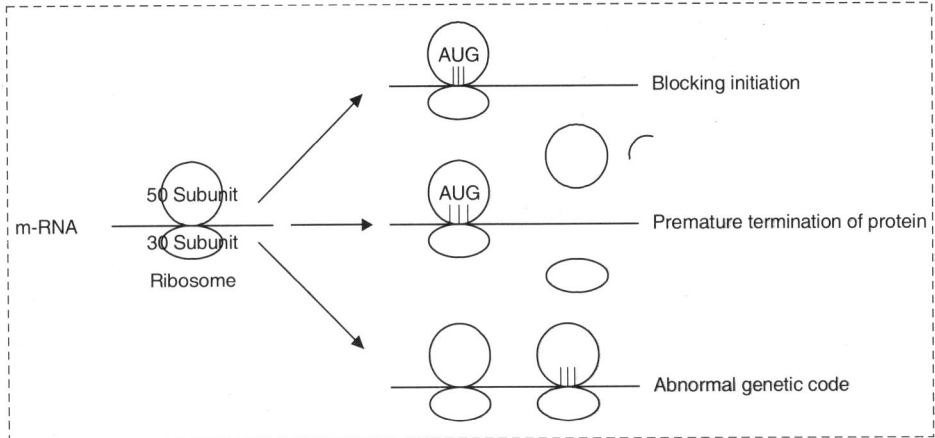

Fig. 56.4.1: Mechanism of action of aminoglycosides

A. Aminoglycoside antibiotics bind to 30S ribosomal subunit and interfere with initiation of protein synthesis by fixing 30S–50S ribosomal complex at the starting codon (AUG of m-RNA) because of which further process of protein synthesis will not occur.

B. This also causes misreading of m-RNA leading to the premature termination of translation with detachment of the ribosomal complex and incompletely synthesized protein.

C. It introduces abnormal codon on m-RNA that result in abnormal attachment of amino acid and hence abnormal protein will synthesize.

▨ BIOLOGICAL EVOLUTION OF AMINOGLYCOSIDES

Streptomycin and Dihydrostreptomycin

- The organism *Streptomyces griseus* was isolated in 1943 by Waksman *et al* as a result of a well-planned scientific research covering more than ten thousand organisms. Other substances like, hydroxy streptomycin, mannisido streptomycin and cycloheximide are also released by the organism but do not height up to the required activity/potency level.

- The development of resistant strains of bacteria and chronic toxicity constitutes major drawbacks of this category.

Neomycins

- Neomycin, kanamycin, gentamicin and paromomycin are among the most stable antibiotics known. Neomycin is a group of six antibiotics (A, B, C, D E, and F) which are produced by certain strains of *Streptomyces fradiae*.
- While neomycin A is a degradation product of Neomycin B and C. Neomycin B is still utilized as topically employed antibiotic.
- It has a broad-spectrum of activity. However, it causes severe renal toxicity and ototoxicity when administered parenterally. It is also known for its effect on the bowel flora.

Kanamycins

- These are produced by *S. kanamyceticus* and have properties and actions similar to streptomycin and neomycin. The mixture consists of three related structures, i.e. kanamycins A, B, and C.
- The kanamycin does not possess D-ribose molecule that is present in neomycins and paromomycin. The use of kanamycin is restricted to infections of the intestinal tract and to systemic infections which are not responding to other antibiotics.
- Due to the toxicity and development of resistant strains of bacteria, kanamycin are largely replaced by the newer agents from this class.

Gentamicins

- These are the metabolic products of *Micromonospora purpurea* and constitute a group of closely related broad-spectrum aminoglycosides that have structures similar to those of neomycins and kanamycins.
- Gentamicin is effective in the treatment of various skin infections and urinary tract infections caused by gram-negative bacteria. The high potency, relatively low toxicity and a virtual absence of resistant strains highlight the clinical utility of these agents.

Paromomycins

- The isolation of drug was first reported in 1956. Paromomycin is similar to neomycin except that it contains D-glucosamine instead of the 6-amino-6-deoxy-D-glucosamine found in neomycin B.
- In addition to inhibiting gram- positive, gram-negative and mycobacteria, it is very active against *Entamoeba histolytica*. The antibiotic mixture consists of paromomycin I and paromomycin II is employed in the treatment of amoebic dysentery and for the elimination of tape worms.

Semisynthetic Aminoglycosides

- Introduced into clinical practice in the 1970s these antibiotics are categorised into semisynthetic aminoglycosides. Biologically derived as one of several components of a complex of aminoglycoside mixture released by *Streptomyces tenebranus*, chemically tobramycin is characterized as 3'-deoxykanamycin B.
- It resembles with gentamicins in its activity and toxicities. Amikacin, on the other hand, has a substituted amino-butyryl in the C-1 amino group and is considered as a derivative of kanamycin. It was identified by Kawaguchi et al in 1972. Netilmicin is a semisynthetic N-ethylsisomicin.

Bacteria Resistance and Recent Trends in Drugs design of Aminoglycoside Antibiotics

- Based upon the common structural features antibiotic shares, these antibiotics are grouped under:

  1. Streptomycin family: It includes streptomycin and dihydrostreptomycin.
  2. Neomycin family: It includes neomycins and paromomycin.
  3. Kanamycin family: It includes kanamycin A, kanamycin B, amikacin and tobramycin.
  4. Gentamicin family: It includes gentamicins, sisomicin and netilmicin.

- A new wave of hope propagated in medical profession with the introduction of aminoglycoside antibiotics. They have broad-spectrum of activity. They are featured by projection of polar groups (like hydroxyl or amino groups) upon a basic carbohydrate skeleton. These structural features unfortunately then served as a platform for enzymatic deactivation of antibiotics resulting into development of microbial resistance to therapy. These polar groups may be phosphorylated, adenylated or acetylated by microbial enzymes present in the periplastic space of gram-negative bacteria. Unfortunately, the resistance can be transmitted from one generation to another due to extra chromosomal R-factors which are self replicative and transferred by direct contact. The R-factor genetically controls the biosynthesis of microbial enzymes. Strains that carry R-factor are resistant to streptomycin, kanamycin and other aminoglycoside antibiotics.

- Attempts were made to find out or synthesize such antibiotics in which target site or functional group is either removed or sterically hindered. Examples can be quoted, like gentamicins do not possess the specific target sites at which streptomycin and kanamycins are deactivated. Amikacin, derivative of kanamycin A, presents another example of antibiotic resistant to most of microbial enzymes. In this case, the susceptible site in kanamycin is sterically hindered. The same principle is stretched and set as a guideline for future trends.

56.5

Polypeptide Antibiotics

As the name indicates, structurally they are peptides containing both lipid moiety (fatty acids) and amino acids. Imino and N-methyl amino acids occur frequently. They also usually have D-amino acids and sometimes D and L forms of the same amino acids. Due to their amphoteric nature they are of three main types: (1) neutral, acidic, and basic. Except gramicidin D, most of these peptides are cyclic in nature.

SPECTRUM OF ACTION

- Their activity spectra is also widespread. For example, the polymyxins are dealing specifically with many types of gram-negative bacteria and seem least interested in gram-positive. Bacitracin holds charge of gram-negative bacteria.

- While capreomycin and viomycin are designated as antitubercular candidates on clinical profile. A drawback common to all these agents is their undesirable side effects, particularly renal toxicity.

- They are highly toxic with low therapeutic indexes and hence too toxic for the systemic use. Individual agents are described below.

Mechanism of Action (Fig. 56.5.1)

- Next to the cell wall, cytoplasmic membrane serves the purpose of protecting the vital bacterial cell constituents from damage. If this membrane is disorganized due to any reason, it results into rapid killing of that microorganism. In contrast to bacteria, the fungal membrane contains sterol as the membrane constituents. The main sterol is ergosterol.

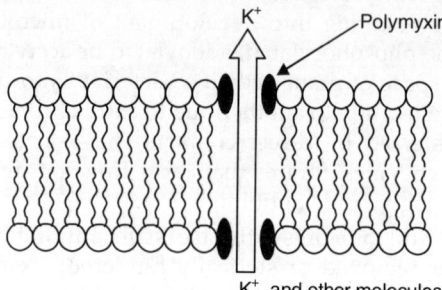

Fig. 56.5.1: Mechanism of action of polymyxin antibiotic

- Antibiotics, like polymyxins, may damage the integrity of the cytoplasmic membrane by disorienting the lipophilic groups present in the membrane. This leads to the leakage of intracellular components. They combine with the membrane sterols and thus create pores or channels in the fungal membranes. They are ineffective against bacteria since bacteria do not have sterols as their membrane constituents.

- Unfortunately mammalian cell membranes also consist of sterols. This is the reason why the margin of safety of antifungal antibiotics is uncomfortably narrow.

Amphomycin

The structural elucidation by Bodanszky et al figured out its typical peptide appearance. It exhibits activity mainly against gram-positive bacteria and occasionally is combined with anti-inflammatory agents for topical use.

Bacitracin

- The antibiotic was discovered in 1943 by Johnson, Anker and Melenecy from *Bacillus lichen informis* a strain of *Bacillus subtilis*. It is found to be a complex mixture of at least ten polypeptides (A, A ', B, C, D, E, F1, F_2, F_3, and G) of which bacitracin A fraction is believed to be most abundant and most potent. A divalent ion Zn^{++} enhances its activity.

- Although bacitracin has been occasionally employed by topical application (often in combination with neomycin, polymyxin and tyrothricin) for the treatment of burns, ulcer, and wounds, can cause serious necrosis of the kidney tubules, if it is given systemically (i.e. IV route). An oral administration is paralysed due to its lack of absorption from GI tract.

Bacitracin

- A variety of gram-positive cocci and bacilli are sensitive to bacitracin. It is to be stored in tight containers due to its hygroscopic nature.

Tyrothricin

- Tyrothricin is a mixture of polypeptides obtained by extraction of cultures of *Bacillus brevis*. Gramicidin and tyrocidine are ingredients which shoulder the activity. First time reported in 1939 by Dubos, tyrothricin now refers to a partially purified antibiotic, which usually contains 1 part of gramicidin and 4 parts of tyrocidine. It is effective primarily against gram-positive organisms. Since its systemic use may lead to lysis of erythrocytes, it is restricted to local applications.
- Gramicidin itself is made up of at least four components and measures 10-20% of tyrothricin. It is more active than tyrocidine fraction. Tyrocidine is made up of tyrocidines A, B, C and D. Both gramicidin and tyrocidines are cyclic decapeptides.
- Tyrothricin is not a drug of choice due to its limited clinical utility. It demanded a place in this section merely due to its historical seniority.

Polymyxin

- The polymyxins are cyclic peptides holding a fatty acid side chain. This is a group of relatively simple basic, cationic, detergent peptides, first isolated in 1947 from various strains of *Bacillus polymyxa*. At least five polymyxins (A, B, C, D, and E) are known but only polymyxin B and polymyxin E are of clinical utility. Both polymyxin B and polymyxin E (colistin) are mixtures of two components.
- Both can be used in the treatment of infection of bacterial meningitis, urinary tract, infected burns and wounds and gastroenteritis. They are active against almost all gram-negative bacilli. In topical applications for local infections, polymyxin B is usually combined with bacitracin which is effective against gram-positive organisms. Colistin is much less toxic than polymyxin B.

Polymyxin

- Polymyxins may affect renal tubules and CNS. Because of their nephrotoxicity associated with their systemic use, they are primarily employed to treat topical infections.

Vancomycin

- It is obtained from *Streptomyces orientalis* in 1956 by McCormick et al. It has a potency against gram-positive bacteria including streptococci, staphylococci and pneumococci.

- It is an amphoteric compound in which the presence of glucose, aspartic acid, N-methyleucine, levulinic acid and 3-chloro-4-hydroxybenzoic acid moieties has been recognised. It did not exhibit cross-resistance.
- Avoparcin and restocetin are other glycopeptide antibiotics of vancomycin family. While avoparcin finds a role of animal growth promotant, restocetin could not be assigned any clinical use.

56.6

Macrolide Antibiotics

The research glamour created by the discovery of penicillins still then, continued its way resulting into identification of a totally new class, i.e. macrolide antibiotics. Isolated from actinomycetes, it is a group of chemically related compounds distinguished by three common structural features as:

1. A many membered large lactone ring (hence the name, macrolide).
2. Various ketonic and hydroxyl functions.
3. Glycosidically linked 6-deoxy sugars.

- More often the lactone ring has 12, 14, or 16 atoms in it and is partially unsaturated with the presence of a double bond in conjugation with a ketone function.
- At present more than 70 such antibiotics are reported. The presence of a dimethylamino group on the sugar moiety credited basic properties to the macrolides.
- These antibiotics are called as penicillin substitutes. They are employed to treat infections due to penicillin resistant organism or where patient feels allergic towards penicillin analogs.
- They are, generally effective against gram-positive bacteria, both cocci and bacilli. They exhibit low spectrum of activity against gram-negative organisms.
- They are not influenced by *Penicillinase* enzymes but organisms may develop resistance by other route.

Mode of Action (Fig. 56.6.1)

Macrolide antibiotics are bacteriostatic agents that inhibit protein synthesis by binding irreversibly to a site on the 50S subunits of the bacterial ribosome, thus inhibiting the translocation steps of protein synthesis.

Erythromycin
History

- It received the most wide clinical acceptance amongst the macrolides. Its isolation was reported by McGuire *et al* in 1952 from *Streptomyces erythreus*.
- It is treated as a drug of choice for the treatment of variety of upper respiratory and soft-tissue infections due to gram-positive bacteria.

Chemistry

- The amino sugar, desosamine is attached to C-5 while another carbohydrate skeleton, i.e. cladinose is linked glycosidically to C-3.

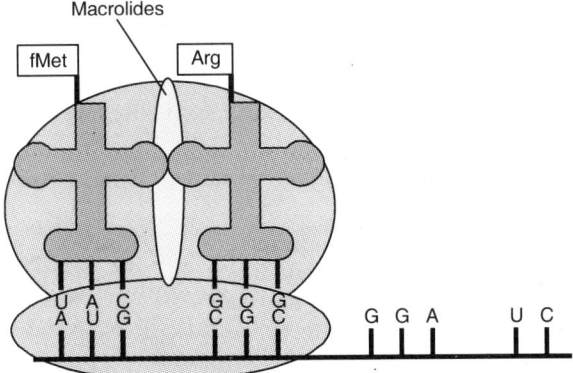

Fig. 56.6.1: Mode of action of macrolide antibiotics

- The large lactone structure is known as erythronolide. Two structures closely related to erythromycin have been isolated from *S. erythreus*.
- They are identified as erythromycins B and C. The B analog does not possess C-12 hydroxyl group and is more stable but less active than erythromycin A. Erythromycin C lacks cladinose methoxy group and is equipotent with A.
- The clinical grade erythromycin contains 90% erythromycin A and about 10% erythromycin B with minute quantity of analog C.
- Its activity shows pH dependence, increasing with pH up to about 8.5. A number of derivatives are designed to improve:
  1. Either its water or lipid solubility necessary to develop more acceptable dosage form,
  2. Its acid stability to increase oral absorption.
  3. The acceptance by masking its bitter taste.
- The basic nature of the dimethylamino group of the desosamine moiety was utilized to prepare its acid salts, like the lactobionate, glucoheptonate and the stearate, and esters of the 2'-hydroxyl group of the desosamine, including the ethyl carbonate, ethylsuccinate and the estolate, e.g. erythromycin estolate being more acid-stable, promotes high oral absorption.
- While due to good water solubility, lactobionate and glucoheptonate forms are used in parenterals. The 2'-esters as such do not possess antibiotic activity and hence efficacy of particular ester depends upon the in vivo rate of ester hydrolysis to release the free base.

Resistance

Bacterial resistance gradually develops to erythromycin. In resistant strains, the affinity of drug to bacterial ribosomal binding sites is modified towards negative side. The latter then, no longer binds erythromycin.

Oleandomycin

- It bears similar structural features as that of erythromycin and stands as an alternative to erythromycin for limited indications. It was obtained from *S. antibioticus* by Sobin et al.

- It loses its claim in gram-positive bacterial treatment due to a bit less activity and high incidence of side effects. It differs chemically from erythromycin in having:
  1. L-oleandrose instead of cladinose moiety.
  2. A 14-membered lactone ring possessing an exocyclic methylene epoxide on C-8, designated as oleandolide instead of erythronolide.
- The position of linkage of both the sugars remained same, i.e. desosamine at C-5 and L-oleandrose at C-3.
- The triacetyl ester derivative, a more preferred form of oleandomycin is prepared by acetylating 3 hydroxyl groups one in each of the sugars and one in the oleandolide. The preference is due to:
  1. Retention of *in vivo* antibiotic activity.
  2. Superior pharmacokinetic properties.
  3. Its tasteless nature.

Oleandomycin

Spiramycin and Josamycin

- They are well established clinically in Europe and Japan and now are clinical newcomers in United States. They are mainly indicated for the gram-positive bacterial infections.
- Both have similar range of activity as erythromycin but are less active. Resistance develops very gradually. However, cross-resistance among above four discussed members is reported.

Spiramycin

Lincomycins

History

- The antibiotic lincomycin is obtained from *Actinomycete, Streptomyces lincolnensis* (so named because found in Lincoln, Nebraska) stood as the first example of sulfur-containing antibiotics. Released in 1963, the antibiotic is followed by its synthetic derivative clindamycin in 1967.
- Later has an improved antibacterial and pharmacokinetic profile lincomycins, in general, possess similar topological, antibacterial spectrum, biochemical mechanism of action, pattern of bacterial resistance and cross-resistance with that of erythromycin analogs.
- They exert bactericidal action on gram-positive bacteria particularly *Staphylococcus aureus*. The activity shows concentration dependence pattern.

Lincomycin

Structure Activity Relationship

1. Variation of the substituents on pyrrolidine portion and C-5 side chain affects the activity.
2. N-demethylation imparts activity against gram-negative bacteria.
3. Increase in chain length of the propyl substituent at 4 positions in pyrrolidine moiety up to n-hexyl increases *in vivo* activity about 1.5 times than parent compound. The thiomethyl ether of α-thiolincosamide moiety is essential for activity.
4. Structural modifications at C-7, like introduction of 7S chloro or 7R-OCH$_3$ changes the physicochemical parameters of the drug (i.e. partition coefficient) and thus alters activity spectrum and pharmacokinetic properties.

Side effect

- The usual side effects include skin rashes, nausea, vomiting and diarrhea. A number of patients developed gastrointestinal complaints ranging into severity from diarrhea to pseudomembranous colitis.
- The latter characterized by diarrhea, abdominal pain, fever, and mucous and blood in the stools, may turn out to be lethal.

Uses

- The ability of lincomycin to penetrate into bone, adds to its qualifications and it gets promoted in chemotherapy of bone and joint infections by penicillin resistant strains of *Staphylococcus aureus*.

56.7

Unclassified Antibiotics (Chloramphenicol)

These antibiotics retain their reputation in the chemotherapy, though do not retain common structural features with any other antibiotic. Due to their high clinical utility, they deserve special attention.

CHLORAMPHENICOL

History

- Originally isolated from *Streptomyces venezuelae* by Ehlrich et al in 1947, chloramphenicol (chloromycetin) is now produced totally by a synthetic route. It contains chlorine and is obtained from an actinomycete so named as chloromycetin.

Spectrum of Action

- Chloramphenicol has a spectrum of activity resembling with that of the tetracyclines except that it exhibits a bit less activity against some gram-positive bacteria.
- It is specifically recommended for the treatment of serious infections caused by *Hemophilus influenzae, Salmonella typhi* (typhoid), *Streptococcus pneumoniae* and *Neisseria meningitidis*.
- It possesses marked effectiveness against several gram-negative bacteria and also exhibits antirickettsial activity. Its ability to penetrate into CNS presents an alternative therapy for meningitis.

SAR of Chloramphenicol

SAR of Paranitrophenyl Group

1. Replacement of the nitro group by other substituents leads to reduction in activity.
2. Shifting of the nitro group from the para positions also reduces the antibacterial activity.
3. Replacement of phenyl group by the alicylic moieties results in less potent compounds.
4. The p-nitrophenyl group may be replaced by other aryl structures without appreciable loss of activity.

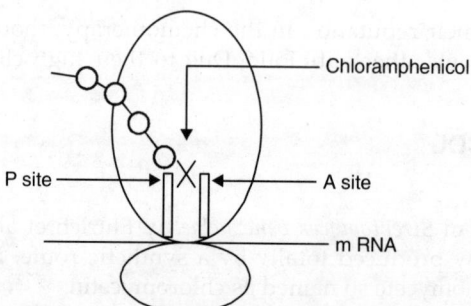

Chloramphenicol

SAR of Dichloroacetatamido side chain

1. Other dihalo derivatives of the side chain are less potent though major activities are retained.
2. While in case of trihalo derivatives, Hanch et al in the light of QSAR calculations claimed that the 2 -$NHCOCF_3$ derivative would be about 1.7 times as active as the chloramphenicol.

SAR of 1, 3-propanediol

1. The primary alcoholic group on C-1 atom if modified, results in a decrease in activity hence the alcoholic group seems to be essential for activity.
2. Of the four stereoisomers of chloramphenicol the antibacterial activity resides in only D-threo compound. Other isomers are inactive compounds.

Mode of Action (Fig. 56.7.1)

- Chloramphenicol inhibits protein synthesis in bacteria. It acts primarily by binding to the 50S ribosomal subunit and appears to prevent the binding of the amino acid containing end of aminoacyl t-RNA to the acceptor site on the 50S ribosomal subunit.
- The interaction between peptidyl transferase and its amino acid substrate cannot occur, and peptide bond formation is inhibited.

Mechanism of inhibition of bacterial protein synthesis

Fig. 56.7.1: Mode of action of chloramphenicol

Side Effects

- Chloramphenicol is a broad-spectrum antibiotic unfortunately instances of serious hematological abnormalities resulting in aplastic anemia occurred which established the needs to re-audit the clinical position of it. The nitrobenzene moiety of the chloramphenicol molecule is supposed to depress the bone marrow and to affect the elements of blood resulting into a fatal outcome.

Chloramphenicol

4'-nitro-acetophenone → (Br₂ bromine) → 2-bromo-4'-nitro-acetophenone → (1. (CH₂)₆N₄, 2. HCl; 1. hexamethylene tetramine) → 2-bromo-4'-nitroaceto-phenone hydrochloride (I)

I + Acetic anhydride → 2-acetomido-4'-nitro-acetophenone → (HCHO)ₙ → 2-acetomido-3-hydroxy-4'-nitropropiophenone (II)

II → (Al[OCH(CH₃)₂]₃, HO–CH(CH₃)₂ Aluminum isopropoxide) → DL-threo-2-acetamido-1-(4-nitrophenyl)-1, 3-propanediol → HCl → DL-threo-2-amino-1-(4-nitrophenyl)-1, 3-propanediol (III)

III → (D–camphorsulfonic acid) → D(−)-threo-2-amino-1-(4-nitrophenyl)-1,3-propanediol → (methyl dichloroacetate) → Chloramphenicol

56.8

Ansamycins (Rifampin)

The rifamycin is a group of structurally similar, complex macrocyclic antibiotics obtained from *Streptomyces mediterrani*. They belong to a new class of antibiotics called as ansamycins. All the members (i.e. rifamycins A, B, C, D, and E) are found to be active on pharmacological screen. Out of hundreds of semisynthetic derivatives prepared of these members, rifampicin, rifamide (rifamycin B diethylamide) and rifamycin SV are most effective and least toxic analogs.

Rifampicin is a broad-spectrum bactericidal antibiotic released in 1971 in United States. It is the most active against gram-positive and many viruses. Its greatest therapeutic success is as antituberculosis drug. It penetrates well into cerebrospinal fluid and is thus of use in the treatment of tuberculous meningitis. Rifampicin is also used in the antileprotic treatment and against infections caused by staphylococci resistant to other antibiotics.

During rifampicin therapy, bacterial resistance develops rapidly. This is the reason why rifampicin in most of the prescriptions is accompanied by other antitubercular drugs.

SAR of rifampins has a scattered and vague pattern. It can be summarized under following lines.

Rifampin

Structure–Activity Relationship

1. Aliphatic modifications do not help to retain the activity.
2. Whereas in the naphthalene ring positions 3 and 4 are bioactive.

Side effect

- Rifampicin is a safe drug. Toxic effects encountered with it are relatively infrequent. A few incidences of hepatotoxicity are documented in literature.

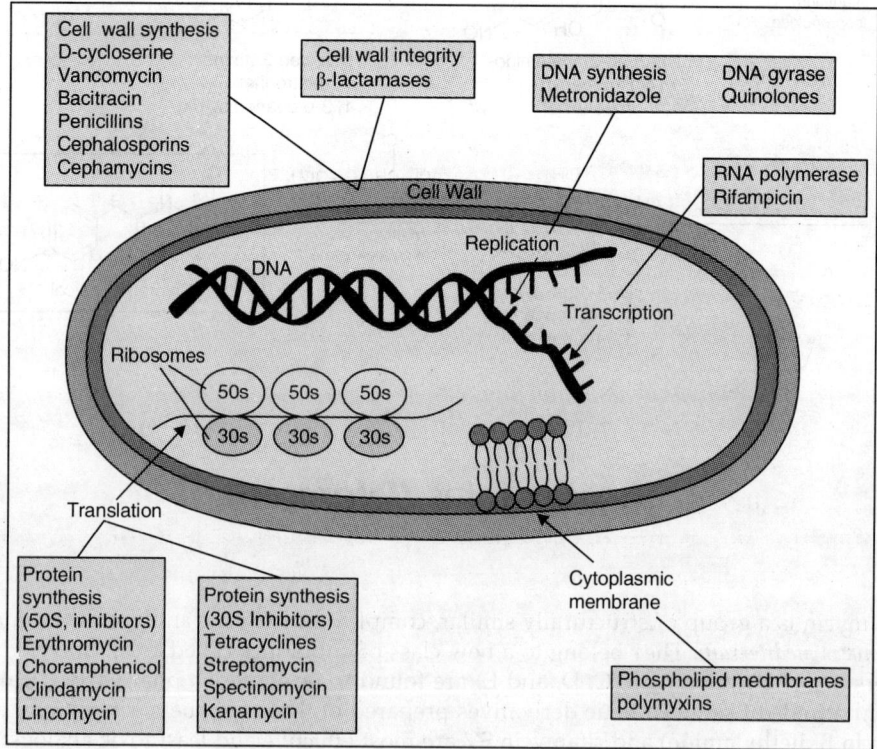

Fig. 56.8.1: Different mode of action of antibiotics

Sulfonamides

The modern chemotherapy and the concept of prodrug was successfully utilized with the introduction of sulfonamides. They were the first effective chemotherapeutic agents to be employed systemically.

- Paul Ehrlich (1854–1915) is regarded as the father of modern chemotherapy due to his pioneer work in this field. He synthesized and successfully used atoxyl in the treatment of sleeping sickness.
- The next major achievement in the field of chemotherapy is credited to Gerhard Domagk, a research director of Bayer laboratories, who in 1932 recognized the antibacterial activity of an azo dye, prontosil red. It was found to be effective in the treatment of haemolytic streptococcal infections in the mice. For this work, he was awarded Nobel Prize in Medicine in 1938. Though synthesized first in 1908, sulfonamides did not receive much attention till 1937—when it was proved by some workers at Pasteur Institute in France that prontosil is a prodrug and the active drug, sulfanilamide gets released into the body after in vivo cleavage of the azo linkage.

Prontosil

Sulfanilamide

- This discovery leads to the synthesis of at least 5500 congeneric substances which are known as sulfonamides. However, only few of them have attained the place in therapeutics.

PHYSICAL PROPERTIES

- Sulfonamides are all white crystalline powder, mostly poorly soluble in water.
- Their sodium salts are usually used because of aqueous solubility.
- The solubility parameter is greatly influenced upon by the nature of the substituents on—SO_2NH_2 group. These substituents modify the chemical features of the molecule. Hence they play an important role in governing the rates of absorption and excretion of sulfonamides.
- They are weak and form salts, which are more water soluble than free sulfonamides. The minus charge on nitrogen is greatly delocalized in sulfonamides making them stable.

691

- The substitution of electron withdrawing heterocyclic rings lowers the pKa of sulfonamides. The sulfonamides and their metabolite are excreted almost entirely in the urine (pH – 6) and the sulfonamides are not water soluble. They crystallize in kidney, thus damaging them. One way to overcome this problem is to raise pH of the urine by oral sodium bicarbonate closer to pH 10.4 (above pKa). The sulfonamides form salts that are water soluble. Many sulfonamides have been synthesized whose pKa is closer to pH of urine.

SPECTRUM OF ACTION

- The term sulfonamide is usually employed as a generic name for the derivatives of para-amino benzene sulfonamides.
- Sulfonamides are bacteriostatic agents but in the rare circumstances where bacteria are exposed to thymine less medium, they may act as bactericidal. Sulfanilamide is the basic skeleton of this category.
- The successful exploitation of this lead nucleus opened up new avenues in the field of chemotherapy. Presence of free amino group ($-NH_2$) is essential for antibacterial activity. However, it can be replaced only by groups which can be reconverted in body back to free amino group. Examples include acetamido ($NHCOCH_3$), succinylamido, and pthalylamido groups. The compounds, in which these groups are present, may undergo metabolism to regenerate free amino functional group.
- Pharmacologically, all sulfonamides exert similar actions. However, they differ from one another in solubility, rate of absorption, distribution, metabolism and excretion and in protein binding behaviour. These differences served as the basis of their clinical classification. For example, relatively insoluble sulfonamides largely remain unabsorbed in GIT after oral administration. Hence such agents may be of value in the treatment of GIT-infections. While the sulfonamides with rapid excretion feature may be used in the treatment of urinary tract infections.
- Sulfonamides are less potent antibacterial than most antibiotics. Their antibacterial potential gradually drops by the presence of pus, tissue fluids and such drugs which contain para-amino benzoic acid (PABA) as a basic skeleton (e.g. local anesthetics). Moreover many staphylococci, enterococci, clostridia and pseudomonas species remain highly resistant to their sulfonamide action. The popularity of sulfonamides as antibacterial agents declined after 1945 because of following reasons:
  a. Publications of reports regarding sulfonamide toxicity in some patients.
  b. Development of sulfonamide-resistant bacterial strains.
  c. Introduction of clinically more effective antibiotics.
- However, the impression as the wonder drugs created by penicillins in their early days unfortunately could not be maintained. Many factors contributed for their clinical devaluation. Acid-instability and microbial resistance are top amongst such factors. Attempts to synthesize new sulfonamides with improved qualities thus began in 1957 after realizing clinical deficiencies associated with the use of antibiotics. The high clinical merits associated with the combination of trimethoprim and sulphamethoxazole re-awakened interest in sulfonamides. Many are still employed in the treatment of various bacterial, protozoal and viral infections.

NOMENCLATURE

- Sulfonamides can be considered as the derivatives of para-amino benzene sulfonamide (i.e. sulfanilamide) skeleton. Since the sulfamyl (SO_2NH_2) group is the most important moiety for the antibacterial activity of sulfonamides, the amide nitrogen is designated as N^1 while nitrogen of para-amino functional group is designated as N_4. Most of the clinically used sulfonamides belong to the class of N'-substituted sulfonamides.

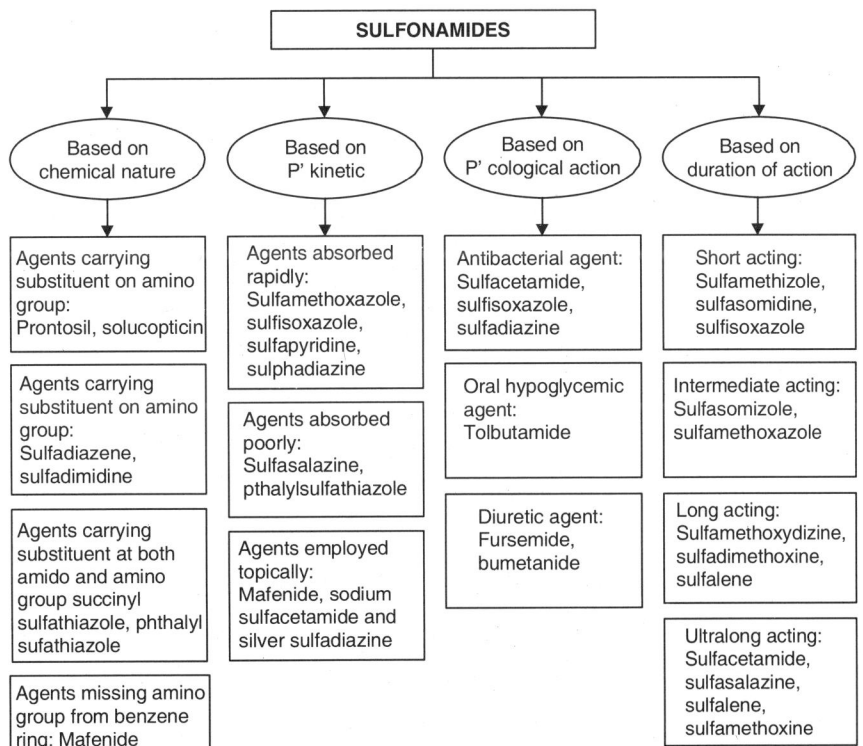

Sulphapyridine

1. By considering the derivatives of sulfanilamide.
   N^1-2-pyridinyl-sulfanilamide.
2. By considering the derivatives of benzene sulfonamide.
   4-amino N^1-2 pyridinyl benzene sulfonamide

- A third but separate category is described by the term, sulphones where the basic nucleus is 4, 4 diaminodiphenylsulphone, rather than sulfanilamide.

4, 4'-diaminophenyl sulphone

- Sulfonamides can be classified by various criteria. (Flow chart 57.1)

Flow chart 57.1: Classification of sulfonamides

SULFONAMIDES

Based on chemical nature	Based on P' kinetic	Based on P' cological action	Based on duration of action
Agents carrying substituent on amino group: Prontosil, solucopticin	Agents absorbed rapidly: Sulfamethoxazole, sulfisoxazole, sulfapyridine, sulphadiazine	Antibacterial agent: Sulfacetamide, sulfisoxazole, sulfadiazine	Short acting: Sulfamethizole, sulfasomidine, sulfisoxazole
Agents carrying substituent on amino group: Sulfadiazene, sulfadimidine	Agents absorbed poorly: Sulfasalazine, pthalylsulfathiazole	Oral hypoglycemic agent: Tolbutamide	Intermediate acting: Sulfasomizole, sulfamethoxazole
Agents carrying substituent at both amido and amino group succinyl sulfathiazole, phthalyl sufathiazole	Agents employed topically: Mafenide, sodium sulfacetamide and silver sulfadiazine	Diuretic agent: Fursemide, bumetanide	Long acting: Sulfamethoxydizine, sulfadimethoxine, sulfalene
Agents missing amino group from benzene ring: Mafenide			Ultralong acting: Sulfacetamide, sulfasalazine, sulfalene, sulfamethoxine

Based on Pharmacokinetic Parameter

Agents which are rapidly absorbed

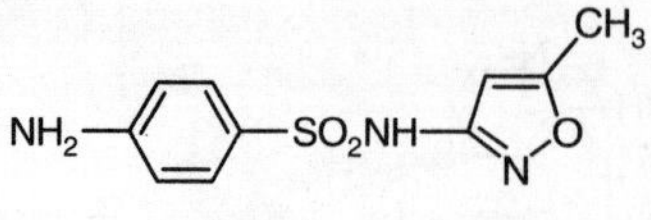

Sulfamethoxazole

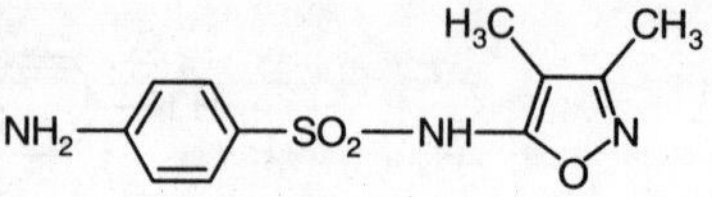

Sulfisoxazole

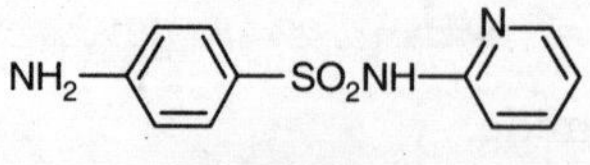

Sulfapyridine

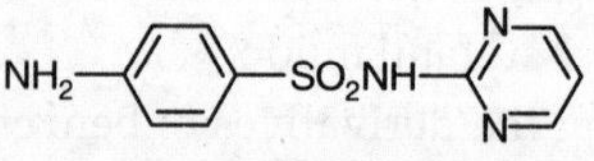

Sulfadiazine

Agents which are poorly absorbed

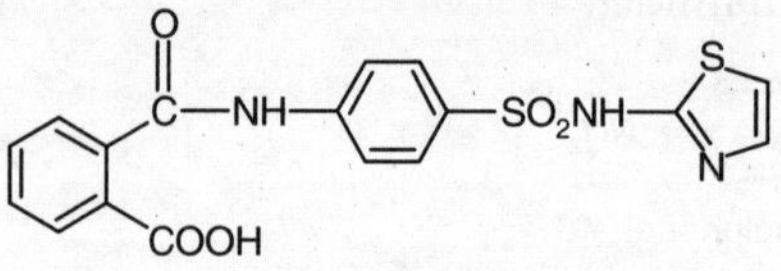

Phthalylsulfathiazole

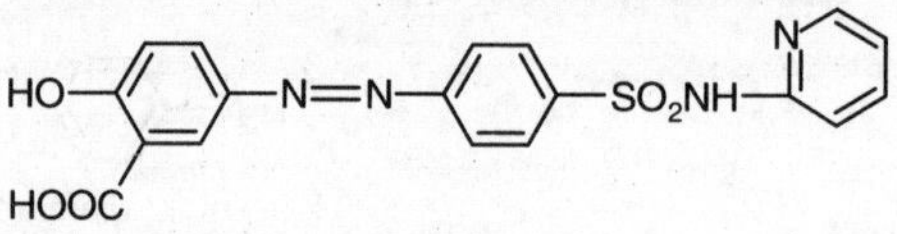

Sulfasalazine

Agents which are applied topically

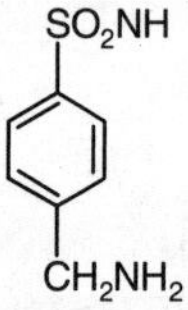

Mafenide

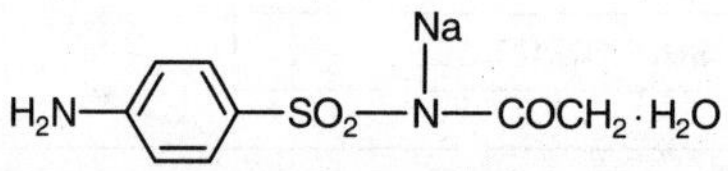

Sodium sulfacetamide

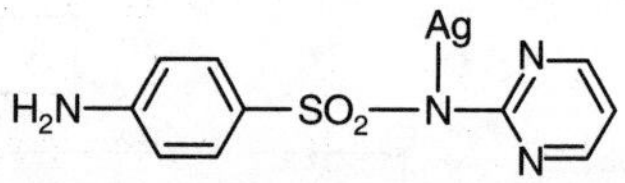

Silver sulfadiazine

Based Upon Chemical Nature

Agents carrying substitution on amino group

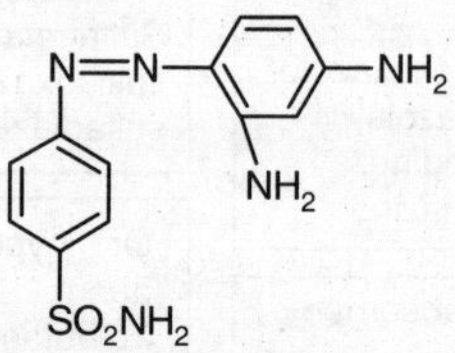

Prontosil

Agents carrying substitution amido group

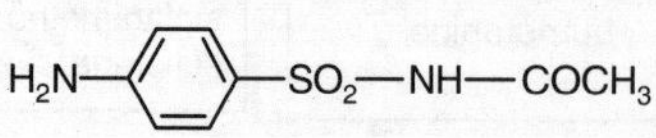

Sulfacetamide

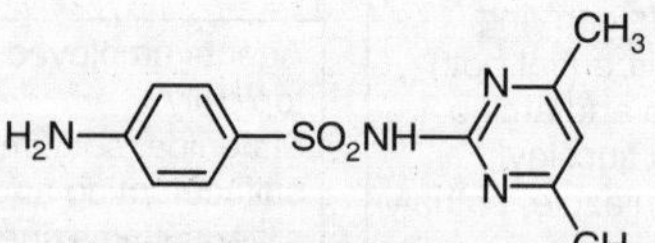

Sulfadimidine

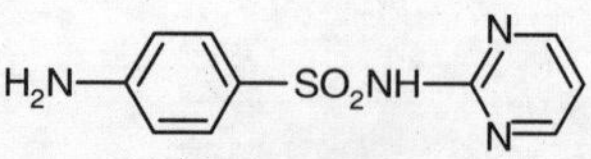

Sulfadiazine

Agents carrying substitution at both amino and amido group

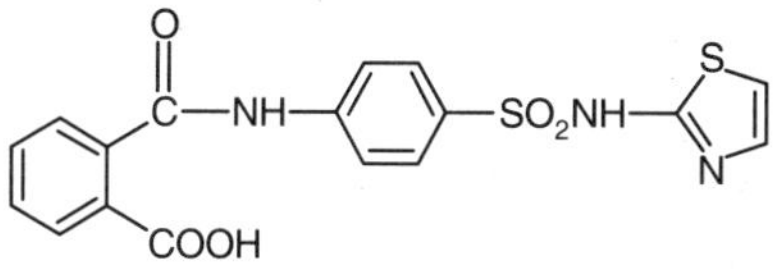

Phthalylsulfathiazole

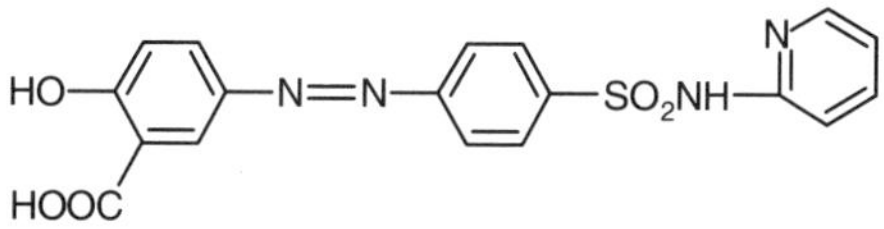

Sulfasalazine

Agents missing the amino functional group from benzene nucleus

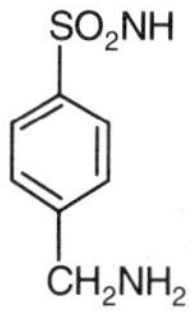

Mafenide

Based on Pharmacological Action

Antibacterial agent

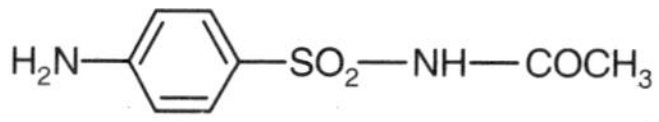

Sulfacetamide

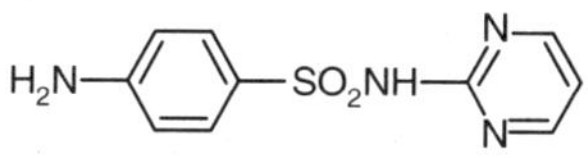

Sulfadiazine

Oral hypoglycemic agent

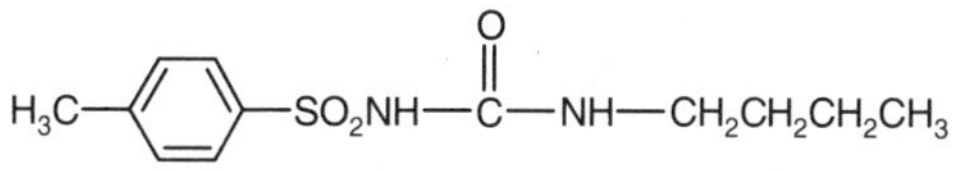

Tolbutamide

Diuretic agent

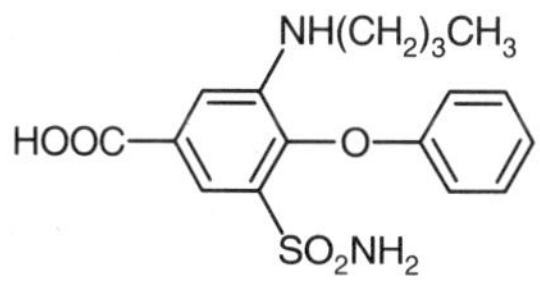

Bumetanide

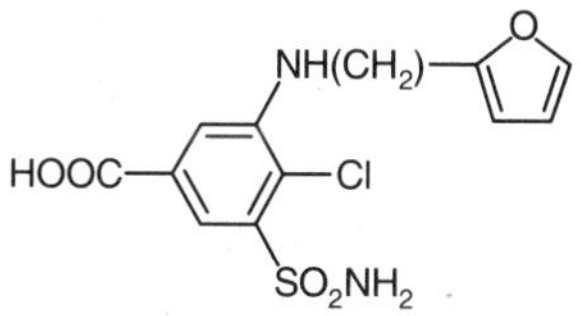

Furosemide

Based on Duration of Action

Short acting sulfonamides

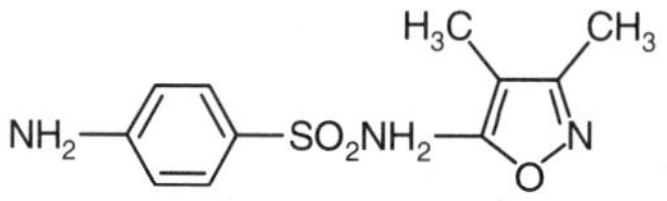

Sulfisoxazole

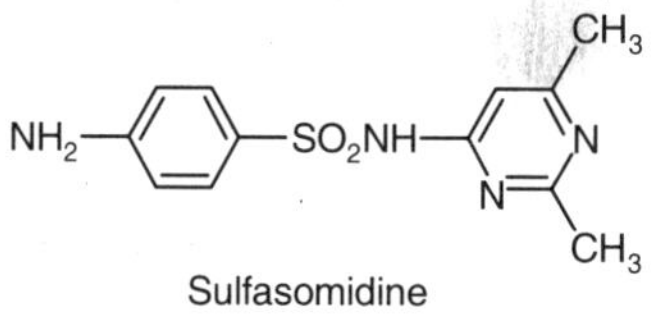

Sulfasomidine

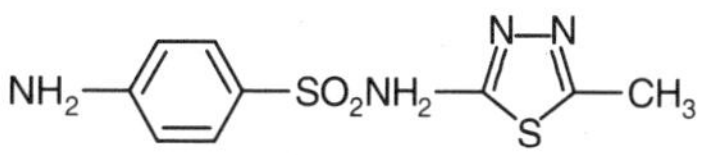

Sulfamethizole

Intermediate acting

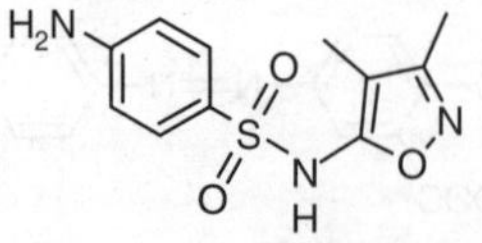

Sulfisoxazole

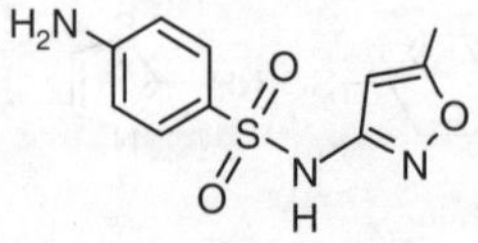

Sulfamethoxazole

Long acting

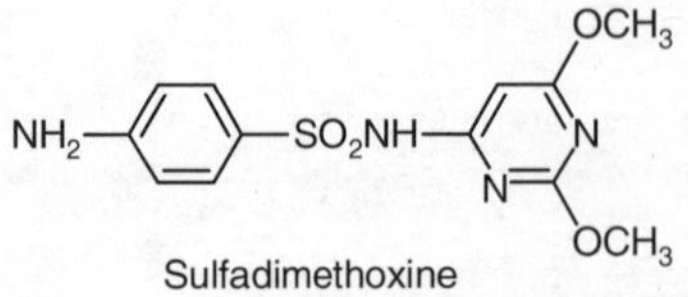

Sulfadimethoxine

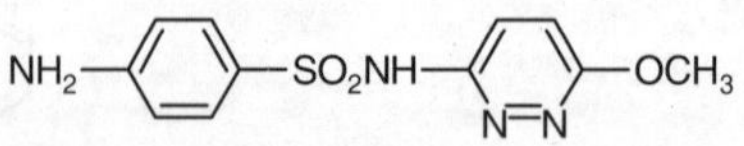

Sulfamethoxypyridiazine

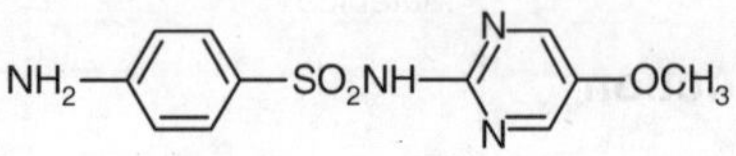

Sulfamethoxydiazine

Ultralong acting

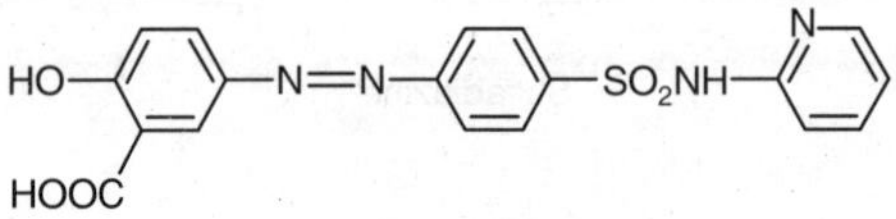

Sulphasalazine

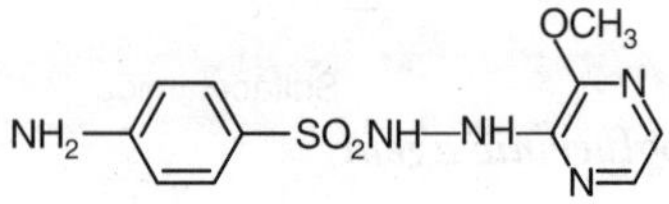

Sulfalene

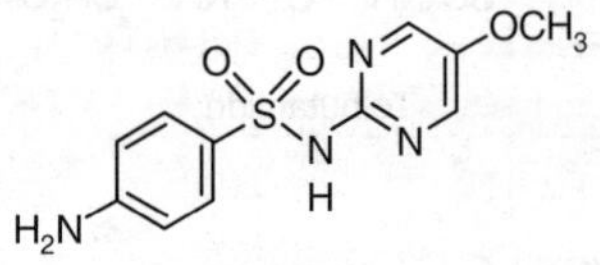

Sulphamethoxine

Classification on the Basis of Pharmacokinetic Properties

- **Agents which are rapidly absorbed rapidly excreted:** They are also known as sulfonamides. Examples include– sulfamethoxazole, sulfisoxazole, sulfapyridine, sulfadiazine.
- **Agents, which are poorly absorbed in GIT:** They are known as locally acting drugs. Their use is intended to exert local antibacterial effect in bowel lumen either to treat specific intestinal disease or to reduce luminal bacterial population prior to surgery. This helps to reduce the changes of postoperative wound infection after colon surgery. Examples include sulfasalazine, phthalylsulfathiazole, etc.
- **Agents which are employed topically:** They are applied only in conjunctiva and vagina to treat bacterial infections. They may also be used topically to abolish bacterial colonization of burns. Examples include mafenide, sodium sulfacetamide and silver sulfadiazine.

Classification Based on Chemical Nature

- **Agents carrying substituent on amino group:** These are N^4-substituted sulfonamides, which undergo metabolism in body to release free amino group. Hence they may be considered as prodrugs. Examples include prontosil, solucopticin.

- **Agents having substituent on amido group:** These are N^1-substituted sulfonamides. Most of the clinically used sulfonamides belong to this category. Examples include: sulfadiazine, sulfacetamide, sulfadimidine, etc.
- **Agents having substituents at both, amino and amido nitrogens:** They are also known as N^1, N^4 disubstituted sulfonamides. Examples include succinyl sulfathiazole, phthalylsulfathiazole, etc.
- **Agents missing the amino functional group from the benzene nucleus:** They are also known as non-amino sulfonamides. Example includes mafenide.

Classification Based on Pharmacological Activity

- **Antibacterial agents:** Examples include sulfacetamide, sulfadiazine, sulfisoxazole, etc.
- **Oral hypoglycemic agents:** Examples include tolbutamide.
- **Diuretics:** Examples include furosemide, chlorthalidone, bumetanide, etc.

Classification Based on Duration of Action

- **Long-acting sulfonamides:** They have plasma half-life greater than 24 hours. They have a greater ability to cause hypersensitivity reactions. Examples include, sulfamethoxypyridazine, sulfamethoxydiazine, sulfadimethoxine.
- **Intermediate-acting sulfonamides:** They have plasma half-life between 10–24 hours. Examples include sulfasomizole, sulfamethoxazole.
- **Short-acting sulfonamides:** They have plasma half-life less than 10 hours. Examples include sulfamethizole, sulfasomidine, sulfisoxazole, etc.
- **Ultra-long-acting sulfonamides:** These agents have plasma half-life greater than 50 hours. Examples include sulfalene, sulfamethoxine, sulfasalazine, sulfamethopyrazine, sulfadoxine (plasma half-life =150 hours). These agents should never be used in patients with renal insufficiency. Recently a new broad-spectrum sulfa drug, sulfaclomide has been introduced. It is found to achieve higher serum level than all presently available sulfa drugs.

PHARMACOKINETIC FEATURES OF SULFONAMIDES

- All sulfonamides in systemic use are well absorbed primarily in small intestine. Upon absorption, they are widely distributed to all organs and to pleural, peritoneal and articular body fluids.
- They can also cross placental barrier. They are also found to appear in cerebrospinal fluid. These agents vary in their ability to bind with plasma proteins. For example, sulfadiazine is poorly bound (20%) while sulfamerazine is 85% bound to the plasma proteins.
- Usually acetylated derivatives are extensively bound to plasma proteins. Protein binding of sulfonamides is directly proportional to plasma albumin concentration. Hence renal adverse effects are more pronounced in patients having hypoalbuminemia due to higher concentration of free drug in the plasma.
- The main metabolic pathways for sulfonamides include acetylation and oxidation. Acetylated metabolites do not retain antibacterial activity. They are usually more toxic and less water-soluble than the parent drugs. The extent of acetylation for any sulfonamide is proportional to the duration of stay of that agent in the body.
- Most of the metabolites and active drugs are excreted in the urine in free or glucuronide form. Some loss may also occur in sweat, tears, saliva, milk and feces. Sulfonamides accumulate in the patients suffering from renal failure.

SAR STUDIES OF SULFONAMIDES

Sulfonamide being an important chemical class several thousand sulfonamides had been investigated for their activity on infective organisms. In antibacterial therapy, they are placed next to antibiotics, sometimes even preferred over the later. The major features of SAR of sulfonamides include:

1. Sulfanilamide skeleton is the minimum structural requirement for antibacterial activity.
2. Sulfur atom should be directly linked to the benzene ring.
3. In N^1-substituted, sulfonamides activity varies with the nature of the substituent at amido group. With substituents, imparting electron rich character to SO_2 group, bacteriostatic activity increases. Heterocyclic substituents lead to highly potent derivatives. While sulfonamides that contain a single benzene ring at N^1 – position, are considerably more toxic than heterocyclic ring analogs.
4. N_1-disubstituted in general leads to inactive compounds. Because one hydrogen is essential for ionization of the ring.
5. The free aromatic group should reside para to the sulfonamido group. Its placement at ortho or meta position results in compounds devoid of antibacterial activity.
6. The presence of free amino group is very essential for the activity. Any substitution of amino group either result in prodrug nature or in the loss of activity.
7. The free amino group could be modified to produce prodrug, which are converted to free amino function *in vivo*, e.g. phthalylsulfathiazole.

Phthalylsulfathiazole

8. The antibacterial activity of sulfonamides is related to pKa. Maximal activity would be found in those having a pKa value between 6.0–7.5.
9. Substitutions in the benzene ring of sulfonamides have also been tried. All attempts ended up in formation of inactive compounds.
10. Substitution of free sulfonic acid (-SO_3H) group for sulfonamido function, destroys the activity but replacement by a sulfamic acid group (-SO_2H) and acetylation of N^4-position retains back the activity.
11. The lipid solubility influences the pharmacokinetic and antibacterial activity. In general, as the lipid solubility increases, so do the half-life and antibacterial activity.
12. The sulfonamides bind to the basic centers of arginine, histidine and lysine site of protein. The binding groups are alkyl, alkoxy, and halo. The binding affects the activity of the drug and its half-life.

ADVERSE EFFECTS

The toxicities of sulfonamides vary considerably and may have little relationship to the drug. Adverse effects of sulfonamides are studied as per the organ involved.

Gastrointestinal Tract

Adverse effects include nausea, vomiting, anorexia, diarrhea, hepatitis, etc.

Urinary Tract (Crystalluria)

- Sulfonamides, although revolutionary in early 1930s often cause severe kidney damage by forming crystal in kidney. Sulfonamides and their derivatives usually acylated at N^4 position because of which water solubility has been decreased. On the other hand, sulfonamides and their metabolites are excreted entirely in the urine. Unfortunately, sulfonamides are not very water soluble, unless pH is above pKa, i.e. above pH 10.4. But we know very well that pH of urine is 6 and often slightly lowered during bacterial infection and that results all sulfonamides is in the insoluble non-ionized form in the kidney.

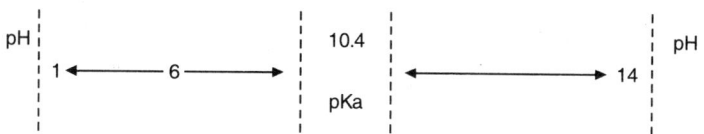

All sulfonamides are poorly water soluble and remain in non-ionized form

Nearly all sulfonamides are in highly water-soluble form

- More effective sulfonamides are usually less soluble in acidic urine. Moreover, acetylated metabolites of most of the sulfonamides are poor water soluble. This leads to the deposition of crystalline aggregates of parent drug and/or its metabolites in the kidney, ureters or bladders. Oliguria, crystalluria and other renal complications may thus result. Such damage can result in epithelial irritability, bleeding and/or complete obstruction of kidneys.

- Hence at pH = pKa, i.e. at pH 10.4 for sulfonamides, there will be a 1:1 mixture of non-ionized and salt forms. Apart from it there are several other ways are also available by which we can increase water solubility of sulfonamides.

1. *Greatly increased urine flow*: During the early days of sulfonamides, patients were warned to take force fluids, *viz* plenty of water.

2. *Raise the pH of the urine*: The closer the pH of the urine to 10.4, the more of the highly water-soluble salt form will be present. Thus, sometimes oral sodium bicarbonate was, and occasionally still is, given to raise the urine pH.

3. Make derivatives of the sulfanilamide that have lower pKa values, closer to the pH of the urine.

Table 57.1: pKa values of some sulfonamides

Sulfone	pka
Sulfadiazine	6.5
Sulfamerazine	7.1
Sulfamethazine	7.4
Sulfisoxazole	5.0
Sulfamethoxazole	6.1

4. Use the mixture of sulfonamides to reach the total dose, since solubilities of sulfonamides are independent, more mixture of sulfonamides can stay in water solution at particular pH than single sulfonamide thus tri-sulfonamides contain mixture of:

Sulfadiazine + Sulfamerazine + Sulfamethazine.

Nervous System

Effects on nervous system include headache, dizziness, confusion, mental depression, peripheral neuritis (motor and sensory neuropathy) and optic neuritis.

Hematopoietic System

Effects include leukopenia, thrombocytopenia, agranulocytosis and marked decrease in erythrocytes and haemoglobin contents. Sulfonamides cause acute hemolytic anemia in patients with glucose-6-phosphate dehydrogenase enzyme deficiency in their erythrocytes.

Hypersensitivity Reactions

These include, skin and mucous membrane eruptions, fever, headache, vascular lesions and serum sickness. Jaundice, hematuria or sore throat is the indications to withdraw the drug immediately.

Effects on Fetus and Neonate

- Sulfonamides compete with bilirubin for the binding sites on plasma proteins (specifically on albumin). As a result, the unbound bilirubin concentration increases in patients under sulfonamide therapy.
- If sulfonamide is given to a pregnant woman, the unbound bilirubin may get deposited in basal ganglia and subthalamic nuclei in CNS of the fetus or newborn, causing kernicterus, a toxic encephalopathy. Hence it should not be given to newborns or pregnant women.

Miscellaneous Effects

- These include conjunctivitis, porphyria, arthralgia and pulmonary eosinophilia. Sulfonamides also compete for binding sites on plasma albumin with many drugs like aspirin, phenylbutazone, coumarins and methotrexate.
- Hence sulfonamides may cause sudden and unexpected rise in the plasma concentration of these drugs by displacing them from plasma proteins. This results into appearance of adverse effects characteristic of displaced drug.

■ MECHANISM OF ACTION (FIGS 57.2 and 57.2)

- The therapeutic effect of sulfonamides is achieved by arresting the growth and multiplication of the infectious organism and thus allowing the host to eradicate the infection by its cellular and humoral defense mechanisms.

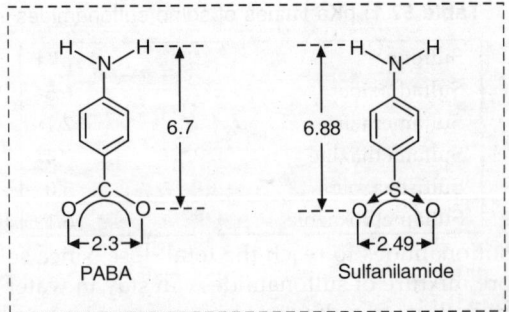

Fig. 57.1: Structural similarities between PABA and sulfanilamide

- Various folate derivatives like, folinic acid; N^5, N^{10}-methylenetetrahydrofolic acid and N^{10}- formyltetrahydrofolic acid act as coenzymes in transport of one-carbon units in several biochemical reactions in human and microorganisms. These one carbon transfer reactions are necessary for the synthesis of purines, thymidine and some amino acids.

- One of the products of these folate dependent biochemical reactions is deoxythymidine monophosphate which is involved in nucleic acid synthesis. Sulfonamides block the biosynthesis of these folate coenzymes resulting into the arrest of bacterial growth and cell division.

- Filds and Woods independently suggested in 1940, that the para-amino benzoic acid (PABA) is essential in the biosynthesis of various folate

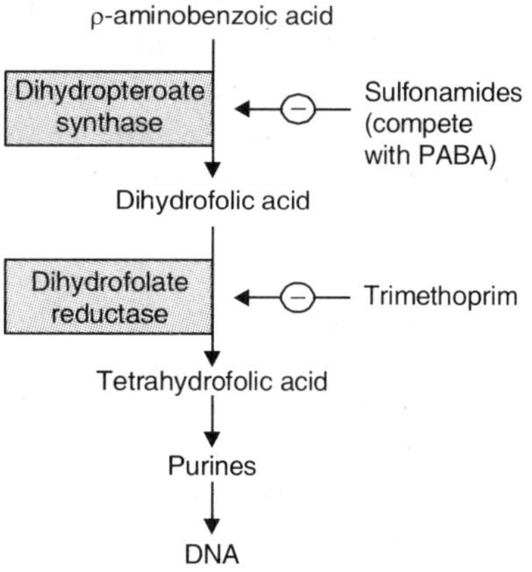

Fig. 57.2: Mode of action of sulfonamides and trimethoprim

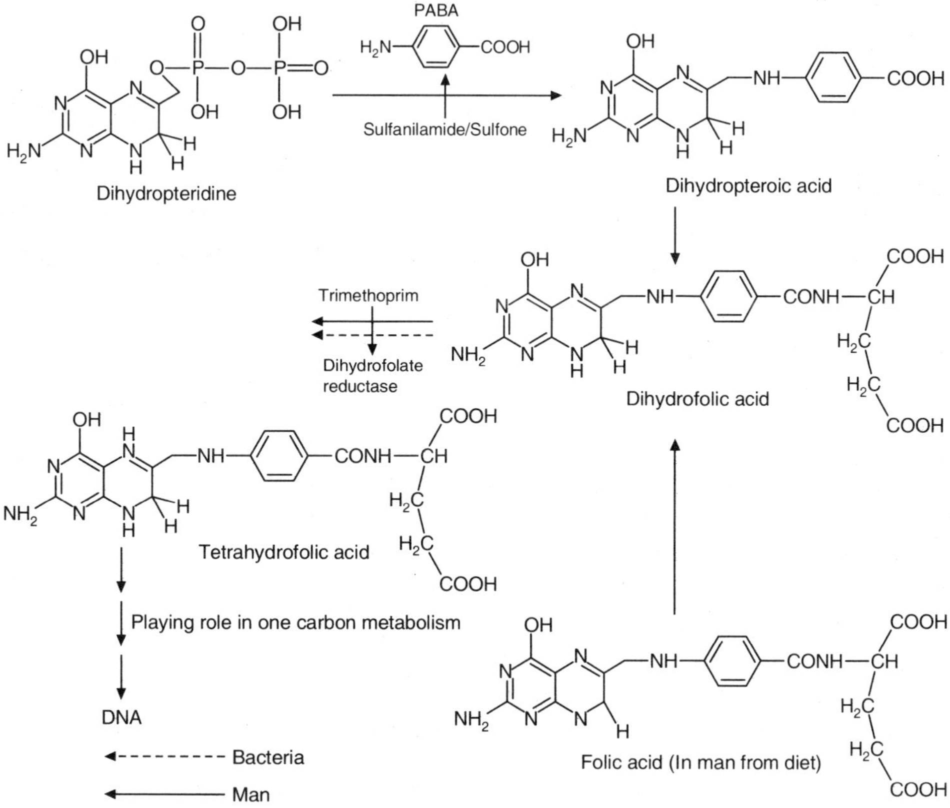

enzymes and cofactors. The structural similarity with PABA results into competitive inhibition and take-up of PABA in microorganisms by sulfonamides. Sulfonamides inhibit the incorporation of PABA in dihydropteroic acid which is a precursor of folic acid needed for the synthesis of DNA and 1-carbon fragments.

Fig. 57.3: Structural mode of action of sulfonamides

- Thus by acting as antimetabolite, sulfonamides prevent the formation of pteroylglutomic acid (PGA). Cells can utilize the preformed PGA present in the diet while bacterial cells can not utilize preformed PGA and they have to synthesize PGA from PABA. Hence sulfonamides do not affect mammalian cells (Fig. 57.3) The antibacterial action of sulfonamides depends upon.

    i. The form (ionized/unionized) in which they are circulated in the body

    ii. The dose of sulfonamide. Greater the concentration of drug in the plasma, greater will be the activity.

- PABA has much greater affinity for the bacterial enzyme system. Since sulfonamide activity based on the principle of competitive antagonism it is necessary to maintain always a high concentration of sulpha drug in the tissue to achieve the desired effect. Hence certain drugs having PABA as the basic skeleton (e.g. procaine) will antagonize the action of sulfonamides *in vivo*.

- Sulfonamides exert only bacteriostatic effect in the body. They possess a wide range of antimicrobial activity against both, gram-positive and gram-negative bacteria. These include, *Mycobacterium tuberculosis, Pneumoniae, Haemophilus influenzae, Corynebacterium diphtheriae, Nocardia, Actinomyces, E. coil, Meningococai*, etc. Sulfonamides therefore have applications in the treatment of tonsillitis, septicaemia, pneumonia, meningococal meningitis and a number of infections of urinary tract.

- The conversion of dihydrofolic acid to tetrahydrofolic acid is catalyzed by the enzyme, folate reductase. Trimethoprim is a potent and competitive inhibitor of this enzyme. It is to be the most active agent that exerts antibacterial activity when combined with a drug. Combination of sulpha drug with other bacteriostatic agent (e.g. tetracycline) may also give synergistic effect.

▨ BACTERIAL RESISTANCE

- Wide and unselective use of sulpha drugs leads to the development of drug-resistant bacterial strains. First seen in *N. gonorrhoeae*, resistance to sulpha drugs then rapidly developed in the variety of streptococci, hemolytic streptococci, meningococci, pneumococci and shigellae.

The bacterial resistance may be:

    a. Natural (intrinsic) resistance or

    b. Acquired resistance.

- Bacterial resistance develops mainly due to mutation process. Bacterial plasmids can cause production of altered enzyme that can bypass the sulfonamide block due to affinity for sulfonamides other possible mechanisms of bacterial resistance include.

    a. An increased production of PABA in the bacterial cell.

    b. An increased ability of bacterial cell to destroy or inactivate the sulfa drug.

    c. Production of sulpha drug antagonist by the bacterial cell.

    d. Decreased bacterial permeability to sulpha drug.

    e. Production of an altered dihydrofolate reductase.

- The development of drug resistance severely limits the therapeutic efficacy of the drug, if a microorganism is resistant to one sulfonamide; it develops resistance against all sulfonamides. Similarly the sulfonamide-sensitive species may develop drug resistance when it comes in contact with a resistant bacterial species. The use of trimethoprim with sulphamethoxazole may reduce development of resistance to sulpha drugs.

TRIMETHOPRIM – SULFONAMIDE COMBINATION (CO-TRIMOXAZOLE) (FIG. 57.4)

- The synergistic effect achieved by the combination of trimethoprim and sulfamethoxazole is recognized as the major advance in the field of chemotherapy.

- Bacteriostatic activity is observed due to the inhibition of two prominent steps in bacterial enzymatic pathway involved in folate synthesis. Sulfamethoxazole inhibits utilization of PABA in the formation of dihydrofolate, while trimethoprim is a potent and selective inhibitor of the enzyme that catalyzes the conversion of dihydrofolate to tetrahydrofolate. Thus a synergistic antimicrobial effect is observed due to the double sequential effects on the bacterial metabolism.

- Originally, introduced as antimalarial agent, trimethoprim has also shown significant bacteriostatic activity. It is effective against most of gram-positive and gram-negative organisms with exceptions of *P. aeruginosa* and *S. faecalis*.

Sulfamethoxazole   Trimethoprim

- Sulfamethoxazole was selected from systemic sulfonamide class on the basis that it has similar pharmacokinetic features (i.e. rates of absorption, and elimination) to that of trimethoprim. It is hence coadministered with trimethoprim in a fixed dose ratio of 5:1. This dose ratio yields a fairly constant plasma concentration of sulfamethoxazole – trimethoprim as 20:1 ratio which is found to be most effective concentration range to exhibit a synergistic effect against most of the pathogenic microorganisms.

- Cotrimoxazole is thus effective against most gram positive cocci and gram-negative bacteria. *Neisseria meningitidis* and gonococci are also susceptible. It is used in the treatment of infections of urinary, intestinal and lower respiratory tracts. It is also effective in the treatment of chronic bacterial prostatis, meningococcal infections, gonorrhea, nocardiosis and antibiotic resistant salmonellae and shigellae infections (Fig. 57.4).

- This combination preparation is preferably used in the treatment of acute and recurrent urinary tract infections, typhoid fever, brucellosis, endocarditis, salmonella sepsis, acute bacterial exacerbations of chronic bronchitis and pneumocystitis.

- Adverse effects of this combination arise as the summation of adverse effects of individual components; however most of the adverse effects of cotrimoxazole are mainly due to sulfamethoxazole moiety. Trimethoprim just helps to intensify some of these (e.g. hematologic adverse effects) toxicities.

THERAPEUTIC USES

Depending upon solubility, sulfonamides may be used systemically, topically or may be used orally for local effects. Following are some principal uses of sulfonamides.

a. Uncomplicated urinary tract infections.

b. Intestinal infections, e.g. sulfaguanidine.

c. Ophthalmic infections, e.g. sulfacetamide.

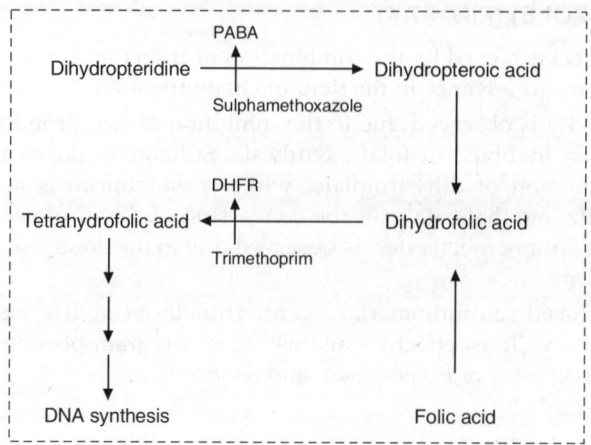

Fig. 57.4: Mode of action of cotrimoxazole

d. Ulcerative colitis, e.g. salicylazosulfapyridine.

e. Rheumatic fever, e.g. sulfadiazine, sulfisoxazole.

f. Nocardiasis, e.g. sulfadiazine, sulfisoxazole.

g. Chancroid (a venereal infection caused by *Haemophilus ducreyi*): sulfasalazine.

h. Toxoplasmosis, e.g. sulpha drug with pyrimethamine.

i. Respiratory tract infections, e.g. cotrimoxazole.

j. Otitis media: sulpha drug is used in combination with erythromycin.

k. Dermatitis herpetiformis, e.g. sulfapyridine.

l. Vaginal infections, e.g. sulfisoxazole diethanolamine.

m. Infected burns, e.g. silver sulfadiazine.

n. Meningococcal meningitis, e.g. sulfadiazine.

o. Trachoma and inclusion conjunctivitis, e.g. sulfisoxazole, sulfadiazine, sulfacetamide.

Systemic Sulfonamides

• These agents are rapidly absorbed into the circulation when given orally. They can also be given parenterally. They are readily removed from the body by the efficient excretion process. Depending upon their duration of action, they can be further sub-divided into:

  a. Short-acting sulfonamides.

  b. Intermediate-acting sulfonamides.

  c. Long-acting sulfonamides.

• Along with the therapy of systemic sulfonamides, an adequate fluid intake is necessary to minimize the risk of crystalluria. In certain cases, urinary alkalinizer may also be tried to help rapid excretion of the drug and/or its metabolites.

Sulfisoxazole

- It is an example of short-acting sulfonamide. Other examples of this group include sulfamethizole, sulfacetamide, sulfanierazine, sulfamethazine, sulfisomidine and sulfadiazine. All they have an ability to cause crystalurea. A mixture of sulfamerazine, sulfamethazine and sulphacetamide is marketed under the name of trisulfapyrmidine. It has an advantage of low potential to cause crystalurea.
- Sulfisoxazole is an orally effective agent. About 91–93% of administered dose is bound to the plasma proteins. It has a plasma half-life of 7.0 hours. About 40% dose appears unchanged in the urine along with 20–30% dose in acetylated form.
- Adverse effects include nausea, vomiting, anorexia, diarrhea, dizziness, hypersensitivity reactions, crystalluria and blood dyscrasias.
- It is available in a fixed dose combination (sulfisoxazole, 500 mg and phenazopyridine, 50 mg) form which is used in the treatment of urinary tract infections caused by the susceptible strains of *E. coli, Klebsiella, S. aureus, P. mirabilis* and *Proteus vulgaris*. It may also be used along with erythromycin, ethylsuccmate in the treatment of otitis media, specifically in children. Sulfisoxazole and sulfadiazine may be used prophylactically to control streptococcal infections in rheumatic fever patients who are hypersensitive to penicillins. It may be used as alternative drug for the treatment of meliodiosis caused by *Pseudomonas pseudomallei* and for the infections caused by nocardiae. It may also be used topically as a 10% cream in the treatment of infections of eye, ear, nose or vagina.

Sulfadiazone

- It is an orally active sulfonamide used in the treatment of nocardiasis and other infections caused by *Chlamydia* and *Toxoplasma gondii*. Optimal antibacterial activity was probably achieved in 1908 with the introduction of this agent. About 54–58% of administered dose is bound to the plasma proteins. It has a plasma half-life of 7–10 hours. About 30–40% dose is acetylated during metabolism. It is excreted in the urine along with about 55–60% dose in unchanged form. Its relative insolubility in acidic urine exposes the patient to the high risk of crystalluria. Hence adequate sodium bicarbonate (a urine alkaline) may be given.
- It may be used intravenously in the therapy of meningitis and as a prophylactic against *meningococcal meningitis*, if *Neisseria* is the basic cause. It is also used as an antimalarial agent when given in combination with pyrimethamine.

Locally Acting Sulfonamides

- These agents are poorly absorbed from GIT when they are given orally. Hence they are intended to be used for exerting local sterilizing effect on the bowel. Examples of such agents include, phthalyl sulfathiazole, succinyl sulfathiazole, phthalyl sulfacetamide and salicylazosulfapyridine. All are the examples of N^1, N^4-disubstituted sulfonamides in which an organic acid is conjugated at N^4-position.

Salicylazosulfapyridine (Sulfasalazine)

- It is a poor orally absorbed sulfonamide that does not have antibacterial activity. It splits in the gut into sulfapyridine and 5-aminosalicyIic acid moieties. The former is absorbed systemically and appear in the urine while the later is excreted in the feces. The enzymes responsible for splitting of sulfasalazine include:
  - Azoreductases.
  - Amidases.
  - Glycosidases.

- Hence it is effective in inflammatory bowel disease. Part of its effectiveness is attributed anti-inflammatory effects of 5-aminosalicylate inhibits prostaglandin synthesis.
- Adverse effects include nausea, vomiting, anorexia, gastric distress, pancreatitis, headache, rashes, fever, arthralgia, anemia, agranulocytosis, thrombocytopenia.
- It is effective in the long-term treatment of ulcerative colitis, granulamatous colitis and regional enteritis. It may also be used in the therapy of malaria. Conjunctivitis, meningococcal meningitis, nocardiasis, otitis media, toxoplasmosis and chancroid (a venereal infection caused by *Haemophilus ducreyi*).

Topically Used Sulfonamides

These agents are extremely useful in decreasing the bacterial colonization of burned skin and thereby preventing burn-wound sepsis. For antibacterial effect, they may also be applied topically to eye, ear, nose, and vagina. Examples include mafenide, silver sulfadiazine, sulfapyridine, sulfisoxazole and sodium sulphacetamide.

Mefenide acetate

- It is a sulfonamide antibacterial agent effective against *pseudomonas aeruginosa*, an organism that colonizes the burns. It is effective in the presence of necrotic tissue and also inhibits other gram-positive and gram-negative bacteria. It is partly absorbed systemically upon topical application and is converted to P-carboxyl benzene sulfonamide. In the form of acetate, it may act as carbonic anhydrase inhibitor and cause either alkalosis or acidosis.
- Adverse effects include skin rashes, eczema, urticaria, exfoliative dermatitis, metabolic acidosis, intense pain at the site of application and chances of super infection with Candida.
- It is available as a cream containing 85 mg/g of mafenide and is applied once or twice a day over burned skin till desired response is obtained, occasional cleansing of wound and removal of debris necessary.

Silver sulfadiazine

- Silver ions are especially effective against gonococci and Pseudomonas species. Silver salts are highly germicidal. Silver sulfadiazine is available in microionized form. It may be used topically in the form of cream (10 mg/g) to inhibit the growth of most bacteria, yeast, some fungi and herpes simplex. It is effectively used to treat extensive burns and burn infections.
- Sulfapyridine is relatively toxic and less effective antibacterial agent. It may be of some value in the treatment of dermatitis herpetiformis. While in the form of eye-drops, sodium sulfacetamide may be used to treat blepharitis and conjunctivitis. It may also be used as prophylaxis against trachoma and conjunctivitis. It penetrates into the ocular tissues in high concentration. Hence it is suitable for local management of ophthalmic infections.

Sulfacitine

3-ethylamino-propionitrile + Potassium cyanate → 1-(2-cyanoethyl)-1-ethylurea → I

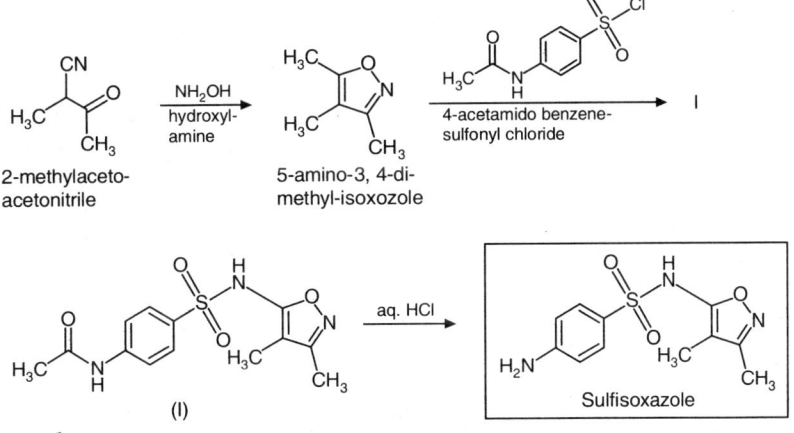

Sulfacetamide

Sulfisoxazole

Sulfamethoxazole

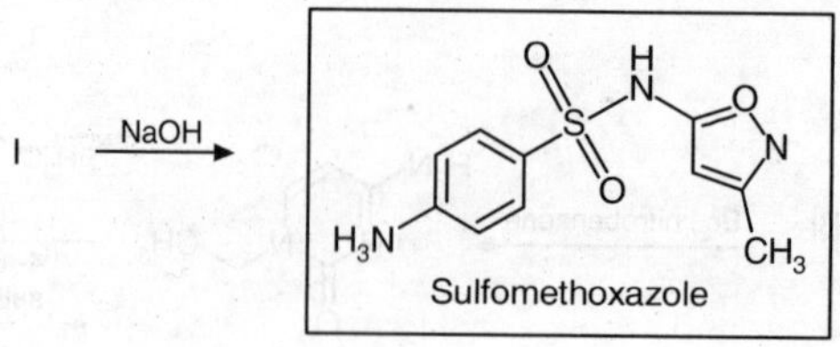
I
NaOH
Sulfomethoxazole

Sulfadiazine

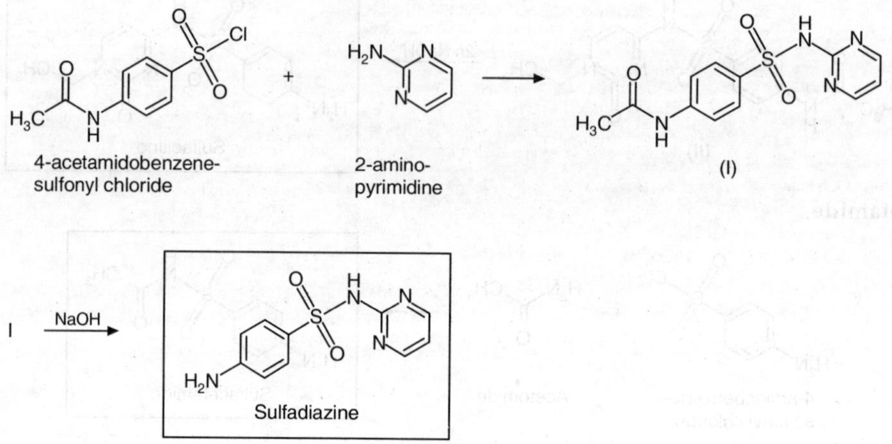
4-acetamidobenzene-sulfonyl chloride
2-amino-pyrimidine
(I)
I
NaOH
Sulfadiazine

Sulfamethoxydiazine

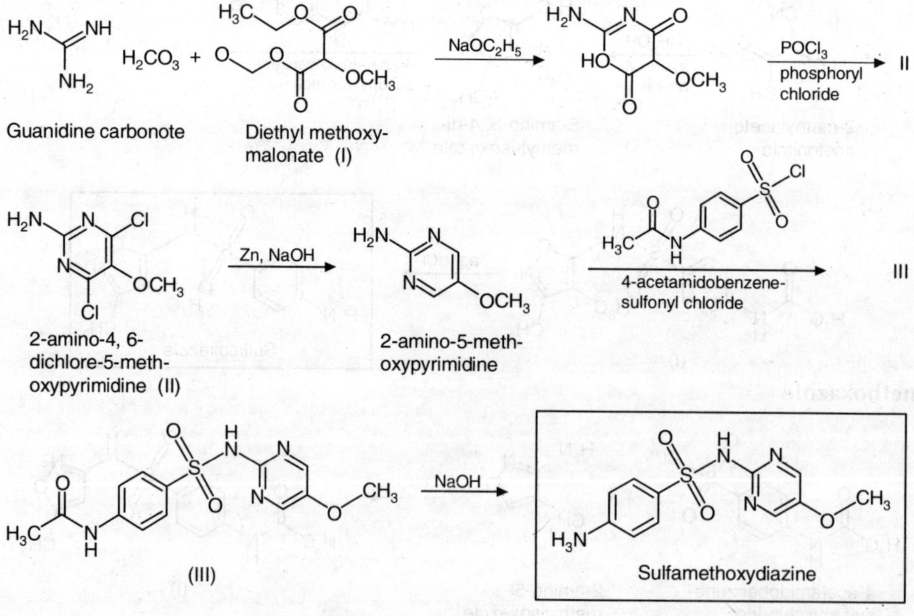
Guanidine carbonote
Diethyl methoxy-malonate (I)
$NaOC_2H_5$
$POCl_3$
phosphoryl chloride
II
2-amino-4, 6-dichlore-5-meth-oxypyrimidine (II)
Zn, NaOH
2-amino-5-meth-oxypyrimidine
4-acetamidobenzene-sulfonyl chloride
III
(III)
NaOH
Sulfamethoxydiazine

Sulfanilamide

Acetanilide → (CISO₃H, chlorosulfonic acid) → 4-acetomidobenzene-sulfonamide (I) → (NH₃) →

I → (NaOH) → Sulfanilamide

Sulfalene

2-amino-pyrazine → (Br₂, CH₃COOH) → (H₃C—Ona (I)) → (H₂, Pd–C) → 3-amino-2-methoxy-pyrazine (II)

II + 4-acetomidobenzene-sulfonyl chloride → → (NaOH) → Sulfalene

Sulfaguanidine

4-aminobenzene-sulfonamide + Guanidine carbonate → (200°C) → Sulfaguanidine

Sulfamethoxypyridiazine

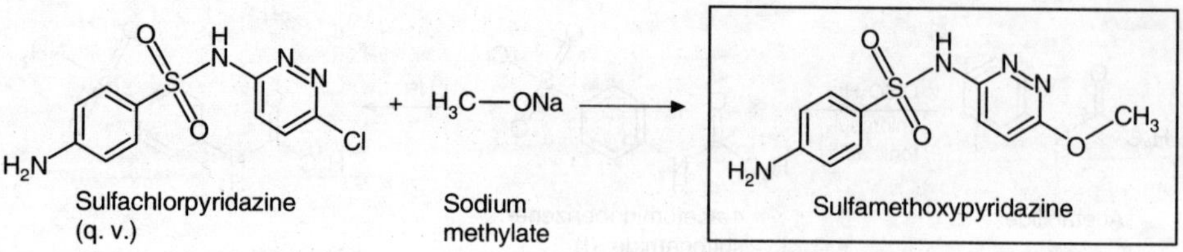
Sulfachlorpyridazine
(q. v.)
Sodium
methylate
Sulfamethoxypyridazine

Sulfamethizole

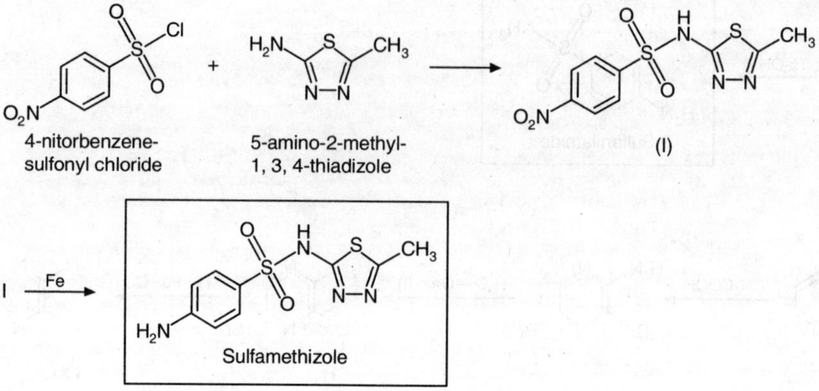
4-nitorbenzene-
sulfonyl chloride
5-amino-2-methyl-
1, 3, 4-thiadizole
(I)
Fe
Sulfamethizole

Sulfamerazine

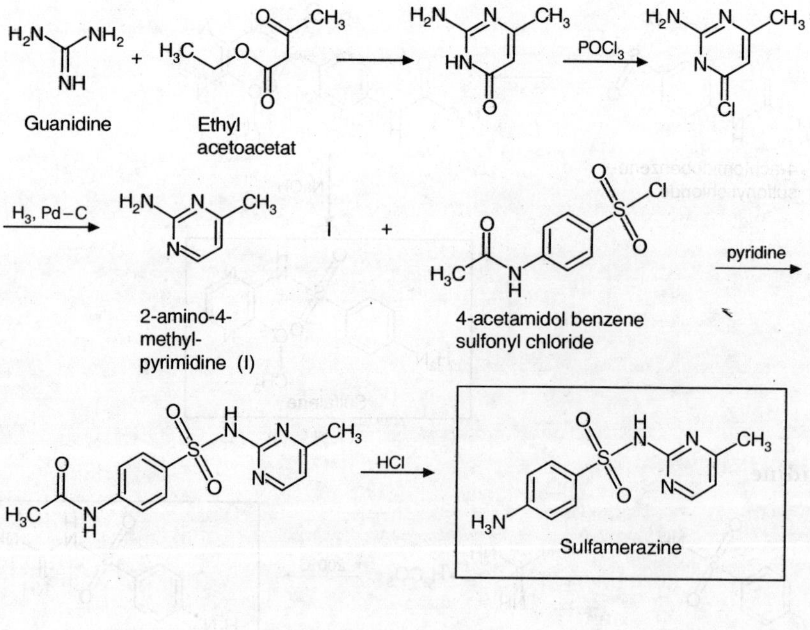
Guanidine
Ethyl
acetoacetat
POCl3
H3, Pd–C
2-amino-4-
methyl-
pyrimidine (I)
4-acetamidol benzene
sulfonyl chloride
pyridine
HCl
Sulfamerazine

58

Antitubercular Agents

Tuberculosis and leprosy are the diseases caused by mycobacterium species. Tuberculosis is caused by either *Mycobacterium tuberculosis* (in man) or by *Mycobacterium bovis* (in animals) while leprosy is caused by *Mycobacterium leprae*.

- Tuberculosis is a disease of respiratory transmission. A person gets infected when he comes in contact with the environment contaminated with viable tubercle bacilli. These bacilli are expelled by coughing, sneezing, shouting and singing of a patient with active tuberculosis. When these bacilli are inhaled by a person, they are inoculated into his respiratory bronchioles and alveoli usually towards the apex of the lung (Fig. 58.1)

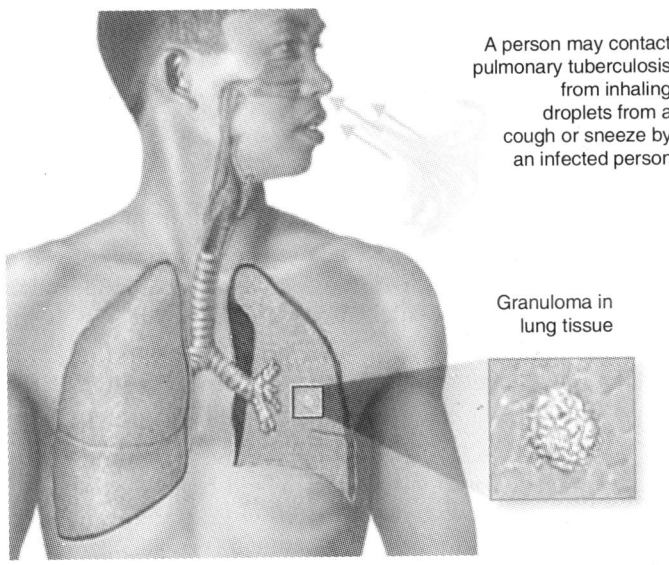

A person may contact pulmonary tuberculosis from inhaling droplets from a cough or sneeze by an infected person

Granuloma in lung tissue

Fig. 58.1: Mechanism of TB infection

- When these microorganisms are multiplied to the sufficient extent, an antigen–antibody interaction is evoked by the cell-mediated T lymphocytes. Tubercles (foci) are then formed due to accumulation of macrophages at the site of infection. This may lead to either permanent suppression of the infection or some microbes may survive in the foci and may become the source of postprimary infection when these foci breakdown under the conditions of weak host defence mechanisms.

- This may occur immediately or months or years later. The hilar lymph nodes may get easily infected due to spreading of some macrophages containing active bacilli. The released microorganisms from the foci are circulated through lymph and blood to different part of the body and infect: (i) reticuloendothelial system (e.g. liver, spleen and lymph nodes), (ii) serosal surfaces and sites with high oxygen pressure (e.g. apices of lungs, renal cortex and epiphyses of growing bones). Due to the multiplication of microorganisms at these sites, numerous small foci develop throughout the body. This type of wide-spread infection is known as miliary tuberculosis (Fig. 58.2)

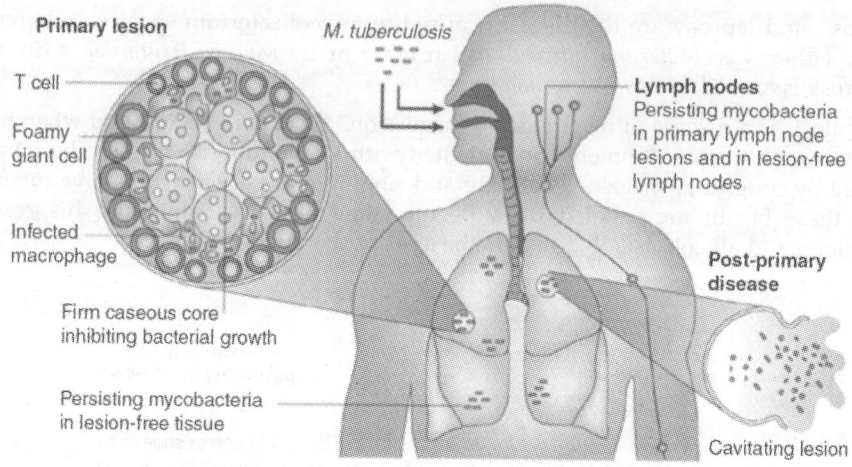

Fig. 58.2: Pathological changes in tuberculosis

- In some patients, the formation of foci leads to temporary suppression of the infection. Microorganisms may still be present in the foci. During coughing, the caseous material containing live microorganisms is expelled out leaving cavities in the lungs. These active bacilli may then either be:
1. Swallowed by the same patient resulting into infection of his alimentary tract, or
2. Inhaled by a healthy adult resulting into infection of his trachea, larynx or bronchi.
3. Such cases are more possible in the conditions of overcrowding and poor personal and public hygiene infections of oropharynx, larynx and tracheobronchial tree respond fairly well to antituberculosis therapy while infections in gastrointestinal tract, urinary tract or lymph nodes respond partially to the drug treatment (Fig. 58.3).
- Tubercles are formed in the infected organs during the course of the disease. Hence the disease is known as tuberculosis. The main symptoms are cough, tachycardia, cyanosis and respiratory failure. Depending upon the site of infection, the disease is known as;
  i. Pulmonary tuberculosis (respiratory tract).
  ii. Genitourinary tuberculosis (genitourinary tract).
  iii. Tuberculous meningitis (nervous system).
  iv. Miliary tuberculosis (a widespread infection).

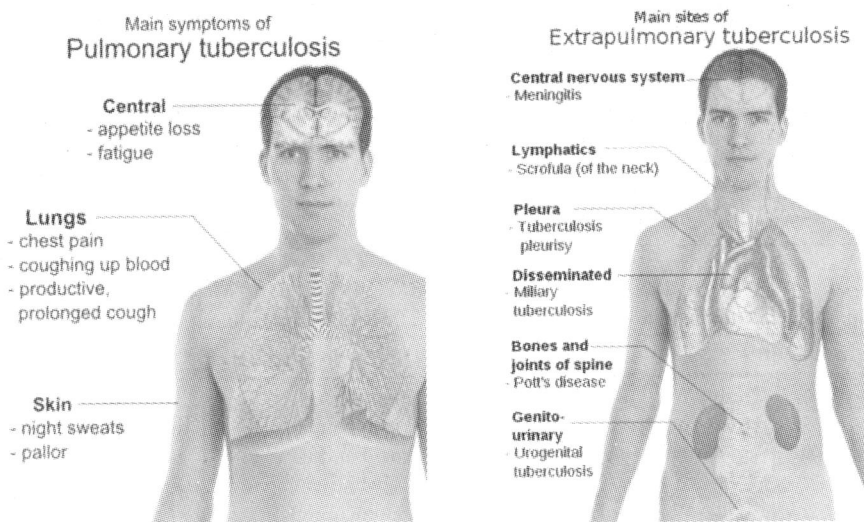

Fig. 58.3: Symptoms of pulmonary and extra pulmonary tuberculosis

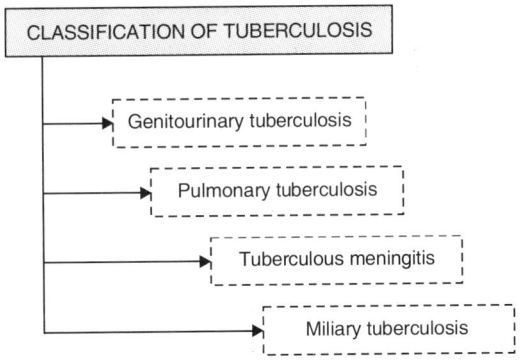

History

A wide variety of drugs are clinically available for the treatment of tuberculosis. Efforts began in 1938 when sulfanilamide and dapsone did not satisfy the clinical requirements of antituberculosis therapy. The major breakthrough was given by Waksman and his coworkers by the introduction of streptomycin in 1944. The story then continued with the introduction of p-amino salicylic acid, isoniazid, ethambutol and rifampin.

▨ PROBLEMS IN CHEMOTHERAPY OF TB

1. Chemotherapy of tuberculosis faced some special problems because of slow growth rate of mycobacteria and their intracellular location.
2. Since the disease is chronic by its nature, the therapy needs to be continued for at least about 1–2 years in most of the cases.
3. In such a chronic treatment, if only single drug is used, the risk of development of drug-resistant strains of mycobacteria is always high. This is coupled with the risk of drug toxicity due to high doses of a single drug needed.

4. The obvious solution to this problem is to use combination therapy. When two or more effective drugs are used in combination, resistance will not develop. However drugs with similar toxological profiles should not be used together.

5. The drugs used in the combination therapy are usually selected from ethambutol, isoniazid and rifampin. The choice is dependent upon the type of disease and some patient-related factors.

Table 58.1: Clinically used antituberculosis agents

Drug	Route of administration	Plasma protein-bound(%)	Plasma half-life (hour)	Principal metabolites	Prominent adverse effects
I. First-line agents					
1. Isoniazid	Orally parenterally	Nil	1-1.5	Acetylisoniazid, isonicotinic acid and its glycine conjugate, isonicotinyl hydrazones, and N-methylisoniazid	Hepatitis, peripheral neuropathy and hypersensitivity
2. Streptomycin	Intramuscularly intrathecally	50-60	5-7	Nil metabolism	Ototoxicity and nephrotoxicity
3. Ethambutol	Orally	20-30	3-4	An aldehyde and dicarboxylic acid derivative	Optic neuritis and hypersensitivity
4. Rifampin	Orally	90	3.5-4.0	25 - 0 - desacetyl -rifamycin and 3-formyl -rifamycin	Hepatitis, fever, thrombocytopenia
II. Second-line agents					
1. p- amino salicylic acid	Orally	60	1.0	N-acetyl derivative	GI-intolerance, hepatotoxicity, hypersensitivity, fluid retention
2. Kanamycin	Intramuscularly	1-3	2.5	Nil metabolism	Ototoxicity and nephrotoxicity
3. Ethionamide	Orally	10	1-1.5	Carbomoyl, thiocarbomoyl and s-oxocarbomoyl derivative	GI-intolerance, hepatotoxicity and hypersensitivity
4. Pyrazinamide	Orally	50-60	9-10	Pyrazinoic acid and 5-hydroxy-pyrazinoic acid	Hepatotoxicity and hyperuricemia
5. Cycloserme	Orally	-	-	Minor metabolism	Rash, seizures, and psychoses
6. Capreomycin	Intramuscularly	-	-	Minor metabolism	Ototoxicity and nephrotoxicity
7. Viomycin	Intramuscularly	-	-	Minor metabolism	Ototoxicity and nephrotoxicity

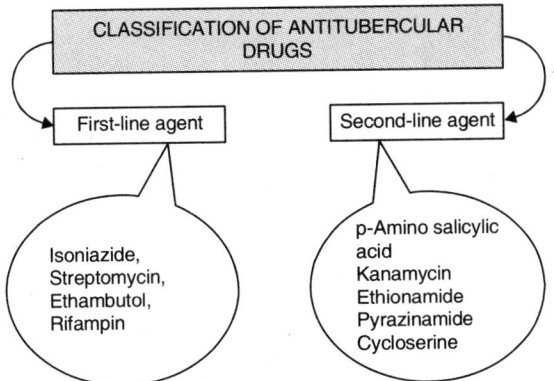

First-line Agents

Isoniazide

Ethambutol

Streptomycin

3.H₂SO₄

Rifampin

Second-line Agents

p-Amino salicylic acid

Ethionamide

Prothionamide

Pyrazinamide

Thiacetazone

Cycloserine

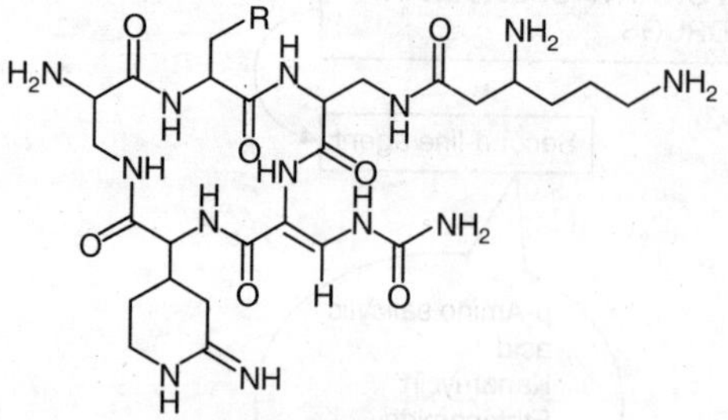

Capreomycin IA R = OH
Capreomycin IB R = H

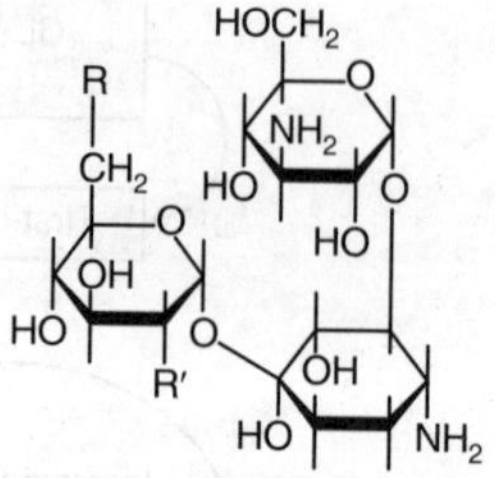

Kanamycin A   NH₂   OH
Kanamycin B   NH₂   NH₂
Kanamycin C   OH   NH₂

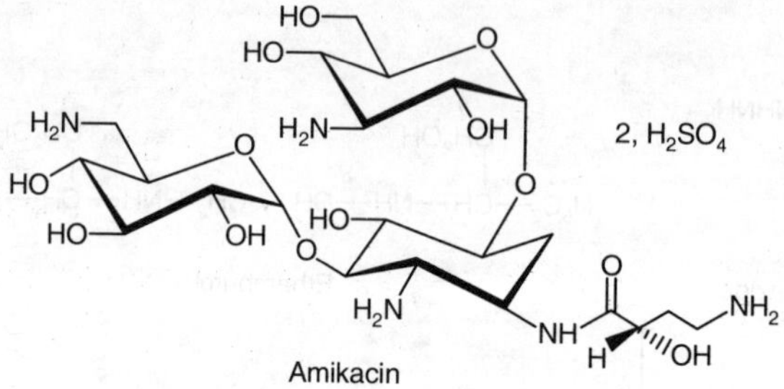

Amikacin

For the sake of clinical convenience, these drugs are categorised into:

i. First-line agents: These are the drugs having high activity and reduced or minimal toxicities. Examples include streptomycin, isoniazid, ethambutol and rifampin.

ii. Second-line agents:

- These are the drugs having less efficiency and significant toxicity. Examples include pyrazinamide, ethionamide, amino salicylic acid, kanamycin, capreomycin, viomycin, amikacin and cycloserine. These drugs are relatively toxic. Hence they should be used only when the organism develops resistance to the first-line agents.

- The above scheme of classification of antituberculosis agents is made by taking into account efficacy, organism susceptibility and spectrum of adverse reactions of the drug.

▨ FIRST-LINE AGENTS

Streptomycin

History

- Amikacin, kanamycin and streptomycin are aminoglycoside antibiotics, which are having in vitro bactericidal and in vivo baceriostatic activity against *Mycobacterium tuberculosis*. All these agents exhibit more or less similar pharmacological and toxicological properties.

- Streptomycin reported in 1944, was the first clinically effective antituberculosis agent. Its introduction radically changed the handling and prognosis of patients with these diseases. It is administered by IM route and very occasionally by intrathecal route. Initially, it was given in large doses.

- The development of drug-resistant strains and incidences of severe adverse effects then aroused the awareness about its dosecalculations. Presently, it is given in the combination with other drugs.

- It is more preferred agent in the treatment of tuberculous meningitis than that of pulmonary tuberculosis. It helps to suppress the disease but does not help to eradicate it. This preventive action may result due to, its inventory action on the bacterial protein synthesis.

Structure–activity relationship

- Reduction of the aldehyde group to alcohol results in compound, which has greater potential as that of initial one.
- Oxidation of the aldehyde to a carbonyl group or conversion to oxime, semicarbazone results in inactive compound.
- Oxidation of methyl group in L-streptose to methylene hydroxyl group gives an active analogue but no advantage over streptomycine.
- Modification of aminomethyl group in the glucosamine portion of the molecule reduces the activity.
- Modification of guanidine in streptidine nucleus results in decrease in activity.

Mechanism of action

Refer chapter Antibiotic.

Side effect

It may cause nephrotoxicity, ototoxicity and blood dyscrasias in patients. Its potential to cause these adverse effects is dose and duration of the treatment-related. Streptomycin resistant strains are usually treated with' kanamycin. If resistance develops to kanamycin then viomycin may be tried.

Isoniazid (Fig. 58.4)

History

Introduced in 1952, isoniazid is an extremely effective and safe antimycobacterial agent. Chemically, it is a hydrazide of isonicotinic acid. It exhibits baceriostatic action on the resting bacilli. Though its single agent therapy is approved, rifampin–isoniazid combination is the most favoured antituberculosis therapy.

Mechanism of action

- Isoniazid inhibits mycolase synthatase, an enzyme necessary for the biosynthesis of mycolic acids. The latter are the important constituents of mycobacterial cell wall. Since mycolic acids are present only in mycobacteria, isoniazid exhibits such a high degree of antimycobacterial action.
- Because of its ability to complex essential metals such as copper or iron present in mycobacterial enzyme; it interferes with various enzyme systems requiring pyridoxal phosphate as a cofactor. This results in changes in the metabolism of lipids, proteins and carbohydrates. Nucleic acid synthesis is also affected.

Structure–activity relationship

1. Movement of the hydrazide function to a position 2 or 3 resulted in reduction of activity.

Iproniazid

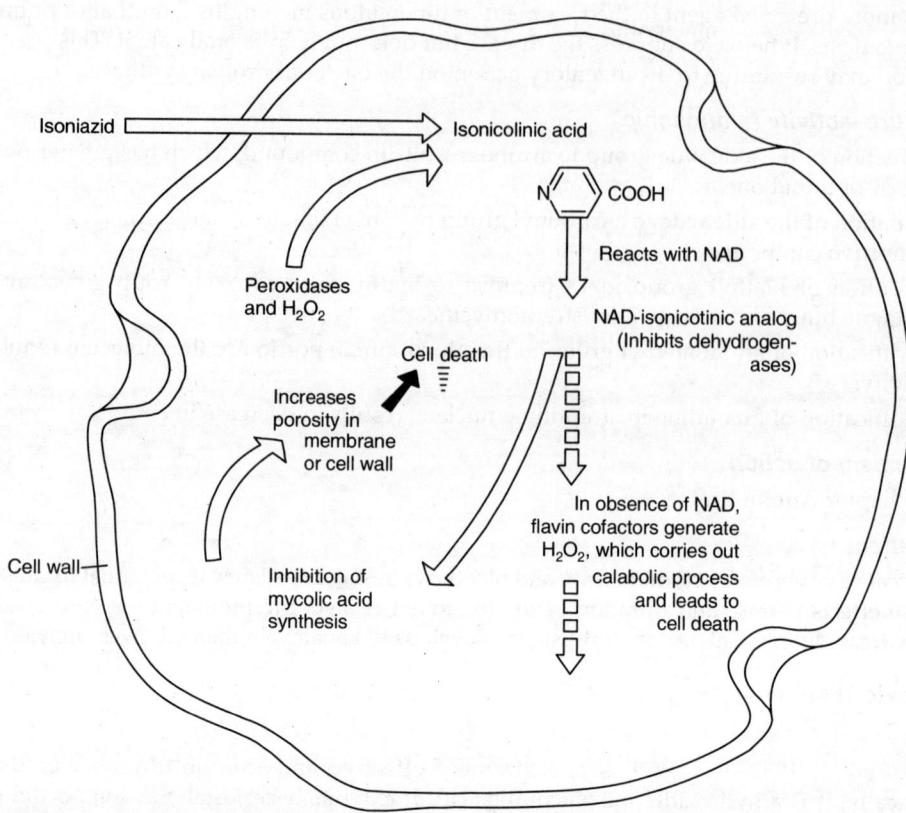

Fig. 58.4: One of the possible mechanism of action of isoniazid

2. Conversion of the hydrazide to other carbonyl group or to amide also resulted in inactive compound.

3. Alkyl substitution on the hydrazide function produced various effects; the trialkylated hydrazides were inactive, whereas the 2,2-dialkylhydrazides showed good activity, e.g. iproniazid, this is disubstituted isoniazid, which show greater effect than the isoniazid.

4. A large number of hydrazones have been made by reacting isoniazid with various aldehyde and ketone. These compound show activity similar to that of isoniazid.

Adverse effects

1. Most of the isoniazid undergoes metabolism by N-acetylation process in the liver. The latter depends on the transfer of acetyl group from coenzyme A by an N-acetyl-transferase. Since the rate of acetylation is under genetic control, patients may be categorised as slow acetylators and rapid acetylators. In slow acetylators, the rate of isoniazid metabolism is slow resulting into more prolonged plasma levels of isoniazid than in rapid acetylators. Hence slow acetylators are more susceptible to the adverse effects than the rapid acetylators.

2. The most common adverse effects of isoniazid include dryness of mouth, epigastric distress, allergic reactions, peripheral neuritis, mental abnormalities, methaemoglobinemia, and hepatotoxicity.

3. The most significant adverse reaction is hepatotoxicity that may arise due to acetyl hydrazine, a toxic metabolite of acetyl isoniazid. It is characterized by fatigue, malaise, weakness, anorexia, fever arthralgia and increased serum glutamic-oxaloa-cetic acid transaminase (SCOT) level.

4. While the neurotoxicity specifically is seen in malnourished patients, chronic alcoholics or slow acetylators. It usually occurs in the form of peripheral neuritis which is characterized by numbness and tingling in lower extremities and paresthesias in the hands and fingers. A supplementary dose of pyridoxal phosphate (vitamin B_6) of 10 mg daily (for 50–100 mg isoniazid dose) corrects the neurotoxic effects of isoniazid.

Pharmacokinetic

It is orally active agent. Its oral absorption is reduced by the presence of food and antacids. It is nil bound to plasma proteins. It has a plasma half-life of 1–1.5 hours. It is well distributed to different body tissues and fluids including cerebrospinal fluid. Because of its wide-spread distribution in the body, it is equally effective against all types of tuberculosis. It undergoes significant first pass hepatic metabolism. The principal metabolites include acetyl isoniazid, isonicotinic acid and its glycine conju-gate, isonicotinyl hydrazones and N-methyl-isoniazid. They are excreted in the urine along with 10 – 25% dose in unchanged form.

Ethambutol

Spectrum of action

It is an orally effective bacteriostatic agent active against most strains of *M. tuberculosis*, *M. kansas* and *M. marinum*. However, *M. avium* and *M. intracellulare* are usually resistant to its action.

$$CH_2OH \qquad\qquad CH2OH$$
$$H_5C_2—CH—NH—CH_2—CH_2—NH—CH—C_2H_5$$

Ethambutol

Structure–activity relationship

1. When the distance between two nitrogen is increased by an inserting oxygen, carbon or sulfur atom that results in loss of activity.

2. Replacement of the secondary butyl group with hydroxy substituted isopropyl or hydroxyl substituted tertiary butyl group, eliminates the activity.

3. Moving of the hydroxyl group to position 3 or 4 of the secondary butyl group results in inactive compounds.

4. Replacements of alcohol function with that of the phenoxy, thio or amino results in loss of activity.

5. The greatest activity is seen into the dextrorotatory isomer, which is 200 to 500 times more active than the levorotatory isomer.

Mechanism of action

Ethambutol prevents the synthesis of the protein, DNA and RNA. It has been proposed that it forms complex with divalent cation and inhibits the functions of amines such as spermidine and spermine; both of which are involved in maintaining integrity of DNA.

Pharmacokinetic

- Chemically, it is ethylene diamino-di-1-butanol. Activity is stereospecific. Dextro isomer is having the maximum antimycobacterium activity. Upon oral administration, it is well distributed in most of the body tissues and fluids except cerebrospinal fluid.
- Because of drug-retention ability, erythrocytes may serve the function of slow drug releasing depots. About 20–30% administered dose is bound to the plasma-proteins.
- It has a plasma half-life of about 3-4 hours. Major metabolites include an aldehyde and a dicarboxylic acid derivative which is excreted in the urine along with about 70% dose in unchanged form.

Adverse effects

- It includes nausea, vomiting, abdominal pain, optic neuritis, headache, fever, mala-ise, diminished visual activity, dermatitis, joint pain, dizziness, confusion, hallucination and peripheral neuritis.
- It is contradicted in pregnancy and in children below 13 years of age. Monthly eye-examination of patients is necessary.

Uses

It is the most favoured drug used in combination therapy with rifampin or isoniazid against streptomycin-resistant strains of tubercle bacilli.

Rifampin

Structure–activity relationship

1. Modifications of the aliphatic portion of the rifamycin molecule normally decrease the activity.
2. N, N-disubstituted acetoxy amide at C-4 results in active compound.
3. A number of 3-substituted aldehyde derivatives have been prepared, giving equal activity.

Mechanism of action

DNA-dependent RNA polymerase is an enzyme necessary for RNA synthesis. Rifampin acts on β-subunit of this enzyme resulting into formation of stable complex. This in turn, causes inhibition of bacterial RNA synthesis. However, mammalian enzymes are not affected by this drug.

Pharmacokinetic

It is an orally active bactericidal semisynthetic derivative of rifamycin B, a macrocylic antibiotic. Its oral absorption is impaired in the presence of food and p-amino salicylic acid. It is well distributed to almost every body tissue and fluid including cerebrospinal fluid. About 90% administered dose is bound to the plasma proteins. It has a plasma half-life of 3.5 – 4.0 hours. The principal metabolites include 25-desacetyl rifamycin (active) and 3-formylrifamycin (inactive). They are excreted in the urine along with 7–10 % dose in unchanged form. About 60–65% dose appears in the faeces through the bile circulation.

Adverse effects

Adverse effects include nausea, vomiting, headache, erythema, nervousness, restlessness, emotional disturbances, tremors, pulmonary edema, hyperglycemia, hypokalemia, increased cardiac output and cardiac arrhythmias.

Uses

Rifampin is a first-line agent. Since bacterial resistance develops rapidly if rifampin is taken alone, its combination with either isoniazid or ethambutol are preferably used. However, combined use of isoniazid and rifampin may increase the risk of hepatotoxicity.

▓ SECOND–LINE AGENTS

A number of second-line agents are available that may be used specifically when bacterial resistance or severe drug toxicity develops with first-line agents.

Ethionamide, Prothionamide

Structure–activity relationship

1. Conversion of thioamide into an amide, amidine or thiourea results in inactive compounds.
2. Moving the thioamide to position 2 or 3 also decreases the activity.
3. Replacement of pyridine ring with pyrazine or benzene causes loss of activity.

Mechanism of action

1. It may interfere in peptide synthesis by acting as antimetabolite and inhibits the incorporation of sulfur-containing amino acids.
2. It may inhibit mycobacterial mycolic acid synthesis.
3. It may affect dehydrogenase systems in tubercle bacilli.
4. It may form a substituted isonicotinic acid derivative that may interfere with NAD-dependent systems.

Pharmacokinetic

It is orally elective agent. However to minimize mucosal irritation, it is usually given in the form of enteric-coated capsules. It is well distributed to various body tissues and fluids including cerebrospinal fluid. About 10% administered dose is bound to the plasma proteins. It has a plasma half-life of 1–1.5 hours. Principle metabolites include carbamoyl, thiocarbomoyl and 5-oxocarbomoyl analogs which are excreted in the urine along with < 1% dose in unchanged form.

Adverse effects

Adverse effects include nausea, vomiting, anorexia, diarrhea, headache, skin rashes, blurred vision, drowsiness, depression, asthenia, olfactory disturbances, restlessness, tremors, impotence and postural hypotension. Because of structural similarity, it blocks hepatic acetylation of isoniazid by acting as alternative substrate for acetylation.

Uses

It is used in combination of other antimycobacterial agent in the treatment of pulmonary tuberculosis resistant to isoniazid.

Para-aminosalicylic Acid (PAS)

Structure–activity relationship

1. Modification in the structure of PAS normally results into the loss of activity.
2. Replacement of the primary amino group with alkoxy, hydroxyl, tertiary amines or results in inactive compounds.
3. Masking the hydroxyl group as the ether or ester or replacing it with a thiol or an amino group results in loss of activity.

4. Conversion of the carboxylic acid group to alkyl esters, amidines, amide or nitrates results in loss of activity.

5. Calcium salts shows less GIT irritation than acid or Nasalt.

6. Conversion of the acid functional group to phenyl esters result into the same active compound (PAS) because this slowly hydrolysed to the free acid.

Mechanism of action

Its structural similarity with PABA suggests its possible role in folate biosynthesis. It interferes with the transfer of one carbon units (Refer Sulfonamide, Chapter 57).

Pharmacokinetic

- It is orally active. It is widely distributed in various body tissues and fluids. About 60% administered dose is bound to the plasma proteins. It has a plasma half-life of 1.0 hour. The principal metabolites include acetylated derivative, free and acetylated p amino salicyluric and 2, 4-dihydroxybenzoic acid which are excreted in the urine along with about 40% dose in unchanged form. Probenecid prolongs its duration of action by inhibiting its tubular excretion.

- Because of its sour taste and irritant properties, this drug is mainly used in the form of its sodium, potassium or calcium salts. In the salt form, it is more water-soluble and less irritant to gastrointestinal mucosa. Moreover, aluminium hydroxide is usually included in its formulation to further reduce GIT-irritation caused by the drug. It is also available in the form of its phenyl and benzoyl esters.

Adverse effects

It includes nausea, abdominal distress, diarrhea, anorexia, eosinophilia, leukopenia, agranulocytosis, thrombocytopenia, hemolytic anemia and allergic reactions. Crystalluria may develop due to poor solubility of free drug and its metabolites in acidic urine. In children, it develops acidosis because of its strongly acidic nature.

Uses

It, however, is effective against only certain mycobacteria. Like ethionamide, it inhibits isoniazid metabolism by competing for hepatic enzymes involved in isonia-zid acetylation. Hence, it elevates the serum isoniazid level when concomitantly administered. It also delays the development of bacterial resistance to streptomycin and isoniazid.

Pyrazinamide

Structure–activity relationship

- Substitution on the pyrazine ring with amino, hydroxyl, chloro or methyl group produced inactive compound.
- Replacement of carboxamide group with an acid, ester, thioamide, nitrile or hydroxamic acid results in compound with no bacteriostatic activity.
- Replacement into the pyrazine ring with other heterocyclic ring such as furan, thiophene, thiazole or pyrimidine results in inactive compound.
- In short any substitution results in loss of activity.

Mechanism of action

Its mechanism of action is still unclear. It acts probably by depressing bacterial protein synthesis. Pyrazinamide is reserved mainly for the treatment of resistant   strains of tubercle bacilli, where it is used along with isoniazid.

Pharmacokinetic

It is orally effective agent. About 50–60% administered dose is bound to the plasma proteins. It has a plasma half-life of 9–10 hours. Principal metabolites include pyrazinoic acid and 5 – hydroxy pyrazinoic acid. They appear in the urine along with 4–14% dose in unchanged form.

Adverse effects

- Adverse effects include nausea, vomiting, urinary retention, anorexia, dysuria, drug rash, fever, malaise, arthralgia, jaundice, hepatic necrosis and decreased urate excretion.
- The pyrazinoic acid metabolites decrease the renal tubular excretion of urate and may induce hyperuricemia and acute gouty arthritis.
- The concomitant administration of para amino salicylic acid was found to prevent or delay.
- The appearance of hyperuricemia. The drug is contraindicated in patients with gouty conditions or hepatic dysfunction.

Thioacetazone (Amithiozone)

MOA: Chemically, it is a thio-semicarbazone. Because of the structural similarity with heterocyclic sulfonamides, it may have sulfonamide-like action. It forms a copper complex that interferes with the biochemical carriers for copper in Mycobacteria

Adverse effect: Adverse effects include nausea, vomiting, skin rashes, leukopenia, hemolytic anemia, thrombocytopenia, hepatotoxicity and renal damage.

Uses: It is now rarely used to treat pulmonary tuberculosis and tuberculoid leprosy. It is, however, effective in delaying the emergence of isoniazid-resistant tubercle bacilli. It may also be used in some combination regimens for leprosy. The drug is given in the daily dose of 50 mg which may then gradually be increased to 300 mg and then is continued for many months.

Cycloserine

Spectrum of action: It is an analog of D-alanine having broad-spectrum antimicrobial profile. It inhibits the growth of some gram-positive and gram-negative bacteria. It is obtained from *Streptomyces orchidaceus*. Chemically, it is D-4-amino-3-isoxazolidone.

MOA: Because of structural similarity with D-alanine, cycloserine prevents the synthesis of cross-linking dipeptide which is necessary in the formation of bacterial cell wall.

Pharmacokinetic: It is orally effective drug. It is widely distributed in various body tissues and a fluid, including cerebrospinal fluid. It is excreted in the form of its metabolites and 50% unchanged drug in the urine.

Adverse effects: Adverse effects include headache, visual disturbances, nervousness, irritability, depression, confusion, tremors and psychoses. The concomitant administration of vitamin B_6 (100 mg three times a day) will reduce its neurotoxicity.

Uses: Cycloserine is now rarely used in the treatment of tuberculosis. It is, however, used in the treatment and long-term suppression of urinarytract infections.

Capreomycin and Viomycin
Spectrum of action

Both these antibiotics are strongly basic peptides having close structural resemblance. Capreomycin is produced by *Streptomyces capreolus* while viomycin is produced by *Streptomyces pumiceus*. Both share similar pharmacological and toxological properties. Capreomycin is more potent but less toxic antimycobacterial agent than viomycin. The crude capreomycin is a mixture of four cyclic polypeptides, IA, IB, IIA and IIB. The clinically used drug consists mainly IA and IB.

MOA

Both these agents act by binding to both 30 S and 50 S ribosomal subunits resulting into inhibition of bacterial protein synthesis.

Adverse effect

- Adverse effects include skin rashes, drug fever, blood dyscrasias, ototoxicity, nephrotoxicity and severe pain at the site of injection.
- Nephrotoxicity is characterized by pyuria, proteinurea, hematuria, nitrogen retention, and electrolyte disturbances. Viomycin is rarely indicated in children.

Uses

Capreomycin is mainly used in combination with ethionamide or ethambutol against streptomycin-resistant strains of M. tuberculosis. Sometimes isoniazid or amino salicylic acid may also be used in the combination with capreomycin.

▦ PROBLEMS IN CHEMOTHERAPY OF TB

1. Chemotherapy of tuberculosis faced some special problems because of slow growth rate of mycobacteria and their intracellular location.
2. Since the disease is chronic by its nature, the therapy needs to be continued for at least about 1–2 years in most of the cases.
3. In such a chronic treatment, if only single drug is used, the risk of development of drug-resistant strains of Mycobacteria is always high. This is coupled with the risk of drug toxicity due to high doses of a single drug needed.
4. The obvious solution to this problem is to use combination therapy. When two or more effective drugs are used in combination, resistance will not develop. However, drugs with similar toxological profiles should not be used together.
5. The drugs used in the combination therapy are usually selected from ethambutol, isoniazid and rifampin. The choice is dependent upon the type of disease and some patient-related factors.

▦ COMBINATION THERAPY

- Chemotherapy of tuberculosis faced some problems because of slow growth rate of the mycobacteria and their intracellular location. Since the disease is chronic by its nature, the therapy needs to be continued for at least 1 to 2 years in most of the cases. In such a chronic treatment, if only single drug is used, the risk of the development of drug resistance strain of mycobacterial is always high. This is coupled with the drug toxicity due to high doses of the single drug. The obvious solution to this problem is to use combination therapy. When two or more effective drugs are used in combination, resistance will not develop. However, in combination therapy, drugs with similar toxicological profile should not be used.

Method (Fig. 58.5)

- As we have discussed in above passage that single drug may cause resistance as well drug toxicity, to avoid such problem, different combination is used.
- In 1952, the combination drug used are: Isoniazid + Streptomycin + PAS

- These drugs are given in three phases— Intensive phase, stabilization phase and consolidation phase.

1. *Intensive phase*

All three drugs are administered simultaneously for 6 to 7 days in a week in order to achieve as rapid as the quickest possible elimination of the resistant organism. This phase lasted for 3 to 6 month.

2. *Stabilization Phase*

During this phase only two drugs has been given, these are isoniazid + PAS were given for 6 to 9 months, the main purpose behind this is that reduction in bacterial count and total elimination of the resistant mutants.

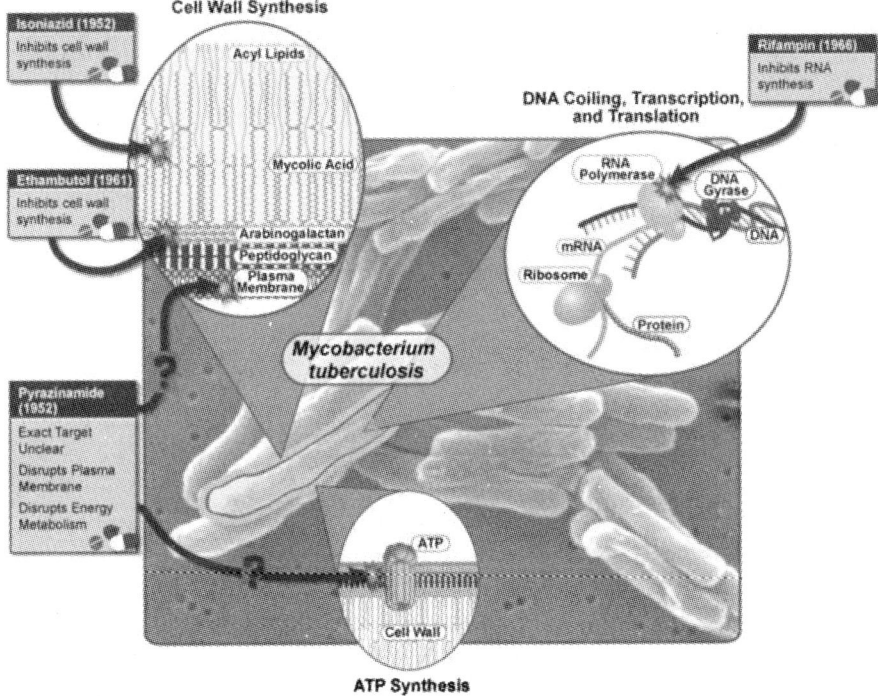

Fig. 58.5: Different mode of action of antitubercular agents

3. *Consolidation phase*

- This phase is lasted up to the two years. Isoniazide was given as mono therapy in order to destroy persisting organism and so to provide greater protection against micro-organism.
- This combination therapy change according to the invention of the new drug.

  In 1962.

  Isoniazid + Streptomycin + Ethambutol.

  Later

  Isoniazid + Rifampicin + Ethambutol

Isoniazid

Ethyl isonicotinate → (H₂N–NH₂, hydrazine) → Isoniazid

Pyrazinamide

Glyoxal + o-phenylene-diamine → Quinoxaline → (KMnO₄) → Pyrazine-2, 3-dicarboxylic acid → (Δ, −CO₂) → Pyrazine-2, carboxylic acid (I)

I + HO—CH₃ → (HCl) → Methyl pyroxine-2-carboxylate → (NH₃, CH₃OH) → Pyrazinamide

Ethionamide

Diethyl oxolate + Butanone → (NaOC₃H₅) → Ethyl 2, 4-dioxo-hexanoate → (cyaoacetomide, pyridine) → I

(I) → (HCl) → 6-ethyl-1, 2-dihydro-2-oxo-4-pyridine-carboxylic acid → (1. POCl₃, PCl₅; 2. HO CH₃) → Ethyl 2-chloro-6-ethyl-iso-nicotinate (II)

II → (H₂, Pd) → Ethyl 2-ethyliso-nicothinate → (1. NH₃; 2. P₂O₅) → 2-ethyl-isonicotino-nitrile → (H₂S) → Ethionamide

ρ-Aminosalicylic Acid

3-amino-phenol + Carbon dioxide → KHCO₃, S–10 atm → p-aminosalicylic acid

Cycloserine

D-serine + H₃C—OH → HCl → D-serine methyl ester hydrochloride → PCl₅ → I

(I) → NH₂OH, OH⁻ hydroxylamine → D-cycloserine

59

Antileprotic Agents

LEPROSY

Leprosy or Hansen's disease is a chronic human disease caused due to an acid-fast bacillus which produces nodules in the skin and loss of sensation in the affected region. This dermatological infection is caused by *Mycobacterium leprae* (Fig. 59.1) and the disease develops very slowly over a period of years.

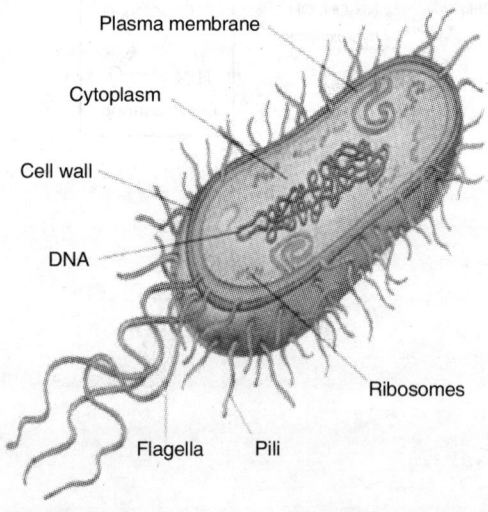

Plasma membrane

Cytoplasm

Cell wall

DNA

Ribosomes

Flagella   Pili

Fig. 59.1: Structure of *Mycobacterium leprae*

- Once the bacilli are multiplied to the sufficient extent, antigen–antibody reactions are evoked by the cell-mediated immunity. These reactions may occur either suddenly in the absence of drug or during the anti-leprotic treatment. These hypersensitivity reactions are occurring not as a result of allergy to the drugs but they should be considered as allergic reactions to the metabolic products of the infecting organism. These reactions are called as lepra reactions. To control these reactions, usually a glucocorticoid is added in the antileprotic drug regimen.

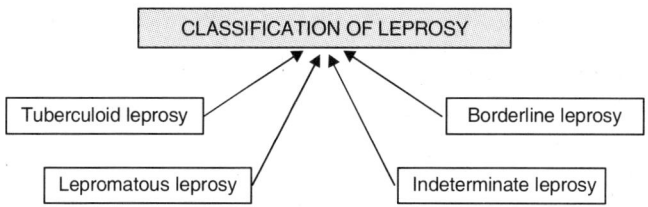

- Based upon the area under infection and intensity of lepra reactions, leprosy can be categorised into:
  1. **Tuberculoid leprosy:** It is characterized by the presence of infection in restricted area and less pronounced lepra reaction. The latter indicates that very few numbers of microorganisms are present in the infected area of the skin. Hence dapsone alone may be effective.
  2. **Lepromatous leprosy:** It is characterized by a widely disseminated disease with a high number of infecting micro-organisms. Hence this form needs more drastic (i.e. multidrug) and prolonged treatment.
  3. **Indeterminate leprosy:** In very early stages of the disease, microorganisms are not multiplied to the extent to induce lepra reactions. This early form of the disease is known as indeterminate leprosy.
  4. **Borderline leprosy:** Tuberculoid leprosy and lepromatous leprosy are the two extremities of the active form of the disease. All other forms that lie in between these two extremities are known as borderline forms of leprosy.

TREATMENT OF LEPROSY

Relatively few drugs are available to treat this chronic dermatological disease. These drugs include dapsone, clofazimine, thiacetazone, ethionamide, prothionamide and rifampin. An ideal antileprotic agent should serve two important objectives. It should be able to control lepra reactions and it should eliminate viable bacilli from the blood and nasal secretions by stopping their multiplication. Because of the vascular nature of the lesions and slow growth of bacilli, a prolonged treatment of about 1–5 years is necessary to prevent relapse of the disease. Along with main drug, adjunct therapy with corticosteroids (to suppress the lepra reaction), amino glycosides or antimalarial agents may be useful.

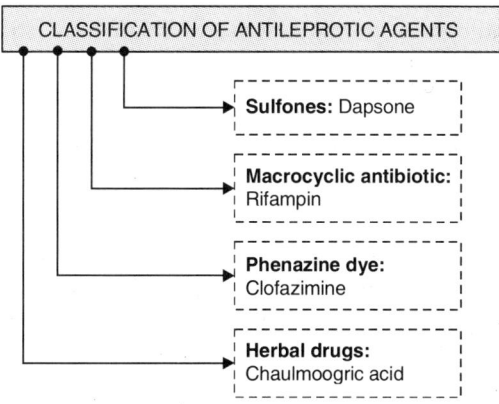

SULFONES

Dapsone

Structure–activity relationship

1. Replacement of one of the amino group by the hydroxy, nitro or hydroxyl amino group results in minimal activity.
2. When both amino groups are replicated with hydroxyl group, it results in inactive compound.

$$H_2N-\text{⟨⟩}-SO_2-\text{⟨⟩}-NH_2$$

Dapsone

3. Reduction of the sulfone group to the sulfoxide reduces the activity; further reduction to thio ether eliminates the activity.
4. An aldehyde-bisulfite complex of the amine functions produces the active compound, such as glucosulfone sodium and sulfoxone sodium. This compound breaks down in vivo to regenerate dapsone.
5. Substitution on dapsone ring by hydroxyl, amino, chloro, methoxy results in inactive compound.

MOA

It is having mode of action like sulfonamide because of structural similarities. (Refer sulfonamide chapter)

Pharmacokinetic

They are orally active and are well-distributed in different body tissues and fluids. Many sulfones are in vivo converted to dapsone. Acetylation and glucuronide conjugation are the main pathways for their metabolic activation. They are mainly excreted in the bile and reabsorbed from the intestine.

Adverse effects

Adverse effects of sulfones include nausea, vomiting, anorexia, insomnia, drug fever, skin rashes, anemia and methemoglobinemia. The latter two effects are more pronounced in patients deficient in glucose-6-phosphate dehydrogenase enzyme. Burning sensation in hands and feet and hepatitis may also occur.

Uses

Besides their use in antileprotic therapy, some of them have shown good results in the treatment of malarial and ricketsial infections. Dapsone itself is used in treatment of both, lepromatous and tuberculoid types of leprosy.

MACROCYCLIC ANTIBIOTIC

Rifampin

Chemistry

The semisynthetic antibiotic rifampicin is the 3-(4-methyl-1-piperazinyl-iminomethyl) derivatives of rifamycin, which though also displaying therapeutic activity, is less potent and has been given parenterally. Like rifamycin, rifampin has an aromatic ring systeme with a long aliphatic bridge called as ansa ring. The ansa ring determines the mechanism of action of rifampin.

Rifampin

MOA

By forming complexes with RNA polymerase, rifampin inhibits RNA synthesis thereby blocking bacterial protein synthesis. Rifampin thus interferes with at a very early stage in the process by which information stored in DNA is transformed, via transcription and translation, into proteins, thereby becoming functionally active in the cell.

Uses

This drug has bactericidal action on the growth of *Mycobacterium leprae* in a dose of 600 mg per day. It is used in combination with other antileprotic agent in the treatment of sulfone-resislant leprotic disease.

▨ PHENAZINE DYE DERIVATIVES

Clofazimine

MOA

It acts mainly by interfering with the replication of bacterial DNA. Beside antibacterial activities, it also possesses anti-inflammatory activity that provides additional benefit to relieve the patient from leprae reactions. Because of its anti-inflammatory activity, the appearance of erythema nodosum leprosum is found to be delayed. It is often used in combination with other potent antileprotic agents to potentiate antileprotic activity. It may also be used to treat Buruli ulcer caused due to *Mycobacterium ulcerans*. It is also used to treat pyoderma gangrenosum.

Pharmacokinetic

It is widely distributed in different body tissues and fluids. It is accumulated specifically in liver, spleen and lymph nodes. It has a plasma half-life of about 2 months. It is insignificantly metabolized and is excreted mainly in unchanged form in urine and faeces. Minor amount is excreted in sweat, tears, saliva and milk.

Clofazimine

Adverse effect

Adverse effects include nausea, vomiting, eosinophilic enteritis, anorexia, diarrhea, crampy abdominal pain, weight loss and red discoloration of the skin.

Uses

It may also be used to treat Buruli ulcer caused due to *Mycobacterium ulcerans*. It is also used to treat pyoderma gangrenosum.

▨ NATURAL PRODUCT

Chaulmoogric Acid

- The oils of chaulmoogra and hydnocarpus are used since from ancient time in the treatment of leprosy. These oils are extracted from the riped seeds of *Hydnocarpus anthelmintica; H. heterophylla* and other species of *Hydnocarpus*. It contains glycerides of chaulmoogric acid and hydnocarpic acid.

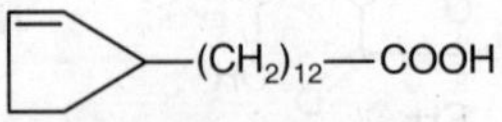

$$\text{Chaulmoorgic acid} \quad \triangleright\!-(CH_2)_{12}-COOH$$

Chaulmoorgic acid

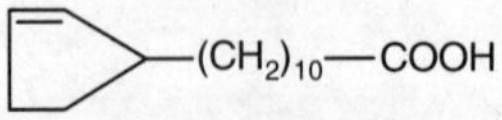

$$\triangleright\!-(CH_2)_{10}-COOH$$

Hydnocarpic acid

- Various derivatives of these acids have been prepared and may be topically employed in the therapy of leprosy, psoriasis, rheumatism and tuberculosis.

Dapsone

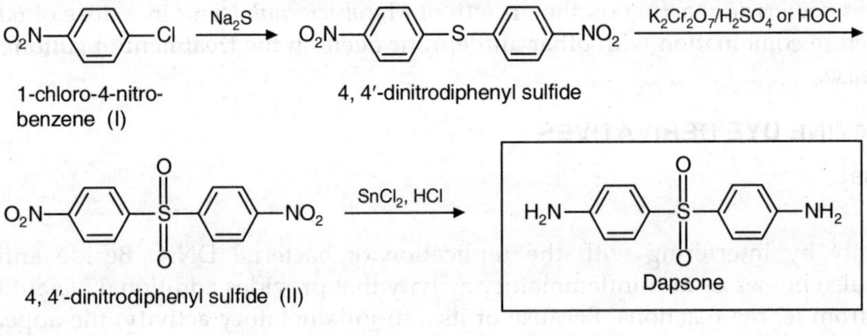

$$O_2N\!-\!\langle\ \rangle\!-\!Cl \xrightarrow{Na_2S} O_2N\!-\!\langle\ \rangle\!-\!S\!-\!\langle\ \rangle\!-\!NO_2 \xrightarrow{K_2Cr_2O_7/H_2SO_4 \text{ or HOCl}} II$$

1-chloro-4-nitro-
benzene (I)

4, 4'-dinitrodiphenyl sulfide

$$O_2N\!-\!\langle\ \rangle\!-\!\overset{O}{\underset{O}{S}}\!-\!\langle\ \rangle\!-\!NO_2 \xrightarrow{SnCl_2, HCl} H_2N\!-\!\langle\ \rangle\!-\!\overset{O}{\underset{O}{S}}\!-\!\langle\ \rangle\!-\!NH_2$$

4, 4'-dinitrodiphenyl sulfide (II)

Dapsone

Antifungal Agents

Fungus is a parasite. The human fungi parasitic relationship results in mycotic illnesses, the majority of which involve superficial invasion of skin or the mucous membranes of body orifices. Fungi have different shapes and sizes. Some are large while others are minute parasitic and saprophytic cells. They differ from:

   a. Algae by lack of photosynthetic ability.

   b. Protozoa by the lack of motility, possession of chitinious cell-wall.

   c. Bacteria by greater size and having certain intracellular structure like mitochondria, nuclear membrane.

- Depending upon some basic differences, fungi may be classified as:

   a. Phycomycetes (algae-like).

   b. Ascomycetes (sac-like).

   c. Basidiomycetes (mushrooms).

   d. Dueteromycetes.

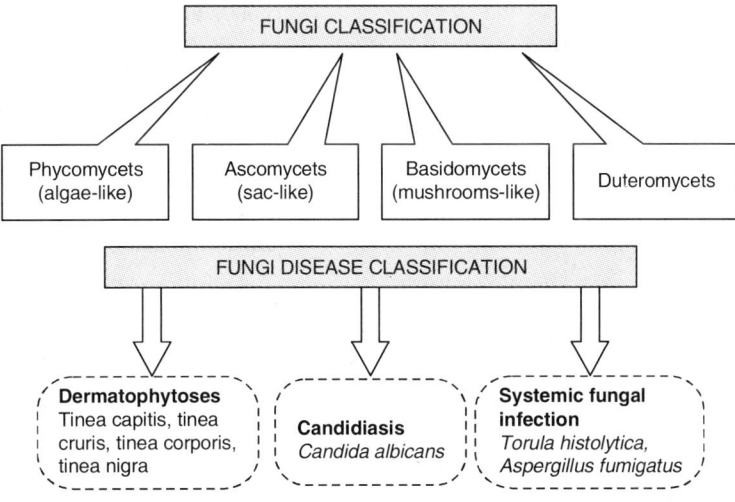

- In addition, the 'higher bacteria' like Actinomyces and Nocardia are sometimes grouped with the fungi.

- Fungal diseases are generally called as mycoses. These mycotic infections may be categorised broadly as given below.

DERMATOPHYTOSES

• Skin infections of contagious nature, caused by various Trichophyton, and Microsporum species. These include superficial infections of keratinized tissues like, stratum corneum, hair, nails, etc. *Tinea capitis, Tinea corporis, Tinea cruris, Tinea unguium, Tinea versicolor* and, *Tinea nigrand* are all grouped under superficial fungal infections. Topical antifungal agents are effective here.

• However, to treat deeper infections (e.g. systemic antifungal, e.g. griseofulvin) may also be given along with topical antifungal agents. Because of the keratolytic action of salicylate, it may often be used along with the topical antifungal agent to improve the drug penetration. Salicylic acid helps the drug to reach the site deep within the hyperkeratotic epidermis.

Table 60.1: Drugs of choice in the treatment of systemic fungal infections

Sr. No	Disease	Fungus	Effective antifungal agents
1.	Actinomycosis	*Actinomyces israelii*	Penicillin G, cephalosporin, tetracycline,
2.	Aspergillosis	*Aspergillus fumigatus, aspergillus niger*	Amphotericin B, rifampin
3.	Blastomycosis (North American type)	*Blastomyces dermatitidis*	Amphotericin B, rifampin and hydroxystibamidine
4.	Blastomycosis (South American type)	*Blastomyces brasiliensis*	Amphotericin B, miconazole
5.	Candidiasis	*Candida albicans*	Amphotericin B, nystatin
6.	Chromoblastomycosis	*Cladsporium*	Flucytosine, amphotericin B, potassium iodide
7.	Coccidioidomycosis	*Coccidioides immitis*	Amphotericin B, miconazole, ketoconazole
8.	Cryptococcosis	*Cryptococcus neofrmans*	Amphotericin B, flucytosine
9.	Histoplasmosis	*Histoplasma capsulatum*	Amphotericin B, hydroxystillbamidine, rifampin
10.	Phycomycosis (mucormycosis	*Mucor species*	Amphotericin B, hydroxystillbamidine
11.	Nocardiasis	*Nocadria asterodies*	Amoxicillin, cotrimoxazole, minocycline
13.	Sporotrichosis amphotericin	*Sporothrix schenckii*	Potassium iodide,

CANDIDIASIS

It affects mainly the skin and mucous membrane. It is caused by *Candida albicans*. These infections mainly develop in the mouth, bowel or vagina and are called as local infections. They may sometimes become systemic and contagious.

SYSTEMIC FUNGAL INFECTION

• Systemic fungal infection is the third major category that involves fungal infections of bones, viscera, lungs and meninges.

- Many fungal infections occur either on skin (a vascular region) or in poorly vascularized area (e.g. nails and hair) are such places where the drug cannot build up its therapeutic concentration necessary to exhibit antifungal activity. Besides this, clinical utility of many drugs is hampered mainly because of poor solubility and poor penetration ability.

- Currently there exist neither clinically available vaccines nor effective antisera for mycotic diseases. Due to various reasons (e.g. differences in solubility, diffusibility or inactivation by serum components) the agents showing excellent antifungal activity in vitro studies, disappointed us when tested in vivo. For example, miconazole and clotrimazole are inactivated by phospholipids and triglycerides.

- To cover such a broad range of systemic fungal infections, very few antifungal agents are available. These include polyene antibiotics (e.g. amphotericin B, nystatin), antimetabolites (e.g. flucytosine), griseofulvin and imidazoles (e.g. ketoconazole, miconazole and clotrimazole).

CLASSIFICATION

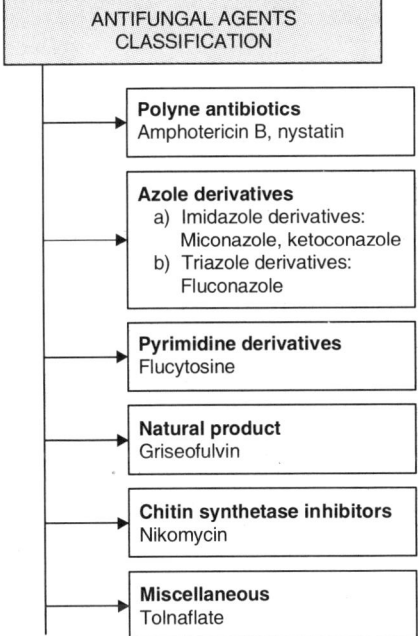

On the chemical basis, currently used antifungal agents can be categorised as:

   a. Polynes antibiotic.

   b. Pyrimidines derivatives.

   c. Azole derivatives.

   d. Natural product.

   e. Chitin synthetase inhibitors.

   f. Miscellaneous agents.

   Due to diversified structures of various antifungal agents, attempts to define SAR also failed. In such cases, interpretation of the activity in terms of drugs physicochemical parameters projects better understanding of SAR studies.

[A] Polyne Antibiotics

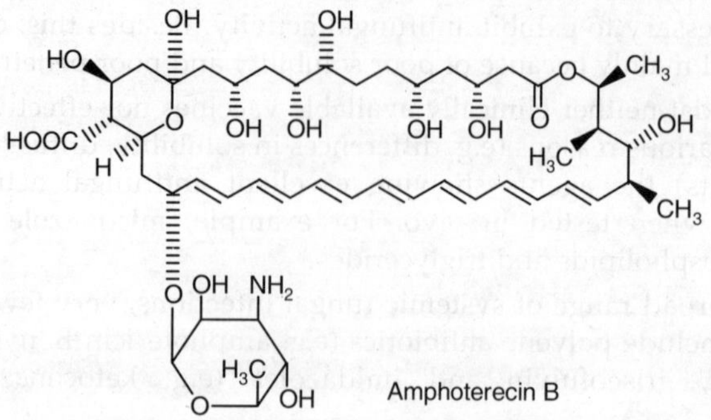

Amphoterecin B

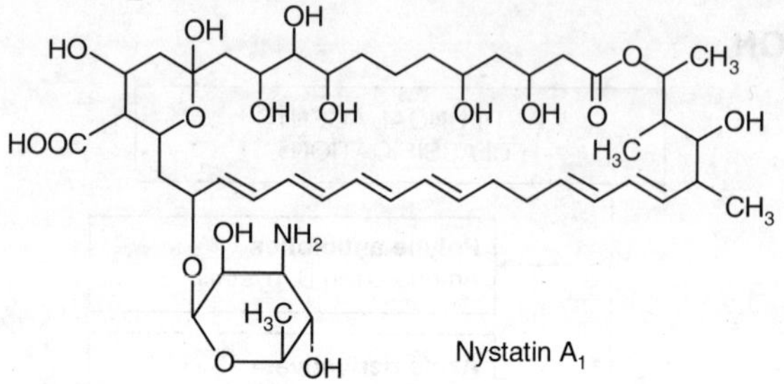

Nystatin A₁

[B] Pyrimidine Derivatives

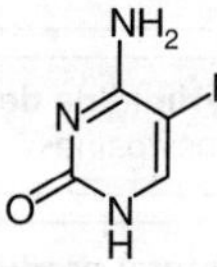

Flucytosine

[C] Azole Derivatives

1. Imidazole Derivatives

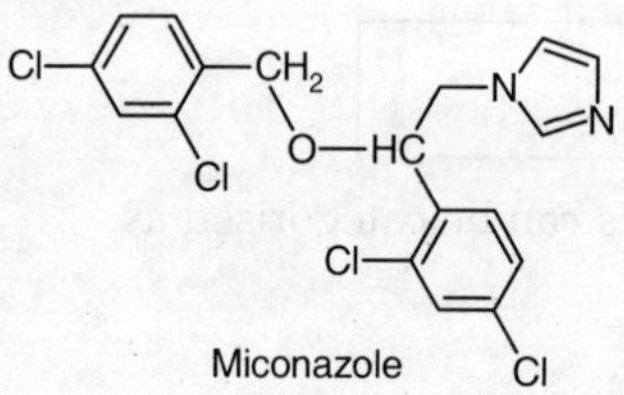

Miconazole

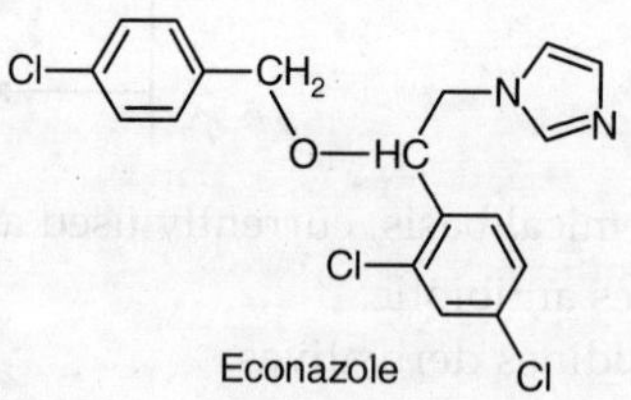

Econazole

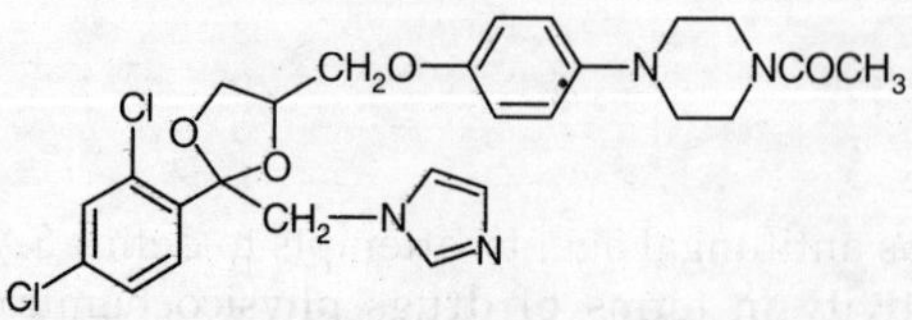

Ketoconazole

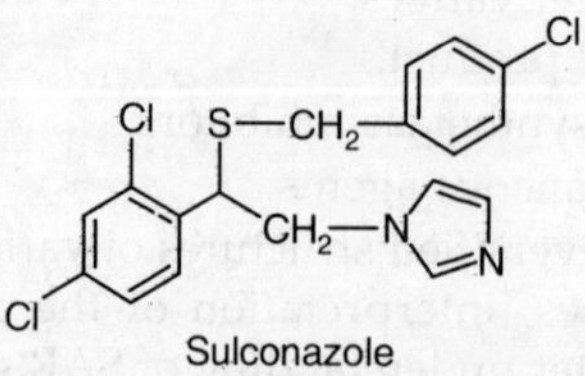

Sulconazole

Clotrimazole

Orconazole

Bifonazole

2. Triazole Derivatives

Itraconazole

Fluconazole

Saperconazole

[D] Natural Product

Griseofulvin

[E] Chitin Synthetase Inhibitors

Nikomycin

[F] Miscellaneous Agent

Tolnaflate

ANTIFUNGAL ANTIBIOTICS

History

In the early 1950s, polyene antibiotics were first identified. As the name implies, these compounds contain, unsaturated carbon rings or chains. About 60 polyene antibiotics (all produced by actinomycetes) have been reported in the literature.

Chemistry

- They all are characterized by the presence of a large ring containing a lactone group (i.e. macrocyclic lactone) and a hydrophobic region coupled with conjugated polyene system of four to seven double bonds. Many of them, contain a glycosidically linked amino sugars. For example, an aminodesoxy hexose (i.e. mycosarnine) is present in amphotericin B and nystatin. The polyene antibiotics are poorly soluble in water. The number of double bonds present in the skeleton serves as a basis of classification of polyenes. For example, they may be categorised as tetraenes (nystatin), pentaenes (filipin), hexaenes (endomycin) and heptaenes (amphotericin B). The most important polyeues are amphotericin B and nystatin. The former being an important therapeutic agent against most of the systemic antifungal diseases. Depending upon die concentration employed, polyene antibiotics exert either fungistatic or fungicidal effects.

MOA (Fig. 60.1)

- **The primary mechanism of action of the polynes:** Amphotericin B binds to the ergosterol, the principal sterol present in the cell membrane of sensitive fungi. This binding alters membrane permeability, causing leakage of sodium, potassium and hydrogen ions, eventually leading to cell death. Binding to ergosterol form pores or channel that involve hydrophobic bond between the lipophilic segment of the polyne antibiotic and the sterol. Amphotericin B also binds to a lesser extent to other sterols, such as cholesterol which accounts for much of the toxicity associated with its usage.
- **Another proposed mechanism:** It is supposed that amphotericin B is going to stimulate to the macrophages.

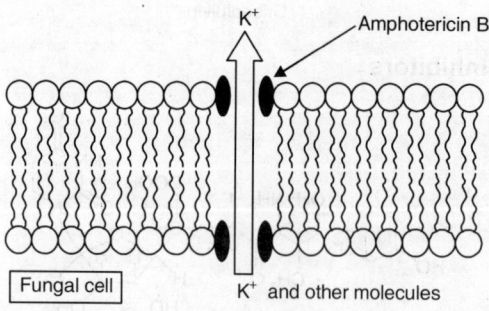

Pore formed by amphoterecin in lipid bilayer

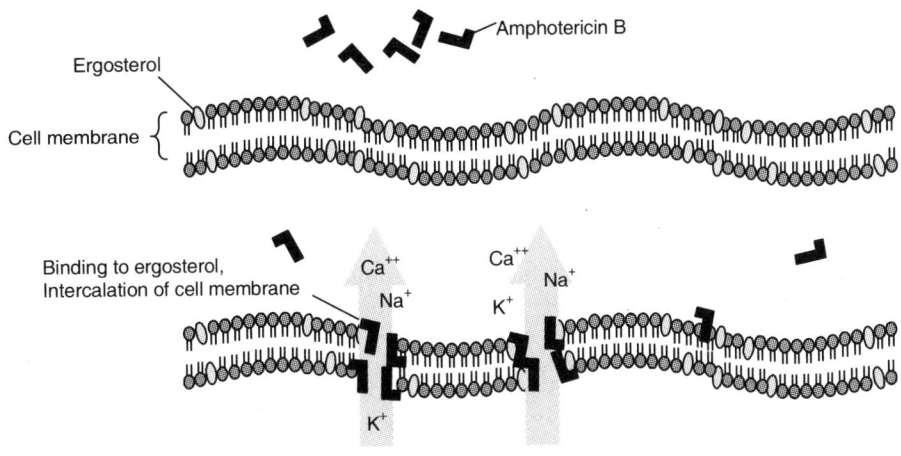

Fig. 60.1: Formation of pore by amphotericin B in cell wall of fungus

Amphotericin B

Amphotericin is a mixture of two compounds A and B, obtained from *Streptomyces nodosus*, a soil *Actinomycete* reported in 1956. As the name suggests, amphotericins are amphoteric in nature. Amphotericin B is a more potent and possesses a broad-spectrum of activity.

Uses

- Amphotericin B is more potent and possesses a broad-spectrum of activity. It is effective against *Aspergillus fumigates, B. dermatitidis, Candida* species, *C. neoformans, H. capsulatum, Coccidioides immitis, M. audouinii, Paracoccidiodes brasiliensis, Rhodotorula* species, *Sporothrix schenckii, Torulopsis glabrata, Trichophyton* species and *mycobacterum leprae*. It exerts maximum antifungal effect between the pH range of 6.0 – 7.5.

- It is available in the form of mixture, lozenges and ointment. It has poor oral absorption pattern. It is effective against a number of fungal infections including aspergillosis, blastomycosis, Candida infections, leishmaniasis, histoplasmosis, sporotrichosis and coccidioidomycosis. It is used topically to treat external ocular infections (i.e. mycotic conjunctivities). For topical use, amphotericin B is available in a 3% concentration as a cream, lotion and ointment. It may be used intravenously or subconjunctivally in the treatment of fungal corneal ulcers or endophthalmitis. In cryptococcal meningitis, it is usually combined with 5-fluorocytosine to get a synergistic action. It may also be given intra-articularly especially in sporotrichosis and coccidioidomycosis.

- In many occasions, flucytosine or rifampin in fact may be added to the regimen in order to reduce the minimum antifungal concentration of amphotericin B. Since the latter is one of the most toxic antimicrobial agent which is in use today, the reduction in the dose of amphotericin B, helps to improve the patient comfort. Amphotericin B methyl ester has equipotent antifungal activity but has better pharmacokinetic features. However, it could not reach to the market because of its ability to cause leukoencephalopathy.

Nystatin

History

It is first isolated from *Streptomyces noursei* in 1951 by Hazen and Brown. The name of this antibiotic was derived from New York state from where it was discovered. It is only slightly soluble in water and is unstable to moisture, heat, light and air. It exerts no effect on bacteria, protozoa or viruses. When used topically, nystatin may sometimes be combined with *iodo-chloro-hydroxyquin*.

Uses

- It is effective specifically against *Candida, Microsporum, Trichophyton, Leishmania, B. denuatitidis, C. neoformans, H. capsulatum, T. vaginalis* and *dermatophytes*. It is often combined with gention violet, procaine hydrochloride, antibiotics or hydrocortisone and is used topically in the treatment of candidiasis of skin, mouth, intestine, conjunctival sac, nails and vagina. It may be given as aerosol or instilled into conjunctival sac. However, it should not be used parenterally due to severe systemic toxicities.

Natamycin

It is yet another tetraene antifungal antibiotic obtained from *Streptomyces natalensis* in 1958. It is a broad-spectrum antifungal agent specifically effective against ocular infections caused by *Fusarium solani* and *Myceliating fungi*. It is used to treat fungal keratitis, fungal blepharitis and fungal conjunctivitis. It may also be inhaled into the respiratory tract to cure bronchopulmonary aspergillosis and candidiasis.

Hamycin and Candicidin

Thses are the examples of other antifungal polyene antibiotics. Candicidin was isolated in 1953 from *Streptomyces griseus* and is used topically in the treatment of vaginal candidiasis. While hamycin is isolated from *Streptomyces pimprima* and is effective against *Blastomyces dermatitidis, Histoplasma capsulatum, Aspergillus fumigatus, Cryptococcus neoformans* and *Candida albicans*. It may be used topically to control vaginal candidiasis.

▓ NATURAL PRODUCT

Griseofulvin

History

It is isolated in 1939 by Oxford, Raistrick and Simonart. Since it was ineffective against bacteria, its appearance on the clinical screen was delayed by almost about 20 years merely due to ignorance about its antifungal activity. It is obtained from the yeast, *Penicillium griseofulvuni*. Gentles in 1958, first reported its antifungal activity.

Mechanism of Action (Fig. 60.2)

Griseofulvin affects only fungi with chitinious cellwall. The drug is fungistatic rather than fungicidal. It is ineffective in the treatment of systemic mycosis. It may be used orally or topically in the treatment of superficial mycosis of skin, hair and nails caused by most strains of Microsporum, Trichophyton and Epidermophyton. It does not have effect on bacteria, yeasts or other fungi. Its antifungal activity is mainly due to its interaction with the polymerized microtubules. Microtubules are the protein structures found in eukaryotic cells that are responsible for the formation of mitotic spindles. The drug induced disruption of mitotic spindles slows down the oxidative phosphorylation and nucleic acid synthesis in the fungal cells.

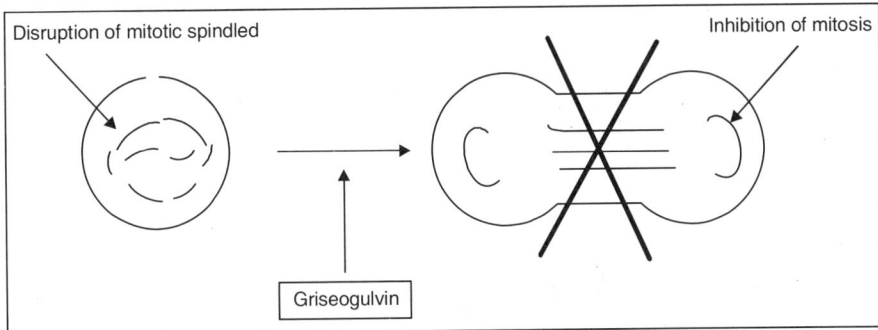

Fig.60.2: Mode of action of griseofulvin

Pharmacokinetic

Major metabolite is 6-methyl-griseofulvin that is excreted in the urine. Some fraction also appears unchanged in the feces. It is also showed promising results in lichen planus, anginal attacks and Raynaud's syndrome.

PYRIMIDINE DERIVATIVES

5-Fluorocytosine

History

- 5-Fluorocytosine is a fluorinated pyrimidine and is related in structure to fluorouracil and flouridine. First introduced in 1957, it failed to build up its career as an effective antineoplastic drug. Ten years thereafter when tested for antifungal activity, it proved its potential against Candida species and *Cryptococcus neoformans* infections.

Mechanism of Action (Fig. 60.3)

The antifungal activity of 5-fluorocytosine is attributed to the formation of 5-fluorouracil an active metabolite is further converted to 5-fluro-2-deoxyuridilic acid which interrupts the fungal DNA synthesis by inhbiting thymidylate synthetase, which is essential for the synthesis of thymidylic acid, an essential DNA component.

- Since mammalians do not contain cytosine deaminase, their function is not affected by flucytosine. Beside this, it is also suspected to interfere in protein synthesis.

Adverse effects

It includes nausea, vomiting, diarrhea, enterocolitis, headache, skin rashes, vertigo, anemia, sedation, hepatomegaly, hepatic necrosis, leukopenia, agranulocytosis and thrombocytopenia.

Uses

- It is not used topically. When used orally, about 4% of administered dose is bound to the plasma proteins. It has a plasma half-life of 4.2–4.5 hours. It is rapidly deaminated in fungal cells to the antimetabolite, 5-fluorouracil. About 80% dose appears in the urine in unchanged form.

- Flucytosine is effective against infections caused by *C. neoformans*, *C. albicans*, *T. glabrata* and *S. schenckii*. It is also effective against chromomycosis caused by cladosporium species and phialophora species. It is used in combination with amphotericin B for the treatment of infections due to yeasts and yeast-like fungi. Amphotericin renders the yeast cell membrane

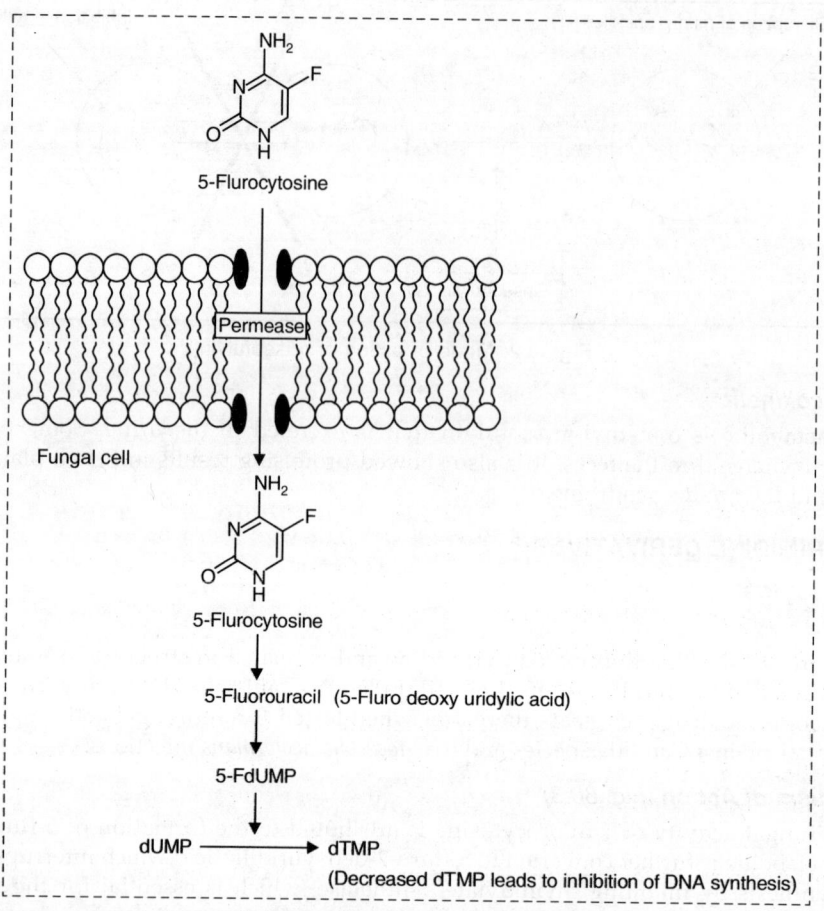

Fig. 60.3: Mode of action of 5-flurocytosine

more permeable to flucytosine. Hence both drugs are used in the treatment of cryptococcal meningitis, Candida endocarditis, pulmonary and urinary tract infection.

- It may also be used in the treatment of chromoblastomycosis.

AZOLE DERIVATIVES (FIG. 60.4)

- Imidazole derivatives are associated with many therapeutic fields. Some have been employed as anthelmintics. Antibacterial and antiprotozoal activities are also observed in some analogs. Miconazole, clotrimazole, ketoconazole, econazole, tioconazole, bifonazole and terconazole are some currently used antifungal imidazole derivatives. They all have activity against a broad range of microorganisms including both fungi and bacteria. Clotrimazole, econazole and tioconazole are effective against superficial fungal infections while bifonazole and terconazole are effective in vulvovaginal. Candidiasis. Other imidazoles like, ketoconazole and raiconazole are effective against both, superficial and systemic infections.

- The cell wall of the fungi mainly contains ergosterol while human contains as cholesterol. For inhibiting the cell wall synthesis in fungi, first we should know about the path by which it is synthesizing ergosterol in it. Let's see that below.

Cell Wall Synthesis in Fungi (Fig. 60.4)

- Azole derivatives act by damaging the fungal cell membrane. They enhance the membrane permeability by inhibiting the synthesis of ergosterol which is the primary cellular sterol of fungi.

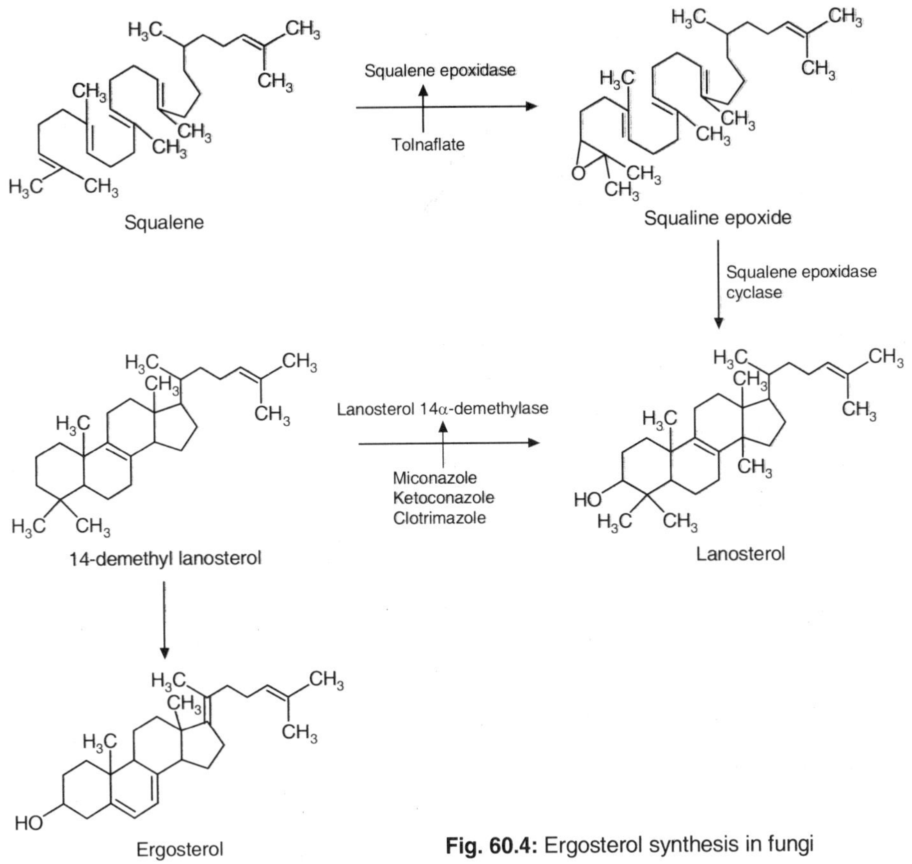

Fig. 60.4: Ergosterol synthesis in fungi

IMIDAZOLE DERIVATIVES

Clotrimazole

Mechanism of action

This is suppose to inhibit the enzyme Lanosterol 14 α-demethylase, which is responsible for demethylation of lanosterol and conversion to ergosterol. The N-3 atom of the azole ring binds to the ferric ion atom in the heme prosthetic group to prevent the activation of oxygen for insertion into lanosterol. Fungal Cyt.P-450 enzymes are 1000 times more sensitive to the azole drug than mammalian enzymes.

Pharmacokinetic

It shows poor oral absorption. Whatever amount absorbed gets rapidly inactivated by cytochrome P-450 enzymes in the liver. It is a broad-spectrum antifungal agent having fungistatic activity against dermatophytes, *C. albicans*, *C. neoformans*, *S. scbenckii* and *B. dermatitidis*. It is used topically in 1–2% concentration as cream, lotion and vaginal preparation to treat cutaneous candidiasis, vulvovaginal candidiasis and dermatophyte infections. It may sometimes be combined with an antibacterial agent in some regimen. Miconazole is a potent antifungal imidazole derivative that may be used topically, intravenously or intrathecally. About 90% of administered dose is bound to the plasma proteins. It has a plasma half-life of 24 hours. It is extensively metabolized in the liver.

Adverse effect

Adverse effects include nausea, vomiting, headache, blurred vision, skin rash, burning, itching, irritation, weakness, arthralgia, seizures, confusion, anemia and thrombocytopenia.

Uses

- It is effectively used topically in the treatment of tinea pedis, tinea cruris, tinea versicolor, onychomycosis, cutaneous candidiasis, pruritus and other superficial dermatomycoses (2% cream, spray, powder or lotion may be applied topically twice a day for 1–2 weeks). To treat vulvovaginal candidiasis and vaginal infections caused by *T. glabratus*, it may be used in the form of a 2% vaginal cream or 100 mg suppositories. The latter may be applied deep in vagina at bedtime for 7 days and in the case of 200 mg vaginal suppositories, a three-day treatment is usually advised. Parenterally, it may be used to control systemic fungal infections like, coccidioidomycosis, paracoccidioidomycosis, cryptococcosis, systemic candidiasis and mucocutaneous candidiasis. In patients with coccidioidal meningitis and urinary bladder infections, the IV route must be supplemented by intrathecal and intrabladder irrigation routes respectively. The free base may also be used topically to treat ophthalmic mycoses.

Ketoconazole

MOA

Same as that of clotrimazole.

Pharmacokinetic

It is an orally active, broad-spectrum antifungal agent that is chemically related with miconazole. About 99% of administered dose is bound to the plasma proteins. It has a plasma half-life of 2–4 hours. It is extensively metabolized in the liver primarily by oxidative dealkylation and aromatic hydroxylation to various inactive metabolites that are excreted (85–90%) in the bile.

Uses

It is effective antifungal agent in the treatment of mucocutaneous candidiasis, vaginitis, oral thrush, blastomycosis, coccidioidomycosis, nonmeningeal cryptococcal disease, histoplasmosis and some dermatomycoses. It may also be concomitantly administered with flucytosine in the treatment of cryptococcal meningitis.

Econazole Nitrate

It is used topically for the treatment of superficial fungal infections of the skin. Mode of action is like clotrimazole.

Tioconazole

It is used in the treatment of dermatophyte infections and candidiasis.

TRIAZOLE DERIVATIVES

Triazole is structurally related to imidazoles and share the same antifungal spectrum and mechanism of action. The triazoles are more slowly metabolized and have less effect on human sterol synthesis than do the imidazole.

Fluconazole

MOA: Same as that of the clotrimazole

Pharmacokinetic: It has increased water solubility and metabolically stable. Absorption is neither pH dependant nor food dependant. It has low protein. binding, and excellent penetration into the central nervous system.

Uses: This is mainly used in candida infection and cryptococcal meningitis. Both of these are serious infectins occur in the AIDS.

Itraconazole

MOA: Same as that of clotrimazole.

Pharmacokinetic: It is water insoluble, lipophilic triazoles analogue that exhibits excellent activity against most human fungal pathogens.

Uses: Recently, it has been found effective in histoplasmosisin HIV infected patient.

CHITIN SYNTHETASE INHIBITORS

Nikomycin

MOA: This is suppose to inhibit chitin synthetase enzyme, which is essential for chitin synthesis.

Chitin is responsible for fungal cell wall synthesis.

MISCELLANEOUS AGENTS

Tolnaflate

MOA

It is suppose to inhibit the squalene epoxidase enzyme, which converts squalene to squalene epoxide in the process of ergosterol synthesis in fungi.

Uses

It is a topical antifungal agent available as cream, solution and powder and aerosol in 1% concentration. It is a thiocarbamate derivative. It is used in the treatment of cutaneous mycoses or ring worm infections. When used against other fungal or bacterial infections, it remains ineffective. It is topically applied to the affected area twice a day. However, relapses may occur after cessation of therapy.

Cyclopirox Olamine

It is a topically used broad-spectrum fungicidal agent effective against dermatophytes. Its antifungal activity may be related to its ability to interfere in uptake of precursors needed for the synthesis of proteins and nucleic acid core. Adverse effects are few and include pruritis and burning at the site of appliction.

Potassium Iodide

In the form of saturated solution of 1 g/ml, it may be used orally as an effective antifungal agent in the treatment of cutaneous and lymphatic forms of sporotrichosis, caused by S. schenckii. It is excreted in the urine. It probably acts by iodination of proteins in fungus cell membrane. Adverse effects include nausea, vomiting, diarrhea, heart burn, sneezing, tearing, metallic taste, acne form skin lesions and swelling of parotid gland. Iodism is frequently encountered during , the therapy.

Whitfield's Ointment

It contains a mixture of benzoic acid (fungistatic agent) and salicylic acid (keratolytic agent). The keratolytic action of salicylic acid helps for desquamation of stratum corneum. This promotes the removal of offending fungus resulting into better penetration of antifungal agent.

Antibiotics

Many antibiotics like, minocycline, tetracyclines have antifungal potential. They may enhance activity of antifungal agent (e.g. amphotericin B) when concomitantly used.

Other Organic Compounds

Salicylic acid, aminacrine, acrisorcin, halopragin, p-chloro-metaxylenol, salicylamide, salicylanilide, iodochlorhydroxyquin, m-cresyl acetate, diamethazole, chlordantoin, gention violet, pecilocin, diiodohydroxy quinoline, iodine, phenylmercuric nitrate, thymol and zinc pyrithione possess significant antifungal activity. Most of them may be used in the treatment of ringworm infections of scalp, feet and groin.

- Haloprogin is a synthetic iodinated trichlorophenol available as a 1% cream. It is effective against various candidal and ringworm infections of the skin. Thymol in 1–2% concentration may be added to Whitfield's ointment to enhance its antifungal potential.

- Zinc pyrithione may be used as 1% solution to control infections due to the *Pityrosporum ovale* and *Tinea versicolor*. While salicylanilide may be used along with undecylenic acid in the form of 5% ointment to exhibit antifungal activity.

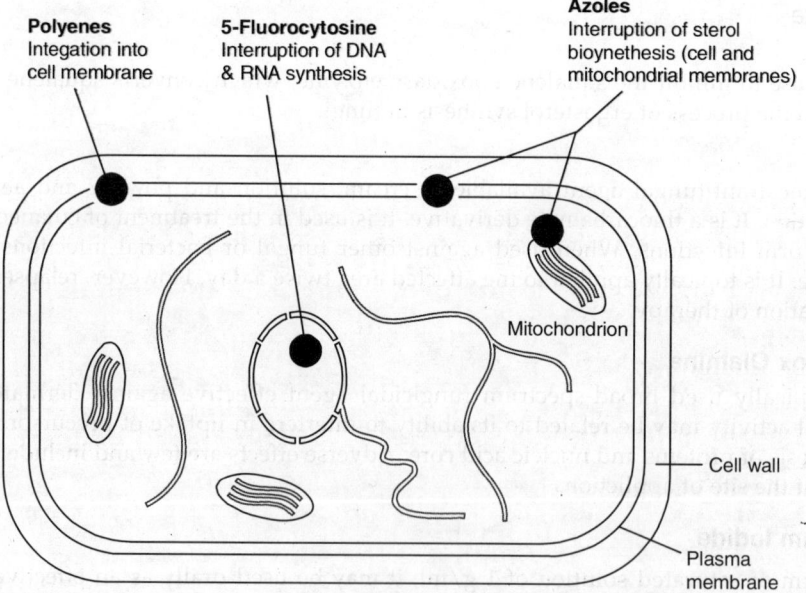

Fig. 60.5: Mechanism of action of polynes, azoles and 5-fluorocytosine

Miconazole

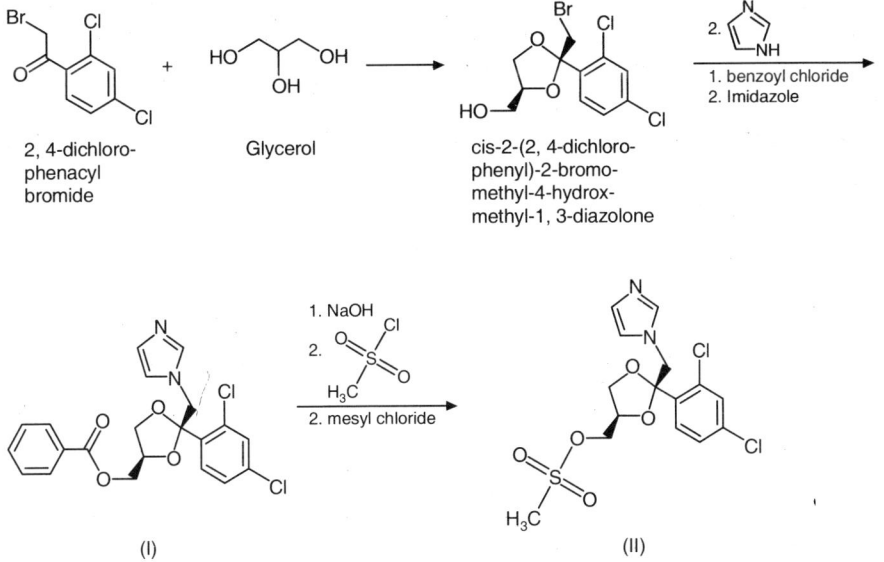

Ketoconazole

II + 1-acetyl-4-(4-hydroxyphenyl)-piperazine

$\xrightarrow{\text{NaH sodium hydride}}$ Ketoconazole

Clotrimazole

2-chloro-toluene $\xrightarrow{\text{Cl}_2,\ Hv}$ 2-chlorobenzo-trichloride $\xrightarrow[\text{benzene (I)}]{,\ AlCl_3}$ 2-chlorotriphenyl-methyl chloride (II)

Clotrimazole $\xleftarrow{}$ Imidazotriethyl amine

Econazole

1-(2, 4-dichlorophenyl)-2-(1H-imidazol-1-yl)ethanol

1. NaH
2. Cl—

1. sodium hydride
2. 4-chlorobenzyl chloride

Econazole

Fluconazole

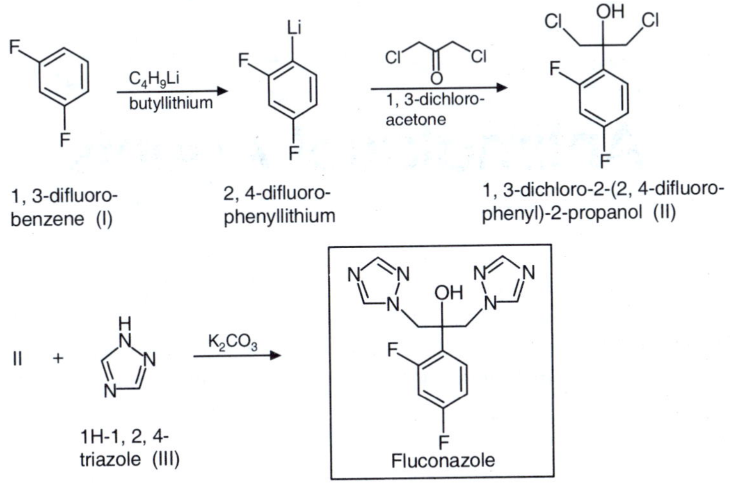

1, 3-difluoro-benzene (I) → 2, 4-difluoro-phenyllithium → 1, 3-dichloro-2-(2, 4-difluoro-phenyl)-2-propanol (II)

C₄H₉Li butyllithium

1, 3-dichloro-acetone

II + 1H-1, 2, 4-triazole (III)

K₂CO₃

Fluconazole

Flucytosine

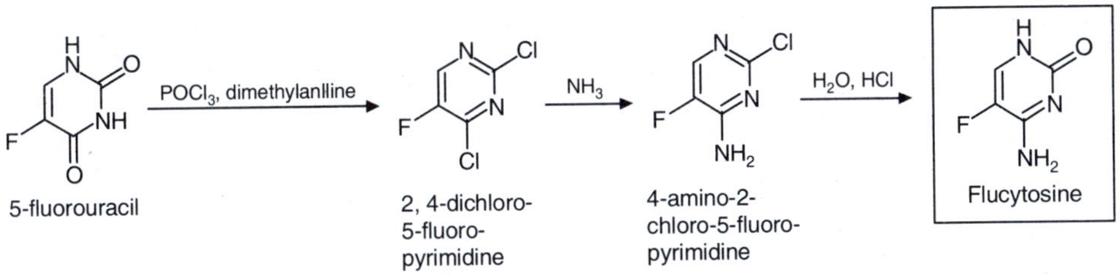

5-fluorouracil → 2, 4-dichloro-5-fluoro-pyrimidine → 4-amino-2-chloro-5-fluoro-pyrimidine → Flucytosine

POCl₃, dimethylanlline

NH₃

H₂O, HCl

61

Antimalarial Agents

In developing countries, the paramount needs are still related to nutrition, communicable diseases and poverty. The messianic call for "health for all by the year 2000", however emotionally attractive, is very difficult to achieve, in the surroundings of hard realities—unhealthy economic system influences the standards of both, health and education in the country.

- Malaria is one of such diseases whose appearance may be related with the socio-economic status of the society. Malaria is mainly a disease of tropic and sub-tropic countries. Though on large scale, malaria eradication program was initiated since from 1957, this disease still affects about 200 million people and causes at least 2 million deaths per year.

- Malaria in humans is caused by the infection with protozoan parasites of the genus, Plasmodium. These parasites spend an asexual phase in a man and a sexual phase in female Anopheles mosquitos. Out of several hundred known Anopheles species, four species infect man.

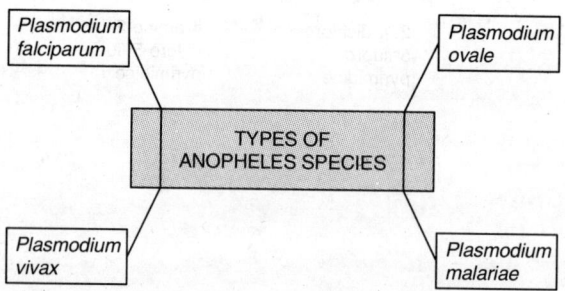

1. **Plasmodium falciparum:** It causes malignant tertian or subtertian form of malaria, which may cause death by invading the CNS. About half of the cases of malaria are caused by this species. In this type, the attacks are more severe and relapses do not occur.

2. **Plasmodium vivax:** It causes benign tertian malaria in which fever revisits patient every 48 hours or on the third day. About 40% of the cases of malaria are caused by this species.

3. **Plasmodium malariae:** It is responsible for the occurrence of quartan malaria in which fever repeats after every 72 hours. It is a milder form of infection. *Plasmodium falciparum* and *P. malariae* do not persist within the liver cells after erythrocytes have become infected.

4. **Plasmodium ovale:** It is responsible for the mild tertian malaria which is most commonly seen in West Africa. Except *P. falciparum*, all three species of Anopheles have a secondary exoerythrocytic stage. *Plasmodium vivax* and *P. ovale* do persist within the liver cells even after erythrocytes become infected and may produce true relapses months or even years after.

▨ LIFE CYCLE OF MALARIAL PARASITE (FIG. 61.1)

Pre-erythrocytic Phase

The female Anopheles mosquito feeds on vertebrate blood. Malaria infection is initiated through the bite of infected female Anopheles mosquito which releases motile sporozoites into the human bloodstream. Within 1–2 hours the sporozoites get entry into the parenchymal cells of the liver. Through repeated nuclear divisions sporozoites multiply and develop into schizonts. After the period of 10–16 days, liver cells rupture due to multiple repeated divisions of schizonts. This results in the release of approximately 20,000 merozoites into circulation. This stage is known as pre-erythrocytic or exo-erythrocytic phase of infection.

Erythrocytic Phase

Merozoites now enter into the circulation and invade erythrocytes. Some merozoites invade fresh liver cells and repeat erythrocytic cycle. Erythrocytes are invaded by merozoites for the following reasons.

1. The plasma constituents and hemoglobin serve as a source of several amino acids necessary for the survival of the parasite.
2. For rapid multiplication of merozoites, the purine bases (i.e. adenine and guanine) are obtained from erythrocytes which are then utilized to synthesize parasitic DNA and RNA molecules.
3. Pentoses and phosphates are necessary for nucleic acid synthesis. The protozoal parasites do not have any means to get these raw materials. Obviously it is the host who is going to suffer.

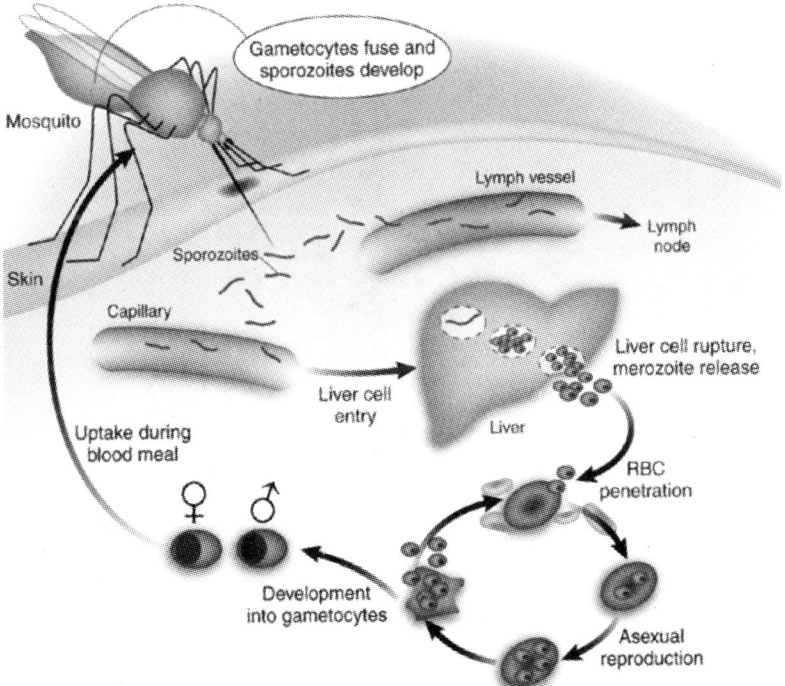

Fig. 61.1: Life cycle of malarial parasite

Schizogony Phase

- Inside erythrocytes, the merozoites continue to grow. In erythrocytes, the merozoites undergo asexual "multiplication, which results into formation of daughter cells, schizonts. Due to the repeated multiplication of the latter, erythrocyte ruptures and releases about 6–24 merozoites into the circulation.
- Each merozoites again invades fresh erythrocyte and the cycle of asexual multiplication is repeated again. This stage is known as schizogony phase of infection. It continues for 48–72 hours. Febrile clinical manifestations are witnessed due to schizogony phase.

Sexual Phase

- After schizogony phase, some of the erythrocytic merozoites develop into male and female gametocytes by some unidentified mechanisms. Such infected blood when ingested by female mosquito, the sexual forms (i.e. gametocytes) undergoes sexual reproduction within the gut of the insect.
- The resulting zygote, through various stages of development gives rise to the infective sporozoites. The latter gets localized in the salivary glands of the insect and enters the host blood circulation when the infected mosquito bites a healthy person. The story thus goes on repeating.

▨ SYMPTOMS OF MALARIA (FIG. 61.2)

The life cycle of malaria protozoa is dependent on the erythrocytes of the human host, where the parasite undergoes main morphological changes. The symptoms of malaria, however, are reported

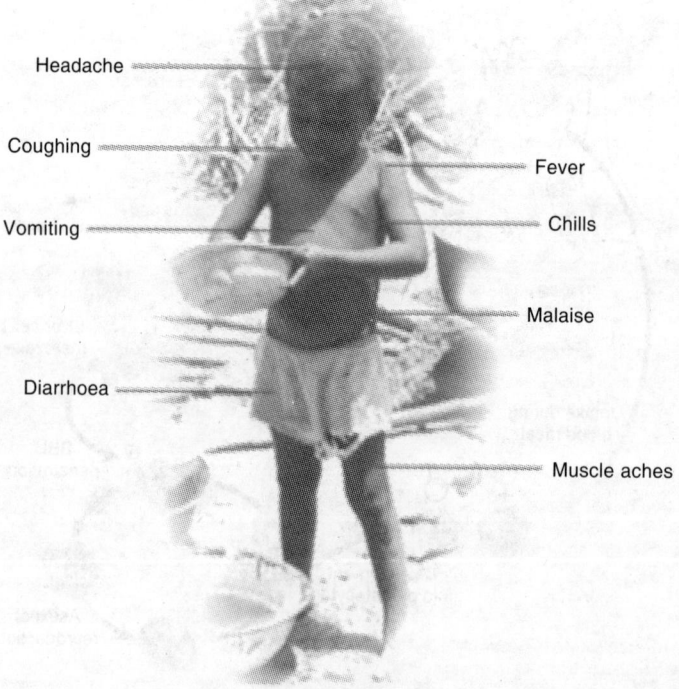

Fig. 61.2: Symptoms of malaria

to occur about 12–16 days after the mosquito bite. It means that the pre-erythrocytic phase is free of any symptoms. It is the erythrocytic phase, which is responsible for the occurrence of various symptoms of malaria. These symptoms can be grouped together as follows.

1. Symptoms like nausea, vomiting, severe chills delirium and fever may reappear after every 3 to 4 days depending upon the species of protozoa and hence upon the type of malaria.

2. As the erythrocytic phase continues, increasing number of erythrocytes undergo destruction, resulting into severe form of anemia.

3. To provide necessary amino acids for the multiplication of parasite, haemoglobin undergoes breakdown process. If this process continues, it leads to jaundice because of accumulated bilirubin.

CHEMOTHERAPY OF MALARIA

Two different attempts have been made to design new or modern antimalarial drugs. After studying the lifestyle of malaria parasite in human, many drugs were designed and their target selectivity was tested for various phases of plasmodium lifecycle (Flow chart 61.1).

Flow chart 61.1: Classification of antimalarial

Classification Based Upon Pharmacological Action

a. **Drugs effective against primary tissue schizonts or pre-erythrocytic phase:** These drugs are also known as prophylactic agents. Since no drug is effective at this stage, true prophylaxis does not exist for malarial parasites. Example includes primaquine.

b. **Drugs active against erythrocyte phase:** These drugs are also known as schizontocidal agents. Examples include modiaquine, chloroquine, mefloquine, quinine, pyrimethamine, etc.

c. **Drugs active against gametocy phase:** These drugs are also known gametocytocidal agents, e.g. primaquine. Gametocyte of *P. falciparum* may remain in the circulation for prolonged period, even after the patient receives the treatment with chloroquine. These gametocytes are rapidly killed by a single dose 79 mg of primaquine phosphate.

- In second approach, the host-parasite relationship was thoroughly examined to point-out biochemical differences. For example, mammalian cells are capable of utilizing preformed folates while bacteria and protozoa are unable to do so. Hence they must synthesize folates of their own. Hence such drugs that selectively inhibit folate biosynthesis in the protozoa blocking the enzymes involved therein can be used for suppression or radical cure of malaria.

- Certain antimalarial drugs are not capable of destroying plasmodium merozoites. They just inhibit the erythrocytic stage of development of malarial parasite and thus prevent the onset of symptoms, the treatment with such drugs is known as suppressive treatment. It may be used to prevent maturation of the erythrocytic infection but it may not have any effect on the stages in liver cells. It serves as a prophylactic measure before entering the area susceptible to malarial infection. Drugs commonly employed in suppressive treatment are chloroquine, amodiaquine, pyrimethamine and proguanil. While some antimalarial drugs completely destroy the plasmodium merozoites and thus terminate the malarial attack. Such agents are said to provide clinical cure of the disease. Examples include, chloroquine, amodiaquine.

- However, the patients treated with these agents may show the relapse of the disease due to the presence of gametocytes in the circulation for prolonged period even after the drug treatment. Radical cure is the third category in which a combination therapy is generally used to eradicate both, the developed parasites and those still developing in the erythrocytes and other tissues. Generally primaquine is used in combination with chloroquine or amodiaquine.

Quinolines

a. Cinchona alkaloids

Cinchonin (+) isomer
Cinchonidine (−) isomer

Quinin (+) isomer
Quinidine (−) isomer

b. 4-Aminoquinoline

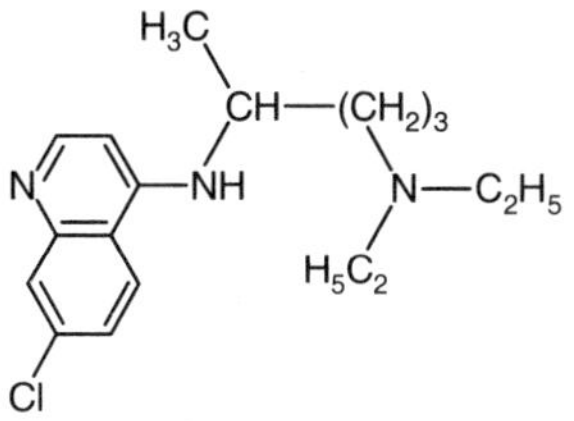

Chloroquine

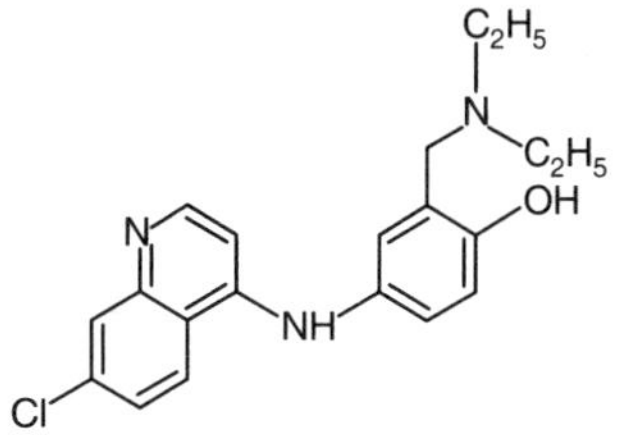

Amodiquine

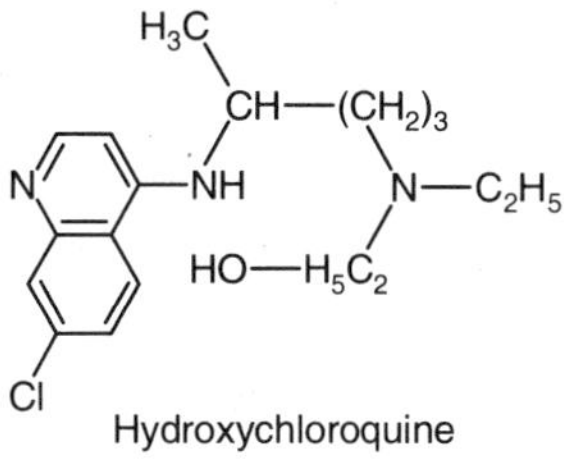

Hydroxychloroquine

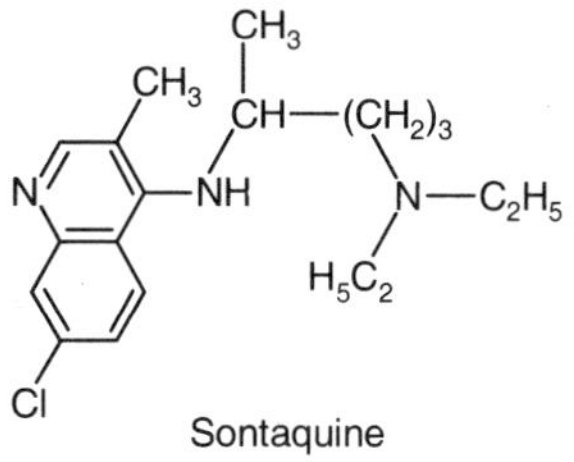

Sontaquine

c. 8-Aminoquinoline

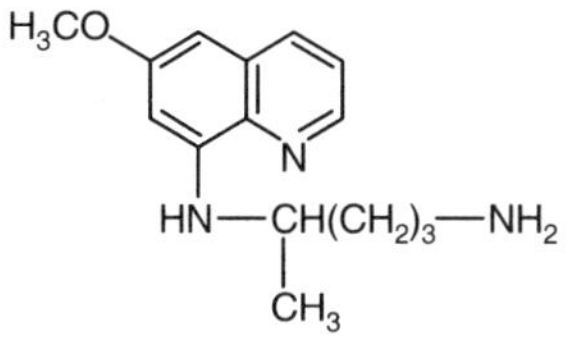

Primaquine

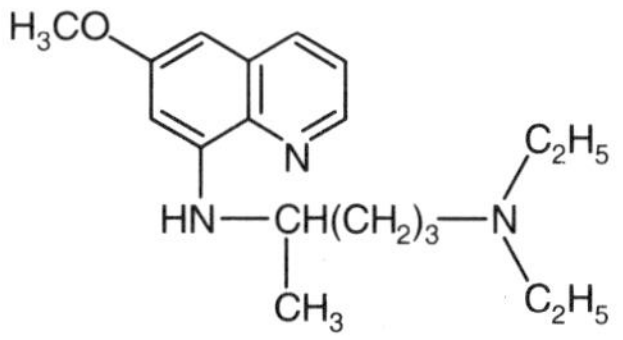

Pamaquine

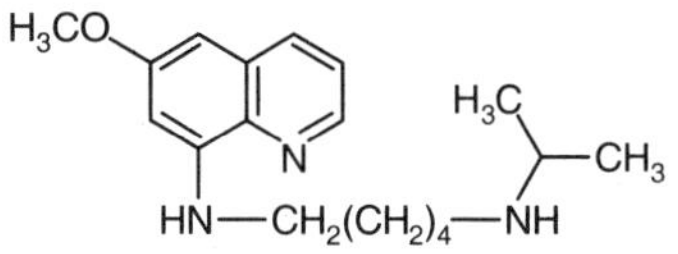

Pentaquine

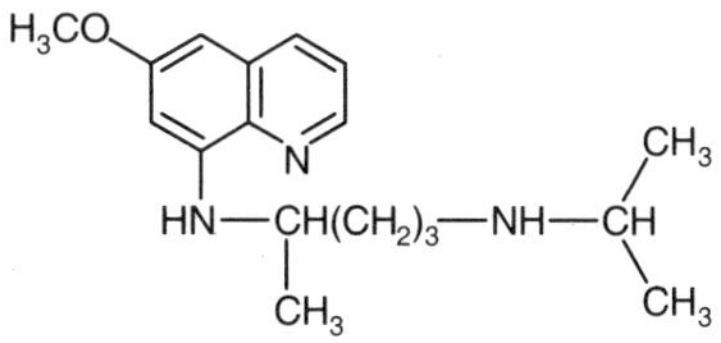

Isopentaquine

9-Aminoacridines

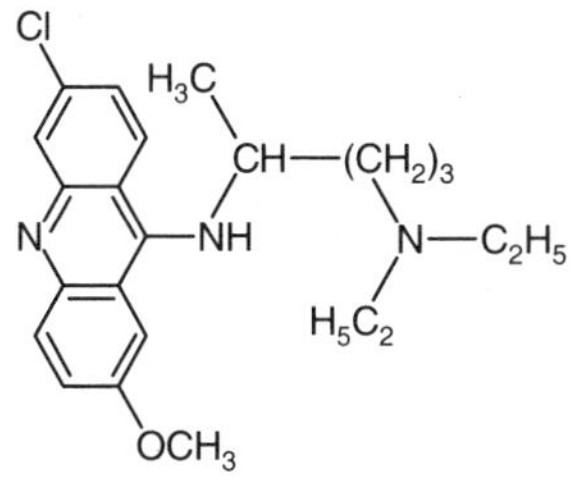

Quinacrine

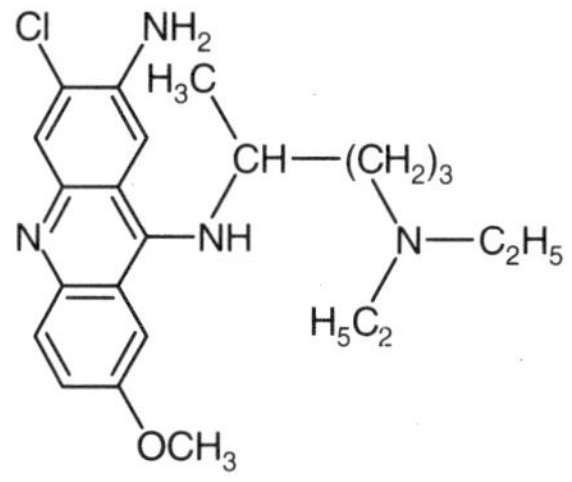

Aminoacriquine

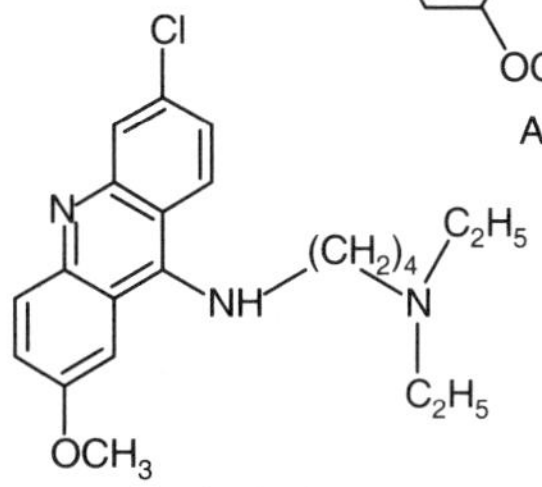

Acriquine

2, 4-Diaminopyrimidines

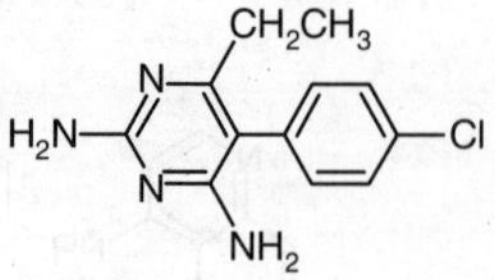

Pyrimethamine

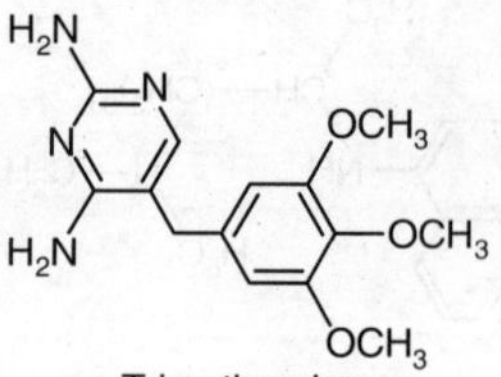

Trimethoprime

Biguanides

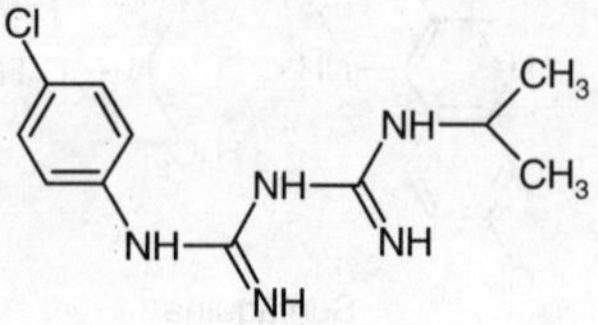

Proguanil

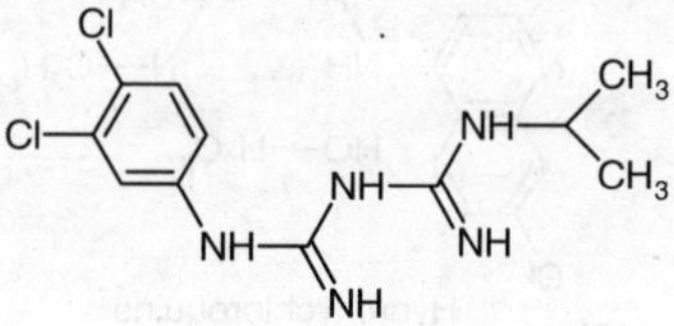

Chlorproguanil

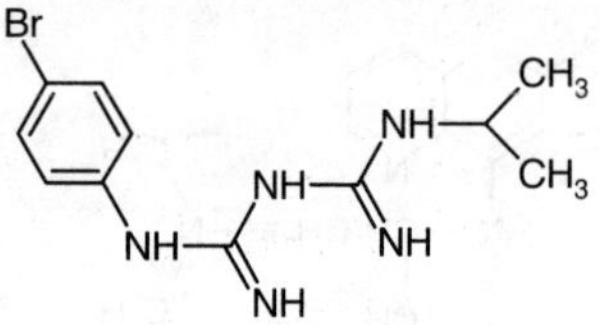

Bromoguanil

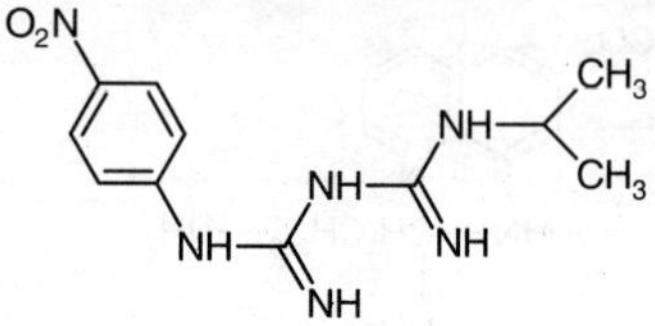

Nitroguanil

Sulfones and Sulfonamides

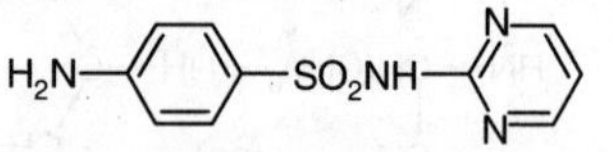

Sulfadiazine

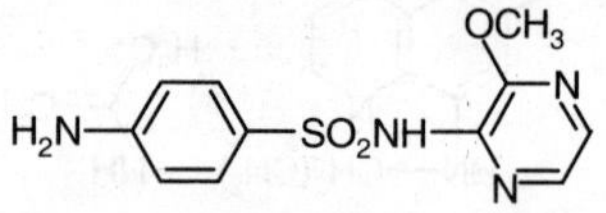

Sulfalene

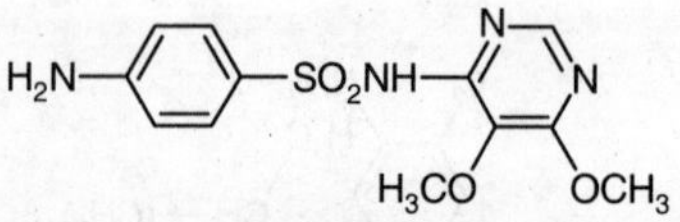

Sulfadoxine

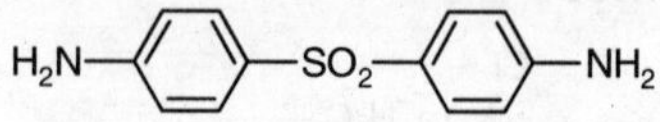

Dapsone

Miscellaneous

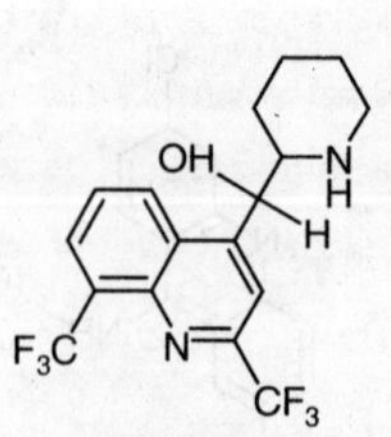

Mefloquine

▓ CLASSIFICATION BASED ON CHEMICAL STRUCTURE

Early discoveries of Paul Ehrlich with organic dyes and organoarsenicals gave new dimensions to the traditional methods of treating malaria. Presently available various antimalarials are the direct outcome of Ehrlich outstanding pioneering efforts. On the chemical basis, antimalarial drugs are classified as:

1. Quinolines.
   a. Cinchona alkaloids.
   b. 4-aminoquinolines.
   c. 8-aminoquinolines.
2. 9-aminoacridines.
3. 2 4-diaminopyrimidines.
4. Biguanides.
5. Sulfones and sulfonamides.
6. Miscellaneous agents.

Cinchone Alkaloids

Chemistry

- Cinchona bark contains a mixture of more than 20 alkaloids. Four major alkaloids are isolated from the cinchona bark. They are effective against erythrocytic merozoites and constitute a part of suppressive treatment of malaria. All four are derivatives of a 4-quinolinemethanol which is linked with a substituted quinuclidine moiety.
- Quinine and its d-isomer, quinidine are the only cinchona alkaloids currently in the use. Quinine is the most active antimalarial ingredient of the cinchona bark and is present in highest concentration to the extent of about 5.0%. It is schizonticidal and gametocytocidal for *P. vivax and P. malariae*. It is orally active in the form of sulfate while quinine dihydrochloride may be used for intravenous administration. The antimalarial activity is mainly associated with the levorotatory form, subcutaneous or intramuscular administration is not usually recommended due to local tissue damage.

Structure–activity relationship

1. Antimalarial activity is usually enhanced by the introduction of Halogen at position C-8.
2. Asymmetry at carbon 3 and 4 is not essential for activity.
3. Addition of phenyl at position 2 increases the antimalarial activity. But such 2-phenyl derivatives were found to be phototoxic.
4. More recently, it was found that high activity without phototoxicity could be obtained by blocking position C-2 with trifluromethyl.
5. Presence of methoxy group in quinine is not essential for the activity. Replacement of methoxy group by a halogen, especially chlorine, enhances the activity.
6. Modification of alcohol at C-9, through oxidation or esterification diminishes the activity.
7. The distance between the oxygen (of OH group) and non-aromatic nitrogen should be about 3Å. Any change in this distance may lead to inactivation of compound.
8. Antimalarial activity was found only when there is proper orientation possible between hydroxyl hydrogen and amine hydrogen in such a way that hydrogen bonding should be possible.
9. Quinaclindine portion is not essential for activity.

Uses

- It is extremely useful in treating chloroquine-resistant *P. falciparum* infections. High doses of quinine may produce a quinidine like depressant effect on the heart. It causes vasodilation and may cause hypotension.
- Since it antagonizes the actions of physostigmine on the skeletal muscles by exerting curare-like effect, it may be beneficial in the symptomatic relief of nocturnal muscle cramps or myotonia congenita. Toxic doses of quinine may induce abortion.
- It has analgesic, antipyretic and local anaesthetic properties.
- Due to its low therapeutic index, quinine is not used alone. It may be used along with primaquine, pyrimethamine or a sulphonamide in the combination therapy,

4-Aminoquinolines

History

During the period 1940–1944, very limited number of antimalarials was available in the market. They were associated with a high toxicity profile and a low therapeutic index. To overcome this situation, 4-aminoquinolines were investigated in United States through a research program. Chloroquine, hydroxychloroquine and amodiaquine are the most important members of this series.

Chemistry

Chemically, chloroquine is 7-chloro-4 (4-diethylamino-1-methylbutylamino) quinoline. Due to the presence of asymmetric carbon in the side chain, it exists in isomers. The chemical name of amodiaquine is 7-chloro-4-(3-diethylamino-4-hydroxyanilino) quinoline. Both these drugs are effective against a sexual erythrocytic form of all four plasmodium species.

Structure–activity relationship

1. A dialkylaminoalkyl side chain, having 2, 5 carbon atoms between the nitrogen atoms, particularly 4-dimethylamino 1-methyl butyl amino side chain is optimal for chloroquine and quinacrine.

2. The tertiary amino group in side chain is very important for antimalarial activity.

3. The introduction of an unsaturated bond in the side chain was not determental of activity.

4. The 7-chlorogroup in the quinoline nucleus is optimal and methyl group in position C-3, reduces the activity and an additional methyl group in position C-8 completely abolishes the activity.

5. The substitution of a hydroxy on one of the ethyl groups on the tertiary amine (hydroxyl quinoline) generally reduces the toxicity and increases the plasma concentration.

6. Incorporation of an aromatic ring in the side chain, e.g. in amodiquine, gives a compound with reduced toxicity and activity.

7. The d-isomer of chloroquine is somewhat less toxic than levo-isomer.

8. The quinoline ring system seems to be inherently more active than the acridine for a given side chains.

Pharmacokinetic

Principal metabolites include desethylchloroquine, bisdesethylchloroquine and a carboxylic acid analog which are excreted in the urine along with 52–53% dose in unchanged form.

Adverse effect

Chloroquine and amodiaquine have some depressant effects on the bone marrow. Both these agents cause hemolysis in patients with glucose-6-phosphate dehydrogenase deficiency. The toxicity profiles of these agents are less severe and include nausea, vomiting, headache, blurred vision and dermatitis. Chloroquine is more prone to cause photoallergic dermatitis since 'it accumulates in the skin to the greater extent than amodiaquine. Hence it must be used with caution in children.

Uses

- Chloroquine also has antihistaminic and anti-inflammatory properties. It is used to treat hepatic amoebiasis, rheumatoid arthritis, discoid lupus erythematosus, solar urticaria and polymorphous light erruptions.
- It is a drug of choice for the suppressive prophylaxis and for the treatment of acute clinical attacks in all types of malaria except chloroquine-resistant falciparum strains. For the treatment of chloroquine-resistant falciparum malaria, a combination therapy comprising of quinine pyrimethamine and sulfadiazine may be given. The combination of a 2-day course of quinine and a single dose of mefloquine is even more effective.
- In chloroquine sensitive strains, response in adults is rapid when 1.5 g of chloroquine is given over 2 days. If parenteral administration is required, the intramuscular route should be preferred. However to prevent relapsing malaria, a single dose of 79 mg of primaquine phosphate may also be given to the patient Amodiaquine hydrochloride and hydroxy chloroquine sulfate are other clinically used members of this group having uses and adverse effects similar to chloroquine.

8-Aminoquinolines

Spectrum of action

- Primaquine was the first synthetic antimalarial agent to be introduced into the clinical practice in 1929. Principal agents from this class include primaquine, pamaquine and quinocide.
- In contrast to 4-aminoquinolines, these agents lack activity against erythrocytic merozoites. In fact they attack both, the pre-erythrocytic phase of the disease and also show gametocidal activity to some extent. Obviously then, if used alone, they can only be used for prophylactic purposes. They produce radical cure of vivax malarias when they are used along with chloroquine.

Structure–activity relationship

1. Compounds with high chemotherapeutic index had a 6-methoxy group in quinoline nucleus and it may be substituted by H, OH or low OR group.
2. The 2, 4 or 6-methoxy analogue of 8-diethylamino-propyl-aminoquino-line were all active.
3. The introduction of a second methoxy group at position 2 or 5 increases therapeutic index.
4. Optimal activity was obtained with 2, 6-methylene group between the two nitrogen of the side chain. Homologs with an even number of methylene group were found to be less active than those odd numbers.
5. The extent of the substitution of the terminal amine is not as critical as in 4-aminoquinolines and the terminal aliphatic amino group may be primary, secondary or tertiary. But the aromatic amine must be secondary.
6. Additional substituents is in the quinoline nucleus at the C-5 and C-5 position may be beneficial, such as 5-phenoxy derivatives

Adverse effect

Their toxic effects are much more severe than those of 4-aminoquinolines and are related principally to the central nervous system and circulatory system. These include nausea, vomiting, anorexia, headache, hemolytic anemia, leukopenia and methemoglobinemia. Because of its relative safety and lower toxicity, primaquine is the only member of this series which is clinically used.

Pharmacokinetic

In the form of its diphosphate, primaquine is completely observed by oral route. It is rapidly metabolized to various metabolities that include 5-hydroxyprimaquine, 5-hydroxy-6-desmethyl primaquine and 8-(3-carboxyl-1-methyl-propylamino)-6-methoxy quinoline. They all appear in the urine along with small amount of unchanged drug. The parenteral form of primaquine is not available.

Uses

- It is usually given along with a 4-aminoquinoline schizontocide (e.g. chloroquine) to prevent relapses in *P. vivax* and *P. ovale* infections and to reduce the chances of development of chloroquine resistant strains of plasmodium.

- It may also be used against primary exoerythrocytic forms of *P. falciparum*. Besides this, it also depresses myocardial excitability and possesses antiarrhythmic actions.

9-Aminoacridines

- Quinacrine, acriquine and aminoacrichin are the clinically useful agents from this class.

- Quinacrine is the most active compound of the series. In general, this derivative poses a high degree of risk with low activity profile. Hence after the development of 4-aminoquinolines, they are used rarely for the treatment of malaria.

- Yellow pigmentation of the skin and yellow colour appears in the urine during the treatment with quinacrine. These signs disappear with the discontinuation of therapy. Nausea, vomiting, headache, convulsions, aplastic anemia and sychomimetic reactions are the adverse effects associated with these drugs.

▨ MODE OF ACTION OF ABOVE MENTIONED CLASSES

Interaction with DNA (Fig. 61.3)

- The quinoline ring containing agents are thought to attach to DNA. The flat ring system intercalates between base pairs in double helical DNA and the side chains in their charged tertiary amino group bind ionically to the negatively charged phosphate group of the deoxyribose phosphate backbone.

- The other interactions mentioned are alcoholic hydroxyl group of quinolonemethanols form hydrogen bonds with one of the DNA bases, and the 7-chloro atom in chloroquine and analogs is electrostatically attracted to the guanine 2-amino group (guanidine specificity). These bindings considerably hamper the required separation of complementary strands of the parent double-helical DNA. Mefloquine does not act by this mechanism. But the current view is that the antimalarial alkaloid blood schizontocides concentrate in and raise the pH of acidic vesicle within sensitive malarial parasite. There, they interfere with lysosomal degradation of haemoglobin and cause clumping of pigments. The plasmodia selectively concentrate these drugs. However, inhibition of the function of Ca^{2+} dependant proteins such as calmodulin has also been implicated.

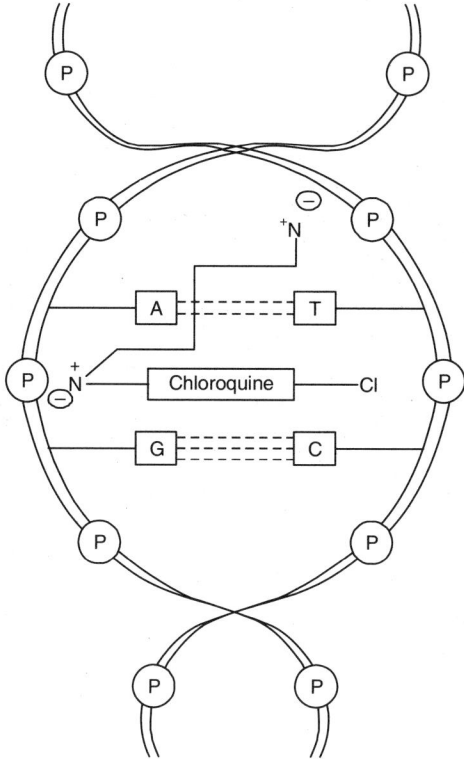

Fig. 61.3: Interacalation of chloroquine between the two strands of DNA

Inhibition of Polymerase Enzyme (Fig. 61.4)

- A recent mechanism of action of chloroquine, amodiaquine and other 4-aminoquinolines has been suggested. This involves interaction between feriprotoporphyrin IX (FP) and chloroquine. Upon digestion of haemoglobin, the heme is released as FP. FP has been shown to induce hemolysis of erythrocytes, lysis of malarial parasites.

- The FP released upon hemoglobin digestion is detoxified by the parasite through conversion to hemozoin, a non-toxic by product. A complex form between chloroquine and FP that itself is toxic to the cell. Thus chloroquine prevents the conversion of FP (a toxic) to non-toxic hemozoin.

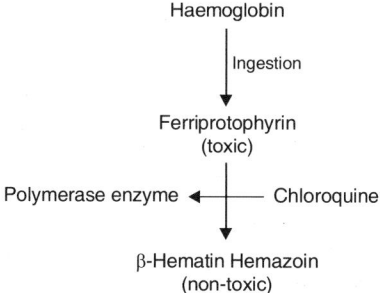

Fig. 61.4: One of the possible mechanism of action of chloroquine

2, 4-Diaminopyrimidines

Mechanism of action

- Tetrahydrofolate (FAH_4) is required for the biosynthesis of purines, pyrimidines and certain amino acids (needed for protozoal DNA synthesis). It is obtained by the reduction of dihydrofolate (FAH_2) catalyzed by the enzyme, dihydrofolate reductase. Mammalian cells are permeable to folates whereas bacteria and protozoa are unable to transport preformed folates. Hence they must synthesize their own folates. Thus any attempt to inhibit protozoal biosynthesis of FAH_2 (e.g. sulfonamide) or a selective inhibition of the protozoal enzyme, dihydrofolate reductase (e.g. pyrimethamine) will lead to the disturbances in the protozoal DNA synthesis. This leads to the death of protozoal cells. Pyrimethamine inhibits malarial dihydrofolate reductase at concentration far lower than needed to inhibit the mammalian enzymes.

- Due to the structural similarity with part of FAH_2 structure, pyrimethamine competitively tries to block the action of dihydrofolate reductase enzyme. However, parasites can develop drug resistance due to utilization of alternative metabolic pathways. Sulfonamides inhibit the conversion of folinic acid to dihydrofolate. Hence the combination of pyrimethamine with a long-acting sulpha drug, (e.g. sutfadoxine, sulfamethoxazole, etc.) gives supradditive therapeutic effect and reduce the chances for developing drug-resistant strains. Pyrimethamine is more potent antimalarial agent chloroguanide and has a much longer duration of action because of its slow rate of excretion.

Structure–activity relationship

1. An electron releasing substituent is present at position six.
2. Chlorine atom is present at para position.
3. Two rings are not separated by carbon or other atom.

Pyrimethamine

Uses

- In this series, pyrimethamine and trimethoprim are the effective antimalarial agents. After establishing itself as a good antibacterial agent, trimethoprim secured a place in the chemotherapy of malaria. These derivatives are effective against both the exoerythrocytic and erythrocytic phases of the disease.

Trimethoprime

Pyrimethamine is very effective in the chemoprophylaxis and treatment of chloroquine-resistant falciparum malaria. It is also used in the treatment of toxoplasmosis and pneumocytosis. Diaminopyrimidines, biguanides and dihydrotriazines are the drugs which are designed through the studies of biochemical differences between the host and parasites.

- Due to non-selectivity in bacterial enzyme inhibition and shorter half-life, trimethoprim is never used alone in the treatment of malaria. It is usually combined with another antimalarial agent.

Biguanides

Structure–activity relationship

1. The presence of an N_1-aryl is important, but the introduction of a second group decreased the activity.
2. Dihalogen substitution in position 3 and 4 of the benzene ring yields potent drugs.
3. Alkyl substitution on N_1, N_2 or N_4 leads to decrease in activity.

4. Replacement of isopropyl group by normal propyl group at N$_5$ gives essentially equal activity.

5. The introduction of shorter or longer alkyl chains resulted in decreased activity.

Mechanism of action

- The antimalarial activity of cycloguanil is due to its structural and functional similarity with pyrimethamine. Due to this similarity, the parasites which are resistant to the action of pyrimethamine, also exhibits resistance to the action of chloroguanide. It inhibits dihydrofolate reductase enzyme and interferes in the folic acid metabolism. This leads to inhibition of nuclear division in malarial parasites. Cycloguanil has duration of action of several weeks. The drug damages gametocytes so that they fail to complete their cycle in mosquito.

- Chloroguanide acts slowly and is effective against susceptible strains of plasmodium. However, the development of drug resistant strains limits its clinical utility, in the form of hydrochloride, it is used orally. While in the form of cyclo-guanil embonate or pamoate, it is used intramuscularly. It provides a longer duration of action.

Sulfones and Sulfonamides

History

Though the antimalarial potency of sulfonamides was proved long back in 1943, they were neglected because of their low therapeutic index. Later on, due to the development of chloroquine resistant strains of *P. faliciparum*, long-acting sulfonamides were tried in combination with pyrimethamine or trimethoprim. Dapsone, in combination with pyrimethamine can also be effectively used as a chemoprophylactic agent against drug-resistant strains of malarial parasites.

MOA

Refer Sulfonamide Chapter 57.

Pharmacokinetic

Dapsone is found to possess mild toxicity and prolonged duration of action. Both, sulfonamides and sulfones are active only against erythrocytic stages of malarial parasite. They are ineffective in the treatment of *P. vivax* infections.

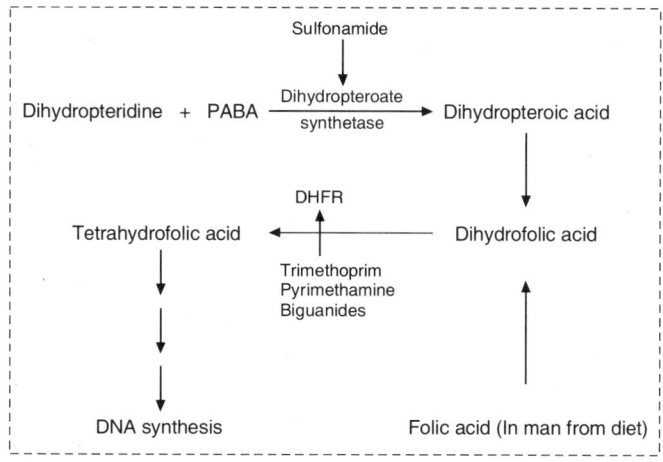

Miscellaneous Agents

Mefloquine

Pharmacokinetic: It bears some degree of structural similarity with quinine. Chemically, it is a 4-quinoline-carbinolamine. It is marketed in the form of its racemic mixture where the erythro form is more active than threo isomer. It is an orally active derivative of 4-quinoline – methanol. About 95–98% of administered dose is bound to the plasma proteins. It has a plasma half-life of 17 days. Principal metabolites include 2, 8-bis-trifluoromethyl quinoline-4-methanol and a carboxylic acid analog. They are excreted in the faeces. Presence of trifluoromethyl moiety at position 2 lowers down the rate of metabolism and precludes the phototoxic effects commonly associated with other carbinolamines.

Mechanism of action: Very little is known about its mechanism of action. It is predicted that it may be acting at erythrocytic stage in the lifecycle of plasmodium. It may affect the ring stages of *P. faciparum* and *P. vivax* by inducing morphological changes. To potentiate its spectrum of activity, it may also be used in combination with pyrimethamine, trimethoprim or sulfadoxine. However, it should not be used in infants, children and during pregnancy.

Uses: It can be used in both, chemosuppressive and radical cure of infections caused by resistant strains of parasites. Adverse effects are mild and mainly include its effects on CVS and pulmonary systems.

Other Antibacterials like Tetracyclines, Clindamycin, Linocomycin and Chloramphenicol

- These are found to possess antimalarial activity. A combination of quinine and tetracycline has been used to treat clinical attacks of chloroquine-resistant *P. falciparum* infection. However, the use of antibiotics may produce antibiotic-resistant pathogenic bacteria, if continued for long-term.

- Shortly after the discovery of mefloquine, a new drug, halofantrine has been developed as a promising alternative to mefloquine.

- Inactivated parasitized red blood cells or their fractions and more recently extracellular erythrocytic merozoites have been tested as vaccines in various forms of experimental procedures. In 1976, Trager and Jensen became successful in demonstrating immunogenicity of small amounts of merozoites antigen isolated in high yield and relative purity from cultured parasites. It was a milestone in the history of malariology.

- Red blood cells, however, are used for culture which exposes the risk of inclusion of red blood cells antigens in the vaccine. This may develop a severe autoimmune hemolytic anemia in patients receiving this vaccine.

DRUG RESISTANCE

- Over 16,000 agents were synthesized and tested for their antimalarial potential just between 1941–46. Similarly 250,000 compounds were screened during the decade 1968–78. Due to the extensive and liberal use of currently available antimalarial drug resistance to most of these drugs has developed in the strains of *P. falciparum* (this species is responsible for about 85% cases of human malaria). The progress, development of drug-resistance in Plasmodium strains may over burden the research programs to yield new synthetic antimalarials.

- Beside the chloroquine resistant strains, incidences of resistance development to pyrimethamine sulfadoxine combinations are also accumulating. The increased number of cases of appearance of multi-drug resistant strains of *P. falciparum* and failure of quinine to re-exhibit its clinical potency are the problems of severe concern. It is for this reason, mefloquine should be reserved only for the treatment of multi-drug resistant strains and it should not be over exposed. The parasites would not need much time to develop mefioquine-resistant strains, if misuse of this drug is permitted.

• Unfortunately, the underlying principles of acquired resistance to antimalarial drugs still remain unclear and demand further investigations.

Mefloquine

2-trifluoro-methyl-aniline (I)	Ethyl γ, γ, γ-trifluoroaceto-acetate	2, 6-bis(trifluoro-methyl)-4-hydroxy-quinoline	2, 6-bis(trifluoro-methyl)-4-bromo-quinoline (II)

2, 8-bis(trifluoro-methyl)-4-lithio-quinoline (III)	2, 8-bis(trifluoro-methyl)-4-quinoline-carboxylic acid (IV)	2-pyridyllithium (from 2-bromo pyridine)

(V)   Mefloquine

Amodiquine

4, 7-dichloro-quinoline	4-aminophenol	7-chloro-4-(4-hydroxy-phenylamino) quinoline (I)

Formaldehyde   Diethylamine   Amodiquine

Primaquine

4-methoxy-2-nitroaniline + Glycerol → (H₂SO₄, Skraup synthesis) → 6-methoxy-8-nitro-quinoline → (Fe, HCl) → 8-amino-6-methoxy-quinoline (I)

I + 4-bromo-1-phthalimidopentane → (intermediate) → (H₂N—NH₂, hydrazine) → Primaquine

Pyrimethamine

4-chlorobenzyl cyanide + Methyl propionate → (NaOCH₃) → (chloro intermediate with CN) → (trimethyl orthoformate) → I

(I) + Guanidine → Pyrimethamine

Dapsone

O_2N—⟨⟩—Cl (1-chloro-4-nitrobenzene (I)) → (Na_2S) → O_2N—⟨⟩—S—⟨⟩—NO_2 (4, 4'-dinitrodiphenyl sulfide) → ($K_2Cr_2O_7/H_2SO_4$ or HOCl) → II

4, 4'-dinitrodiphenyl sulfide (II) → ($SnCl_2$, HCl) → Dapsone

Trimethoprim

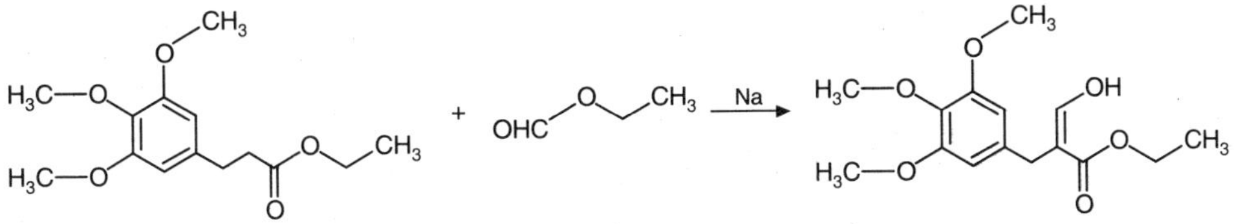

Ethyl 3-(3, 4, 5-tri-
methoxyphenyl) propionate

Ethyl
formate

(I)

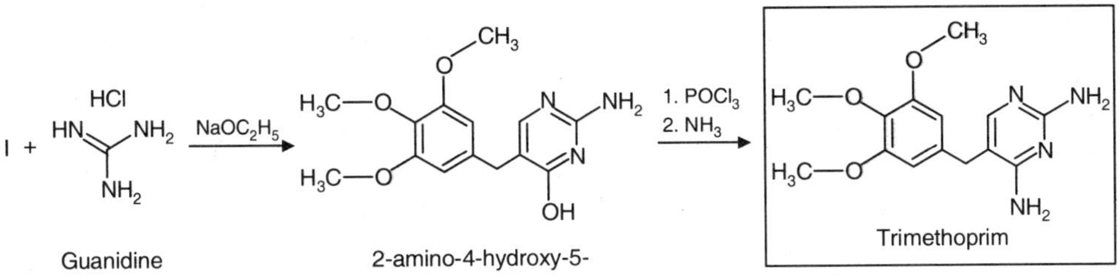

Guanidine
hydro-
chloride (II)

2-amino-4-hydroxy-5-
(3, 4, 5-trimethoxy-
benzyl) pyrimidine

Trimethoprim

62

Antiamoebic Agents

This is an infection caused by *Entamoeba histolytica*. It is an invasion of gastrointestinal mucosa, liver and other tissue by the negative trophozoite forms of the protozoan.

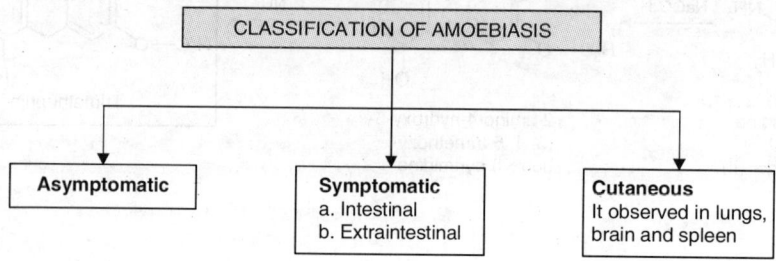

LIFE CYCLE OF *ENTAMOEBA HISTOLYTICA*

- Amoebiasis is an infection of the mucous membrane of the large intestine where *Entamoeba histolytica* is the causative organism. This organism occurs in the intestine in the form of trophozoites and cysts. In most infections, trophozoites (vegetative form) appear to feed on intestinal bacterial flora and multiply in the lumen without causing any symptom. But under certain circumstances, trophozoites may get activated and invade the intestinal mucosa, causing tissue lysis and producing dysentery or diarrhea.

- Under unfavorable atmosphere, however, trophozoites are encysted and the vast form is excreted in the feces. In majority of cases, infected persons do not show any symptom and create both cysts and trophozoites in the feces.

- The cyst form of the organism is ineffective and the infection is acquired by ingestion of amoebic cysts in food or water contaminated due to handling by such asymptomatic infected person, ingested cysts liberate trophozoites in the intestine and continue the process in the new host. The infection usually prevails in the areas of poor hygienic conditions and inadequate sanitation.

- Invasive intestinal amoebiasis may vary in its symptoms from a mild illness to severe amoebic dysentery with blood and mucus in the stool. Trophozoites may spread to the liver through portal vein and produce either an acute amoebic hepatitis or may encyst and produce amoebic liver abscess. The later may be complicated by rupture or extension of infection to adjacent organs. It may be associated with chronic colonic dysfunction, acute colonic perforation, insidious peritonitis and amoebic granuloma.

- Amoebic abscess of the liver is the most common extraintestinal manifestation of invasive amoebiasis. It may be characterized by abdominal pain, anorexia, fever, weight loss and hepatomegaly. In the mild amoebiasis, the symptoms are mainly of intestinal origin which appears due to invasion of the intestinal wall by the multiplying trophozoites. In more severe form, other vital organs like liver, lungs, brain, and genitourinary tract may get affected. This constitutes the cause of extra-intestinal symptoms.

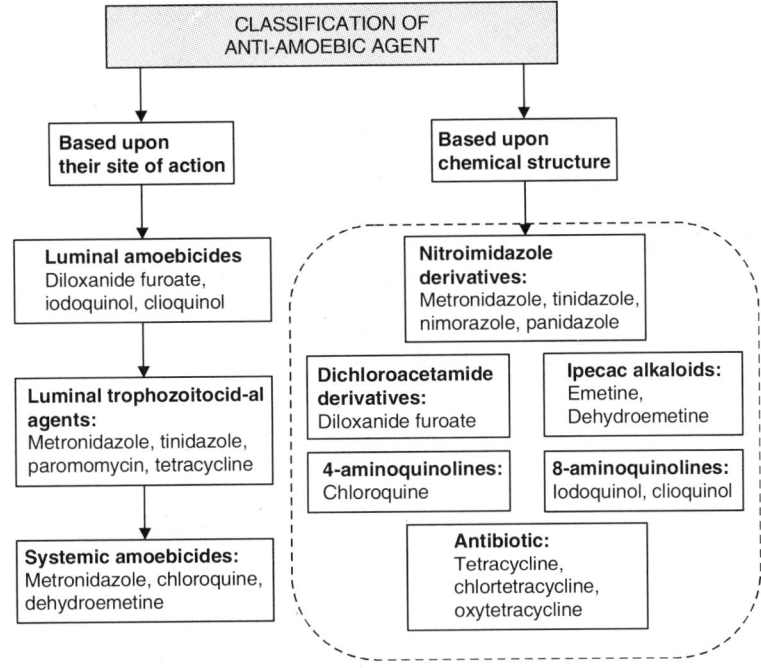

Based Upon Chemical Structure

1. Nitroimidazole Derivatives

2. Dichloro-acetamide Derivatives

3. Ipecac Alkaloids

Emetine

Dehydroemetine

4. 4-Aminoquinoline

Chloroquine

5. 8-Aminoquinoline

Iodoquinol

6. Antibiotic

Tetracycline

Oxytetracycline

- Various drugs used in the treatment of amoebiasis can be categorised on the basis of their site of action.

Luminal Amoebicides

These drugs are effective against the organism present in the bowel lumen. Most of them owe their effectiveness due to their poor oral absorption. This helps the drug to stay more time in the intestine. They are highly effective in eliminating cysts in asymptomatic carriers. Examples include diloxanide furate, iodoquinol, clioquinol, etc.

Luminal Trophozoitocidal

These agents mainly attack intestinal trophozoites and are effectively used to treat invasive intestinal amoebiasis. Examples include metronidazole, tinidazole, paromomycin, tetracycline and erythromycin.

Systemic Amoebicides

- As the name indicates, these drugs are not acting locally in the intestine. When trophozoites spread into liver, brain or lungs, these drugs may be used to treat extra-intestinal manifestations of invasive amoebiasis. Examples include metronidazole, tinidazole, chloroquine and dehydroemetine. Metronidazole and tinidazole thus not only eliminate trophozoites present in the intestine but are also effective at extra-intestinal sites.
- In addition to the chemotherapeutic measures, the large liver abscesses may be aspirated percutaneously for better results.

Nitroimidazole Derivatives

History

- First report of study on nitroimidazole derivatives appeared in 1955 by Nakamura and coworkers. Four such active members of the series include metroimidazole, tinidazole, nimorazole and ornidazole.
- Out of these, metronidazole was introduced in 1959 for the systemic treatment of trichomonal infections of urinogenital tract. It has exhibited a high degree of activity against amoebiasis, trichomoniasis, giardiasis and balantidiasis. It has been found to possess extremely broad-spectrum of both antibacterial and antiprotozoal activities.

Mechanism of action

1. Nitroimidazole derivatives act as an artificial electron acceptor after accumulating within the cell as the reduced compound. This diverts electron from normal pathways of protozoan. Nitro group accepts electron from electron-transport proteins such as FAD and diverts the normal energy yielding pathway.

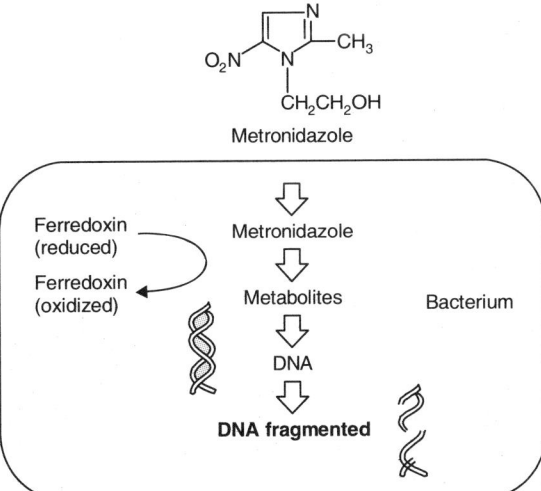

Fig. 62.1: Showing how nitroimidazole group causes DNA helical disturbance

2. This may be possible that a nitroimidazole derivative impairs the ability of DNA to function as template. The reduced nitroimidazole derivatives cause the loss of the helical structure of DNA strand, strand breakage and an accompanying impairment of its function resulting into the cell death (Figs. 62.1 and 62.2)

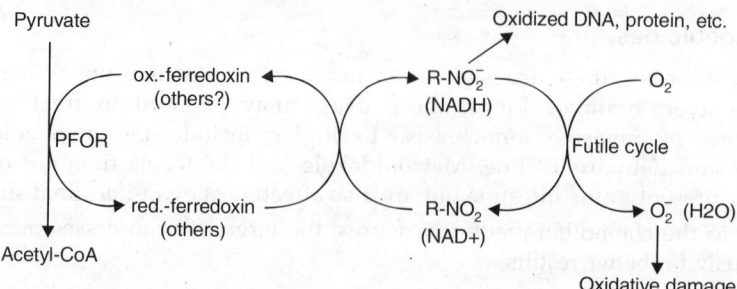

Fig. 62.2: Showing how nitroimidazole group causes DNA helical disturbance by oxidative way.

Pharmacokinetics

Metronidazole is an orally active drug. About 10% of administered dose is bound to the plasma proteins. It has a plasma half-life of 8.5 to 10.0 hours. The 2-hydroxy methyl metabolite and several inactive metabolites appear in the urine.

Adverse effects

It includes nausea, vomiting, anorexia, metallic taste, stomatitis, glossitis, vertigo, dizziness, flushing, and lombophlebitis. It is effectively used in the treatment of amoebiasis, giardiasis and trichomoniasis. However, ornidazole alone may not always eradicate the intestinal phase.

Uses

It is also effective against a number of aerobic bacteria (e.g. *Bactericides, Eubacterium, Clostridium, Fusobacterium, Peptococcus*, etc.). It may be used with other antibiotics to control the infection caused by aerobic microorganisms. It is contraindicated in patients with blood dyscrasias and alcoholic drinks (because of its disulfiram like effects). In children, a tasteless oral suspension of metronidazole is usually preferred.

Dichloroacetamide Derivatives

Diloxamide furoate

MOA: Little is known about its mechanism of action. It appears to interfere with protein synthesis and with the activity of some essential enzymes of protozoa. It is used in the treatment of cyst-passing patients. In the treatment of extraintestinal amoebiasis, it may be used along with a systemic amoebicidal agent.

Pharmacokinetic: It is a cheap, relatively nontoxic dichloroacetamide derivative, mainly used in the treatment of chronic amoebiasis. It is less effective in the treatment of acute intestinal amoebiasis. Studies of diloxanide ester showed that, in the form of furoate, the drug is less soluble and hence more effective locally. This ester undergoes hydrolysis in upper intestine to release diloxanide which is then absorbed. Major amount of drug is excreted in the urine in the form of its inactive glucuronide. About 4–10% dose appears unchanged in the feces.

Adverse Effects: It includes vomiting abdominal cramps, flatulence, diarrhea, urticaria and pruritus. It is contraindicated during pregnancy and in children less than 2 years of age.

Ipecac Alkaloids

Emetine and dehydroemetine

Chemistry: The latter is a synthetic analog of emetine, an alkaloid obtained from the roots of ipecac plant (*Cephaelis ipecacuanha*). Emetine is highly effective agent in systemic amoebiasis but it fails to act as luminal amoebicide because of poor concentration of the drug in that area. However, it may be used as luminal amoebicide in the form of emetine bismuth iodide which contains about 25% anhydrous emetine and 20% bismuth. It releases emetine slowly in the intestinal lumen.

MOA:

- Dehydroemetine is a better chemotherapeutic agent than emetine. Both are more effective against motile trophozoites than cysts. They affect protein synthesis by inhibiting the translocation of peptidyl t-RNA on ribosomes resulting into inhibition of polypeptide chain elongation.
- In severe cases of amoebiasis, emetine is used in combination with either chloroquine, tetracycline. While dehydroemetine may be used for rapid relief of symptoms in patients with severe amoebic dysentery; emetine is not a safe drug. Administration of either drug needs close medical supervision.

Adverse effect: A number of adverse effects affecting gastrointestinal, neuromuscular, cardiovascular systems are reported with their use. Dehydroemetine is less toxic than emetine.

4-Aminoquinoline Derivatives

Chloroquine

- It is an effective agent in the treatment of systemic amoebiasis. It is used only in the cases where other drugs either fail or are contraindicated. It is highly effective drug when used along with quinine, in the treatment of hepatic amoebic abscesses or amoebic hepatitis because of its preferential localization in the liver. To achieve complete cure, it should be given along with intestinal amoebicide.
- It is not much effective in the treatment of colonic amoebiasis in which its only function is to prevent development of liver abscesses.

8-Hydroxyquinolines

Iodoquinol and Clioquinol

MOA:

- It kills trophozoites and cysts in intestinal track by chelating ferrous ions which are essential for the protozoal metabolism. As a luminal amoebicide, it is used in the dose of 2 g daily for 20 days.
- These are examples of halogenated derivatives of 8-hydroxyquinoline having luminal amoebicidal activity. They are used alone in the treatment of chronic intestinal amoebiasis. In acute amoebiasis, they are generally used in combination with emetine and metronidazole. Since the drug therapy increases plasma iodine levels, these agents must be used with caution in patients hypersensitive to iodine or with thyroid dysfunction.

Uses: In long-term therapy, these agents are reported to cause optic neuritis and may prove to be dangerous.

Adverse effect: Iodoquinol is excreted mainly through the feces. Adverse effects include nausea, vomiting, diarrhea, stomach pain, chills, muscle pain, weakness, headache and peripheral neuropathy.

Antibiotics

• Tetracycline, chlortetracycline, oxytetracycline, erythromycin and paromomycin are the examples of antibiotics which can be used in the treatment of amoebiasis. Since amoebicidal action is not their main activity, they are usually used in combination with the principal amoebicidal agents in the treatment of mild to severe stages of intestinal amoebiasis.

• Most of the trophozoites, present in the lumen, feed the intestinal bacterial flora and then multiply. Except paromomycin, rest of the antibiotics exert an indirect trophozoitocidal action by destroying the enteric bacterial necessary for amoebic proliferation. Paromomycin is an aminoglycoside antibiotic obtained from *Streptomyces rimosus*.

MOA

It has a direct effect on the amoebae present in the lumen. It interferes in the protozoal DNA and RNA synthesis. It is generally used as a supplementary therapy in amoebiasis and in the treatment of various tapeworm infections. Adverse effects include diarrhea and anorexia.

Miscellaneous Agents

Many compounds exhibit amoebicidal activity when used orally. Important examples of such clinically used agents include chlorbetamide, chlorphenoxamine, chlorphenoxamine ethyl ether, phanquone and teclozan. These agents are used as luminal amoebicide.

Metronidazole

2-methyl-imidazole → 2-methyl-5-nitroimidazole (I) → Metronidazole

I + Ethylene oxide → Metronidazole

Tinidazole

p-toluenesulfonyl chloride + 2-(ethylsulfonyl)-ethanol → 2-(ethylsulfonyl) ethyl p-toluenesulfonate

I + 2-methyl-5-nitromidazole → Tinidazole

Nimorazole

2-morpholino-
ethyl chloride
+
4-nitroimidazole
sodium salt
Pyridine
Nimorazole

Diloxanide Furoate

Diloxanide
+
2-furancarbonyl
chloride
Pyridine
Diloxanide furoate

63

Anthelmintic Agents

Infestation with the parasitic worms is the most common disease in many tropical and subtropical countries. These parasitic worms firmly hold the intestinal mucosa and continue their reproduction by egg production.

- Worms parasitic to man can be categorised as cestodes (tapeworm), nematodes (round worms) and trematodes (flukes). Anthelmintics are the agents which are used to destroy or eliminate this parasitic worm from the gastrointestinal tract.
- They act by killing or paralyzing the worms so that such worms could be easily expelled out of gut. Some anthelmintic agents also impair the egg production process in worms.

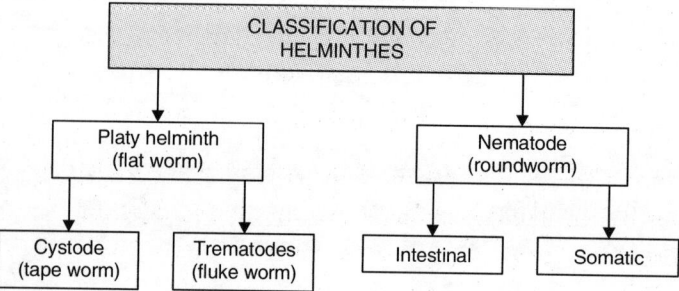

PLATY HELMINTHES (FLAT WORM)

A. Cestodes (Tap Worm)

1. *Tenia saginata.*
2. *Tenia solium.*
3. *Diphyllobothrium latum.*
4. *Rheinococcus granulosis.*
5. *Hymenolepis nana.*

Drugs in Cystode

1. Niclosamide.
2. Praziquantle pamoate.
3. Albendazole.
4. Mebendazole.
5. Paramomycin.

B. Trematodes

a. **Blood Fluke**

1. *Schistosoma haematobium.*
2. *Schistosoma mansoni.*
3. *Schistosoma japonicum.*

b. **Liver Fluke**

1. *Clonorchis sinesis.*
2. *Fasciola hepatica.*

c. **Lung Fluke:** *Paragominus westermani.*

d. **Intestinal Fluke:** *Buski.*

Drugs in Trematodes

1. Antimoney sodium tartarate.
2. Sodium stibogluconate.

NEMATODES (ROUND WORM)

A. Intestinal Nematodes

1. *Ascaris lumbricoids.*
2. *Ancylostoma duodenale.*
3. *Nectarate Americans.*
4. *Enterobius vermicularis.*
5. *Trichuris trichuria.*
6. *Strongaloids stercoralis.*
7. *Trichinella spiralis.*

Drugs in Intestinal Nematodes

1. Albendazole.
2. Levimisole.
3. Piperazine citrate.
4. Bephenium hydroxyl napthoate.

B. Somatic Species

1. *Wucheraria bancrofti.*
2. *Loa-loa.*
3. *Draccuulus medinensis.*
4. *Onichocera volvulus.*

Drugs

1. Diethylcarbamazine citrate.
2. Antimoney sodium tartarate.
3. Urea.
4. Stebamine.

DISEASE

1. River Blindness (Onchoceriasis)

Causative agent: *Onchocera volvulus.*

Symptoms:

1. Skin rashesh.
2. Blindness.

Therapy:

1. Diethylcarbamazine citrate.
2. Avermectin.
3. Pyrantel pamoate.

2. Ascariasis (Round Worm Disease)

Causative agent: *Ascaris lumbricoids.*

Symptoms:

1. Intestinal obstruction.
2. Lung damage.

Therapy:

1. Pyrantel pamoate.
2. Mebendazole.
3. Albendazole.
4. Thiobendazole.
5. Piperazine citrate.
6. Diethyl carbamazine.

3. Enterbiasis

Causative agent: *Enterobius vermicularis.*

Symptoms: GI tract disturbance.

Therapy:

1. Mebendazole.
2. Thiobendazole.
3. Albendazole.
4. Piperazine citrate.

4. Trichuriasis

Causative agent: *Trichuris trichuria.*

Symptoms:

1. Abdominal pain.
2. Diarrhea.

Therapy: Mebendazole.

5. Filariasis

Causative agent: *Wuchereria bancrofti.*

Symptoms:

1. Lymph flow blockage.
2. Arms and legs infection.

Therapy:

1. Avermectin.
2. Diethylcarbamazine.

6. Strongyloidiasis

Causative agent: *Strongyloids stercoralis.*

Symptoms: GI tract disturbance.

Therapy:

1. Thiobendazole.

2. Albendazole.

7. Trichinosis

Causative agent: *Trichenella spiraliss.*

Symptoms: GI tract disturbance.

Therapy: Thiobendazole.

CLASSIFICATION OF ANTHELMINTICS

Benzimidazoles:
Albendazol, melebendazole, thiabendazole

Quinoline and isoquinilines:
Praziquantel, qxamniquine

Vinylpyrimidines:
Pyrantel pamoate

Piperazine derivatives:
Piperazine citrate,
Diethyl carbamazine citrate

Amides:-
Niclosamide

Natural products:
Avermectins

Imidazothiazoles:
Levamisole

Nitro derivatives:
Niridazole

Organophosphorus:
Metrifonate

1. Benzimidazole Derivatives

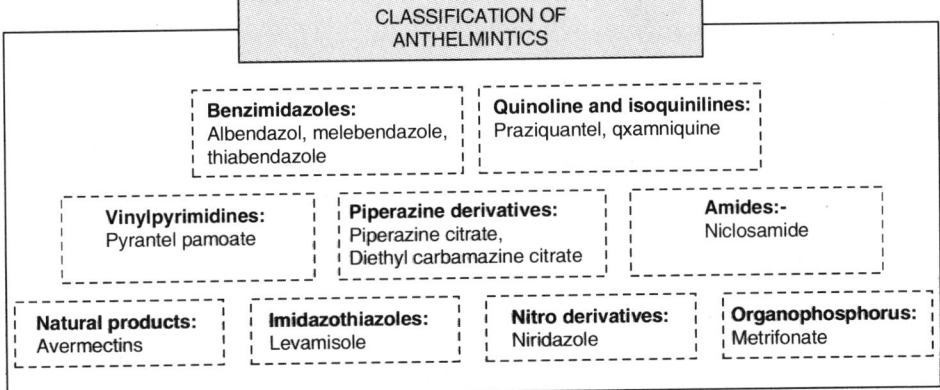

Albendazole

Mebendazole

Flubendazole

Cyclobendazole

Dribendazole

Fenbendazole

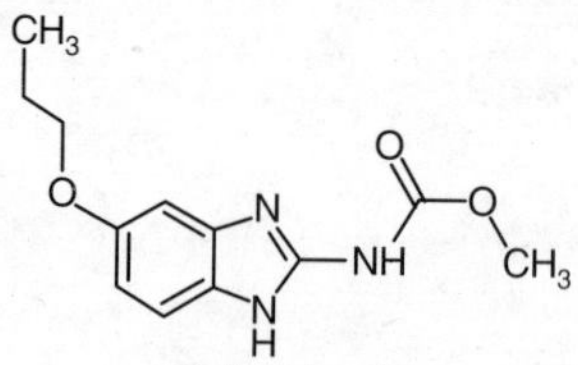

Oxibendazole

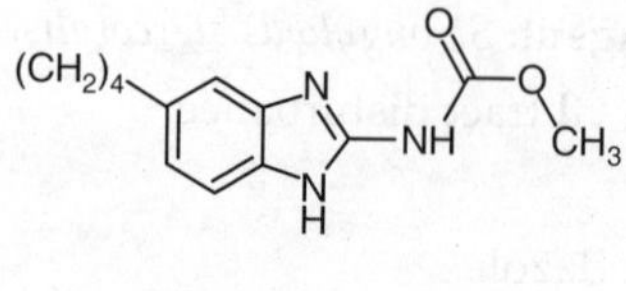

Parbendazole

2. Quinoline and Isoquinoline

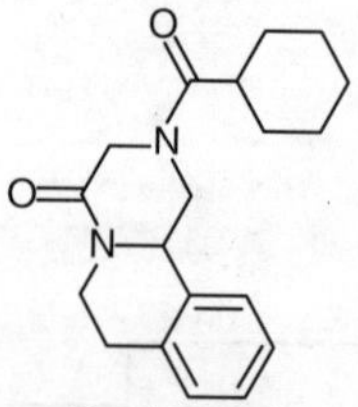

Praziquantel

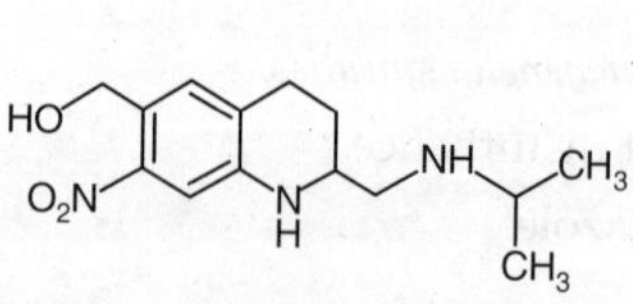

Oxamniquine

3. Piperazine Derivatives

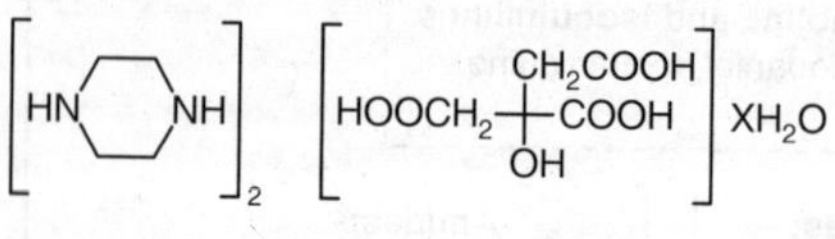

Piperazine citrate

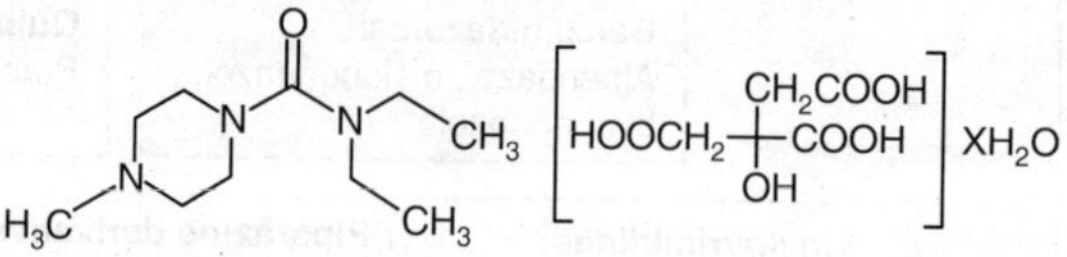

Diethylcarbamazine citrate

4. Vinylpyrimidines

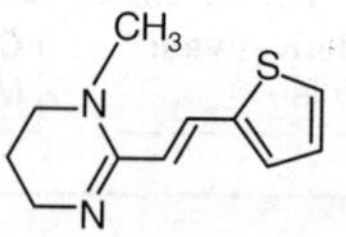

Pyrantel

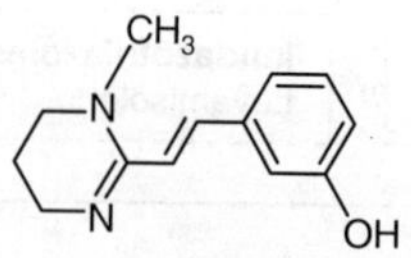

Oxantle

5. Amides

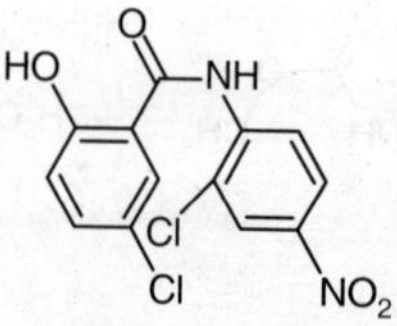

Niclosamide

6. Imidazothiazoles

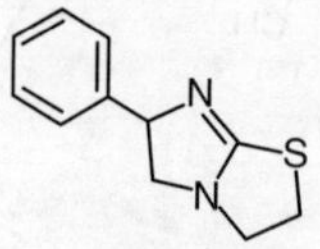

Levamisole

7. Nitro Derivatives

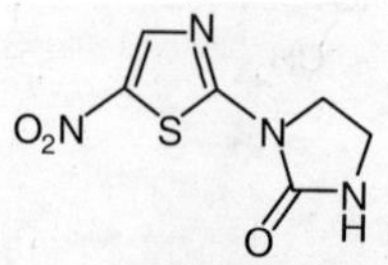

Niridazole

8. Organophosphorus

Metrifonate

Table 63.1: Clinically used anthelmintic agents

Sr. No.	Worm infection	Drugs commonly used
1.	Ascariasis	Mebendazole, piperazine, pyrantel, bephenium
2.	Cestode infection	Paromomycin
3.	Cutaneous larva migrans	Thiabendazole
4.	Dracunculiasis	Niridazole
5.	Enterobiasis	Piperazine, pyrantel, pyrvinium
6.	Filariasis	Diethylcarbamazine
7.	Fascioliasis	Bithionol, hexylresorcinol
8.	Nematode (round worm) infection	Bephenium, mebendazole, pyrantel, hexyl resorcinol
9.	Onchocerciasis	Diethylcarbamazine, suramin
10.	Paragonimiasis	Bithionol
11.	Schistosomiasis	Lucanthrone, niridazole, metrifonate, praziquantel
12.	S. haematobium	Hycanthone, niridazole, oxamniquine, praziquantel
13.	S. mansoni	Praziquantel, niridazole, tartar emetic
14.	S. japonicum	Pyrvinium, thiabendazole
15.	Strongyloidiasis	Bithionol
16.	Trematode(fluke)infections	Mebendazole
17.	Trichuriasis	Mebendazole, corticosteroids
18.	Trichiniasis	

▓ CLASSIFICATION

Presently available anthelmintic agents are structurally diversified. On the chemical basis, they can be classified as:

    a. Benzimidazole.
    b. Quinoline and isoquinoline.
    c. Vinylpyrimidines.
    d. Amides
    e. Piperazine analogs.
    f. Imidazothiazoles.
    g. Alkaloids and plant extracts.
    h. Nitro derivatives.
    i. Organophosphorus.

BENZIMIDAZOLE DERIVATIVES

Thiabendazole

MOA:

1. This inhibits the mitochondrial fumarate reductase enzyme, which is essential for the ATP production.

2. Another proposed mechanism is that it supposes to inhibit the acetylcholinestrases, which is hydrolyzing enzyme of acetylcholine, leading to paralysis in worm.

SAR:

1. Replacement of the 4-thiazolyl ring system by a methyl carbamate grouping gave interesting group of anthelmintics.

2. Substitution at 5-position were introduced to prevent metabolic inactivation.

Pharmacokinetics: It has a plasma half-life of 1.2 hours. It is excreted in urine mainly as 5 - hydroxy thiabendazole either in the form of glucuronide or sulfate.

Adverse effects: It includes nausea, vomiting, epigastric distress, anorexia, diarrhea, numbness, skin rash, hyperglycemia, crystalluria and transient leukopenia.

Uses: Thiabendazole is effective in the treatment of *A. duodenal* (common hookworm), *E. vermicularis* (pin worm), *A. lumbricoides* (round worm) and *S. stercoralis* infections. Adult oral dose is 3 g per day. In early trichinosis, treatment may be continued for 2 – 3 additional days while in disseminated strongyloidiasis, treatment may be continued for at least 5 days.

Mebendazole

MOA:

1. This irreversibly blocks the uptake of exogenous glucose (from outside) leading to glycogen depletion and reduced generation of ATP, which are essential for parasite survival.

2. It also suppose to inhibit tubulin polymerization by binding to β-tubulin in several intestinal and tissue membranes and in some cestodes.

Pharmacokinetics:

- It is a benzimidazole derivative having broad-spectrum anthelmintic activity. It is poorly absorbed orally. About 78–80% administered dose is bound to the plasma proteins.

- It has a plasma-half-life of 2.5–5.5 hours. About 95% dose is excreted unchanged or as 2-amino-5-benzoyl-benzimidazole (primary metabolite) in the feces. Up to 2–5% dose appears in the urine unchanged or as primary metabolite.

Uses: It is effective in the treatment of ascariasis, trichuriasis, and hookworm infections in the oral dose of 100 mg twice a day for 3 days. In enterobiasis, a single oral dose of 100 mg is given. After 2 weeks, second dose of 100 mg may be given.

Albendazole

MOA: This irreversibly blocks the uptake of exogenous glucose (from outside) leading to glycogen depletion and reduced generation of ATP, which are essential for parasite survival.

SAR:

1. Variation in the position of C-5 resulted in very active compound, with low toxicity.

2. Replacement of $NHCOCH_3$ by aromatic ring, heteroaromatic ring prevents the metabolic inactivation.

Side effect: Insomnia, dizziness, diarrhea, headache, etc.

Uses: It is mainly used in ascariasis, trichuriasis and strongyloidiasis

▨ QUINOLINE AND ISOQUINOLINES

Oxamniquine

MOA: The exact mode of action is not clear, indirect evidences shows that susceptible parasites converts this drug into unstable ester, which is decomposed to yield reactive electrophile intermediates, which alkylate DNA and stops further process of protein synthesis.

Pharmacokinetics:

- It is an orally active yellow dye having anthelmintic activity. Chemically, it is 2-amino methyl tetra-hydroquinoline derivative. It is especially effective against *Schistsoma mansoni*.
- It has a plasma half-life of 1 – 2.5 hours. Principal metabolites include 6-carboxyl and 2-carboxylic acid derivatives which are excreted in the urine along with traces (0.4 – 1.9% dose) of parent drug.

Uses:

- It is effective schistosomicidal agent used against *Schistosoma mansoni*. It is also used in combination with metrifonate in the treatment of mixed mansoni and haematobium infections.
- Adult oral dose is 15 – 60 mg/kg body weight as a single dose given at bedtime.

Praziquantel

MOA: It increases the permeability of helminth cell membranes to calcium (Ca^{2+}); calcium diffuses from the cells, the entire worm contracts, and become paralysed. The worm is eventually disintegrated.

Side effect: Side effects thus far have been mild sedtion, headache and nausea.

Uses: It is mainly used in the treatment of schistomiasis.

▨ PIPERAZINE DERIVATIVES

Diethylcarbamazine

MOA:

- The drug causes a hyperpolarization effect which decreases the muscular activity and consequently immobilizing organism and dislodging organism from GI tract.
- It also alters the microfilarial surface membranes, thereby rendering them more susceptible to destruction by host defence mechanism.

Pharmacokinetics: It is orally well absorbed and has a plasma half life of 12 hours. Upon extensive metabolism, variety d inactive metabolites are excreted in the urine along with 10% dose as unchanged drug.

Uses:

- It is used to treat infections caused *by W. bancrofti, W. malayi and O. volvulus*. It is a drug of choice for the treatment of filariasis due to *Tetrapetalonema perstans* or *Tetrapetalonei streptocerca*.
- It may also be used in tropic eosinophilia and Ascaris infections. Adult oral dose is 2 mg/kg body weight three times the day after meal for 1 – 3 weeks.

Piperazine Citrate

MOA:

- The drug blocks the response of *Ascaris* muscle to acetylcholine, apparently by altering the permeability of the cell membrane to ions that are responsible for the maintenance of the resting potential.
- It causes hyperpolarization and suppression of spontaneous spike potentials with peristalsis.

Side effects: It causes nausea, vomiting, convulsion, confusion, seizure and epilepsy.

Uses: It is mainly used in ascariasis.

VINYLPYRIMIDINE DERIVATIVES

Pyrantel Pamoate

MOA: It depolarizes and paralyzes worm muscle by persistent nicotinic activation. Intestinal nematodes can then no longer maintain the tone necessary to attach to host tissue and are expelled by host peristalsis. Pyrantel causes depolarization, on the other hand piperazine citrate causes hyperpolarization with mutually antagonistic effects, and therefore simultaneous use should be avoided.

Side effects: Anorexia, vomiting, nausea.

Uses: It is used in the treatment of enterobiasis caused by pin worm (*E. vermicularis*).

Adverse effects: These are few and include gastric irritation, photo sensitization, nausea, vomiting, diarrhea, cramps and skin rash.

AMIDES

Niclosamide

MOA: The drug inhibits anaerobic phosphorylation of adenosine diphosphate by the mitochondrial of the parasite, an energy producing process that is dependent on carbon dioxide fixation. It acts by inhibiting respiration and blocking glucose absorption by the intestinal adult worms.

SAR: For maximum activity, the hydroxyl group in the benzoic acid moiety had to be in the 2-position.

Uses:

- It is used in the treatment of diphyllobothriasis (*Diphyllobothrium latum*), hymenolepiasis (*H. nana*), taeniasis (*T. saginata*) and dipylidiasis (*Dipylidium conium*). *Enterobium vermicularis* is also susceptible.

- For destruction of tapeworm, niclosamide is the most effective and safe drug.

- Adult oral dose is 500 mg usually in the fasting condition 3–4 times a day. Antiemetic may be given one hour before and purgative about 2 hours, after the treatment.

NITRODERIVATIVES

Niridazole

MOA: It interferes with egg formation process of female parasite.

Pharmacokinetics: It undergoes an extensive first pass hepatic metabolism. 1-Thiocarbamoyl-2-imidazolidinone is the active metabolite. The metabolites appear both, in urine and faeces.

Uses: It is used in the treatment of *D. medinensis*. It may also be used for the therapy of schistosomiasis due to *S. japonicum*.

ORGANOPHOSPHORUS

Metrifonate

MOA: This metabolite is probably responsible for inhibition of acetylcholinestrases to explain one of the causes of its anthelmintic activity.

Pharmacokinetics: It has a plasma half-life of 1.5 hours. It is extensively metabolized by plasma and schistosomal arylesterases. Principal metabolites include dichlorvos (2, 2-dichlorovinyl dimethyl phosphate) and various inactive products.

Adverse effects: Adverse effects include nausea, vomiting, colic, abdominal pain, mild vertigo, lassitude, decreased sperm count and some intestinal nematodes.

Uses: It is used for the treatment of urinary schistosomiasis and of *S. haematobium* infections. Adult oral dose is 5–15 mg/kg body weight 3 times after every 2 weeks.

IMIDAZOTHIAZOLES

Levamisole

MOA: It is levorotatory isomer and a potent stereospecific inhibitor to fumarate reductase in many nematodes.

Adverse effect: GI tract disturbances.

Uses: It is drug of choice for round worm and hook worm infections.

NATURAL PRODUCT

Avermictin

MOA: This increases the concentration of GABA, which control over the release of different neurotransmitter. In this way, it blocks the motor neuron transmission.

Adverse effect: Fever, joint pain is the side effects.

Mebendazole

4-chloro-benzophenone → (HNO$_3$, < –5°C) → 4-chloro-3-nitro-benzophenone → (NH$_3$, CH$_3$OH, sulfolane, 125°C) → I

4-amino-3-nitro-benzophenone (I) → (H$_2$, Pd–C) → 3, 4-diamino-benzophenone (II)

S-methylthiouronium-sulfate + H$_2$SO$_4$ + Methyl chloroformate → (NaOH, pH B) → Methyl S-methyl-isothiourea-N-carboxylate (III)

II + III → (CH$_3$COONa) → Mebendazole

Praziquantel

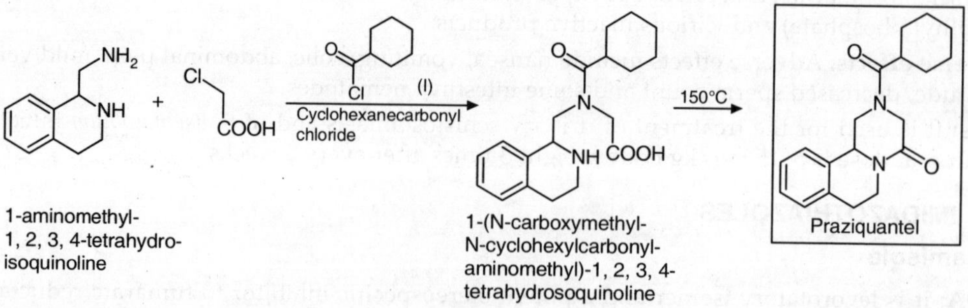
NH2
NH
+
Cl
COOH
O
Cl
(I)
Cyclohexanecarbonyl chloride
N
NH COOH
150°C
N
N
O
Praziquantel
1-aminomethyl-1, 2, 3, 4-tetrahydro-isoquinoline
1-(N-carboxymethyl-N-cyclohexylcarbonyl-aminomethyl)-1, 2, 3, 4-tetrahydrosoquinoline

Piperazine

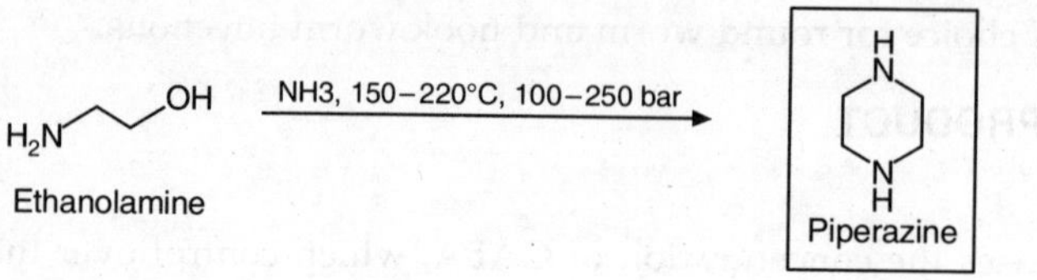
H2N
OH
Ethanolamine
NH3, 150–220°C, 100–250 bar
H
N
N
H
Piperazine

Diethylcarbamazine

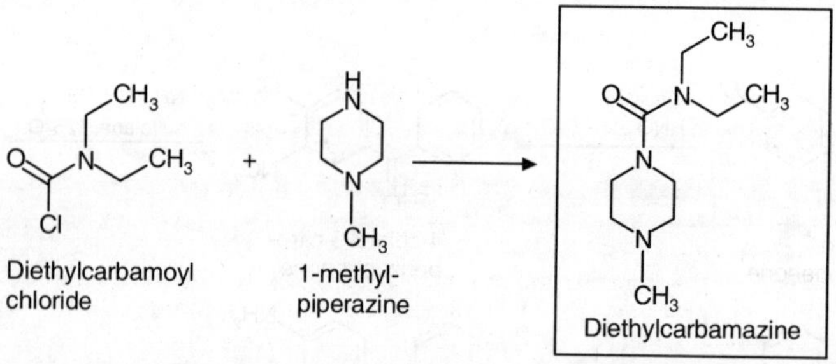
CH3
O
N
CH3
Cl
Diethylcarbamoyl chloride
+
H
N
N
CH3
1-methyl-piperazine
CH3
O
N
CH3
N
N
CH3
Diethylcarbamazine

Niclosamide

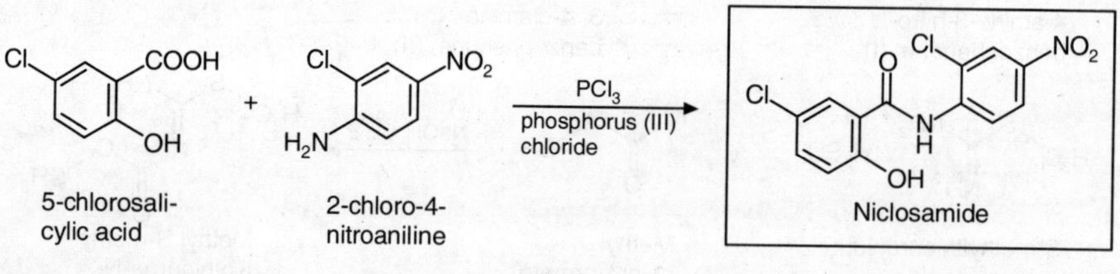
Cl
COOH
OH
5-chlorosali-cylic acid
+
Cl
NO2
H2N
2-chloro-4-nitroaniline
PCl3
phosphorus (III) chloride
Cl
O
NO2
Cl
N
H
OH
Niclosamide

Levamisole

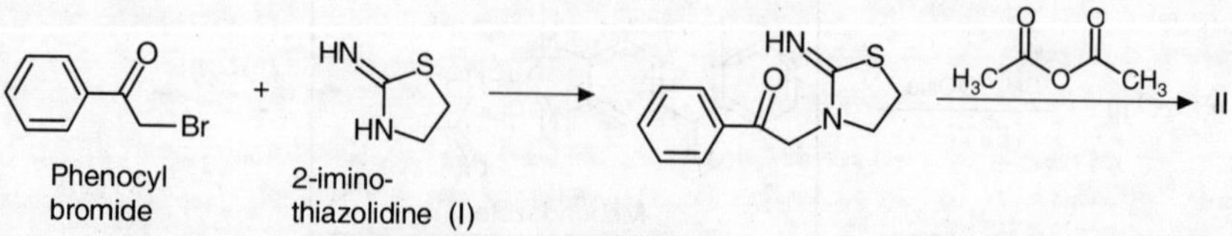
O
Br
Phenocyl bromide
+
HN
S
HN
2-imino-thiazolidine (I)
HN
S
O
N
O
O
H3C
O
CH3
II

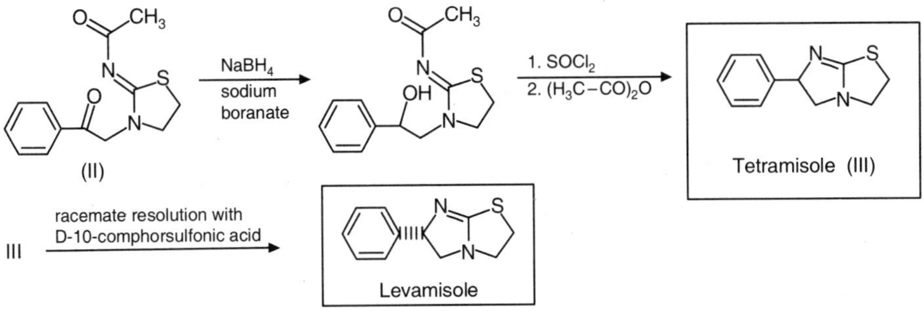

(II)

NaBH$_4$ sodium boranate

1. SOCl$_2$
2. (H$_3$C−CO)$_2$O

Tetramisole (III)

III → racemate resolution with D-10-comphorsulfonic acid

Levamisole

Niridazole

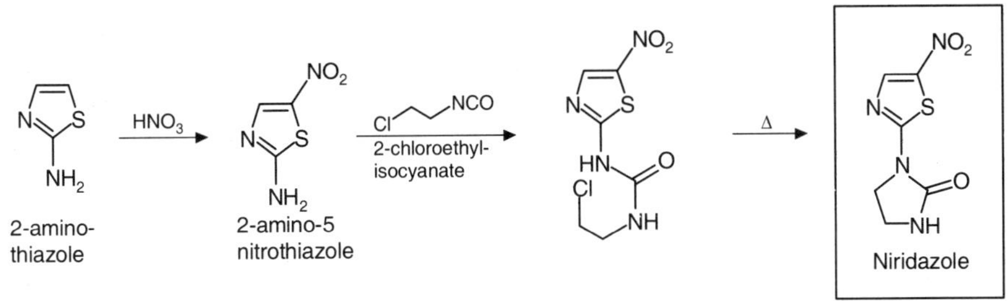

2-amino-thiazole

HNO$_3$

2-amino-5 nitrothiazole

Cl〜NCO
2-chloroethyl-isocyanate

Δ

Niridazole

Antiviral Agents

Viruses represent a separate and unique class of infectious agents. The smallest viruses possess a diameter of not more than 20 mm while in the large viruses, diameter may go up to 300 mm. The constitution of a virus is much simpler as compared to the bacteria. According to Lwoff, an infectious agent is that;

1. Possesses simple chemical composition.
2. Lacks the metabolic enzyme machinery.
3. Lacks the protein-synthesizing system.
4. Contain only one type of nucleic acid (i.e. either DNA or RNA).
5. Possesses host-cell dependent machinery for multiplication can be named as virus.

- Unlike bacteria, viruses do not possess cell wall. Viruses consist of one or more strands of linear or helical strands of either DNA or RNA enclosed in a shell of protein known as the capsid. The capsid is composed of several sub-units known as capsomeres that decide the shape of the capsid. Though often be spherical, capsid may possess different shapes. In certain cases, capsid may be surrounded by an outer protein or lipoprotein envelope. This encirculating membrane may be called as an envelope (Fig. 64.1).

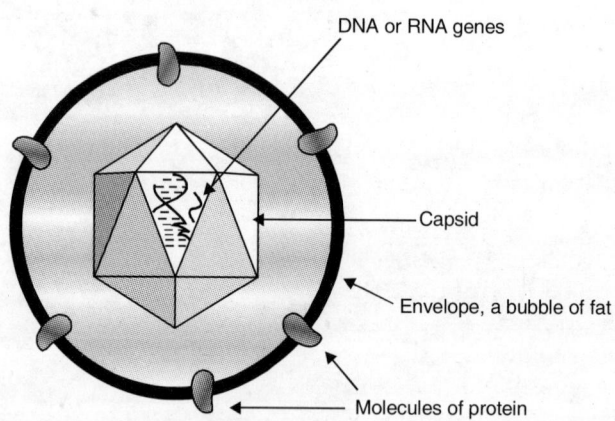

Fig. 64.1: Structure of virus

- Since the biology of viral replication is dependent on the host cell metabolic machinery (e.g. protein synthesis, various enzyme systems), unlike bacteria, viruses will not grow on the nutrient media. They can replicate only in the host cell which may be a bacteria, animal or plant cell. Hence viruses are considered as obligatory intracellular parasites that utilize many of biochemical machinery products of host cell to sustain their viability.

- Viral diseases include influenza, smallpox, rabbies, poliomyelitis, yellow fever, ornithosis, psittacosis and lymphogranuloma venereum.

THE VIRAL REPLICATION CYCLE

Adsorption

The virion invades the host cell membrane. The reactive sites on the capsid firmly bind with their complimentary sites on the host cell. The viral particle is encapsulated by host cell cytoplasm, forming a vacuole.

Uncoating

- The genetic material or viral genome (DNA or RNA) passes into the host cell, leaving the capsid covering outside the host cell. Sometimes uncovering of viral genome occurs within the host cell. This step is referred to as penetration into host cell.
- Only the viral genome is infectious to the host cell and the capsid of the protein coat determines the site of the attacks of virus within the host.
- The viral genome is different from the host nucleic acids and hence it is infectious. Sometimes due to its proteinous nature, capsid contents may turn to be antigenic to the host cell and initiates a number of immunological reactions to the host.

Synthesis of Viral Components

Viral genome enters the cytoplasm or neoplasm and directs or utilises the host nucleic acid machinery for the synthesis of new viral protein and the production of more viral genome. Thus it not only consumes the actual material for its own use from the host-cell but also enjoys the services of the biochemical systems of the host to get incorporated this material into the several proteinous subunits needed for its replication.

Release of the Virus

- Viral nucleic acid and capsid protein materials are synthesized in different parts of the host cell by the host cell ribosomes.
- The m-RNA is synthesized from the viral genome. The host cell machinery, however, fails to differentiate between viral and cell directed orders. The large numbers of newly synthesized particles then have to be brought together for assembling into new virions.
- The later are released from the cell by budding process. They may acquire the lipoprotein envelope at the time of their release. The new virions then invade fresh host cell and repeat the whole process. Since the host cell machinery is totally utilized for production of new virions, the normal cell function ceases at the time of replication (Fig. 64.2).
- Some viruses induce the production of toxic intermediates that adds to their pathogenicity. Viruses are composed of one or more strands of a linear or helical nucleic acid core, consisting of either DNA or RNA, but not both. Viruses thus can be classified as per the type of nucleic acid present in them. For example:

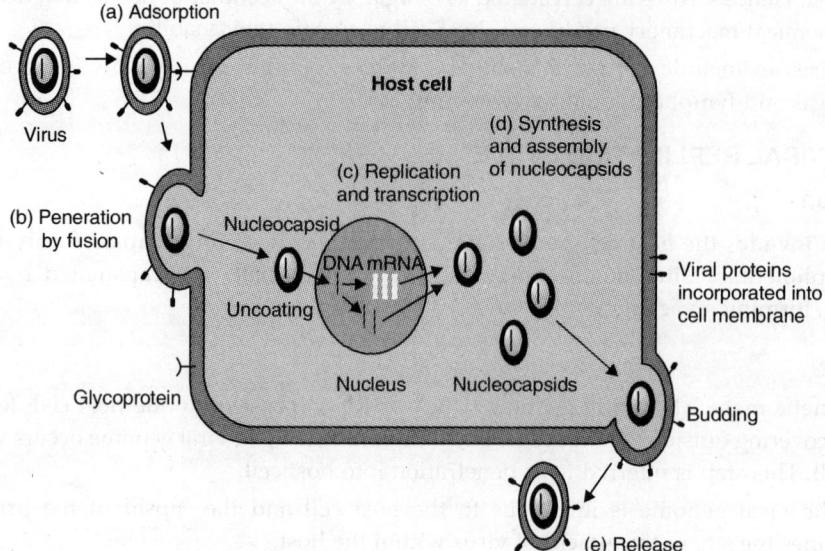

Fig. 64.2: Replication of DNA virus

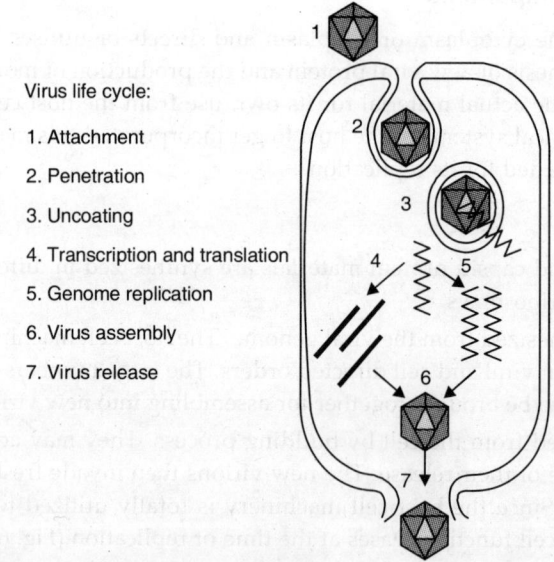

Virus life cycle:

1. Attachment
2. Penetration
3. Uncoating
4. Transcription and translation
5. Genome replication
6. Virus assembly
7. Virus release

Fig. 64.3: Different stages of life cycle of virus

DNA viruses: This class includes pox viruses, papoviruses, adenoviruses and herpes viruses.

RNA Viruses: This class includes arboviruses, myxoviruses, picornaviruses and rhinoviruses.

▨ CLASSIFICATION OF ANTIVIRAL AGENTS (Flow chart 64.1)

Flow chart 64.1: Classification of antiviral agents

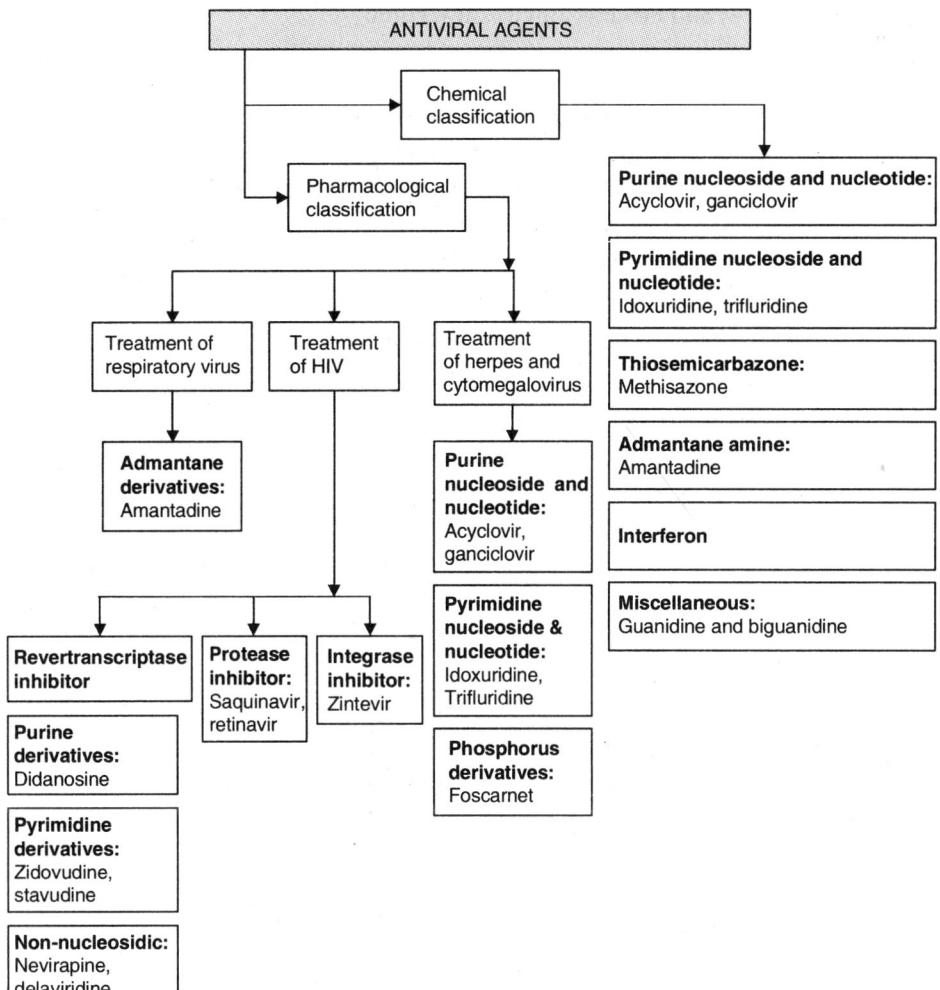

- **The currently available antiviral drugs can be chemically classified as:**
  - a. Purine nucleosides and nucleotides.
  - b. Pyrimidine nucleosides and nucleotides.
  - c. Thiosemicarbazones.
  - d. Benzimidazoles.
  - e. Adamantane amines.
  - f. Interferons.
  - g. Miscellaneous agents.

- **According to treatment protocol:**
- **a. Treatment of respiratory virus infection:** Admantine derivative— amantadine, rimantadine.
- **b. Treatment of herpes and cytomegalovirus infection:**
  1. Purine nucleotide— acyclovir, ganciclovir, vidarbine.
  2. Pyrimidine nucleotides— trifluridine, idoxuridine.
  3. Phosphorus derivatives— foscarnet.
- **c. Treatment of human immunodefeciency virus (HIV):**
  1. **Reverse transcriptase inhibitors:**
     –Purine derivatives— didanosine.
     –Pyrimidine derivatives— zidovudin, stavudin.
     –Non-nucleosidic— nevirapine, delaverdine.
  2. **Protease inhibitors—** saquinavir, indinavir, ritonavir.
  3. **Integrase inhibitor—** zintevir.

CHEMICAL CLASSIFICATION

Purine Nucleoside and Nucleotide

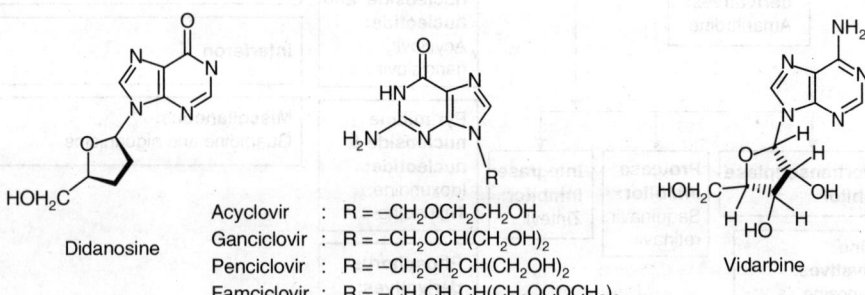

Didanosine

Acyclovir : R = –CH$_2$OCH$_2$CH$_2$OH
Ganciclovir : R = –CH$_2$OCH(CH$_2$OH)$_2$
Penciclovir : R = –CH$_2$CH$_2$CH(CH$_2$OH)$_2$
Famciclovir : R = –CH$_2$CH$_2$CH(CH$_2$OCOCH$_3$)$_2$

Vidarbine

Pyrimidine Nucleoside and Nucleotide

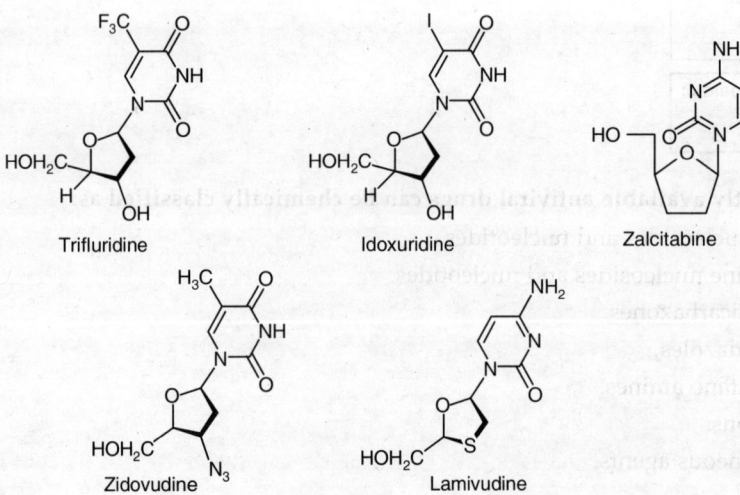

Trifluridine

Idoxuridine

Zalcitabine

Zidovudine

Lamivudine

Thiosemicarbazone Derivatives

Isatin-β-thiosemicarbazone   Methisazone

Admantane Amine Derivatives

Amantadine   Rimantadine   1-amantyl-guanidine

PHARMACOLOGICAL CLASSIFICATION

Treatment of HIV Infection

1. Reverse Transcriptase Inhibitor

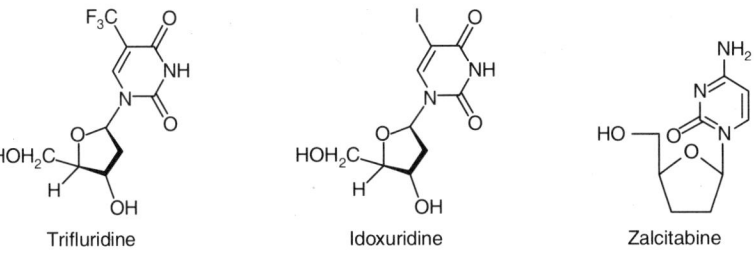

Trifluridine   Idoxuridine   Zalcitabine

(a) Purine derivatives

Stavudine

(b) Pyrimidine derivatives

Didanosine

(c) Non-nucleoside Reverse Transcriptase Inhibitors

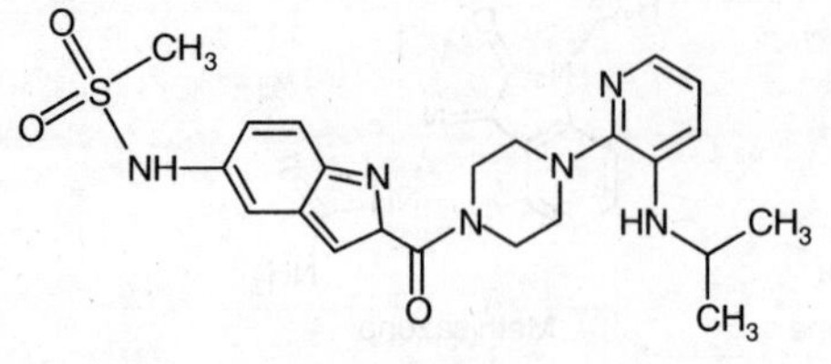

Delavirdine

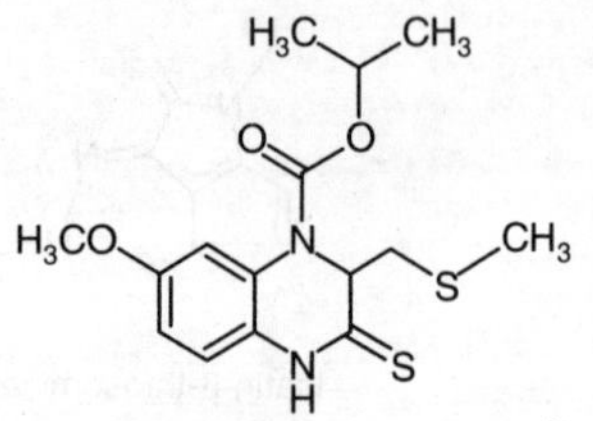

Talviraline

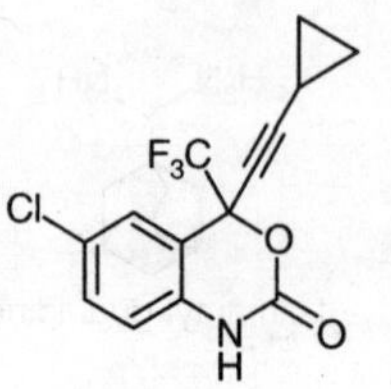

Efavirenz

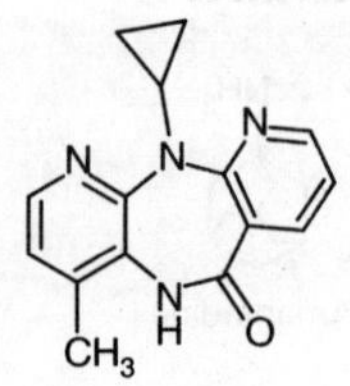

Nevirapine

2. HIV Protease Inhibitor

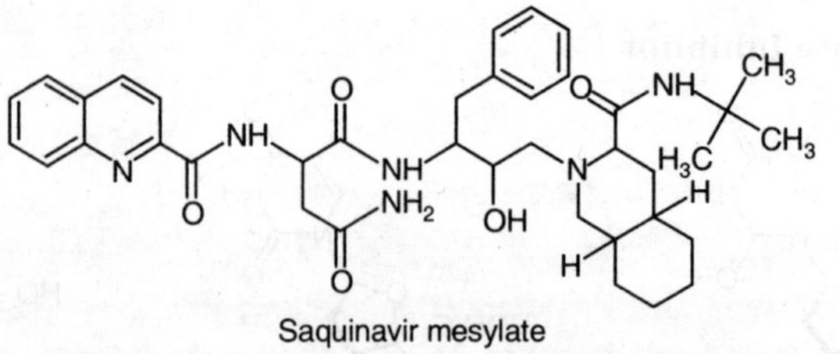

Saquinavir mesylate

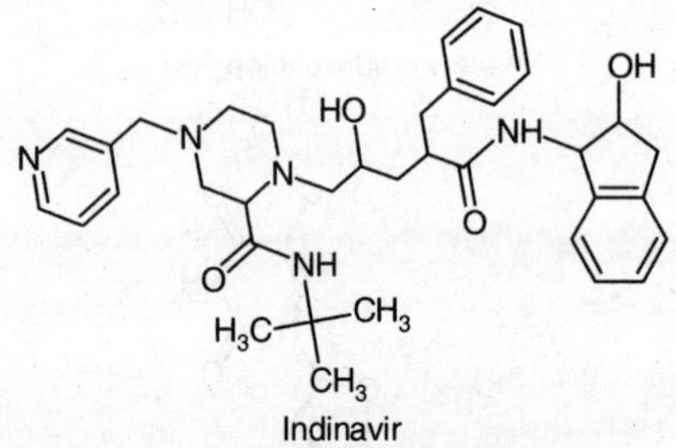

Indinavir

■ PURINE NUCLEOSIDES AND NUCLEOTIDES

Acyclovir Triphosphate (Acycloguanosine)

Chemistry

It is a synthetic purine nucleoside analog in which a linear side chain (i.e., -CH$_2$OCH$_2$CH$_2$OH) is attached at 9-position instead of the cyclic sugar present in the guanosine molecule.

MOA

Acyclovir undergoes phosphorylation process with the help of viral thymidine kinase enzymes to form acyclovir trisphosphate. The later selectively inhibits herpes virus DNA polymerase.

The faulty transcription in viral DNA leads to inhibition of virus replication process. The affinity of viral thymidine kinase enzymes for acyclovir is about 200 times greater than that of mammalian enzymes for the drug. This explains the selectivity of attack on the viruses.

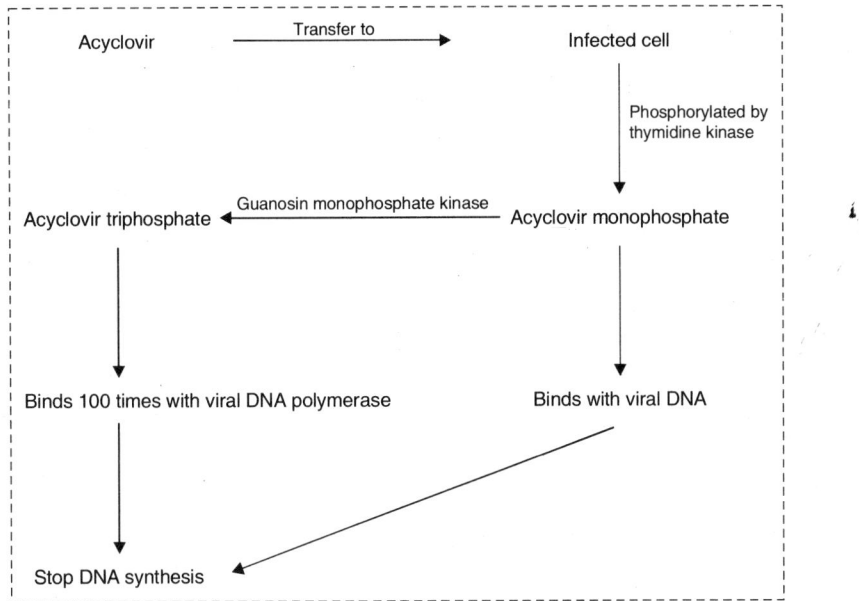

Pharmacokinetics

It can be used orally, topically and intravenously. About 15% of administered dose is bound to the plasma proteins. It has plasma half-life of about 2.5 hours. It is excreted in urine mostly in unchanged form along with minor amount of inactive metabolite, 9-carboxy methoxy methylguanine.

Adverse effects

Adverse effects include nausea, headache, amnesia, hypotension, tremors and coma. Local irritation, ulceration and burning may occur when it is applied to genital lesions.

Uses

- It is effective against herpes virus infections, herpes zoster infections and infections caused by varicella-zoster and cytomegalovirus. It may be used orally for the treatment of both initial and recurrent episodes of genital herpes.
- A 3% acyclovir ointment may be used for the treatment of ocular herpetic infection and herpes keratoconjunctivitis.
- It may also be used intravenously in the treatment of herpes simplex encephalitis. However, development of resistance to acyclovir may limit its clinical utility.

Vidarabine (Adenine Arabinoside)

MOA

It is a purine nucleoside. This antiviral agent is isolated from the bacteria, *Streptomyces antibiotics*. It is an analog of adenosine originally developed for the treatment of leukemia. It is converted *in vivo* enzymatically to ara-ATP. The later impairs early steps in viral DNA synthesis, presumably by inhibiting viral DNA polymerase. It exhibits considerable host toxicity due to partly inhibition of cellular DNA polymerase enzymes.

Pharmacokinetic

About 20–30% administered dose is bound to the plasma–proteins. It has a plasma half-life of 1.5 hours. In the cornea and in the plasma, it metabolizes to ara-hypoxanthine (active; half-life is 3.3 hours) by xanthine oxidase enzyme through a process of deamination.

Uses

- It is effective against vaccine, herpes simplex virus, cytomegalovirus, varicella-zoster, pseudorabies and myxoma virus. It may be given topically as a 3% ophthalmic ointment or as IV infusion.

- It is used to treat herpes simplex infections in neonates. It is also used to treat herpes simplex encephalitis and herpes zoster infections in immunocompromised patients. It may have activity in cytomegalovirus infections and in type B virus hepatitis. In the form of 3% ophthalmic ointment, it may be used topically to control recurrent epithelial keratitis and keratoconjunctivitis.

- However, it remains ineffective against bacterial, fungal and adenovirus infections. Its antineoplastic potential is under investigations.

- Vidarabine-5'-monophosphate and vidarabine-hypoxanthine-5' monophosphate are the vidarabine derivatives that are currently under investigation for their utility in antiviral therapy.

PYRIMIDINE NUCLEOSIDES AND NUCLEOTIDES

Idoxuridine

MOA

Idoxuridine is chemically very similar to thymidine, a compound which in the normal cell undergoes phosphorylation and then gets incorporated into DNA molecule. Due to the structural similarity with thymidine, with the help of thymidine kinase and thymidine monophosphate kinase enzymes, it is converted to the active triphosphorylated derivative. The later blocks DNA polymerase enzyme resulting into interference in nucleic acid and protein synthesis in DNA viruses. It also prevents the assembling of viral components by inhibiting the synthesis of a protein required for their assembling. Since the host cell-DNA synthesis is also affected, it produces host cytotoxicity. Hence its systemic use is not recommended. It is thus usually given topically. Hence serious side effects rarely attend its use.

Adverse effects

Adverse effects include pain, irritation, pruritus, inflammation or edema of conjunctiva and eyelids, corneal, vascularization, lacrimation, stomatitis, neutropenia and thrombocytopenia. It is effective in the treatment of herpes simplex infections of eyelid, conjunctiva and cornea.

Uses

It is a topically used antiviral agent chemically related with trifluridine. It is effective against vaccine and herpes simplex virus, pseudorabies, myxoma virus, polyoma virus and some papovaviruses.

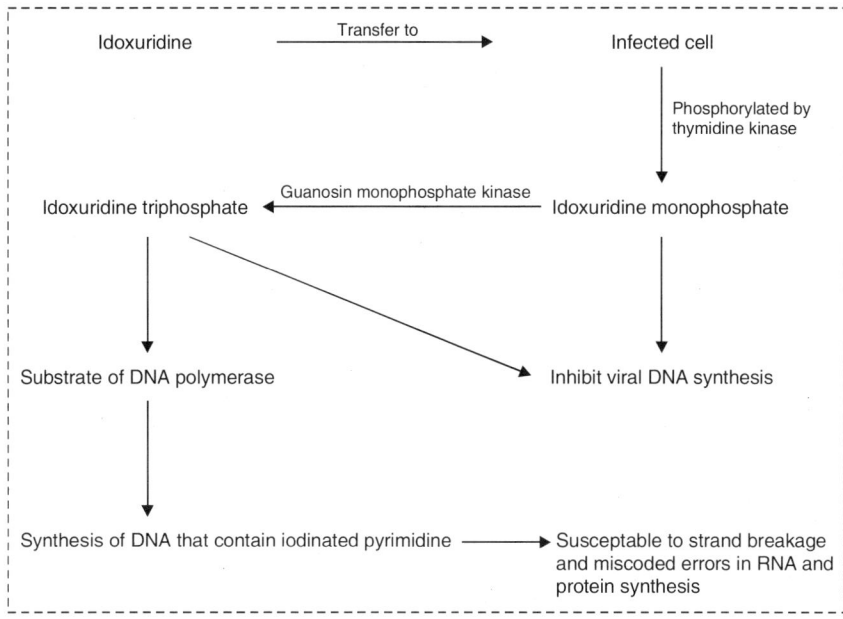

Trifluridine

MOA

It is converted to the active 5-monophosphate form. Due to the structural similarity with thymidine, it gets incorporated, instead of thymidine phosphorylated form, into replicating viral DNA. This results into wrong expression of genetic information due to abnormal base pairing. It also blocks thymidylate synthatase and deoxythymidine kinase enzymes in the viruses. The overall biological effects may get reflected into

a. Increased rate of mutation.

b. Inhibition of viral replication process.

Uses

- It is a halogenated thymidine analog used as a topical antiviral agent. It is effective against herpes simplex virus, vaccine and adenovirus

- In the form of 1% ophthalmic solution, it is used to treat certain ocular infections (e.g. ocular keratitis and keratoconjunctivitis). It exhibits effectiveness in cases where idoxuridine treatment fails.

Ribavirin

MOA

It is a synthetic nucleoside chemically related to inosine, guanosine and xanthosine. It is a broad-spectrum antiviral agent effective against nearly all major viruses. It has virustatic properties. It is *in vivo* converted to ribavirin-5'-monophosphate which acts as a competitive inhibitor of inosine 5'-monophosphate dehydrogenase. This results into inhibition of guanine monophosphate synthesis followed by inhibition of viral RNA synthesis.

Pharmacokinetics

It has a plasma half-life of 9 hours. It is extensively metabolized in the liver. Principal metabolites include mono-, di- and trisphosphate derivatives, tricarboxylic acid analog and 1, 2, 4-triazole carboxamide metabolite. De ribosylation and breakdown of triazole ring is also reported to occur.

Uses

- It is an investigational antiviral agent used in the treatment of infections due to respiratory viruses. It is used in the form of aerosol to treat severe lower respiratory tract infections due to respiratory syncytial virus (RSV). It is also undergoing evaluation in the treatment of human immunodeficiency virus (HIV) infections, like AIDS.

- Adenine arabinoside and cytosine arabinoside are other examples from this category. Cytosine arabinoside (cytarabine) is effective against herpes viruses. It is presently used in cancer chemotherapy.

▓ THIOSEMICARBAZONES

Methisazone

History

In 1947, Domagk (sulfonamide fame) reported that some derivatives of benzaldehyde thiosemicarbazone protected laboratory animals against tuberculosis. This initiated an extensive investigation of the thiosemicarbazone during which the activity of methisazone (N-methylisatin-p-thiosemicarbazone) was discovered. It is effective against a variety of poxviruses and some RNA viruses.

MOA

The antiviral action of thiosemicarbazone is perhaps due to the formation of metal chelate with various metal ions including Cu, Zn, Ni, ferrous and magnese. Methisazone thus acts by interacting with metalloenzymes that are necessary for the replication of certain viruses. The thiosemicarbazone may also react directly and specifically with viral nucleic acid.

Pharmacokinetic

Methisazone prevents replication of vaccine viruses. It is poorly absorbed by oral route. Major metabolic pathways include demethylation, replacement of sulfur by oxygen in the side chain and hydroxylation in the aromatic ring. Isatin-3-thiosemicarbazone is the active metabolite retaining half the activity of parent drug.

Uses

It is used as a prophylactic agent against smallpox and for the prevention and treatment of generalised vaccine or vaccine encephalitis.

▓ TREATMENT OF RESPIRATORY VIRUS INFECTION

Adamantane Amines

Amantadine hydrochloride

SAR:

1. N-alkylated and N, N-dialkyl derivatives possess some antiviral activity as that of the amantadine.

2. N-acyl derivative shows reduced antiviral activity.

3. Replacement of amino group by OH, SH, CN, halogen produce inactive compound.

4. Optical isomers and racemic mixtures of rimatadine are equally active.

5. Pyrolidine derivatives are more potent and active than admantane HCl.

MOA:

- Amantadine allows viral adsorption to the host cell but inhibits the uncoating of the influenza virus and prohibits penetration of viral genome into the host cell. Because the virion remains adsorbed to host cell surface, it becomes susceptible to attack by host antibodies.

- Besides its antiviral potential, it may also be employed in the therapy of Parkinsonism. Rimantadine is the better tolerated and less toxic analog of amantadine which is currently undergoing clinical evaluation. It has similar actions and uses.

Uses: It was first reported by Davies et al in 1964. It is a synthetic antiviral agent effective against infections caused by influenza A viruses including H_3N_2, Hsw INI and H_1N_1 subtypes. In higher concentrations, it is also effective against influenza B, rubella and other viruses.

Interferons (Antiviral Proteins)

Introduction

- The presence of interferons was first reported in 1957 by scientists Issaes and Lindermann at the National Institute for Medical Research, U.K. The term is applied to a class of glycoproteins of molecular weights from about 20,000 to 50,000.

- Each contains approximately 150 amino acids. Interferons are produced from the host cell when it is infected or is exposed to an inactive virus.

- The endogenous synthesis of interferons is under the control of host cell RNA. There are three major types of human interferons that are designated a, p and y according to antigen specifications. The preferred abbreviation of interferon is IFN. Interferons can also be designated as per the source, e.g. human (Hu IFN), bovine (Bov. IFN) murine (Mu IFN), etc.

- Currently major source of human interferons is from white blood cells that have been cultured and then exposed to appropriate viruses. In body, after their release, they may attach to surface receptors of the adjacent cells and initiate the production of additional interferons.

Mechanism of viral interference (Fig. 64.4)

- Viruses differ in their ability to induce the synthesis and/or liberation of interferons. The adsorption of a virus to the host cell or the full infected condition of the host cell induces the formation and release of interferons.

- This is a sort of immunization process. The release of interferon imparts resistance to the person against the attack of viral infection. Generally, a person once infected with one virus, develops a resistance against other viral infections. This phenomenon is known as viral interference. In non-infected cells, it can induce the formation of second inhibitory protein which has an ability to prevent the transcription of any viral m-RNA that might subsequently be produced in that cell.

Interferons are characterized by the following features:

1. Nontoxic substances to the host cell.

2. Exhibit antiviral activity in extremely low concentrations.

3. Do not possess antigenic activity.

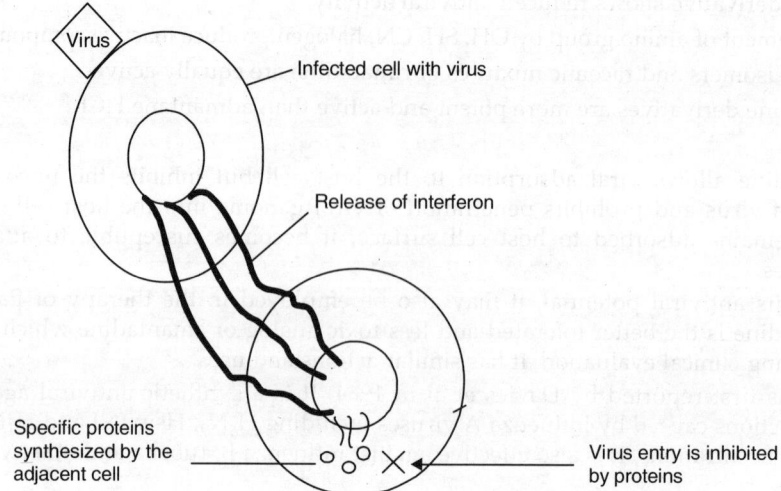

Fig. 64.4: Mechanism of viral interference

- Interferons appear very soon and sometimes within seconds after the viral attack. However, they lack specificity. Once released from the infected host cell, interferons induce the synthesis of translational inhibitory proteins in other, non-infected cells. These proteins impair the translation of viral m-RNAs and thus interfere in the viral replications. The synthesis of viral RNA polymerase and viral thymidine kinase is inhibited. The transcription of viral genome is also found to be inhibited.

- Interferon preparations may contain more than one type of interferon. Interferons have a unique broad-spectrum of antiviral activity in vitro and show promising effects when used in combination with vidarabine. Interferon preparations are effective against infections caused by varicella-zoster, encephalo-myocarditis virus, vesicular stomatitis virus, rabies, vaccine, influenza B and cytomegalovirus.

- Interferons are not orally absorbed. They are usually given by IV infusion. They have plasma half-life of about 15–20 minutes. Metabolic pathways for interferons are not still known.

Adverse effects

- Adverse effects mainly include fever, reticulocytopenia, neutropenia and thrombocytopenia. They are clinically effective against chronic active hepatitis B viral infection, cytomegaloviral infection, congenital rubella infections and respiratory viral infections.

- Interferons are also showing promising results in the therapy of some cancers like, melanoma, multiple myeloma, osteogenic sarcoma, certain leukemias and breast cancer.

- Their use in organ transplantation is also being extensively studied.

Interferon synthesis and liberation in animals

1. **Biological inducers:** These include human leukocytes, fibroblasts or lymphoblastoid cells.

2. **Chemical Inducers:** These include:

   1. Polyriboinosinic polyribocytidilic acid, which is a complex of polyinosinic and polycytidilic acids. Structurally, this complex is a synthetic analog of double stranded RNA.

   2. A new group of 6-phenylpyrimidine derivatives induces the host cell to produce interferons.

   3. Tilorone hydrochloride.

All these interferon inducers including viral infections produce diminished response upon re-exposure. It was proved difficult to make interferon in sufficient quantities for trials due to limitations of human tissue culture techniques. Recently recombinant DNA technology has been employed as an alternative method of producing large quantities of interferon in prokaryotic (bacteria) cells. In this technique, genes for human interferon are inserted into *E. coli* genome. The interferon thus produced could be used to perform extensive clinical trials against a variety of human viral infections.

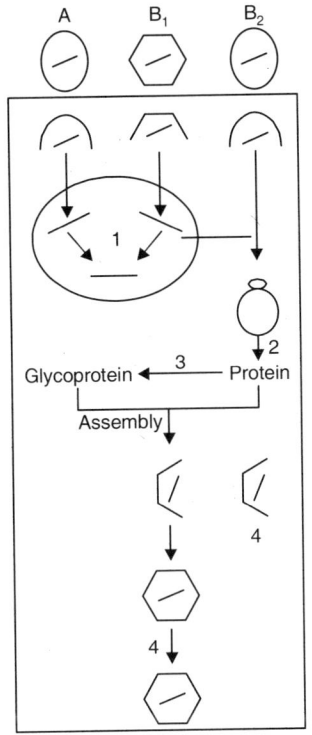

Viruses

A. DNA
B. RNA

MOA of interferon
1. Transcription inhibition
2. Translation inhibition
3. Protein processing inhibition
4. Virus maturation ibhibition

Fig. 64.5: Mode of action of interferon

The major drawbacks of interferon therapy

1. Interferon will have to be obtained from human subjects, if it is to be used in the treatment of human viral disease.

2. In human subjects, its serum half-life is not more than 15–20 minutes. The brief survival of interferon in body may be attributed to its rapid distribution and excretion from the body.

3. Numerous clinical trials of interferon utility suggested that it is not as useful in the therapy of viral infections as initially suspected.

▓ TREATMENT OF ACQUIRED IMMUMODEFICIENCY SYNDROME (AIDS)

Over 30 million people were infected with HIV. The basic difficulty experienced with this viral infection is the ability of the virus to mutate leading to rapid drug résistance. AIDS patient can prolong their life if early diagnosis and treatments are started. Initial HIV treatment requires specific drugs that inhibit reverse transcriptase and HIV protease.

Structure of HIV (Fig. 64.6)

HIV is a typical retrovirus with a small RNA genome of 9300 base pairs. Two copies of the genome are contained in a nucleocapsid core surrounded by a lipid bilayer, or envelope, that is derived from the host cell plasma membrane. The viral genome encodes three major open reading frames: *gag* encodes a polyprotein that is processed to release the major structural proteins of the virus; *pol* overlaps *gag* and encodes three important enzyme activities an RNA-dependent DNA polymerase or reverse transcriptase with RNAase activity, protease, and the viral integrase; and *env* encodes the large transmembrane envelope protein responsible for cell binding and entry. Several small genes encode regulatory proteins that enhance virion production or combat host defenses. These include *tat, rev, nef,* and *vpr*.

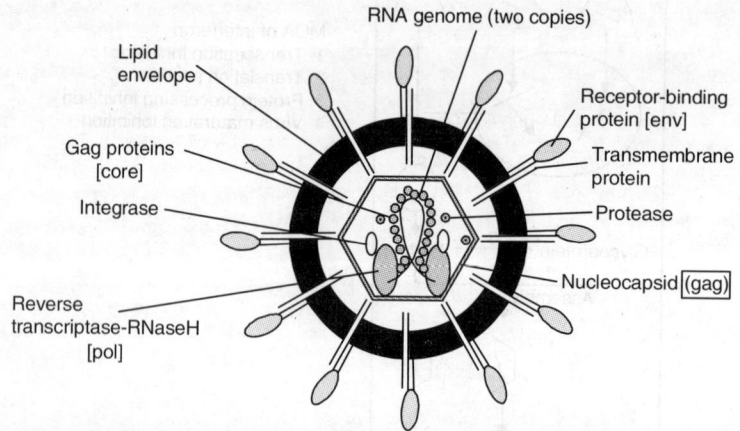

Fig. 64.6: Structure of HIV

Life Cycle of Human Immune Virus (HIV) (Fig. 64.7)

• HIV tropism is controlled by the envelope protein gp160 (env). The major target for env binding is the CD4 receptor present on lymphocytes and macrophages, although cell entry also requires binding to a coreceptor, generally the chemokine receptor CCR5 or CXCR4. CCR5 is present on macrophage lineage cells.

• Most infected individuals harbor predominately the CCR5-tropic virus; it is believed that this virus is responsible for sexual transmission of HIV and that the initial cells infected in sexual transmission express this coreceptor. A shift from CCR5 to CXCR4 utilization is associated with advancing disease, and the affinity of HIV-1 for CXCR4 allows infection of Tlymphocytes. A phenotypic switch from CCR5 to CXCR4 heralds accelerated loss of CD4+ helper T cells and increased risk of immunosuppression.

• Whether coreceptor switch is a cause or a consequence of advancing disease is still unknown. The gp41 domain of env controls the fusion of the virus lipid bilayer with that of the host cell. Following fusion, full-length viral RNA enters the cytoplasm, where it undergoes replication to a short-lived RNA-DNA duplex; the original RNA is degraded by RNase H to allow creation of a full-length double-stranded DNA copy of the virus. Because the HIV reverse transcriptase is error-prone and lacks a proofreading function, mutation is quite frequent and estimated to occur at approximately three bases out of every full-length (9300-base-pair) replication.

- Virus DNA is transported into the nucleus, where it is integrated into a host chromosome by the viral integrase in a random or quasi-random location. Following integration, the virus may remain in a quiescent state, not producing RNA or protein but replicating as the cell divides. When a cell that harbors the virus is activated, viral RNA and proteins are produced. Structural proteins assemble around full-length genomic RNA to form a nucleocapsid.

- The transmembrane envelope and other structural proteins assemble at the cell surface, concentrated in cholesterol-rich lipid rafts. The nucleocapsid cores are directed to these sites and bud through the cell membrane, creating a new enveloped HIV particle containing two complete single-stranded RNA genomes. Reverse transcriptase is incorporated into this particle so that replication can begin immediately after the virus enters cell.

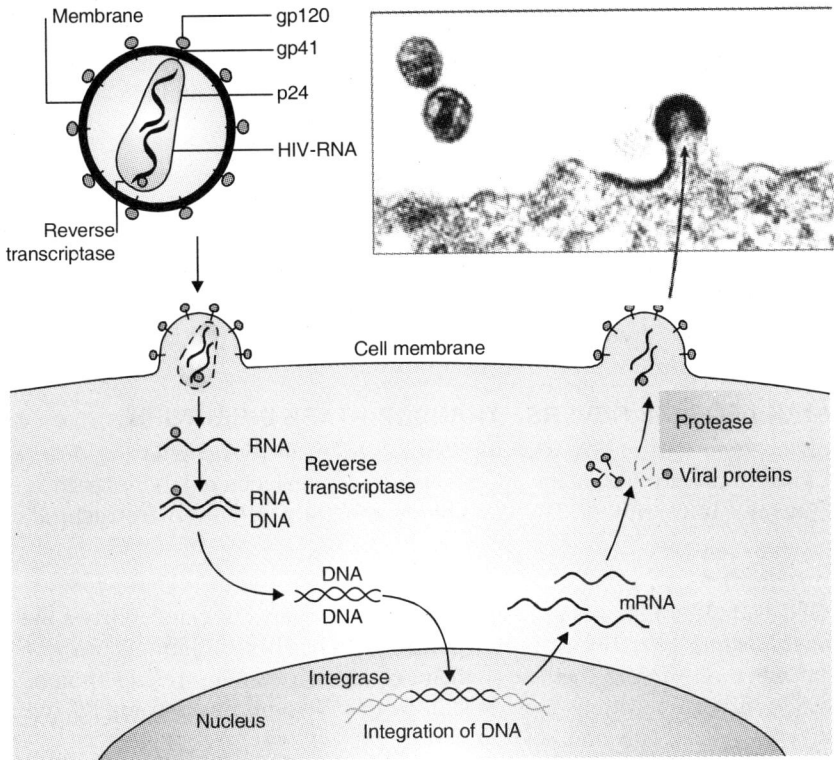

Fig. 64.7: Life cycle of HIV

▓ REVERSE TRANSCRIPTASE INHIBITORS

Zidovudine

MOA: The active trisphosphate metabolite inhibits viral RNA-dependant DNA polymerase (reverse transcriptase, RT). This enzyme is essential for the life cycle of the retrovirus. Zidovudine trisphosphate has greater selectivity affinity for reverse transcriptase than for human DNA polymerase. This causes chain termination and reverse transcriptase inhibition.

Pharmacokinetic: The oral bioavailability of zidovudine is 60 to 65%. The half-life is about 1 hour and metabolized to inactive 5′-glucuronide.

Adverse effect: Serious side effects, such as granulocytopenia and anemia, severe headache, nausea, insomnia and myalgias.

Zalcitabine

MOA: The principle mechanism of action involves phosphorylation to the trisphosphate and then inhibition of the reverse transcriptase and proviral DNA chain termination.

Adverse effect: Most severe side effects are peripheral neuropathy, pancreatitis, rash, oral ulcers, decreased blood platelet counts and abnormal liver function.

Didanosine

MOA: Didanosine undergoes intracellular conversion to the purative active trisphosphate metabolite. The active metabolite appears to inhibit viral reverse transcriptase and terminate the proviral DNA, and produces viustatic inhibition of actively replicating HIV.

Adverse effect: Didanosine is generally well tolerated with minimal haematological toxicity. Peripheral neuropathy and pancreatitis are the predominant dose-limiting adverse events.

Stavudine

MOA: Stavudine is a drug that resembles zidovudine and didanosine both structurally and mechanistically. It is phosphorylated and the phosphate is belived to be the active form of stavudine, which inhibit the enzyme reverse transcriptase.

Adverse effect: Nausea and vomiting and sensory peripheral neuropathy have been reported as adverse effect.

Uses: It is given for the treatment of patient with AIDS who are intolerant of refractory to approved therapies.

▓ NON-NUCLEOSIDIC REVERSE TRANSCRIPTASE INHIBITORS

Since the discovery in 1981 of HIV, the virus causing AIDS, the development of drugs to treat HIV infection has been a priority. One of the principal targets for inhibition of HIV has been the blockade of the enzyme, reverse transcriptase. These inhibitors generally fall into two structural classes:

1. Nucleoside analogue
2. Non-nucleosides

The non-nucleoside RT inhibitors are a structurally heterogeneous class of drugs that selectively inhibit HIV-1variants but lack activity against HIV-2. These inhibitors do not undergo a intracellular metabolism, and their mechanism of anti-viral action relates to non-competitive binding to RT. Adverse reactions include skin rashes. Two non-nucleoside RT inhibitors have been marketed— delavirdine and nevirapine.

▓ HIV PROTEASE INHIBITORS

- HIV, encodes an aspartate protease consisting in its active form of two symmetric subunits. This enzyme is required for cleavage of polypeptide precursors that generate the structural proteins and enzymes of the virus, including reverse transcriptase, integrase, and the protease itself. This aspartate proteinase is essential for the final step of viral proliferation. It is translated as part of the large gag-pol 160-KDA precursor proteins and undergoes autocatalytic cleavage from this precursor.

- The active enzyme then hydrolytically affects the precursor proteins to generate proteins which are necessary to the virus. The HIV protease inhibitors interfere in this process and lead to the assembly of non-functional virions.

- Recently, three HIV protease inhibitors have been approved— saquinavir, ritonavir, and indinavir. All are very specific for the vital enzyme and generally much higher concentrations are required to inhibit mammalian proteases. They are orally effective but, nausea, vomiting and diarrhea do occur.
- Examples, saquinavir, indinavir, ritonavir.

HIV INTEGRASE INHIBITOR

HIV integrase is a new target for therapeutic intervention in HIV-1 infection. HIV integrase is the enzyme responsible for catalyzing the insertion of the viral cDNA into the host-cell chromosome, an essential step for the replication of this virus.

Zintervir

MOA: Zintevir binds strongly to the HIV second receptor, chemokine receptors, thus preventing binding and fusion of the HIV virus with the host cells.

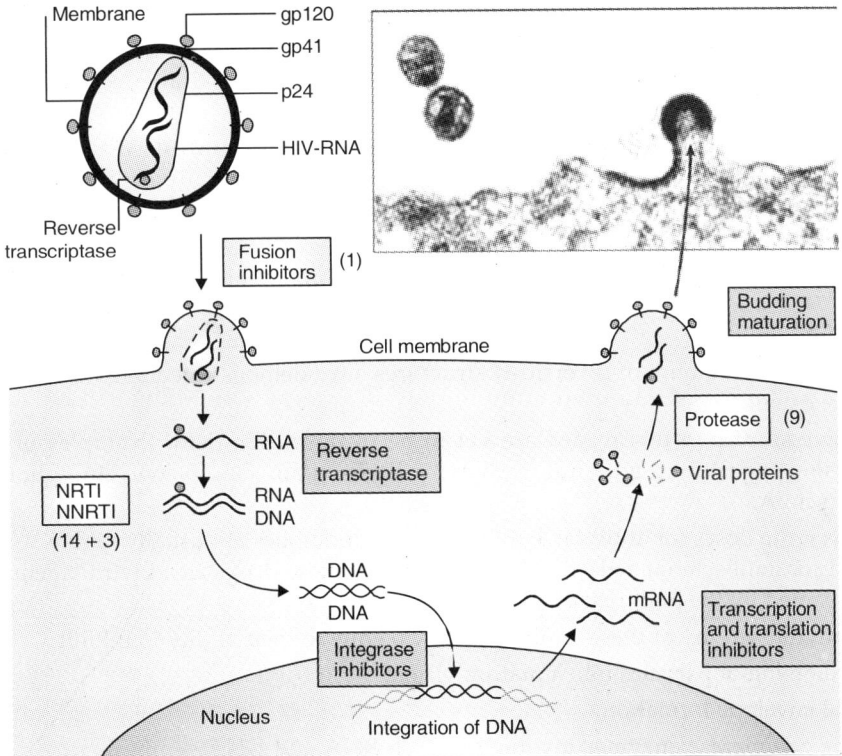

Fig. 64.8: Possible targets for HIV

MISCELLANEOUS AGENTS

Ureas and Thioureas

Members of this class exhibited good antiviral activity but they could not be evaluated further because of their immunosuppressive side effects.

Guanidines and Biguanidines

Guanidine hydrochloride shows selective inhibition of enteroviruses and more specifically polioviruses. But probably due to its rapid urinary excretion, the drug failed to achieve a clinical status. The mode of action involves the selective inhibition of viral RNA polymerases. An extensive investigation in this class is still going on.

Heterocyclic Dyes

- The members of this series having antiviral potential include proflavin and neutral red. The herpetic lesions are painted with 0.1% solution of these dyes and then the painted area is exposed to 16–30 W fluorescent light for 15 minutes.
- This results into breakdown of viral DNA and death of the virus. The painted area may be re-exposed to the light at the interval of 6–8 hours.

Gamma Globulin (Immune Globulin)

- It is the antibody-rich fraction of the plasma which contains a variety of antiviral antibodies. It is thought to act by preventing the penetration of virus into the host cell. It is orally ineffective. After a single injection, it offers protection against viral infection for about 2 – 3 weeks.
- These immunoglobulins are derived from p-lymphocytes and plasma cells in very low amounts. Usually only one class of immunoglobulins is initially synthesized by a given immunocyte and a clone of immunocytes synthesizes a specific type of immunoglobulins.
- Details about the fate of immunoglobulins are not available. Liver serves as a major site where they are degraded. Rarely immunoglobulines are eliminated through the urine.

Antibiotics

- A number of antibiotics of diversified structures have demonstrated antiviral activity to less or more extent.
- Extensive studies in this regard are yet to be made in this field. Examples of antibiotics possessing significant antiviral activity include rifamycin, bleomycin, gliotoxins and clistamycin A.
- However, the doses for antiviral activity of these antibiotics are usually higher than the dose needed for antibacterial activity. Hence the use of these drugs as antiviral agents is always accompanied by the high risk of adverse effects.
- The antiviral activity of these antibiotics may be due to their ability to inhibit
  1. Assembling of particles into a mature virion.
  2. Viral envelope formation.
- Various polymerase enzymes involved in both RNA and DNA synthesis in viruses are the principal target sites of action of these antibiotics.

▨ DESIGN OF ANTIVIRAL AGENTS

- Viral chemotherapy is still in the phase of infancy. Although a great deal of work has been done, it has resulted in the development of only 3–4 clinically used agents. Presently immunization, public health measures and physical and chemical disinfection procedures play a vital role in the prevention of spread of viral diseases.

- Viruses are essentially intracellular parasites. Unlike bacteria, the viral replication is totally dependent upon the energy, proteins and enzymatic machinery of the host cell. Bacteria have self-contained biosynthetic machinery. Hence the drug in bacterial chemotherapy enjoys the advantage of selective attack on bacteria due to many metabolic and molecular differences between the pathogen and the host cell.

- Since viruses literally take over the metabolic machinery of the infected human cell, a close relationship exists between the multiplying virus and the host cell. Virus replication is intimately dependent upon the host cell metabolism. This fact severely limits the usual opportunities to design antiviral agent having selective effect on the viral cell. Attempts to inhibit viral growth without damaging the host cells became fruitless.

- Even the host cell is infected by a virus; the announcement of its presence is received so late that extensive viral multiplication and tissue damage has been already occurred. The late diagnosis and recognition of the disease state projects almost negligible chances for effective therapy. The drugs become useless, even if they are made available.

- The important key events in the viral replication are diagrammatically shown in the figure of virus multiplication.

- It is apparent that various steps involved in the viral replication could be successfully utilized as the basis of designing antiviral agents. For example, the following sites in viral replication offered promising points for the attack of antiviral agents.

  1. Adsorption of virus on the host cell.
  2. Penetration of virus in host cell.
  3. Synthesis of viral genetic material.

- Amantadine hydrochloride inhibits viral penetration and prevents influenza while methisazone and idoxuridine inhibit viral DNA synthesis. Due to one or more reasons (e.g. narrow activity spectra or toxicity) not a single drug in this area, enjoyed clinical popularity. The development of antiviral agent having selective toxicity to viral cells leaving host cells unaffected still remained a dream for the medicinal chemists.

- Antiviral agents have often been proved to be disappointing due to the following problems in their development:

  1. Lack of satisfactory experimental models.
  2. Use of wrong virus in the laboratory.
  3. Narrow spectrum of activity.
  4. Limitations on uses due to their toxicity.
  5. Difficulties in their clinical assessment.

- These disappointing features of antiviral therapy force us to accept vaccines as the best prophylactic agents in the treatment of viral diseases. There are four forms of antigen used in vaccines. These include:

  1. Attenuated living.
  2. Killed by the chemicals, such as formalin.
  3. Toxoids (i.e. toxins which through the application of heat or formalin are converted to non-toxic).
  4. Subunits prepared by purifying important antigens of microorganisms.

- Vaccination can be effectively used to prevent measles, rubella, mumps, poliomyelitis, yellow fever, smallpox and hepatitis B. They have only prophylactic utility. They remain ineffective once the infection has occurred and spreaded within the host.

Zidovoudine

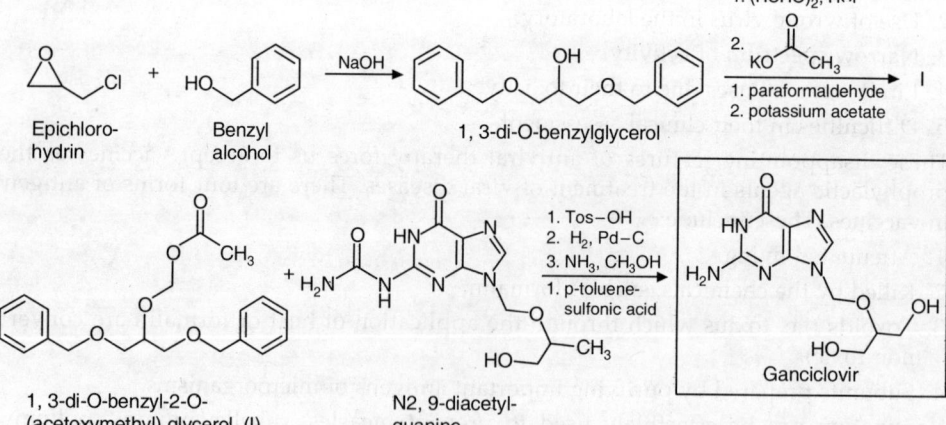

Thymidine (I)

1. Trt—Cl, pyridine
2. H₃C—S—Cl, pyridine
1. triphenylmethyl

(II)

Trt: triphenylmethyl

II

Phthalimide potassium

5'-O-trityl-2-3'-anhydrothymidine

1. NaN₃, DMF
2. aq. CH₃COOH, Δ
1. sodium azide

Zidovudine

Didanosine

2', 3'-dideoxy-odenosine

Fermentation with Acinetobacter lwoffi (ATCC 9036)

Didonosine

Ganciclovir

Epichloro-hydrin

Benzyl alcohol

NaOH

1, 3-di-O-benzylglycerol

1. (HCHO)₂, HCl
2. KO—C(=O)—CH₃
1. paraformaldehyde
2. potassium acetate

I

1, 3-di-O-benzyl-2-O-(acetoxymethyl) glycerol (I)

+ H₂N—C(=O)—NH—

N2, 9-diacetyl-guanine

1. Tos—OH
2. H₂, Pd—C
3. NH₃, CH₃OH
1. p-toluene-sulfonic acid

Ganciclovir

Stavudine

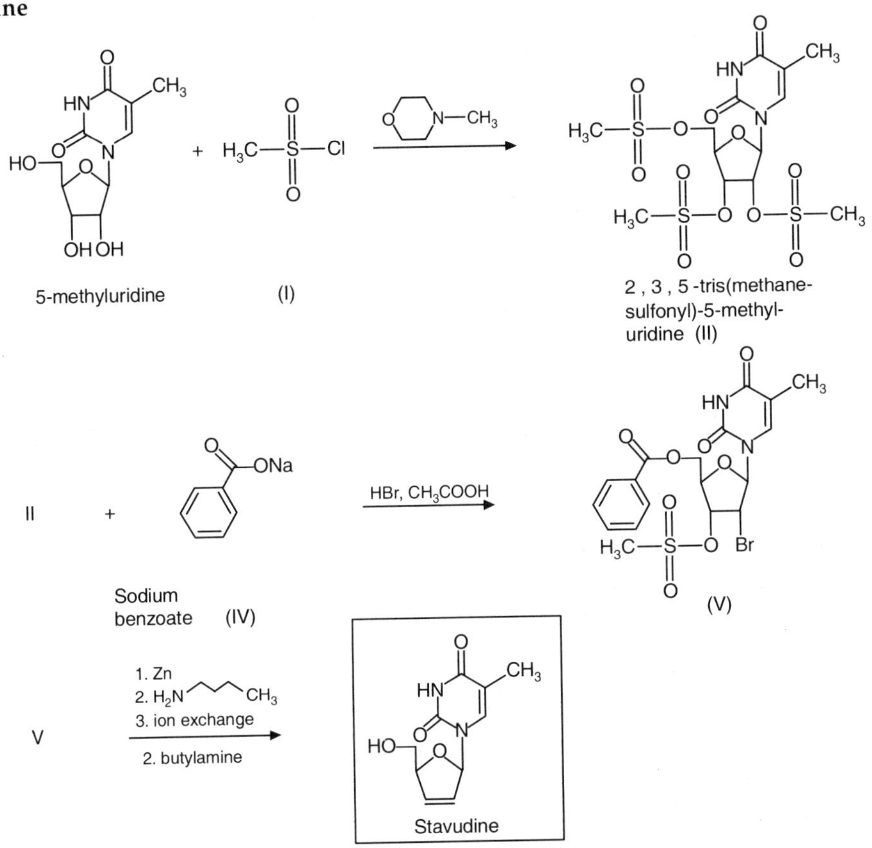

5-methyluridine   (I)

2,3,5-tris(methane-
sulfonyl)-5-methyl-
uridine (II)

II   +

Sodium
benzoate   (IV)

HBr, CH₃COOH

(V)

V

1. Zn
2. H₂N   CH₃
3. ion exchange

2. butylamine

Stavudine

Amantadine

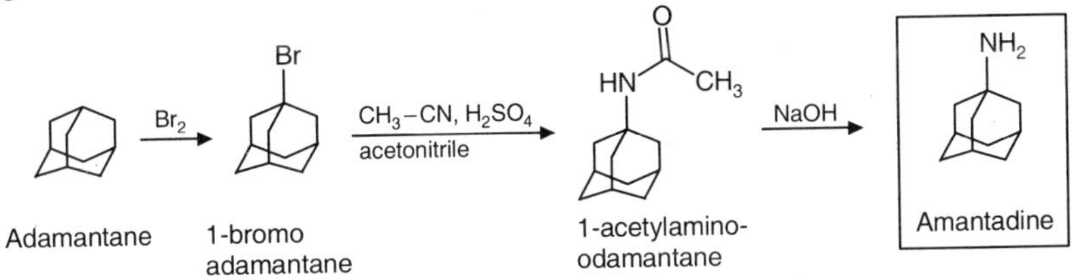

Adamantane   1-bromo
adamantane

Br₂

CH₃–CN, H₂SO₄
acetonitrile

HN   CH₃

1-acetylamino-
odamantane

NaOH

NH₂

Amantadine

Rimantadine

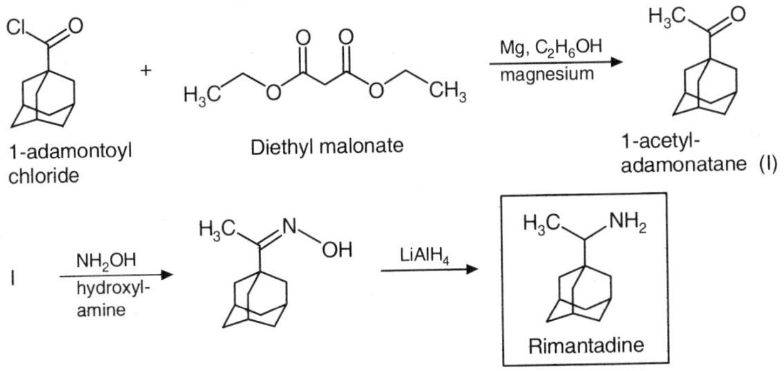

1-adamontoyl
chloride

+   Diethyl malonate

Mg, C₂H₆OH
magnesium

1-acetyl-
adamonatane (I)

I

NH₂OH
hydroxyl-
amine

LiAlH₄

Rimantadine

Anticancer Agents

Cancer means uncontrolled growth of the cell. Tumour is a general term indicating proliferation of the cells which is no longer under the control of the organism. This unwanted proliferation of cells consumes a significant portion of the body's supply of food material and metabolic energy thereby leaving the patient progressively weaker.

TYPES OF CARCINOMA

On the basis of tissue involved, cancer can be classified into the following types:

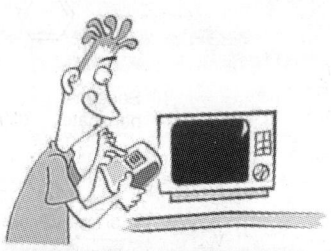

1. **Carcinoma:** This type of cancer originated from epithelial cells e.g. breast cancer, skin cancer, lungs cancer.

2. **Sarcoma:** This type of cancer originated from connective tissue and from mesodermal tissue, e.g. bones cancer, lymph cancer.

3. **Lymphoma:** It is developed in lymph nodes, e.g. lymphoma.

Cook for 3 minutes stir, wait 30 years to discover if the contaminated ingredient gives you stomach cancer.

4. **Leukemias:** It is suppose to develop from blood tissue and bone marrow, e.g. blood cancer. The advances that have occurred in the treatment of neoplastic disorders have placed clinical cures within reach. As knowledge has been accumulated in the areas of pharmacology, tumor biology, cytokinetics and drug-resistance, therapeutic strategies have been developed that maximize the tumor-cell kill, decrease the resistance and enhance the potential for cure by chemotherapy. Chemotherapy plays a significant role in the treatment of macrometastatis along with surgery or radiation.

CAUSES OF CANCER (FIG. 65.1)

Many factors are implicated in the induction of cancer. These factors may include:

1. Exposure to the carcinogenic hydrocarbons or to excessive radiation.

2. A cancer family syndrome has been described by Lynch et al. The hereditary factors involved in the causation of cancer include cromosomal abnormality, enzymes, immune defence system and hormonal imbalances. For example, the susceptibility to the lung cancer is associated with high inducible levels of the enzyme, aryl hydrocarbon hydroxylase.

3. Culture factors play a dominant role by causing about 70% of all cancers. Such important cultural factors include diet, smoking, drinking and sexual habits.

4. Occupational factors like, ionizing radiation, chemicals and other carcinogenic substances play an important role. For example, coal tar, mustard gas, chromium, hematite, nickel and

asbestos can trigger lung cancer in employees working in chemical, insulation and gas factories.

5. Though it is known that viruses cause cancer in animals, their role in human cancers has not been proved.

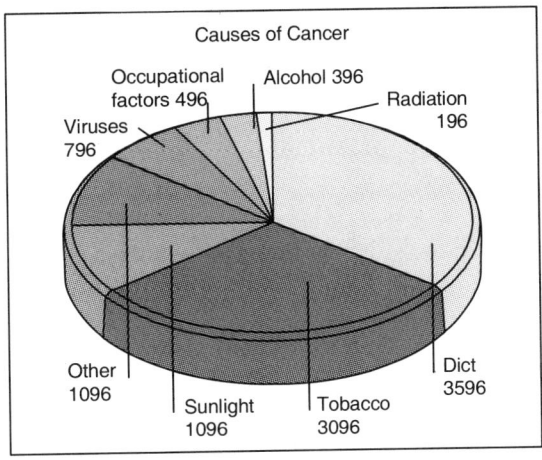

Fig. 65.1: Causes of cancer

▨ CELL-CYCLE KINETICS (FIG. 65.2)

- During cell cycle, each cell divides into two daughter cells having identical genetic material. Each of these cells may immediately re-enter a new cell cycle or pass into a non-proliferative resting state. The growth and division of cells can be defined into four prominent phases of cell cycle. These include:

  1. **S-phase:** This phase is a phase of DNA synthesis. In human tumour, it is approximately of 10 to 20 hours.

  2. **G_2-phase:** This period last for 1 to 3 hours during which the cell is made ready for mitosis. In this phase, the cells contain a tetraploid number of chromosomes. This phase is followed by mitosis.

  3. **M-phase:** It is a phase of mitosis that involves chromosomal condensation, spindle formation and cell division. It lasts for approximately one hour. The resulting two daughter cells may either immediately enter into G_1-phase (post-mitotic rest) or pass into a non-proliferative resting phase.

  4. **G_0-phase:**

- Since proliferating cells are usually more' sensitive to chemotherapy, the cells in G_0 -phase are least affected by chemotherapeutic agent.

- The cells readily pass into G_0-phase, if they are far away from the blood vessels through which nutrients are supplied. The growth of a tumor usually follows exponential pattern that is growth occurs initially at much higher rate which is then followed by a plateau region.

- The decrease in the growth rate with increasing tumor size may be, corelated with an increase in the rate of cell loss due to hypoxic necrosis, immunological defence mechanism and poor nutrient supply.

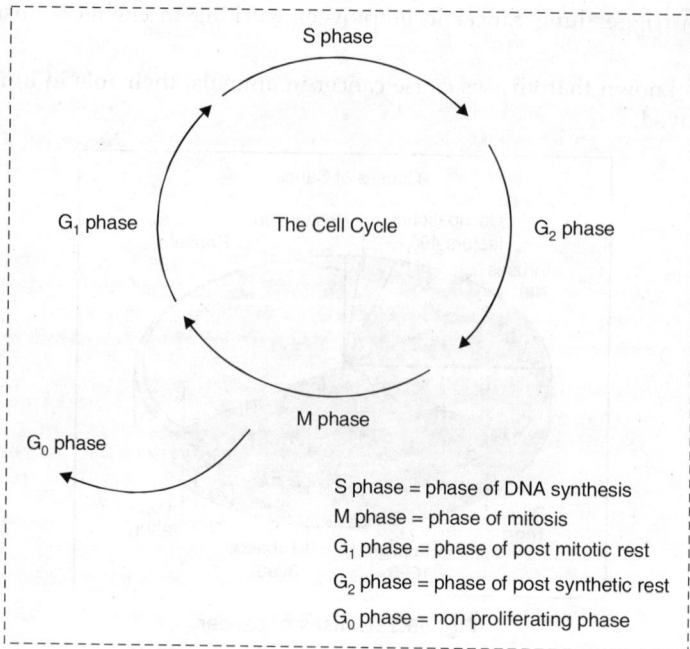

Fig. 65.2: Cell cycle with different phases

- Since proliferating cells are generally more sensitive to chemotherapy, smaller tumors (i.e. tumors with high growth rate) will be more sensitive to chemotherapy than the large solid tumors (i.e. tumors with slow growth rate).

PROBLEMS FACED IN CHEMOTHERAPY OF CANCER

1. Cell parameters like morphology, immunogenicity, rate of multiplication, metastatic property significantly govern the responsiveness to antineoplastic agents. In case of individual heterogenic tumors which contain many submasses of different types of neoplastic cells.

2. In infections, the invading of micro-organism is biologically foreign to the host and its distinct metabolic reaction can selectively be attacked by chemotherapeutic agents without disturbing the normal body metabolic processes. In addition, the immune mechanism and other host defence system offer major contribution to chemotherapy but since malignant cell is no way different to the normal cell the host defence plays a negligible role in the therapy of neoplastic diseases. The addition of immunostimulants, to the therapeutic regimen helps the body's natural defence mechanisms to identify the cancer cells.

3. Neoplastic cells may develop resistance to drugs. Amplification of various genes usually occurs due to rapid proliferating rate in cancer cells. This serves as an important genetic mechanism for developing resistance to drugs. Hence smaller tumors are more susceptible to the action of antineoplastic drugs than large tumors because of increased probability of drug resistant materials in large tumors.

4. Antineoplastic drugs kill a constant fraction of tumor cells rather than a fixed number of cells at a given dose. Such killing pattern is known as log-cell kill pattern. Because of such

first order cell kill kinetic, several dose schedules of therapy would be required to decrease the size of tumor to such an extent which would no longer be detectable clinically.

5. Since many dose schedules of antineoplastic agents are to be repeated in order to get complete remission, the use of these agents is associated with high risk of adverse effects. These chemotherapeutic agents are more effective on the malignant cells with high proliferating rate. But since malignant cell is no way different to the normal cell, many normal tissues having high proliferating rate are also affected by antineoplastic agents. The toxicity of these agents hence may be observed on rapidly proliferating normal tissues such as bone marrow, hair follicles, germinal tissues, lymphoidal tissues and intestinal epithelium. On the other hand, slow growing tumors and cells in the resting state are often unresponsive to these agents.

6. Most of the quantitative differences between normal and cancer cells relate to biochemical pathways, transport processes and DNA repair mechanism. Since differences between normal and malignant cells are merely quantitative rather than qualitative, it leads to certain degree of drug-induced toxicity to normal tissues. Individual agent may produce its own distinctive adverse effects on heart, lungs, kidneys and other organs.

ADVERSE EFFECTS

The prominent adverse effects of antineoplastic drugs are exerted on rapidly proliferating normal tissues in addition to their chronic and cumulative toxicities.

Bone Marrow Toxicity

- Bone marrow is an example of site where a rapid proliferation of hematopoietic precursor cells usually takes place. The toxicity is reflected in terms of myelo-suppression which is characterised by leucopenia, thrombocytopenia and hemorrhage.
- Since white blood cells and platelet count are decreased in the presence of antineoplastic drugs, this results into increased chances of life-threatening infections and bleeding.
- However, few antineoplastic agents (e.g. bleomycin, L-asparginase and certain hormonal agents) have minimal myelosuppressive activity.

GI tract

- Anorexia, nausea, vomiting, stomatitis, dysphagia, oesphagitis, peptic ulcer and diarrhea are some of the few common adverse effects associated with the use of antineoplastic agents.
- Most of these effects appear as a result of damage to normally proliferating mucosa of GIT. However, nausea or vomiting occurs due to the stimulatory effects of these drugs on chemoreceptor trigger zone in the CNS.

Hair Folical Toxicity

Alopecia or loss of hair is a common adverse effect specifically with methotrexate, vincristine, cyclophosphamide and doxorubicin. However, hair regrows if the therapy is discontinued.

CNS Toxicity

- These effects are of reversible nature which disappears after some days of therapy. They include headache, weakness, disorientation, somnolence, myalgias and parasthesias of hands and feet.

- Orthostatic hypertension and chronic constipation are also reported to occur as a result of impairment of autonomic functions.

Nephrotoxicity

- Uric acid production increases because of increased metabolism of nucleic acids released from destruction of tumor cells by anticancer drugs. This uric acid is a source of nephrotoxicity which can be minimized by either: (1) adequate hydration of patient and alkalinization of urine and/or (2) by prior administration of allopurinol.
- The nephrotoxicity is characterised by inappropriate anti-diuretic hormone secretion, hyponatremia, renal tubular damage, bladder fibrosis and electrolyte problems.

Hepatotoxicity

It is mainly caused by drugs like azathioprim, mercaptopurin, L-asparaginase, etc. The extent of liver damage ranges from minimal elevation of transaminases, cirrhotic changes to even necrosis.

Skin Rashes

- Some of the antineoplastic agents (e.g. vinca alkaloids, nitrosouria, anthracyclins, mitomycin C, etc.) are potent irritant.
- They must not be injected by s.c. or i.m. route, since they cause local tissue necrosis. Most of these agents may cause hyperpigmentation, flushing, hyperkeratosis, dermatitis or urticaria.

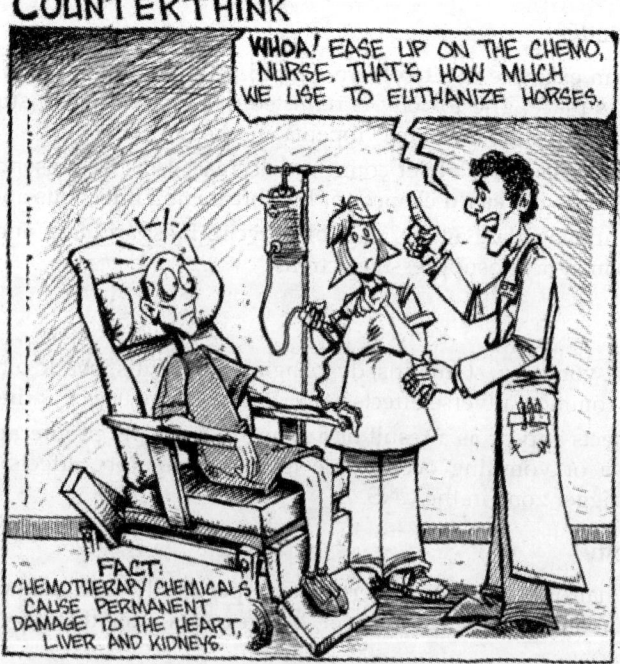

Pulmonary Toxicity

Many drugs like bleomycin, methotrexate, busulfan, etc. exert adverse effects on the lung function. These effects include allergic intestitial pneumonia and chronic pulmonary fibrosis.

Cardiac Toxicity

Severe cardiac damage is reported to be induced by chronic administration of doxorubicin, daunorubicin and anthracyclins.

Immunosuppression

- Most of the antineoplastic agents have an ability to suppress natural defence mechanism. These effects may be helpful in patients undergoing organ transplantation surgery.
- However, in normal patients, the immunosuppressive effect of these drugs exposes the patient to the risk of various infections.

Miscellaneous Effects

These effects include fever, anaphylaxis, cataracts, hemolytic anemia, pancreatitis, pituitary insufficiency, adrenal insufficiency, coagulation problems, suppression of growth and carcinogenicity. Methotrexate is the potent teratogen.

Germinal Tissue

- Since germinal tissue is an example of rapidly proliferating tissues, its functioning is adversely affected by antineoplastic drug therapy.
- The prominent effects include impaired spermatogenesis and impaired oogenesis.

▓ DRUG RESISTANCE

- The cell-kill exhibited by antineoplastic agents follows first order kinetics. It means that a constant fraction of tumor cells rather than a fixed number of tumor cells are killed by antineoplastic agents at a given dose. Hence in order to achieve complete clinical remission of the tumor, several cycles of therapy would be required. For example, most curable tumors require at least six to eight cycles of therapy. Development of resistance to the drug action is thus quite obvious that results into regrowth of tumor cells.
- Tumor grows as a result of amplification of various genes. The increasing number of mutations that occur during the growth of a tumor results into development of subpopulations of heterogenous cells within the tumor. Hence, the tumors of same size and type will vary in their responsiveness to the drug therapy. The large tumors are usually less susceptible to the chemotherapeutic agents because of increased probability of drug resistant mutations. Various mechanisms used to explain the emergence of drug resistant tumor cells are discussed below.

1. Pleotropic resistance, this type of resistance develops due to decreased drug transportation or drug retention within the tumor cells. Due to the spontaneous mutations over production of high molecular weight membrane glycoprotein, gp - 180 occurs resulting into alterations in the cell membrane permeability to the drug. This type of resistance is seen with the use of dactinomycin, vinca alkaloids and anthracyclins.

2. Many antineoplastic agents should undergo metabolic activation in order to exhibit therapeutic effectiveness. They would be ineffective, if they are not converted to their active metabolites. Some tumour cells develop resistance to the action of such antineoplastic agents by lowering down the concentration of enzymes which are involved in metabolic activation of such anti-tumor agents.

3. In some tumors, resistance to the action of antineoplastic agents emerges because of their rapid inactivation.

4. L-asparaginase acts by decreasing the concentration of aspargin in the concerned tumors. Resistance to its action can be developed due to drug-related induction of enzyme aspargin synthetase. This enzyme increases the rate of formation of aspargin and compensate the loss made by L-asparaginase.

5. Increased production of the target molecule is an important mechanism by which resistance can develop. For example, in the treatment with alkylating agents an increase in cell thiol content serves as alternate target of alkylation.

COMBINATION THERAPY

- Because of heterogenic nature of the tumor cells and the chronic nature of the therapy, the use of single chemotherapeutic agent would be less effective and more toxic.
- The use of drug combination therapy would also be helpful to suppress the emergence of drug resistant tumor cells. The drugs which are included in combination therapy should have:
  1. Dissimilar modes of action.
  2. Different spectra of adverse effects.
  3. Additive or synergistic antitumor activity.
- Acute leukemia, carcinoma of breast, advanced ovarian carcinoma, soft tissue sarcoma, neuroblastoma, advanced small cell carcinoma of lungs and stage III and IV of Hodgkin's disease are few examples where combination therapy provides better results. For example, in the treatment of stage III – IV of epithelial ovarian cancer PAC (i.e. cisplatin, adriamycin and cyclophosphamide) combination therapy is prescribed. In the treatment of ovarian cancer CHAD (i.e. cyclophosphamide, hexa-methyl melanin, adriamycin and cisplatin) combination is commonly used while PVB (i.e. cisplatin, vinblastin and bleomycin) provides better results in the treatment of dissiminated testicular cancer.
- While CMF (cyclophosphamide, methotrexate and 5-flourouracil) combination therapy is commonly used in the treatment of breast cancer. A complete remission of acute lymphocytic leukemia can be achieved by using VAMP (vincristin, methotrexate, mercaptopurine and prednisone) combination.

PHASE SPECIFIC AGENTS

- These drugs act at a particular phase of cell cycle. They are more effective on proliferating cells. For sample, bleomycin attacks cells in G_2-and early M-phase. Cytarabine kills cells only in the S-phase by inhibiting DNA synthesis. The effectiveness of phase specific antineoplastic agents is maintained by giving them through continuous infusion. Dactinomycin is more effective against cells in G_1-phase while doxorubicin kills cells in late S-phase. Many antimetabolit are specifically effective against cells in G_1 and G_2 phases where they act by inhibiting RNA synthesis.
- Some antineoplastic agents exert their effect on both normal and malignant cells. Their activity is not influenced by the degree of proliferation. Even non-proliferating cells are also killed to the same extent. Examples include carmustine and mechlorethamine.

1. **S-phase-specific agents:** These include alkylating agents, cisplatin, hydroxyurea, daxorubicin and daunorubicin.

2. **G_1-phase-specific agents:** These include agents like bleomycin and doxorubicin.

3. **M-phase specific agents:** These include vincristine, vinblastine and colchicine.

4. **G_2-phase specific agents:** These include prednisone, daunorubicin and L-asparaginase.

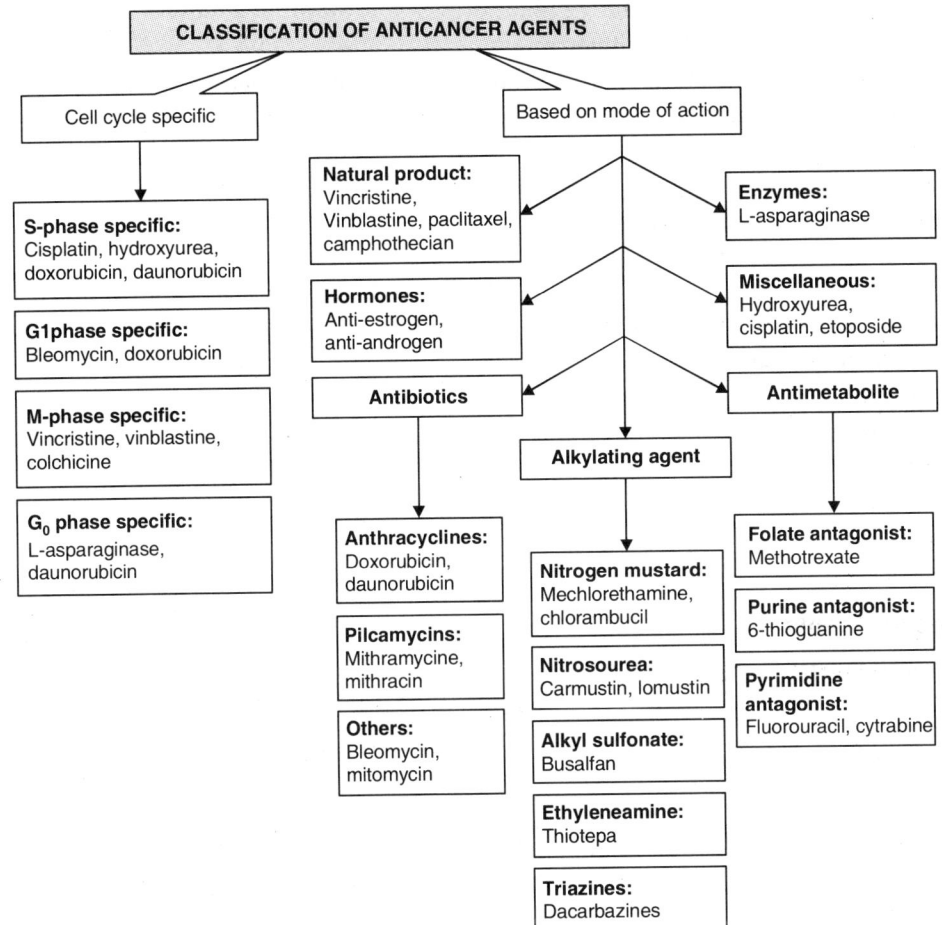

BASED UPON THEIR SITE OF ACTION

1. **Alkylating agents:**
- Nitrogen mustards— cyclophosphamide, chlorambucil.
- Alkyl sulfonates— busulfan
- Nitrosoureas— carmustine, streptozocin
- Ethylenimines— thiotepa, triazenes, dacarbazines

2. **Antimetabolites:**
- Folate antagonists— methotrexate
- Purine analogues— 6-thioguanine.
- Pyrimidine analogues— cytarabine, fluorouracil

3. **Antibiotics**
- Anthracyclines— doxorubicin, daunorubicin
- Bleomycins— bleomycin
- Mitomycin C

- Dactinomycins (actinomycin-D)
- Plicamycins— mithramycin, mithracin
4. **Natural product:** Vincristine, vinblastine, paclitaxel, camphothecian
5. **Enzymes:** L-asparaginase
6. **Hormones**
- Glucocorticoids
- Estrogens/antiestrogens— tomoxifen, estramustine
- Androgens/antiandrogens— eyproteron
- Progestins
- LH-RH antagonists— buserelin, leuprolide
7. **Miscellaneous**
- Hydroxyurea
- Procarbazine
- Mitotane
- Hexamethyl melamine
- Cisplatin
- Etoposide

Alkylating Agents

a. Nitrogen mustard

Cyclophosphamide   Mechlorethamine   Chlorambucil   Melphalan

b. Nitrosourea

Lomustine   Carmustine

c. Aziridines

1-(2, 4-dinitrophenyl) aziridines   Triethylene melamine

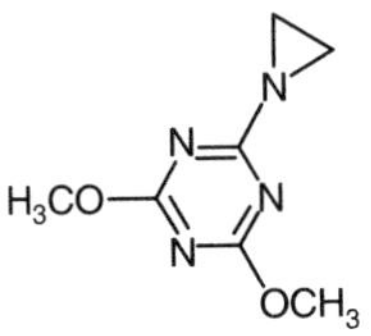

4(1-aziridinyl)-2, 6-dimethoxy triazine 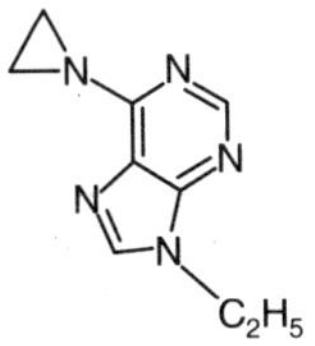   6-(aziridinh-1-yl)-9-ethyl-9H-purine

d. Methane sulfonate ester

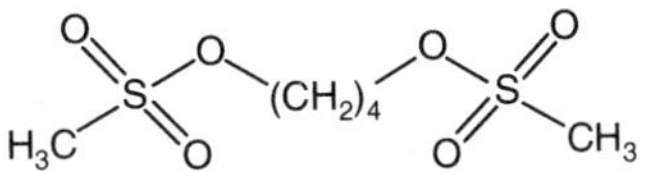

Busulfan

Antimetabolites

a. Folate antagonist

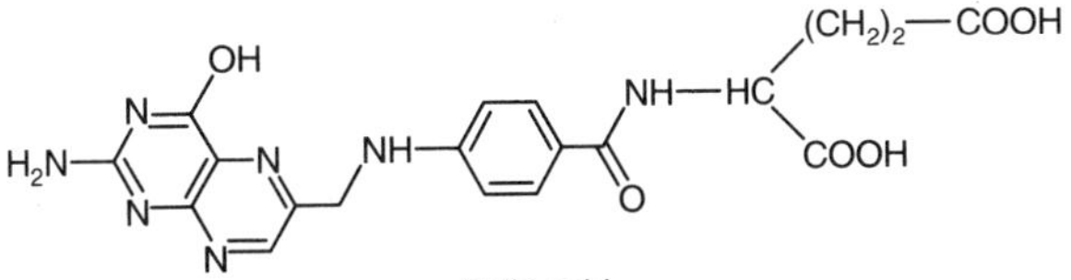

Folic acid

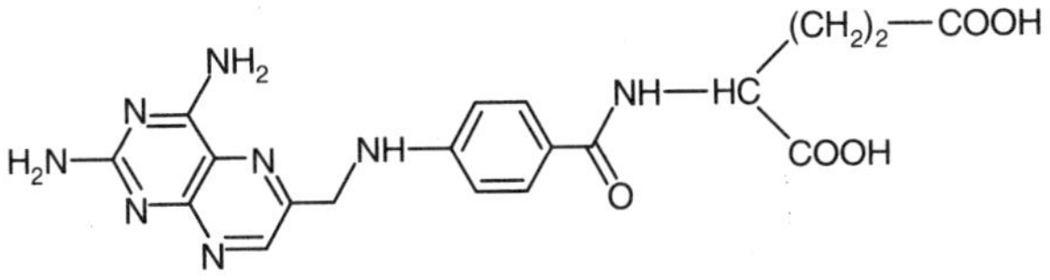

Aminopterin

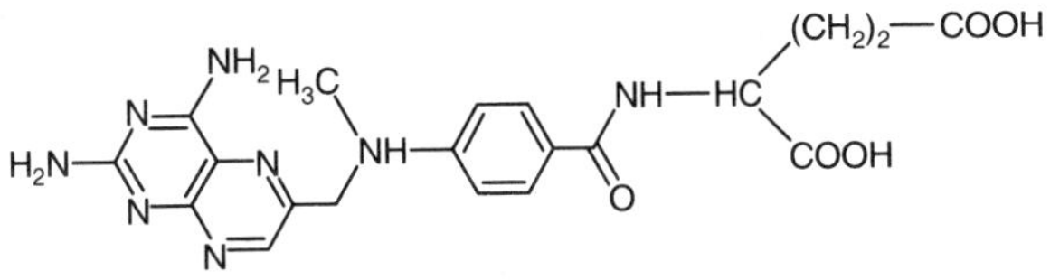

Methotrexate

b. Purine antagonist

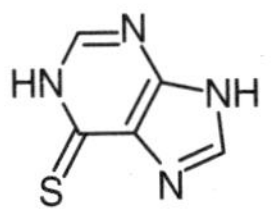

6-mercaptopurine 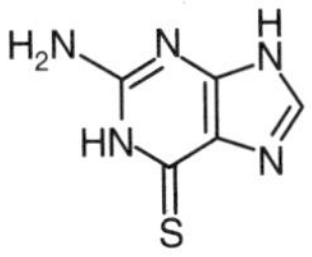   6-thioguanine 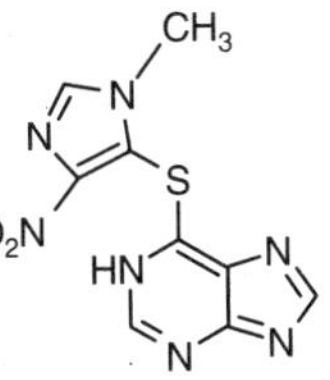   Azathioprine

c. Pyrimidine antagonist

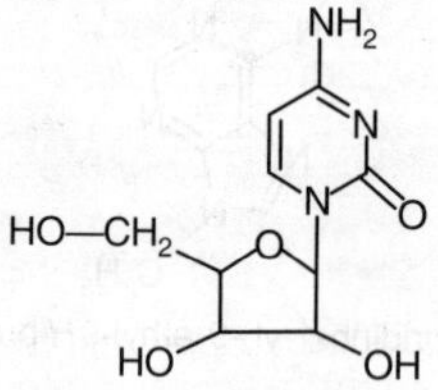

Cytrabine

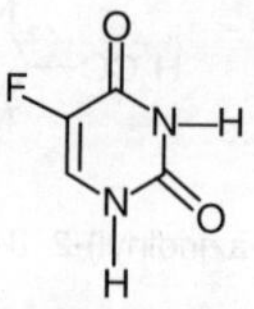

5-fluro-uracil

d. Amino acid antagonist

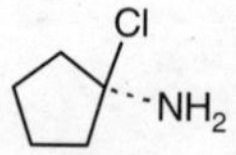

1-amino cyclopentanecarboxylic acid

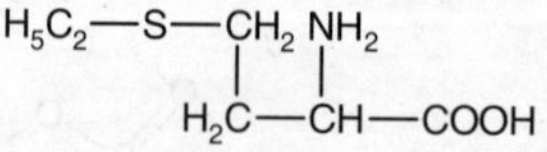

DL-2-amino (ethylthio) -butyric acid

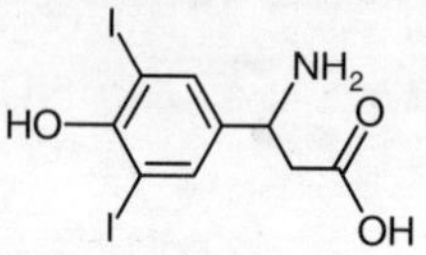

Tyrosine analogue

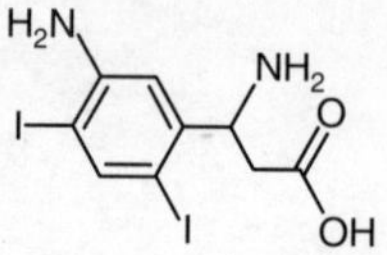

Tyrosine analogue

e. Vitamin and coenzyme antagonist

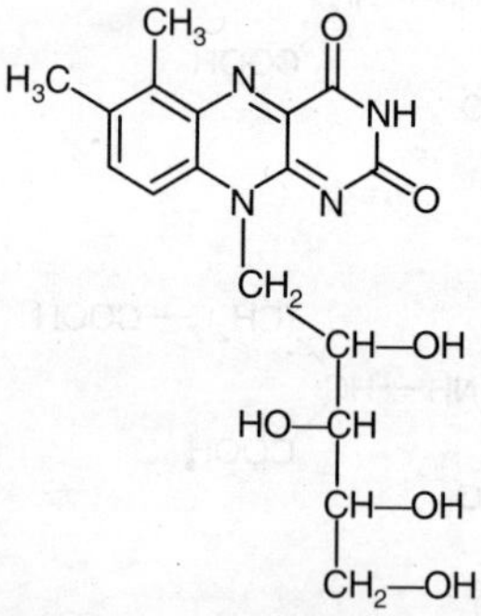

Isoriboflavin

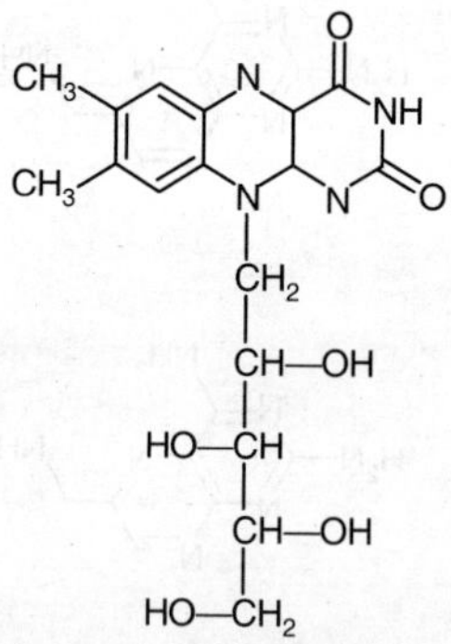

Galactoflavin

Antibiotics
a. Bleomycins

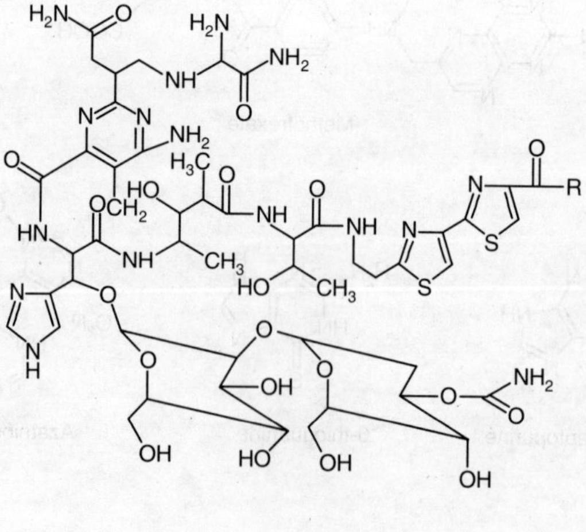

Antibiotics	R
Bleomycinic acid	OH
Bleomycin A$_2$	
Bleomycin B$_2$	

b. Dactinomycin

Dactinomycin

c. Mitomycin

Mitomycin C

d. Anthracycline antibiotics

	R$_1$	R$_2$	R$_3$	R$_4$
Doxorubicin	OCH$_3$	H	OH	OH
Daunorubicin	OCH$_3$	H	OH	H
Idarubicin	H	H	OH	H
Epirubicin	OCH$_3$	OH	H	OH

Hormones

17-β-estradiol

Progesteron

Testosteron

Prednisone

Ethinyl estradiol

Tamoxifen

O(CH₂)₂N(C₂H₅)₂

Clomiphen

Diethylstilbesterol

Natural Product

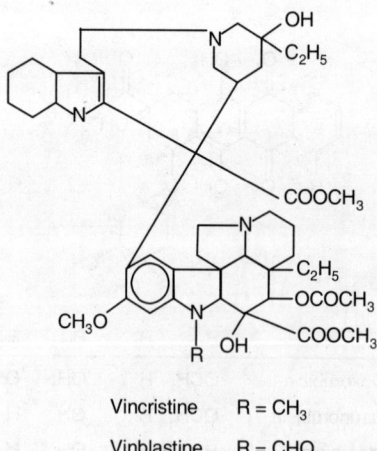

Vincristine   R = CH₃

Vinblastine   R = CHO

Miscellaneous

Hexamethylmelamine

Cisplatin

Carboplatin

Oxaliplatin

Ormaplatin

CHEMOTHERAPY

- Chemotherapy plays a significant role in the treatment of early stage disease, in the preoperative period and as adjuvant therapy for the treatment of micrometastasis. As knowledge has been accumulating in the area of pharmacology, tumor biology, cytokinetics and resistance, therapeutic strategies have been developed that maximize the tumor-cell kill, decrease resistance and enhance the potential for cure by chemotherapy.

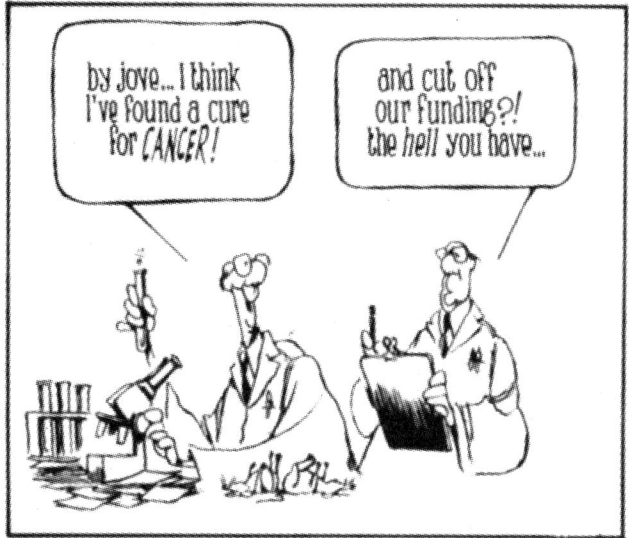

- The antineoplastic armamentarium currently contains over 30 drugs, with many additional agents under investigation. Human pituitary growth hormone, prostaglandins, cyclic-AMP, RNA-dependent DNA polymerase, etc. also show promising results.

- Since the differences between normal and neoplastic human cells are merely quantitative rather than qualitative, most antineoplastic drugs are associated with certain side effects.
- The toxicity usually involves attack of drugs on rapidly proliferating normal body tissues such as bone marrow, hair follicles and intestinal epithelium.
- In addition, individual drug may produce its own distinctive toxic effects on heart, lungs, kidneys and other organs. Hence with some exceptions, it can be said that the antineoplastic agents are generally palliative and not curative.

1. ALKYLATING AGENTS

MOA (In general) (Fig. 65.3)

1. Alkylating agents act by the transfer of alkyl groups to biologically important cell constituents such as amino sulfhydryl or phosphate groups whose function is then impaired. Under physiological conditions, alkylating agents are positively charged and they react with any molecules that are negatively charged or have regions of high electron density (nucleophile). It is thought that DNA is the main target site for alkylating agents and protein or RNA synthesis is least affected by them at that dose levels.

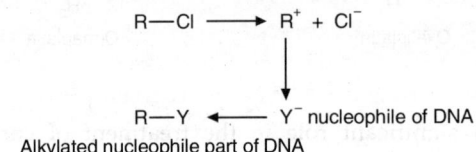

Fig. 65.3: General mode of action of alkylating agents

2. Most alkylating agents are bifunctional (have two alkylating arms). The cross-linking of DNA base pairs resulting due to the bifunctional nature of alkylating agents may develop cytotoxicity. Alkylating agents may also interfere with the activity of ATP-NMN adenyl transferase, the enzyme required for the biosynthesis of NAD. As a result, there occurs inhibition of glycolysis (Figs. 65.4 and 65.5).

Various alkylating agents can be studied by grouping them as under:

a. **Nitrogen mustards:** Chlorambucil, cyclophosphamide, mechlorethamine, melphalan.

b. **Aziridines:** Azotepa, thiotepa, benzotepa.

c. **Methane sulfonic esters:** Busalfan

d. **1, 2-epoxides:** Epoxypiperazine

e. **Nitrosoureas:** Carmustine, lomustine

f. **Triazenoimidazoles:** Dacarbazine

g. **Hydrazine derivative:** Procarbazine

Nitrogen Mustards

Mechlorethamine

MOA (Fig. 65.6):

- These are toxic, vesicant and unstable compounds. At physiological pH, aliphatic mustard hydrochlorides are readily and unimolecularly converted via the free base to a relatively stable aziridinium ion, which once produced reacts biomolecularly with available nucleophilic centers.

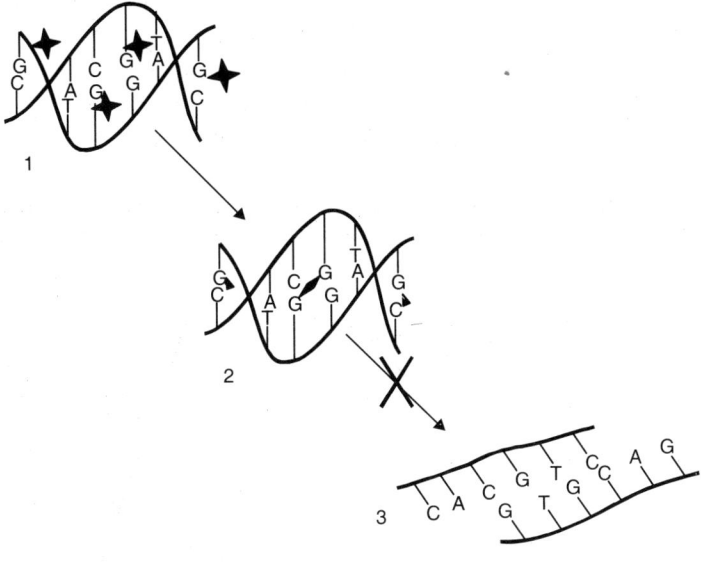

Fig. 65.4: Mode of action of alkylating agent

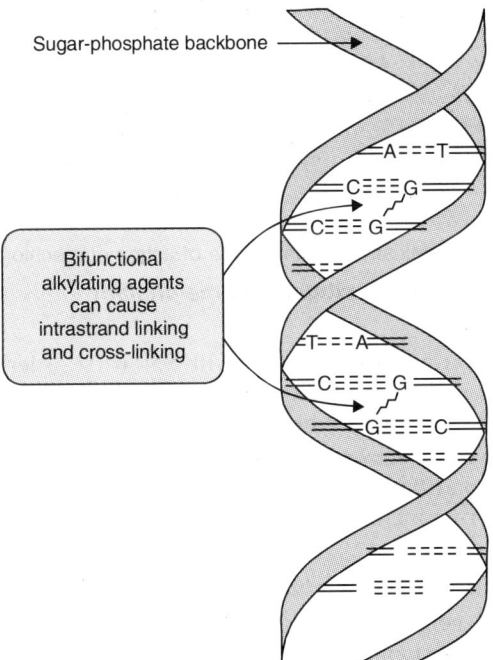

Sugar-phosphate backbone

Bifunctional alkylating agents can cause intrastrand linking and cross-linking

Fig. 65.5: Alkylation at 7th Guanine base of DNA by alkylating agent

- These agents act by alkylating the N^7 of guanine in DNA which leads to
  1. Alteration of guanine so that it forms an abnormal base pair with thymidine (miscoding);
  2. Cleavage of the imidazole ring of guanine thus destroying guanine;
  3. Linking of guanine pairs, producing cross-linked DNA strands which can not replicate; and
  4. Deprivation of DNA causing actual breakage of the DNA strands.
- The prototype of nitrogen mustards is mechlorethamine which was first synthesized in 1935 and still remains the alkylating agent of choice.

Adverse effect: Severe nausea and vomiting of rather short duration is seen regularly following nitrogen mustard treatment and hair loss is also usual. For these reasons, many protocols are now utilizing chlorambucil in place of nitrogen mustard.

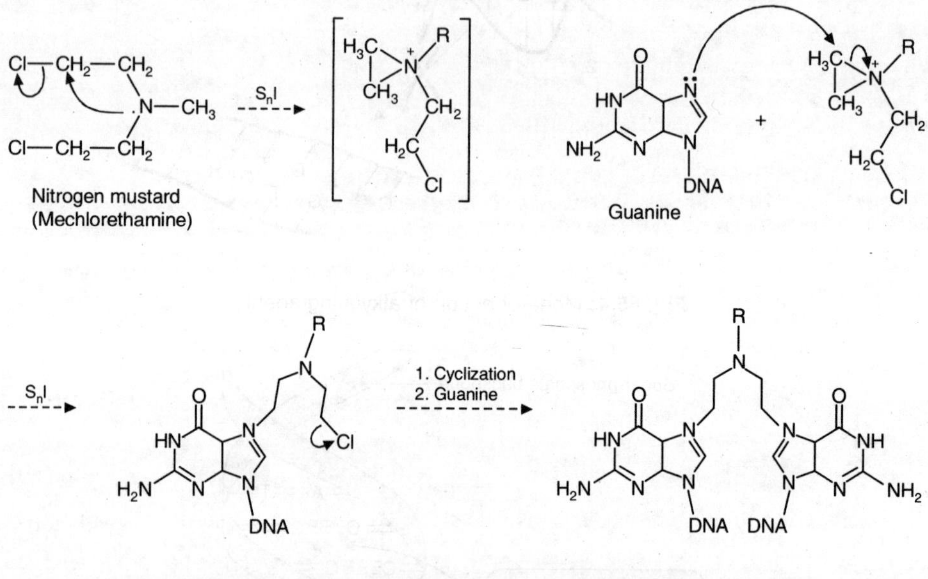

Fig. 65.6: Chemically showing mode of action of mechlorethamine

Aromatic nitrogen mustard (chlorambucil and melphalan)

MOA:

- Aromatic nitrogen mustards generally react with SN^1 (first order nucleophilic substitution reaction) kinetics, i.e. here the rate of alkylation mainly depends only upon the concentration of nitrogen mustard. These drugs are highly selective cytotoxic against malignant cells.
- Those compounds having electron withdrawing substituents apparently do not alkylate under physiological conditions and hence are less effective. While electron donating substituents on phenyl ring increase the activity of the drug.

SAR:

1. Attempts were also made to get favourable activity by varying the halogen atom.
2. The iodo-derivatives generally exhibit low order, activity which may be due to a complexity of reaction mechanism involved.
3. Attempts were also made to incorporate carbohydrate, hydroquinone and steroid systems in nitrogen mustard.

Uses: Both these drugs have long-standing clinical utility and are safer, more convenient constituents of multidose therapy. Chlorambucil is used extensively in chronic lymphocytic leukaemia and ovarian cancer while Melphalan is prescribed in the treatment of breast cancer, malignant melanoma and ovarian carcinoma.

Cyclophosphamide

MOA (Fig. 65.7):

- The *in vivo* release of biologically active compound from a suitably derivatized form is known as latentiation. Cyclophosphamide is an example of this concept.

- The phosphoramidase is more abundant in neoplastic cells than in normal cells, and hence, above drug is developed by phosphorylating the nitrogen mustard. The drug might be hyrdrolysed in tumor cells by the enzyme phosphoamidase.

- The current view about mode of action of cyclophosphamide is that liver converts the drug to 4-hydroxy derivative, which is in equilibrium with aldophosphamide. The later is cleaved to phosphoramide mustard and acrolein, both of which are cytotoxic. The lower levels of enzymes in tumor cells that prevent this cleavage may be the basis of the tumor selectivity of cyclophosphamide. It effectively inhibits a variety of human carcinoma and sarcomas as well as leukemia and lymphomas.

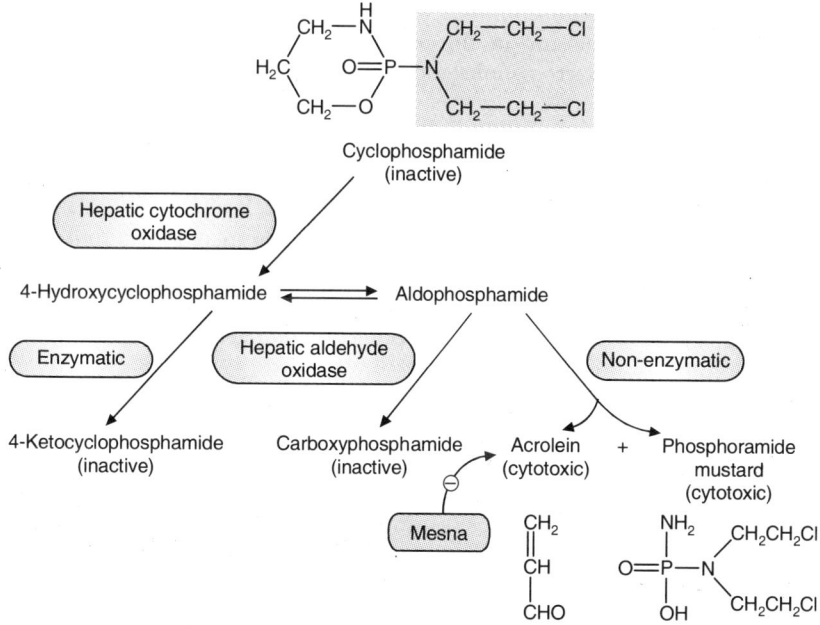

Fig. 65.7: Mode of action of cyclophosphamide

Pharmacokinetics: Suppression of cell membrane transport plays a role in the resistance of nitrogen mustard (HN_2). Metabolism of cyclophosphamide results into active metabolites and 4-ketocyclophosphamide (inactive).

Uses: It effectively inhibits a variety of human carcinoma and sarcomas as well as leukemia and lymphomas.

Aziridines

Azotepa and thiotepa

MOA:

- At physiological pH, aliphatic nitrogen mustards get readily and unimolecularly converted to a relatively more stable aziridinium ion.

Nitrogen mustard   Physiologica pH   Aziridinium ion

- This observation then leads to the development of aziridines as biological alkylating agents. Heterocyclic rings like purine, pyrimidine and quinone were also used as a carrier for aziridim moiety.
- Just similar to the phosphorylated nitrogen mustard derivatives, phosphorylated aziridines were also prepared and found clinically effective.

SAR: When oxygen from TEPA, is replaced with sulfur, the compound having greater stability results which is named as thio-TEPA.

Methanesulfonic Acid Esteres

MOA: It produces clinical remission in chronic myelogenous leukemia. It acts through SN^2 nucleophilic displacement and cross-links the DNA, since the methane sulfonate ion is an excellent leaving group.

SAR:

1. This class is represented by the general formula CH_3SO_2 or where R may be CH_3, C_2H_5, CH_2, CH_2Cl or CH_2CH_2F.
2. Symmetrical nature (bifunctionality) of the drug results in increased activity e.g., CH_3SO_2O — $(CH_2)_4$ - OSO_2 CH_3 (busulfan).

Uses: Busulfan is the most potent member of the drug homologus series. It is mainly used in the treatment of chronic granulocytic leukemia and polycythemia vera.

Nitrosoureas

Carmustine and lomustine

MOA: Under physiological conditions chemically, reactive entities are produced. The nitrosoureas may act as alkylating agents. The isocyanate portion of the molecule causes carbamylation of amino acids and proteins resulting in inhibition of DNA repair. They may also inhibit several key enzymes of DNA synthesis and repair.

Adverse effect: Acute nausea, vomiting and delayed myelosuppression while renal toxic effects have also been noted.

■ 2. ANTIMETABOLITES

- Chemical substances which take part in cellular metabolism are called metabolites. Antimetabolites are derived by incorporating one or two bioisosteric groups or other minor changes in the structure of metabolites. They interfere with the utilization of natural metabolites by virtue of similarity of chemical structure.

- The structural similarity between the naturally occurring compounds (metabolite) and antimetabolite (drugs).

Classification:

    a. Amino acid inhibitors.

    b. Vitamin and coenzyme inhibitors.

    c. Antagonists of metabolites involved in nucleic acid synthesis.

    d. Folic acid antagonists.

    e. Purine bases antagonists.

    f. Pyrimidine base antagonists.

(a) Amino Acid Inhibitors

Because of their resemblance with natural amino acids (valine, alanine, serine, etc.), these amino acid inhibitors are thought to interfere with amino acid metabolism but little definite results have been reported.

(b) Vitamin and Coenzyme Antagonists

Riboflavin analogs

MOA:

- Isoriboflavin and galactoflavin cause deficiency of riboflavin and control lymphosarcomas.
- The above compound was active due to its conversion to an inhibitory analog of niacinamide.

Pyridoxine analog

MOA: These compounds do not interfere with the formation or the metabolism of vitamin B_6. Rather they form inactive conjugates of coenzyme pyridoxal phosphate.

(c) Antagonists of Metabolites Involved in Nucleic Acid Synthesis

Azaserine

MOA: They interfere with the conversion of 5-phospho-ribosyl pyrophosphate to 5-phosphoribosylamine, cytidine triphosphate from uridine triphosphate and various other biologically important metabolic processes in which glutamine is cofactor.

Uses: Both these drugs are effective against sarcoma and leukemias.

(d) Folic Acid Antagonists

Folic acid must be reduced to L-tetrahydrofolic acid before it can serve as a coenzyme. The reduction takes place stepwise via dihydrofolic acid and both steps are generally thought to be carried out by the enzymes, folic reductase and dihydrofolic reductase. Folic acid coenzyme participates at three phases in nucleic acid biosynthesis. Probably the last phase is most sensitive to the inhibitory action of folic acid antagonists.

Methotrexate

Mechanism of action (Fig. 65.8):

- Methotrexate acts as an antifolate by binding almost irreversibly to the enzyme dihydrofolate reductase, and preventing the formation of the coenzyme tetrahydrofolic acid, essential for DNA synthesis and for replication of animal cell.

- These agents competitively inhibit dihydrofolate reductase thus restricting the availability of tetrahydrofolic acid (THF) to cells. THF is critically important to the metabolic transfer of one-carbon units in a variety of biochemical reactions. These include the biosynthesis of thymidylic acid (for DNA synthesis) and inosinic acid (needed for RNA synthesis).

Toxicities:

- Stomatitis, diarrhea, hepatic dysfunction, anemia and thrombocytopenia.
- In certain cells, incorporation of the C-8 carbon into 4-amino imidazole-5-carboxamide ribotide is inhibited by folic acid antagonists. Methotrexate, homofolic acid or tetrahydrohomofolic acid nonselectively inhibit DNA synthesis.

Major Indication:

- Breast carcinoma.
- Testicular carcinoma.
- Medullablastoma.
- Bronchogenic carcinoma.
- Acute lymphocytic leukemia.

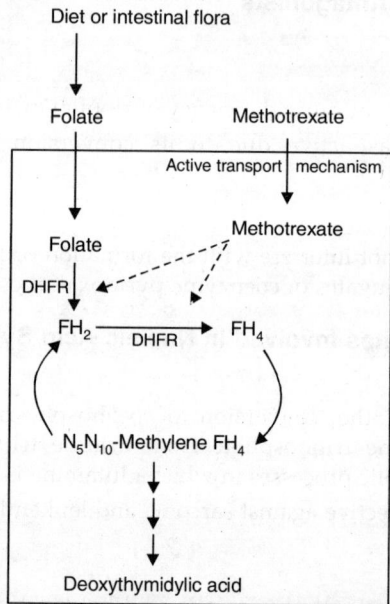

Fig. 65.8: Mode of action of methotrexate

Pharmacokinetics:

- Methotrexate is not extensively metabolized in man ar 1 the bulk of the compound is excreted in the urine within a few hours of administration. The enzymatic block produced by methotrexate can be bypassed by giving a folate (folinic acid). This reversal of the action is commonly referred to as rescue.
- In certain cells, methotrexate (MTX), homofolic acid or tetrahydrohomofolic acid inhibit the incorporation of the C-8 carbon into 4-aminoimidazole-5-carboxamide ribotide. Inhibition of DNA synthesis by MTX and related antagonist is not selective but is balanced by concurrent inhibition of RNA and/or protein synthesis. A therapeutic advantage with reduced toxicity

is achieved by the administration of high doses of MTX, followed by "rescue" with folinic acid as an antidote.

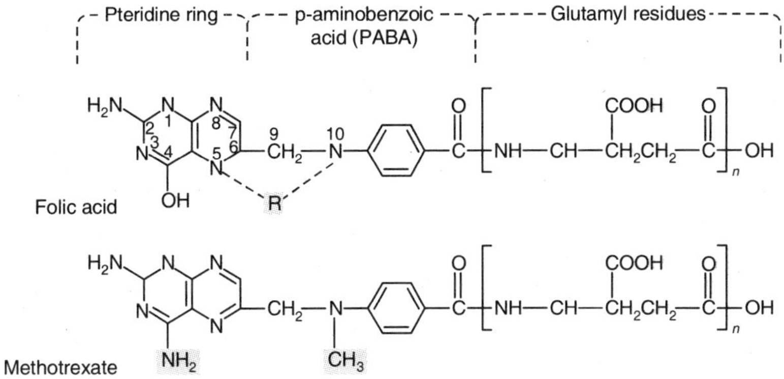

Fig. 65.9: Structure similarities between folic acid and methotrexate

(e) Purine Antagonist
6-Mercaptopurine
MOA: It is converted to 6-thioinosinate by the enzyme hypoxanthine phosphoribosyl transeferase. 6-Thioinosinate is a potent inhibitor of the conversion of inosinic acid to adenylic acid. 6-Thiosinate is a potent inhibitor of the conversion of 5-phosphoribosyl pyrophosphate into 5-phosphoribosylamine. It acts as a substrate for a methyl transferase, requiring 5-adenosyl methionine, that converts it in to 6-methyltoinosinate.

6-Thioguanine
MOA: Thioguanine is converted into its ribonucleotide which inhibits the enzymes into synthesis of purines. Thioguanine is incorporated into RNA and its 2-deoxy-metabolite is incorporated into DNA.

Azathioprine
MOA: Its mode of action is similar to 6-mercaptopurine, as it is converting in it inside the liver.

Toxicities:
- Gastrointestinal— nausea, vomiting.
- Hematologic— leukopenia, thrombocytopenia, anemia.

Major indications:
- Acute granulocytic leukemia.
- Acute lymphocytic leukemia.

(f) Pyrimidine Base Antagonists
Azapyrimidines
Azacytidine and azuridine: The azacytidine plays a role in the treatment of acute myeloblastic leukemia while the later blocks the enzyme, orotidylate decarboxylase and may have a specific role in combination chemotherapy with other pyrimidine antimetabolites.

MOA:

- Azacytidine is an analog of cytidine and is rapidly phosphorylated and incorporated in both RNA and DNA. By disrupting the process of translation of nucleic acid sequences into protein, protein synthesis is inhibited. Moreover, it affects de novo pyrimidine synthesis by inhibiting orotidylic acid decarboxylase enzyme.
- 5-azacytidine inhibits the incorporation of tritiated thymidine or deoxyadenosine into DNA to a greater extent than it does tritiated uridine into RNA. It inhibits the S-phase (DNA synthesis) of the cell cycle by reducing the activity of uridine kinase, the enzyme that catalyzes the initial phosphorylation step of uridine, cytidine and 5-azacytidine.

Fluropyrimidines (5-Flurouracil)

MOA:

- 5-Fluorouracil metabolises to fluorodeoxyuridine monophosphate which is a potent competitive inhibitor of the enzyme, thymidylate synthetase. Thus the primary cytoxic action of the drug is to block thymidylate (and thereby DNA) synthesis.
- In addition, 5-fluorouracil may also be incorporated as the nucleotide into RNA, probably depressing RNA synthesis directly by blocking incorporation of uracil and orotic acid into RNA. 5-FU might be more effective in patients with liver metastases when given orally, due to high drug concentrations in the portal system.

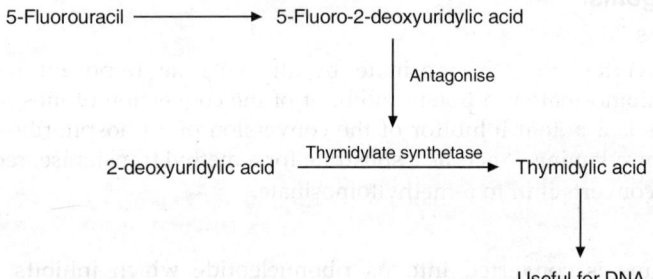

Uses: 5-FU enhances the antitumor effect of radiation in bronchogenic carcinoma. The antitumor effect is also increased when it is combined with an anticoagulant (e.g. warfarin).

▓ 3. DNA COMPLEXORS (ANTIBIOTICS)

This is a class of antibiotics which were thought to be useful in cancer chemotherapy due to their cytotoxic properties. They differ from each other in individual's capacity to interfere in protein. RNA and DNA synthesis at various stages and hence may be given alone or in combination with other antineoplastic drugs.

Actinomycin D

MOA: It is a powerful bacteriostatic antibiotic isolated from Actinomycetes. Both, the lactone ring and polypeptide chain are essential for biological effect. It intercalates between DNA base pairs and inhibits DNA dependent RNA synthesis especially that of ribosomal RNA. It is found to inhibit the DNA-polymerase activity.

Uses: It is mainly used in the treatment of sarcomas, Wilms' tumor and testicular carcinoma. A single dose of actinomycin D provides cytotoxic concentrations for up to 24 hours. Actinomycin D enhances the toxicity of morphine probably by increasing brain permeability. It also stimulates isoperoxidase activity at low concentration and represses it at higher concentration.

Mithramycin

- It is a Streptomyces antibiotic. It forms complexes with DNA, probably with guanine, in the presence of divalent cations especially magnesium.
- It also inhibits DNA dependent RNA synthesis without affecting DNA synthesis. It is mainly prescribed in the treatment of testicular carcinoma.

Bleomycins

MOA: These are relatively high molecular weight peptide antibiotics. Bleomycin A2 is more potent than bleomycin B in antitumor activity. They inhibit DNA synthesis, produce scission of single stranded DNA and also inhibit cell DNA repair by a marked inhibition of DNA ligase.

Adverse Effect: All bleomycins (i.e. A1, A2, B1, and, B2) contain a sulfur containing chromospheres. Bleomycin A2 exhibits very low renal toxicity and may inhibit ATP dependent DNA ligase activity.

Uses:

- Bleomycin A2 is clinically useful in the treatment of human epidermal cancer, squamous cell carcinoma of the head and neck, lymphosarcoma, Hodgkin's disease, Kaposi's sarcoma, carcinoma of the thyroid and brain tumors.
- It exhibits low renal toxicity and rarely causes leukopenia, thrombocytopenia or hepatopoiesis in patients. Bleomycin A2 frequently causes pulmonary toxicities.

Anthracyclines

MOA

Following three mechanism of actions are possible

1. Intercalation in The DNA: The drugs insert nonspecifically between adjacent base pairs and bind to the sugar-phosphate backbone of DNA causing a local uncoiling thus blocking DNA and RNA synthesis. Intercalation can interfere with the topoisomerase II catalysed breakage reunion reaction of DNA strands to cause unrepairable breaks.

2. Generation of oxygen free radicals:

- Cytochrome P-450 reductase (present in cell nuclear membranes) catalyzes reduction of the anthracyclines to semiquinone free radicals.
- These in turn reduce molecular O_2, producing superoxide ion and hydrogen peroxide that mediate simple strand scission of DNA.
- Tissue with ample superoxide dismutase (SOD) or glutathione peroxidase activity is protected. Tumors and the heart are generally low in SOD. In addition, cardiac tissue lacks catalase and this cannot dispose of hydrogen peroxide. This may explain the cardiotoxicity of anthracyclines.

3. Binding of cell membranes: This action alters the function of transport proteases coupled to phosphatidylinositol activation.

SAR:

1. When the amino sugar of these anitibiotics is masked or exchanged for x-D-glucos-amine, it results in the loss of activity.
2. The ability of these antibiotics to, bind DNA is found to be associated with the structure of the amino sugar. Both antibiotics possess immunosuppressive properties.

Uses: Daunorubicin rapidly metabolizes to daunorubicinol R = CH(OH)CH₃ and aglycones'of parent compound and this metabolite. Adriamycin is useful for acute lymphoblastic and chronic myelogenous leukemias, transitional cell carcinoma, squamous cell carcinoma and adenocarcinoma of breast.

4. NATURAL PRODUCTS (MITOTIC INHIBITORS)

- These agents cause reversible or irreversible metaphase arrest of the mitotic sequence, probably by damaging the spindle apparatus.
- In addition to this, they may cause morphological and motility changes in the proteins of the microtubules. Aggregations of ribosomes and polysomes have also been noted.

Vinca Alkaloids

Vincristine and vinblastine

MOA (Fig. 65.10): Both are having broad anti-tumor activity and there is an evidence of cross-resistance in cell culture. These cause mitotic arrest, by promoting dissolution of microtubule in cells. These drugs arrest the cell in metaphase and interfere with the synthesis of transfer RNA, possibly by acting as acylating agent.

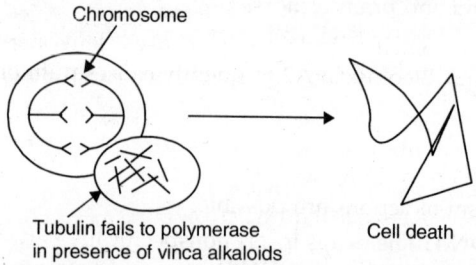

Fig. 65.10: Mechanism of action of vinca alkaloids

Paclitaxel

MOA (Fig. 65.11): The mode of action of taxol is somewhat different than the vinca alkaloids, it makes tubulin more stable so that cell remain in frozen state in metaphase.

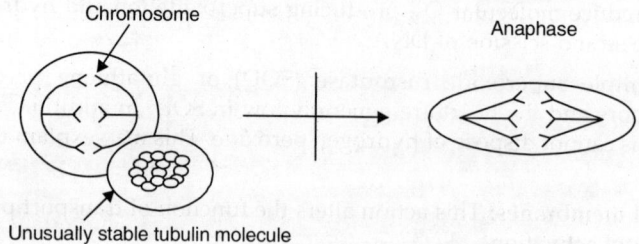

Fig. 65.11: Mechanism of action of paclitaxel

Epipodophyllotoxins

- VM 26 and VP 16-213 are epipodophyllotoxin analogues extracted from the plant, *Podophyllum pelatum.*

- Cells exposed to these drugs are arrested in metaphase but no alteration of microtubules has been demonstrated.

Colchicine

It is an alkaloid from *Colchicum autumnale*. The colchicine analog demecolcine is somewhat effective in chronimyclocytic leukemia but it shows its antitumor activity at toxic dose only, which can cause bone marrow depression.

Campothecin

- It is an alkaloid from the tree *Camptotheca acuminata*. It exhibits antineoplastic activity against leukemias.
- The primary effect of this alkaloid is on DNA synthesis. It affects cells in S phase and the capacity of these cells to go through G_0 phase.
- It inhibits ribosomal RNA synthesis without affecting transfer-RNA or protein synthesis. The RNA synthesis inhibition is rapidly reversible upon removal of the drug.

5. ENZYMES

L-Asparaginase

MOA

The asparaginase used clinically is extracted from bacterial cultures of *Escherchia coli*. It is observed that the enzyme hydrolyzes asparagine into aspartic acid and ammonia; thus tumour cells are deprived of this essential nutrient. The enzyme also shows glutaminase activity causing a decrease in plasma glutamine and an increase in glutaminic acid. The reduced aspargine and glutamine levels cause immediate inhibition of protein synthesis and a delayed inhibition of DNA and RNA synthesis.

Adverse effect

Asparaginase treatment is not myelosuppressive but nausea, vomiting, transient pyrexia and anorexia are frequent.

6. HORMONES (FIG. 65.12)

- Cancer of certain organs (such organs whose functioning is mainly controlled by hormones) may respond favourably to the hormonal therapy, e.g. alteration of the hormonal levels causes remission of some cases of cancer of breast, prostate and endometrium and hormonal therapy to tumors of other organs like kidney, may also produce the favourable results.
- Mechanism of hormone action: All hormonally sensitive tissues contain either cytoplasmic or cell-surface receptors. Steriodal hormones bind to cytoplasmic receptors and get translocated into the cell nucleus where they interact with the DNA.
- The hormone is thus able to modulate gene function and may alter cellular growth control. While, the polypeptide hormones (e.g. insulin, prolactin, adreno-corticotrophic hormone (ACTH), etc. do not have affinity for cytoplasmic receptor but they blind to cell surface receptors and mediate their response via a second messenger i.e. cyclic 3', 5'- adenosine triphosphate or cyclic AMP. Some cancers also contain nuclear estrogen receptors.
- The anti-neoplastic hormone can be broadly classified into—estrogen derivatives, testosterone derivatives and steroidal anti-inflammatory agents.

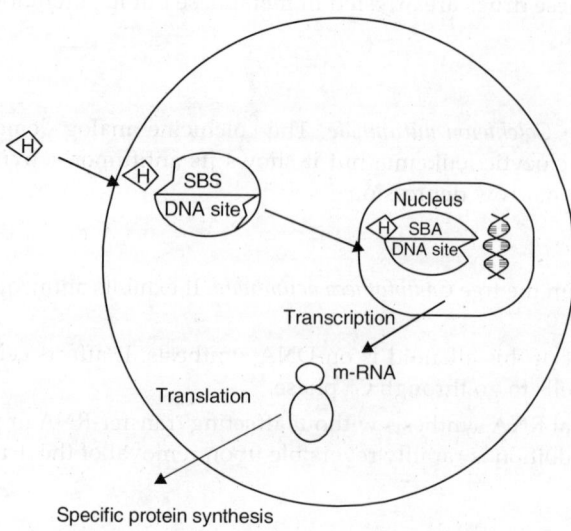

Fig. 65.12: Mode of action of hormone

Estrogen Derivatives

Large doses of estrogen inhibit prolactin stimulation of mammary tumor growth. Estrogen may be involved in transport of RNA from nucleus cytoplasm.

| Estradiol | Progesteron | Testosterone | Prednisolone |

MOA

- Estrogens are used in the treamtent of prostatic cancer, breast cancer in post-menopausal women. Estrogens are potent inhibitors of gonadotropic secretion and it is believed that they exert their major effect in prostatic cancer by suppressing LH (luteinizing hormone) released by pituitary gland thereby inhibiting testicular testosterone production.
- More recently still, a new class of hormone analogues has been synthesized which appeared to bind to the cytoplasmic hormone receptor and in some cases, block normal hormone responsiveness. These drugs include the antiestrogens, e.g. tamoxifen, clomifen.

Ethinyl estradiol

Diethyl stilbesterol

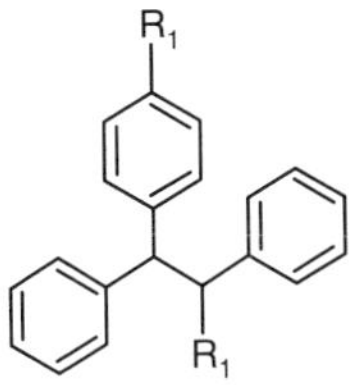

Tamoxifen

$R_1 = O(CH_2)_2N(CH_3)_2$

$R_2 = -CH_2CH_3$

Clomiphen

$R_1 = O(CH_2)_2N(C_2H_5)_2$

$R_3 = Cl$

- Antiestrogens antagonise estrogen-induced responses of one or more target organs (e.g. uterus, vagina, breast or pituitary gland).
- On the similar line, a number of drugs which interfere with the normal synthesis of hormones in the adrenal gland or pituitary have also been synthesized, e.g. O, P - ODD and aminoglutethimide, both of which block adrenal steroid synthesis and perform the purpose of a medical adrenalectomy.

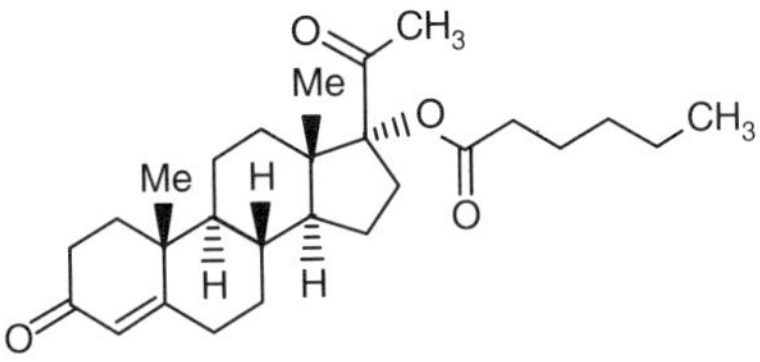

Hydroxyprogesteron captroate

$R_1 = H$ $R_2 = -COC_5H_{11}$

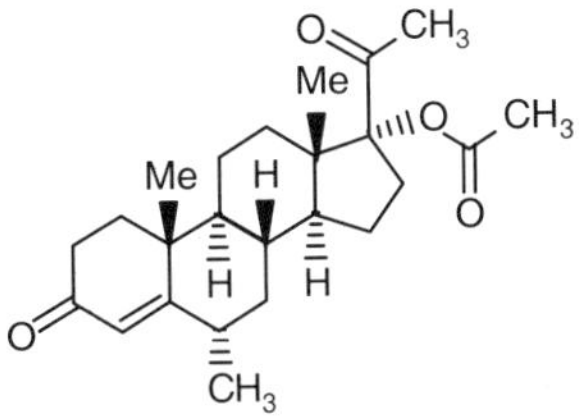

Medroxyprogesteron acetate

$R_1 = CH_3$ $R_2 = -COCH_3$

- Advanced carcinoma of uterine endometrium or diseminated endometrial cancer may respond to progestational agents. The effective progestins in this category are pituitary.
- Hydroxyprogesterone caproate gave excellent responses in adenocarcinoma of the uterine corpus.

Testosterone Derivatives

- The effective anticancer agents from this class are— testolactone and testolactone propionate.

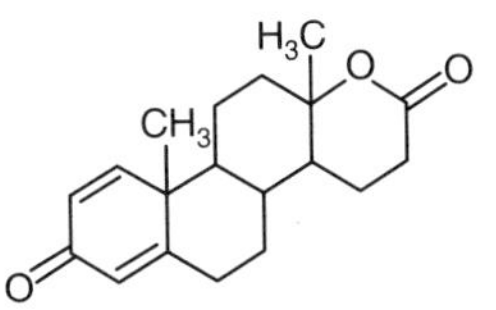

Testolactone

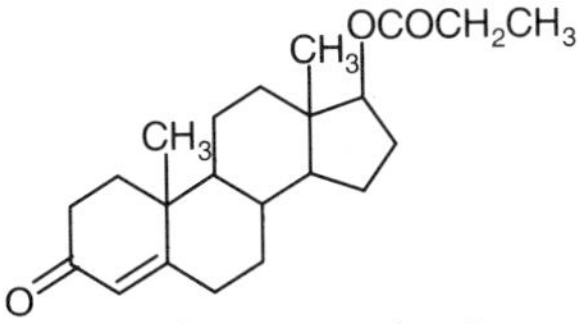

Testolactone propionate

- Just similar to antiestrogens, antiandrogens interfere with the action of androgens at the target organ. The antiandrogen, cyproterone acetate has elicited symptomatic improvement in advanced prostatic carcinoma.

Flutamide

Cyproterone acetate

Steroidal Anti-inflammatory Agents (Corticosteroids)

- These agents are useful in the treatment of acute chronic and lymphocytic leukemia, breast cancer, brain tumors and Hodgkin's disease.
- They are also useful in palliative management of major complications like hypercalcemia (breast cancer) and brain edema (brain tumor).
- They act by suppressing the adrenal and pituitary glands. They also inhibit lymphoid proliferation and have lymphocytic effects. The clinically used agents from this class are dexamethasone, prednisolone and triamcinolone.

Dexamethasone

Prednisolone

Triamcinolone

Side Effects of Steroidal Hormone Therapy

1. Oestrogens:
   1. Metabolic effects
   2. Fluid retention
   3. Hypercalcemia
   4. Coronary occlusion.

2. Estrogenic effects:
   1. Feminization
   2. Uterine bleeding.

3. Progestins:
   1. Occasional nausea,
   2. Fluid retention.

4. Testosterone derivatives:
   1. Hypercalcemia
   2. Fluid retention
   3. Musculinization
   4. Cholestatic jaundice.

Hormone–cytotoxic Drug Combinations

- Because the action of hormones seems to be related to receptors present in the cancer cell, the hormones if linked to chemotherapeutic agents might be useful in directing the cytotoxic drug to the cancer cell, e.g. in breast cancer the addition of prednisolone to cyclophosphamide, methotrexate or 5-fluorouracil results in an increase in the potency.
- Similarly, the combination of estradiol and nitrogen mustard has been synthesized and is used clinically in prostatic cancer, e.g. estramustine phosphate.

▓ 7. MISCELLANEOUS AGENTS

Hexamethylamine

MOA: It is used to treat ovarian carcinoma and bronchogenic carcinoma. It is a nonpolar derivative of EDTA. It is a potent inhibitor of DNA synthesis but does not affect RNA or protein synthesis. It is used to treat acute lymphocytic leukemia and lymphoma.

Cis-dichloridiamine platinum

MOA:

- It may undergo sequential transformation with loss of chloride and the resultant platinum species may act bifunctionally to cross-link adjacent nucleophilic centers of DNA through covalent binding. Deafness was noted in preclinical trials.
- It inhibits DNA synthesis by cross-linking complementary strands of DNA and therefore acts like a bifunctional alkylating agents. The preferred binding site for cis-platin in DNA is guanine. The drug is accompanied by many side effects.

Carboplatin

Efforts to improve the therapeutic index of cisplatin (platinol) have focused primarily on decreasing the drug-induced toxicity. Carboplatin is a second generation platinum analog that may prove to reduce toxicity while maintaining the antitumor effects of cisplatin.

MOA

It may act by direct binding of DNA that results in the formation of both inter- and intrastrand crosslinking. Platinum administered as carboplatin binds to proteins much more slowly than does platinum administered as cis-platin. Clinical trials were initiated in 1981. It showed reduced toxicities and spectrum of activities very similar to cisplatin. It has received PDA approval in Feb 1989 for the palliative treatment of patients with ovarian carcinoma recurrent after prior chemotherapy.

Amacrine

MOA

It is 4'-(9 Acridinyl amino)-methanesulfon-m-anisidide. It is also immunosuppr-essive and shows evidence of antiviral activity. It is thought that m-AMSA inhibits DNA synthesis probably by intercalation between DNA strands.

Emetine

MOA:

As an inhibitor of protein synthesis at the transcription level, emetine is also active against leukemias L-1210 and P-3880, B168, B16 melanomas, Ehrlich ascites carcinoma and Yoshida sarcoma. Pharmacologic studies showed that it effects a sympathetic blockade, antagonizes hyaluronidase, inhibits oxydative N-demethylation of aminopyrine and N-ethyl-morphine as well as the S-demethylation of 6-MP riboside *in vitro*.

Side effects

- Preliminary clinical trials indicated that emetine reduced lung tumor size and purulent bloody vaginal discharge; severe muscle weakness is the most important dose-limiting toxic effect. Emetine is not myelosuppressive and may be useful in patients with poor marrow reserve.
- Cardiotoxic effects of this alkaloid and its 2dehydro analog were noted in rabbit heart. The observed cardiopathy compares with those not accompanied by vascular symptoms but associated with necroses due to electrolyte and steroid disturbance. N-substituted 1-emetine derivatives have also been found to inhibit growth of Ehrlich ascites carcinoma.

t-RNA methyltransferase

MOA:

- Abnormally high levels of methyltransferase enzymes and methyltransferase activity were found in neoplastic tissues including virally induced, chemically induced and spontaneous tumors.
- The t-RNAs of many tumors contain highly elevated amounts of N-methylated, C-methylated, and the 2'-0-methylated nucleosides. t-RNA from solid human tumors with t-RNAs from normal tissues was compared chromatographically. t-RNAs are associated with the regulation of protein synthesis at the translation level and since alkylating carcinogens were found to alkylate t-RNA in vivo, the aberrancy of methyltransferase could be involved in the initiation of tumor induction and neoplasia.
- Inhibitors of methyl transferase are postulated to be of potential value in cancer chemotherapy.

Vitamin A Acid

- Vitamin A acid is capable of inducing regressions in a benign as well as malignant epithelial tumor.
- It has a therapeutic effect on established skin papillomas and skin carcinomas induced by 7, 12 dimethylbenzanthracene and croton oil. Initial clinical trial has established the effect of topically applied vitamin A acid on basal cell carcinomas on the skin in man.

Ricin

- A phytotoxic protein from *Ricinus communis* and has inhibitory effect on DNA synthesis leaving RNA sythesis unaffected.
- It is inhibitory towards protein synthesis in experimental tumor cells. It has a moderate inhibitory effect on DNA synthesis without affecting RNA synthesis. Its mode of action is not known, but is not due to impairment of glucose metabolism nor amino acid uptake in tumor cells.

Gallium Salts

- With a special affinity for malignant tumors, gallium salts are used as diagnostic tools for detection of neoplastic bone metabolism and allied neoplastic diseases.
- Gallium bromide, chloride, citrate, iodide, and nitrate as well as ammonium gallium chloride have antitumor activity against walker carcinosarcoma and P-1798 lymphosarcoma.

Alpha-interferons

- The alpha-interferons and Intron A were approved for the treatment of hairy cell leukemia in 1986. The proposed mechanisms of action include antiviral, anti-proliferative, and immunomodulatory plus phenotypic reversion and inhibition of oncogene expression.

- It has an elimination half-life of 2.2 hours following IM administration and 2.9 hours when administered s.c.
- The toxicities include fever, chills, myalgias and headaches. Nausea, vomiting, fatigue, and alopecia are also reported occasionally.
- Alpha-interferons represent the first of a series of biological products that may become the "fourth arm" of cancer treatment in addition to surgery, radiation and chemotherapy. They have shown activity in hairy cell leukemia, AIDS-related Kaposi's sarcoma, lymphoma, multiple myeloma, renal cell carcinoma and melanoma.

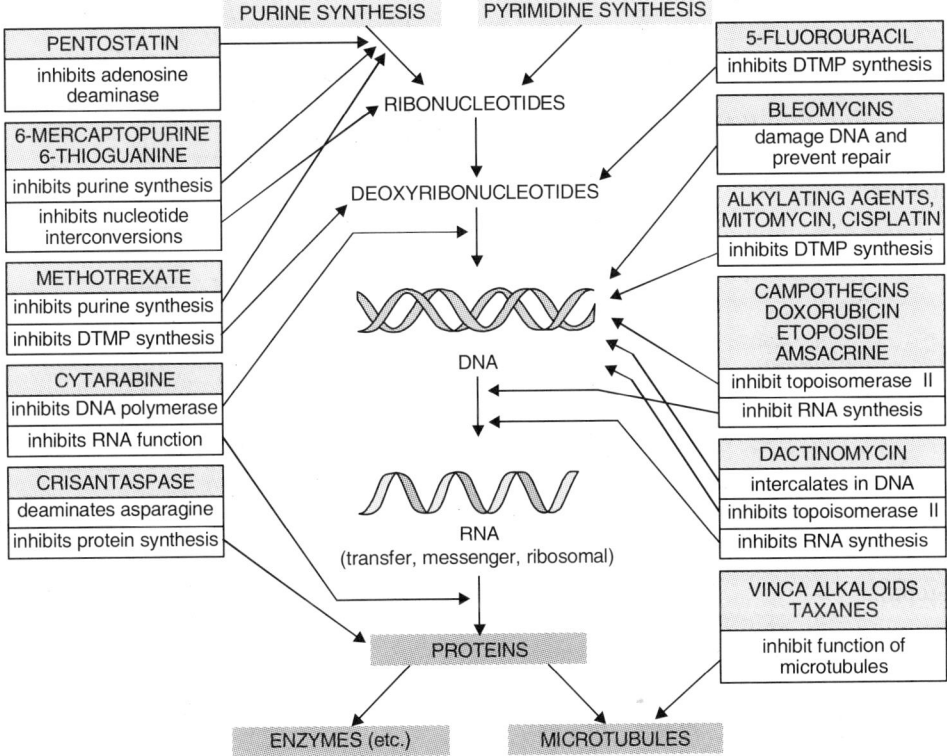

Fig. 65.13: Mode of action of anticancer agents

Cyclophosphamide

Ifosamide

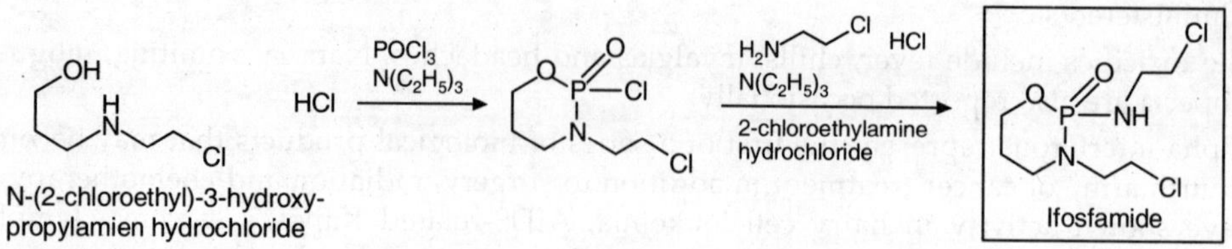

N-(2-chloroethyl)-3-hydroxy-
propylamien hydrochloride

POCl₃
N(C₂H₅)₃

HCl

H₂N
N(C₂H₅)₃

2-chloroethylamine
hydrochloride

Ifosfamide

Carmustine

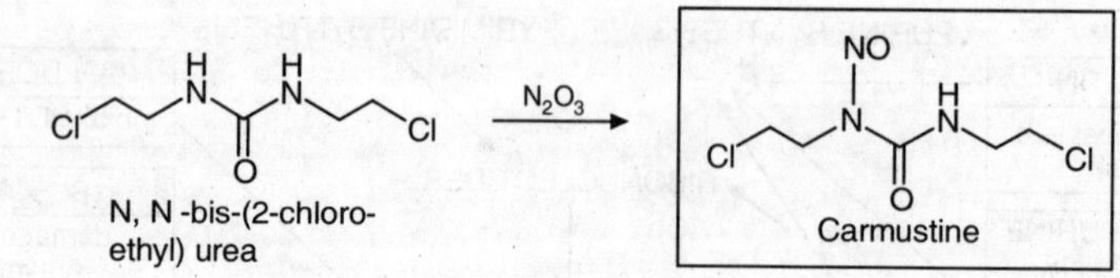

N, N -bis-(2-chloro-
ethyl) urea

N₂O₃

Carmustine

Lomustine

Cyclohexyl
isocyanate

Ethanolamine

SOCl₂

I

1-(2-chloroethyl)-3-
cyclohexylurea (I)

HCOOH, anhydrous NaNO₂

Lomustine

Thiotepa

Aziridine

Thiophosphoryl
chloride

N(C₂H₅)₃

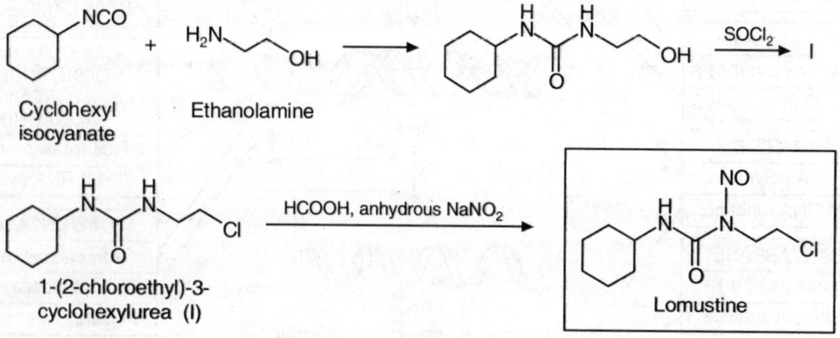

Thiotepa

Busulfan

1, 4-butanediol

Methane sulfonyl
chloride

pyridine

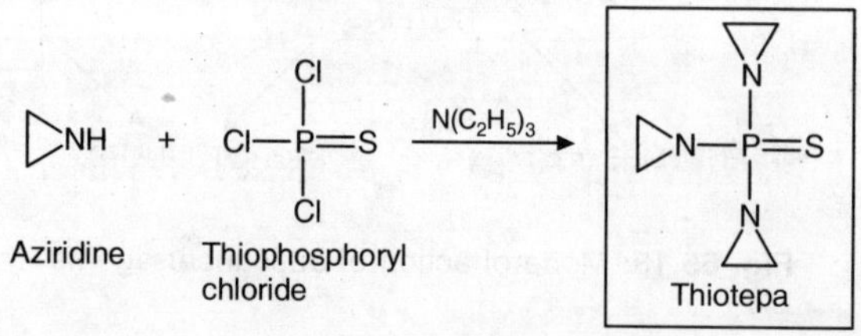

Busulfan

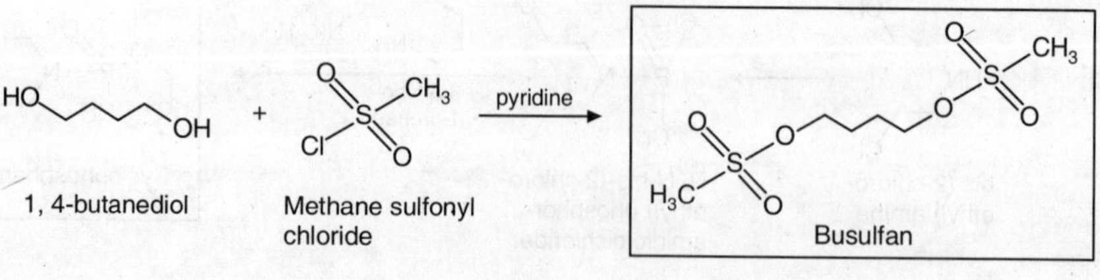

Dacarbazine

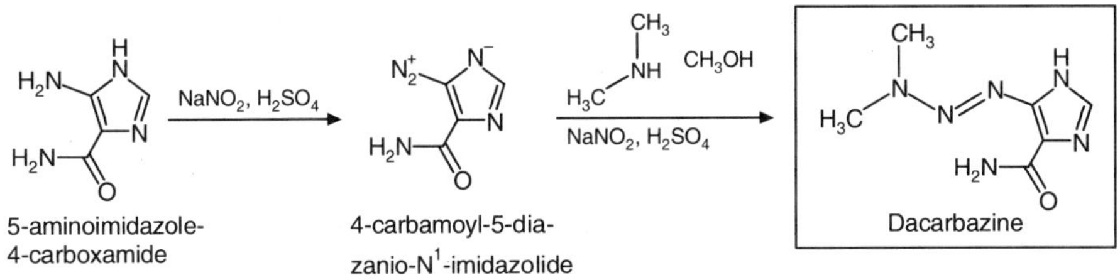

5-aminoimidazole-
4-carboxamide

NaNO$_2$, H$_2$SO$_4$

4-carbamoyl-5-dia-
zanio-N^1-imidazolide

CH$_3$OH
NaNO$_2$, H$_2$SO$_4$

Dacarbazine

Mercaptopurine

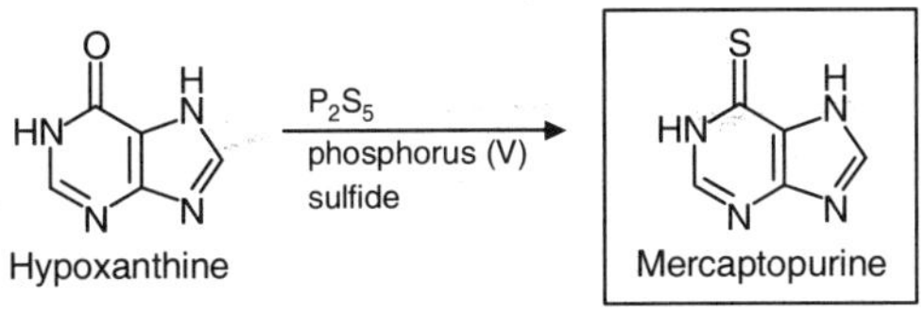

Hypoxanthine

P$_2$S$_5$
phosphorus (V)
sulfide

Mercaptopurine

Methotrexate

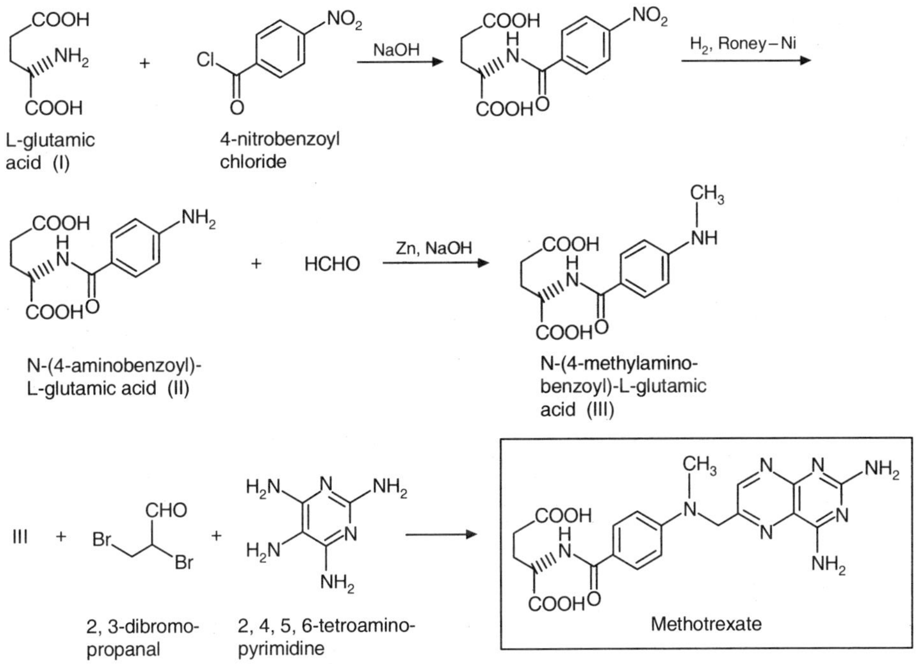

L-glutamic
acid (I)

+

4-nitrobenzoyl
chloride

NaOH

H$_2$, Roney–Ni

N-(4-aminobenzoyl)-
L-glutamic acid (II)

+ HCHO

Zn, NaOH

N-(4-methylamino-
benzoyl)-L-glutamic
acid (III)

III +

2, 3-dibromo-
propanal

+

2, 4, 5, 6-tetroamino-
pyrimidine

Methotrexate

Flutamide

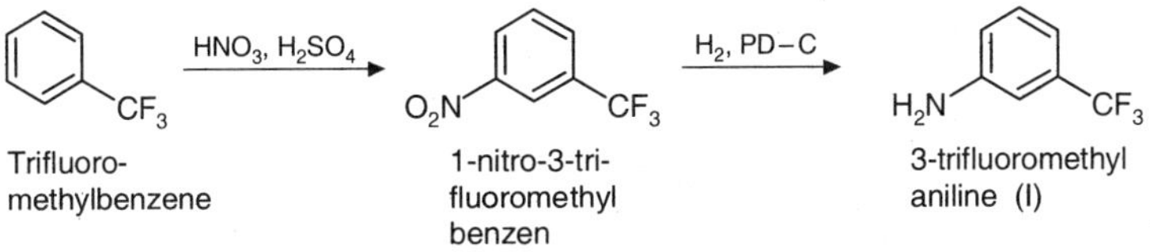

Trifluoro-
methylbenzene

HNO$_3$, H$_2$SO$_4$

1-nitro-3-tri-
fluoromethyl
benzen

H$_2$, PD–C

3-trifluoromethyl
aniline (I)

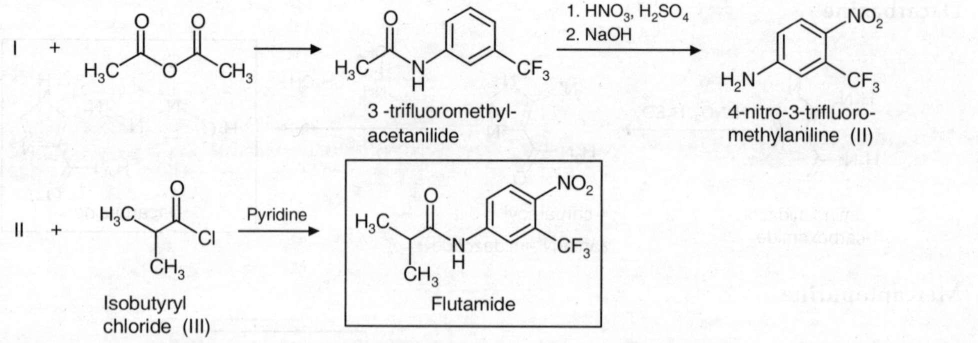
I +
1. HNO3, H2SO4
2. NaOH
3 -trifluoromethyl-
acetanilide
4-nitro-3-trifluoro-
methylaniline (II)
II +
Pyridine
Isobutyryl
chloride (III)
Flutamide

Azathioprine

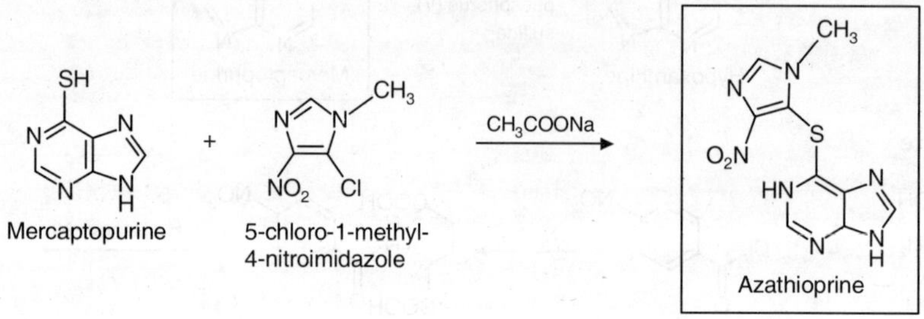
CH3COONa
Mercaptopurine
5-chloro-1-methyl-
4-nitroimidazole
Azathioprine

Cytarabine

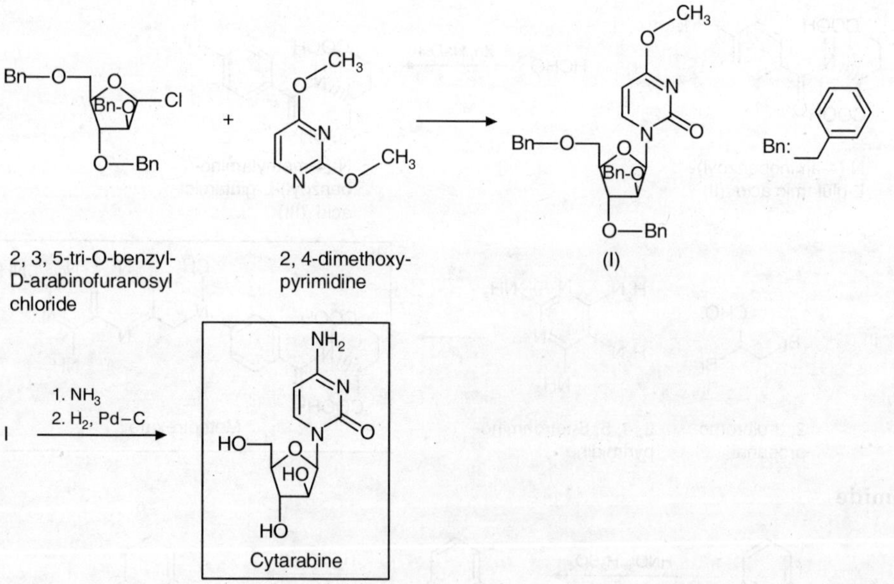
Bn:
(I)
2, 3, 5-tri-O-benzyl-
D-arabinofuranosyl
chloride
2, 4-dimethoxy-
pyrimidine
1. NH3
2. H2, Pd–C
Cytarabine

Anti-infective Agents

Skin is the largest organ of the body. Hospital disinfection, sterilization of instruments and the surgical handwash are the general measures which are being routinely used to reduce the risk of hospital-acquired infections and to minimize the transfer of microorganisms to the susceptible patients. Topical anti-infective agents are applied to intact cutaneous and mucous surfaces before surgery and to treat minor cuts, abrasions or burns. Koch (1865) had established the relationship of infection and microorganisms. The pathogenic manifestation may be limited to skin or systemic symptoms may also appear in some cases.

- Until it was discovered that microorganisms cause the pathogenic conditions, the need for topical anti-infective agents was not realised. Thereafter, they are extensively used in surgical, public health, hospital and laboratory techniques to destroy both, pathogenic as well as non-pathogenic micro-organisms.
- Lister was first to employ phenolic solution to treat infections in surgery. Early attempts of disinfection relied largely on aromatic substances and on chemical deodorants, which still continue today. Alcohols, cationic detergents or chlorine were the drugs of choice when only disinfection is desired. Beside this, UV radiation and heat are also preferred. For example saturated steam at 2 atmospheres pressure (120° C) for 20 minutes is successfully used to destroy microorganisms. While for sterilization of heat-labile materials, UV radiation can be used frequently.
- Topical anti-infective agents may be categorised into Flow chart 66.1:

Flow chart 66.1: Classification of anti-infective agents

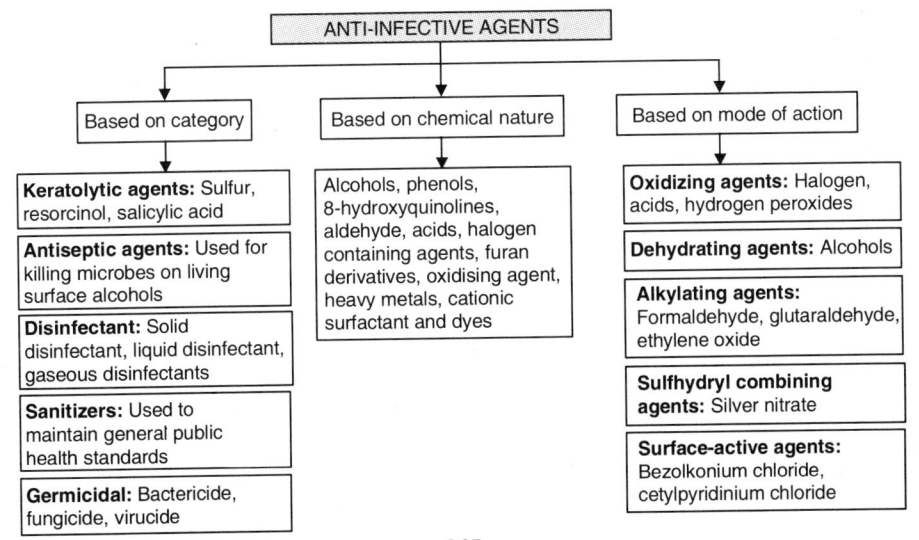

1. Keratolytic agents
2. Antiseptic agents
3. Disinfectants
4. Sanitizers
5. Germicides

KERATOLYTIC AGENTS

They include sulfur (2–10%), resorcinol (2–6%) and salicylic acid. They may be used alone or in combination with one another depending upon the situation. Salicylic acid is usually combined with sulfur to get synergistic effect. Pumice, aluminium oxide or polyethylene granules may also be employed for this action. Keratolytics act by removing surface oils and causing drying and peeling of surface skin. This leads to suppression of the spread of skin lesions.

ANTISEPTIC AGENTS

They oppose the sepsis, putrefaction or decay of the damaged or exposed tissue by inhibiting microbial multiplication and metabolic activities or by killing the pathogenic microorganisms. An ideal antiseptic should destroy bacteria, spores, fungi, viruses or any other infective agent without causing any harm to the tissues of the host. They can be applied to almost all tissues of the body and may be used in the form of mouthwashes, soaps, deodorants, throat and nasal sprays and vaginal douches. In general, all antiseptics are protein denaturants and act on enzymes, etc. in the bacteria. This accounts for the reduced effectiveness of most antiseptics in serum, blood or pus. Out of so many antiseptic agents, only intestinal and urinary tract antiseptics are pharmacologically important.

DISINFECTANTS

- These are widely used for home and hospital sanitation. They are bactericidal and rapidly produce irreversible lethal effects. Disinfection may be accomplished by heat, irradiation or chemicals. They are non-selective and destroy non-pathogens as well. They are applied only to inanimate objects. These include the substances which remove bacterial contaminants from dishes and bed pans or substances which are used in water treatment and public health sanitation. All disinfectant solutions undergo deterioration under storage and elevated temperature conditions.

- Some powerful disinfectants are too irritant, corrosive or toxic to be applied to the skin or to tissues. The chemical disinfectants can be subclassified as:

a. Solid disinfectants, e.g. bleaching powder

b. Liquid disinfectants, e.g. phenol, formalin

c. Gaseous disinfectants, e.g. formaldehyde gas.

SANITIZERS

Disinfectants that are used to maintain general public health standards are known as sanitizers. Sanitation is the process commonly used in the restaurants and at similar places for cleaning the dishes. It is mainly concerned with cleaning or washing away the organic matter (e.g. saliva, mucous, etc.). An infection may re-occur, if the pathogenic organism is not killed. Hence the anti-infective agent used should have power to destroy (-cidal properties) the microorganisms.

GERMICIDAL

- A germicidal agent may further be subcategorized as bactericide, fungicide, virucide or amoebicide. Many agents at higher concentration exhibit germicidal activity. This concentration should not produce local cellular damage. Similarly, it should not interfere with the body defenses or impair the healthy process. Upon topical application, if absorbed it should not produce systemic toxicities.

- The rate of germicidal action is dependent upon the concentration of the drug, local pH and temperature. The germicidal action of anti-infective agents is usually defined by the phenol coefficient of the agent. This parameter is obtained by following expression.

$$\text{Phenol coefficient} = \frac{\text{Dilution of chemical agent}}{\text{Dilution of phenol}}$$

- It is a ratio between minimal effective concentrations of phenol and test compound under standardized conditions against bacteria usually *Salmonella typhi* and *Staphylococcus aureus*. If the coefficient is greater than 1, it is assumed that the substance is having better germicidal activity than phenol. The germicidal activity of these agents is brought about due to their ability to alter proteins through oxidation, alkylation, and dehydration or by inactivation of the sulfhydryl group. They may also affect the bacterial cell permeability.

CLASSIFICATION

- The topical anti-infective agents can be classified on chemical basis as:

(a) Alcohols	(b) Phenols	(c) 8-Hydroxyquinolines
(d) Aldehyde	(e) Acids	(f) Halogen-containing agents
(g) Furan derivatives	(h) Oxidising agents	(i) Heavy metals
(j) Cationic surfactants	(k) Dyes	(l) Miscellaneous agents.

- These agents can also be categorized on the basis of their mechanism of action. For example:
  a. Oxidizing agents: Examples include halogens, hydrogen peroxide, acids, etc.
  b. Dehydrating agents: Examples include alcohols.
  c. Alkylating agents:Examples include formaldehyde, glutaraldehyde and ethylene oxide.
  d. Sulfhydryl combining agents: Examples include silver nitrate.
  e. Surface-active agents: Examples include benzalkonium chloride, cetylpyridinium chloride.

Alcohols

Since long back, alcohols have been used as antiseptic agents in the dressing of the wounds. Germicidal potency in the aliphatic alcohol runs parallel with its lipophilicity value. Branching and additional hydroxy groups cause the decrease in the potency. Ethyl and isopropyl alcohols are most commonly used agents in the concentration range of 30–70%. Benzyl alcohol is also used as a baceriostatic agent in a number of parenteral preparations

MOA

The antibacterial action is due to their ability to denature the bacterial proteins. In addition to this, alcohols also inhibit phosphorylation systems. They give synergistic effect when used with chlorhexidine iodine or hexachlorophene. Ethyl and isopropyl alcohols are also used as cleansers and rubefacients. They do not irritate the tissues. However, they lack antibacterial effect on spores. Ethanol may coagulate the proteins present in the wound that results into formation of protective layer over microorganisms. Alcohols that are currently being used for anti-infective activity include:

C₂H₅—OH

Ethanol

Isopropyl alcohol

Chlorobutanol

Phenyl ethyl alcohol

Phenols

- The first aseptic surgery was demonstrated by Lister in 1867 with the use of phenol. The bacteriostatic concentration of phenol is 0.5% while it is bactericidal in the concentration of 1.0% and fungicidal in the concentration of 1.5%. In fact, phenol coefficient is used as the parameter to judge the anti-infective activity of the new drugs. Although phenol is no longer used clinically, it still remains a component (0.1–4.5%) of various gels, liquids, ointments, throat sprays and lozenges. Because of its penetrability, it is used as an effective fecal disinfectant.

- A large number of phenolic derivatives have been synthesized and are used as germicides. These include alkyl and aryl phenols, parabens, halophenols and bisphenols. In all these series, activity is related to the number of free hydroxy groups. Halogenation, especially para to the hydroxy group potentiates the activity.

- Phenols and their derivatives have antiseptic, anthelmintic, anesthetic, keratolytic, vesicant and protein precipitant properties. For example, thymol may be used as:

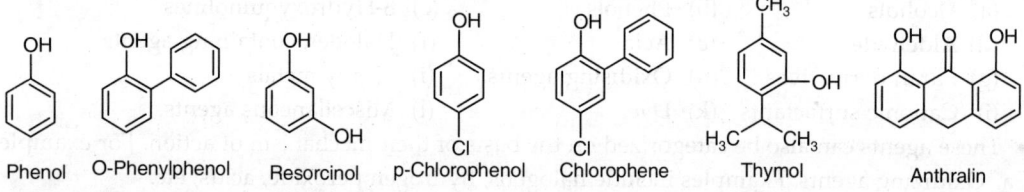

Phenol   O-Phenylphenol   Resorcinol   p-Chlorophenol   Chlorophene   Thymol   Anthralin

- Anthelmintic agent while hexylresorcinol is frequently used in throat lozenges due to its spreading and penetrating properties. It is also used in mouth washes and for cleaning the skin wounds. Parachlorometaxylenol is an effective bactericidal agent used for acne, seborrhea and ear infection. The antiseptic action of coal tar and coal tar solution is because of their various phenolic components.

- Hexachlorophene a chlorinated bisphenols is commonly used for hand washing by hospital personnel and for preoperative skin preparation.

SAR

1. The activity of alcohols increases with increasing molecular weight and chain length.
2. In phenols bisphenolic compounds are far more effective than the monomer.
3. Increase in the lipophilic nature of the aliphatic substituents in phenol increases the activity so as the increase in molecular weight.
4. Increase in chlorine content of phenols further increases the activity. The halogen para to hydroxyl group increases the potency.

MOA

It exhibits germicidal activity mainly due to their ability to denature bacterial proteins. At higher concentration, phenols cause cell-membrane lysis.

8-HYDROXYQUINOLINES

- The members of this series have antibacterial, antifungal and antiamoebic properties. The mechanism of their anti-infective action involves a transfer of iron or copper ions into bacterial cell via a chelation process This leads to an interference in the normal bacterial enzyme functioning.

8-Hydroxyquinolines   Chloroxine

Aldehydes

- Several aldehydes possess bactericidal, sporicidal and virucidal acitivites. Following are some of the examples of effective anti-infective agents.

HCHO   Formaldehyde

$(CH_2O)n$ Paraformaldehyde

Glutaraldehyde

- Formaldehyde is an excellent germicide but having unpleasant odor. It is highly effective antimicrobial agent and is used as a vapor or as an aqueous solution in the concentration range of 1–10%. Because of its irritant nature and poor penetrability in the tissues it cannot be used as an antiseptic. Hence it is widely used as a disinfectant for surface sterilization. For example, rooms can be sterilized by the use of formaldehyde gas.

MOA

- The mechanism of action involves denaturation of proteins by the replacement of labile H-atoms in amino, carboxyl, hydroxy or thiol groups of component amino acids. Ethylene oxide also acts as anti-infective agent by the same mechanism. It reacts with water and chloride to form ethylene glycol and ethylene chlorohydrin. Both are active germicides. Because of its explosive nature, ethylene oxide should not be used in the concentration above 3%. It is mainly used for sterilization of plastic equipments. It is mutagenic, carcinogenic and causes irritation to eyes and mucous membranes.
- Glutaraldehyde (glutefal) is effective dialdehyde against almost all microorganisms when its 2% aqueous solution buffered at pH 7.5–8.0 is employed. It has the broad-spectrum antimicrobial and sporicidal activities. It is mainly used to sterilize equipments, surgical instruments and surfaces contaminated with hepatitis virus. Beside this succinic dialdehyde is also sometimes used as a disinfectant.

Acids

Benzoic acid, undecylenic acid, mandelic acid, acetic acid and other organic acids and their ester forms are often used for their antiseptic, fungicidal and spermatocidal activities. Benzoic acid and its few derivatives (e.g. methyl paraben) are used extensively as preservative in food

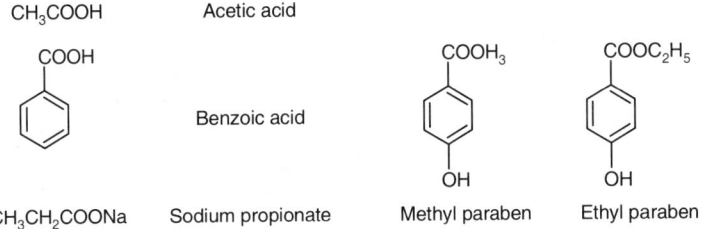

CH₃COOH   Acetic acid

Benzoic acid

CH₃CH₂COONa   Sodium propionate

Methyl paraben   Ethyl paraben

and drinks in a concentration of 0.1%. It is also used to treat ringworm and other skin infections. Acetic acid is bactericidal to many microorganisms. While mandelic acid is used in the form of its sodium salt to treat urinary tract infection in the oral dose of 8–12 g per day.

Beside this, boric acid, lactic acid, propionic acid and salicylic acid also possess anti-microbial activity. However, the use of boric acid should be limited to only ophthalmic ointment.

Halogen Containing Compounds

Chlorine is well known for the sterilization of community water supplies and for other sanitation purposes. Halogen containing compounds include both, chlorine, iodine and their complexes with organic compounds (i.e. chlorophores and iodophores). They act by oxidizing sulfhydryl groups to S – S form and thereby affecting the protein structure and function. Bromine and fluorine are not used for this purpose.

MOA (Fig. 66.1)

- Elemental chlorine and chlorophores are the potent germicidal agents having broad-spectrum of activity. When necessary, rooms can be sterilized by chlorine washing. Chlorine also has fungicidal and virucidal activities. Chlorophores serve as a depot from which is slowly released. Chlorine and its derivatives are popularly used as disinfectants. Their bactericidal activity is due to the formation of hypochlorous acid (HOCl). The ease and extent of hypochlorous acid liberation determine the efficacy of chlorophores. Some examples of effective chlorophores include:

$$ClO_2 \qquad\qquad \text{Chlorinated lime}$$

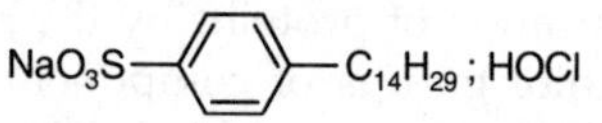

$$NaO_3S-\!\!\left\langle\bigcirc\right\rangle\!\!-C_{14}H_{29}\,;\,HOCl \qquad \text{Oxychlorosene sodium}$$

Chlorophores are usually less volatile, less irritant and longer-acting compounds. Chlorinated lime is an unstable form of chlorine that forms hypochlorite upon dissolution. While oxychlorosene is a mixture of alkyl benzene sulfonates and hypochlorous acid, from which the later is slowly released to produce germicidal activity. All these chlorophores were thought to act by:

  i. Releasing chlorine which then oxidizes the sulfhydryl groups of bacterial enzymes.
 ii. Deactivating certain bacterial proteins, or
iii. Releasing HOCl which then generates nascent oxygen to destroy the vital cellular machinery of micro-organism.

$$\underset{\text{Chlorinated lime}}{ClO_2} + HOH \longrightarrow \underset{\text{Hypochlorous acid}}{HClO} + HO_2$$

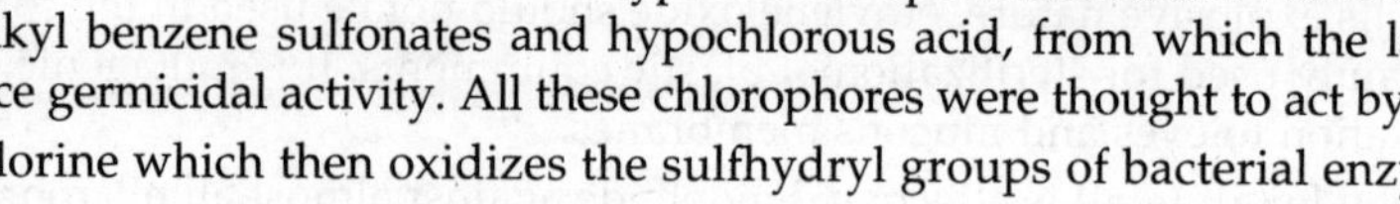

$$\underset{\text{Protein}}{R-\overset{\overset{\displaystyle O}{\|}}{C}-\overset{\overset{\displaystyle H}{|}}{N}-CH_2-R} + \underset{\text{Hypochlorous acid}}{HClO} \longrightarrow R-\overset{\overset{\displaystyle O}{\|}}{C}-\overset{\overset{\displaystyle H}{|}}{N}-CH_2-R + H_2O$$

Fig. 66.1: Mechanism of action of halogens

Furan Derivatives

- Nitrofurazone (furacin) is the most effective anti-infective agent in this class. The essential features of this class include a nitro group at 5 positions and an amine group at 2 position. The effective members of this class include:

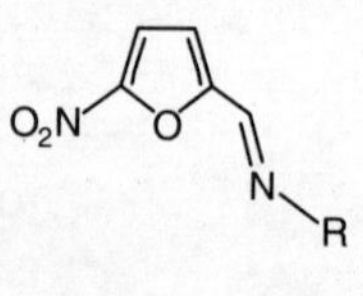

Compound	R
Nitrofurazone	—N(H)—C(=O)—NH₂
Nifuroxime	— OH
Furazolidone	—N(ring oxazolidinone)
Nitrofurantoin	—N(ring hydantoin)

- First studied in 1944, nitrofurazone is used topically in the form of a 0.2 % cream, solution ointments and powder on superficial wounds and surgical dressings. It is highly effective in the treatment of burns. It is effective against a wide variety of gram-positive and gram-negative bacteria and some protozoa. It lacks fungistatic properties.

MOA

The bactericidal action of these furan derivatives may be due to:
  i. Cessation of cell division due to the blockage of energy transfer processes.
  ii. Inhibition of bacterial respiratory enzymes.

Oxidizing Agents

Oxidizing agents are mainly having germicidal activity and of value in the treatment of infections caused by anaerobic microorganisms. They are also known for their wound cleanser and deodorant properties.

MOA

- Oxidation of the sulfhydryl group of bacteria enzymes and other vital groups present in the bacteria along with the lysis of bacterial cell-wall contribute to their germicidal activity. In the concentration range of 2–3%, hydrogen peroxide is a good disinfectant and sterilant rapidly decomposes into oxygen and water. The liberated oxygen then mechanically loosens pus and tissue debris and kills bacteria. Its ability to generate free radicals, adds further to its bactericidal activity. A 3% solution may be instilled in ears to loosen and remove cerumen.
- Although hydrogen peroxide is having a broad antibacterial spectrum, it is not stable. It undergoes decomposition upon storage. To overcome this problem, hydrogen peroxide is used in the form of carbamide peroxide and hydrous benzoyl peroxide. These preparations slowly release hydrogen peroxide when they come in contact with water. Carbamide peroxide is marketed as a 12.6% carbamide peroxide solution in anhydrous glycerin. Topical benzoyl peroxide is used mainly in the therapy of mild to moderate acne vulgaris. It also functions as exfoliant, sebostatic and comedolytic agent. It is available in 5 and 10% concentrations as creams, lotions and cleanser and as 5 and 10% concentration as washes and 2.5, 5 and 10% concentration as gels.

$$NH_2-C(=O)-O-O-C(=O)-NH_2$$

Cabamide peroxide

Benzoyl peroxide

- Sodium perborate releases oxygen when it comes in contact with tissues. As a 2% solution, it is used as a mouthwash. A 40% suspension of zinc peroxide may also be used against anaerobic infections of oral cavity. Ozone and potassium permanganate solutions are germicidal due to their oxidizing properties.

Heavy Metals

MOA

They are also known as sulfhydryl-combining agents due to their ability to react principally with -SH (sulfhydryl) group of bacterial enzyme. This results into bacterial enzymatic inactivation. Metals can be conveniently studied under the following heads.

1. Mercurials

- From early days, mercurials were used locally to treat skin infections and syphilis. They can be used as antiseptics, disinfectants and diuretics. Mercuric chloride was the first mercurial which was used as an antiseptic and disinfectant.

Nitromersol   Phenylmercuric nitrate   Merbromin

- Mercurials are neither bactericidal nor sporicides. Due to the reversible nature of sulfhydryl group blockage by these agents, they are only baceriostatic and fungistatic. Hence mercurial status is less preferred. The currently used mercurials from this category include merbromin, thiomersal, nitromersol and ammoniated mercury. Thiomersal is an organic complex that contains about 50% mercury. Though they are less toxic than the inorganic salts, they are potential contact allergens.

2. Silver compounds

Silver ions combine with sulfhydryl, carboxyl, phosphate and amino groups of the bacterial cell constituents. Hence silver salts are highly germicidal. Silver nitrate, at a concentration of 1% is often used to control gonococcal ophthalmia neonatorum. It may also be used in the treatment of extensive burns. However, it may stain tissue black due to the deposition of reduced form of silver upon exposure to sunlight. Similarly silver sulfadiazine, 1% cream may be used to treat burns and chronic pressure ulcers. Because of its ability to release silver and sulfadiazine, it effectively suppresses microbial flora. The colloidal silver preparations (e.g. mild silver protein) also act by slowly releasing the silver ions.

3. Zinc compounds

Zinc ions are effective antibacterial because of their astringent (i.e. precipitate the proteins) ability. Inorganic zinc salts are mild antiseptic and may be used in eye and skin infections. Examples include zinc sulfate, zinc oxide, zinc stearate, zinc oleate and zinc pynthione. Calamine powder consists of not less than 98% zinc oxide along with small amount of ferric oxide.

Cationic Surfactants

- The anionic surfactants (common soaps) exhibit activity against only gram-positive organisms, while gram-negative organisms are not affected; they emulsify the sebaceous matter and remove them along with dirt and microbes. Hence to increase the efficacy, other antiseptics like, phenols or mercuric iodide may be incorporated in the soaps. In comparison to anionic surfactants, cationic surfactants are more effective and have a broader antibacterial spectrum.

- They are effective against a broad range of gram-positive and gram-negative bacteria, many fungi, lipid containing viruses and spermatozoa.

- However, they do not kill spores. They have been employed either as 10% solution or as 0.1% tincture for detergent, antiseptic and disinfectant purposes. They wet the surfaces, penetrate the skin and have emulsifying, keratolytic and detergent properties. In aqueous solution, these agents undergo ionization to form cations which then react with negatively charged phosphate groups on membrane phospholipids. This leads to an increase in the permeability of bacterial cell-membrane and a change in the cell-wall integrity.

- Benzalkonium chloride is the prototype agent of quaternary ammonium compounds. It may be used to reduce infection in the wounds.

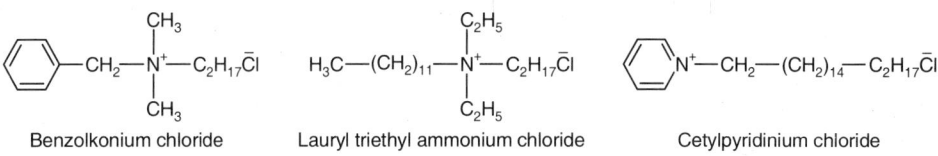

Benzolkonium chloride   Lauryl triethyl ammonium chloride   Cetylpyridinium chloride

Dyes

- Ehrlich was first to notice the antimicrobial potential of dyes. Before 1930, they were employed topically for controlling various skin infections. These dyes can be categorised into:

  o Azo dyes

  o Thiazine dyes

  o Triphenylmethane dyes, and

  o Acridine dyes

9-aminoacridine   3, 6 diaminoacridine   Methylene blue

Malachite green

- These dyes exert their bacteriostatic and bactericidal actions by enzyme inhibition and denaturation of proteins. Bacteria cannot survive due to the dysfunctioning of important biological processes.

BIS-Biguanides

- The biguanides are strongly basic compounds. They are very much similar with cationic surfactants in many aspects. Chlorhexidine is the most effective member of the series of antiseptic biguanides. This chlorophenyl biguanide has effectiveness against a broad range of gram-positive and gram-negative bacteria but it remains ineffective against some gram-negative bacilli, spores and viruses.

- Since from last 25 years, it is being marketed in Europe. It is one of the three most important surgical antiseptics. At low concentrations, it disrupts cytoplasmic membrane of bacterial cells and causes cellular constituents to leak out from the cell. At high concentrations, it causes the precipitation of cell membrane and the cytoplasmic constituents. It is most commonly used as mouth wash, general sanitation, dental antiseptic and in the treatment of superficial infections. In the form of heat sterilized fresh solution of 0.1% in water, it can also be used to rinse the wounds.

- The bactericidal concentration of chlorhexidine is estimated to be about 200 ug/ml. It is marketed in the form of 4% aqueous emulsion and as a 0.5% tincture in 70% isopropyl alcohol.

Miscellaneous Agents

Lactones

- From this series, the most effective gaseous sterilizing agent is β-propiolactone. Chemically, it is a lactone of β-hydroxy propionic acid.

β-propiolactone

- The practical drawbacks of this agent include its toxicity and the lack of penetrating ability. It acts in the similar manner to that of ethylene oxide. The probable site of action is adenine in the DNA structure. Alkylation of adenine results in the death of the cell.

Sulfur

Sublimed sulfur, precipitated sulfur, colloidal sulfur are the forms in which sulfur constitutes the part of germicidal soaps, gels, lotions and creams.

Amides

- Combination with other keratolytic agents in the treatment of cutaneous disorders.
- Tribromsalan and dibromsalan are the examples of antibacterial amides. Both are the derivatives of salicylamide

Essential oils

Pine oil was extensively studied for its disinfectant property against many pathogens. Borneol, and fenchyl alcohol are amongst the main constituents of pine oil.

Urinary tract antiseptic agents

In urinary tract infections, many drugs are used to kill or to inhibit the growth of pathogenic organisms. These agents are retained in the renal tubules. They are effective antiseptics due to their localized actions in the urinary bladder, ureters and kidneys. The list of urinary antiseptics includes mandelic acid, methenamine mandelate, nitrofurantoin, nalidixic acid and hexylresorcinol. (Discussed in Sulphonamides).

Topical camedolytic agents

Many compounds may be used as because of their sebostatic, keratolytic and anti-infective properties. These include sulfur, resorcinol salicylic acid, benzoyl peroxide, tretinoin (vitamin A acid), isotretinoin (i.e. 13-cis tretinoic acid), etc. Tretinoin is the most effective topical comedolytic agent available today. It is marketed as a 0.1 and 0.5% cream, 0.025 and 0.01% gel and 0.05% solution. A synthetic derivative of vitamin. A is isotretinoin. Adverse effects of these agents include eye irritation, xerosis, pain, stiffness and arthralgia.

Table 66.1: Mechanism of action of topical anti-infective agents

S. No.	Class	Mechansim of action	Examples
1	Alcohols	Protein precipitation	Ethanol, isopropyl alcohol
2	Alkylating agents (aldehydes)	Protein denaturation	Formaldehyde, glutaraldehyde
3	Surface-active agents (Quaternary ammonium compounds)	Alteration of cellular membrane Denaturation of lipoprotein membrane	Benzalkonium, benzethonium cetylpyridinium
4	Halogens	Coagulation of proteins Interference with enzyme action	Iodine solution, povidone iodine, halazone
5	Heavy metals	Denaturation of proteins Inactivation of SH group	Nitromersol, thiomersol, Merbromin, silver nitrate
6	Organic dyes	Denaturation of proteins Enzyme inhibition	Gention violet, methylene blue
7	Oxidizing compounds	Oxidation of organic matter	Hydrogen peroxide, zinc peroxide, potassium permanganate
8	Phenolic compounds	Protein precipitation	Phenol, cresol, resorcinol, hexylresorcinol, hexachlorophene, methyl paraben, thymol

Hexylresorcinol

Resorcinol   Hexanoic acid   4-hexanoyl-resorcinol   Hexylresorcinol

Nitrofurantoin

Hydrazine (hydrote)   Chloroacetic acid   2-hydrazino acetic acid (I)   Potassium cyanate

Semicarbazide acetic acid   1-aminohydantoin (II)   2-diacetoxymethyl-5-nitrofuran   Nitrofurantoin

Agents for Urinary Tract Infection

Many drugs are used to control urinary tract infections mainly because of their ability to develop concentration in urinary bladder, adequate to inhibit the growth of infective organisms. Examples include nitrofurantoin, nalidixic acid, oxolinic acid, resoxacin, norfloxacin, cinoxacin and methenamine. Several other 4-quinolones, such as ciprofloxacin, amifloxacin, enoxacin, etc. are under clinical investigations (Flow chart 67.1).

Flow chart 67.1: Classification of urinary tract anti-infective agents

```
┌──────────────────────────────────────────────┐
│   URINARY TRACT ANTI-INFECTIVE AGENTS          │
└──────────────────────────────────────────────┘
        ┌───► ┌──────────────────────────────────┐
        │     │ Quinolone:Nalidixic acid,          │
        │     │ oxolinic acid, resoxacin, norfloxacin │
        │     └──────────────────────────────────┘
        ├───► ┌──────────────────────┐
        │     │ Nitrofurantoin        │
        │     └──────────────────────┘
        ├───► ┌──────────────────────┐
        │     │ Mandelic acid         │
        │     └──────────────────────┘
        └───► ┌──────────────────────┐
              │ Methenamine           │
              └──────────────────────┘
```

A. Quinolone

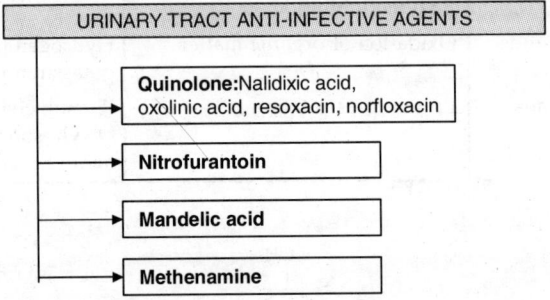

Nalidixic acid Oxolinic acid Cinoxacin

Resoxacin Norfloxacin

B. Nitrofurantoin

Nitrofurantoin

856

C. Mandelic Acid

OH
COOH

D. Methenamine

N
N N
N
Methenamine

- Nalidixic acid is effective against *E. coli, P. mirabilis, Klebsiella, Coliform bacteria* and some shigellae. Hence it is used as a bactericidal agent in the treatment of urinary tract infections caused by all above gram-negative bacteria.

Quinolone

It is an orally active antibacterial agent belonging to 4-quinolone series. Its introduction in 1962 was followed by development of other agents from this class. These include cinoxacin, oxolinic acid, resoxacin, norfloxacin, ciprofloxacin amifloxacin. All they are found to be effective against most gram-positive staphylococci and *P. aeruginosa.*

MOA

- It acts by inhibiting DNA-gyrase enzyme that is responsible for unwinding of super coiled bacterial DNA prior to its replication and transcription (Figs. 67.1 to 67.3).

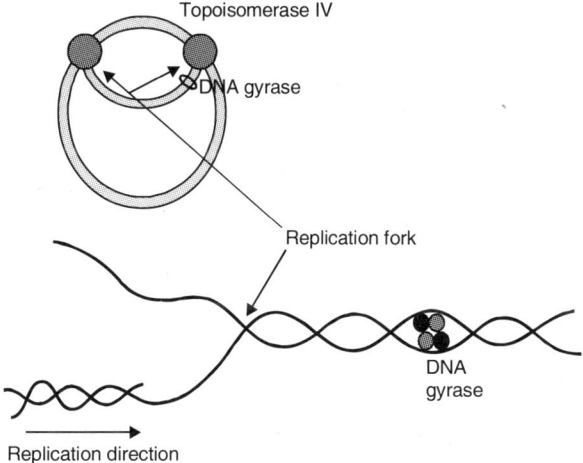

Fig. 67.1: Role of DNA gyrase in fork separation of DNA

- Bacteria, however, can readily develop resistance to its action. About 93-97% of administered dose is bound to the plasma proteins. It has a plasma half-life of 8 hours. Active hydroxynalidixic acid metabolite is excreted as conjugated form in the urine along with 2–3% dose in unchanged form. About 4–5 % dose also appears unchanged in the feces.

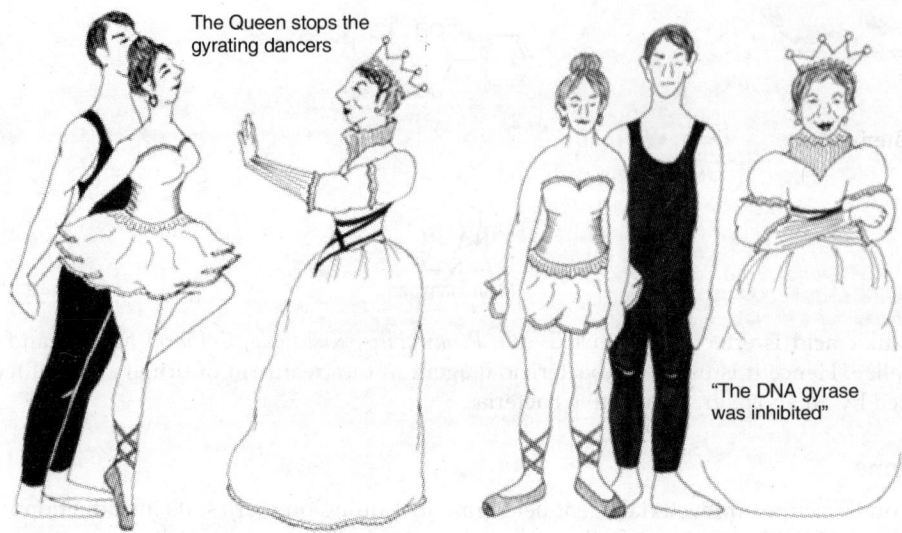

Fig. 67.2: Cartoons showing mode of action of quinolone

Adverse effects

It includes nausea, vomiting, abdominal pain, urticaria, eosinophilia, photo-sensitivity, headache, vertigo, dizziness, weakness, drowsiness, visual disturbances, hallucinations, hemolytic anemia, leucopenia and thrombocytopenia. It should not be used in infants under 3 months of age because of their inability to metabolize or excrete nalidixic acid efficiently. It may also be useful in the treatment of mild to moderate forms of gastroenteritis.

Cinoxacin: It is an orally active antibacterial agent having structural similarity with nalidixic acid. About 63% of administered dose is bound to the plasma proteins It has a plasma half-life of 1.5 hours.

Oxolinic acid: It is yet another 4-quinolone having potent antibacterial activity. It is extensively metabolized in the liver. Inactive metabolites in the form of glucuronide appear in the urine along with 5% in unchanged form. Adverse effects and therapeutic uses are similar to those of nalidixic acid.

Ciprofloxacin and norfloxacin: They are the examples of other active quinolone antibacterial agents used in treatment of urinary tract infections. Resoxacin is the member of same class but it is not used in the treatment of urinary tract infections.

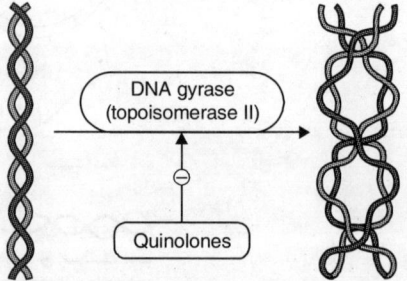

Fig. 67.3: Mode of action of quinolone

Nitrofurantoin

It is an orally active nitrofuran antibacterial agent effective against various trains of *E. coli*, *Klebsiella*, *Proteus* species and *S. faecalis*.

MOA

- The antibacterial activity is due to the presence of 5-nitro group, which helps to generate the super and other toxic oxygen compound by undergoing conversion to nitro anion. The latter undergoes interaction with molecular oxygen leading to formation of superoxide and the original nitro group. The former interferes with the carbohydrate metabolism in bacteria. It does not affect the functioning of human cell because of its low serum concentration rapid rate of drug in metabolism in liver. Antibacterial activity can be potentiated in acid pH range. Alkalinization of urine enhances the rate of excretion urine and also lowers down its antibacterial efficacy. It is a bacteriostatic in low concentrations while exerts bactericidal effect at higher concentrations.

- It exhibits antibacterial activity against most of organisms that cause lower urinary tract infection may also be used to prevent recurrence infections. It may also be used to prevent infection after prostatectomy. It is contraindicated in children one month of age and in patients with renal dysfunction.

Methenamine

It is an orally active urinary tract antiseptic agent, administered in the form of normal tablet; a considerable amount (about 10–30%) of methenamine decomposes in the stomach due to acidic pH. Hence it is to be supplied in the form of enteric-coated tablet.

MOA

In acidic urine of pH 5.5 or lower, it spontaneously decomposes to ammonia and formaldehyde. The latter agent (alleviating agent) denatures bacterial protein and acts as a nonspecific antibacterial agent effective against both gram-positive and gram-negative bacteria. Acidic urine is must for the liberation of formaldehyde. However, some bacteria (e.g. Proteus species) prevent normal urinary acidification by releasing ammonia from urea. Hence methenamine is usually administered as a salt of mandelic, hippuric or ascorbic acid to impart acidic pH to the urine. Beside this function, all these acids also exert antibacterial property.

Adverse effects

- It includes nausea, stomach upset, epigastric distress, bladder irritation, pruritus, albuminurea, crystal urea and painful and frequent micturition. It is contraindicated in renal dysfunctioning.

Nitrofurantoin

Hydrazine hydrate + Chloroacetic acid ⟶ 2-hydrozinoacetic acid (I) + Potassium cyanate ⟶ Semicarbazida acetic acid

⟶ 1-aminohydantoin (II) + 2-diacetoxymethyl-5-nitrofuran ⟶ Nitrofurantoin

Anti-Leishmanial Agents

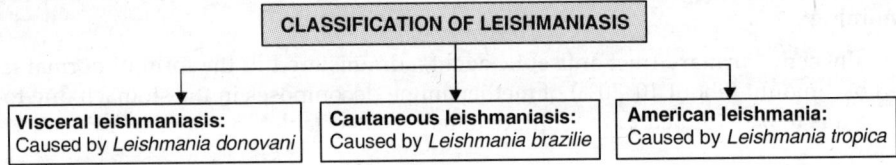

This infection is transmitted to the humans by the bites of infected female flies which are pre-infected by biting the cats, dogs or rodents, the non-human mammalian reservoirs (Fig. 68.1). Depending upon the protozoa involved and the organ affected, leishmaniasis may be of three different types.

```
                    CLASSIFICATION OF LEISHMANIASIS

  Visceral leishmaniasis:      Cautaneous leishmaniasis:    American leishmania:
  Caused by Leishmania donovani  Caused by Leishmania brazilie  Caused by Leishmania tropica
```

Visceral Leishmaniasis (Kala-azar)

It is caused by *Leishmania donovani*. This protozoa parasitizes the reticuloendothelial cells that results into an enlargement of lymph nodes, liver and spleen. The main symptoms of the disease include fever, dysentery, severe anemia and spleen become massive.

Cutaneous Leishmaniasis

It is caused by *Leishmania brazilie* involves ulceration of skin and formation of lesions.

American Leishmaniasis

It is caused by *Leishmania tropica*. The infection is characterized by the ulceration of mucous membranes of nose, mouth and pharynx, skin lesions may also appear. Of all the types, visceral leishmaniasis (kala-azar) is the commonly occurring form of infection, other two forms are rarely occurring. The occurrence localized or systemic (kala-azar) form of disease depends on the type of the infecting protozoa and the host immunological system.

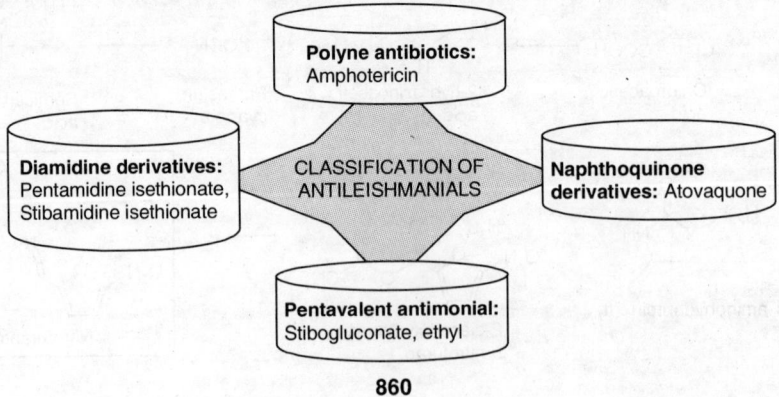

1. Pentavalent Antimonial

Sodium stibogluconate

Sitbamine

Phenyl sitbonic acid

2. Naphthoquinone Derivatives

Atovaquone

3. Diamidine Derivatives

Stilbamidine isethionate

Pentamidine isethionate

4. Polyne Antibiotics

Amphotericin B

Pentavalent Antimonial

Most of the drugs used in the treatment of leishmaniasis belong to pentavalent antimonial category. These include sodium stibogluconate urea, stibogluconate, ethyl stibamine, dihydroxy-stibisethionate and meglumine antimonate.

MOA

These pentavalent antimonial get in vivo converted to trivalent antimonial latter it inhibits phosphofructokinase, which catalyses a rate limiting step in glycolysis. Hence the organisms whose growth is dependent upon the anaerobic metabolism of glucose, cannot survive in the kick of energy source. Beside this, these agents were also reported to inhibit several enzyme systems of the protozoa. The effectiveness of sodium stibogluconate in treatment of visceral leishmaniasis is due to its ability to concentrate in liver and spleen.

Pentamidine Derivatives

Pentamidine isethionate

MOA: Their mode of action is not properly understood. It probably interacts with kinetoplast DNA and inhibits topoisomerase II or interferes with aerobic glycolysis.

Pharmacokinetics: Pentamidine isethionate is a poor orally absorbed aromatic diamidine having antiprotozoal and fungicidal activities. About 80% of administered dose is bound to the plasma proteins. It is excreted unchanged in the urine at much slow rate.

Adverse effects: It includes nausea, vomiting, anorexia, headache, fever, rash, pancreatitis, leukopenia, thrombocytopenia, dizziness, confusion, hypotension and hypoglycemia. It is used as a prophylactic agent in systemic blastomycosis, trypanosomiasis, cutaneous leishmaniasis and in pneumonia due to *P. carimi*. The later infection may be associated with acquired immune deficiency syndrome (AIDS).

Polyne Antibiotics

Amphotericin B

It is also reported to be effective in the cases of leishmaniasis, not responding to other drugs.

69

Anti-Trypanosomal Agents

Trypanosomes are mobile protozoan parasites that require two host including man (vertebrate) and insect (invertebrate). The parasites may be found in the blood and spinal fluid of the infected person. Some trypanosomes are non-pathogenic and live silently in the body of the host. Trypanosomiasis may be of two types based upon the species of trypanosomes involved.

```
              CLASSIFICATION OF TRYPANOSOMIASIS

        African trypanosomiasis          American trypanosomiasis
```

African Trypanosomiasis

It is caused by the bite of the fly belonging to Glossina species. The infective protozoa may be *T. gambiense* or *T. rhodesiense*. The disease is known as sleeping sickness which is characterise by fever, headache, lymph node enlargement, drowsiness, lethargy, weakness and mental disturbances. Since protozoans enter into the cerebrospinal fluid the signs of mental disturbances are seen.

American Trypanosomiasis

- It is caused by *T. cruzi* and is transmitted by kissing bugs.

```
              CLASSIFICATION OF TRYPANOCIDAL AGENT

  Non-metallic        Dimercaprol        Nitrofuran         Pentavalent
  dye derivatives:    derivatives:       derivatives:       arsenical derivatives:
  Suramin sodium      Melarsoprol        Nifurtimox         Tryparsamide
```

1. Non-metallic Dye Derivatives

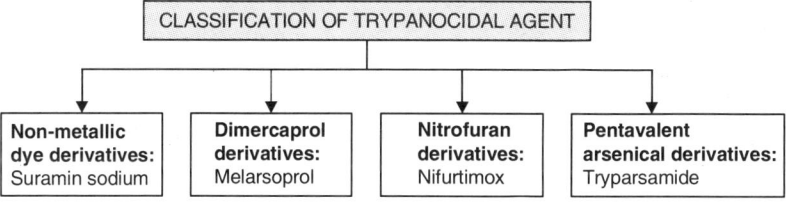

Suramin sodium

863

2. Dimercaprol Derivatives

Melarsoprol

3. Pentavalent Arsenical Derivatives

Typarsamide

4. Nitrofuran Derivatives

Nifurtimox

Non-metallic Dye

Suramin sodium

MOA:

- Because of its anionic nature, it may bind with the cationic sites present of proteins and enzymes in glycolytic pathways and inhibit their functioning.
- Protozoa may die due to the lack of energy source. It does not readily penetrate mammalian cells. This explains its selectivity of action.

Pharmacokinetics:

- It is a non-metallic dye derivative having trypanocidal activity. Freshly prepared solution should always be used for IV administration. About 99% of administered dose is bound to the plasma proteins. It has a plasma half-life of 48–49 days.
- It does not undergo metabolism and is excreted slowly in urine in unchanged form over a period of months. Since a single injection provides adequate blood concentration for several months.

Uses:

- It may be used in both, prophylaxis and treatment of African trypanosomiasis. It may also be effective in treatment of onchocerciasis either alone or along with arsenicals.
- It is also effective in the prophylaxis of Rhodesian and Gambian trypanosomiasis.

Dimercaprol Derivative

Melarsoprol

MOA:

- It is a dimercaprol derivative of melarsen oxide used as antiprotozoal agent. Trimelarsan is a water soluble derivative of melarsoprol which may be used intramuscularly. The activity is due to the arsenic content which inhibits the essential sulfhydryl group containing enzymes.

- This inhibitory action of arsenic is of non-specific and non-selective nature which explains the severe adverse effects associated with the use of this drug. Drug-resistant strain of protozoa is less permeable to the drug.

Uses: It is marketed as a 3.6 % w/v sterile solution in propylene glycol. It is used to treat African trypanosomiasis involving CNS symptoms.

Pentavalent Arsenical Derivatives

Typarsamide

- It is a pentavalent arsenical, once used in the treatment of advance cases of trypanosomiasis. It contains about 25% antimony.
- It may be used along with suramin in the treatment of West African trypanosomiasis. Because of drug-induced optic nerve damage, it is a less preferred agent.

Nitrofuran Derivatives

Nifurtimox

MOA:

- The nitro group of nifurtimox is converted to nitro anion radical in the presence of pyridine nucleotides. This anion produces superoxide by reaction with molecular oxygen, resulting into regeneration of nifurtimox.
- This superoxide then may interfere in the synthesis of proteins and in the functioning of protozoal enzymes.

Pharmacokinetics: It is a nitrofuran derivative, effective specifically against *T. cruzi* infections. It is orally effective drug. It has a plasma half-life of about 8 hours. Inactive metabolites appear in the urine along with 5% dose in unchanged form.

Adverse effects: It includes nausea, vomiting, headache, weight loss, euphoria, tremors, insomnia, drowsiness, psychic disturbances and peripheral neuropathy.

Uses:

- Nitrofurazone is a topical antibacterial agent effective against many gram-positive and gram-negative bacteria and some protozoa.
- It is used to treat special cases of American trypanosomiasis which are resistant to other drugs. The adult oral dose in the treatment of trypanosomiasis is 500 mg daily for 3 days and then 500 mg every 8 hours for a week. This dose schedule may be repeated thrice with a week interval each time.

70

Anti-Trichomonal Agents

Trichomonas are unicellular, flagellated protozoal parasites. Most of them are nonpathogenic in nature. In humans, the pathogenic parasites reside in the urogenital tract. The pathogenic species include *Trichomonas vaginalis* in humans and *T. foetus* in animals.

PATHOPHYSIOLOGY

- Males are asymptomatic carriers but females often develop severe vaginitis and cervicitis. *T. vaginalis* infection in male appears as a symptom-free urethritis while in female, it occurs as vaginitis which is characterised by a frothy pale yellow discharge.
- Age of the female, pH at vaginal region and period of her menstrual cycle are some of the factors that affect her susceptibility to the infection. Since the transmission of disease is affected due to sexual contacts, the male sexual partner should be treated simultaneously to prevent occurrence of relapses in the female.

```
CLASSIFICATION OF TRICHOMONICIDAL AGENT
```

Nitroimidazole derivatives: Nimorazole, tinidazole, metronidazole, niridazole, aminitrozole	Pentavalent arsenicals: Acetarsol	Nitrofuran derivatives: Furazolidone, nifurtimox	8-hydroxyquinoline: Iodoquinol	Polyne antibiotics: Pimaricin, hachimycin

1. Nitroimidazole Derivatives

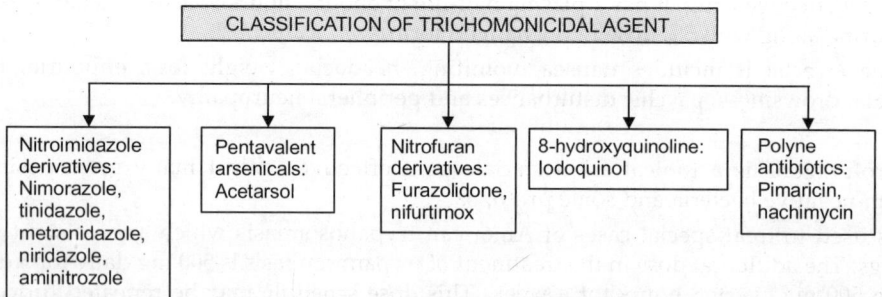

Metronidazole   Tinidazole   Panidazole   Nimorazole

Aminitrozole   Niridazole

866

2. Nitrofuran Derivatives

Nifurtimox

Furazolidone

3. Pentavalent Arsenicals

Acetarsol

4. 8-Hydroxyquinoline

Iodoquinol

- Aminitrozole, niridazole, acetarsol, furazolidone and nifurtimox are the agents which may be used in the treatment of vaginitis. Along with these agents, metronidazole, nimorazole, tinidazole, arsenicals, 8-hydroxyquinolines (for fetail refer Anti-amoebic chapter) and certain polyene antibiotics (e.g. pimaricin and hachimycin) may also be used. A single dose of 2 g of either metronidazole or tinidazole has been shown to be effective, if the patient is not re-infected.

Anti-Giardial Agents

Giardiasis is an intestinal protozoal infection caused by *Giardia lamblia*. Unhygienic conditions, low socio-economic status and homosexuality are some factors that contribute in the spread of giardiasis. The asymptomatic patients may release protozoal parasites in the form of cysts in the feces. Transmission then occurs after ingestion of cysts in contaminated food or water. The main symptoms include diarrhea, anorexia, bloating, flatulence and weight loss.

- Though all amebicidal drugs can be used in the treatment of giardiasis, metronidazole, tinidazole and quinacrine are more preferred agent.

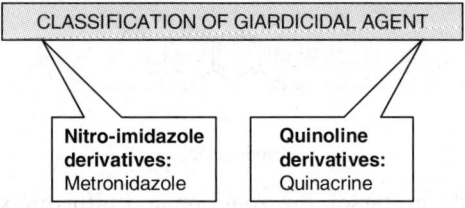

Quinacrine

MOA

- It binds to DNA through an intercalation mechanism, and strongly inhibits DNA replication and RNA transcription process. It also interferes with protein synthesis and functioning of various enzyme systems. It is also used as anticonvulsant agent in certain cases. It exerts quinidine-like effects on the heart.

- Though it is no longer used in the prophylaxis and treatment of malaria but still it is used as an important agent in the treatment of giardiasis. It is an orally acridine derivative which is very slowly excreted in the urine. The metabolic pathways for quinacrine are poorly understood.

Adverse effects

It includes nausea, vomiting, anorexia, diarrhea, headache, ocular toxicity, discoloration of nails, dizziness, anxiety, restlessness, blood dyscrasias and psychosis. It is contraindicated during pregnancy and in patients receiving antimalarial therapy with primaquine.

Uses

It is a drug of choice in the treatment of giardiasis and is used in the oral dose of 100 mg three times a day for 5 – 7 days. The dose-schedule may be repeated, if necessary about 2 weeks later. Beside furazolidone and paromomycin may also be used for treatment of giardiasis.

Toxoplasmosis and Balantidiasis

Toxoplasmosis

Toxoplasmosis is caused by the ingestion of cysts of *Plasma gondii* from the feces of infected, ingestion of cysts from affected raw meat. Active toxoplasmosis, systemic toxoplasmosis and cotoxoplasmosis (in newborns) are the important in this infection.

Drugs

- Drugs like pyrimethamine, sulfadiazine, piramycin (a macrolide antibiotic) may be used alone or in combination with corticosteroids in the treatment of infection.
- Folinic acid (leukovorin calcium) may be administered along with pyrimethamine to minimize the adverse effects of pyrimethamine on folic acid metabolism.

Balantidiasis

This intestinal infection is caused by *Balantidium coli*, which is normally a parasite of pigs. Trophozoites may induce either a superficial necrosis or a deep ulceration in mucosa and submucosa of large intestine. This results into a variety of symptoms including nausea, vomiting, abdominal pain, diarrhea or severe dysentery.

Drugs

- The infection may be treated by giving tetracycline, 500 mg four times daily for 10 days. Iodoquinol, 650 mg 3 times a day is also effective in the treatment of balantidiasis.
- Other pathogenic intestinal protozoan infections include isosporiasis (*Isospora belli* and *I. hominis*) and *Pneumocystis carinii* infection—both are treated with either pyrimethamine-sulphonamide or cotrimoxazole combination preparations. Pentamidine may be given intramuscularly to control pneumocystosis.

Miscellaneous

Immunomodulators

Diseases in humans are caused by a variety of reasons. Most of the pathological diseases in humans are caused by three most important groups of microorganisms namely, bacteria, rickettsia and viruses. Skin provides a barrier for the easy entry of microorganisms in the body. The intact skin is virtually impregnable to microorganisms and only when a tissue injury occurs, microorganisms enter the blood circulation.

A continuous chain of natural defence barriers exists in our body that restricts microorganisms to areas where they can be tolerated. Bactericidal action is exerted by many of the body secretions. For example, tears, nasal secretions and saliva contain the enzyme, lysozyme; hydrochloric acid is released from the gastric mucosa or a basic polypeptide like spermine which is present in the semen. These nonspecific endogenous antimicrobial systems are operative at all times against the entry of pathogenic microorganisms. Besides this phagocytosis (Fig. 73.1) is an important tool for the engulfment and digestion of microorganisms.

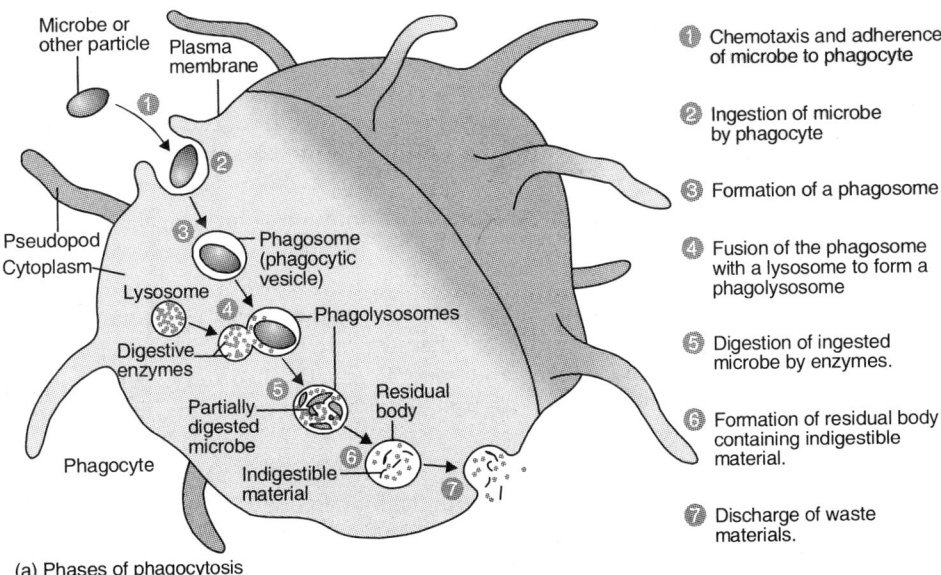

(a) Phases of phagocytosis

Fig. 73.1: Mechanism of phagocytosis

FIRST-LINE DEFENCE

- In fact the first-line of body defence mechanisms consists of phagocytes and lymphocytes. Polymorphonuclear leucocyte is a short-lived, non-dividing white blood cell derived from the totipotent bone marrow stem cell. It is an actively phagocytic, motile cell that can pass through capillary walls and ingest foreign material, microorganisms or antigens.

- The foreign material is ingested and is fused with lysosomal granules present within the cell. Destruction of infectious agent usually occurs after the release of lysosomal enzymes from the lysosomal granules.

- It provides the major line of defence against pyogenic (pus-forming) bacteria. Thus polymorphonuclear leucocytes are the mobile phagocytes while macrophages are the long lived tissue-fixed phagocytes. Though macrophages are scattered throughout all body organs, they are present in higher concentrations mainly in lung, liver, spleen and lymph nodes.

- They have an ability to take up and concentrate inert particulate matter, including microorganisms and tissue debris. In these organs, macrophages function as filters to remove foreign material from the circulating lymph and blood. The macrophage system is also known as reticuloendothelial system.

- When polymorphonuclear leukocytes fail to inhibit the entry of bacteria in the body, bacteria escape into blood vessels and lymphatics and are carried to lymph nodes and spleen. At this place, they are trapped by macrophages.

- When microorganisms escape from the attack of both the tissue-fixed phagocytes and mobile phagocytes, they enter the tissues which are normally inaccessible. This results into failure of the primary defences and development of infection. If remains untreated, a pathological condition may arise because of invasion and multiplication of microorganisms in the body organs. The term virulence is used to indicate the degree of pathogenicity of a given strain of microorganism.

SECOND LINE DEFENCE MECHANISM

- In presence of virulent bacteria species, phagocytosis alone, is inadequate and the second line of defence including antibody and complement must act in concert to exert antimicrobial action. This combination of phagocytosis (i.e. nonspecific) and antibody-complement system (i.e. specific) constitutes body's natural defence mechanism, known as immunity.

- The word immunity is derived from a latin word immunis which means 'exempt from'. Immunity is usually defined as a state of relative resistance to an infection. Substances capable of stimulating immune mechanism are known as antigens.

- Chemically, they are mostly proteins, polysaccharides and complex lipids having molecular weight greater than 5000. Immunological mechanisms are found to be more pronounced in certain disease conditions like cancer and several genetic disorders. Many allergic and autoimmune disorders develop due to functional impairments in the immunological mechanisms.

- Polymorphonuclear leukocytes (neutrophils), macrophages, and lymphocytes are the important categories of immune cells present in the human body. They are all obtained from the stem cells present in the bone marrow which is a site of continual proliferation and turnover of immature blood cells. Formation of particular immune cell occurs through differentiation of stem cells (Fig. 73.2). This depends upon the demand for cells in peripheral immune organs.

- A sort of coordination and interconnection is seen between all these types of immune cells. For example, one of the types of monokines secreted from macrophages is interleucin-1 (IL-1) which, in the presence of antigen induces T lymphocytes to proliferate.

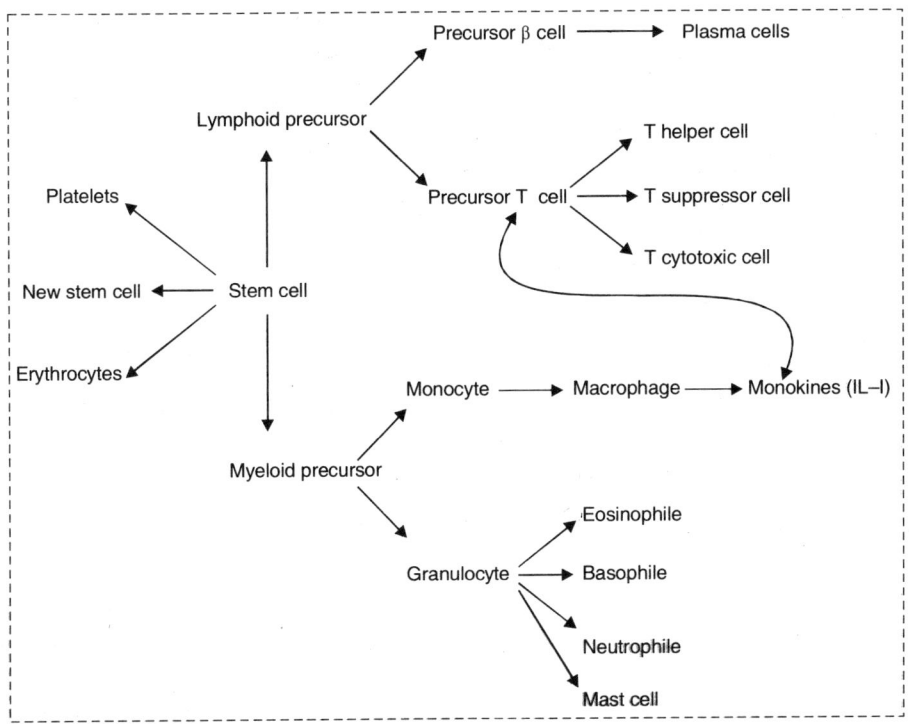

Fig. 73.2: Differentiation of stem cell in bone marrow

COMPONENT OF IMMUNE SYSTEM

Lymphocytes

- They are an integral part of specific immune mechanisms and are mainly formed in the bone marrow through proliferation and differentiation of stem cells. Some stem cells also migrate to thymus gland where they proliferate to give lymphocytes.

- Thus depending upon the site of formation, they can be classified into two major types, namely T lymphocytes (thymus-derived) and B lymphocytes (bone marrow-derived). Both types are found in the blood.

- T lymphocytes are concerned with cellular immunity (i.e. phagocytosis) while B lymphocytes are concerned with humoral immunity (i.e. antibodies production). Under certain conditions like stress or administration of corticosteroids, production of lymphocytes is inhibited.

Cellular Immunity

- The effector substances in cell-mediated immunity include lymphokines, interferon and monokines. T lymphocytes protect the tissue from intracellular diseases and cellular neoplasms.

- These lymphocytes are responsible for the immunity to those microorganisms that have an ability to live and multiply within the cells of the host, e.g. tubercle bacillus, viruses and protozoal parasites.

- They react directly with foreign material. This interaction leads to the production of lymphokines by lymphocytes. These lymphokines either destroy the foreign material through phagocytosis or react with receptor sites present on B lymphocytes to induce humoral immunity.
- The cellular immunity (T lymphocytes) plays an important role against bacterial, fungal and viral infections, in transplant rejection, in neoplasms and in some autoimmune processes.

Humoral Immunity

- Humoral immunity involves the production of specific antibodies from B lymphocytes upon antigenic stimulation. Small populations of B lymphocytes are specifically concerned with retaining of memory of antigens.
- They are known as memory cells. Re-exposure to same antigen at a later time causes activation of memory cells to proliferate and secrete antibody at much faster rate. Upon antigenic stimulation, B lymphocytes proliferate and differentiate into protein molecules having specific antibody activity.
- These molecules are known as immunoglobulins (Ig) or gamma globulins. They are categorized into five major classes like:
  a. Immunoglobulin G
  b. Immunoglobulin M
  c. Immunoglobulin A
  d. Immunoglobulin D
  e. Immunoglobulin E
- For every antigen, there is a specific clone of B lymphocytes that secretes an antibody capable of neutralizing only that antigen.
- Since the secreted antibodies circulate throughout the body, the immune responses associated with antibody production are called humoral immune responses.
- The high specificity antigen–antibody interaction is due to differences in the chemical composition of the outer surfaces of the microorganisms.

Immunoglobulins (Antibodies)

- Synthesis of various immunoglobulins occurs after the primary antigenic stimulation. They are extremely effective agglutinating agents that appear early in the response to infection.
- Immunoglobulin G is the most abundant immunoglobulin synthesized during antigen activation. It contains 4 polypeptide chains (i.e. two heavy chains and two light chains) which are joined together by disulfide bonds. It has a molecular weight of about 150,000. This type of antibodies is found throughout the body and is effective against a large variety of antigens. Most virus antibodies and antitoxins belong to this class of immunoglobulins. Because of their ability to cross the placenta, they are effective against infections seen in newborn.
- Immunoglobulin A appears mainly in saliva, tears, nasal secretions, sweat, in secretions of the lungs, urinogenital and gastrointestinal tracts where it protects the surface of mucosal cells from microbial attack. In all these secretions, it appears as a dimer.
- Immunoglobulin D does not have any precise function. However, their role in the control of lymphocyte activation and suppression is suspected. They may serve as lymphocyte antigen receptor.

- Immunoglobulin E sensitizes the mast cells after its interaction with antigens present on the surface of mast cells. As many as 500,000 IgE receptor sites are present on each mast cell. Thus this type of antibody is involved in degranulation of mast cells resulting into release of histamine, serotonin, plasmakinins, platelet activating factor, eosinophil chemotactic factor and slow releasing substance of anaphylaxis. While immunoglobulin M participates in agglutinating and cytolytic reactions.

Lymph Nodes

- Lymph has same composition of salts as interstitial fluid and plasma. The lymph vessels possess numerous valves and the flow of lymph from the periphery to thoracic duct is brought about in the same way as the flow of blood in the vein.
- Lymph contains large number of lymphocytes, mainly T lymphocytes. Particulate matter which is being collected by the lymph is brought into close contact with these lymphocytes in the lymph nodes. This results into fixation of particulate matter with the lymphocytes.

Spleen

- Because of the slow circulation through the spleen, macrophages get opportunity to sequester and ingest the aged red cells or other foreign substances.
- Beside this, foreign particles are brought into close contact with lymphocytes resulting into their fixation.

Thymus

- It is a 'master' lymphoid tissue which controls other lymphoid tissues (like, lymph node and thymus). This control is mediated through the release of hormones.
- Thymus consists of a peripheral cortex densely packed with lymphocytes and a central medula containing less numerous lymphocytes.
- After adolescence, thymus becomes less active. This results into decrease in the effectiveness of cell-mediated immunity in old aged persons.

▬ TYPES OF IMMUNITY

"Immunity is defined as resistance exhibited by host towards injury caused by micro-organism and their product."

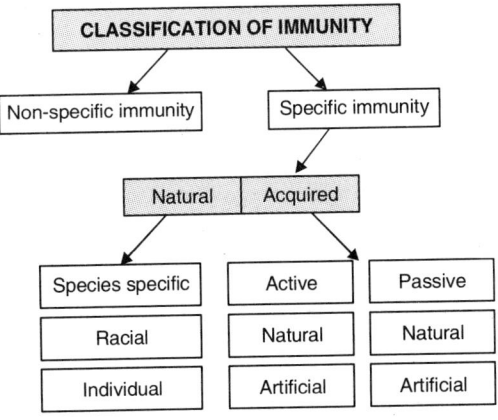

Specific Immunity

Natural immunity

It is defined as the resistance to infection, which is possessed by individual because of its genetic and constitutional make up. It does not depend upon the prior contact with the micro-organism or immunization.

1. Species specific immunity: This is the natural resistance to infection observed in particular species, e.g. human beings are totally insusceptible to the plant pathogen and to the many pathogen of animals. Like humans are immune to chicken cholera while many of the lower species are resistant to variety of human infection just like typhoid, syphilis, etc.

2. Racial specific immunity: This is the natural resistance to infection observed in particular races, e.g. the high resistance Algerian race of sheep to the Anthrax.

3. Individual immunity: This is the natural resistance to infection observed in to the individual e.g. individual of blood group 'O' and 'B' are more resistant to small pox than those of blood group 'A'.

Acquired immunity

It is defined as the resistance that an individual can acquire during lifespan is known as the acquired immunity.

1. Active immunity: It can be imparted either naturally by means of a clinical or subclinical infection or artificially by injection of appropriate antigen in the form of a vaccine or toxoid. These vaccines contain microbial strains of abnormally low pathogenicity. Their administration leads to antigenic stimulus and formation of antibodies at much faster rate. This type of immunity is normally long-lasting.

2. Passive immunity: This type of immunity can be imparted either naturally by placental transfer of mother antibodies to their child (and also through breast milk) or artificially by means of administration of antibodies preformed in another actively immunized human being (e.g. human, gamma globulins) or in an animal like horse. Examples include antitoxic sera such as tetanus, diphtheria, etc.

Human gamma globulin thus may be used in the prevention of infectious hepatitis. Passive immunity offers protection immediately but such protection is usually of short duration. Horses are chiefly used for the production of immunosera but cattle, goats and sheep are alternative sources. Responses to vaccines against poliomyelitis and smallpox have markedly reduced impact of these diseases on humankind.

▨ HYPERSENSITIVITY

- Antigen recognition leads to activation of immune mechanisms. This results into clonal proliferation of specific B lymphocytes or T lymphocytes. The interaction of antigen with the immune system can give rise to two types of responses.

  1. During the interaction, the antigen may damage immune system functionally. An immunodeficiency thus develops. Body's natural resistance to infection is decreased and person can easily be affected by infections. The immuno-suppression may or may not be reversible. The immunosuppression leads to an increased susceptibility to bacterial, fungal or a viral infection. For example, patients under a long-term cortisone therapy are more prone to certain diseases including rheumatoid arthritis, Hodgkin's disease, etc.

  2. During the interaction, the antigen provokes the typical manifestations of allergy. Under certain conditions, the antigen–antibody interaction may provide an unusual and

exaggerated reaction, damaging the host body tissues. This altered response of the host tissues is known as hypersensitivity or allergy. The details about types of antibodies that are found to be involved in immune reactions are tabulated in Table 73.1.

Table 73.1: Antibodies present in human immune system

Type of antibody	Molecular weight (nx 10^3)	Half-life T ½(days)	Normal serum concentration (mg)
IgA	170	6.0	275
IgD	150	2.8	5
IgE	196	1.5	0.03
IgG	150	23	1200
IgM	890	5.0	120

- "This is the improper immune response that results in tissue damage and it is manifested into the individual on second or subsequent contact with the antigen"
- This is known as the allergy and is caused by allergens. Allergens may be pollen grains, dust particles and sometime it may be component of bacteria. Although pollengrains and dust particles are inactive form but the reaction which they carry out are is much exaggerated.
- Hypersensitivity reaction can be classified as either immediate or delayed. Obviously the immediate reaction appears faster than delayed ones. But the main difference between them is in the nature of the immune response to the antigen. Realizing this concept, hypersensitivity is classified in Table 73.2.

Table 73.2: Classification of allergic responses

Type	Antibody involved	Target tissues	Symptoms
Type I (Anaphylactic reaction or immediate hypersensitivity)	IgE	Respiratory tract (asthma), vasculature (anaphylactic shock), skin (urticaria.)	Edema and vasodilation
Type II (Cytotoxic reactions)	IgG and IgM	Circulatory system	Hemolytic anemia Granulocytopema
Type III (Immune complex reactions)	IgG	Vascular endothelium	Urticaria, arthritis, lymphadenopathy, fever, serum sickness
Type IV (Delayed hypersensitivity)	These reactions are mediated by sensitized T lymphocytes and macrophages		

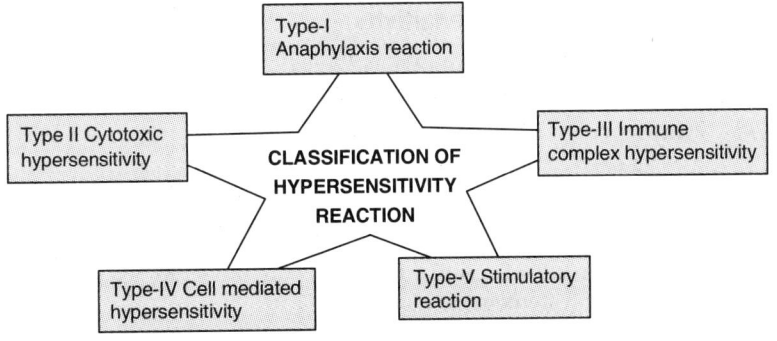

Type I: Anaphylaxis Reaction

Whenever allergen enters in our body, it induces antibodies IgE production only restricted to anaphylaxis reaction.

Mechanism (Fig. 73.3)

- Upon initial exposure to an allergen, β-cell is stimulated, which upon differentiation gives rise to plasma cell and IgE antibody.
- This synthesized IgE binds to the several Fc receptors of mast cells which are characterized by granules. This phenomenon occurs when primary exposure of allergen takes place. When secondary exposure of the same allergen occurs, the allergen attaches to the surface of bounded IgE on the sensitized mast cells causing degranulation.
- Degranulation releases physiological mediators such as histamine, prostaglandins, heparin and proteolytic enzyme that leads to edema, erythroma, smooth muscle contraction, vasodilation, vascular permeability, etc.

Example

1. Asthma: It is characterized by paroxysmal attacks of difficult respiration. The symptoms include bronchoconstriction, edema of bronchial mucosa and cyanosis.

2. Hay fever: It is a type of hypersensitivity that occurs in persons sensitive to a variety of pollens. Symptoms of hay fever include sneezing, running nose, itching and irritation of the nose and eyes, perfused lacrymation and photophobia.

3. Urticaria: It is one of the commonest adverse drug reaction which is characterized by localized patchy or generalised erythematous lesions. These lesions are accompanied by an intense itching. This reaction is short-lived and disappears within few hours. Lesion is dose-dependent and high incidence of rash, fever, eosinophilia and other blood dyscrasias is associated.

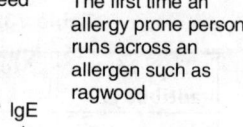

Fig. 73.3: Mechanism of anaphylactic reaction

The first time an allergy prone person runs across an allergen such as ragwood

he or she makes large amounts of regweed IgE antibody.

These IgE molecules attach themselves to mast cells.

The second time that person has a brush with regweed,

The IgE primed mast cells release granules and powerful chemical mediators, such as histamine and cytokines, into the environment.

These chemical mediators cause the characteristic symptoms of allergy.

Type II Reactions (Cytotoxic Hypersensitivity)

- This type of hypersensitivity is also known as the cytotoxic reaction because it results into the destruction of host cells either by lysis or toxic mediators.

Mechanism (Fig. 73.4)

- In this reaction IgG or IgM antibodies are directed against the cell surface or tissue antigens. They usually stimulate the complement pathway and variety of effector cells. The antibodies interact with the complement (1q) and effector cells through their Fc region.
- The damage mechanism is a reflection of the normal physiological process involved in interaction of the immune systeme with pathogen.

Example

Thrombocytopenia purpura: Blood platelets (thrombocytes) are minute cell that are essential for blood clotting. They are destroyed by antibodies and complement, in the disease called thrombocytopenia purpura.

In this condition, the platelets have become coated with molecule of drug, such as aspirin and some antibodies which act as hapten, because of which these platelets are recognized as allergen and body will start producing antibodies against it and this results in destruction of platelet. As platelets are essential for blood clotting, their loss results in hemorrhages that appear on the skin as purple spot (purpura).

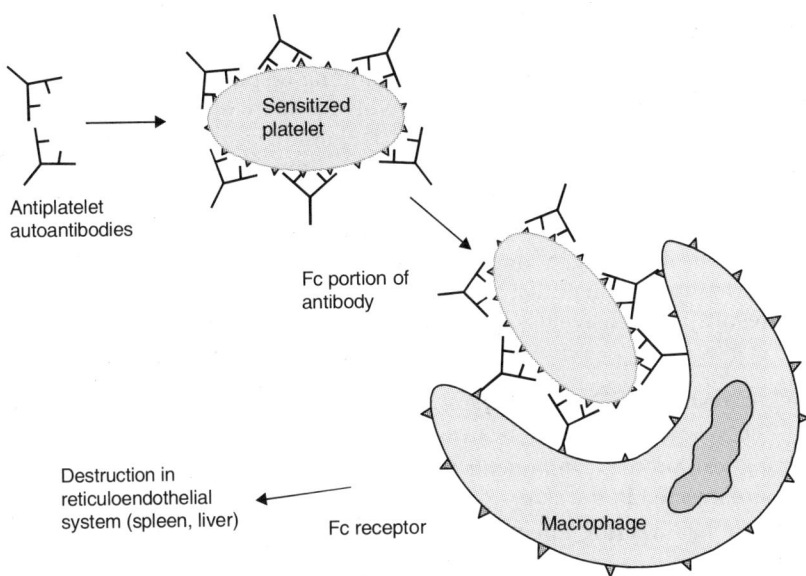

Fig. 73.4: Mechanism of action of thrombocytopenia purpura

Type III Reaction (Immune Complex Hypersensitivity)

- Many times immune-complex reactions are responsible to cause hypersensitivity reaction. Normally, these complexes are removed effectively by monocytes of the reticuloendothelial systeme. In the presence of excess of amounts of some antigen, the antigen–antibody complex may not be efficiently removed. Their accumulation can lead to a hypersensitivity reaction from complement that triggers a variety of responses (Fig. 73.5).

- These complexes circulate in the blood vessels and become trapped in the basement membranes beneath the cell. In this location, they may activate compliment and cause

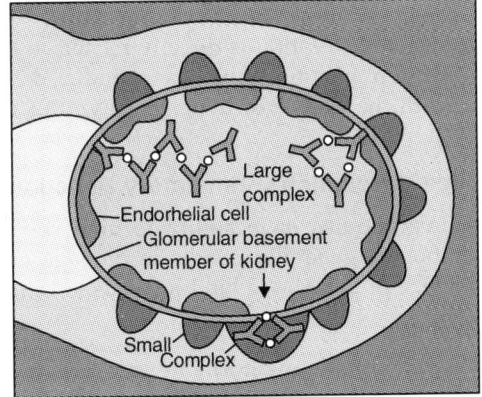

Fig. 73.5: Mechanism of immune complex hypersensitivity

transient inflammatory reaction. Repeated introduction of the same antigen can lead to serious inflammatory reaction.

Example

Rheumatoid arthritis: It is a disease in which immune complex of IgM and IgG and complement are deposited into the joints. In fact there is evidence that immune complexes called rheumatid factors may be formed by IgM binding to Fc region of normal IgG. These factors are found in 70% of persons suffering from rheumatoid arthritis. The chronic inflammation caused by this deposition eventually leads to severe damage to the cartilage and to the bone.

Type IV (Cell Mediated Hypersensitivity)

- This type of reaction involves cell-mediated immune response and is caused mainly by T cells, although macrophages may also be involved. It involves delayed T cell mediated immune reaction. A major factor in this delay is the time required for a special subset of T cells called delayed type of hypersensitivity. Such type of reaction occurs, when antigens especially those binding to tissue cells, are phagocytosized by macrophages and then presented to receptors on the T cell surface.
- Contract between the antigen and T cell causes the cell to proliferate and release lymphokinins. Lymphokinin attract lymphocytes, macrophages and basophils to the affected tissue. This results in extensive tissue damage.

Example

Tuberculin skin test (Fig. 73.6): As *Mycobacterium tuberculosis* is often located within the macrophages, this disease can stimulate a cell-mediated immune response.

- As a screening test, protein components of the bacteria are injected in the skin.
- If the recipient has a prior infection by tuberculosis bacteria, an inflammatory reaction by tuberculosis bacteria, an inflammatory reaction to the injection of these antigens will appear on the skin in one or two days, this interval is typical of delayed hypersensitivity reactions. The size and duration is directly related to the amount of antigen that was introduced and with the degree of hypersensitivity of the individual.

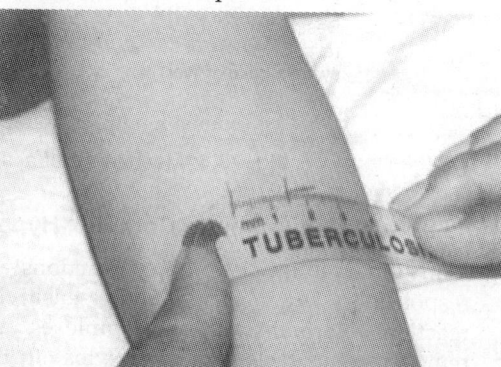

Fig. 73.6: Tuberculin skin test

Type V Reaction (Stimulatory Reaction)

Autoantibodies have ability to bind self-antigen associated with cell. The binding of such antibodies generally results in damage of tissues, cell or organ. In several cases instead of damage of the Ab-Ag binding leads to "stimulatory action" on functioning of organ.

Example

Thyroid stimulating hormone promotes functioning of thyroid gland. Normally on thyroid cell, a receptor is present for binding of TSH. The TSH binding to thyroid gland triggers adenyl cyclase, which further leads to cAMP formation. cAMP activates the thyroid gland. In abnormal condition, autoantibodies were produced which also can bind to TSH-receptor of thyroid gland. Binding of autoantibody to TSH receptor stimulates the function of thyroid gland.

Table 73.3: Mediators of anaphylactic reaction

Mediator	Responses
1. Histamine	H$_1$ receptor mediated responses: Smooth muscle contraction, vascular permeability, pruritus and prostaglandin release H$_2$ receptor mediated responses: Gastric acid release, mucus secretion, vasodilation and inhibition of lymphokine release.
2. Prostaglandins and thromboxanes	Vasodilation (PGE), increased pain sensation (PGE), mucus secretion (PGD$_2$ PGF$_{2a}$, TxA, bronchospasm (PGD$_2$, PGF$_{2a}$, TxA) and bronchodilation (PGE, and PGI)
3. Acetylcholine	Mucus secretion and bronchospasm
4. Heparin	Anticoagulant and modulator of complement activation
5. Bradykinin	Bronchospasm, vasodilation and vascular leakage
6. Eosinophil chemotactic factor of anaphylaxis	Eosinophil chemotaxis
7. Leukotrienes (SRS-A)	Mucus secretion, bronchospasm and vascular leakage
8. Unspecified inflammatory factors	Neutrophil chemotaxis followed by mononuclear infiltration
9. Chymase	Chymotrypsin-like activity
10. Acetyl glycerophosphoryl choline (PAF)	Platelet aggregation, bronchospasm and vascular leakage.

- In such cases, TSH not alone determine the activity of thyroid gland but autoimmunity also interfere with its functioning.

▒ INTERLEUKINS

These are the lymphokinins released from lymphocytes during immune activation process. The important interleukins released during immune mechanism are given below.

a. Interleukin-1 (IL-1): It is a protease-sensitive molecule having a molecular weight of 12000 – 16000. It mainly acts by induction of interleukin-2 production.

b. Interleukin-2 (IL-2): Since it induces proliferation of T lymphocytes in response to stimulation by antigens, it is also called as T cell growth factor. It is a protein having a molecular weight of 14500. Interleukin-2 is also suspected to play a role in the regulation of growth of B lymphocytes.

c. Interleukin-3 (IL-3): It is a lymphokine that induces mast cell proliferation in vitro. It also offers resistance to T lymphocytes from the action of corticosteroids, by inducing 20 α- steroid dehydrogenase enzyme.

d. Lymphotoxins (LTS): It is a strong inducer of influx of Ca^{++} ions. Its lytic effects on the cell are produced within minutes by rapid shrinkage of the cells.

▒ IMMUNOMODULATORS

- The important components of immune system include:
  1. Granulocytes.
  2. Complement synthesis and antibody formation.
  3. Cellular immunity.
  4. Mucocutaneous barriers.

- The overall immunological pattern may be influenced either by the administration of certain drugs by infection with viruses or because of inherited disorders of immune system. Under such conditions, defects may be seen in the essential components of immune system resulting into immunomodulation.

CLASSIFICATION OF IMMUNOMODULATORS
Antihistaminic
Indomethacin
Interferons
Levamisole
Isoprinosine
Transfer factor
Thymic hormones
Lymphokines

- Since neutrophiles are synthesized from granulocytes, as the total granulocyte count falls below 1000 cells/mm^3, the rate of bacterial infection increases. The common organisms affecting granulocytopenic patients include *E. coli, Pseudomonas aeruginosa, Klebsiella pneumomae* and *Staphylococcus aureus.* The chances of fungal, viral or protozoal infections are also significantly high.

- An increase in the infection rate is also seen when the defect occurs in complement synthesis and antibody production. Such defects are usually encountered through the chronic treatment with chemotherapeutic agents.

- Cellular immunity provides protection against fungal, bacterial, viral and protozoal infections. Certain drugs (e.g. corticosteroids, cyclosporine, etc.), neoplastic diseases (e.g. Hodgkin's disease, lymphoma) and organ transplantation procedures paralyze cellular immunity.

- Mucocutaneous barriers present in our body prohibit pathogenic organisms to take entry into the internal vital organs. However, these barriers are damaged by a number of medical devices, procedures, endotracheal tubes or chemotherapy. This leads to easy access of pathogens to the internal organs resulting into infectious state. Important immunomodulators used clinically are summarized below.

Antihistaminic agents

Histamine-binding lymphocytes have immuino-suppressive activities. By inhibiting the activation of these lymphocytes, antihistaminic agents improve cell-mediated immune responses.

Indomethacin

- It is a non-narcotic analgesic agent that relieves pain sensation by inhibiting prostaglandin biosynthesis.

- The impairment of prostaglandin production results in the significant improvement in the functioning of T lymphocytes.

- It may be used to improve immune response in leishmaniasis, coccidioidomycosis and mycobacterial infections which cause deficient cell-mediated immunity.

Interferons

- These are the endogenous substances having immunopotentiating activity. They have potent antiviral and antitumor activities.

- Interferon specifically has a potent macrophage-stimulating activity. Beside this, bestatin and lentinan are other natural products having immunopotentiating activity.

Isoprinosine

Chemically, it is a complex of inosine and an organic salt. Though it was originally developed as an antiviral agent, latter it was found to possess a stimulant activity on a number of immunological and inflammatory processes. It enhances T cell proliferation, phagocytosis and chemotaxis through unknown mechanism

Levamisole

- It improves chemotactic responses and immune mechanisms in patients with diseases associated with immunodeficiency.
- It probably acts by inducing the release of c-GMP.

Lymphokines

Only two such lymphokinins known as IL-1 (i.e. T lymphocyte activating factor) and IL-2 (i.e. T lymphocyte growth factor) were found to stimulate the patient's cellular immunity.

Thymic hormones

- These are the polypeptides isolated from epithelial cells of thymus gland. They induce formation of mature T cells by unknown mechanisms.
- They may be used to improve immunity in patients with immunodeficiency. These preparations consist of thymic humoral factor, thymosin fractions, serum thymic factor, a nonapeptide secreted by thymic epithelium, a dialyzable fraction of calf thymus extract and a protein with molecular weight of 5260 daltons.
- They are usually given in saline IM, in doses between 0.5 mg/kg and 1.0 mg/kg per day for 2–3 weeks and then reduced to 1–3 doses per week.

▓ DRUGS AFFECTING IMMUNE RESPONSE

Many drugs upon chronic administration influence body's immune responses by affecting these vital elements of immune mechanisms. Depending upon the suppressant and stimulant effects exerted by these drugs on immune system, they are categorised as:

  i. Immunosuppressants,
  ii. Immunoenhancers.

Table 73.4: Drug affecting immune responses

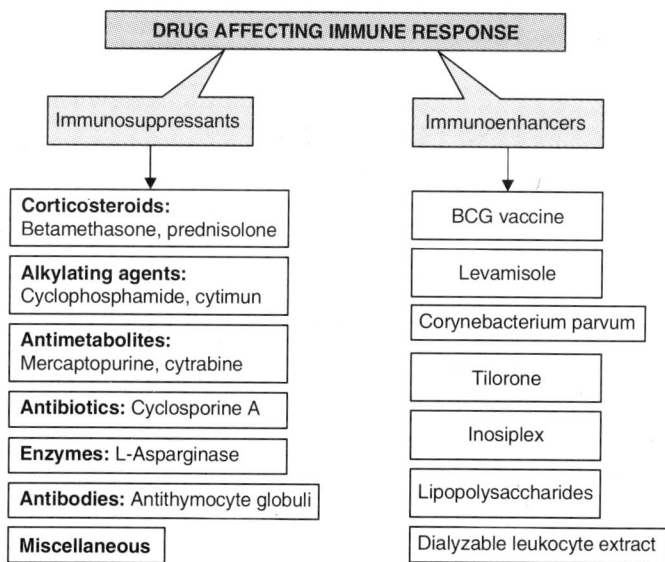

Immunosuppressors

Azathioprene   Cyclophosphamide   Methotrexate

Immunostimulant

Levamisole   Tilorone   Inosiplex

Phases of immune response	Suppressants	Enhancers
1. Antigen recognition and processing	Corticosteroids Cyclophosphamide Cytimun	BCG vaccine C. *parvum* Tetramisole
2. Amplification	L-asparaginase Corticosteroids Cyclophosphamide Cytimun 5-fluorouraci 16-mercaptopurine	Concanavalin A Tetramisole
3. Antibody formation	Corticosteroids Cyclophosphamide Cyclosporin A cytimun	Lipopolysaccharide Tetramisole
4. Immune effector responses	Corticosteroids Cyclophosphamide Cyclosporin A Cytarabine cytimun Methotrexate	C. *parvum* Tetramisole

▨ IMMUNOSUPPRESSANTS (FIG. 73.7)

- During organ transplantation, certain complex antigens or allografts activate the cytotoxic T lymphocytes.
- Their activation results into development of cellular (and in some cases, humoral immunity also) immunity that rejects organ transplants. Immunosuppressive agents exert beneficial effects in such conditions by suppressing the cellular immunity.
- They are also used to treat some autoimmune disorders like, myasthenia gravis, rheumatoid arthritis, systemic lupus erythematosus, cranial arteritis, membranous glomerulonephritis and ulcerative colitis.

- Most of these agents are primarily used as antineoplastic agents since these drugs also possess anti-inflammatory activity; they are useful in conditions where inflammation accompanies exaggerated immune response.
  1. Glucocorticoid inhibit MHC expression and IL-1,IL-2,IL-6 production so that helper T cell are not activated .
  2. Cytotoxic drugs block proliferation and differentiation of T and B cells.
  3. Cyclosporine and tacrolimus inhibit antigen stimulated activation and proliferation of helper T cells as well as expression of IL-2 and other cytokinines by them.
  4. Antibodies like muromonab CD3, antithymocyte globulin specifically bind to helper T cells, prevent their response and deplete them.

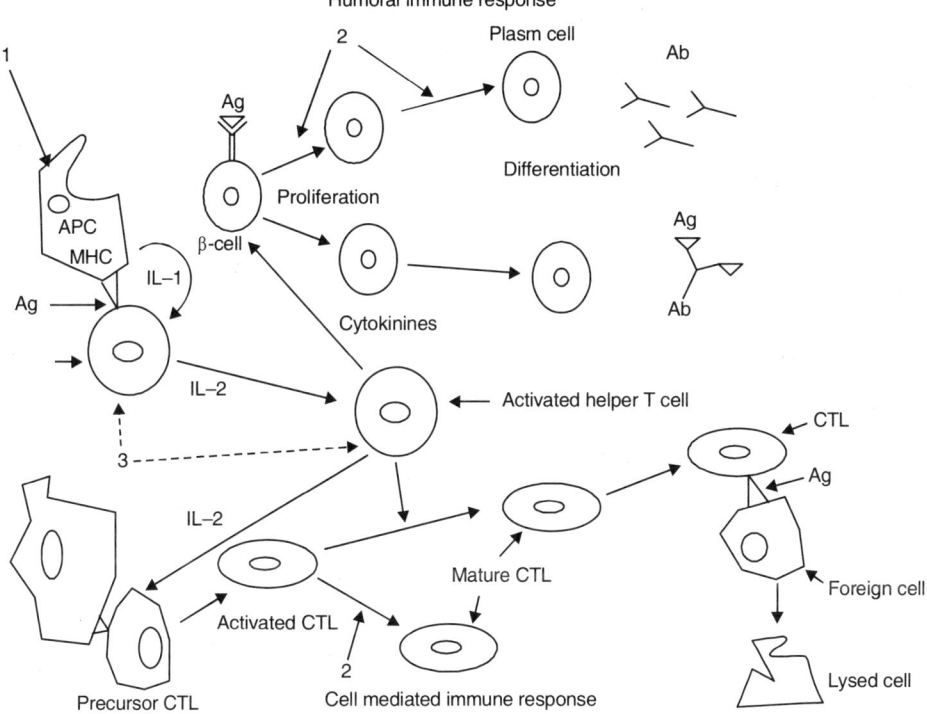

Fig. 73.7: Immune response and site of action of immunosuppressant drugs
APC– antigen presenting cell, CTL– cytotoxic lymphocytes, APC– antigen presenting cell
MHC– major histocompatbility complex, Ag– antigen, Ab– antibodies

Immune Responese

Humoral immune response

Whenever any antigen enters inside the body, it is processed by macrophages or other antigen presenting cells (APC), coupled with class II major histocompatibility complex (MHC) and presented to the CD4 helper cell which are activated by interleukin-1 (IL-1), proliferate and secrete cytokinines these in turn promote proliferation and differentiation of antigen activated β cells into antibody secreting plasma cells. Antibodies finally bind and inactivate the antigen.

Cellular response

In cell mediated immunity foreign antigen is processed and presented to CD4 helper T cell, which elaborate IL-2 and other cytokines that in turn stimulate proliferation and maturation of precursor cytotoxic lymphocytes (CTL) that have been activated by antigen presented with class I MHC. The mature CTL (killer cell) recognize cells carrying the antigen and lyse them.

Classification

a. Corticosteroids: Betamethasone, prednisolone.

b. Alkylating agents: Cyclophosphamide, cytimun.

c. Antimetabolites: Mercaptopurine, cytarabine.

d. Antibiotics: Cyclosporin A.

e. Enzymes: L-Asparaginase.

f. Antibodies: Antithymocyte globulin.

g. Miscellaneous agents.

Corticosteroids

MOA:

- Examples of immunosuppressive corticosteroids include betamethasone, dexamethasone, hydrocortisone, paramethasone, prednisolone, methyl-prednisolone, triamcinolone. They all possess antiallergic, anti-inflammatory and immunosuppressive activities.

- They affect almost all phases of immune response. T lymphocytes are more susceptible to the action of corticosteroids resulting into lymphopenia (i.e. reduction in blood lymphocytes).

- They also interfere with binding of antibodies to target cells and affect humoral immune responses by inhibiting antibody synthesis.

Adverse effect:

- Adverse effects usually result from the use of high doses and include osteoporosis, hyperglycemia, ulcer formation and increased susceptibility for fungal infections.

- By using combination therapy, one can lower down the dose of the drug and hence the frequency and intensity of these adverse effects.

Uses: Corticosteroids are used either alone or in combination with other cytotoxic agents in the treatment of autoimmune disorders and for the prevention of allograft rejection. They are usually given in the dose range of 2–10 mg/kg per day for few weeks or months.

Alkylating agents

- These are the examples of cytotoxic drugs that kill the components of immune responses of the body.

- Since bone marrow is tissue having a high rate of proliferation, their immuno-suppressive action results in toxic effects on rapidly proliferating cells.

- They exert cytotoxic effects to lymphocytes by alkylating their nucleic acids. Examples include cyclophosphamide and cytimun.

a. Cyclophosphamide

MOA:

- It is nitrogen mustard having broad-spectrum of antineoplastic and immunosupp-ressive activities. Though it affects all phases of immune response, it is more effective suppressant of humoral immune mechanisms

- It exerts cytotoxic action on both T cells and on B cells. However, its effects on B cells are more pronounced. Its many active metabolites (e.g., 4-hydroxycyclophos-phamide, acrolein and nornitrogen mustard) are responsible for its antineoplastic and immunosuppressant effects.

Uses: It is usually used in combination with corticosteroids in the treatment of several autoimmune diseases, including Wegener's granulomatosis, idiopathic thrombocyto-penia purpura, childhood nephrosis and severe rheumatoid arthritis. For this purposes, it is used orally in the dose of 2 mg/kg per day.

b. Cytimun

- It is an analogue of cyclophosphamide having better therapeutic index. It is specifically effective against B cells.

Antimetabolites

- These drugs act by exerting cytotoxic effects on rapidly proliferating cells like, those of bone marrow, myeloid tissues, gonadal tissues and gastrointestinal tract.
- Hence they can be used as immunosuppressant. Methotrexate, 6-mercaptopurine and azathioprine are the examples of phase-specific cytotoxic drugs which are more toxic to S-phase, when DNA synthesis is occurring.
- Their nonselectivity of action leads to appearance of serious side effects including bone marrow suppression, more susceptibility to infection and sterility. Azathioprine and mercaptopurine are the most extensively studied immuno-suppressive agents.

a. Azathioprine

MOA:

- It is an imidazolyl derivative of 6-mercaptopurine. It has an anti-rheumatic activity along with cytotoxic effect. It is orally effective drug having plasma half-life of about 16 hours. It is metabolised to 6-mercaptopurine.
- Xanthine oxidase enzyme converts much of this active drug in liver and erythrocytes to 6-thiouric acid, thioinosinic acid and various other metabolites.
- Thioinosinic acid competitively inhibits the synthesis of inosinic acid, the precursor of adenylic acid and guanylic acid. This results into inhibition of DNA synthesis.
- Thus upon metabolic activation, azathioprine suppresses both cell-mediated and humoral immune responses and depresses antibody proliferative responses. It also possesses powerful anti-inflammatory activity.

Uses:

- Azathioprine is thus most effective suppressant of phase II of immune responses. It is used orally in the treatment of acute glomerulonephritis, systemic lupus erythematosus.
- Wegener's granulomatosis, temporal-cranial arteritis and polymyalgia rheumatica. It is also used in the management of organ transplantation and delayed hyper-sensitivity reactions. Adult oral dose is 1–3 mg/kg per day.

b. Methotrexate

MOA:

- It is an orally active folic acid analog having antineoplastic, antipsoriatic and mild immunosuppressant activity. It has a plasma half-life of 7.2–9.0 hours. It acts by inhibiting folate metabolism and affects phase II of immune responses.
- It, however, does not block the expression of established delayed hypersensitivity reactions but may alter the intensity of these reactions.

Uses: It is used to treat severe psoriasis, dermatomyositis and rheumatoid arthritis. It is also used in organ transplantation procedures.

Antibiotics

Example from this category includes cyclosporine A. It is a cyclic undecapeptide having immunosuppressive activity and is isolated from tin soil fungus, *Tolypocladium inflatum*. It is an orally effective antibiotic having plasma half-life of 10–12 hours. It possesses more marked immunosuppressant effects than its antibiotic potential.

MOA:

- It specifically inhibits generation of effector T lymphocytes without affecting expression of suppressor lymphocytes and impairing B cell activity.
- It impairs proliferative response of T cells to antigens. Once T cells are stimulated by antigens, they synthesize interleukin-2 that exerts growth promoting effects on T lymphocytes.
- Hence to be effective, cyclosporine must be administered before proliferations of T cells occur.

Adverse effect: Cyclosporine possesses specificity and low toxicity profile. Commonly associated adverse effects include gum hypertrophy, tremor, hirsutism, neurasthesia, depressive psychosis, nephrotoxicity and benign breast tumors.

Uses:

- It is used along with glucocorticoids for prophylaxis and treatment of organ rejection specifically in patients with kidney, liver, pancreas, bone marrow and heart transplants.
- It also exerts beneficial effects when used in the treatment of autoimmune diseases like rheumatic arthritis, psoriatic arthropathies, etc. Adult oral dose is 10–15 mg/kg per day. Intravenously 50 mg diluted with normal saline may be given by slow infusion.

Enzymes

- L-Asparaginase is a drug of choice in the treatment of acute lymphoblastic leukemia. It has a plasma half-life of about 11–23 hours.
- The enzyme is usually given either intravenously or intramuscularly. When combined together with methotrexate, it lowers down the adverse effects and intensifies therapeutic effects of the methotrexate.

Antibodies

MOA:

- These are produced in significant concentration into an appropriate recipient, usually a horse by repeated injection of human cells. This results into formation of specific antibodies against lymphocytes or thymocytes.
- These antibodies are then used in the form of antiserum to produce immunosuppressant. These monoclonal antibodies have great potential to be used against lymphocytes. Example of this category includes antithymocyte globulin (ATG).

Uses: ATG is used alone or in combination with azathioprine and corticosteroids in the prevention of renal allograft rejection in the dose of 1–5 mg per day. However, in some patients, allergic reactions have been reported to occur leading to serum sickness and nephritis.

Miscellaneous agents

a. Adenosine deaminase inhibitors:

- The immunosuppressive examples from this category include, erytliro-9-(2-hydroxy-3-nonyl) adenine hydrochloride and 2'-deoxy-coformycin (pentostatin).

- The former agent selectively exerts toxic effects against T lymphocytes while pentostatin has synergistic effect with vidarabine and is used as antimetabolite in treatment of certain neoplastic diseases.
- Pentostatin causes pronounced lymphoidal depletion, especially in spleen. It has a plasma half-life of 25 – 30 hours.

b. Bredinin: It is an imidazole nucleoside having antimetabolite antineoplastic activity. It is used as an immunosuppressant in human kidney transplantation.

c. Cycloimmun: It is an analog of cyclosporine, undergoing clinical trials for its immunosuppressant activity. It has shown promising activity to suppress tissue rejecting ability of patients in organ transplantation procedures.

Niridazole: It is an orally active nitrothiazole derivative having anthelmintic, antibacterial (against a variety of anaerobic bacteria) and immunosuppressive activities. It is used to suppress cell-mediated immunity responses.

IMMUNOENHANCERS

- This category of drugs is used to overcome immunodeficiency or immunosuppression arising as a result of either inherited or acquired disorders of immune system. A gamma globulinemia and severe combined immune deficiency syndrome (SCIDs) are the examples of inherited disorders of immune system.
- While chemotherapy, therapy with immunosuppressive agents, radiation or viral infection (e.g. AIDS) may cause immunosuppression. Besides this certain autoimmune disorders and some types of fungal infections may require therapy with immunoenhancers.
- This category of drugs may either cause a generalized, nonspecific stimulation of immune mechanisms or may enhance only specific phases of immune responses. Examples of this category are given below.

Bacillus Calmette Guerin (BCG) Vaccine

MOA

- It is used as an immunological enhancer to stimulate intact immune system (i.e. a nonspecific immunoenhancer) of the body. BCG and its methanol extracted residue (MER) contain muramyl dipeptide as an active immune stimulant ingredient.
- T lymphocytes are the principal target cells for the action of BCG vaccine. It causes stimulation of macrophage functions, phagocytic activity, lysosomal enzyme activity and chemotaxis mechanisms. It induces the production of lymphocyte-activating factor resulting into stimulation of phase I of the immune responses.

Uses

- Because of its reactivity against tumor cell antigen, its use is beneficial in the treatment of malignant melanoma, acute lymphocytic leukemia, lung cancer, breast cancer, acute and chronic myelogenous leukemia, lymphomas and colorectal cancer.
- It is available either as live unlyophilized, live lyophilized or in killed lyophilized form. It may be administered by oral, intradermal, intrapleural, intralesional or intravenous route. Adult dose depends upon the route of administration chosen.

Tetramisole (Levamisole)

MOA

- Levamisole is orally active S (-) isomer of tetramisole. Besides anthelmintic agent, it may be used as immunostimulant in the therapy of certain infections, rheumatoid arthritis and in immunosuppressive conditions.

- It has a plasma half-life of 4.0 hours. Upon hepatic metabolism, it is converted to DL-2-oxo-3-(2-mercaptoethyl)-5-phenylimidazolidine, an active metabolite and several other inactive metabolites.
- It mainly acts by raising the c-GMP levels through interacting with thymopoietin receptor sites. This leads to decrease in metabolic inactivation of c-GMP accompanied with increased breakdown of c-AMP. This increase in c-GMP level induces lymphocyte proliferation and augmentation of chemotactic responses. This reflects into increased antibody production, lymphokine production, proliferative responses of lymphocytes and increased phagocytosis by macrophages. Tetramisole is also a potent inhibitor of mammalian alkaline phosphatase and diamine oxidase enzymes.

Uses

- Certain chronic and recurrent bacterial and viral infections including acute hepatitis, herpes labialis, herpes genitalis, recurrent furunculosis, influenza, upper respiratory tract infections, acne conglobata and chronic pyogenic skin infections.
- Certain diseases with immunodeficiency like, Wiskott-Aldrich syndrome, chronic granulomatous disease, lazy leukocyte syndrome, ataxia telangectasis, Job's syndrome (i.e. hyperimmunoglobin E syndrome) and cyclic neutropenia.
- Autoimmune diseases like, rheumatoid arthritis, Crohn's disease, aphthous stomatitis and systemic lupus erythematosus.

Cocynebacterium Parvum

MOA

It has pronounced stimulatory effect on phase I of immune responses. The humoral immune response is intensified by an increase in the antibody production against both, the T cell dependent and independent antigens. This reflects into increased macrophage proliferation, accumulation of lysosomal enzymes, activation of phospholipase A and accelerated phagocytosis.

Adverse effect

Adverse effects include chills, fever and changes in blood pressure. It is used as adjuvant in cancer chemotherapy.

Uses

It may also be used to depress allograft rejection. It may be administered intravenously or intraperitoneally.

Tilorone

- It is a synthetic immunoenhancer that stimulate T lymphocytes originating in the thymus. It also possesses antiviral activity because of its stability to induce interferon production. Adverse effects are few and include nausea, vomiting, epigastric discomfort dizziness and headache.

Inosiplex

MOA

- Chemically, it is the p-acetamidobenzoic acid salt of inosine dimethylamino-isopropanol. It is orally active synthetic drug that activates the cellular immunity through stimulation of interleukin-1 (i.e., T lymphocyte growth factor).

- This results into an increase in macrophage activity and population of T-lymphocytes. It also has an ability to inhibit replication of both RNA and DNA viruses.

- Since upon its metabolism, uric acid is formed, it induces gouty arthritis upon chronic administration.

Uses

- It is used as immunoenhancer to treat cancer-induced immunosuppression in the dose of 50 mg/kg per day in divided doses.

- Because of its antiviral property, it may also be used in the treatment of infections due to herpes virus, rhinovirus, influenza virus and chronic measles virus.

Lipopolysaccharides (IPSS)

MOA

The lipopolysaccharides possess antitumor and immunostimulant effects. They mainly activate phase III of immune response.

Dialyzable Leukocyte Extract (Transfer Factor)

MOA

- It is obtained from peripheral leukocytes of individuals who have been sensitized or are immune to certain pathogens. The extract contains ascorbic acid. Chemo-attractants for monocytes and neutrophil immobilizers, thymic factors, nicotinamide, serotonin, histamine and prostaglandins along with several moieties composed of proteins and RNA.

- The extract contains polyribonucleotide which is known as transfer factors. These factors potentiate antigen-specific cellular immunity responses. However, minimum required number of T lymphocytes must be present in patient receiving the treatment with transfer factor.

Adverse effect

Adverse effects are few and include transient fever, occasional pain or erythema at the site of injection.

Uses

- Transfer factor is used in the treatment of sarcoidosis. Hodgkin's disease, mycobactenal infections, fungal infections, viral infections and autoimmune diseases.

- The solution of transfer factor is prepared in salin. Each one ml of this solution is equivalent to the extract obtained from $1 \times 10^8 – 1 \times 10^9$ leukocytes. Adult dose is 1 ml either s.c. weekly or monthly.

▨ DISORDER OF IMMUNE SYSTEM

Immunodeficiency

- Because of certain inherited or acquired diseases, the natural immune response gets paralyzed. Besides this, a variety of factors such as malnutrition, metabolic disorders, malignancy and cytotoxic drugs may lead to immunodeficiency.

- Defects may be seen in particular phase of immune mechanism or immune system as a whole gets impaired. There may be a failure of humoral (antibody) immune response or a failure of cellular immunity or a combination of both.

Myeloma (Excessive Production of Immunoglobulins)

- This condition arises because of an increase in immunoglobulin (antibody) production. This occurs; specifically in patients in whom malignant change in the clone of plasma cells is reported.
- As the number of immunoglobulins increases, their metabolic turnover also gets increased. This results into appearance of light chains (Bence -Jones protein) into the urine of the patient.

Autoimmune Diseases

- In normal person, complex network of feedback loops exist to make a smooth coordinations between different components of immune responses.
- Control is lost and the aberrant immune reaction will result in a disease. Antibodies are secreted against a component of an individual's own immunoglobulins.
- These circulating immune complexes (e.g. DNA, anti-DNA antibodies) fix with complements and lodge in certain tissues (e.g. skin, neuromuscular junction, joints of affected individuals and kidney). Autoimmune diseases of thyroid gland, stomach (pernicious anemia) and adrenal gland are also reported.

Table 73.5: Classification of primary immunodeficiency syndrome

Disorders of specific immunity	Disorders of complement
Humoral immunodeficiencies (B cell defects):	**Disorders of phagocytosis**
a. X-linked agammaglobulinemia	a. Chronic granulomatous disease
b. Selective immunoglobulin deficiencies (IgA,IgM or IgG)	b. Myeloperoxidase deficiency
c. Immunodeficiencies with hyper-IgM	c. Leukocyte G 6 PD deficiency
d. Transcobalamin II deficiency	d. Job's syndrome
Cellular immunodeficiencies (T cell defects):	e. Lazy leukocyte syndrome
a. Thymic hypoplasia (Di George's syndrome)	f. Hyper-IgE syndrome
b. Chronic mucocutaneous candidiasis	g. Actin-binding protein deficiency
c. Purine nucleoside phosphorylase (PNP) deficiency	
Combined immunodeficiencies (B and T cell defects):	
a. Cellular immunodeficiencies with abnormal Ig synthesis	
b. Wiskott-Aldrich syndrome	
c. Immunodeficiency with thymoma	
d. Severe combined immunodeficiency, e.g. adenosine deaminase (ADA) deficiency	

Myasthenia gravis

- In which antibodies are produced against cholinergic nicotinic receptors present in neuromuscular junction.
- The breakdown of this junctional cholinergic receptor makes the patient weak and unable to move voluntary muscles.

Rheumatoid arthritis

- In this disease, antibodies are secreted against a component of body's own immunoglobulins. These antibody-immunoglobulin complexes get deposited in the joints of affected persons.

- The local tissue necrosis and inflammation of joints are caused by lysosomal enzymes released during phagocytosis process.

Systemic lupus erythematosus (SLE)

- In this disease, many organs are affected because of the production of autoantibodies. It is a chronic multiorgan inflammatory disorder that affects skin, lungs, joints, kidneys, heart and brain. The characteristic symptoms include fatigue, fever, weight loss, skin lesions, dyspnea, joint pain and swelling, renal damage (i.e. nephritis, proteinurea, hematuria, hypertension), abdominal pain and neurological manifestations.

- The immune complexes after fixing with complement get deposited into various organs and produce tissue damage by inflammatory reactions. Patients show B lymphocyte hyperactivity and impairment in T cell immunoregulation.

- Aspirin like drugs (e.g. aspirin, sulindac, ibuprofen or naproxen) may be used orally in the dose of 3.5 g per day to treat systemic lupus erythematosus.

Pernicious anemia

- The disease involves appearance of two types of auto-antibodies. One type of antibody causes achlorhydria and atrophic gastritis by affecting the functioning of gastric parietal cells.

- While second type of antibodies bind with gastric intrinsic factor and inhibit its uptake by intestinal mucosa. This results into inhibition of absorption of vitamin B_{12}.

Mechanisms Involved in Autoimmune Diseases

- The breakdown of feedback inhibitory loops of immune system leads to emergence of forbidden clones of antibodies. These antibodies then evoke immune responses against self-antigens.

- Under physical, chemical or biological influences, antigenic alterations are reported to occur. Such altered antigen may then evoke immune responses by inducing the release of antibodies.

- In some pathogenic conditions, defects are incorporated in a variety of T lymphocytes. (e.g. enhanced helper T cells and decreased concentration of suppressor T cells) and B lymphocytes. These defects may then lead to autoimmune responses. Besides this, defects in stem cell development, thymus and macrophage functioning may also contribute for the occurrence of autoimmune diseases.

▓ ACQUIRED IMMUNE DEFICIENCY SYNDROME (AIDS)

Introduction

- AIDS is the end stage disease representing the irreversible breakdown of immune defence mechanisms.

- The immune competence of the patient is completely lost. As a result, chemotaxis, antigen identification and the functioning of monocytes and macrophages are gradually diminished.

- The patient is susceptible to the attack of infections with relatively virulent microorganisms as well as to lymphoid and other malignancies.

- The commonly seen infections in AIDS patients include oral candidiasis, herpes zoster, hairy cell leukoplakia, salmonellosis, *P. carinii* pneumonia, toxoplasmosis or tuberculosis. Lymphoid and other malignancies may also be present.

History

- The first case of AIDS patient was identified in 1981 in New York. Thereafter efforts were directed to isolate the infecting agent of AIDS. The first report about isolation of infecting agent appeared in 1983 from the Pasteur Institute, Paris.

- It was isolated from West African patient. It was found to be a retrovirus. It was named as lymphadenopathy associated virus (LAV). This was followed by many reports describing the isolation of etiological agents in AIDS.

- All these agents were described under the term, AIDS-related viruses (ARV). In 1986, the International Committee on Virus Nomenclature had coined the term human immunodeficiency virus (HIV) for these infective agents, in order to avoid confusion.

Structure (Fig. 73.8)

- The virus, HIV belongs to the Lentivirus subgroup of the family Retroviridae. It is an example of a thermolabile enveloped virus having a diameter of 90–120 mm.

- It survives for about 7 days at room temperature. It withstands lyophilization. Structurally, it is a nucleoprotein core that contains single-stranded RNA genome along with proteins.

- Minor antigenic differences in both core and envelope antigens are reported between isolates from different patients as well as from the same patient.

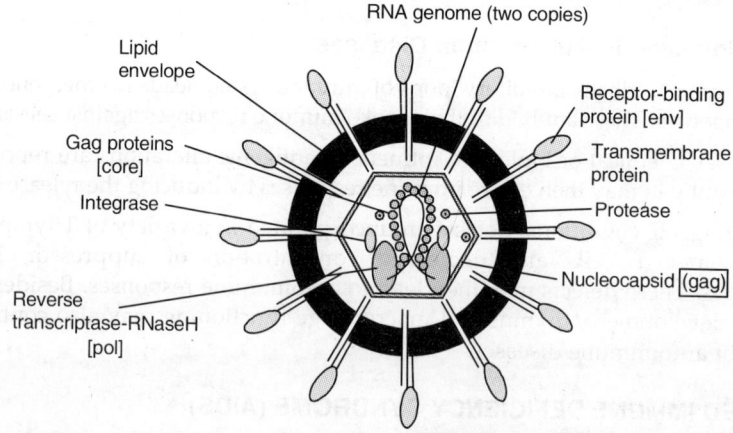

Fig. 73.8: Structure of HIV

- The HIV can remain silent over a long period of time. Under favourable conditions, viral replication occurs by increased rate of synthesis of viral RNA and other components.

- Since HIV affects the functioning of immune system, the symptoms associated are mainly due to the failure of immune responses rather than due to viral cytotoxicity. The T_4 lymphocytes serve as suitable host cell for HIV viruses.

- The major damage occurs to T_4 lymphocytes. T cells decrease in the number. This results into a lack of secretion of activating factors from T lyrnphocytes. This is a contributing factor for the failure of immune system.

Way of Transmission

- In an infected person, HIV can be detected in the saliva, tears, urine, cervical secretions, semen, breast milk, blood, lymphocytes and cell-free plasma. It can be transmitted by following possible routes:
  1. Through sexual contacts in both homosexuals and heterosexuals,
  2. Through the transfer of blood, blood products or other body fluids,
  3. Through the donation of tissue or organ
  4. Through certain infections and/or injuries
  5. From infected mother to baby. About half of the number of babies born to infected mothers is infected with HIV.
- However, HIV are not transmitted through air, water or insect bite. Within a few weeks of infections with HIV, the patient experiences mild symptoms like fever, malaise, headache, rash, arthropathy, lymphadenopathy, etc.
- Due to the paralyzed immune system, patient may get attacked by many infections and malignancies like lymphomas, Kaposi's sarcoma, Hodgkin's and non-Hodgkin's types. AIDS is the last stage in the wide-spectrum of clinical features of HIV infection.
- Depending upon the type of infection and the organ most affected, different patients may complain about different symptoms.

Symptoms

Gastrointestinal tract

- It is most susceptible for the attack of organisms like mycobacteria, salmonellae, cryptosporidium, adenoviruses and isospora.
- Prominent symptoms include mouth thrush, dysphagia, abdominal pain, diarrhea, gingivitis, herpetic stomatitis, and hairy leukoplakia. Chronic colitis is seen mainly in male homosexuals.

Cutaneous signs: These include candidiasis, impetigo, herpes lesions, prurigo, xeroderma, folliculitis, seborrheic dermatitis and mulluscum contagiosum.

Respiratory system: This system becomes vulnerable for the attack of *P. carinii*, *M. tuberculosis* and *M. avium intracellulare*. Major symptoms include fever, dyspnea, dry cough and pneumonia.

Central nervous system

Dementia and impairment of CNS functions are reported to occur because of the ability of HIV to enter into CNS. Besides this toxoplasmosis, cryptococcosis and lymphomas of CNS are also reported to occur.

Treatment

The first phase

- It deals with control of infections and malignancies associated with the patient. The treatment is infection specific. For example, in AIDS patients with *Pneumocystis carinii* infection, cotrimoxazole is given orally. Pentamidine may also be used either IM or IV in the dose of 4 mg/kg body weight per day.
- *Toxoplasma gondii* is a protozoal organism that affects mainly heart, lung, liver, spleen and CNS. Drugs of choice include pyrimethamine (25 mg/day) and sulfadiazine (2 g per day) orally. Folinic acid may be used in the dose of 10 mg per day to prevent hematologic abnormalities.

- Besides this, *Mycobacterium avium-intracellulare* is found in 50% patients with AIDS. It affects mainly GIT, lung and other tissues. To correct most of these infections, interleukin-2 is commonly used agent. It is a potent lymphokine responsible for the activation of various components of immune system.

The second phase

- The second phase of the treatment consists of employing general measures to cool down imaginary anxiety and fear experienced by the patients.
- The infected person must be reassured that he can resume a normal life if proper precautions and treatment are taken. The high-risk factors must be identified and eliminated. This is to be supported by health education.

The third phase

- The third phase of the treatment deals with measures to improve the functioning of immune system.
- A large number of antiviral agents (e.g. α-interferon, ribavirin, suramin, etc.). This can be supplemented by administration of immunoenhancer interleukin-2, thymic factor, leukocyte transfusion or by the transplantation of bone marrow.

The fourth phase

- The last phase of the treatment consists of administration of anti-HIV agent. Zidovudine (azidothymidine) is the only drug available. It is an orally effective antiviral agent beneficial in the treatment of AIDS and AIDS related syndromes. Adverse effects include headache, leukopenia and macrocytic anemia.
- Efforts are being continued to develop a vaccine effective in the treatment of AIDS. However, prospects for such a vaccine in the near future are unfortunately dim.

Adverse Effect

Human body is a complex multicompartmental living system. Naturally any drug that has been given; for a specific purpose, does not exert selectively that action alone. To more or less extent, the desired action is always associated with undesired effects or side effects. Since these effects are not necessary for that therapeutic indication, their occurrence may place limitations on the use of the drug. The study of such undesired effects which occur with the therapeutic dose (and not with overdose) of the drug is included in this chapter.

ADVERSE EFFECTS

- The unintended effects of the substances employed in the diagnosis or treatment of diseases are known as adverse effects. The prominent adverse effects of some clinically used categories of drugs are given in Table 74.1.

- Adverse reactions have been reported ever since the drugs have been used. However, public awareness in this regard was first aroused with the sulphanilamide diethylene glycol complications in United States in 1937. The use of any therapeutic agent is inevitably attended by a small risk that the patient may react adversely to the prescribed agent. No drug is free from the adverse effects. The right dose differentiates a poison from a remedy. Hence if the beneficial effects dominate the side effects, then that drug is of clinical utility. In some drugs, the beneficial effects are so obvious (i.e. benefit to risk ratio is high) that the drug must be made available despite the fact that adverse reactions are predictable.

- In some cases, side effects of the drug may function in mutual beneficial manner with the therapeutic main effect and thus assist the later to achieve its objectives. Due to the beneficial nature of side effects in certain instance, side effects cannot always be called adverse effects. Sometimes, the adverse effects of a drug may be wrongly interpreted as the symptoms of the diseases. Adverse effects can also be called as iatrogenic (physician-caused) reactions. There is a wide-spread availability of potent drugs in the market; iatrogenic reaction may be considered as an offspring of unskilled use of the drug and its high potency. However, presently there is an increased inclination to find out opportunities for the conversion of side-effects of the drugs into therapeutic innovations. For example, the hair growth promoting activity of minoxidil (an antihypertensive agent) was exploited clinically to correct baldness. Similarly Iatrogenic galactorrhea may be used to induce milk production in adopting mothers for a better mother–child relationship.

- Until 1961, the importance of adverse effects was not acknowledged during the process of drug development. In 1960-61 in West Germany, many cases of phocomelia (i.e. seal extremities) were reported. It is a congenital deformity of long bones of limbs in the newborn fetus. On 26 November 1961, an article appeared in the newspaper Welt am Sonntag, blaming the drug Contergan (thalidomide, a recently introduced hypnotic) responsible for this teratogenecity. This shocking experience of thalidomide diaster aroused public awareness and forced the government to impose certain restrictions over the process of drug introduction. As a result, thalidomide was withdrawn from W. Germany in November 1961, followed by the same type of announcement from British market in December, 1961.

Table 74.1: Prominent adverse effects of some clinically used categories of drugs

Category of drug	Prominent adverse effects
1. Antidibetic agents	Nausea, vomiting anorexia, diarrhea, stomach pain, headache, chills, cold sweat, dizziness, weakness, anxiety, confusion, heartburn and difficulty in breathing.
2. Antihistaminic agents	Dry mouth, anorexia, stomach upset, urinary retention, constipation, blurred vision, skin rash, weakness, drowsiness, confusion, and difficulty in breathing.
3. Anticholinergic agents	Nausea, vomiting, constipation, mydriasis, urinay retention, headache, dry mouth, slurred speech, decreased sweating, blurred vision, dizziness, weakness and confusion.
4. Antipsychotic agents	Skin rash, dry mouth, constipation, difficulty in urination, decreased sweating, nasal congestion, blurred vision, dizziness, hypotension and extrapyramidal symptoms.
5. Beta blockers	Skin rash, diarrhea, sweating, chest pain, headache, anxiety, weakness, dizziness, depression, seizures, slow heartbeat, hypotension and decreased sexual activity.
6. Bronchodilators	Nausea, vomiting, dry mouth, chest pain, headache, anxiety, weakness, dizziness, nervousness, trembling, fast heartbeats and hypertension.
7. CNS depressants	Nausea, vomiting, slurred speech, staggering, dizziness, weakness, drowsiness, confusion, depression and hangover.
8. CNS stimulators	Nausea, vomiting, headache, blurred vision, skin rash, dizziness, anxiety and increased blood pressure, insomnia, nervousness, restlessness, irritability and rapid heartbeats.
9. Diuretics	Nausea, vomiting, stomach cramps, diarrhea, headache, dizziness, weakness, itching, clumsiness, lack of energy and decreased sexual ability.
10. Local anesthetics	Nausea, vomiting, headache, blurred vision, skin rash, dizziness, anxiety and increased blood pressure.
11. Neuromuscular blockers	Increased sweating increased intraocular pressure, muscle pain, decreased blood pressure and tachycardia.
12. Nonsteroidal anti-inflammatory agents	Constipation, anorexia, ulcerative stomatitis, soreness of mouth, ringing in ears, skin rash, itching, headache, dizziness and drowsiness.
13. Opioid analgesics	Vomiting, stomach cramps, anorexia, diarrhoea, sneezing, dizziness, drowsiness, weakness and seizures.
14. Oral contraceptive agents	Vomiting, diarrhea, slurred speech, headache, pain in chest, vision changes, painful urination, skin rash, alopecia, irritability, fainting and mental depression.
15. Progestins	Nausea, vomiting, slurred speech, headache, changes in vision, weakness, depression, acne, alopecia, increased breast tenderness and changes in vaginal bleeding pattern.
16. Anabolic agents	Nausea, vomiting, bone pain, weight gain, acne, deepening of voice, virilism, enlarged clitoris, increased frequency of erection and irregular menstrual bleeding.
17. Sympathomimetic agents	Insomnia, sweating, agitation, tremors and tachycardia.
18. Psychotomimetic agents	Dilated pupils, reactivity to light, disruption of thought and uncontrolled behavioral disturbances.

- Iatrogenic reactions of a drug may be manifested either due to an extension of its pharmacological response or may remain totally unrelated to its pharmacological properties. The former categories of iatrogenic reactions hence, are easily predictable because of their pharmacodynamically related nature. Predictable toxicity is mostly of reversible nature, and causes a temporary inconvenience. The later category of adverse effects is totally detached from the drug's pharmacological profile. This is of unpredictable nature and may lead to permanent disability or discomfort in the patient. The unexpected toxicity is more likely to occur when several drugs are given in the combination. It may also occur in patients having either genetic defects or having liver or renal dysfunction. Under such circumstances, the accumulation of drug or its metabolites may rapidly built up to the toxic levels in the body, even if the drug is administered at therapeutic concentration. Similarly, very young and very old patients may lack in having efficient drug metabolizing machinery. This may lead to intolerance of such patients to the usual therapeutic doses of the drug.

- Unexpected adverse reactions are completely unrelated to the known toxicity of the drug. A chemically active, structurally different drug metabolite may be responsible, rather than the parent drug, for such iatrogenic effects. For example, paracetamol is converted into toxic hydroxylamine metabolite or isoniazid may be converted into acetyl hydrazine metabolite, as shown below:

Paracetamol → N-hydroxylamine derivatives

Isoniazid → N-Acetylisoniazid → Acetylhydrazine

- These highly reactive metabolites induce biochemical damage to vital cellular ingredients like; proteins, genetic material or phospholipids present in the cellular membranes. The toxicity may become more pronounced in patients with genetic defect either in the metabolic (i.e. liver) or excretory (i.e. kidney) machinery. Then resulting accumulation of reactive metabolites in the body may induce hypersensitivity in some individual even after a small dose of the drug. In some cases, the drug metabolite itself may not be harmful for the endogenous vital cellular components. However, it may form a sort of immunogenic conjugate with the endogenous macromolecule (e.g. protein) resulting into formation of an antigen. This antigen then evokes allergic responses by interacting with the antibodies and thus sensitizes the patient for that particular drug. Skin rashes and eruptions are the most common symptoms of this type of sensitization.

- Beside this, in normal adult, the only causative factor in inducing iatrogenic reactions may be the overdose of the drug. The drug may cross the therapeutic concentration level and may be present in blood at higher concentration enough to evoke adverse reactions Table 74.2.

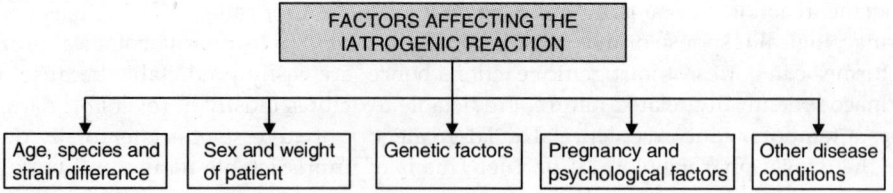

FACTORS AFFECTING THE IATROGENIC REACTION

Prominent factors that exert influence over the biological responses of the drug in general, include;

1. Age, species and strain differences.
2. Sex and weight of the patient.
3. Genetic factors.
4. Pregnancy and psychological abnormalities.
5. Other diseased conditions.

Age and Racial Differences

- Age of the patient exerts an influence over the pattern of drug metabolism and its excretion from the body.
- Usually infants, children and elderly patients have less efficient machinery for drug metabolism. In old patients, diminished renal function is reported even that patient is free from any diseased condition.

Table 74.2: Toxic blood concentrations of some clinically used drugs

Drug	mg/L	Drug	mg/L
Aminophylline	20	Ibuprofen	100–150
Amitriptyline	0.5–3.4	Imipramine	0.5–1.5
Amoxapine	0.2–0.5	Isoniazid	20
Amphetamine	0.1–0.3	Lidocaine	7–10
Bromoamphetamine	0.05–0.1	Lithium	13–15
Caffeine	40–65	Lorazepam	0.2–0.4
Carbamazepine	20–60	Maprotiline	0.5–0.8
Carbromal	25–80	Meperidine	4–6
Carisoprodol	25–30	Paracetamol	30–150
Chlordiazepoxide	5–60	Phenobarbital	40–60
Chlorpromazine	0.3–0.5	Phenytoin	20–50
Chloroquine	0.4–0.8	Meprobamate	60–100
Desipramine	0.5–0.8	Methaqualone	2–10
Diazepam	5–8	Morphine	-5.2–0.3
Diphenhydramine	1–3	Nortriptyline	0.2–0.3
Ethosuximide	150–200	Oxazepam	2.0–2.5
Fenfluramine	0.3–0.8	Pentazocine	0.4–0.6
Fentanyl	0.02–0.05	Propranolol	2.0–2.5
Flurazepam	0.2–0.4	Quinidine	10–25
Glutethimide	10–75	Trifluoperazine	1–3
Haloperidol	0.01	Valproic acid	200

- There may be decreased glomerular filtration and/or tubula, function which leads to accumulation of drug or its active metabolite.
- The toxicity of that drug may further be aggreviate in the presence of diabetic nephropathy or congestive heart failure (Table 74.2).
- The treatment of grand mal epilepsy in adults mainly includes a combination of both, barbiturate and phenytoin. The combination, however, may aggreviate the situation, if used in children:
- Hence in such cases, phenytoin may be used alone to control the seizures. The susceptibility to adverse reactions varies in persons secondary to the racial difference.

Sex

- Some drugs produce side effects whose intensity and duration of action is sex-dependent. For example, phenylbutazone induces agranulocytosis more frequently in females than in males.
- Similarly, females are more susceptible to pancytopenia induced by chloramphenicol. Sex hormones are well known for their sex-dependent effects.

Genetic Factors

- Some people are sensitive to even a low dose of a drug. While others remain unaffected by adverse effects, even quite large dose of same drugs is ingested.
- This may be attributed to the inborn genetic defect in the patient which results into either enzyme deficiencies or abnormal enzyme systems. For example, acetylation is an important conjugation reaction for the drugs containing free amino functional group. People may be categorised broadly as either slow acetylators or fast acetylators depending upon the rate of *in vivo* acetylation reaction. Patients from formal category, if kept on long-term treatment with isoniazid, are more susceptible to peripheral neuritis than patients known as fast acetylators.
- The enzyme, glucose-6-phosphate dehydrogenase [G-6-PD] is involved in the production of NADPH. The later plays a role of cofactor for glutathione reductase which is necessary for formation of reduced glutathione.
- Glutathione protects the vital cellular constituents from the attack of toxic (i.e. free radicals, endoperoxide, etc.) metabolic intermediates. Some patients are genetically deficient in G-6-PD. Since the deficiency of G-6-PD ultimately leads to the deficiency of reduced glutathione; the vital cellular constituents are less effectively protected. Such patients, specifically when kept under antimalarial therapy, are likely to develop hemolytic anemia.
- Porphyrins are red coloured pigments involved in the synthesis of heme (i.e. hemoglobin, myoglobin and the cytochrome). Due to the genetic defect, the liver porphyrin metabolism may be altered resulting into increased porphyrin excretion from the body.
- The symptoms of acute porphyria appear in patients who are carriers of such genetic defect. Beside this, the excretion of porphyrins is also found to be enhanced in patients with hemolytic anemia or impaired liver function.

Pregnancy and Psychological Factors

- After the thalidomide disaster tragedy, government agencies and medical profession became alert about the safety of drug when given to a pregnant woman. The extent of structural malformations in the fetus depends upon the stage of fetal development during which the drug is administered. For example, the liver of newborn does not contain sufficient glucuronyl transferase enzymes needed to conjugate chloramphenicol.

- The use of this drug before labour, thus may lead to toxicity in neonates due to inadequate renal excretion of the drug. The shocking experience with thalidomide led to a widespread reappraisal of many other drugs in clinical use and the discovery of other agents with appreciable teratogenicity in man.

- This made people to realize a need for routine teratogenicity studies on potential new drugs in order to avoid congenital defects. However, the present tests for teratogenicity are not much reliable. Hence new drugs are usually released into the market with the caution that they should be avoided during the pregnancy unless it is essential.

Other Diseased Conditions

- The prominent organs of metabolism and excretion of the drugs include GIT, liver, lungs and kidney. An impairment of functioning of any other organs leads to an interference in the rate of drug metabolism and its excretion from the body.

- Hence toxicity manifestations of the drug may be prolonged or potentiated in presence of liver dysfunction, renal failure or pulmonary diseases. For example, morphine may precipitate coma in patients with liver cirrhosis while paraldehyde induces a profound sleep in patients with liver disease. Ethacrynic acid and furosemide are reported to induce deafness in some patients with renal failure.

■ CLASSIFICATION OF ADVERSE EFFECTS

Pharmacological Effects (Secondary Effects)

- These effects are the indirect consequences of the primary drug action. Hence such side effects may be considered as an extension of pharmacological activities of the drug. For example, barbiturates when used as the anticonvulsants, CNS depression may be the expected side effect.

- These effects occur either due to overdose of the drug or patient's intolerance for the drug. Hence the selection of right dose of the drug for the particular patient is important in order to avoid the occurrence of these secondary effects.

Biochemical Effects (Hypersensitivity Reactions)

- These include allergic reactions and blood dyscrasias or disorders. The word allergy is derived from the Greek literature, meaning 'different work'. These reactions originate due to antigen–antibody interactions.

- The drug, if not already a protein, may combine with protein in the body to form an antigen which then induces adverse effects belonging to this category.

- When patient develops sensitivity to one drug, there may be chances of development of sensitivity to other structurally related drugs. This is termed as cross-sensitivity reactions.

Pathological Effects

- These are the adverse effects of unexpected nature. They are not the indirect consequences of the drug action.

- They mainly occur due to the formation of cytotoxic, unstable, reactive, structurally unrelated metabolites form the parent drug during *in vivo* metabolism.

- Many drugs belonging to this category usually exhibit hepatotoxicity and/or nephrotoxicity. Examples include paracetamol, isoniazid, etc.

Genotoxic Effects

- These effects involve an alteration of genetic material. These effects are more likely to be associated with antineoplastic agents.
- Idiosyncrasy then may follow in such patients. It is an inborn predisposition to respond to a drug action in totally abnormal fashion, independent of antigen-antibody interactions. For example, mepacrine-induced hemolytic anemia in glucose-6-phosphate dehydrogenase deficient subjects is an idiosyncratic reaction.

Pharmacokinetic Effects

- Adverse effects belonging to this category arise due to sudden fluctuations in the plasma concentration of drugs. This is possibly due to alterations in the mode of absorption, distribution, metabolism and excretion of the drug by other concomitantly administered agent.
- These reactions are more evident in polypharmacy where the toxicities not exhibited by the single drug may arise when used in the combination therapy. For example, a MAO inhibitor may induce severe hypertensive crisis when used together with sympathomimetic amines.
- Such toxicities may develop due to interference of one drug in the various pharmacokinetic processes of other drug. Hence these reactions are known as drug interactions. Some drugs may get fastly absorbed in the presence of other drug. For example, certain drugs (e.g. procainamide) exhibit short biological half-life due to their extensive first-pass metabolism in the liver.
- If their absorption is retarded due to the influence of another drug, their therapeutic plasma level could not be achieved. On the contrary, the activity of many catecholamines decreases due to their oxidation in IV solutions. Antacids alter the pH at the absorption sites in GIT and affect the absorption of many drugs.
- Some drugs may compete with each other for the binding sites present on the plasma proteins. While doing so, they may displace other drugs from the plasma proteins. This results into an unexpected rise in the plasma concentration of the displaced drug. Naturally, the pharmacological activity and metabolism of such displaced drug is also amplified.
- Similar type of events may also occur during the metabolic processes. The drugs having higher affinity for metabolizing enzymes may inhibit or lower down the rate of metabolism of other drug. This results in the activity (or toxicity) of the later drug. This phenomenon is also known as drug synergism, For example, allopurinol, a xanthine oxidase inhibitor, inhibits the metabolism of antipyrine, 6-mercaptopurine and azathioprine. Profound bone marrow toxicity occurs with the intensification of the effects of the later drugs. The metabolism of tolbutamide is inhibited by many drugs, including bishydroxycoumarin and some sulphonamides.
- Similarly, during urinary excretion, the chances of tubular reabsorption of drug are more if the favourable pH condition is not present. For example, basic drugs or metabolites can easily be excreted through the urine, if the urinary pH is in the acidic range. While acidic drugs (or metabolites) can easily be excreted through the urine, if the urine pH is in the basic range.

- Since urine is the important vehicle for excretion of majority of drugs, the influence of urinary pH over the rate of drug clearance is a determinant factor in the control of the adverse effect.
- Similarly, many acidic drugs compete for the same transport system in the proximal tubules and reduce excretion of each other. For example, phenylbutazone reduces the excretion of acetohexamide and chlorpropamide resulting into an intense hypoglycemia.

Miscellaneous Reactions

These are the reactions unrelated to the administration of the drug into the body. Sometimes an untoward reaction may be falsely reported to occur due to the drug. However, that reaction is arising from other unrecognized sources and the drug is not at all responsible for its occurrence.

■ HYPERSENSITIVITY REACTIONS

- The interaction of a drug with the immune system can give rise to two types of toxicities:

1. During the interaction, the drug may damage immune system–functionally. An immunodeficiency thus develops. Body's natural resistance to infection is decreased and the person can easily be affected by infections. The immunosuppression may or may not be reversible. The immunosuppression leads to an increased susceptibility to bacterial, fungal or a viral infection. For example, patients under a long-term cortisone therapy are more prone to certain diseases including rheumatoid arthritis, Hodgkin's disease, etc.

2. The immune system is activated due to the presence of a drug (allergen). The allergen is responsible for the antigen–antibody interactions that provoke the typical manifestations of allergy. Drugs may be degraded to reactive immunogen. Drug or its metabolites serve as a hapten via covalent binding to an endogenous protein as a carrier which interact with T lymphocytes initiating response. Once T cells are activated, antihapten antibodies are formed. The drug or its metabolite, combines with an endogenous protein to form antigen. In most of the cases, antigens are of proteinious nature. The antibodies are produced in response to the presence of antigen in the body (exceptions isoantibodies which are naturally occurring antibodies in the human circulation). For one molecule of immunogen or antigen, millions of specific antibodies are formed and released into the body fluids. The antibodies produced by the host defence mechanisms, protect the host against the action of antigen by neutralizing the antigen-toxins. However, with response to specific agents or under certain conditions, the antigen–antibody interaction may provoke an unusual and exaggerated reaction, damaging the host body tissues. This altered response of the host tissues is known as hypersensitivity or allergy.

- Based on the mechanism of immunological involvement, the allergic response have been divided into four types, as shown in Table 74.3.

Type I Reactions

Type I reactions include anaphylactic shock and atopic diseases. They are mediated by humoral antibodies and depend primarily on the interaction of antigen with IgE antibodies (reagin antibodies). The term, anaphylaxis (which means 'removal of protection') was first coined by Richet and Port in 1902 to describe a hypersensitivity reaction which was in exaggerated form. It leads to an intense systemic and general reactivity resulting into urticarial rash, swelling of the soft tissues, bronchoconstriction, pulmonary air way obstruction, and hypotension. It is a sudden and life-threatening reaction which may lead to the death of a patient due to bronchoconstriction and cardiovascular collapse.

Table 74.3: Classification of allergic responses

Type	Antibody Involved	Target Tissues	Symptoms
Type I(anaphylactic reactions) or immediate hypersensitivity	IgE	Respiratory tract (asthma) Vasculature (anaphylactic shock)	
Type II (cytotoxic reactions)	IgG and IgM	Skin (urticaria)	
Type III (immune toxic complex reactions)	IgG	Circulatory system Vascular endothelium	Edema/vasodilation Hemolytic anemia Granulocytopenia
Type IV (delayed hypersensitivity)	These reactions are mediated by sensitized Tlymphocytes and macrophases		Urticaria, arthritis, lymphadenopathy, fever, serum sickness

- Drugs that cause anaphylactic reactions include organic mercurials, opiates, organic, iodides, dextran, amphotericin B, etc. Chemical mediators which play an important role in anaphylaxis include histamine, SRS-A (i.e. slow releasing substance of anaphylaxis), plasmakinins, prostaglandins, heparin, ECF-A (i.e. eosinophil— chemotactic factor of anaphylaxis) and platelet activating factor.

- Hence adrenergic agonist (e.g. terbutaline, salbutamol which induce bronchodilation), antihistaminic agents (e.g. ketotifen, cromoiyn sodium), theophylline, diethylcarbamazine and corticosteroids may be used to reduce the frequency and severity of anaphylactic attacks. Anaphylactic shock attacks almost all vital organs of the body and can be considered as a state of systemic anaphylaxis whereas in atoptic diseases, the functioning of only restricted areas of the body is affected. Hence atopic diseases, in simple words can be considered as state of local anaphylaxis.

- A strong hereditary predisposition, eosinophilia (i.e. an increase in the blood eosinophil count) and a natural tendency to disappear with time are some of the characteristic of atopic diseases. Examples include asthma, hey fever and urticaria dermatitis.

Asthma: It is characterized by paroxysmal attacks of difficult respiration. The symptoms include bronchoconstriction, edema of bronchial mucosa and cyanosis.

Hay fever: It is a type of hypersensitivity that occurs in persons sensitive to a variety of pollens. Symptoms of hay fever include sneezing, running nose, itching and irritation of the nose and eyes, profuse lachrymation and photophobia.

Urticaria (means 'Nettle'):

- It is one of the commonest adverse drug reaction which is characterized by localized patchy or generalized erythematous lesions. These lesions are accompanied by an intense itching. This adverse effect is short-lived and disappears within few hours.

- In type-II reactions, antigen–antibody interaction not only results into the destruction of antigen but also that of host cells. Therefore, type II reactions are known as cytotoxic reactions. For example, hypersensitivity reactions, if occurred during blood transfusions, can be categorised under type-II reactions.

Type II Reactions

Hemolytic anemia: Penicillin, quinine, quinidine, dipyrone RAS, mephenytoin, stibophen, cephalothin and phenacetin.

Thrombocytopenia: Quinine, quinidine, meprobamate, chlorothiazide, thiouracite, chloramphenicol, sulphonamides

Granulocytopenia: Aminopyrine, phenylbutazone, thiouracils, sulphonamides, anticonvulsants and tolbutamide.

Type III Reactions

Type III reactions are classified in to:

1. Reactions in which antigen is in excess. Example is serum sickness, and
2. Reactions in which antibodies are in excess.

Serum Sickness

- In this reaction, antigen in excess, leads to the production of soluble type of immune (i.e. antigen–antibody) complexes. These complexes fix on the complement and get deposited during their circulation, in the blood vessels. This results into acute inflammatory and tissue damaging type of response. Symptoms vary according to the severity.
- They include fever, urticaria, maculopapular eruptions, painful and swollen joints, lymphadenopathy and glomerulonephritis with albuminuria. The myocardium is also vulnerable to attack of inflammatory origin. The immunoglobulines, IgM, IgG1, and IgG2 have ability to produce serum sickness, in the descending order. Drugs involved include penicillins, sulphonamides, thiouracils, cholecystographic dyes, phenytoin, PAS and streptomycin.

Type I, type II, and type Ill reactions occur immediately after the introduction of an antigen. All these reactions are mediated by humoral antibodies. On the contrary, type IV reaction is mediated by sensitized lymphoidal cells (specific T lymphocytes). As this reaction is provoked after long time lag it is also called as a delayed type of hypersensitivity response (DHR) or tuberculin type hypersensitivity. Examples of this type include, contact dermatitis, transplant rejection, etc.

Contact Dermatitis

- It is characterized by skin eruptions induced by the topical application of the drug. Depending upon the drug applied, the nature of skin eruption varies. For example, many drugs including isoniazid, rifampicin, corticosteroids, anticonvulsants induce acne-form eruptions.
- Vesicular or bullous eruptions are found to be associated with the use of sulphonamides and frusemide. Bromides and iodides cause verrucous eruptions while lichenoid eruptions are induced by p-amino salicylic acid and chloroquine. Sometimes pigmented eruptions may occur especially with mepacrine and griseofulvin.

▓ IATROGENIC DERMATOLOGICAL REACTIONS (TABLE 74.4)

- Adverse reactions affecting the skin may be produced by topical as well as systemic administration of drugs. They vary considerably in site, extent and severity.
- The severity of reaction is related to the dose of the drug. Cutaneous eruptions can be considered as the most guaranteed signs of untoward reaction by the body to the drugs. These reactions may be categorised into allergic, idiosyncratic or photosensitivity types.

Erythema Nodosum

- Many drugs (e.g. salicylates, thiouracil, sulphonylurea—oral hypoglycemic agents) may induce an appearance of tender and nodular erythematous lesions generally on the shins of legs.
- These lesions may have a diameter range between 1–4 cm. A gradual colour change over a period of few weeks is reported to occur with these lesions.

Exfoliative Dermatitis

- Drugs like antibiotics, anticonvulsants and sulphonamides may induce reddening and drying of some skin patches.
- This is accompanied by itching and irritation. The skin lesion appears to be attacked by inflammatory disease. In some cases, loss or damage to hair and nails is also reported to occur.

Acne Vulgaris

- Acne-form lesions are produced due to inflammatory changes in the subjacent pilosebaceous follicle. These are characterized by swelling and pitting of the skin surface.

Table 74.4: Iatrogenic dermatological reactions

Dermatological reactions	Causative drugs (examples)
Urticaria	Cephalosporins, griseofulvin, penicillins
Eczematous dermatitis	Allopurinol, warfarin
Erythema multiforme .	Barbiturates, salicylates
Erythema nodosum	Barbiturates, sulphonamides
Exfoliative dermatitis	Phenylbutazone, cimetidine, phenytoin
Lupus erythematosus	Hydrallazine, griseofulvin, sulphonamide, procainamide, propylthiouracil
Generalized toxic erythema	Sulphonamides and non-steroidal anti-inflammatory agents
Psoriasis	Chloroquine, p-blockers, lithium
Stevens-Johnson syndrome (An exagarated form of erythema multiforme)	Sulphonamide, phenylbutazone
	Isoniazid, glucocorticoids, ethionamide
Acne vulgaris	Rifampicin, frusemide, chloroquine
Contact dermatitis	Tetracyclines
Pruritus	Phenothiazines, sulphonamides, thiazide
Photosensitivity	diuretics, sulphonylurea derivative and nalidixic acid

Pruritus

- It occurs partly due to the drug allergy and partly due to overgrowth of *Candida* (candidiasis) species.
- It is characterised by an intense itch, generalised exfoliative dermatitis and superinfection with Candida. The itch may persist long even after drug discontinuation.

Photosensitivity

- In the malpighian layer of epidermis, the drug or its metabolite is conjugated with a protein to form a photosensitizing substance.

- It induces photosensitization, phototoxicity or photoallergy when that part of the body is exposed to the sunlight. Photosensitivity usually disappears after the withdrawal of the drug.

BLOOD DYSCRASIAS (BLOOD DISORDERS)

The drug-induced blood disorders mainly include hemolytic anemia, aplastic anemia, megaloblastic anemia, granulocytopenia, agranulocytosis, throm-bocytopenia, leukopenia, methemoglobinemia, erythroid hypoplasia, thrombosis, thrombophlebitis and capillary purpura.

Hemolytic Anemia

- It may occur either due to the genetic deficiency of glucose-6-phosphate dehydrogenase (G-6-PD) enzymes or due to autoimmunological reaction. During the deficiency of G-6-PD, the red cell is not protected against oxidant damage and is destroyed prematurely.
- While the possible mechanism of hemolytic anemia induced by methyldopa involves the formation of autoantibodies. Excretion of porphyrins in urine and feces increases in patients with hemolytic anemia.
- Drugs that induce hemolytic anemia include antimalarial agents, antibiotics, methyldopa, dapsone, nitrofurantoin, sulfisoxazole, furazolidone, mefenamic acid, nalidixic acid, etc.

Aplastic Anemia (Pancytopenia)

- In this disorder, the precursors of red cells, granulocytes and platelets get damaged. Aplastic or hypoplastic conditions of the bone marrow may affect the formation and development of these cells.
- Drugs that induce pancytopenia include, salicylates, indomethacin, mepacrine, chloramphenicol, phenyl-butazone, tolbutamide, propyl thiouracil, phenytoin, etc.

Megaloblastic Anemia

- Vitamin B_{12} and folic acid are necessary for DNA synthesis and cell proliferation. Deficiency of these essential factors will principally affect the tissues (e.g. bone marrow and GIT) where the rapid cell turnover occurs.
- One of the symptoms of deficiency is megaloblastic anemia in which there is a marked disorder of erythroblast proliferation and defective erythropoiesis.
- It is characterized by an increase in the number of large abnormal erythrocyte precursors (macrocytes) with an increased susceptibility to destruction. Megaloblastic anemia is usually accompanied by some degree of leukopenia and thrombocytopenia.
- Many drugs lead to megaloblastic anemia by causing a disturbance in the folic acid metabolism pattern. Examples include phenobarbitone, primidone, nitrofurantoin, phenytoin, etc.

Leukopenia and Agranulocytosis (Granulocytopenia)

- These reactions are characterized by a fall in leukocyte count induced by either antigen–antibody interaction or a failure in cell division involving DNA synthesis. They may also occur as a part of a general pancytopenia.
- Drugs which induce these reactions include aspirin, phenytoin, phenylbutazone, meprobamate, chloramphenicol, imipramine, chlorpromazine, thiouracil, methimazole.

- These effects are of reversible nature and disappear upon drug-withdrawal. Antibody-mediated leukocyte destruction must be distinguished from the direct effect of cytotoxic drugs, most of which cause granulocytopenia. Leukocytic lysis releases such products which then cause fever and severe sore-throat. In some cases, even the early precursors of granulocytes are eliminated.

Thrombocytopenia

- It is a relatively common manifestation associated with the administration of drugs that cause a severe pancytopenia. It is characterized by a profound fall in the platelet count.
- It appears to be mediated by a drug-induced immunological mechanism exerting a toxic effect on megakaryocytes in the bone marrow. Some drugs may cause direct disintegration of platelets at periphery. Neonatal thrombocytopenia is induced by the antepartum administration of drugs like, aspirin, quinine or thiazide diuretics.
- Drugs that induce thrombocytopenia include, aspirin, propranolol, penicillins, sulphonamides, rifampin, meprobamate, furosemide, methyldopa, dextran, alprenolol, trimethoprim, valproic acid, phenylbutazone, etc.

Leukemia

- A variety of so-called oncogenic viruses such as leukemia, sarcoma, polyoma, SV40 and papilloma viruses invades the host cells.
- As a result, the affected cells continue to multiply in an uncontrolled, unabated fashion. Normally there are 5000–10,000 leukocytes per cubic millimeter, in leukemias, there is an increase in the number of leukocyte count.
- This may arise due to either appearance of malignant clones of the cell or due to attack of oncogenic viruses.

Methemoglobinemia

- Methemoglobin is an oxidised form of hemoglobin in which the iron is in the ferric state. It cannot combine with and transport oxygen, since its iron is in the ferric state.
- A small amount of methemoglobin is present in the blood of normal individuals. Methemoglobinemia results due to failure in the normal reconversion of methemoglobin to hemoglobin or by a more rapid production of methemoglobin induced by certain drugs or oxidizing agents.
- The condition is attributed to the deficiency of the enzyme, methemoglobin reductase or more specifically cytochrome B_5 reductase. Examples of drugs that induce methemoglobinemia include acetanilid, iodine, nitrites, phenacetina, sulfonethyl-methane, pamaquine, primaquine, sulfones, etc.
- Prominent signs of methemoglobinemia include headache, acute hypoxia, cyanosis, dizziness and deterioration of mental functions. Reducing agents (e.g., methylene blue, ascorbic acid) may be used to convert back methemoglobin to oxyhemoglobine.

Thrombophlebitis and Thrombosis

- Thromophlebitis is the condition in which intravascular clot formation process is induced by an inflammation of a vein.
- While thrombosis is condition in which intravascular coagulation occurs that results into start of bloodstream followed death of the organ cells.

Capillary Purpura

It is characterized by the minor local hemorrhage due to the drug-induced damage to the capillary cells.

▨ IATROGENIC REACTIONS AFFECTING LIVER

Majority of drugs are metabolized to less or more extent in the liver. Some drugs may produce hepatotoxicity by forming highly reactive unstable free radicals or peroxides during the metabolism in liver. These toxic intermediate induced biochemical dysfunctioning in the liver. The main intense form of hepatotoxicity is liver necrosis while fatty liver syndrome is the milder form.

Deficiencies of Vitamins and Nutrients

- Deficiency of vitamins and nutrients or a variety of drugs when administered, may lead to the inhibition of hepatic protein synthesis.
- This results into abnormalities in lipid metabolism in the liver. Accumulation of fats and other lipids occurs in the liver, causing fatty acid syndrome.
- If remains untreated, this condition may lead to enlargement of the liver, fibrotic changes, cirrhosis and several impaired liver functions.

Hepatic Jaundice

- The bile pigments (e.g. bilirubin and biliverdin) are derived from the heme of hemoglobin from worn out red blood cells and from other heme proteins.
- It is transported to the liver for excretion. Bilirubin predominates in the human bile. In the liver, bilirubin is conjugated with glucuronic acid to form bile diglucuronide which is then readily excreted by way in bile into the intestine and eliminated in the feces. The term 'jaundice' means an elevation of bilirubin concentration in the plasma. In hemolytic jaundice, the excessive erythrocyte destruction liberates bilirubin in the amounts much higher than the conjugation ability of the liver.
- This results in an increase in the unconjugated bilirubin amounts in the plasma. In hepatic or obstructive jaundice, the conjugated bilirubin is prevented from being excreted into the intestine due to the partial or complete blocking of the bile ducts. It may also occur, in some cases, due to increased viscosity of the bile associated with excessive permeability of the bile canaliculi.
- This results into an increased plasma level of conjugated bilirubin. Enlargement of liver, as in acute hepatitis; may also lead to an obstruction in the internal bile duct.
- In the hepatocellular jaundice, certain drugs or chronic disease conditions may impair the liver's capacity to conjugate bilirubin. For example, rifampicin interferes with the clearance of bilirubin from the liver by competitive inhibition. While novobiocin may interfere with conjugation of bilirubin.
- This results into an increased plasma concentration of unconjugated bilirubin. In patients with a hereditary deficiency of the hepatic enzyme, bilirubin-UDP- glucuronyl transferase, the conjugation of bilirubin gets impaired.

Hepatic Cirrhosis (Fibrosis of the Liver)

- It occurs due to progressive fibrous tissue over growth resulting into toughening and atrophy of liver. It may be associated with a high incidence of hepatic carcinoma.

- It usually follows upon chronic active hepatitis. Main functions of liver involve, its role in the protein, carbohydrate and fat metabolism and its detoxification and excretion abilities for foreign substances.
- Hence when due to degenerative effects of drug and or its metabolites, large number of hepatic cells are damaged, lipid can accumulate in the liver mainly in the form of triacylglycerol. When accumulation of lipid in liver becomes chronic, fibrotic changes occur in the hepatic cells. This leads to cirrhosis and impaired liver function. It may occur due to chronic intake of certain drugs, ethanol, excess of copper, excess of iron or a deficiency of antitrypsin.

Hepatic Coma

- Ammonia is released in the large intestine as a result of microbial attack on nitrogenous substrates.
- This is absorbed into the portal circulation, but under normal conditions it is rapidly removed from the blood by the liver.
- In liver dysfunction, the ammonia level crosses the toxic limits. The elevated plasma ammonia concentration then leads to hepatic coma.

Hepatitis (Inflammation of the Liver)

- Drugs which are reported to induce hepatitis include paracetamol, aspirin, halothane, daunorubicin, phenothiazines, tetracyclines, isoniazid, isocarboxazid, etc.
- It may occur due to hepatic biochemical damage due to highly reactive free radicals or other unstable intermediates which are released during, drug metabolism. It may also occur due to the viral infection.

IATROGENIC REACTIONS AFFECTING THE RENAL FUNCTION

- Urine serves as an important vehicle for excretion of majority of drugs and/or their metabolites. Naturally then the toxic metabolites may exert adverse effects upon the kidney leading to degenerative lesions of the renal parenchyma.
- When substantial renal parenchyma is lost or diseased, clinical symptoms of renal impairment begin to appear. This results into varying degrees of tubular dysfunction and progressive renal insufficiency. In acute tubular necrosis, damage to proximal tubules is reported to occur by drugs like, cephaloridine, cephalothin, gentamicin, streptomycin and aminoglycoside antibiotics.
- While amphotericin may damage the distal tubules as well. Sometimes due to involvement of immunological mechanisms, the basement membrane of glomerular capillaries may also get damaged.
- Because of the high concentration of solutes in renal papilla, this region is more susceptible to get affected. This leads to acute papillary necrosis. Renal tubules passing into necrotic papillae are obstructed resulting into their degeneration.

Pyelonephritis

It is an inflammatory condition mainly affecting the kidney and pelvis of the ureter, due to blood-borne infection from the renal parenchyma or ascending infection when there is an obstruction of the lower urinary channels.

Crystalluria

- Acetylation is an important conjugation reaction for the drugs containing a free amino group. The acetylated metabolites, in general, are less water soluble than the parent drugs. This is specifically true for sulphonamides.

- If a large amount of insoluble acetylated sulphonamide is excreted in relatively small volume of acidic urine, the danger of deposition and solidification of this acetylated derivative in the kidney becomes more evident. This if remains untreated, may lead to crystalluria.

IATROGENIC REACTIONS AFFECTING THE GIT FUNCTION

- Most of the common adverse reactions associated with the oral administration of the drug include nausea, vomiting, anorexia, constipation, diarrhea, achlorhydria (absence of gastric acid secretion), hyperchlorhydria (excess gastric acid secretion) and gastric or peptic ulceration. These effects appear due to structural and functional changes in the GIT mucosal membrane induced by the drugs. For example, caffeine and theophylline enhance gastric acid secretion by potentiating vagal tone.

- This results into ulcerogenicity due to drug-induced erosion of the mucous membrane. Similarly by inhibiting prostaglandin biosynthesis, aspirin-like drugs destroy the protective layer over the gastric mucosa and cause erosions of epithelium together with the capillary thrombosis and hemorrhage.

- Besides certain drugs, some diseased conditions may also create favorable opportunities for certain GIT effects. For example, achlorhydria is associated with pernicious anemia, in gastric carcinomas and a number of other conditions. Some drugs also induce pancreatic dysfunction which is characterised by pain, steatorrhea, protein malabsorption and raised serum amylase level.

IATROGENIC REACTIONS AFFECTING PULMONARY FUNCTION

- Regardless of the route of administration, there are significant chances of occurrence of iatrogenic reactions affecting the pulmonary function. In majority of cases, pulmonary reactions to drugs are due to the idiosyncrasies.

- Since certain drugs are mainly excreted through the exhaled air, toxic drug metabolite may induce pulmonary fibrosis. Upon chronic administration of such drugs (e.g. busulphan, methysergide, nitrofurantoin, etc.) the respiratory collapse may occur. Certain drugs may induce hypersensitivity reactions in the alveolar walls, resulting into pulmonary eosinophilia.

- Later is characterized by cough, fever and severe dysponea usually without wheeze. Examples of such drugs include penicillin, sulphonamides, tetracyclines, imipramine, mephenesin, nitrofurantoin, etc. Pulmonary edema may occur from overloading with IV fluids. Similarly few drugs like, amiodarone (i.e. antiarrhythmic drug) may cause pulmonary alveolitis. Other common drug-induced pulmonary effects include bronchoconstriction, bronchospasm, bronchodilation and decreased bronchial secretion.

IATROGENIC REACTIONS AFFECTING THE OPTIC SYSTEM

- The drug-induced ocular changes are more prominent, when drug comes in direct contact with the ocular components. Though all ocular structures are delicate in nature, the most frequently affected ocular components include conjunctiva, cornea, sclera, lens, retina and optic nerve. The signs of ocular damage may be reflected into the appearance of photophobia, panconjunctivitis, subconjunctival fibrosis, cornea ulcer or blindness.

- The most common side-effects of systemically absorbed drug include miosis (constriction of pupil), mydriasis (dilation of pupil), glaucoma (an increase in the intraocular pressure), cycloplegia (paralysis of accommodation,) blurred vission and photophobia.

- All these effects are reversible in nature and may disappear upon withdrawal of the drug. However, some agents (e.g. chloroquine) may induce relatively irreversible damage to retina and optic nerve resulting into blindness. Similarly ethambutol, upon chronic treatment, may cause optic neuritis. Corticosteroids may increase intraocular pressure and may induce posterior subcapsular cataracts upon chronic treatment.

- Some drugs may cause myopia which is characterized by a progressive blurring of distance vision resulting due to a myopic shift in refractive index of the patient. Antibiotics, specifically from aminoglycoside category, damage 8th cranial nerve resulting into vestibular and/or auditor toxicities. For example, streptomycin and gentamicin attack mainly vestibular branch while neomycin and kanamycin attack the auditory function.

IATROGENIC REACTIONS AFFECTING SEXUAL FUNCTIONS

- Adverse effects may induce sexual impairments by:
  1. Causing a decrease or loss of libido.
  2. Causing erectile dysfunction (i.e. impotence).
  3. Causing ejaculation problems.
  4. Causing hormonal imbalance.
  5. Orgasmic dysfunction.

- Hormonal alteration is involved in a variety of iatrogenic reactions. Examples include menstrual irregularities, vaginal lubrication, breast enlargement in women, galactorrhea, (prolactogenic or increased milk secretion from the breast), gynecomastia in men, deepening of voice, hirsutism and virilizing effect.

- Hirsutism (the condition of excessive hairiness.) usually is used in relation to female in which hair grows in such area where normally it is absent in the female but present in the males. Virilism differs from hirsutism in that in addition to excessive hair growth, other signs of male characteristics (e.g. deepening of voice, clitoral hypertrophy) are present in female.

- Anabolic steroids may disturb the menstrual pattern, may increase libido and may cause failure of spermatogenesis upon chronic treatment. Virilization of voice is also reported to occur.

- Galactorrhea effect promotes the milk production and induces lactation. Drugs causing galactorrhea include neuroleptic agents, tricyclic antidepressants, methyl-dopa, verapamil, cimetidine, metoclopramide, sulpiride, etc. Both hair loss and hypertrichosis (i.e. hair growth promoting activity) are seen during the use of oral contraceptives. Hypertrichosis occurs frequently during the systemic administration of corticosteroids. The virilizing effects may be seen in neonates after the use of phenytoin by the pregnant women.

- Antihypertensive and antipsychotic agents have a high potential for causing sexual dysfunction.

- Other examples of drugs which induce sexual dysfunction include amitriptyline, baclofen, clonidine, barbiturates, benzodiazepine, chlorpromazine, cimetidine, clofibrate, diphenhydramine, doxepine, guanethidine, haloperidol, hydroxyzine, imipramine, labetalol, methadone, morphine, methyldopa, oral contraceptives, propranolol, spiranolactone, thioridazine, tranylcypromine, etc.

OTHER IATROGENIC EFFECTS

Extrapyramidal Symptoms

Most of the narcoleptic (i.e. antipsychotic) agents exhibit extrapyramidal effects at varying degree. These effects are characterized by:

1. **Akinesia:** It is an inability to lie or to sit due to the muscular weakness and fatigue.

2. **Acathisia:** It is characterized by motor restlessness.

3. **Dyskinesia or dystonic reactions:** These are characterized by rhythmic purposeless involuntary muscle movements occurring over face, mouth and tongue. It is accompanied by difficult breathing and disturbed gait. Examples of antipsychotic agents that induce extrapyramidal effects include chlorpromazine, promazine, prochlorperazine, perphenazine, fluphenazine and trifluoraperazine.

4. **Alopecia:** Many drugs upon chronic treatment may affect hair growth and may lead to the hair fall. Both, hair loss (alopecia) and hypertrichosis have been reported during the use of oral contraceptives. Drugs which may cause alopecia include warfarin, lithium, gold, carbimazole, methyldopa, heparin, propranolol, oral contraceptives.

5. **Paraesthesia:** It is characterized by numbness and tingling sensation. Many drugs regardless of route of administration, cause numbness of extremities.

6. **Myopathy (muscle weakness):** It usually results due to hypokalemia. Drugs which may cause myopathy include bumetanide, ethacrynic acid and furosemide.

7. **Myxoedema:** It results due to antithyroid action of some drugs. Certain drugs may cause myxoedema by inhibiting iodine uptake by thyroid.

8. **Immunosuppression:** Many drugs (e.g. corticosteroids, purine flogues, folic acid analogues, alkylating agents, promethazine, cyclosporine A, etc. may cause immunosuppression. The immunosuppression may or may not be reversible. It is increased susceptibility of the patient to bacterial, fungal and viral infections. Such drugs may be used clinically to suppress immune system of the patient undergoing organ transplantation.

9. **Teratogenicity:** Drugs that have a capacity to cross the placenta barrier eventually pose a potential threat to the sloping fetus, if used during pregnancy. Thalidomide diaster caused public awareness and since teratogenicity testing for every new drug was made compulsory. Drugs that can cross the placenta and may endanger the fetus (if taken during pregnancy) include antithyroid drugs, steroidal sex hormones, cytotoxic drugs (e.g. chlorambucil, cyclophosphamide, etc.), folate antagonists, tetracyclines, coumarin anticoagulants, phenytoin, trimethadione, cyclizine, meclozine, halothane, etc. Barbiturates can induce hemorrhagic disease in the newborn.

10. **Carcinogenicity:** It is the capacity of the drug to induce a tumorous or cancerous growth in any of the body organ in the subjects under treatment. This property is more linked with the repeated (i.e. chronic) administration.

TREATMENT OF DRUG POISONING

- The treatment of toxic symptoms arising due to the overdose of any drug, primarily involves maintenance of respiration and cardiovascular function. Measures should also be taken to treat imbalances in fluid and electrolyte levels.

- Antidote therapy plays an important role in the management of poisoning. Unfortunately, it does not give positive results in the treatment of all poisoning cases. Hence, beside antidote treatment, supportive therapy is also utilised in the treatment of poisoning cases. It includes the followings.

Vomiting

- If the poisoning occurs due to orally ingested substance, a logical approach is to clear off that substance from the stomach. Vomiting is generally induced by either taking syrup of ipecac or by injecting apomorphine, 0.066 mg/kg subcutaneously. In absence of emetics, vomiting can be induced mechanically by stroking the posterior pharynx. For prompt emesis, it is better to take 1–2 glasses of water before hand.
- Emesis is contraindicated, if corrosives, strychnine, petroleum distillates are ingested and during coma.

Gastric Lavage

- It is used in the cases where emesis does not work. It involves the insertion of a tube into the stomach of the patient and washing the stomach in order to remove the unabsorbed poison.
- Oral passage is easier but in adults, nasal route may also be utilised. The fluid generally used for lavage may be water, normal saline or one-half saline solution. The process is effective as long as six hours after the ingestion of a poison and should be repeated until the washing conies free from poison.

Chemical Adsorption

- Once the poison has been removed maximally from the stomach by emesis, the traces of poison left in stomach can be removed by using activated charcoal. It easily adsorbs into the surface through irreversible fashion, thereby preventing its further absorption and poisoning.
- It is administered usually as slurry, suspended in water. It may either be given orally or by lavage. The amount of activated charcoal to be used is determined in such a way to achieve a charcoal: drug ratio of 10:1.

Purgation

- An aim of every therapy used in the treatment of poisoning is to neutralise or reduce the manifestations arising due to such poisoning.
- Purgatives are also employed in order to reduce absorption of the poison by hastening its passage through GIT. Saline cathartics are usually preferred due to their prompt action and less side effects.

Forced Diuresis

To treat barbiturate and other intoxications, other options are also open. These include forced osmotic diuresis and alkalinization of the urine.

Antagonism

- The drugs having the capacity to block the action of the poison can be utilized. Such drugs are known as antidotes. They are broadly divided into categories on the basis of their mechanism of action.
  1. Some antidotes have opposite physical, chemical or pharmacological property to nullify the effect of the poison. In such cases, problem arises if the duration of action of poison and antidote, does not match each other. If duration of action of antidote is more, it may lead to poisoning with the antidote.

2. Some antidotes fix-up the poison molecules by forming a complex with it. They are also known as chelating agents. Chelating agents possess a high degree of selective affinity for certain metallic ions.

- Heavy metals cannot be metabolized in the body. During their stay, they combine with vital functional groups, necessary for normal physiological functions. The toxicity arising due to this ligand formation may be deal with chelating agents. Chelating agents can prevent or reverse toxic effects by forming soluble chelates (complexes) with the heavy metals. Thus they enhance the excretion of the metals.

Dialysis

- Peritoneal dialysis and hemodialysis are usually employed techniques in the life-threatening intoxication. In the blood, the poison may bind to several cells and plasma proteins. The rate of elimination of such poison therefore, is governed by the rate of dissociation of the poison from its binding sites.

1. Hemodialysis (artificial kidney): It is much more effective dialysing technique than peritoneal dialysis. It can be used to treat intoxication due to barbiturates, glutethimide, salicylates, etc.

2. Peritoneal dialysis: Though it is less effective than the hemodialysis, it is generally used to enhance the rate of elimination of the toxic elements from the body. The poisoning resulting due to overdoses of many exogenous poisons may be treated using this technique.

Blood Transfusion

- When all the approaches to remove poison from the blood fail then blood transfusion remains the only solution.
- Similarly, if hemoglobin is converted to methemoglobin due to the toxic action of drug present, the life of the patient comes in danger.
- In such cases of methemoglobinemia, the circulating blood has to be replaced. Blood transfusion is an effective therapy to supply normal hemoglobin that can train oxygen to the tissues at required rate.

▨ HEAVY METAL POISONING

- To function various physiological activities smoothly and in coordinated fashion, a number of metals are essential. Depending upon their need, some are required in appreciable quantity whereas some metals are needed in trace amounts.
- Due to some reasons, if the concentration of metals in the biophase exceeds than that is required, toxic effects start appearing. These toxic effects can be accounted on the basic of interaction of the metal with specific functional groups (ligands) present on' the macromolecules (i.e. enzymes or receptors) in the cells.
- Due to this interaction, macromolecule cannot catalyse the functions, vital to the existence of the cell. Metal generally interacts with functional groups like, amino, carboxyl, phenolic, phosphoric and sulfhydryl moieties. The interaction with such vital functional groups (ligands) leads to disruption of energy production and ion regulation. Adverse reactions of metals are also reported. For example, the heavy metals like, cadmium, lead, mercury, arsenic, tin and cobalt can lead to immunosuppressive effects. Similarly arsenic, chromium and nickel may cause cancer in humans.
- In the treatment of intoxication due to heavy metals, chelating agents play a dominating role. All such compounds that can form complexes (chelates) with the heavy metals and have a

common property to prevent or to reverse the binding of metallic cations to body ligands, are collectively referred under the term, chelating agents.

- The ligand atoms entrap the metal ion and form a complex with it by co-ordinate bonds. The bond is often indicated by an arrow. The head of an arrow is directed away from the atom (ligand) which donates the electron pair needed for formation of the bond. The stability of chelate (complex) formed varies with the metal and ligand atoms. A large number of drugs can form metal chelates.
- Chelate formation may be a part of their mechanism of action against the diseases for which they are intened.

Arsenic Poisoning

- Arsenic as such is not needed for the body. It does not catalyse any biological function. It is the trioxide form in which arsenic is usually present. The most severe form of arsenic toxicity involves erythrocyte hemolysis. Similarly kidney and liver damage may occur. Dimercaprol, a chelating agent, may be used in the treatment of arsenic poisoning.
- In toxic symptoms, arsenic can cause uncoupling of mitochondrial oxidative phosphorylation. This uncoupling is known as arsenolysis.
- Since it inhibits the functioning of many vital enzymes, almost every important organ is affected by arsenic poisoning. Besides dimercaprol, oral penicillamine may also be given to treat the poisoning. But to treat severe arsenic induced nephropathy, renal dialysis is the only solution.

Mercury Poisoning

- Mercury constitues as an important part of the chemical structure of many diuretics, antiseptics, antibacterials and laxatives. It has a high affinity for sulfur. Hence mercury readily forms covalent bonds with sulfhydryl groups and inactivates the enzymes containing sulfhydryl group. Thus, presence of mercury can easily retard the normal cell metabolism.
- Dimercaprol and penicillamine which contain a sulfhydryl group can be routinely used to treat intoxication due to either inorganic or elemental mercury. N-acetyl-D, L-penicillamine appears to be more potent and safer than the former agents. In severe case, hemodialysis may also be employed.

Lead Poisoning

- Human exposure to lead is primarily from food, environmental and industrial sources. It is mainly absorbed into the circulation from GIT and respiratory system. In body, lead is mainly deposited in liver, kidney and bones. The chronic exposure to lead results into gastrointestinal, neuromuscular, CNS, hematological and renal toxicities.
- Lead as such is not essential for life. The intoxication due to lead can be treated by using one of the three chelating agents— edetate calcium disodium ($CaNa_2$ EDTA), dimercaprol and D-penicillamine. The lead-EDTA complex is non-toxic, water soluble and hence is rapidly excreted. Usually at the start, the combination of edetate calcium disodium and dimercaprol is used. This is followed by oral penicillamine, continued for a long term.

Cadmium Poisoning

- It occurs in nature in association with zinc and lead. After absorption, kidney retains higher concentration of cadmium than do any other tissue. This accumulation leads to renal tubular damage. Liver also shoulders considerable deposition of cadmium.

- Intoxication leads to nausea, dizziness, diarrhea, chest pain and irritation of the upper respiratory tract. Treatment commences with respiratory support and steroidal therapy. Chelating agent like, edetate calcium disodium can be used whereas; dimercaprol should not be used, due to its nephrotoxicity. Vitamin D is recommended for the treatment of associated orthopedic problems.

Iron Poisoning

- Body has a considerable amount of iron, circulating in the plasma. The plasma circulating iron cannot exhibit toxic reactions because of the presence of natural chelating agent, transferrin in the blood.
- It protects the body from the toxic actions of the circulating iron. Iron, if absorbed into circulation in excess amounts, may lead to toxic manifestations. These include irritation of GIT, pneumonitis, convulsions and coma. Hepatic damage is also reported to occur. Deferoxamine is an effective chelating agent in treating the systemic iron toxicity.

Cyanide Poisoning

- Even though cyanide does not come under the term 'heavy metals' the treatment of cyanide poisoning deserves a special attention. Cyanogenic compounds, if ingested orally, may release hydrogen cyanide due to their hydrolysis in GIT. The cyanide ion impairs several vital cellular functions. For example, there occurs impairment of tissue oxygen utilization due to inhibition of cytochrome oxidase enzyme. The blood runs deficient of oxygen. The patient suffers from hypoxia followed by ataxis, coma and death.
- There is a need of two fold therapy in the treatment of cyanide poisoning, i.e.
  1. The cyanide ions present in the circulation should immediately be converted into a nontoxic form.
  2. Attempts should be made to reverse the condition of hypoxia i.e. placing the patient in the oxygen-riched atmosphere and a quick conversion of methemoglobin to hemoglobin should be affected.
- The treatment involves the use of amyl nitrite by inhalation or sodium nitrite by injection. These agents serve the second purpose. The subsequent intravenous administration of sodium thiosulfate facilitates the conversion of free cyanide ions to nontoxic thiocyanate form. Thiocyanate can readily by excreted in the urine.

Pharmaceutical Aids

The substances which are used in the manufacture or compounding (formulating) of various pharmaceutical preparation are called as pharmaceutical aids. They have very little or no therapeutic value of their own.

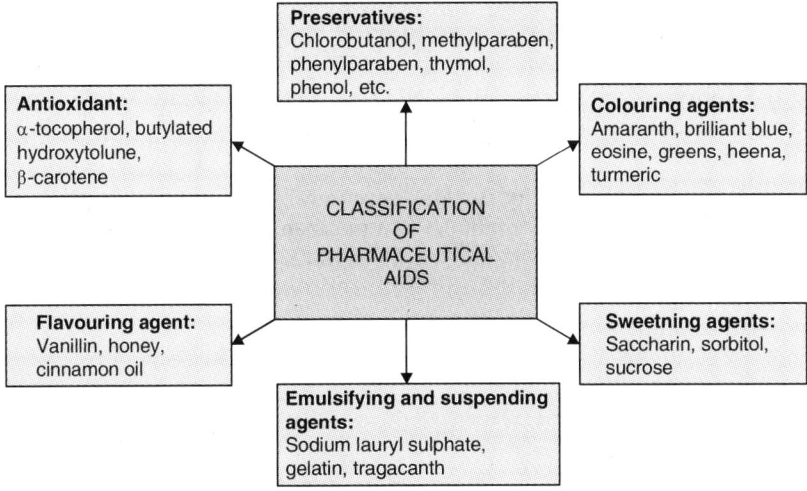

Preservatives:
Chlorobutanol, methylparaben, phenylparaben, thymol, phenol, etc.

Antioxidant:
α-tocopherol, butylated hydroxytolune, β-carotene

Colouring agents:
Amaranth, brilliant blue, eosine, greens, heena, turmeric

CLASSIFICATION
OF
PHARMACEUTICAL
AIDS

Flavouring agent:
Vanillin, honey, cinnamon oil

Sweetning agents:
Saccharin, sorbitol, sucrose

Emulsifying and suspending agents:
Sodium lauryl sulphate, gelatin, tragacanth

PRESERVATIVES

- A preservative is in the common pharmaceutical sense, a substance that prevents or inhibits microbial growth and may be added to pharmaceutical preparation for this purpose to avoid consequent spoilage of the preparation by micro-organisms.
- The choice of suitable preservative for a preparation depends on pH, compatibility with other ingredients, the route, dose and frequency of administration of the preparation, partition coefficient with ingredients contamination, or closures, degree and type of contamination, concentration, and rate of antimicrobial effects.

Chlorobutanol

Properties: White crystalline with camphoreceous odour, melts about 95° C, sparingly soluble in chloroform and alcohol.

Identification:

- On reaction with aniline in presence of base, gives phenyl isocyanides.
- On addition of iodine in presence of a sodium hydroxide, it gives a yellow precipates of iodoform.

Uses:
- It has antibacterial, germicidal properties and is chiefly used as a preservative in solution of epinephrine, posterior pituitary.
- It has local anaesthetic potency and used topically as a dental analgesic. It has sedative-hypnotic property.

Synthesis:

$$H_3C-\overset{O}{\underset{}{C}}-CH_3 + CHCl_3 \longrightarrow Cl-\underset{Cl}{\overset{Cl}{\underset{|}{C}}}-\underset{CH_3}{\overset{CH_3}{\underset{|}{C}}}-OH$$

Acetone   Chloroform   Chlorobutanol

Methylparaben

Identification:
- In boiling with water and subsequent addition of ferric chloride solution, a reddish-voilet colour is produced.
- Dissolve the substance in alcohol and boil, add mercury nitrate solution a precipate is formed and the liquid is coloured red.

Uses:
- This is used as preservative in certain parenteral preparation. Topical antibiotic or corticosteroid preparation may contain 0.3% of paraben.
- Methylparaben is used in combination with propylparaben as a preservative in artificial tears.

Storage: In closed containers.

Synthesis:

4-hydroxy benzoic acid $+$ H_3C-OH $\xrightarrow{H_2SO_4}$ methylparaben

Phenol

Uses:
- It is used as a caustic disinfectant, topical anesthetic and pharmaceutical necessity as a preservative for injection.
- It is used in several proprietary antiseptic mouth washers and burn remedies.

Synthesis:

Chlorobenzene $\xrightarrow[\text{Steam}]{H_2O}$ Phenol $+ HCl$

Storage: In well closed, light resistant containers, in a cool place.

Thymol

Uses: It is used as antifungal and antibacterial agents. Thymol is included in mouth washes for its antiseptic action and in perfumery.

Identification: A sample is dissolved in glacial acetic acid, sulfuric acid and nitric acid are added, a deep bluish green colour is produced.

Storage: In well closed, light resistant containers.

Synthesis:

3-methylphenol   2-chloropropane   Thymol

Thiomersal

Uses: It is used as a weak bacteriostatic and mild fungistatic agent. It is used in a concentration of 1:10,000 in whole blood, plasma or serum as a preservative.

Identification:

- A sample is dissolved in water. On addition of silver nitrate solution, a white precipitate is produced.
- An aqueous solution of the substance on treatment with dilute HCl, gives a white precipitate which melts at 110° C.

Storage: In well closed, light resistant containers.

Synthesis:

Thiosalicylic acid   Thiomersal

Sodium Benzoate

Uses: It has been extensively used as a food and pharmaceutical preservative, the only one permitted to be used for many classes of food products.

Identification: Sample solution in water on addition of ferric chloride solution, a buff coloured precipate is produced.

Storage: In well closed, light resistant containers.

Synthesis:

Benzoic acid   Sodium benzoate

Chloroform

Uses: It is used as a preservative during the aqueous percolation of vegetable drugs to prevent bacterial decomposition in the process of manufacture.

Identification: Chloroform is warmed with aniline in presence of sodium hydroxide, which gives phenyl isocyanide with a characteristic odour.

ANTIOXIDANT

- An antioxidant is a substance capable of inhibiting oxidation and this may be added for this purpose to pharmaceutical products subject to deterioration by oxidative process, as for example, the development of rancidity in oils and fats or the inactivation of some medicinal in the environment of their dosage forms. These function as reducing agent and capable of inhibiting oxidation.

Ascorbyl palmitate

α-Tocopherol

β-Carotene

- Antioxidants are among the most important variables in controlling or preventing the free radical reaction. Antioxidant, if present in low concentration, can prevent oxidation of substances like proteins, lipids and DNA. The major biological anti-oxidants are ascorbyl palmitate, tocopherol, β-carotene, plant phenolic and thiol containing compounds.
- These antioxidants act by preventing the initial loss of allylic hydrogen from methylene carbon inhibiting the cleavage of hydroperoxides or peroxide or scavenging the radicals. Alpha tocopherol reduces O_2, HO together with lipid peroxy radicals.
- β-carotene is another lipid soluble molecule, which is an efficient singlet oxygen scavenger. A large number of phenolic compounds are used as antioxidant. The mechanism of free radicals scavenging effect of phenolic is given below.

- The selection of antioxidant is made by taking into consideration the following points:
  1. Possible physiological and chemical incompabilities. The antioxidant should be physiologically inert and employed at sufficiently low concentration.
  2. Consideration of possible solubility problems between the reducing agent and the drug. In preparation containing calcium, it should be adjusted to an acidic pH if a sulphite ion is going to be used. Because sulfite ions will cause the precipitation of calcium from solution of neutral to alkaline pH.
  3. Handling of oxidants while mixing of strong oxidizing agents with very strong reducing agents will form excessive mixture. So caution should be observed.

- Most recently, the use of antioxidants has been enlarged to greater areas of therapeutic importance. They have been used to treat neurodegenerative disorders such as Alzheimer's and Parkinson's disease and also cognition dysfunction.

Butylated Hydroxytolune

Uses: It is used as an antioxidant employed to retard oxidative degradation of oils and fats in various cosmetics and pharmaceuticals.

Identification: An alcohol solution of the compound is reacted with potassium ferrocyanide and ferric ammonium sulphate in sulphuric acid. A green to blue colour is formed.

Storage: In well closed containers.

Synthesis:

Butylated hydroxytolune

Butylated Hydroxyanisole

Uses: It is used as an antioxidant employed to retard oxidative degradation of oils and fats in various cosmetics and pharmaceuticals.

Identification: An alcoholic solution of the compound is reacted with borax and 2,6-dichloroquinone chloramide, a blue colour is produced.

Storage: In well closed, light resistant containers.

Synthesis:

Butylated hydroxyanisole

Propyl Gallate

Uses: It is used as antioxidant and preservative.

Identification:

1. Test for phenol with ferric chloride.

2. The compound is dissolved in hot water. On addition of dilute ammonia solution, a red colour is produced.

Storage: In well closed containers free from contacts with metals.

Propyl gallate

Maleic Acid

It is used in preparation of ergometrine maleate injection, as rancidity retardants in fats and oils.

Maleic acid

Ascorbyl Palmitate

It is used as an antioxidant in foods and pharmaceuticals. It is also used to prevent rancidity, in meat curing and in the prevention of canned or frozen foods.

■ COLOURING AGENTS

- Colouring agents may be defined as compounds employed in pharmacy solely for the purpose of imparting colour. Colouring agents have long been used in food and cosmetics in an attempt to improve the appearance of the product or subjects.
- Two subdivisions can be made.
  1. Natural colouring principles.
  2. Synthetic colouring principles.
- The use of colours has to be certified by FDA or government agency. The certified colours are obtained into three groups as follows:
  1. FD and C dyes which may be legally used in foods, drugs and cosmetics.
  2. DLC dyes which may legally be used in drugs and cosmetics.
  3. External D and C dyes which may legally be used only in externally applied drugs and cosmetics.

Synthetic Colouring Agents

Allura red: It is used as colouring agents to foods, medicines and cosmetics.

Allura red

Amaranth: It is used as colouring agents in medicines, foodstuffs and cosmetics. It is incompatible with cetrimide.

Black PN: It is used as a colouring agent in medicinal, cosmetics and foods. Acceptable daily intake is up to 1 mg per body weight.

Bordeaux B: It was used as a colouring agent for medicines and foods.

Bordeaux B

Brilliant blue FCF: It is used as a colouring agent in medicines, cosmetics and foods. Acceptable daily intake of 12.5 mg per kg body weight.

Brown HT

Brown HT: It is used as colouring agents for food stuffs. Acceptable daily intake is 1.5 mg per kg body weight.

Carmoisine: It is used as colouring agents in foods and cosmetics.

Carmoisine

Erythrosine:
Uses:

1. It is used as colouring agents for medicines and foods.
2. It is also used in cosmetics as discolouring agents for plaque on teeth.

Storage: In well closed, light resistant containers.

Erythrosine

Green S: It is used as a colouring agent in medicines, cosmetics and foodstuffs. Staining of the conjunctiva with green S was found to be reasonably specific test diagnosing early xerophthalmia.

Green S

Ponceau 4R: It is used as a colouring agent in medicines and foods. Acceptable daily intake up to 4 mg per kg body weight.

Ponaceau 4R

Qunoline yellow: It is the mixture of sodium salts of the mono-and di-sulphonates of quinolone or 2-quinoyl) indanedione. It is used as a colouring agent in medicine, cosmetics and food stuffs. Acceptable daily intake is up to 10 mg per kg body weight.

Red 2G: It is used as a coloring agent in medicines, foods and cosmetics. Acceptable daily intake is up to 0.1 mg per kg body weight.

Red 2G

Sunset yellow: It is used as a colouring agent in cosmetics, medicines and foods. Acceptable daily intake is up to 2–5 mg per kg body weight.

Sunset yellow

Natural Colouring Agents

Caramel:

Properties: It is a thick, but free flowing dark brown liquid with pleasant bitter taste. It is miscible with water in all proportion.

Uses: It is used as a colouring agent to produce pale yellow to dark brown colour in elixirs, syrups and other preparation.

Chlorophyll: It is green colouring matter of plants. It is a mixture of chlorophyll A and chlorophyll B. It is employed principally as a colouring agent in foods, medicines and cosmetics. Externally, it can be used in the treatment of wounds and ulcers.

Cochineal: It is obtained from dried female insect, *Dactylopius cocus*, containing eggs and larvae. It is used as red colouring agent in food, medicines and cosmetics.

Henna: The dried leaves of *Lasonia insermis* containing lawsone. It is used for dying the hair and skin.

Raspberry: The fresh ripe fruit of *Rubus idaeus* gives raspberry juice, is used as a colouring and flavouring agent in medicine and food stuffs.

Red cherry: The fresh ripe fruit of varieties of the red cherry, *Prunus cerassus* gives the juice. It is used as a colouring and flavouring agent.

Red poppy petal: The dried petals of *Papaver rhoeas* have been used as colouring agent and as mild astringent.

Saffron: The dried stigmas and tops of the styles of *Crocus sativus* have been used as a food and cosmetic dye and flavouring agent.

Turmeric: The dried rhizome of *Curcuma longa* is used principally as a constituent of curry powders and the condiments. Turmeric and its main ingredient curcumin are used as a yellow colouring agent in foods.

FLAVOURING AGENTS

- The word flavours refers to a mixed sensation of taste, touch, smell, sight and sound, all of which continue to produce an infinite number of gradations in the perception of a substance. The proper selection of flavor for disguising nauseating medicines aids in their ingestion.
- Flavours used by the pharmacist in compounding prescriptions, may be divided into four main categories according to the type of taste which is to be masked as follows.

1. Salty taste, cinnamon syrup has been found to be the best vehicle for ammonium chloride and other salty drugs such as sodium salicylates and ferric ammonium citrate.

2. Bitter taste, cocoa syrup was found to be the best vehicle for disguising the bitter taste of quinine bisulfate. Other like raspberry syrup, cherry syrup and orange syrup.

3. Acrid or sour taste, raspberry syrup and other fruit syrups are especially efficient in making the taste of sour substances such as hydrochloric acid.

4. Oily taste, castor oil may be made palatable by emulsifying with an equal volume of aromatic rhubarb syrup.

Methyl Salicylate

Uses: It is used to flavor the official aromatic cascara sagrada fluid extract. As a counter irritant, it is used as ointment or cream.

Storage: In well-closed, light-resistant container.

Synthesis:

Vanillin

Identification:

- An aqueous solution of the substances gives a white, precipates with lead acetate solution.
- With ferric chloride, a blue colour is produced.

Uses: It is used as a flavor for foods.

Synthesis:

Vanillin

Other examples

Acacia syrup	Anethol	Anise oil	Aromatic elixir
Benzaldehyde	Caraway oil	Cardamom oil	Cardamom tincture
Cinnamon	Cinnamon oil	Cinnamon water	Cherry syrup
Citric acid	Clove oil	Cocoa	Coriander oil
Ginger	Glucose	Glycerin	Glycyrrhiza

■ SWEETNING AGENT

- Sweetning agents are substances added to pharmaceutical products in order to mask the obnoxious taste of certain drugs and thereby render them acceptable to patients.

Saccharin

Identification:

- A sample is mixed with resorcinol and the mixture heated, it produces a dark colour.
- The substances is treated with aqueous sodium hydroxide, a fluorescent green liquid is produced.

Uses: It is an intensely sweet substance. It is used as a sweetning agent in vehicles, canned foods, beverages and in diets of diabetic to replace sucrose.

Sucrose

Identification: The substance is hydrolsed by boiling in sulfuric acid. Neutralize the acid with sodium hydroxide. Add potassium cupritartarate solution a red precipate is formed.

Uses: It is used principally for making syrups and lozenges. It gives viscocity and consistency to fluids.

Sorbitol

Identification: A sample is dissolved in water. Catechol solution is mixed. The mixture is poured in sulfuric acid, a pink colour is formed.

Uses:

- It is used as a sweetner. It is also used as an osmotic diuretic given intravenously in 5% (W/V) solution.
- Other uses include laxative, humectants and plasticizer.

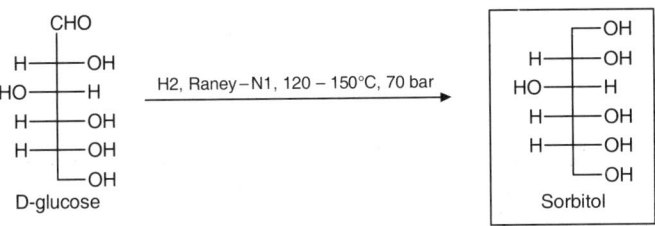

EMULSIFYING AND SUSPENDING AGENTS

- An emulsion is a two-phase systeme in which one liquid is dispersed in the form of small globules throughout another liquid that is immiscible with the first liquid. Emulsion are formed and stabilized with the help of emulsifying agents, which are surfactant and/or viscosity producing agents.
- A suspension is defined a preparation containing finely divided insoluble material suspended in a liquid medium. The presence of suspending agent is required to overcome agglomeration of the dispersed particles and to increase the viscosity of the medium so that the particles settle more slowly.
- Emulsifying and suspending agents are used extensively in the formation of elegant pharmaceutical preparation for oral, parenteral and external use. Some of the agents are also used in the manufacture of tablets as disintegration, binding and granulating agents and for film or enteric coating.

Sodium Lauryl Sulfate

Identification: Mix a small quantity of the sample with methylene blue and H_2SO_4 solution, add 2 ml of chloroform and shake, the chloroform layer is coloured dark blue.

Storage: In well-closed containers.

Carboxymethyl Cellulose Sodium

Identification:

- A sample is dissolved in water after stirring. The solution taken in a test tube and few drops of a menthol solution is added; then sulfuric acid is added slowly to form two layers; a red purple colour is developed at the interface.
- Further on addition of barium chloride solution to an aqueous solution, a white precipitate is formed.

Storage: In well-closed containers.

Stearic Acid

Uses: Sodium stearate is used in enteric tablet coating, toilet creams, vanishing creams and emulsion.

Storage: In well-closed containers.

Glyceryl Monostearate

Identification: A sample is heated with potassium bisulfate; the fumes evolved darken the filter paper impregnated with alkaline potassium mercury iodide solution.

Uses: It is used as thickening and emulsifying agents for ointment.

Storage: In well-closed containers.

Tragacanth

Identification: The substance is added in alcohol and mucilage is prepared with water. On addition of barium hydroxide solution, a flocculent precipitate is formed, which on heating gives an intense yellow colour.

Uses: It is used as pharmaceutical jellies, in various confection products, pill excipient and as demulcent in sore throat.

Storage: In well-closed containers.

Pectin

Identification: A sample is mixed with equal volume of alcohol, a translucent gelatinous precipitate is produced.

Uses: It is used as an emulsifying agents and thickening agent. It is also used in the treatment of diarrhea in infants.

Storage: In well-closed containers.

Acacia

Identification: A gelatin is formed on addition of lead acetate solution to an aqueous solution of acacia.

Uses:

- It is extensively used as a suspending agent for insoluble substance in water, in the preparation of emulsion and for making pills and troches.
- It is also used as a demulcent in inflammation of throat or stomach.

Storage: In well-closed containers, protected from moisture.

Gelatin

Identification:

- On addition of picric acid/tannic acid to an aqueous solution of gelatin gives a precipitate
- On heating with soda lime, it gives ammonia.

Uses:

- It is used to coat pills and form capsules (encapsulating agent) and as a vehicle for suppositories.
- It is also recommended as an emulsifying agent and absorbable gelatin sponge.

Storage: In well-closed containers, in dry place.

Polyvinyl Pyrrolidone

Identification:

- An aqueous solution with iodine produces a deep red colour.
- An aqueous solution is treated with hydrochloric acid. On addition of potassium dichromate solution, an orange-yellow precipates is produced.

Uses:

- It is used a dispersing and suspending agent in pharmaceutical preparation.
- It is also used as tablet binder and coating agent.

Storage: In tightly-closed containers.

Diagnostic Agents

The concept of nuclear pharmacy was first put forward by captain Willis H. Briner in 1960. The term radioactivity was first coined by Curies in 1898 to describe the radioactive decay of radium and polonium. Alpha, beta and gamma rays are the types of radiation obtained through radioactive decay. Some of the characteristic rays are known as X-rays.

In recent times, the role played by the radiation technology in various fields has assumed considerable significance. The applications of various types of radiation have been well established and have been successfully demonstrated in areas of technical and with economic effectiveness of potential benefits to the public health and diagnostic field. They can also be used in the treatment of cancer and in radioimmunoassay. On the diagnostic side, they are used to trace the defective functioning of the body organs or to detect the abnormalities in the tissue structure. Hence they are known as radiotracers or radioactive pharmaceuticals or radiopharmaceuticals or diagnostic agents.

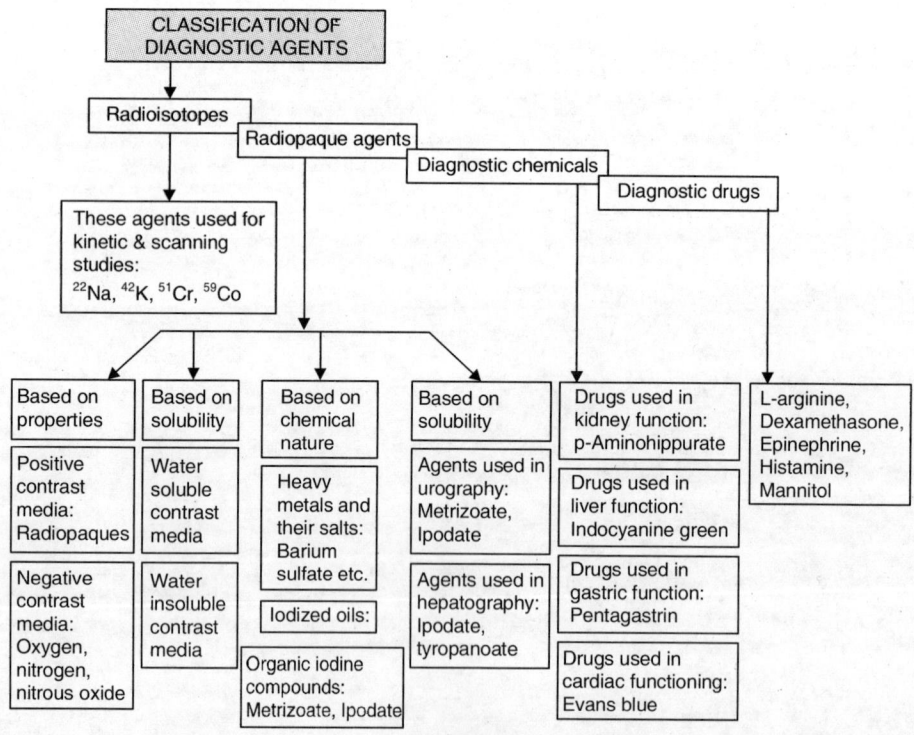

▩ MECHANISM

- These agents are all X-ray opaque (i.e. X-rays do not pass through them). Naturally, when such agent is injected into the body to fill up a specific organ which is to be examined, the organ would not allow X-rays to pass through.
- If in such situation, the X-ray film is placed behind at the site concerned, the shape of the organ will be clearly outlined on the film.
- Thus radiopaque substances help in delineation of body organs and tissues against their immediate environment during fluoroscopic or roentgen graphic amination.
- The bio-distribution of these agents is known as scintiphotos and is obtained with a radiation detective device known as scintillation camera.

▩ RADIO-OPAQUE AGENTS

Water soluble contrast media

Iodohippurate sodium

Metrizoic acid

Iothalmic acid

Iodipamide

Ipodate

Sodium acetrizoate

Metrizamide

Water Insoluble Contrast Media

Iophendylate

Iocetamic acid

Idoxamate

Iopanic acid

Propyliodone H₃CH₂CH₂COOCH₂C

Tyropanoate sodium

DIAGNOSTIC CHEMICALS

A. Drugs used in kidney function

p-Aminohippuric acid

Indigotindisulfonate sodium

Phenolsulfonaphthalein

B. Drugs used to test liver functioning

Rose bengal

Indocyanine green

Sulfobromophthalein sodium

C. Drugs used to test gastric function

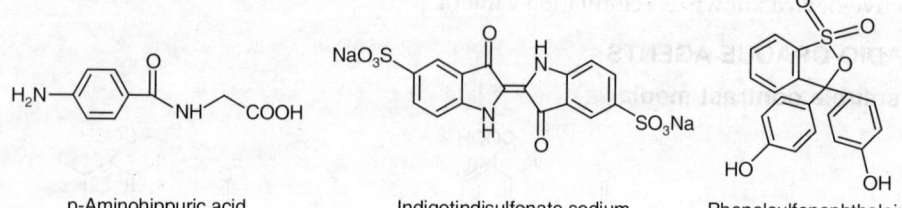

β—Ala—Trp—Met—Asp—Phe—NH₂

Pentagastrin

D. Agents used to test cardiac functioning

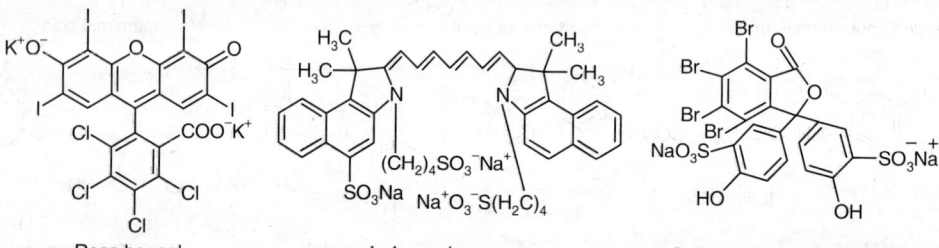

Evans blue

E. Miscellaneous

Fluorescein sodium

Metyrapone

- These agents are either radioactive forms (radioisotopes) of stable elements (like, iodine) or radioactive analogues of stable elements. They cannot categorized under the term, drug, since they usually are devoid of any pharmacological effects. The structure of any radiopharmaceutical agent consists of:

a. Radioactive part: It is an essential part. It gives off the radiations necessary for tracer activity.

b. Nonradioactive part: It has a very little effect upon the tracer activity of the agent. It is of complex nature and governs the tissue distribution or localization in a particular organ through its distinctive chemical or physical properties.

CLASSIFICATION OF DIAGNOSTIC AGENTS

RADIOISOTOPES

- These agents may be used for kinetic studies (i.e. radioisotopes I) or for scanning studies (i.e. radioisotopes II). Kinetic studies include determination of total blood volume, plasma volume, and the excretion pattern of the drug and/or its metabolites through bile, faeces and urine.

- While the scanning studies may be utilized to know the localization or uptake or particular ion into certain tissues or organs. Thus examination of bone, brain, kidney, lung, thyroid, spleen and liver can be done by the use of radioisotopes II.

- Some commonly used radioisotopes include ^{22}Na (sodium chloride form) ^{42}K (potassium chloride), ^{51}Cr (sodium chromate), ^{59}Co (cyanocobalamin), ^{125}I (various forms), ^{197}Hg (chloromerodrin), etc.

RADIO-OPAQUE AGENTS (CONTRAST MEDIA)

- These agents have in common the property of opacity to X-ray radiations. Hence they are used to facilitate X-ray diagnosis by visualizing specific body organs or systems. They may be further subdivided into following types.

Classification Based on Property

Positive contrast media

- These agents have an ability to absorb X-rays. This leads to appearance of a darker shadow on the fluoroscopic screen and lighter shadow on X-ray film, of the organ to be visualized against its immediate environment, e.g. radiopaque.

Negative contrast media

- These agents are transparent to X-rays. This leads to a lighter shadow on fluoroscopic screen and a darker shadow on the X-ray film. Examples include air, oxygen, nitrogen, carbon dioxide, nitrous oxide, etc.

- Radiopaque or positive contrast media comprise of examples of diversified structures and pharmacological properties. The common feature of all these reagents is that they consist of elements of high molecular weight. These elements impart the property of opacity to these agents. Besides this, localization and concentration of contrast medium in the organ also influence the degree of opacity.

Classification Based on Solubility

Water soluble contrast media

- Most of these preparations contain either citrate or a phosphate buffer and a chelating agent. These agents are used mainly in urography and angiography.

- All the iodinated compounds are usually administered by systemic procedure or by retrograde method (i.e. by mechanical means).
- In all of these methods, toxicity or side effects are mild, if the patient is tested for his sensitivity prior to the administration of contrast media.

Water insoluble contrast media

- These agents have a very slight solubility in water. Agents from this class are used mainly for cholecystography, bronchography and myelography. To aid in diagnosing the disease, the patient should not eat or drink anything for at least six hours before the examination.

Table 76.1: Commonly used terms in radiography

Sr. no.	Procedure	Organ visualized
1.	Radiography	X-ray examination
2.	Angiography	Blood vessels
3.	Arteriography	Arteries
4.	Aortography	Aortas
5.	Arthrography	Joints
6.	Bronchography	Lungs
7.	Cholangiography	Gallbladder and bile ducts
8.	Cholecystography	Gallbladder
9.	Esophagography	Esophagus
10.	Hepatography	Liver
11.	Hepatolienography	Liver and spleen
12.	Hysterosalpingography	Uterus and oviducts
13.	Lymphography	Lymph nodes and vessels
14.	Lymphadenography	Lymph nodes
15.	Myelography	Lumbar, thoracic and cervical regions of the brain and spinal cord
16.	Pelviography	Pelvis
17.	Pyelography	Kidney and ureter
18.	Splenohepatography	Liver and spleen
19.	Urography	Urinary tract
20.	Ventriculography	Ventricles of brain
21.	Salpingography	Fallopian tubes

Classification Based on Chemical Nature

Heavy metals and their salts

Chemistry:

- Heavy metals with high atomic numbers may be used as radiopaque because of their high radiopacity. Tantalum dust is such an example of radiopaque agent used by insufflations in bronchography, esophagography and gastrography.
- It has a particle size of 2.5 m in diameter. It possesses the clearance half-life of 105-817 days. Ciliary activity and coughing help to remove the metal particles from the bronchi.

1. Barium sulfate

Formulation:

- Because of low systemic toxicity, low water solubility and a lack of osmotic activity, barium sulfate is a preferred radiopaque used for X-ray studies of gastrointestinal tract.
- It was introduced by Bachem and Gunter in 1910 to replace toxic bismuth salts for GI roentgenography.
- Sodium citrate is added to stabilize colloidal preparation of barium sulfate while sorbitol is added to enhance the function. Some polybasic acids like tartaric acid may be added to obtain the preparation of specific gravity close to 3.

Uses:

- It is most preferred agent for gastrointestinal roentgenographic examination and inhalation bronchography. It may be used in the form of a paste or a thick cream (esophageal studies) or as a suspension (in gastric or small intestine studies) or as a retention enema (in colon studies).
- The dose ranges from up to 300 g (orally). It is also used for bronchography in infants and in children.

2. Bismuth subnitrate

- Bismuth subnitrate was the first clinically used contrast medium for GI-roentgenographic examination.
- This agent and other bismuth salts are less favoured because of toxicity signs produced by bismuth.

3. Ferrites

Ferrites (Fe_2O_3) possess about 80% opacity than that of barium sulfate. Four ferrites containing copper, zinc nickel, mangnese and magnesium are used as radiopaque for roentgen graphic studies of esophagus, bronchi, stomach and small intestine.

4. Thorium dioxide

Thorium dioxide is used for angiography and cerebral arteriography. However, the long-term radiation effects from thorium 232 induces fibrosis and neoplastic growth in liver and spleen. This results into fibrosis of their efferent lymph nodes. Because of these effects, it is less favoured.

5. Toxicity profile

- The significant toxicity associated with metal ions like, cobalt, nickel, lead and calcium can be lowered down through chelation process.
- Various chelating agents have been tried to sequester heavy metal ions for roentgenographic studies. These include 1,2-diaminocyclohexane-N, N'-tetracetic acid diethylne triamine pentacetic acid; N, N' - (2- hydroxy cyclohexyl) ethylene diamine diacetic acid; 2-hydroxycyclohexyl ethylene diamine triacetic acid and b-hydroxy ethyl ethylene diamine triacetic acid.

Iodized oils

Chemistry:

- These preparations are formed by interaction of vegetable oils with hydroiodic acid. Chemically, they are glyceryl esters and ethyl esters of iodinated fatty acid.
- Usually they are yellow or amber coloured oils that decompose upon exposure to air or light to liberate iodine.

Uses: Upon administration, these oils liberate inorganic iodide in the body which appears in the urine. Pulmonary or systemic embolization is the only adverse effect of serious concern. Iodized oils may be used in lymphography, hepatography and hepatosplenography.

Organic iodine compounds

Chemistry: In general these agents contain either benzene or pyridone nucleus as iodine carrying moiety. Iodine content plays a governing role in determining the intensity of opacity. The nonionic contrast media will be less toxic than ionic ones because of lower osmolality

Uses:

- Members of this series are the most widely used radiopaque agents in angiographic, choreographic, urographic and myelographic studies. Tetraiodophenolphthalein was the first clinically used agent from this series. It was used in 1926 by Graham et al in intravenous cholecystography.

- Based on chemical features, organic iodine compounds can be subcategorized into:

   a. Triodobenzoates, e.g. metrizoate

   b. Tri-iodoisophthalamates, e.g. iothalamic acid

   c. Tri-iodophenyl alkanoates, e.g. ipodate

   d. Tri-iodophenocy alkanoates, e.g. iopronic acid

   e. Tri-iodobenzamides, e.g. metrizamide

   f. Tri-iodoanilides, e.g. iocetamic acid

   g. Dimeric triodobenzoates, e.g. iodipamide

   h. Dimeric tri-iodoisophthalamates, e.g. iosefamic acid

   i. Other dimers and polymers, e.g. iozomic acid

   j. Di-iodophenyl alkanoates, e.g. iodoalphionic acid

   k. Di-iodopyridones, e.g. propylidone

   l. Iodophthaleins, e.g. iodophthalein

   m. Miscellaneous, e.g. iodohippurate sodium

Classification Based on Organ to be Examined

Agents used in urography

Criteria:

- The agents from this category should be readily soluble in water, less readily bind to plasma proteins and should have minimal osmotic activity.

- They should have maximum tubular secretion and minimal tubular reabsorption.

- Examples of such agents include diatriazoate, iodamide, metrizoate, and iodohippurate sodium.

1. Diatrizoate

Chemistry: Diatrizoate is an ionic, monomeric tri-iodinated benzoic acid derivative. It has poor oral absorption. It exhibits very low binding to plasma-proteins. It has a plasma half-life of 30–60 minutes. Major dose appears unchanged in the urine.

Adverse effect:

- Adverse effects include chills, dizziness, headache, nausea, vomiting and sweating.

- It is available as a salt of meglumine as well as of sodium. Combination of both these salts is preferred to lower down intensity of adverse hemodynamic neurotoxic and cardiotoxic effects probably because of the sodium ions.

Uses: Diatrizoate is indicated for cholangiography, brain imaging, gastrointestinal radiography, hysterosalpingography, urography and angiography.

2. Iodohippurate sodium I 123

- Iodohippurate sodium I 123 is an agent of choice to assess renal function, effective renal blood flow and urinary tract obstruction.
- It has a plasma half-life of 20–30 minutes. It is excreted by both tubular secretion and glomerular filtration.

Adverse effects: Adverse effects are few and include nausea, vomiting, fainting and allergic reactions. Adult IV dose is 100–400 microcuries for renography and 1 millicurie for renal imaging.

Agents used in hepatography and cholecystography

Pathophysiology:

- Liver is the main site for metabolic and detoxifying enzymes of the body. It is one of the largest playgrounds for metabolic activities.
- This is the reason why liver damage cannot be recognised at its early stage. The decreased liver function cannot be identified until 70–90% of the liver cells get damaged.
- Agents, whose excretion depends exclusively upon liver function, are used to detect the liver dysfunctioning. The rate of clearance of such agents from the plasma becomes a measure of the excretory capacity of the liver.

Classification: The latter class can be subcategorized as:

1. Agents used to detect gallbladder disorders, e.g. iocetamic acid, ipodate, iopanoic acid and tyropanoate.
2. Agents used to detect biliary tract disorders, e.g. iopanoic acid and ipodate salts.

Criteria:

1. The agents used in cholecystography should pass slowly from blood to liver and then to the bile. These agents should bind strongly to plasma proteins and should not actively secreted in the urine.
2. These agents or their glucuronide conjugates should be excreted largely through biliary secretory pathways.
3. These agents should be effective by both oral and intravenous routes.

Mechanism:

- All above cholecystographic agents belong to the class of organic iodine compounds. They may be used for oral cholangiography to visualize biliary ducts.
- However, IV cholangiography is a method of choice. All they have high binding affinity to the plasma proteins.
- Upon hepatic metabolism, these agents are converted to radiopaque glucuronides. They are mainly excreted through the urine and faecal routes.

Adverse effects: These are few and include nausea, vomiting, diarrhea, skin rash, itching, dizziness and headache.

Miscellaneous Radiopaque Agents

Metrizamide

Chemistry:

- It is a first generation, non-ionic, contrast medium used as a diagnostic aid in cardiac, CNS, CSF and vascular disorders.
- It is a monomeric tri-iodinated benzoic acid derivative commonly used in myelography.

Mechanism:

- After intrathecal administration in subarachnoid space, metrizamide rapid diffuses into cerebrospinal fluid.
- It rapidly penetrates into nerve root, nerve rootlets and narrow areas of subarachnoid space and helps to visualize different regions of head and spinal cord.
- While after IV injection, metrizamide helps to visualize those vessels in its path of flow. Most of the dose administered appears in the urine.

Adverse effect: Adverse effects include nausea, vomiting, skin rash, wheezing, headache, restlessness, and irregular heartbeats.

Dose:

- Since metrizamide is isotonic with cerebrospinal fluid at an approximate concentration of 170 mg of iodine per ml of the solution, dosage of metrizamide is usually expressed in terms of iodine.
- For example, various commercial grades available include 2.5 g of metrizamide with 1.21 g of iodine; 6.75 g of metrizamide with 3.26 g of iodine and 13.5 g of metrizamide with 6.51 of iodine per vial.

Iothalamate

Chemistry: It is available in the forms of iothalamate meglumine and Iothalamate sodium. It is an ionic, monomeric tri-iodinated benzoic acid derivative used in angiography and to trace out brain, pancreas, biliary tract and urinary tract disorders.

Mechanism: In the form of meglumine salt, it binds to plasma protein to the extent of 1–4% while about 8–27% administered dose of iothalamate sodium binds to the plasma proteins. Most of the administered dose appears unchanged in the urine.

Adverse effect: Adverse effects include nausea, vomiting and flushing of the skin, severe hypotension and redness, swelling or pain at the site of injection.

Dose:

- For peripheral arteriography about 20–40 ml of 60% solution may be administered in a single dose rapidly into bronchial artery in the arm or femoral artery in the leg.
- For brain imaging, about 2 ml of 60% solution per kg body weight (not above 150 ml) may be administered intravenously. For urography, about 3 ml of 43% solution per kg body weight not above 200 ml) may be given by IV infusion at a rate of 40–50 ml/min.

Iophendylate

Mechanism: It is a radiopaque agent used to trace out CNS and CSF disorders. After intrathecal administration into subarachnoid space, it gets rapidly distributed in different regions in head and in spinal canal. Hence it is indicated for conventional lumbar, thoracic, cervical and total columnar myelography to determine the presence of abnormalities in CSF circulation or in CNS.

Adverse effects:

- Adverse effects include nausea, vomiting, snuffy nose, headache, blurred vision, chest pain, wheezing, backache, fever and skin rash. In myelography, it may be injected intrathecally in the dose of 3.0–12.0 ml.

Iodipamide meglumine

Mechanism:

- It is an ionic, dimeric, tri-iodinated benzoic acid derivative, used as a diagnostic agent in the disorders of gallbladder and biliary tract.
- It is extensively bound to the plasma proteins. Upon hepatic metabolism, it is mainly excreted through the hepatobiliary system. In the form of iodinated ion, it gets concentrated in the gallbladder bile and allows visualization of gallbladder and biliary ducts.

Uses: In cholangiography and cholecystography, it is given by IV infusion in the dose of 100 ml of 10.3% solution slowly over a period of 30–45 minutes.

Iohecol

Mechanism: It is a second generation nonionic contrast medium used for cardiac, vascular, CNS, CSF and urinary tract disorders. It is insignificantly bound to the plasma-proteins. It has a plasma half-life of 2.0 hours. It is mainly excreted through urine.

Uses: In myelography, it is injected intrathecally in the dose of 10-17 ml of solution containing equivalent of 180 mg of iodine per ml.

Lopamidol

Mechanism

It is a second generation nonionic contrast medium used for cardiac, vascular, CNS and CSF disorders. It has a plasma half-life of 2 hours. It is insignificantly bound to the plasma proteins. It is mainly excreted through the urine.

Uses:

- In myelography, it is injected intrathecally in the dose of 10–15 ml of solution containing equivalent of 200 mg iodine per ml.
- While in arteriography, it may be injected into femoral artery or subclavian artery in the dose of 5.0–40 ml.

Locaglate meglumine

Mechnism: It is also available in the form of its sodium salt. It has an elimination half-life of 61–140 minutes. It has very low binding affinity for plasma proteins. It is primarily excreted in the urine.

Uses:

- It is used mainly for diagnosis of cardiac and vascular diseases. In cerebral angiography, through percutaneous or via catheter, it is administered at a rate not exceeding normal flow in artery (i.e. about 5 ml/sec).
- In left coronary arteriography, it is administered via catheter in the dose of 2–14 ml. In right coronary arteriography, about 1–10 ml of the agent may be administered via catheter while in left ventriculography about 45 ml of the agent may be administered via catheter in a single dose.

Simethicone

Mechanism: It is a surface active agent used as an anti-flatulent. It may also be used as antifoaming agent during gastroscopy to enhance visualization and in radiography of the bowl to reduce gas shadows. Adult oral dose is 67 mg in 2.5 ml of water as a single dose.

Adverse Effect Associated With Contrast Media

- Ionic contrast media are usually more toxic than nonionic contrast media. The high degree of toxicity of ionic contrast media may be attributed to cations as well as anions. The cations commonly present in ionic contrast media include sodium, calcium, magnesium and N-methylglucamine (i.e. meglumine).

- In order to reduce toxicities, usually a combination of sodium, magnesium and N-methylglucamine salts is preferred rather than any single agent. Beside this, toxicity may also be reduced by forming salt of acid form of the contrast medium with a basic amino acid.

- The intensity and frequency of adverse effects of these contrast media are also influenced by the route of administration chosen. For example, the intensity of adverse effects is reported to increase in following order.

Intrathecal > intravascular > oral > topical.

- Nausea, vomiting, headache, mental confusion, cyclic changes in blood pressure, dizziness, blurred vision, flushing, wheezing, chest pain, etc. are the common adverse effects reported to occur. Sometimes severe respiratory, neurological and CVS disturbances may accompany to increase the complexity of adverse effects.

▨ DIAGNOSTIC CHEMICALS

Mechanism Used by Diagnostic Chemicals

- Certain substances are retained or excreted almost exclusively only by a specific organ. Thus depending upon the property of retention of excretion, the impairment in the organ function can be searched out.

- For example, phenol tetrachlorophthalein when administered parenterally, it is found to be excreted only in the bile. Hence the failure to remove the dye through the bile is indicative of impaired functioning of the organ.

Drug Used to Test Kidney Function

Examples from this category include p-aminohippurate, inulin and phenolsulphonphthalein. To test kidney function, the bladder is completely emptied before dye administered. This is done under aseptic conditions by introducing a catheter into the bladder.

p-Aminohippurate

Mechanism: It is administered intravenously in the form of its sodium salt. It is not bound to the plasma-proteins. It distributes primarily in the extra-cellular space. It is exclusively excreted via the active secretory processes of proximal convulated tubules in almost unchanged form. It has clearance rate of more than 600 ml/minute.

Adverse effect: Adverse effects include nausea and feeling of warmth.

Uses:

- It is mainly used to determine the functional capacity of the tubular excretory mechanism.

- The time period during which this agent is excreted in the urine is used to determine renal function.

- It is available as a sterile solution containing 2 g per 10 ml. The adult dose is adjusted to get a plasma concentration of 10–20 mg/litre.

Inulin
Mechanism:

- It is a polyfructosan polysaccharide of plant origin having a molecular weight of 5000. It has a plasma half-life of 2–4 hours. It is rapidly distributed in extracellular space.
- It does not undergo metabolism in the body. It is excreted almost entirely by glomerular filtration. Its renal clearance rate is about 125 ml/min. It is also excreted in trace amount in the bile.

Adverse effect: It is devoid of any adverse effects. However, it may produce osmotic diuresis, if used in larger doses. The loading dose (i.e. 100 ml at 10 ml/min rate) is administered by intravenous route, followed by IV infusion at a rate enough to achieve a stable plasma concentration.

Drug Used to Test Liver Functioning
Indocyanine and sulfobromophthalein
Mechanism:

- Liver is the main site for metabolic and detoxifying enzymes of the body. It is one of the largest playground for metabolic activities.
- This is the reason why liver damage cannot be recognized at its early stage. The decreased liver function cannot be identified until 70–90% of the liver cells get damaged.
- Agents whose excretion depends exclusively upon liver function, are used to detect the liver dysfunctioning. The rate of clearance of such agents from the plasma becomes a measure of the excretory capacity of the liver.

Adverse effect:

- Since these agents are almost exclusively taken up by liver and excreted unchanged in the bile, they are used to assess hepatic blood flow and hepatic (biliary) secretory function.
- The common adverse effects include localized acute thrombophlebitis and delayed hypersensitivity.

Dose:

- Indocyanine green is available as a sterile powder (25 mg and 50 mg vials) which is to be disolved freshly at the time of use. It is given intravenously at a dose of 0.15 mg/kg body weight to test liver function.
- While sulfobromophthalein is available as a sterile ampoules (3.0, 7.5, 10.00 ml) of a concentration of 50 mg/ml. It is given intravenously in the dose of 0.5 – 2.0 mg per kg body weight.

Drug Used to Test Gastric Functioning
Pentagastrin
Mechanism:

- Many gastric stimulants are used to gather the evidence of hyper- or hyposecretion of gastric acid. Proof about the absence of gastric acid in the stomach is necessary for the diagnosis of pernicious anemia.
- While over secretion of gastric acid confirms the case of peptic ulcer or peptic esophagitis. The gastric stimulants mainly used to test gastric function include, alcohol, caffeine, pentagastrin, histamine, phosphate, betazole hydrochloride, etc.

$$(CH_3)_3N-CO-CO-p-ala-Trp-Met-Asp-Phe-NH_2$$
Pentagastrin

Uses:

- Pentagastrin is a potent, short acting, synthetic carboxy terminal pentapeptide derivative of gastrin. It has a plasma half-life of 10 minutes.
- It is used in the diagnosis of pernicious anemia, atropic gastritis, gastric carcinoma or the cases of hypersecretion of gastric acid. Adult s.c. dose is 6 mg/kg body weight.

Drug Used to Test Cardiac Functioning

Evans blue and indocyanine

- Examples from this category include Evans blue. It is extensively bound to the plasma proteins. It has plasma half-life of more than 15 days.
- It is relatively safe agent. In some patients, a blue-green tinge may be imparted to the skin. It is available as a single dose ampoule containing 25 mg (5.0 ml of 0.5% solution) for intravenous route. While indocyanine green may be given intravenously at a dose of 5 mg/ kg body weight to determine cardiac output.

Miscellaneous Diagnostic Chemicals

These include fluorescein sodium, metyrapone, congo red and erythrosine sodium. Fluorescein sodium is mainly use for ophthalmological studies. Metyrapone is primarily used to determine residual pituitary function in patients with hypopituitarism. While erythrosine sodium is used as dental diagnostic agent to detect areas of plaque on the teeth.

▓ DIAGNOSTIC DRUGS

- Table 76.2 enlists the commonly used diagnostic drugs to test the presence of specific disease state of the organ.

Table 76.2: Currently used diagnostic drugs

Drugs	Diagnostic use
1. L-arginine	To test growth hormone secretion response
2. Dexmethasone	To test endocrine gland dysfunction
3. Epinephrine	To test denervation of postganglionic sympathetic pathways in the eyes
4. Histamine	To test gastric acid secretion
5. Mannitol	To test renal function
6. Norepinephrine	To test deneravation of sympathetic pathways
7. Pentagastrin	To test gastric acid secretion
8. Phentolamine	To test a state of pheochromocytoma
9. Tyramine	To test a state of pheochromocytoma

Index